Handbook of Contemporary Neuropharmacology

VOLUME 2

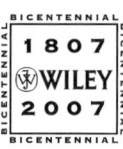

THE WILEY BICENTENNIAL–KNOWLEDGE FOR GENERATIONS

*E*ach generation has its unique needs and aspirations. When Charles Wiley first opened his small printing shop in lower Manhattan in 1807, it was a generation of boundless potential searching for an identity. And we were there, helping to define a new American literary tradition. Over half a century later, in the midst of the Second Industrial Revolution, it was a generation focused on building the future. Once again, we were there, supplying the critical scientific, technical, and engineering knowledge that helped frame the world. Throughout the 20th Century, and into the new millennium, nations began to reach out beyond their own borders and a new international community was born. Wiley was there, expanding its operations around the world to enable a global exchange of ideas, opinions, and know-how.

For 200 years, Wiley has been an integral part of each generation's journey, enabling the flow of information and understanding necessary to meet their needs and fulfill their aspirations. Today, bold new technologies are changing the way we live and learn. Wiley will be there, providing you the must-have knowledge you need to imagine new worlds, new possibilities, and new opportunities.

Generations come and go, but you can always count on Wiley to provide you the knowledge you need, when and where you need it!

WILLIAM J. PESCE
PRESIDENT AND CHIEF EXECUTIVE OFFICER

PETER BOOTH WILEY
CHAIRMAN OF THE BOARD

Handbook of Contemporary Neuropharmacology

VOLUME 2

Editor-in-Chief

David R. Sibley
National Institutes of Health
Bethesda, Maryland

Associate Editors

Israel Hanin
Loyola University Chicago
Maywood, Illinois

Michael Kuhar
Emory University
Atlanta, Georgia

Phil Skolnick
DOV Pharmaceuticals
Somerset, New Jersey

The *Handbook of Contemporary Neuropharmacology* is available online at
www.interscience.wiley.com/reference/hcn

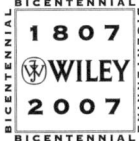

WILEY-INTERSCIENCE
A John Wiley & Sons, Inc., Publication

Copyright © 2007 by John Wiley & Sons, Inc. All rights reserved

Published by John Wiley & Sons, Inc., Hoboken, New Jersey
Published simultaneously in Canada

No part of this publication may be reproduced, stored in retrieval system, or transmitted in any form or by any means, electronic, mechanical, photocopying, recording, scanning, or otherwise, except as permitted under Section 107 or 108 of the 1976 United States Copyright Act, without either the prior written permission of the Publisher, or authorization through payment of the appropriate per-copy fee to the Copyright Clearance Center, Inc., 222 Rosewood Drive, Danvers, MA 01923, (978) 750-8400, fax (978) 750-4470, or on the web at www.copyright.com. Requests to the Publisher for permission should be addressed to the permission Department, John Wiley & Sons, Inc., 111 River Street, Hoboken, NJ 07030, (201) 748-6011, fax (201) 748-6008, or online at http://www.wiley.com/go/permission.

Limit of Liability/Disclaimer of Warranty: While the publisher and author have used their best efforts in preparing this book, they make no representations or warranties with respect to the accuracy or completeness of the contents of this book and specifically disclaim any implied warranties of merchantability or fitness for a particular purpose. No warranty may be created or extended by sales representatives or written sales materials. The advice and strategies contained herein may not be suitable for your situation. You should consult with a professional where appropriate. Neither the publisher nor author shall be liable for any loss of profit or a any other commercial damages, including but not limited to special, incidental, consequential, or other damages.

For general information on our other products and services or for technical support, please contact our Customer Care Department within the United States at (800) 762-2974, outside the United States at (317) 572-3993 or fax (317) 572-4002.

Wiley also publishes its books in a variety of electronic formats. Some content that appears in print may not be available in electronic formats. For more information about Wiley products, visit our web site at www.wiley.com.

Wiley Bicentennial Logo: Richard J. Pacifico

Library of Congress Cataloging-in-Publication Data

Handbook of contemporary neuropharmacology : 3 volume set / editor-in-chief, David R. Sibley; associate editors, Israel Hanin, Michael Kuhar, Phil Skolnick.
   p. cm.
   Includes index.
     ISBN: 978-0-471-66053-8 (cloth)
1. Neuropharmacology. I. Sibley, David Robert, 1954-
   [DNLM: 1. Neuropharmacology. QV 76.5 H2353 2007]
   RM315.H3434 2007
   615'.78–dc22
                                                                              2006030749

Printed in the United States of America

10 9 8 7 6 5 4 3 2 1

Contents

Preface   xi
Contributors   xiii

VOLUME 1

PART I   BASIC NEUROPHARMACOLOGY   1

Chapter 1   Soup or Sparks: The History of Drugs and Synapses   3
William Van der Kloot

Chapter 2   Synaptic Transmission: Intercellular Signaling   39
J. David Jentsch and Robert H. Roth

Chapter 3   Synaptic Transmission: Intracellular Signaling   59
R. Benjamin Free, Lisa A. Hazelwood, Yoon Namkung Michele L. Rankin, Elizabeth B. Rex, and David R. Sibley

Chapter 4   Neuronal Nicotinic Receptors: One Hundred Years of Progress   107
Kenneth J. Kellar and Yingxian Xiao

Chapter 5   Muscarinic Acetylcholine Receptors   147
Jürgen Wess

Chapter 6   Norepinephrine/Epinephrine   193
Megan E. Kozisek and David B. Bylund

Chapter 7   Dopaminergic Neurotransmission   221
John A. Schetz and David R. Sibley

Chapter 8   Serotonin Systems   257
John A. Gray and Bryan L. Roth

Chapter 9   Neuropharmacology of Histamine in Brain   299
Raphaël Faucard and Jean-Charles Schwartz

Chapter 10	Ionotropic Glutamate Receptors	365
	David Bleakman, Andrew Alt, David Lodge, Daniel T. Monaghan, David E. Jane, and Eric S. Nisenbaum	
Chapter 11	Metabotropic Glutamate Receptors	421
	James A. Monn, Michael P. Johnson, and Darryle D. Schoepp	
Chapter 12	Pharmacology of the $GABA_A$ Receptor	465
	Dmytro Berezhnoy, Maria C. Gravielle, and David H. Farb	
Chapter 13	Metabotropic GABA Receptors	569
	Martin Gassmann and Bernhard Bettler	
Chapter 14	Voltage-Gated Ion Channels	617
	Alex Fay, Patrick C. G. Haddick, and Lily Yeh Jan	
Chapter 15	Neuropeptides	669
	Fleur L. Strand	
Chapter 16	Neurotransmitter Transporters	705
	Jia Hu, Katherine Leitzell, Dan Wang, and Michael W. Quick	
Chapter 17	Gaseous Signaling: Nitric Oxide and Carbon Monoxide as Messenger Molecules	743
	Kenny K. K. Chung, Valina L. Dawson, and Ted M. Dawson	

PART II MOOD DISORDERS — 763

Chapter 18	Neurobiology and Treatment of Depression	765
	Alexander Neumeister, Dennis S. Charney, Gerard Sanacora, and John H. Krystal	
Chapter 19	Neurotrophic Factors in Etiology and Treatment of Mood Disorders	789
	Ronald S. Duman	
Chapter 20	Antidepressant Treatment and Hippocampal Neurogenesis: Monoamine and Stress Hypotheses of Depression Converge	821
	Alex Dranovsky and René Hen	
Chapter 21	Neuroendocrine Abnormalities in Women with Depression Linked to the Reproductive Cycle	843
	Barbara L. Parry, Charles J. Meliska, L. Fernando Martinez, Eva L. Maurer, Ana M. Lopez, and Diane L. Sorenson	
Chapter 22	Neurobiology and Pharmacotherapy of Bipolar Disorder	859
	R. H. Belmaker, G. Agam, and R. H. Lenox	

Index — 877

Cumulative Index — 915

VOLUME 2

PART I ANXIETY AND STRESS DISORDERS   1

Chapter 1 Neurobiology of Anxiety   3
Miklos Toth and Bojana Zupan

Chapter 2 Pharmacotherapy of Anxiety   59
Jon R. Nash and David J. Nutt

Chapter 3 Benzodiazepines   93
Hartmut Lüddens and Esa R. Korpi

Chapter 4 Neuroactive Steroids in Anxiety and Stress   133
Deborah A. Finn and Robert H. Purdy

Chapter 5 Emerging Anxiolytics: Corticotropin-Releasing Factor Receptor   177
Antagonists
Dimitri E. Grigoriadis and Samuel R. J. Hoare

Chapter 6 Neurobiology and Pharmacotherapy of Obsessive-Compulsive   215
Disorder
Judith L. Rapoport and Gale Inoff-Germain

PART II SCHIZOPHRENIA AND PSYCHOSIS   249

Chapter 7 Phenomenology and Clinical Science of Schizophrenia   251
Subroto Ghose and Carol Tamminga

Chapter 8 Dopamine and Glutamate Hypotheses of Schizophrenia   283
Bita Moghaddam and Houman Homayoun

Chapter 9 Molecular Genetics of Schizophrenia   321
Liam Carroll, Michael C. O'Donovan, and Michael J. Owen

Chapter 10 Postmortem Brain Studies: Focus on Susceptibility Genes in   343
Schizophrenia
Shiny V. Mathew, Shruti N. Mitkus, Barbara K. Lipska,
Thomas M. Hyde, and Joel E. Kleinman

Chapter 11 Pharmacotherapy of Schizophrenia   369
Zafar Sharif, Seiya Miyamoto, and Jeffrey A. Lieberman

Chapter 12 Atypical Antipsychotic Drugs: Mechanism of Action   411
Herbert Y. Meltzer

PART III SUBSTANCE ABUSE AND ADDICTIVE DISORDERS — 449

Chapter 13 Introduction to Addictive Disorders: Implications for Pharmacotherapies — 451
Mary Jeanne Kreek

Chapter 14 Dopaminergic and GABAergic Regulation of Alcohol-Motivated Behaviors: Novel Neuroanatomical Substrates — 465
Harry L. June and William J. A. Eiler II

Chapter 15 Nicotine — 535
August R. Buchhalter, Reginald V. Fant, and Jack E. Henningfield

Chapter 16 Psychostimulants — 567
Leonard L. Howell and Heather L. Kimmel

Chapter 17 MDMA and Other "Club Drugs" — 613
M. Isabel Colado, Esther O'Shea, and A. Richard Green

Chapter 18 Marijuana: Pharmacology and Interaction with the Endocannabinoid System — 659
Jenny L. Wiley and Billy R. Martin

Chapter 19 Opiates and Addiction — 691
Frank J. Vocci

PART IV PAIN — 707

Chapter 20 Neuronal Pathways for Pain Processing — 709
Gavril W. Pasternak and Yahong Zhang

Chapter 21 Vanilloid Receptor Pathways — 727
Makoto Tominaga

Chapter 22 Opioid Receptors — 745
Gavril W. Pasternak

Chapter 23 Advent of A New Generation of Antimigraine Medications — 757
Ana Recober and Andrew F. Russo

Index — 779

Cumulative Index — 817

VOLUME 3

PART I SLEEP AND AROUSAL — 1

Chapter 1 Function and Pharmacology of Circadian Clocks — 3
Gabriella B. Lundkvist and Gene D. Block

Chapter 2	Melatonin Receptors in Central Nervous System Margarita L. Dubocovich	37
Chapter 3	Narcolepsy: Neuropharmacological Aspects Seiji Nishino	79
Chapter 4	Hypocretin/Orexin System J. Gregor Sutcliffe and Luis de Lecea	125
Chapter 5	Prokineticins: New Pair of Regulatory Peptides Michelle Y. Cheng and Qun-Yong Zhou	163
Chapter 6	Sedatives and Hypnotics Keith A. Wafford and Paul J. Whiting	177

PART II	DEVELOPMENT AND DEVELOPMENTAL DISORDERS	201
Chapter 7	Regulation of Adult Neurogenesis Heather A. Cameron	203
Chapter 8	Neurotrophic Factors Franz F. Hefti and Patricia A. Walicke	221
Chapter 9	Neurotrophins and Their Receptors Mark Bothwell	237
Chapter 10	Tourette's Syndrome and Pharmacotherapy Pieter Joost van Wattum and James F. Leckman	263
Chapter 11	Neuropharmacology of Attention-Deficit/Hyperactivity Disorder Paul E. A. Glaser, F. Xavier Castellanos, and Daniel S. Margulies	291
Chapter 12	Psychopharmacology of Autism Spectrum Disorders Adriana Di Martino, Steven G. Dickstein, Alessandro Zuddas, and F. Xavier Castellanos	319

PART III	NEURODEGENERATIVE AND SEIZURE DISORDERS	345
Chapter 13	Stroke: Mechanisms of Excitotoxicity and Approaches for Therapy Michael J. O'Neill, David Lodge, and James McCulloch	347
Chapter 14	Epilepsy: Mechanisms of Drug Action and Clinical Treatment William H. Theodore and Michael A. Rogawski	403
Chapter 15	Pharmacotherapy for Traumatic Brain Injury Donald G. Stein and Stuart W. Hoffman	443
Chapter 16	Dementia and Pharmacotherapy: Memory Drugs Jerry J. Buccafusco	461

Chapter 17	**Pharmacotherapy and Treatment of Parkinson's Disease** Wing Lok Au and Donald B. Calne	479
Chapter 18	**Parkinson's Disease: Genetics and Pathogenesis** Claudia M. Testa	523
Chapter 19	**Invertebrates as Powerful Genetic Models for Human Neurodegenerative Diseases** Richard Nass and Charles D. Nichols	567

PART IV NEUROIMMUNOLOGY 589

Chapter 20	**Myelin Lipids and Proteins: Structure, Function, and Roles in Neurological Disorders** Richard H. Quarles	591
Chapter 21	**Pharmacology of Inflammation** Carmen Espejo and Roland Martin	621
Chapter 22	**Pharmacological Treatment of Multiple Sclerosis** B. Mark Keegan	671
Chapter 23	**Novel Therapies for Multiple Sclerosis** Martin S. Weber and Scott S. Zamvil	683
Chapter 24	**Neuropharmacology of HIV/AIDS** Sidney A. Houff and Eugene O. Major	693

PART V EATING AND METABOLIC DISORDERS 731

Chapter 25	**Leptin: A Metabolic Perspective** Dawn M. Penn, Cherie R. Rooks, and Ruth B. S. Harris	733
Chapter 26	**Ghrelin: Structural and Functional Properties** Birgitte Holst, Kristoffer Egerod, and Thue W. Schwartz	765
Chapter 27	**Mechanisms Controlling Adipose Tissue Metabolism by the Sympathetic Nervous System: Anatomical and Molecular Aspects** Sheila Collins, Renato H. Migliorini, and Timothy J. Bartness	785
Chapter 28	**Antiobesity Pharmacotherapy: Current Treatment Options and Future Perspectives** Yuguang Shi	815

Index 845

Cumulative Index 881

PREFACE

Neuropharmacology is the study of drugs that affect the nervous system. This includes not only the identification of neuronal drug targets but also the study of basic mechanisms of neural function that may be amenable to pharmacological manipulation. Indeed, neuropharmacological drugs are commonly used as valuable tools to discover how nerve cells function and communicate in addition to therapeutic agents for the treatment of a wide variety of neuropsychiatric disorders. In fact, drugs that are used to treat disorders of the brain and nervous system represent one of the largest groups of approved therapeutic agents. Clearly the demand for drugs to treat disorders of the nervous system will only grow in the face of an aging population. Not surprisingly, almost all major pharmaceutical corporations and many biotechnology companies have extensive drug discovery programs in neuroscience and neuropharmacology. The recent pace of research and discovery in neuropharmacology and associated therapeutics has been quite rapid, as is true for most areas of biomedical research. Given this as well as the extremely broad nature of the field, we felt that it would be timely and important to develop a comprehensive handbook of neuropharmacology that would include state-of-art reviews covering both basic principles and novel approaches for clinical therapeutics.

Our approach for the organization of this handbook was primarily translational (bench to bedside) in nature. The three book volumes consist of 10 clinical sections, each consisting of 4–7 chapters devoted to various neuropsychiatic disorders, including mood, anxiety, and stress disorders, psychosis, pain, neurodegeneration, and many others. In most cases, these sections have introductory chapters providing background information and/or basic principles prior to presenting chapters covering state-of-the-art therapeutics. Volume I also contains a large introductory section consisting of 17 chapters on basic neuropharmacological subjects and principles. These include chapters on the history of neuropharmacology as well as intercellular and intracellular signaling followed by chapters covering all of the major neurotransmitter systems and other important signaling molecules, such as ion channels and transporters. Our objective for this project was to create a high-level reference work that will be useful to all practitioners of neuropharmacology ranging from graduate students, academicians, and clinicians to industrial scientists working in drug discovery. These volumes will be part of the John Wiley & Sons major reference work program and will be published online as well as in print. The online version of this handbook is expected to undergo frequent updates and additions in order to maintain its cutting-edge status.

The editors would like to thank all of the chapter contributors for their hard work and commitment to this project. We would also like to thank our managing editor, Jonathan Rose, at John Wiley & Sons for all of the valuable assistance that he has provided.

David R. Sibley
Israel Hanin
Michael J. Kuhar
Phil Skolnick

CONTRIBUTORS

G. AGAM, *Ben Gurion University, Beersheeva, Israel*, Neurobiology and Pharmacotherapy of Bipolar Disorder

ANDREW ALT, *Lilly Research Laboratories, Eli Lilly and Company, Indianapolis, Indiana*, Ionotropic Glutamate Receptors

WING LOK AU, *Pacific Parkinson's Research Centre, Vancouver, British Columbia, Canada; National Neuroscience Institute, Singapore*, Pharmacotherapy and Treatment of Parkinson's Disease

TIMOTHY J. BARTNESS, *Georgia State University, Atlanta, Georgia*, Mechanisms Controlling Adipose Tissue Metabolism by the Sympathetic Nervous System: Anatomical and Molecular Aspects

R. H. BELMAKER, *Ben Gurion University, Beersheeva, Israel*, Neurobiology and Pharmacotherapy of Bipolar Disorder

DMYTRO BEREZHNOY, *Laboratory of the Molecular Neurobiology, Department of Pharmacology and Therapeutics, Boston University School of Medicine, Boston, Massachusetts*, Pharmacology of the $GABA_A$ Receptor

BERNHARD BETTLER, *University of Basel, Basel, Switzerland*, Metabotropic GABA Receptors

DAVID BLEAKMAN, *Lilly Research Laboratories, Eli Lilly and Company, Indianapolis, Indiana*, Ionotropic Glutamate Receptors

GENE D. BLOCK, *University of Virginia, Charlottesville, Virginia*, Function and Pharmacology of Circadian Clocks

MARK BOTHWELL, *Department of Physiology and Biophysics, University of Washington School of Medicine, Seattle, Washington*, Neurotrophins and their Receptors

JERRY J. BUCCAFUSCO, *Alzheimer's Research Center, Medical College of Georgia, Augusta, Georgia*, Dementia and Pharmacotherapy: Memory Drugs

AUGUST R. BUCHHALTER, *Pinney Associates, Bethesda, Maryland*, Nicotine

DAVID B. BYLUND, *Department of Pharmacology, University of Nebraska Medical Center, Omaha, Nebraska*, Norepinephrine/Epinephrine

DONALD B. CALNE, *Pacific Parkinson's Research Centre, Vancouver, British Columbia, Canada*, Pharmacotherapy and Treatment of Parkinson's Disease

HEATHER A. CAMERON, *Unit on Neuroplasticity, National Institute of Mental Health, National Institutes of Health, Department of Health and Human Services, Bethesda, Maryland*, Regulation of Adult Neurogenesis

LIAM CARROLL, *Department of Psychological Medicine, Wales College of Medicine, Cardiff University, Cardiff, Wales, United Kingdom*, Molecular Genetics of Schizophrenia

F. XAVIER CASTELLANOS, *New York University Child Study Center, New York, New York*, Neuropharmacology of Attention-Deficit/Hyperactivity Disorder; Psychopharmacology of Autism Spectrum Disorders

DENNIS S. CHARNEY, *Department of Psychiatry, Mount Sinai School of Medicine, New York, New York*, Neurobiology and Treatment of Depression

MICHELLE Y. CHENG, *University of California, Irvine, California*, Prokineticins: New Pair of Regulatory Peptides

KENNY K. K. CHUNG, *Institute for Cell Engineering, Department of Neuroscience, Johns Hopkins University School of Medicine, Baltimore, Maryland*, Gaseous Signaling: Nitric Oxide and Carbon Monoxide as Messenger Molecules

M. ISABEL COLADO, *Facultad de Medicina, Universidad Complutense, Madrid, Spain*, MDMA and other "Club Drugs"

SHEILA COLLINS, *CIIT Centers for Health Research, Research Triangle Park, North Carolina and Duke University Medical Center, Durham, North Carolina*, Mechanisms Controlling Adipose Tissue Metabolism by the Sympathetic Nervous System: Anatomical and Molecular Aspects

TED M. DAWSON, *Institute for Cell Engineering, Johns Hopkins University School of Medicine, Baltimore, Maryland*, Gaseous Signaling: Nitric Oxide and Carbon Monoxide as Messenger Molecules

VALINA L. DAWSON, *Institute for Cell Engineering, Departments of Neurology, Neuroscience, and Physiology, Johns Hopkins University School of Medicine, Baltimore, Maryland*, Gaseous Signaling: Nitric Oxide and Carbon Monoxide as Messenger Molecules

LUIS DE LECEA, *Department of Molecular Biology, The Scripps Research Institute, La Jolla, California*, Hypocretin/Orexin System

STEVEN G. DICKSTEIN, *Phyllis Green and Randolph Cowen Institute for Pediatric Neuroscience, New York University Child Study Center, New York, New York*, Psychopharmacology of Autism Spectrum Disorders

ADRIANA DI MARTINO, *Phyllis Green and Randolph Cowen Institute for Pediatric Neuroscience, New York University Child Study Center, New York, New York; University of Cagliari, Italy*, Psychopharmacology of Autism Spectrum Disorders

ALEX DRANOVSKY, *Departments of Psychiatry, Pharmacology, and the Center for Neurobiology and Behavior, Columbia University, New York State Psychiatric Institute, New York, New York*, Antidepressant Treatment and Hippocampal Neurogenesis: Monoamine and Stress Hypotheses of Depression Converge

MARGARITA L. DUBOCOVICH, *Northwestern University Feinberg School of Medicine, Center for Drug Discovery and Chemical Biology, Northwestern University, Chicago, Illinois*, Melatonin Receptors in Central Nervous System

RONALD S. DUMAN, *Division of Molecular Psychiatry, Departments of Psychiatry and Pharmacology, Yale University School of Medicine, New Haven, Connecticut*, Neurotrophic Factors in Etiology and Treatment of Mood Disorders

KRISTOFFER EGEROD, *Laboratory for Molecular Pharmacology, Department of Pharmacology, Panum Institute, Copenhagen, Denmark*, Ghrelin: Structural and Functional Properties

WILLIAM J. A. EILER II, *Psychobiology of Addictions Program, Department of Psychology, Indiana University-Purdue University, Indianapolis, Indiana*, Dopaminergic and GABAergic Regulation of Alcohol-Motivated Behaviors: Novel Neuroanatomical Substrates

CARMEN ESPEJO, *Unitat de Neuroimmunologia Clinica, Hospital Universitari Vall D'Hebron, Barcelona, Spain*, Pharmacology of Inflammation

REGINALD V. FANT, *Pinney Associates, Bethesda, Maryland*, Nicotine

DAVID H. FARB, *Laboratory of Molecular Neurobiology, Department of Pharmacology and Therapeutics, Boston University School of Medicine, Boston, Massachusetts*, Pharmacology of the $GABA_A$ Receptor

RAPHAËL FAUCARD, *Centre de Recherche Bioprojet Biotech, Saint-Grégoire, France*, Neuropharmacology of Histamine in Brain

ALEX FAY, *University of California, San Francisco, California*, Voltage-Gated Ion Channels

DEBORAH A. FINN, *Department of Behavioral Neuroscience, Oregon Health & Science University and Department of Veterans Affairs, Portland, Oregon,* Neuroactive Steroids in Anxiety and Stress

R. BENJAMIN FREE, *National Institute of Neurological Disorders and Stroke, National Institutes of Health, Bethesda, Maryland,* Synaptic Transmission: Intracellular Signaling

MARTIN GASSMANN, *University of Basel, Basel, Switzerland,* Metabotropic GABA Receptors

SUBROTO GHOSE, *University of Texas Southwestern Medical Center, Dallas, Texas,* Phenomenology and Clinical Science of Schizophrenia

PAUL E. A. GLASER, *University of Kentucky Medical Center, Lexington, Kentucky,* Neuropharmacology of Attention-Deficit/Hyperactivity Disorder

MARIA C. GRAVIELLE, *Laboratory of Molecular Neurobiology, Department of Pharmacology and Therapeutics, Boston University School of Medicine, Boston, Massachusetts,* Pharmacology of the $GABA_A$ Receptor

JOHN A. GRAY, *University of California, San Francisco, San Francisco, California,* Serotonin Systems

A. RICHARD GREEN, *Institute of Neuroscience, School of Biomedical Sciences, Queen's Medical Centre, University of Nottingham, Nottingham, United Kingdom,* MDMA and other "Club Drugs"

DIMITRI E. GRIGORIADIS, *Neurocrine Biosciences, San Diego, California,* Emerging Anxiolytics: Corticotropin-Releasing Factor Receptor Antagonists

PATRICK C. G. HADDICK, *University of California, San Francisco, San Francisco, California,* Voltage-Gated Ion Channels

RUTH B. S. HARRIS, *University of Georgia, Athens, Georgia,* Leptin: A Metabolic Perspective

LISA A. HAZELWOOD, *National Institute of Neurological Disorders and Stroke, National Institutes of Health, Bethesda, Maryland,* Synaptic Transmission: Intracellular Signaling

FRANZ F. HEFTI, *Rinat Neuroscience Corporation, Palo Alto, California,* Neurotrophic Factors

RENÉ HEN, *Departments of Psychiatry, Pharmacology, and the Center for Neurobiology and Behavior, Columbia University, New York State Psychiatric Institute, New York, New York,* Antidepressant Treatment and Hippocampal Neurogenesis: Monoamine and Stress Hypotheses of Depression Coverge

JACK E. HENNINGFIELD, *Pinney Associates, Bethesda, Maryland; The Johns Hopkins University School of Medicine, Baltimore, Maryland,* Nicotine

SAMUEL R. J. HOARE, *Neurocrine Biosciences, San Diego, California,* Emerging Anxiolytics: Corticotropin-Releasing Factor Receptor Antagonists

STUART W. HOFFMAN, *Department of Emergency Medicine, Emory University, Atlanta, Georgia,* Pharmacotherapy for Traumatic Brain Injury

BIRGITTE HOLST, *Laboratory for Molecular Pharmacology, Department of Pharmacology, Panum Institute, Copenhagen, Denmark,* Ghrelin: Structural and Functional Properties

HOUMAN HOMAYOUN, *University of Pittsburgh, Pittsburgh, Pennsylvania,* Dopamine and Glutamate Hypotheses of Schizophrenia

SIDNEY A. HOUFF, *Laboratory of Molecular Medicine and Neuroscience, National Institute of Neurological Disorders and Stroke, National Institutes of Health, Bethesda, Maryland,* Neuropharmacology of HIV/AIDS

LEONARD L. HOWELL, *Division of Neuroscience, Emory University, Atlanta, Georgia,* Psychostimulants

JIA HU, *University of Southern California, Los Angeles, California,* Neurotransmitter Transporters

THOMAS M. HYDE, *Section of Neuropathology, Clinical Brain Disorders Branch, Genes, Cognition, and Psychosis Program, Division of Intramural Research Programs, National Institutes of Mental Health, National Institutes of Health, Bethesda, Maryland,* Postmortem Brain Studies: Focus on Susceptibility Genes in Schizophrenia

GALE INOFF-GERMAIN, *Child Psychiatry Branch, National Institute of Mental Health, National Institutes of Health, Bethesda, Maryland*, Neurobiology and Pharmacotherapy of Obsessive-Compulsive Disorder

LILY YEH JAN, *University of California, San Francisco, San Francisco, California*, Voltage-Gated Ion Channels

DAVID E. JANE, *University of Bristol School of Medical Sciences, Bristol, United Kingdom*, Ionotropic Glutamate Receptors

J. DAVID JENTSCH, *Yale University School of Medicine, New Haven, Connecticut*, Synaptic Transmission: Intercellular Signaling

MICHAEL P. JOHNSON, *Lilly Research Laboratories, Eli Lilly and Company, Indianapolis, Indiana*, Metabotropic Glutamate Receptors

HARRY L. JUNE, *Division of Alcohol Abuse, Department of Psychiatry, University of Maryland School of Medicine, Baltimore, Maryland*, Dopaminergic and GABAergic Regulation of Alcohol-Motivated Behaviors: Novel Neuroanatomical Substrates

B. MARK KEEGAN, *Department of Neurology, Mayo Clinic College of Medicine, Rochester, Minnesota*, Pharmacological Treatment of Multiple Sclerosis

KENNETH J. KELLAR, *Georgetown University, Washington, District of Columbia*, Neuronal Nicotinic Receptors: One Hundred Years of Progress

HEATHER L. KIMMEL, *Division of Neuroscience, Emory University, Atlanta, Georgia*, Psychostimulants

JOEL E. KLEINMAN, *Section of Neuropathology, Clinical Brain Disorders Branch, Genes, Cognition, and Psychosis Program, Division of Intramural Research Programs, National Institutes of Mental Health, National Institutes of Health, Bethesda, Maryland*, Postmortem Brain Studies: Focus on Susceptibility Genes in Schizophrenia

ESA R. KORPI, *Institute of Biomedicine/Pharmacology, Biomedicum Helsinki, University of Helsinki, Helsinki, Finland*, Benzodiazepines

MARY JEANNE KREEK, *Rockefeller University, New York, New York*, Introduction to Addictive Disorders: Implications for Pharmacotherapies

MEGAN E. KOZISEK, *Department of Pharmacology, University of Nebraska Medical Center, Omaha, Nebraska*, Norepinephrine/Epinephrine

JOHN H. KRYSTAL, *Department of Psychiatry, Yale University School of Medicine, VA Connecticut Healthcare System, West Haven, Connecticut*, Neurobiology and Treatment of Depression

JAMES F. LECKMAN, *Child Study Center, Yale University School of Medicine, New Haven, Connecticut*, Tourette's Syndrome and Pharmacotherapy

KATHERINE LEITZELL, *University of Southern California, Los Angeles, California*, Neurotransmitter Transporters

R. H. LENOX, *University of Pennsylvania School of Medicine, Philadelphia, Pennsylvania*, Neurobiology and Pharmacotherapy of Bipolar Disorder

JEFFREY A. LIEBERMAN, *College of Physicians and Surgeons, Columbia University, Lieber Center for Schizophrenia Research, New York State Psychiatric Institute; Psychiatrist-in-Chief, New York Presbyterian Hosptial and Columbia University Medical Center, New York, New York*, Pharmacotherapy of Schizophrenia

BARBARA K. LIPSKA, *Section of Neuropathology, Clinical Brain Disorders Branch, Genes, Cognition, and Psychosis Program, Division of Intramural Research Programs, National Institutes of Mental Health, National Institutes of Health, Bethesda, Maryland*, Postmortem Brain Studies: Focus on Susceptibility Genes in Schizophrenia

DAVID LODGE, *University of Bristol School of Medical Sciences, Bristol, United Kingdom*, Ionotropic Glutamate Receptors; Stroke: Mechanisms of Excitotoxicity and Approaches for Therapy

ANA M. LOPEZ, *University of California, San Diego, La Jolla, California*, Neuroendocrine Abnormalities in Women with Depression Linked to Reproductive Cycle

HARTMUT LÜDDENS, *Laboratory of Molecular Biology, Department of Psychiatry, University of Mainz, Mainz, Germany,* Benzodiazepines

GABRIELLA B. LUNDKVIST, *Department of Neuroscience, Karolinska Institutet, Stockholm, Sweden,* Function and Pharmacology of Circadian Clocks

EUGENE O. MAJOR, *Laboratory of Molecular Medicine and Neuroscience, National Institute of Neurological Disorders and Stroke, National Institutes of Health, Bethesda, Maryland,* Neuropharmacology of HIV/AIDS

DANIEL S. MARGULIES, *New York University Child Study Center, New York, New York,* Neuropharmacology of Attention-Deficit/Hyperactivity Disorder

BILLY R. MARTIN, *Department of Pharmacology and Toxicology, Virginia Commonwealth University, Richmond, Virginia,* Marijuana: Pharmacology and Interactions with the Endocannabinoid System

ROLAND MARTIN, *Unitat de Neuroimmunologia Clinica, Hospital Universitari Vall D'Hebron, Barcelona, Spain; Institució Catalana de Recerca i Estudis Avançats (ICREA),* Pharmacology of Inflammation

L. FERNANDO MARTINEZ, *University of California San Diego School of Medicine, La Jolla, California,* Neuroendocrine Abnormalities in Women with Depression Linked to the Reproductive Cycle

SHINY V. MATHEW, *Section of Neuropathology, Clinical Brain Disorders Branch, Genes, Cognition, and Psychosis Program, Division of Intramural Research Programs, National Institutes of Mental Health, National Institutes of Health, Bethesda, Maryland,* Postmortem Brain Studies: Focus on Susceptibility Genes in Schizophrenia

EVA L. MAURER, *University of California San Diego School of Medicine, La Jolla, California,* Neuroendocrine Abnormalities in Women with Depression Linked to the Reproductive Cycle

JAMES MCCULLOCH, *Division of Neuroscience, The University of Edinburgh, Edinburgh, Scotland,* Stroke: Mechanisms of Excitotoxicity and Approaches for Therapy

CHARLES J. MELISKA, *University of California San Diego School of Medicine, La Jolla, California,* Neuroendocrine Abnormalities in Women with Depression Linked to the Reproductive Cycle

HERBERT Y. MELTZER, *Vanderbilt University School of Medicine, Nashville, Tennessee,* Atypical Antipsychotic Drugs: Mechanism of Action

RENATO H. MIGLIORINI, *Universidad do Sao Paulo, Sao Paolo, Brazil,* Mechanisms Controlling Adipose Tissue Metabolism by the Sympathetic Nervous System: Anatomical and Molecular Aspects

SHRUTI N. MITKUS, *Section of Neuropathology, Clinical Brain Disorders Branch, Genes, Cognition, and Psychosis Program, Division of Intramural Research Programs, National Institutes of Mental Health, National Institutes of Health, Bethesda, Maryland,* Postmortem Brain Studies: Focus on Susceptibility Genes in Schizophrenia

SEIYA MIYAMOTO, *Department of Neuropsychiatry, St. Marianna School of Medicine, Kawasaki City, Kanagawa Prefecture, Japan,* Pharmacotherapy of Schizophrenia

BITA MOGHADDAM, *University of Pittsburgh, Pittsburgh, Pennsylvania,* Dopamine and Glutamate Hypotheses of Schizophrenia

DANIEL T. MONAGHAN, *Department of Pharmacology, University of Nebraska Medical Center, Omaha, Nebraska,* Ionotropic Glutamate Receptors

JAMES A. MONN, *Lilly Research Laboratories, Eli Lilly and Company, Indianapolis, Indiana,* Metabotropic Glutamate Receptors

YOON NAMKUNG, *National Institute of Neurological Disorders and Stroke, National Institutes of Health, Bethesda, Maryland,* Synaptic Transmission: Intracellular Signaling

JON R. NASH, *University of Bristol, Bristol, United Kingdom,* Pharmacotherapy of Anxiety

RICHARD NASS, *Vanderbilt University Medical Center, Nashville, Tennessee,* Invertebrates as Powerful Genetic Models for Human Neurodegenerative Diseases

ALEXANDER NEUMEISTER, *Yale University School of Medicine, Molecular Imaging Program of the Clinical Neuroscience Division, West Haven, Connecticut,* Neurobiology and Treatment of Depression

CHARLES D. NICHOLS, *Department of Pharmacology and Experimental Therapeutics, Louisiana State University Health Science Center, New Orleans, Louisiana,* Invertebrates as Powerful Genetic Models for Human Neurodegenerative Diseases

ERIC S. NISENBAUM, *Lilly Research Laboratories, Eli Lilly and Company, Indianapolis, Indiana,* Ionotropic Glutamate Receptors

SEIJI NISHINO, *Sleep and Circadian Neurobiology Laboratory, Center for Narcolepsy, Stanford University School of Medicine, Palo Alto, California,* Narcolepsy: Neuropharmacological Aspects

DAVID J. NUTT, *University of Bristol, School of Medical Science, Bristol, United Kingdom,* Pharmacotherapy of Anxiety

MICHAEL C. O'DONOVAN, *Department of Psychological Medicine, Wales College of Medicine, Cardiff University, Cardiff, United Kingdom,* Molecular Genetics of Schizophrenia

MICHAEL J. O'NEILL, *Eli Lilly, Windlesham, Surrey, United Kingdom,* Stroke: Mechanisms of Excitotoxicity and Approaches for Therapy

ESTHER O'SHEA, *Facultad de Medicina, Universidad Complutense, Madrid, Spain,* MDMA and other "Club Drugs"

MICHAEL J. OWEN, *Department of Psychological Medicine, Wales College of Medicine, Cardiff University, Cardiff, Wales, United Kingdom,* Molecular Genetics of Schizophrenia

BARBARA L. PARRY, *University of California San Diego School of Medicine, La Jolla, California,* Neuroendocrine Abnormalities in Women with Depression Linked to the Reproductive Cycle

GAVRIL W. PASTERNAK, *Memorial Sloan-Kettering Cancer Center, Laboratory of Molecular Neuropharmacology, New York, New York,* Opioid Receptors; Neuronal Pathways for Pain Processing

DAWN M. PENN, *University of Georgia, Athens, Georgia,* Leptin: A Metabolic Perspective

ROBERT H. PURDY, *Department of Neuropharmacology, The Scripps Research Institute, La Jolla, California,* Neuroactive Steroids in Anxiety and Stress

RICHARD H. QUARLES, *Laboratory of Molecular and Cellular Neurobiology, National Institute of Neurological Disorders and Stroke, National Institutes of Health, Bethesda, Maryland,* Myelin Lipids and Proteins: Structure, Function, and Roles in Neurological Disorders

MICHAEL W. QUICK, *University of Southern California, Los Angeles, California,* Neurotransmitter Transporters

MICHELE L. RANKIN, *National Institute of Neurological Disorders and Stroke, National Institutes of Health, Bethesda, Maryland,* Synaptic Transmission: Intracellular Signaling

JUDITH L. RAPOPORT, *Child Psychiatry Branch, National Institute of Mental Health, National Institutes of Health, Bethesda, Maryland,* Neurobiology and Pharmacotherapy of Obsessive-Compulsive Disorder

ANA RECOBER, *Department of Neurology, University of Iowa, Iowa City, Iowa,* Advent of a New Generation of Antimigraine Medications

ELIZABETH B. REX, *National Institute of Neurological Disorders and Stroke, National Institutes of Health, Bethesda, Maryland,* Synaptic Transmission: Intracellular Signaling

MICHAEL A. ROGAWSKI, *National Institute of Neurological Disorders and Stroke, National Institutes of Health, Bethesda, Maryland,* Epilepsy: Mechanisms of Drug Action and Clinical Treatment

CHERIE R. ROOKS, *University of Georgia, Athens, Georgia,* Leptin: A Metabolic Perspective

ROBERT H. ROTH, *Brain Research Institute, University of California, Los Angeles, California,* Synaptic Transmission: Intercellular Signaling

BRYAN L. ROTH, *University of North Carolina, Chapel Hill, North Carolina,* Serotonin Systems

ANDREW F. RUSSO, *Department of Physiology and Biophysics, University of Iowa, Iowa City, Iowa,* Advent of a New Generation of Antimigraine Medications

GERARD SANACORA, *Department of Psychiatry, Connecticut Mental Health Center, Clinical Neuroscience Research Unit, New Haven, Connecticut,* Neurobiology and Treatment of Depression

JOHN A. SCHETZ, *Department of Pharmacology and Neuroscience, University of North Texas Health Science Center, Fort Worth, Texas,* Dopaminergic Neurotransmission

DARRYLE D. SCHOEPP, *Lilly Research Laboratories, Eli Lilly and Company, Indianapolis, Indiana,* Metabotropic Glutamate Receptors

THUE W. SCHWARTZ, *Laboratory for Molecular Pharmacology, Department of Pharmacology, Panum Institute, Copenhagen, Denmark; 7TM Pharma, Hørsholm, Denmark,* Ghrelin: Structural and Functional Properties

JEAN-CHARLES SCHWARTZ, *Centre de Recherche Bioprojet Biotech, Saint-Grégoire, France,* Neuropharmacology of Histamine in Brain

ZAFAR SHARIF, *College of Physicians and Surgeons, Columbia University; Lieber Schizophrenia Research Clinic, New York State Psychiatric Institute, New York, New York,* Pharmacotherapy of Schizophrenia

YUGUANG SHI, *Department of Cellular and Molecular Medicine, Penn State School of Medicine, Hershey, Pennsylvania,* Antiobesity Pharmacotherapy: Current Treatment Options and Future Perspectives

DAVID R. SIBLEY, *National Institute of Neurological Disorders and Stroke, National Institutes of Health, Bethesda, Maryland,* Synaptic Transmission: Intracellular Signaling; Dopaminergic Neurotransmission

DIANE L. SORENSON, *University of California San Diego School of Medicine, La Jolla, California,* Neuroendocrine Abnormalities in Women with Depression Linked to Reproductive Cycle

DONALD G. STEIN, *Emergency Medicine Brain Research Laboratory, Emory University, Atlanta, Georgia,* Pharmacotherapy for Traumatic Brain Injury

FLEUR L. STRAND, *New York University, New York, New York,* Neuropeptides

J. GREGOR SUTCLIFFE, *Department of Molecular Biology, The Scripps Research Institute, La Jolla, California,* Hypocretin/Orexin System

CAROL TAMMINGA, *University of Texas Southwestern Medical Center, Dallas, Texas,* Phenomenology and Clinical Science of Schizophrenia

CLAUDIA M. TESTA, *Emory University, Center for Neurodegenerative Diseases, Atlanta, Georgia,* Parkinson's Disease: Genetics and Pathogenesis

WILLIAM H. THEODORE, *National Institute of Neurological Disorders and Stroke, National Institutes of Health, Bethesda, Maryland,* Epilepsy: Mechanisms of Drug Action and Clinical Treatment

MAKOTO TOMINAGA, *Section of Cell Signaling, Okazaki Institute for Integrative Bioscience, National Institutes of Natural Sciences, Okazaki, Japan,* Vanilloid Receptor Pathways

MIKLOS TOTH, *Department of Pharmacology, Weill Medical College of Cornell University, New York, New York,* Neurobiology of Anxiety

WILLIAM VAN DER KLOOT, *State University of New York, Stony Brook, New York,* Soup or Sparks: The History of Drugs and Synapses

PIETER JOOST VAN WATTUM, *Child Study Center, Yale University School of Medicine, New Haven, Connecticut,* Tourette's Syndrome and Pharmacotherapy

FRANK J. VOCCI, *National Institute on Drug Abuse, National Institutes of Health, Bethesda, Maryland,* Opiates and Addiction

KEITH A. WAFFORD, *Merck Sharp & Dohme Research Laboratories, Harlow, Essex, United Kingdom,* Sedatives and Hypnotics

PATRICIA A. WALICKE, *Rinat Neuroscience Corporation, Palo Alto, California,* Neurotrophic Factors

DAN WANG, *University of Southern California, Los Angeles, California,* Neurotransmitter Transporters

MARTIN S. WEBER, *Department of Neurology, University of California, San Francisco, San Francisco, California,* Novel Therapies of Multiple Sclerosis

JÜRGEN WESS, *National Institute of Diabetes and Digestive and Kidney Diseases, Bethesda, Maryland,* Muscarinic Acetylcholine Receptors

PAUL J. WHITING, *Sandwich Laboratories, Pfizer Limited, Sandwich, Kent, United Kingdom,* Sedatives and Hypnotics

JENNY L. WILEY, *Department of Pharmacology and Toxicology, Virginia Commonwealth University, Richmond, Virginia,* Marijuana: Pharmacology and Interactions with the Endocannabinoid System

YINGXIAN XIAO, *Department of Pharmacology, Georgetown University Medical Center, Washington, DC,* Neuronal Nicotinic Receptors: One Hundred Years of Progress

SCOTT S. ZAMVIL, *Department of Neurology, University of California, San Francisco, San Francisco, California,* Novel Therapies of Multiple Sclerosis

YAHONG ZHANG, *Laboratory of Molecular Neuropharmacology, Memorial Sloan-Kettering Cancer Center, New York, New York,* Neuronal Pathways for Pain Processing

QUN-YONG ZHOU, *Department of Pharmacology, University of California, Irvine, California,* Prokineticins: New Pair of Regulatory Peptides

ALESSANDRO ZUDDAS, *Department of Neuroscience, University of Cagliari, Cagliari, Italy,* Psychopharmacology of Autism Spectrum Disorders

BOJANA ZUPAN, *Department of Pharmacology, Weill Medical College of Cornell University, New York, New York,* Neurobiology of Anxiety

PART I

Anxiety and Stress Disorders

1

NEUROBIOLOGY OF ANXIETY

MIKLOS TOTH AND BOJANA ZUPAN
Weill Medical College of Cornell University, New York, New York

1.1	Introduction	4
1.2	Psychological Traits and their Genetic Basis	4
1.3	Extrapolation of Psychological Trait of Neuroticism to Mouse Behavior	6
	1.3.1 Emotionality as Measure of Avoidance, Behavioral Inhibition/ Activation, and Autonomic Arousal in Animals	6
	1.3.2 Quantifying Emotionality in Animals	6
1.4	Anxiety: Continuous Expression of Normal Human Personality Traits	9
	1.4.1 Anxiety Disorders	9
	1.4.2 Anxiety-Like Behavior in Animals	10
1.5	Fear/Anxiety Circuits	13
	1.5.1 Brain Regions Related to Anxiety Disorders	13
	1.5.2 Brain Regions Related to Emotionality/Anxiety-Like Behavior in Animals	14
1.6	Neurotransmitter Systems and Neuronal Messengers Implicated in Anxiety and Anxiety-like Behavior	15
1.7	Genetic Susceptibility to Anxiety Disorders	18
1.8	Genetic Base of Anxiety-like Behavior in Mice	19
	1.8.1 QTL Studies	19
	1.8.2 Anxiety-Like Behavior in Genetically Altered Mice	19
1.9	Knockout Mice with Disturbances in Neuronal Messengers Exhibiting Alterations in Anxiety-like Behavior	24
1.10	Knockout Mice with Deficits in Neurotransmitter Receptors and Other Cytoplasmic Membrane–associated Proteins Exhibiting Anxiety-like Behavior	26
1.11	Intracellular Regulators Associated with Anxiety-like Phenotype	30
	1.11.1 Modeling Complex Genetics of Anxiety in Mice: Oligogenic Anxiety-Like Conditions in Mice	32
1.12	Effects of Early-Life Environment on Anxiety	33
	1.12.1 Early-Life Experience on Expression of Anxiety in Later Life	33
	1.12.2 Interaction of Environment with Genes in Establishing Level of Anxiety	34
1.13	Conclusions: Neurobiology of Anxiety Disorders	35
	References	37

Handbook of Contemporary Neuropharmacology, Edited by David R. Sibley, Israel Hanin, Michael Kuhar, and Phil Skolnick. Copyright © 2007 John Wiley & Sons, Inc.

1.1 INTRODUCTION

"Anxiety" is the subjective feeling of heightened tension and diffused uneasiness. It is a normal reaction to threatening situations and serves a physiological protective function in eliciting avoidance behaviors. The majority of individuals respond to anxiety-evoking environment appropriately but with some individual differences. The range of appropriate responses to threatening situations can best be described by individual differences in personality traits, in particular in emotional (in)stability/neuroticism [1–3]. Both genetic and environmental factors contribute to emotional (in)stability and to personality traits in general [4]. Approximately 5–10% of individuals display an exaggerated response to real or perceived threat or interpret ambiguous situations as threatening and can be classified as suffering from anxiety disorders [5]. It may be conceptualized that these individuals lie outside of the normal range of individual differences in emotional (in)stability [6]. Indeed, emotional instability and anxiety share common genetic factors.

Although a genetic contribution to emotional instability (neuroticism) and anxiety has long been known, it is only recently that multipoint linkage analysis identified chromosomal regions that may harbor candidate genes [7, 8]. Also, genetic polymorphisms in the serotonin (5-HT) transporter (5-HTT), 5-HT$_{1A}$ receptor, and brain-derived neurotrophic factor (BDNF) have recently been associated with neuroticism and anxiety conditions [9–11]. The slow pace of discovering susceptibility genes in human is largely due to the complex genetics of personality traits and common disorders; thus, individual genes have a relatively small contribution to traits/diseases. The effect of the environment on the expression of anxiety disorders also complicates the elucidation of the underlying pathogenic processes.

Animal models have long been used in the research of anxiety. Quantitative trait locus (QTL) analysis suggests that the genetic basis of "emotionality"/fear reaction in mice can be defined as the variance of a set of few behavioral measures [12–15], such as avoidance of novel environment (abbreviated in this review as Av), behavioral inhibition/activity in highly or moderately threatening situations (Ac) and autonomic arousal (Aa). These dimensions of rodent behavior are reminiscent of the characteristics of emotional instability/neuroticism in humans. In the last decade, a large number of induced mutations have been generated by homologous recombination in the mouse, and some of these strains show a significant deviation from their parental strain in measures of fear response. The abnormal fear response of these mice can be conceptualized as anxiety-like, similar to anxiety disorders in humans. By analyzing a large number of these strains and by classifying them according to the three fundamental dimensions of noncognitive behavior proposed above (AvAcAa), it is possible to implicate multiple neurobiological processes in anxiety-like behavior. Furthermore, these genetic models allow the study of the combined effect of two or more genes as well as the interaction of genes and environment in the expression of anxiety-like behavior in mice. These results may be extrapolated to humans and they eventually could help to better understand the polygenic and multifactorial nature of human anxiety disorders.

1.2 PSYCHOLOGICAL TRAITS AND THEIR GENETIC BASIS

Since anxiety is the continuous expression of normal human personality traits, it is important to briefly summarize a few of the leading personality theories. Personality

PSYCHOLOGICAL TRAITS AND THEIR GENETIC BASIS 5

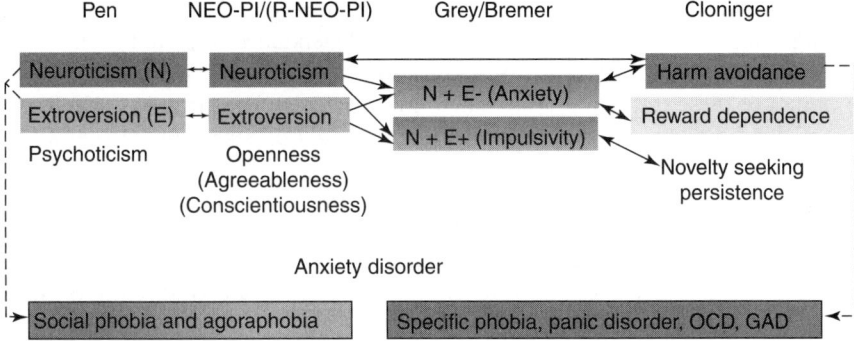

Figure 1.1 Psychological traits and models. According to various models, personality consists of three to five fundamental traits. Arrows indicate corresponding traits in the various models. Traits are highly variable in individuals, but most individuals fall in between the extremes of a trait. Behavior outside of this range can be considered abnormal. For example, higher than normal level of neuroticism (in the PEN model) or harm avoidance (in the Cloninger model) is characteristic for anxiety disorders. (See color insert.)

traits are underlying characteristics of an individual that can explain the major dimensions of human behavior. Traits are dimensions representing a continuum of characters and most people fall in between the extremes. Personality traits have a wide individual variation, but they are relatively stable in individuals over time [16]. Cognitive/intellectual and noncognitive/affective/psychological traits are two fundamental domains of personality. Although the separation of the cognitive and noncognitive domains of personality may be practical, these variables interact and influence each other. Among the psychological traits two, extroversion versus introversion (E) and emotional stability versus instability or neuroticism (N), are probably the most important. An additional dimension is psychoticism (P) in the PEN model [1, 2] (Fig. 1.1). Autonomic arousal is an integral part of neuroticism and it is characterized by increased heart rate and blood pressure, cold hands, sweating, and muscular tension. A similar system based on the broad traits of neuroticism, extroversion, and openness is the NEO personality inventory (NEO-PI) [3]. Other models hypothesize the existence of more than three fundamental traits. The Big 5 (B5) model has three other dimensions in addition to emotional stability and extroversion [17–19]. The revised (R) NEO-PI also has five factors, and besides neuroticism, extroversion, and openness, consists of the factors of agreeableness and conscientiousness [20] (Fig. 1.1). NEO-PI-R is a self-report inventory with a high retest reliability, item validity, longitudinal stability, consistent correlations between self and observer ratings, and robust factor structure that has been validated in a variety of populations and cultures [3]. Gray [21] has modified Eysenck's PEN model by rotating the dimensions of neuroticism and extroversion by 45°, resulting in two new dimensions: anxiety (N+, E−) and impulsivity (N+, E+). Gray's work, however, has been done mostly on animals. Still another personality assessment is Cloninger's biosocial model, which conceptualizes temperament as consisting of the four genetically and biochemically distinct traits of harm avoidance, reward dependence, novelty seeking, and persistence [22] (Fig. 1.1). Harm avoidance is correlated with NEO-PI-R neuroticism. Reward dependence is related to the anxiety/neuroticism/extroversion traits of other classifications (Fig. 1.1). Novelty seeking is also related to these traits and is similar to impulsivity in the Gray hypothesis. Each of these broad dimensions of personality is comprised of a number of smaller traits which are narrower in scope.

Using the techniques of quantitative behavioral genetics, it became clear that roughly 40–60% of the variation in most personality traits has a genetic base. Broad personality traits are under polygenic influence [4, 23]. Recently, genomewide linkage studies have been performed by using the EPQ (Eysenck personality questionnaire) [1, 2] to identify chromosomal regions associated with neuroticism. A two-point and multipoint nonparametric regression identified 1q, 4q, 7p, 8p, 11q, 12q, and 13q [7], while another similar study using multipoint, nonparametric allele sharing and regression identified 1q, 3centr, 6q, 11q, and 12p [8], confirming some of the linkages in the previous study.

1.3 EXTRAPOLATION OF PSYCHOLOGICAL TRAIT OF NEUROTICISM TO MOUSE BEHAVIOR

1.3.1 Emotionality as Measure of Avoidance, Behavioral Inhibition/Activation, and Autonomic Arousal in Animals

Behavioral studies with various rodent strains indicate that a set of a few behavioral measures can describe "emotionality," a behavior similar to the psychological traits of emotional instability/neuroticism in humans [12–15]. To be able to analyze and compare a large number of animal studies, we have selected throughout this review three commonly used measures of emotionality: avoidance of novel environment, activity/behavioral inhibition in highly or moderately threatening situations, and autonomic arousal (Fig. 1.2). Here we refer to this triad of behavioral measures as AvAcAa (avoidance, activity, and arousal).

1.3.2 Quantifying Emotionality in Animals

Attempts to measure emotionality and stress response in rodents have yielded a large number of tests [24–28]. Ten years ago it was estimated that there were over 30 such tests in use [29], and modifications of earlier tests have likely increased this number since then. Initially, the development of these tests was facilitated by the need of preclinical identification and characterization of anxiolytics. Indeed, these tests are often referred to as anxiety tests, anxiety-related tests, or animal models of anxiety, even if most of them actually measure the normal reaction of animals to novelty and stress.

The animal models measure either unconditioned or conditioned fear/anxiety-like behaviors. Another classification is based on more specific behaviors such as social and defensive behavior. Table 1.1 provides a short list of the more commonly used tests while more thorough reviews of the assays can be found elsewhere [28–32]. Unconditioned exploration tests measure the natural conflict experienced by animals to either explore a novel environment for food, water, or social reward or avoid it due

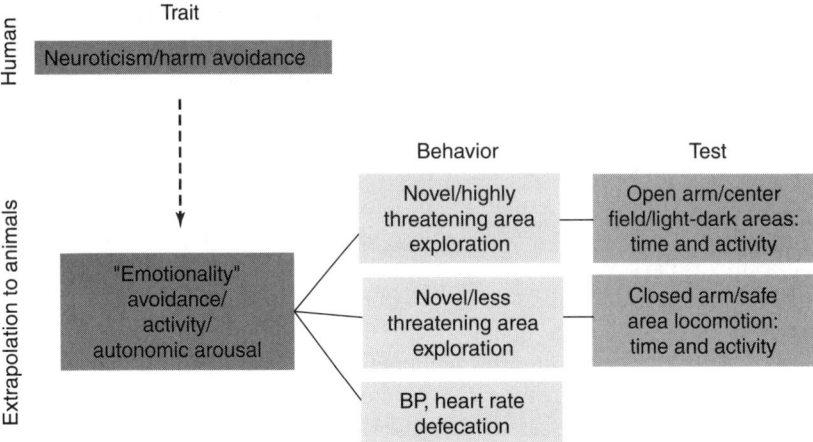

Figure 1.2 Measures of "emotionality" in rodents. The human trait of neuroticism is extrapolated to the measures of emotionality in rodents: avoidance, activity, and autonomic arousal (AvAcAa). AvAcAa can be quantified in well-established behavioral models. Exploration of a low and a moderate to highly threatening environment provides measures of avoidance and activity, while physiological functions provide measurements of autonomic arousal. (See color insert.)

TABLE 1.1 Commonly Used Animal Tests of Anxiety

Conditioned tests	*Punishment-Induced*: Geller–Seifter conflict, Vogel punished drinking	*Fear*: fear-potentiated startle, contextual/cued fear conditioning, passive/active avoidance	
Unconditioned tests	*Exploration*: elevated-plus and zero mazes, open field, light–dark box	*Social Interactions*: maternal separation social competition	*Other*: acoustic startle, hyponeophagia, defense test batteries, shock-probe burrying

to potential unknown dangers. Measurements of avoidant behaviors, such as decreased exploration of a particular region of the testing apparatus, compared to overall locomotor activity provide a quantifiable measure to assess the level of conflict in such novel environments. In a laboratory setting, animals are introduced into a novel and more or less fearful environment and their avoidance, behavioral inhibition/activity, and autonomic responses are measured. For example, the elevated-plus maze (EPM) [33] consists of a cross with opposing pairs of arms which are either open or enclosed and is elevated above the ground. The normal rodent behavior is to prefer the enclosed compartment of the maze, which is less aversive. During normal exploratory activity, however, the animal will enter the open arms. These entries into and the time spent in the open arms are counted and used to assess the level of avoidance, although additional, more complex behaviors can also be recorded [33]. The elevated-zero maze (EZM) is a modification of the EPM where the four arms have been replaced by a circular track separated into four quadrants of alternating open and enclosed regions. Avoidance can also be assessed in the center of a brightly lit open field [34]. Animals tend to stay and move around the periphery of the field, since the open area and bright illumination are aversive. The avoidance measured in an open field is assessed by the number of entries into and the time spent in the center of the open field or the path length in this area. An adaptation of this test is the light–dark crossing task [35], consisting of a two-compartment box in which one area is dark and the other is brightly lit. This test uses the animals' natural tendency to prefer the dark and to avoid the brightly lit area. In this case, the number of crosses into and the time spent in the light compartment reflect the level of avoidance. Most studies compare the open arm/light compartment/center field activity/time as a percent of total activity/time. Also, exploration in the less aversive areas of the test apparatus (closed arm/dark compartment, periphery of the open field) is often regarded as an assessment of general activity levels, and it has been proposed that avoidance in the more stressful areas cannot be interpreted unless locomotor activity in low-stress areas is normal [36]. However, out-of-cage test environments are stressful even if they are moderately threatening. This notion is supported by the finding that a QTL has been linked to both the suppression of general locomotor activity and high-stress-area avoidance in a study involving a large number of mice [15]. Therefore, a number of laboratories, including ours, prefer to score overall locomotor activity separately (e.g., in activity boxes) as one measure of emotionality [37, 38]. The EPM, open field, and light–dark box tests are viewed as straightforward and relatively simple tests to conduct and as such are frequently used. However, more complex methods which highlight different aspects of avoidant behavior are available but are less commonly used. For example, in the social interaction test, behavior such as sniffing, grooming, mounting, and contact are monitored and used to infer changes in emotionality [39].

Conditioned conflict tests assess punishment-induced avoidance of a conditioned behavior. The Geller–Seifter test [40] is based on the conflict between completing an appetitive conditioned response that is unexpectedly paired with an unpleasant stimulus, such as the delivery of a mild electric shock. The Vogel punished drinking test [41] is similar to the Geller–Seifter test but does not require an extensive training period for the conditioning of the measured response. In the Vogel punished drinking test, the subject is water deprived for 12–24 h and then placed into a testing apparatus containing a water bottle with a spigot from which the animal can drink. Thirsty subjects learn quickly that water is available from the spigot and will readily drink from it when repeatedly placed into the testing apparatus. During the test session, however, the water spigot is connected to an electrical source that provides a mild electric shock upon contact with the spigot, placing the animal in conflict of choosing the appetitive reward or avoiding it. The level of avoidance reflects the emotionality of the subject.

Emotionality can also be measured in conditioned fear paradigms [42] such as fear-potentiated startle and contextual fear conditioning. These tests involve the element of emotional learning, as a neutral stimulus such as sound or light is paired with an electric foot shock. After a few trials, the previously neutral stimulus becomes aversive when presented alone. Mobility and freezing time can be used as indices of behavioral inhibition. A similar test is passive/active avoidance, a one-pairing fear-induced avoidance assay. An animal is placed into a compartment and it has to either remain in that compartment to avoid a mild shock (passive avoidance) or go to another compartment (active avoidance, or escape-directed behavior) to avoid the aversive stimulus. Overall, conditioned tests provide less between-subject baseline variability than unconditioned response tests, but most conditioned assays require extensive training and the use of additional groups for controlling potential differences in learning and memory.

1.4 ANXIETY: CONTINUOUS EXPRESSION OF NORMAL HUMAN PERSONALITY TRAITS

It has long been proposed that the underlying structure of normal adaptive traits and the maladaptive personality traits of anxiety are the same [22]. Analysis of normal personality traits by NEO-PI in persons with psychiatrist-ascertained anxiety disorders in a general population showed an association of high neuroticism with lifetime anxiety disorders [simple phobia, social phobia, agoraphobia, panic disorder, obsessive-compulsive disorder (OCD), and generalized anxiety disorder] (Fig. 1.1). Social phobia and agoraphobia were also associated with low extroversion, and OCD was associated with high openness to experience [43]. In the Cloninger model, anxiety incorporates many aspects of harm avoidance [22]. Autonomic arousal, an integral part of neuroticism, is also a characteristic of anxiety disorders and is manifested as tachycardia, increased blood pressure, and elevated core temperature [44].

Recent genetic studies further support the notion that anxiety is the continuous expression of certain personality traits. For example, neuroticism/harm avoidance share a common genetic variant with susceptibility to anxiety disorders. Lesch et al. demonstrated that a functional 5-HTT promoter polymorphism is associated with the NEO-PI-R factor neuroticism and harm avoidance of the Cloninger model [9]. Extension of these genetic studies to anxiety disorders by the same authors showed no differences in 5-HTT genotype distribution between anxiety patients and comparison subjects, but among anxiety patients, carriers of a specific 5-HTT allele exhibited higher neuroticism scores than noncarriers [45]. Over 20 other studies investigated this association, and recent meta-analyses of these studies found a small but significant association between 5-HTT polymorphism and in some but not all measures of neuroticism/anxiety [46]. These studies remind us of the multifactorial nature of anxiety and that individual genes have only a small contribution to the clinical phenotype.

1.4.1 Anxiety Disorders

In the United States, anxiety disorders are most often defined and diagnosed according to a categorical system established by the **Diagnostic and Statistical Manual of Psychiatric Disorders**, currently in its fourth edition (DSM-IV) [5]. The DSM-IV sets the boundary at which a particular level of emotionality becomes an anxiety disorder—a level often based on the number and duration of observable symptoms of anxiety. This categorical model of anxiety, although necessary for the clinical diagnosis of anxiety disorders, is far from being reflective of the biological nature of emotional states. Emotionality and anxiety are more realistically illustrated through a dimensional model that encompasses a continuum of various measures. The subjectivity of diagnosis is further illustrated by the marked differences in the diagnostic criteria of generalized anxiety disorder between the DSM-IV [5] and the ICD-10 Classification of Mental and Behavioral Disorders [47]. Although a core group of symptoms is identical in the two systems, DSM-IV relates these symptoms to vigilance while ICD-10 emphasizes the importance of autonomic arousal/hyperactivity. For the purpose of the present review, a quick overview of the DSM-IV classifications of anxiety disorders will be presented, while further discussions on different diagnostic criteria of DSM-IV and ICD-10 can be found elsewhere [48, 49].

The DSM-IV provides diagnostic criteria for a number of anxiety disorders, including panic disorder, specific and social phobias, OCD, posttraumatic stress disorder (PTSD), and generalized anxiety disorder [5, 50]. Individuals suffering from panic disorder experience recurrent and unexpected panic attacks which lead to discrete periods of intense fear and/or discomfort. Panic attacks are characterized by increased autonomic responses, including increased heart and breathing rates, sweating, nausea, abdominal distress, chills or hot flashes, and lightheadedness. Panic disorder may include agoraphobia, defined as the avoidance of places or situations in which escape may be difficult or embarrassing in the event of a panic attack. Specific and social phobias are marked by persistent fear of either clearly discernible objects or situations or potentially embarrassing social or performance situations, respectively. Exposure to the phobic stimulus almost invariably leads to heightened anxiety that may be expressed as a panic attack. Phobic stimuli are most often actively avoided. OCD features recurrent obsessions and compulsions severe enough to interfere with everyday life. Obsessions are described as persistent and inappropriate anxiogenic ideas, thoughts, or impulses that are unrelated to a real-life problem. Individuals suffering from OCD reduce obsession-induced anxiety by performing repetitive behaviors known as compulsions. These excessive and stereotypic behaviors or mental acts are not realistically connected with what they are designed to neutralize (i.e., washing and cleaning, counting, checking, and rearranging, etc.). PTSD can develop following a traumatic event involving feelings of intense fear, helplessness, or horror (e.g., military combat, rape, assault, and serious accident). Patients experience distressing recollection of the event, numbing of general responsiveness, and persistent arousal. They make deliberate and persistent efforts to avoid trauma-associated stimuli. Finally, generalized anxiety disorder is characterized by persistent (over six months) and excessive worry, inability to control worry, muscle tension, irritability, and sleep disturbance that are not necessarily related to a specific threatening situation. Many individuals also experience somatic symptoms (dry mouth, sweating, nausea, urinary frequency) that are reminiscent of certain symptoms of panic attacks [5].

1.4.2 Anxiety-Like Behavior in Animals

Studying rodent behavior in various anxiety-related test paradigms (see Section 1.3.2) reveals variation in emotionality in these species [51–53]. This includes variability in avoidance of aversive environment (Av), activity/behavioral inhibition in highly or moderately threatening situations (Ac), and autonomic arousal (Aa)

ANXIETY: CONTINUOUS EXPRESSION OF NORMAL HUMAN 11

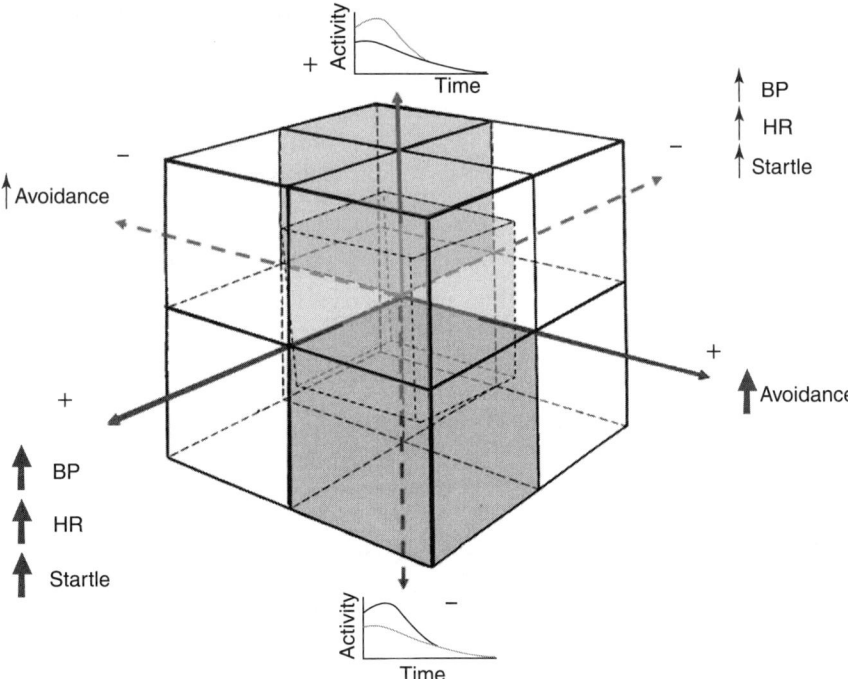

Figure 1.3 The three dimensions (AvAcAa) of emotionality in rodents in three-dimensional representation. Avoidance (Av) is plotted on the x axis, the positive spectrum representing increased levels of avoidance in stress-inducing environments or following stress-inducing stimuli and the negative spectrum representing attenuation of avoidance or even increased risk-taking behavior. Activity (Ac) as a response to stress and fear is plotted on the y axis, with the positive spectrum corresponding to increased levels of activity in a moderate to highly stressful environment. Following habituation, the activity is not different. Decreased activity in such an environment would be plotted in the negative spectrum of the y axis. Finally, the z axis is used for autonomic arousal (Aa) elicited by fearful or stressful stimuli, including increased heart rate, increased blood pressure, heightened levels of muscle tension (as measured by the startle response), defecation, and urination. A positive or negative deviation from the normal level of autonomic arousal can be represented by the positive and negative spectra of this axis, respectively. The normal range of these measures in a population is represented by the grey cube. Increased anxiety-like behavior can be conceptualized as increased avoidance, reduced activity, and increased arousal beyond the normal range of variations, denoted by the red area of the cube. Reduced anxiety-like behavior or increased novelty-seeking/risk-taking behavior is characterized by attenuation of avoidance, increased activity, and reduced autonomic arousal, highlighted by the blue area of the cube. (See color insert.)

(Fig. 1.2). Figure 1.3 displays these three basic characteristics as dimensions that together determine the degree of emotionality (see gray box for the range of normal variation of the three dimensions).

Many selectively bred and genetically modified mouse/rat strains show significant deviations from the normal variability of these dimensions. Once measures of behavior in mutant rodents exceed the threshold of variance of the normal/control population (increased avoidance, reduced activity, and increased autonomic arousal), the resulting condition can be conceptualized as anxiety-like and similar to anxiety disorders in humans (Fig. 1.3; see red area of the cube). Emotionality can also be decreased (attenuation of avoidance, increased activity, and attenuated autonomic arousal) in a novel environment (Fig. 1.3; see blue area of the cube). Indeed, individual animals with higher and lower emotionality have been selected from a population and bred selectively to obtain strains characterized with high and low anxiety-like behavior. The Maudsley reactive inbred rat strain shows a stable and reproducible deficit in exploratory behavior as compared to the Maudsley nonreactive strain [54]. A similar breeding strategy based on behavior in the EPM test (open arm entries and time) resulted in the high-anxiety-related behavior (HAB) and low-anxiety-related behavior (LAB) rat lines [55]. These differences in behavior presumably reflect contributions from multiple genetic loci. Since generating induced mutations in mice has became routine, numerous mutant strains with either increased or decreased anxiety-like phenotype have been identified (see detailed description of these lines in Section 1.8.2).

Mutant mice with increased emotionality/fear reactions can be used as models of anxiety, and it is important to determine if they have construct and face validity. The criterion of construct validity requires that the rationale used to form the animal model is based on the etiology and the biological factors of anxiety. Construct validity criteria are difficult to fulfill because factors underlying the human disorders are largely unknown. However, in a few cases, the animal model has a genetic defect similar to that identified in anxiety disorders. For example, reduced expression of the $5-HT_{1A}$ receptor has been repeatedly shown in anxiety disorders and mice heterozygous for the inactivated $5-HT_{1A}$ receptor have an increased anxiety-like phenotype (see Sections 1.6 and 1.10).

Face validity represents a similarity in the physiological and behavioral measures observed in humans and in the animal model. As with construct validity, some animal models meet this criterion more easily than others. Physiological expressions of fear as well as anticipation of fear are comparable across species as they include easily quantifiable autonomic or endocrine responses such as increases in heart rate, blood pressure, body temperature, and muscle tension or changes in plasma corticosterone.

Predictive validity refers to the sensitivity of the model to clinically effective pharmacotherapeutic drugs. Benzodiazepines, for example, are commonly used in the treatment of anxiety; hence, a proposed animal model with predictive validity should show decreased measures of anxiety following benzodiazepine administration. In contrast, anxiogenic compounds should produce the opposite in physiological and behavioral measures. In addition, compounds with no effect in the clinic should not alter these measures in an animal model. Although predictive validity is an essential criterion for an animal model of anxiety in preclinical research, it has less relevance in studies focusing on the pathogenesis of anxiety disorders. Indeed, sensitivity to anxiolytics such as benzodiazepines varies in the population [56, 57]. For example, it has been shown that subjects high in neuroticism [58] and panic disorder patients [59–61] are less sensitive to benzodiazepines, with true benzodiazepine treatment resistance occurring in up to 24% of panic patients [62]. A similar difference in drug response can also be seen in certain animal models of anxiety such as the $5-HT_{1A}$ receptor–deficient mouse strains on various genetic backgrounds [38].

1.5 FEAR/ANXIETY CIRCUITS

1.5.1 Brain Regions Related to Anxiety Disorders

Anxiety is an emotion involving a complex interaction among many interconnected brain regions, with each component playing a specific role [63]. Most of these brain regions are part of the basic fear network, which is comprised of the prefrontal cortex, hippocampus, thalamus, and amygdala and its projections to brain regions responsible for coordinating the behavioral, autonomic, and endocrine response to fear (i.e., ventral tegmental area, locus ceruleus, dorsal motor nucleus of the vagus, nucleus ambiguus, lateral hypothalamus, paraventricular nucleus of the hypothalamus, etc.). Imaging technologies such as positron emission tomography (PET), magnetic resonance imaging (MRI), and functional MRI (fMRI) have made a large impact on elucidating the roles of various fear pathway structures in anxiety disorders. One of the best characterized limbic structures for its role in processing fear-related stimuli is the amygdala [64–66]. Furthermore, neuroimaging studies have shown that abnormal amygdala function is involved in anxiety disorders. Excess amygdala activation has been observed in PTSD patients in response to stimuli reminiscent of the traumatic event [67, 68] as well as in specific phobia patients when exposed to a phobia-related stimulus [69]. A volumetric MRI study revealed a significantly lower bilateral amygdala volume in panic disorder patients compared to individuals in the healthy control group [70]. Abnormal amygdala volume is not specific to panic disorder, as reduced amygdala volume has also been observed in patients suffering from OCD [71]. In contrast, larger right amygdala volume was measured in generalized anxiety disorder patients [72]. However, this particular study was performed in children; thus age, in addition to different anxiety diagnosis, may explain the contradicting results. Interestingly, the same cohort of children was later followed up with an fMRI study in which an exaggerated right amygdala response to fearful faces was observed in generalized anxiety disorder patients but not in healthy children. These results are suggestive of a relationship between structure and function and indicate that hyperactivity of the amygdala may be a characteristic feature of some anxiety disorders [73].

In addition to the hyperactivity of the amygdala, a number of neuroimaging studies have reported functional abnormalities in other fear pathway substrates in anxiety disorder patients. For example, increased levels of activity were found in the orbitofrontal cortex, hippocampus, and anterior and posterior cingulate in response to directed imagery of strongly emotional personal experiences in subjects suffering from panic disorder compared to healthy individuals [74]. Exaggerated activation of the orbitofrontal cortex has also been documented in specific phobia patients [69]. In contrast, the anterior cingulate gyrus showed lower levels of activity in PTSD during exposure to emotional stimuli by several groups [72, 75–77]. The anterior cingulate abnormality, together with the observed hyperactivity of the amygdala, has been incorporated into a neuroanatomical model of PTSD. Medial prefrontal structures, including the cingulate cortex, are thought to inhibit the activity of brain regions involved in fear responses, and therefore a hypoactive medial prefrontal cortex would fail to inhibit the amygdala in this model of PTSD [77, 78].

The hippocampus has also been extensively studied by neuroimaging techniques. Volumetric imaging studies that have been performed on PTSD patients have yielded conflicting results with regard to hippocampal size. Some have found no differences in hippocampal volume between PTSD patients and non-trauma-exposed controls [79, 80], while others have documented either unilateral or bilateral reduction in hippocampal volume in PTSD patients [81–84]. A fundamental problem with most imaging studies is that the correlation between size of a neural substrate and the disorder in which it is documented may not be causal. In an attempt to address this issue, Wignall et al. [83] measured the hippocampal volume of recent-onset PTSD patients and found a decrease in right-sided hippocampal volume. Although the authors could not exclude the possibility that the hippocampal damage occurred during the time between the traumatic event and the onset of PTSD (mean of 158 days), they leaned toward the interpretation that smaller hippocampal volumes predispose individuals to the development of PTSD. A similar, yet longitudinal MRI study, however, showed that survivors of traumatic events who developed PTSD had no differences in hippocampal volumes at one week and at six months following the trauma when compared to trauma survivors that did not develop PTSD [80]. This particular controversy was somewhat abated by a study that found that monozygotic twins of PTSD combat veterans who themselves were not exposed to combat showed comparable hippocampal volumes to their combat-exposed brothers and that the hippocampi of these twins were significantly smaller than those of both combat veterans without PTSD and their non-combat-exposed twins [81]. These results indicate that a smaller hippocampal volume is a pre existing PTSD predisposing factor rather than a product of the disorder. A reduced hippocampal volume is not, however, a prerequisite for the development of the disorder.

Certain dopaminergic substrates, particularly the ventral striatum, have been found to be both larger in volume [85] and functionally hyperactive in patients suffering from OCD. Other hyperactive regions documented include orbitofrontal cortex, caudate, thalamus, and the anterior cingulate cortex [85, 86]. Based on these data the prevailing hypothesis of OCD pathogenesis proposes that OCD symptoms are mediated in part by a defect in the orbitofrontal-subcortical circuits.

1.5.2 Brain Regions Related to Emotionality/Anxiety-Like Behavior in Animals

Brain regions involved in fear and emotionality in animals are largely the same as those implicated in anxiety disorders (Fig. 1.4). The amygdala has a central importance in the acquisition, retention, and expression of conditioned fear [87–89]. The amygdala seems to function as an emotional/cognitive interface receiving sensory information via projections from the cortex and the thalamus. Outputs from the amygdala to the frontal cortex are related to the conscious perception of fear while outputs to the locus ceruleus, hypothalamus, periaquaductal grey, and striatum mediate autonomic, neuroendocrine, and skeletal-motor responses associated with fear and anxiety.

Although it is widely accepted that the hippocampus plays an important role in certain forms of learning and memory, recent studies have show that the hippocampus is also involved in fear and emotionality. Interestingly, ventral hippocampal lesions affect anxiety while dorsal lesions result in defects in spatial learning. For example, cytotoxic lesions of the ventral hippocampus resulted in reduced aversion in the center of the open field, reduced freezing after footshock, and reduced inhibition in novelty-suppressed feeding [90]. Also, lesion of the ventral but not dorsal

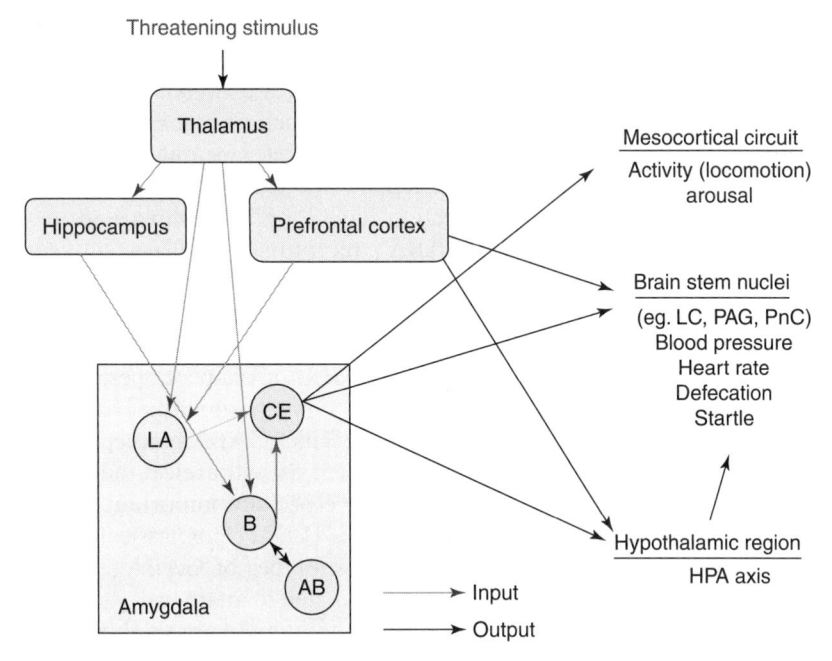

Figure 1.4 Brain regions involved in processing fear, stress, and emotionality in animals. Threatening stimuli are received and processed by brain regions such as the thalamus, hippocampus, prefrontal cortex (PFC), and amygdala. The amygdala sends projections to a number of target regions. These include brain stem nuclei such as the locus ceruleus (LC), periaqueductal gray (PAG), and pontine nucleus caudalis (PnC), which mediate various forms of autonomic arousal. The amygdala is also connected to the mesocortical circuit that mediates arousal and activity (as measured by locomotion in mice) and the hypothalamic region which controls glucocorticoid levels through the hypothalamic–pituitary-adrenal (HPA) axis. The PFC, which is involved in executive functions such as attention, also sends projections directly to the brain stem and the hypothalamus. (See color insert.)

hippocampus increased open-arm exploration in EPM [91, 92]. The septohippocampal system has been identified as being essential for the sensory processing of stimuli based on novelty and punishment [93]. Hippocampus has also been implicated in contextual fear conditioning [94].

Forebrain structures, including the medial prefrontal cortex (MPFC) and septum, are connected to the limbic system and their dysfunction has also been found in anxiety. Also, several studies have shown that lesions (cytotoxic and transection) of the MPFC inhibit fear-related behavior in rats [95–98]. These data indicate that MPFC promotes anxiety-like behavior. Finally, brain stem nuclei are important in the regulation of arousal. Of particular importance in anxiety are the noradrenergic locus ceruleus and the serotonergic raphe nuclei [99, 100].

1.6 NEUROTRANSMITTER SYSTEMS AND NEURONAL MESSENGERS IMPLICATED IN ANXIETY AND ANXIETY-LIKE BEHAVIOR

Traditionally, anxiety disorders have been viewed as disturbances in neurotransmitters, including γ-aminobutyric acid (GABA), 5-HT, norepinephrine (NE), dopamine

(DA), and neuropeptides such as corticotropin-releasing hormone (CRH), cholecystokinin (CCK), and neuropeptide Y (NPY). Many of these neurotransmitters and their receptors have been identified as sites of action for anxiolytic drugs. However, neuronal messengers other than neurotransmitters such as cytokines have recently been implicated in anxiety. Here we summarize the relevant pharmacological data while a later section covers the pertinent genetic studies.

Alterations in $GABA_A$ receptor function have long been implicated in anxiety disorders. For example, a deficit in $GABA_A$ receptors has been identified in the hippocampus and parahippocampus of patients suffering from panic disorder and generalized anxiety disorder [101–103]. Furthermore, $GABA_A$ receptor antagonists can elicit anxiety in patients with panic disorder, thereby mimicking a functional deficit of $GABA_A$ receptors [104]. The $GABA_A$ receptor is a pentameric ion channel typically composed of $2\alpha(\alpha_{1-6})$, $2\beta(\beta_{1-3})$, and $1\gamma(\gamma_{1-3})$ subunits [105, 106], and animal studies suggest that alterations in specific $GABA_A$ receptor subunits are associated with certain forms of anxiety, such as withdrawal-induced anxiety [107, 108]. $GABA_A$ receptor subunits have an especially important relevance in terms of the anxiolytic effect of benzodiazepines [109–111]. Classical benzodiazepines exert their effects by binding to multiple subtypes of $GABA_A$ receptor, the predominant subtypes in the brain being those that contain $\alpha_{1,2,3,5}$ subunits. A recent report using receptor subtype–preferring compounds in nonhuman primate models concluded that α_1 subunits containing receptors do not play a key role in the anxiolytic and muscle-relaxant properties of benzodiazepine-type drugs; instead, these effects involve $\alpha_{2,3,5}$ subunits containing $GABA_A$ receptors [112]. Animal models have recently also been used to determine the $GABA_A$ receptor subtype involved in the anxiolytic action of benzodiazepines (see description of these animals in Section 1.10).

Although lesion of 5-HT neurons in animals suggests a role for 5-HT in the control of anxiety states [113], the evidence for this notion is both conflicting and controversial. On the other hand, pharmacological manipulation of either the 5-HTT or the 5-HT_{1A} receptor can clearly alter 5-HT neurotransmission and anxiety. The level of 5-HT is regulated by both the 5-HTT and the 5-HT_{1A} autoreceptor (in the serotonergic raphe nuclei) [114, 115]. Inhibiting 5-HTT by selective serotonin reuptake inhibitors (SSRIs) has been shown to be very effective in certain anxiety disorders [114, 115]. Also, partial 5-HT_{1A} receptor agonists such as buspirone have an anxiolytic effect [116]. Recently, animals with genetic modifications have significantly contributed to our understanding of the 5-HT system and the possible role of various 5-HT receptors in anxiety (see Section 1.10).

The role of NE in anxiety is based on its well-known involvement in stress reaction. Stress provokes and aggravates anxiety by increasing catecholamine release via the sympathoadrenal system in the periphery. In addition, NE neurons in the locus ceruleus play a critical role in the body's response to alarm and threat. NE is believed to play an especially important role in anxiety disorders, such as panic disorder and PTSD [117, 118].

DA is mostly known as a mediator of reward and locomotor activity. However, these processes are also fundamental in personality traits and emotionality (Figs. 1.1–3), and the pharmacological manipulation of DA receptors have been reported to modulate anxiety-related behaviors. Specifically, agonists and antagonists for the DA D_2 class of receptors (which includes D_2, D_3, and D_4 subtypes) have anxiogenic and anxiolytic properties, respectively [119–121].

A number of neuropeptides have been implicated in anxiety and have been suggested as therapeutic targets [122]. The stress response is mediated partly by the activation of CRH. CRH is produced in the hypothalamus (H), leading to the secretion of the adrenocorticotropin hormone (ACTH) from the pituitary (P), which in turn causes an increase in the synthesis and release of glucocorticoids from the adrenal glands (A) (HPA axis). The activation of the HPA axis is also involved in stress-related psychopathology such anxiety disorders [123–125]. The maladaptive effects of chronic stress on the HPA axis have been extensively studied in both preclinical and clinical settings, and since a number of excellent reviews are available, this topic is not discussed further here [125–129]. In addition to the activation of the HPA axis and the consecutive release of the stress hormones, CRH is present outside of the hypothalamus where it is believed to participate in stress response [130]. Central administration of CRH in rodents produces behavioral effects that correlate with a state of anxiety such as reduced exploration in a novel environment or enhanced fear response [131–134]. Preclinical studies strongly implicate a role for central CRH, probably via the central noradrenergic systems, in the pathophysiology of certain anxiety disorders [125].

Glucocorticoids (corticosterone in rodents and cortisol in humans), the final effectors modulating the physiological response to stress, act via two receptor subtypes: the mineralocorticoid receptor (MR) and the glucocorticoid receptor (GR) [135]. GRs are also the main regulators of a negative-feedback circuit that regulates the HPA axis following stress. Activation of GRs in the pituitary, hypothalamus, hippocampus, and frontal cortex decreases CRH gene expression, leading to a decrease in CRH release and the suppression of the stress-induced endocrine response [136, 137].

Another neuropeptide, NPY, has also been suggested to be involved in the clinical symptoms of anxiety [138]. In rats, central administration of NPY produces effects similar to that of anxiolytic drugs [139] whereas specific inhibition of the NPY-1 receptor by antisense oligonucleotide resulted in an increased anxiety-like behavior [140].

During the last few years, CCK has emerged as an important polypeptide in the central nervous system (CNS). There are several lines of evidence for a role of CCK in anxiety and panic attacks, and data also indicate that specific agonists to brain CCK(2) receptors produce anxiogenic-like effects while CCK(2) antagonists elicit anxiolytic-like responses [141–144].

Substance P has also been suggested to have a modulatory role in anxiety [145]. Substance P is released in response to aversive stimuli [146] and its administration in animal models elicits both anxiogenic and anxiolytic activity, depending on the dose and the specific brain region [122]. The receptor for substance P is the G-protein-coupled tachykinin NK-1 receptor which is expressed in brain areas associated with fear and anxiety [147]. Increasing numbers of reports indicate that specific antagonists of NK-1 receptors produce anxiolytic effects [148].

Although cytokines are not neurotransmitters and their primary role is in the immune system, several lines of evidence indicate that interleukin (IL) 1β, interleukin-6, and tumor necrosis factor (TNF) α modulate anxiety and mood [149].

Specifically, these proinflammatory cytokines elicit symptoms of anxiety/depression that may be attenuated by chronic antidepressant treatment. Also, immunotherapy using IL-2 or interferon (IFN) α, promotes depressive/anxiety symptoms [149]. Interestingly, the effects of cytokines are exacerbated by stressors, and chronic cytokine elevations may act synergistically with stressors [149].

1.7 GENETIC SUSCEPTIBILITY TO ANXIETY DISORDERS

A number of studies have sought to identify chromosomal regions and genes relevant to anxiety disorders. Although the results of linkage and association studies are inconsistent so far (see detailed description of these studies in [150–152]), candidate gene studies have yielded more consistent data. In several studies, a relatively small but significant increase in neuroticism was found in individuals who carry the *s/s* (short promoter repeat) alleles of the 5-HTT as compared to individuals with *s/l* (long) or *l/l* alleles [9, 153]. The *s* allele is associated with decreased transporter activity. Over 20 other studies extended this association to psychopathology, but not all found evidence for an association between 5-HTT polymorphism and anxiety [45]. However, recent meta-analyses of these studies found a moderate but significant association between 5-HTT polymorphism and NEO neuroticism [46] and TPQ (tridimensional personality questionnaire) harm avoidance [154]. The association of decreased transporter activity with anxiety is a rather surprising finding because pharmacological inhibition of the 5-HTT by SSRIs reproducibly results in an anxiolytic effect. However, the genetically determined reduction in 5-HTT activity in patients is present from early prenatal life and may affect brain development leading to anxiety in later life. Consistent with this notion, pharmacological inhibition of 5-HTT in early postnatal life in mice (which corresponds to late prenatal life in human) resulted in increased anxiety-like behavior in later life [155]. In summary, these data suggest that genetic or pharmacological reduction of transporter activity during brain development can lead to increased anxiety in adult life.

The 5-HT$_{1A}$ receptor (5-HT$_{1A}$R) has also been implicated in anxiety because reduced receptor levels were detected in the anterior cingulate, posterior cingulate, and raphe by positron tomography in patients with panic disorder [156]. These recent data complement previous reports that showed a deficit in the 5-HT$_{1A}$R in PTSD and panic disorder patients [157–160]. However, no specific 5-HT$_{1A}$R allele has been associated with anxiety disorders (a promoter polymorphism, on the other hand, has been linked to major depression and suicide [159]).

Although polymorphism in BDNF has primarily been studied in depressive disorder, the *val* allele of the Val66Met substitution polymorphism has recently been shown to be associated with higher mean neuroticism scores in the NEO- five factor inventory (NEO-FFI) in healthy subjects [161]. In another study the self-ratable state-trait anxiety inventory (Spielberger state-trait anxiety inventory) score, which allows anxiety to be quantified as a comparatively stable personality trait, showed a higher level of anxiety in Val/Val compared to Val/Met and Met/Met genotypes [11, 162]. These are surprising findings since it is the *met* allele that is hypofunctional (as a result of alterations in BDNF trafficking and secretion [163]) and because animal studies clearly show that genetic inactivation of BDNF results in anxiety (see Section 1.9).

1.8 GENETIC BASE OF ANXIETY-LIKE BEHAVIOR IN MICE

1.8.1 QTL Studies

QTL analysis of F2 hybrids of two strains of mice (A/J and C57BL/6J) that differ markedly in thigmotaxis and light-to-dark (LD) transition behaviors showed a linkage of LD to chromosome 10 (near D10Mit237; LOD of 9.3) and suggestive QTLs (LOD > 2.8) at chromosomes 6, 15, 19, and X [14]. In the open field, suggestive QTLs were mapped to chromosomes 6 and 14 [13]. These data indicate a lack of shared QTLs of fear/anxiety-associated behavior in various experimental paradigms (avoidance in LD and open field). Another group using multiple measures of avoidance and autonomic arousal found that the various measures are mapped to the same or nearby chromosomal location(s) [12, 15]. These studies used two relatively closely related mouse lines bred for differential anxiety-like behavior; thus a relatively small subset of genes may have changed during breeding. In contrast, the study that concluded a lack of shared QTLs in anxiety-like behavior [13] utilized the more distantly related A/J and C57BL/6J mice which presumably carried different anxiety-related alleles in multiple loci. This study may be easier to extrapolate to human populations characterized by a high degree of heterogeneity. So far, no genes have been identified in anxiety-related QTLs. Since QTLs are in the range of 10–30 cM, a region containing hundreds of genes, identification of linked genes within QTLs is difficult.

1.8.2 Anxiety-Like Behavior in Genetically Altered Mice

Recently, it has become possible to inactivate specific genes routinely in the mouse, and a large number of knockout strains have been generated. Many of the targeted genes have been implicated in anxiety, and the corresponding knockout strains have regularly showed behavioral abnormalities in anxiety-related tests (Tables 1.2 and 1.3). Beyond the mouse strains with inactivated "candidate" anxiety genes, anxiety-like behaviors were sometimes seen in mice with genetic inactivation in genes not obviously related to anxiety. These genes include intracellular signaling molecules and regulators of transcription/translation (Table 1.4). The association of these genes with anxiety-like phenotype indicates that anxiety is not limited to abnormalities of the neurotransmitter systems but can also be related to gene regulatory processes. Analysis of the genomic position of these genes shows that they are distributed throughout many chromosomes with no obvious clustering at any locus (Fig. 1.5).

One caveat of the analysis of anxiety-related knockout mouse strains is that the behavioral phenotypes are not always robust and are sometimes even questionable. Moreover, many variables can alter the interpretation of anxiety-related behavioral tests and tests are not standardized across laboratories and environmental factors. Furthermore, anxiety-like behavior may be part of a complex phenotype and secondary to major developmental or neuroanatomical defects. We limited our

TABLE 1.2 Mice with Genetic Alteration of Neuronal Messengers Exhibiting Altered Anxiety Levels

Targeted Gene/Protein	Behavioral Test	Avoidance (Av)	Activity (Ac)	Arousal (Aa)	Anxiety	Chr	Reference
GAD65 KO	OF, EZM	+	−	n/a	↑	chr2 qA3 (1)	[164]
COMT KO	L/D	+(F only)	−(F only)	n/a	↑	chr16 qA3 (2)	[168]
NET KO	OF	n/a	−	n/a	?	chr8 qC5 (3)	[169]
5-HTT KO	OF, EZM	+	−	+(?)	↑	chr11 qB5 (4)	[171]
CRH overexpressing	OF, EPM, NSF, AA, FPS	+/−	0	n/a	↑/0	—	[172]
CRH KO	OF, EPM	+	−	n/a	↑	chr3 qA2 (5)	[173, 174]
CRH-BP overexpressing	EPM, OF, and other	0	0	−	0	—	[175]
CRH-BP KO	OF, EPM	−	+	0	↓	chr13 qD1 (6)	[180]
NPY KO	EPM, OF and other	+	−	0	↑	—	[179]
ProEnkephalin KO	OF, AS, EPM, PA	0	−	+	↑	chr6 qB2.3 (7)	[181]
OFQ/N KO	OF, EZM	+	−	n/a	↑	chr4 qA1 (8)	[182]
BDNF cond KO	OF, EPM, L/D	+	−	+	↑	chr14 qD1 (9)	[184]
TNFα overexpressing	OF, EPM, L/D	+	n/a	+	↑̃	—	[185]
TNFα KO	OF, L/D	+	+/−	n/a	↑	chr2 qE3 (10)	[190]
Interferon γ KO	L/D	+	−	n/a	↑	chr16 qA1 (11)	[192]
	OF, EPM	+	0	0	↑(?)	—	[194]
	OF, EPM, PA	+	−	+	↑	chr10 qD2 (12)	[195]

Notes: AvAcAa shown as decreased (−), increased (+), or not different (0) from wild-type (WT) controls. n/a = data not obtained by investigator. F = females; Chr = chromosome location and assigned number corresponding to illustration in Figure 1.5; OF = open-field exploration; KO = knockout; EZM = elevated-zero maze; L/D = light-dark box; EPM = elevated-plus maze; NSF = novelty-supressed feeding; AA = active avoidance; FPS = fear-potentiated startle; AS = acoustic startle; PA = passive avoidance; GAD65 = glutamic acid decarboxylase, 65-kD isoform; COMT = catechol-*O*-methyl transferase; NET = norepinephrine transporter; 5-HTT = serotonin transporter; CRH = corticotropin-releasing hormone; CRH-BP = CRH binding protein; NPY = neuropeptide Y; OFQ/N = orphanin FQ/nociceptin; BDNF = brain-derived neurotrohpic factor; TNFα = tumor necrosis factor α.

TABLE 1.3 Mice with Genetic Alteration of Receptors and Other Cell Membrane–Associated Proteins Exhibiting Altered Anxiety Levels

Targeted Gene/Protein	Behavioral Test	Avoidance (Av)	Activity (Ac)	Arousal (Aa)	Anxiety	Chr	Reference
GABA$_A$R:$\gamma_2^{+/-}$	EPM, OF, L/D, PA, FC	+	−	n/a	↑	chr11 qA5 (13)	[196]
5HT$_{1A}$R KO	EPM, OF, EMZ and other	+	−	+	↑	chr13 qD1 (14)	[207–209]
5HT$_{1B}$R KO	OF, EPM, NSF	−	+	n/a	↓	chr9 (15)	[220]
	EPM, FC, and other	0	0	n/a	0	—	[94]
CRH-R1 KO	L/D, EPM	−	0	−	↓	chr11 qE1 (16)	[224]
CRH-R2 KO	EPM, L/D, OF	+/0	0/+	+	↑	chr6 qB3 (17)	[225, 226]
DA D$_3$ KO	OF, EPM	−	+	n/a	↓	chr16 qB4 (18)	[229]
α_{2A}-AR KO	EPM, OF	+	−	n/a	↑	chr19 qD2 (19)	[234]
Adenosine A$_{2a}$ KO	EPM, L/D	+	−	n/a	↑	chr10 qC1 (20)	[236]
nAChR α_7 KO	OF, L/D, AS, FC	0	+	0	0/↓	chr7 qB5 (21)	[243]
nAChR α_4 KO	EPM	+	−	n/a	↑	chr2 qH4 (22)	[244]
trkb overexpressing	EPM, L/D, FC	−	+	n/a	↓	chr13 qB2 (23)	[246]
NCAM KO	EPM, L/D	−	+	n/a	↓	chr9 qA5.3 (24)	[248]
L1 cond KO	EPM, OF	−	+	n/a	↓	chrX qA7.2 (25)	[249]
Cadherin 11 KO	EPM, AS, FC	−	+	−	↓	chr8 qD1 (26)	[250]
GIRK2 KO	EPM, L/D	−	+	n/a	↓	chr16qC4 (27)	[238]

Notes: AvAcAa shown as decreased (−), increased (+), or not different (0) from wild-type (WT) controls. n/a = data not obtained by investigator. Chr = chromosome location and assigned number corresponding to illustration in Figure 1.5; KO = knockout; EZM = elevated-zero maze; L/D = light-dark box; EPM = elevated-plus maze; OF = open-field exploration; PA = passive avoidance; AS = acoustic startle; FC = fear conditioning; GABA$_A$R: γ_2 = γ-aminobutyric acid receptor A, γ_2 subunit; 5-HT$_{1A/1B}$R = serotonin 1A or 1B receptor; CRH-R1/R2 = CRH receptor 1 or 2; DA D$_3$ = dopamine D$_3$ receptor; α_{2A}-AR = α_{2A}-adrenergic receptor; nAChR $\alpha_{7/4}$ = nicotinic acetylcholine receptor α_7 or α_4; trkB = neurotrophin receptor tyrosine kinase B; NCAM = neural cell adhesion molecule; L1 = NCAM L1; GIRK2 = G-protein-coupled inwardly rectifying K$^+$ channel 2.

TABLE 1.4 Mice with Genetic Alteration of Intracellular Signaling Molecules and Transcriptional Regulators Exhibiting Altered Anxiety Levels

Targeted Gene/Protein	Behavioral Test	Avoidance (Av)	Activity (Ac)	Arousal (Aa)	Anxiety	Chr	Reference
αCaMKII KO	FC, OF	−	n/a	−	↓	chr18 qE1 (28)	[252]
PKCγ KO	EPM, L/D and other	−	+	n/a	↓	chr7 (29)	[255]
Fyn trk KO	L/D, PA	+	−	n/a	↑	chr10 qB1 (30)	[256]
NF-kB p50 KO	OF, EPM and other	−	+	n/a	↓	chr3 qG3 (31)	[260]
GR KO	L/D, EZM	−	+	0	↓	chr18 qB3 (32)	[263]
GR overexpressing	EPM, L/D	+	−	0	↑	—	[265]
VDR KO	OF, EPM, L/D	+	−	n/a	↑	chr15 qF4 (33)	[266]
CREB KO	OF, EZM, EPM, L/D	+	−	0	↑	chr1 qC2 (34)	[268]
CREM KO	EPM, OF, EZM, FC	−	+/0	n/a	↓	chr18 qA1 (35)	[270]

Notes: AvAcAa shown as decreased (−), increased (+), or not different (0) from wild-type (WT) controls. n/a = data not obtained by investigator. Chr = chromosome location and assigned number corresponding to illustration in Figure 1.5; OF = open-field exploration; KO = knockout; EZM = elevated-zero maze; L/D = light–dark box; EPM = elevated-plus maze; FC = fear conditioning; PA = passive avoidance; αCaMKII = α-calcium–calmodulin kinase II; PKCγ = protein kinase Cγ; Fyn trk = Fyn tyrosine kinase; NF-kB = nuclear factor kB; GR = glucocorticoid receptor; VDR = nuclear vitamin D receptor; CREB = cAMP-responsive element binding protein; CREM = cAMP-responsive element modulator.

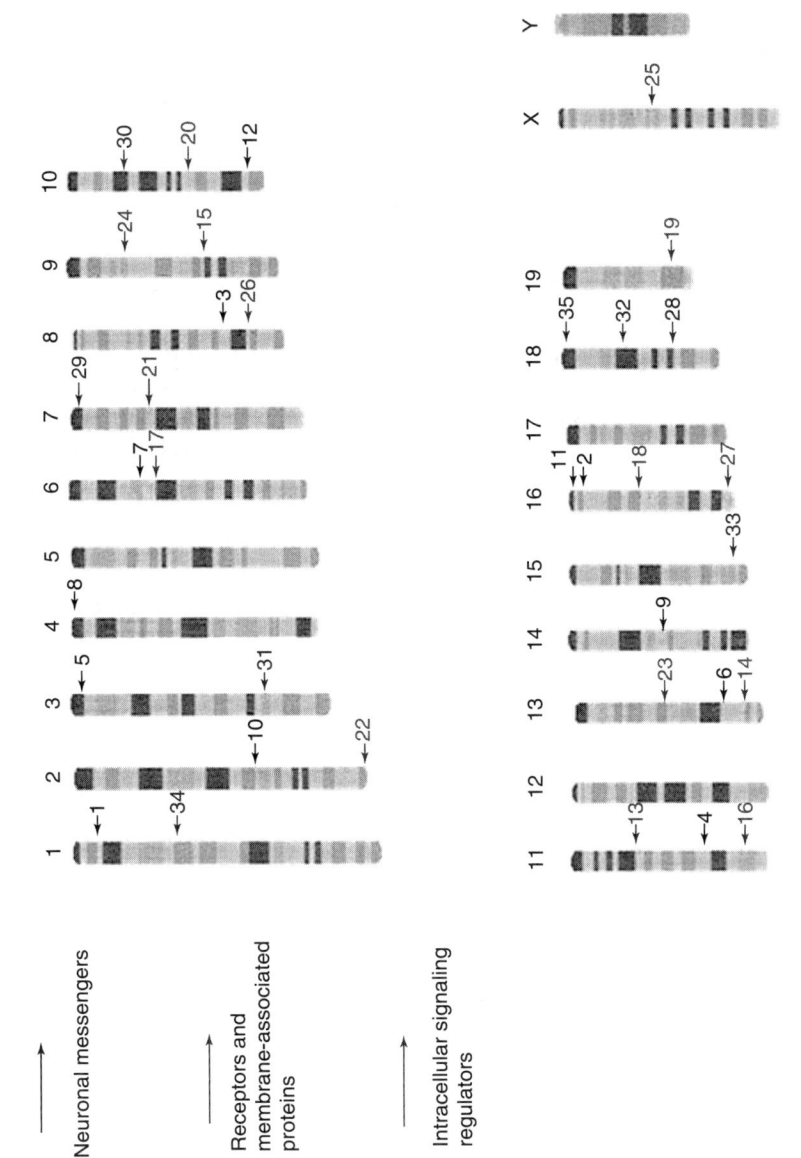

Figure 1.5 Chromosomal location of anxiety-related genes listed in Tables 1.2–4. (See color insert.)

analysis to mutant strains that have been generated and studied by multiple groups and to those that, although analyzed by a single laboratory, showed anxiety-related phenotypes in at least two independent behavior tests.

1.9 KNOCKOUT MICE WITH DISTURBANCES IN NEURONAL MESSENGERS EXHIBITING ALTERATIONS IN ANXIETY-LIKE BEHAVIOR

Classical neurotransmitters (GABA, NE, 5-HT) and neuropeptides have long been implicated in anxiety, so it was not surprising that inactivation of genes encoding enzymes responsible for the synthesis and metabolism of neurotransmitters or encoding neuropeptides alter anxiety levels (Table 1.2).

Glutamic acid decarboxylase (GAD) catalyzes the synthesis of GABA from glutamate and the genetic inactivation of the 65-kDa isoform of GAD (GAD65) results in anxiety-like behavior in mice [164]. Although GAD65 is responsible for the synthesis of a smaller pool of GABA than GAD67 [165, 166], it is associated with nerve terminals and synaptic vesicles and can be rapidly activated in times of high GABA demand. In GAD65$^{-/-}$ tissues the overall GABA content is normal but K^+-stimulated GABA release is reduced. Therefore, GAD65$^{-/-}$ mice show no overt developmental phenotype but the more subtle anxiety-like behavioral phenotype [164] and increased seizure sensitivity [165]. In contrast, GAD67$^{-/-}$ mice, although born at the expected frequency, die of severe cleft palate during the first morning after birth [166]. These data are consistent with reports that enhancing synaptic GABA levels, for example by GABA reuptake inhibitors, has an anxiolytic effect [167] and indicate that an appropriate level of synaptic GABA release is important for maintaining normal behavioral responses in anxiety-inducing situations.

The enzyme catechol-O-methyl transferase (COMT) is involved in the degradation of DA, NE, and epinephrine and its inactivation also leads to anxiety-like behavior [168]. Measurement of tissue catecholamine levels in COMT$^{-/-}$ mice showed a specific increase in DA levels with no change in NE or 5-HT levels. Furthermore, this increase in DA seems to be restricted to the frontal cortex. Although the increased DA levels were evident in both males and females, an increased anxiety behavior was observed only in females.

Genetic inactivation of the NE transporter (NET), as expected, results in a significant increase of extracellular levels of NE [169]. These mice show increased activity in the open field that would be consistent with a reduced level of anxiety. However, no data are available regarding avoidance and autonomic arousal of these mice and hyperactivity can arouse independently of a change in anxiety.

Since 5-HTT (s/s genotype) has been identified as a susceptibility gene for anxiety (see Section 1.7), it was expected that mice with an inactivated copy of the corresponding gene would show elevated levels of anxiety. Initial studies indicated that knockout mice have no obvious behavioral phenotype even if 5-HTT binding sites were completely absent in these animals [170]. However, a later study indicated an increased anxiety-like phenotype in 5-HTT knockout mice which was more pronounced in females [171]. A more recent analysis of these mice found no differences in anxiety-related behaviors in the open-field and EPM tests, but an increase was seen in latency to feed in a novel environment [172]. Lack of a reproducible and robust anxiety-like phenotype in 5-HTT knockout mice raises the question of how a partial reduction in 5-HTT activity in humans (s/s genotype) can be associated with elevated levels of neuroticism and anxiety.

Pharmacological experiments indicate the involvement of neuropeptides in the pathogenesis of anxiety, and this notion has been further supported by genetically modified mouse strains. An anxiety-like phenotype has been described in transgenic mice overexpressing CRH [173, 174]. However, mice with a deleted CRH gene did not differ from wild-type animals in anxiety-related behaviors even if they had significantly decreased basal corticosterone levels [175, 176]. One possible explanation is the redundancy in the central CRH system (e.g., urocortin). Consistent with this notion, stress-induced behavioral effects in CRH mutant mice could be reduced by the administration of a CRH antagonist [177]. Two independent groups have generated mice with a deletion of the urocortin gene [178], but only one study found behavioral abnormalities, namely an increased anxiety-like phenotype [178]. Finally, deletion of the CRH binding protein (BP), which normally binds and inactivates CRH, resulted in increased anxiety [179]. The authors hypothesized that the inactivation of CRH-BP may increase the "free" or unbound levels of CRH or urocortin, which results in anxiety. These data are also consistent with the reduced anxiety-like phenotype of mice constitutively overexpressing CRH-BP in the anterior pituitary gland [180].

Mice lacking the gene for NPY show a decrease in central area activity in the open field and an increased reactivity to acoustic startle [181]. However, no change in EPM was seen in $NPY^{-/-}$ mice compared to controls, suggesting that the absence of the peptide results in a condition characterized by increased stress responsiveness rather than anxiety.

Apart from altered pain responses, preproenkephalin-deficient mice exhibit increased anxiety in the open field and EZM [182]. It is believed that the modulatory role of enkephalins on anxiety behavior may be mediated by the GABA system [183].

Consistent with the anxiolytic activity of orphanin FQ/nociceptin (OFQ/N) or selective synthetic agonists in rodents, OFQ/N knockout mice display increased anxiety in several anxiety-related tests and impaired adaptation to repeated stress [184, 185]. Increased plasma corticosterone levels and a failure to show stress adaptation of OFQ/N knockout mice may suggest that activation of the HPA axis contributes to the anxiety phenotype in these mice.

BDNF, a member of the family of neurotrophins, promotes the formation, maturation, and stabilization of both glutamatergic and GABAergic synapses during CNS development, and it therefore regulates the balance between excitatory and inhibitory transmission, a fundamental step in neural circuit formation [186, 187]. Although homozygote BDNF knockout mice die during the second postnatal week [180, 188], heterozygote or conditional knockout mice show signs of altered emotional behavior. The role of BDNF in emotional reactions is important because the *val* allele has been associated with predisposition to anxiety disorders [10, 11]. Heterozygote BDNF knockout mice showed a slower escape behavior in the learned helplessness paradigm after training as compared to wild-type mice [189]. However, this effect may have been due to reduced sensitivity to centrally mediated pain as BDNF is essential for the survival and maintenance of peripheral sensory neurons [180, 188]. On the other hand, conditional BDNF mutant mice have also shown other signs of anxiety-like behavior [190]. In these conditional knockout mice, BDNF was removed after birth when most neurons are postmitotic, suggesting that the abnormal behaviors are related to neuronal maturation, survival, and/or plasticity rather than to the absence of BDNF during behavioral testing. Recently a mouse strain was generated in which the *val* allele was replaced by the *met* allele [190a]. Met substitution for Val in *BDNF* is a common polymorphism in humans associated with alterations in brain anatomy and memory. In agreement with association studies [10], BDNF(Met/Met) mice exhibited increased anxiety-related behaviors indicating that this variant predisposes to anxiety disorders.

In agreement with the anxiogenic effect of intracerebroventricularly administrered TNFα in the EPM [191], transgenic mice overexpressing TNFα show less exploration in novel environment [192] and increased activity [193]. However, TNFα knockout mice have a similar behavior in the EPM [193, 194]; thus, the role of TNF in the regulation of emotionality is not clear. Lack of another cytokine, IFNγ, has been reported to cause an anxiety-like phenotype [195]. However, the expression of this phenotype was visible only in C57BL/6 but not in the BALB/c mouse strain, indicating that major genetic modifiers play a role in the manifestation of anxiety in these mice. IFNγ is involved in regulating the growth of axodendritic processes, raising the possibility that, similar to the BDNF knockout mice, a neurodevelopmental abnormality underlies the anxiety in these knockout mice.

1.10 KNOCKOUT MICE WITH DEFICITS IN NEUROTRANSMITTER RECEPTORS AND OTHER CYTOPLASMIC MEMBRANE–ASSOCIATED PROTEINS EXHIBITING ANXIETY-LIKE BEHAVIOR

Blocking $GABA_A$ receptor increases anxiety-like behavior and genetic inactivation of some of the subunit genes has a similar effect (Table 1.3). For example, heterozygote $\gamma_2^{+/-}$ mice have reduced numbers of $GABA_A$ receptors and display an anxiety phenotype [107, 196]. The $\gamma_2^{+/-}$ mouse spends less time in the open arms of the EPM and less time in the lit area of the light–dark box, typical of increased anxiety-type behavior. In addition, $\gamma_2^{+/-}$ mice show increased responses in the passive avoidance paradigm. This is consistent with enhanced emotional memory for negative associations, a common feature of several anxiety disorders. These behavioral alterations are associated with a lower single-channel conductance, a pronounced deficit of functional receptors, and a reduction in α_2/gephyrin containing postsynaptic $GABA_A$ receptor clusters in cortex, hippocampus, and thalamus. Transgenic mice overexpressing either the mouse γ_{2L} or γ_{2S} subunits of the $GABA_A$ receptor showed no difference in anxiety-related behavior as compared to wild-type littermates [197]. Since compensation at the level of $GABA_A$ receptor subunit expression and assembly often occurs when subunit expression is disturbed (see below), it would be important to know the expression of all subunits in these mice. Among the α subunits, α_1 is predominant in $GABA_A$ receptors [198]. Two groups have independently generated mice with a deleted α_1 subunit and found no evidence for increased anxiety or other behavioral abnormalities [199–201]. However, an additional study demonstrated that lack of the α_1 subunit is compensated and substituted by other α subunits, presumably during development, mitigating the effect of the genetic deletion [199]. Although α_2-subunit-deficient mice have been generated and a point mutation in this subunit (H101R) abolishes the anxiolytic effect of diazepam [202, 203], no published data exist on the behavior of these mice except a faster habituation to a novel environment of the α_2-subunit-deficient mice (which was interpreted as less activity in a novel environment) [204]. Therefore it is not clear if these mice have an increased anxiety phenotype. An additional complication of the interpretation of the role of the α_2 subunit can be compensation by other α subunits as occurs in the α_1-subunit-deficient mice (see above). "Knockin" mice in the α_5 subunit (H105R) display enhanced trace fear conditioning to threat cues [196]. This is somewhat surprising because similar knockouts in the $\alpha_{1/2}$ subunits have no behavioral problems (see above). Further analysis showed that the knockin mice exhibit a 33% reduction in hippocampal (CA1 and CA3) α_5 receptor subunits; thus, these mice should be considered a partial knockout [196]. Also, α_5 receptor subunit null mutant mice exhibit improved performance in the water maze of spatial learning task but no change in locomotor activity in a novel environment [205]. Although the behavioral characterization of these mice is far from complete, it seems that the α_5 subunit is involved in hippocampal memory rather than in anxiety-related processes. Finally, the genetic inactivation of $\beta 2$, another predominant subunit, resulted in a more than 50% reduction in the total number of $GABA_A$ receptors and increased locomotor activity in the open field, suggesting that these receptors may control motor activity [200].

Besides the $GABA_A$ receptor, the $5\text{-}HT_{1A}$ receptor has long been implicated in the pathogenesis of anxiety disorders. In 1998, three groups reported the generation of $5\text{-}HT_{1A}$ receptor knockout mice on different strain backgrounds [38, 206–209]. All three groups reported that the mutant mice exhibit consistently enhanced anxiety-like behaviors alongside reduced immobility in the forced-swim test [209] or tail suspension test [207, 208], indicating an antidepressant-like effect. Anxiety-related tests in these studies included open field, EPM and EZM, and novelty-induced suppression of feeding as well as fear-conditioning paradigms [207–210]. The consistency in these reports is rather remarkable because of the difference in the targeting constructs and genetic backgrounds. $5\text{-}HT_{1A}$ receptors are expressed both at postsynaptic locations in 5-HT target areas (such as amygdala, hippocampus, and cortex) and presynaptically on 5-HT neurons in the raphe nuclei as somatodendritic autoreceptors. Since autoreceptors control neuronal firing, it was first believed that the anxiety phenotype of the $5\text{-}HT_{1A}$ receptor knockout mice was the result of an increase in 5-HT release and activation of other 5-HT receptor subtypes. However, basal 5-HT levels are not altered, as measured by in vivo microdialysis, in $5\text{-}HT_{1A}$ receptor null mice [47, 211–213], and expression of $5\text{-}HT_{1A}$ receptors in forebrain regions rescued the phenotype of $5\text{-}HT_{1A}$ receptor knockout mice [214], suggesting that the behavioral phenotype results from the absence of postsynaptic $5\text{-}HT_{1A}$ receptors. Another interesting feature of the $5\text{-}HT_{1A}$ receptor knockout mice is that their anxiety-like behavior is likely the result of an irreversible early postnatal developmental abnormality [214]. In addition to increased avoidance, $5\text{-}HT_{1A}$ receptor knockout mice display reduced locomotor activity, another sign of increased anxiety-like behavior [214]. Another characteristic of anxiety, increased autonomic arousal (Figs. 1.2 and 1.3), was also observed in these mice. Specifically, following exposure to injection or novelty-induced stress, $5\text{-}HT_{1A}$ receptor knockout mice exhibited a significantly greater increase in heart rate and body temperature than wild-type mice [215, 216]. Another group reported a similar effect following footshock [37]. Taken together, $5\text{-}HT_{1A}$ receptor knockout mice show abnormalities in three important measures of anxiety: increased avoidance, decreased locomotor activity, and increased autonomic arousal following exposure to a novel environment or stress. Moreover, these behavioral changes are reproducible across laboratories, which makes this genetic anxiety model not only one of the best studied but also the most robust so far in terms of the behavioral phenotype.

Another member of the 5-HT receptor family whose deletion has been associated with an alteration in anxiety levels is the 5-HT_{1B} receptor. 5-HT_{1B} receptors are predominantly localized to nerve terminals and serve as both auto- and hetero-receptors to inhibit neurotransmitter release [217, 218]. The open-field test indicated reduced anxiety-like behavior in 5-HT_{1B} receptor knockout mice [219], suggesting that this receptor may have an opposite function than that of the 5-HT_{1A} receptor (see above). Reduced anxiety was also seen in the novelty-induced suppression of feeding test [219]. However, the light-dark box and EPM tests showed no significant change in anxiety-like behavior in the 5-HT_{1B} receptor knockout mice [94, 220]. A further complication with this strain is that its behavioral phenotype was not reproducible in different laboratories even if the source of the mice was identical [220]. A similar reduced anxiety-like behavior was recently reported in 5-HT_{2A} receptor deficient mice in the EPM, open field and the light-dark box test [220a]. Importantly, the selective cortical re-expression of the 5-HT_{2A} receptor rescued the reduced anxiety-like behavior of 5-HT_{2A} receptor knockout mice indicating a role for cortical 5-HT_{2A} receptors in the modulation of conflict based anxiety-related behavior [220a].

There are two known CRH receptors (R1 and R2) and both have been suggested to be important in regulating anxiety levels. As discussed above, there are two ligands for these receptors: CRH and urocortin. Both CRH and urocortin are potent mediators of the endocrine, autonomic, behavioral, and immune responses to stress [221, 222]. CRH-R1 has a widespread distribution with high levels in anterior pituitary, hippocampus, amygdala, and cerebellum. While in the anterior pituitary CRH-R1 is involved in the activation of the HPA axis, in other regions it is responsible for the central action of CRH/urocortin and its activation is anxiogenic. In contrast to CRH-R1, expression of CRH-R2 in the CNS is restricted to the lateral septum and the ventromedial nucleus of the hypothalamus. While mice lacking CRH-R1 display decreased anxiety in the light-dark box and the EPM [223, 224], CRH-R2-deficient mice, generated independently by three groups, exhibit varying degrees of anxiety-related behavior. Bale et al. reported an increased anxiety in the EPM and open field but not in the light-dark box test in CRH-R2-deficient mice [225]. In the study of Kishimoto et al. [226], only male CRH-R2$^{-/-}$ mice exhibited anxious behavior in the EPM and light-dark box but, paradoxically, spent more time in the center of the open field, which is more consistent with reduced anxiety. However, Coste et al. found no significant change in anxiety behavior in the EPM or open field [227]. Although not all studies are consistent with a simple interpretation, the behavioral data obtained with various CRH-R knockout mice indicate that CRH and/or urocortin mediate a dual modulation of anxiety behavior. Activation of CRH-R1 appears to be anxiogenic while activation of CRH-R2 is anxiolytic. Therefore it may not be surprising that dual CRH-R1/2 knockout mice have only a subtle behavioral phenotype; specifically, females have a reduced anxiety-like behavior in the EPM but not in the open field while males show no behavioral abnormalities related to anxiety at all [228].

As mentioned earlier, DA, presumably by regulating reward and activity, is believed to be involved in anxiety-like behavior. In particular, DA D_2 receptors have been implicated in anxiety-related behavior. Consistent with these data, DA D_3 receptor knockout mice display reduced anxiety in the open field and EPM and increased locomotor activity [229]. In contrast, D_4 knockout mice exhibit enhanced anxiety in the open-field test in the presence of a novel object [230]. While altered anxiety levels were evident, the authors interpreted much of the behavioral phenotype as changes in exploratory behavior.

Although a role for the cannabinoid 1 (CB-1) receptor is less known in anxiety-like behavior, it has been reported that CB-1 knockout mice have increased anxiety-like behavior in the light–dark box [231] and reduced exploration of the open arms of the EPM apparatus [232]. However, evidence for reduced anxiety was found in CB-1 knockout mice in the shock-probe burying test, in which anxiety is reflected by increased burying, corresponding to increased active avoidance [233].

Although the NE system and the locus ceruleus (LC) are clearly significant in the pathogenesis of anxiety as well as in animal models of anxiety, there are relatively few studies that specifically tested the role of adrenergic receptors in these conditions. So far, the α_{2a}-adrenergic receptor has been studied (among the α_{2a}, α_{2b}, and α_{2c} receptors) and mice deficient in this receptor show increased anxiety-like phenotype in various tests [234].

Consistent with the "calming" effects of adenosine and anxiety-inducing nature of caffeine, rats treated with a nonspecific antagonist at adenosine receptors [235] as well as adenosine$_{2a}$ (A_{2a}) receptor null mice exhibit increased avoidance in the EPM and light–dark box, decreased exploratory behavior, and decreased locomotor activity (reduced activity), typical signs of increased emotionality and anxiety [236] (see also Fig. 1.3). The A_{2a} receptor is co expressed with DA D_2 receptors in GABAergic neurons in basal ganglia and striatum and is thought to regulate the expression of the proenkephalin gene [237]. In situ hybridization studies showed a decrease in proenkephalin gene expression in the A_{2a} receptor knockout mice, which may explain the anxiety-like behavior of these mice.

G-protein-gated inwardly rectifying K^+ (GIRK) channels contribute to postsynaptic inhibition triggered by many neurotransmitters, including DA and 5-HT, and GIRK2-deficient mice have been found to display a phenotype consistent with reduced anxiety [238]. Four GIRK subunits (GIRK1 to GIRK4) have been identified, and tetrameric channels formed by various combinations of GIRK1, GIRK2, and GIRK3 mediate inhibition in the nervous system [239, 240]. In addition to less avoidance in the EPM and light–dark box test, GIRK2 knockout mice also display increased locomotor activity satisfying two criteria of reduced emotionality (see Fig. 1.3).

Nicotinic agonists and antagonists can modulate anxiety [241, 242], and mice with a null mutation in the nicotinic acetylcholine receptor (nAChR) α_7 subunit gene have been shown to exhibit decreased anxiety in the open field but not in the light–dark box [243]. In contrast, mice deficient in the nAChR α_4-subunit gene display increased anxiety in the EPM [244], indicating that the subunit composition of the nAChR may determine whether the effect is anxiogenic or anxiolytic.

One of the targets of BDNF is trkB, a receptor tyrosine kinase [245]. Consistent with the increased anxiety-like phenotype of the conditional BDNF mutant mice

[246], transgenic mice overexpressing trkB in postmitotic neurons in a pattern similar to that of the endogenous receptor display less anxiety in the EPM test [246].

Neurotransmitter and neuromodulator receptors are not the only substrates of communicating external signals into neurons. Cell–cell interactions are crucial in regulating neuronal functions and developmental processes. One group of proteins that mediate cell–cell interactions is represented by neuronal adhesion molecules that regulate, among others, synaptic plasticity in both the developing and adult brain. Recent studies indicate that neuronal cell adhesion molecules of the immunoglobulin superfamily (NCAM and L1) are important mediators of the effects of stress. Chronic stress alters the expression pattern of cell adhesion molecules in parallel with their effects on behavior [247]. The connection between neuronal cell adhesion molecules and emotional behavior is also supported by the change in the anxiety-like phenotype of NCAM and L1 null mice. Genetic inactivation of NCAM results in decreased anxiety in the light–dark and EPM tests [248]. In addition, these mice respond to the anxiolytic effect of buspirone in the light–dark test at lower doses than the $NCAM^{+/+}$ mice, suggesting that there may be an alteration in the sensitivity of the 5-HT_{1A} receptors in these knockout mice. However, the authors reported no changes in the density of 5-HT_{1A} receptors or in tissue 5-HT content. Since NCAM has been demonstrated to have a role in CNS development and neuroplasticity, a developmental abnormality may explain the expression of anxiety-like behavior in these mice (similarly to the BDNF, IFNγ, and 5-HT_{1A} knockout mice; see Sections 1.9 and 1.10). Also, conditional inactivation of L1 in the forebrain, mostly from early postnatal life [by cre-recombinase under the control of the calcium/calmodulin-dependent protein kinase II (CaMK II) promoter], resulted in decreased anxiety in the open field and EPM [249]. Conditional expression avoids the severe morphological and behavioral abnormalities associated with the absence of L1 during prenatal development. Finally, the lack of cadherin-11, another cell adhesion molecule, results in reduced fear- or anxiety-related responses [250]. Cadherin-11 is expressed in the limbic system of the brain, most strongly in the hippocampus, and is densely distributed in synaptic neuropil zones. Taken together, the loss of function of three cell adhesion molecules leads to maladaptive behavioral responses that are "opposite" to anxiety and may be characterized as excessive novelty seeking and a lack of appropriate response to danger (see Fig. 1.3, blue region of the cube, and discussion in the accompanying text). It is striking that all three adhesion molecules mentioned above are involved in the regulation of synaptic structure and function [251]. This indicates that the optimal functioning of synapses is essential for mediating appropriate responses to novelty and stress.

1.11 INTRACELLULAR REGULATORS ASSOCIATED WITH ANXIETY-LIKE PHENOTYPE

A number of intracellular signaling molecules and transcription factors have been shown to cause increased or reduced anxiety-like phenotype in mice. The α isoform of CaMKII is an important second messenger, and Chen et al. [252] demonstrated decreased anxiety in CaMKII knockout mice. CaMKII is a major component of the postsynaptic density in glutamatergic synapses [253] and is involved in neuronal functions related to calcium signaling, including the induction of long-term potentiation (LTP) [254]. Therefore, the disruption of CaMKII function could alter many aspects of neuronal function, making it difficult to relate it to a specific anxiety behavior. Indeed these knockout mice also exhibit enhanced aggression and learning impairment.

The serine/threonine kinase protein kinase C γ (PKCγ) has recently been shown to be a regulator of anxiety behaviors [255]. PKCγ is restricted to the CNS and is highly expressed in limbic areas of the brain. In three different behavioral tests (EPM, light–dark test, mirrored chamber) PKCγ knockout mice consistently showed reduced anxiety-like behavior. Bowers et al. [255] proposed that PKCγ modulates anxiety by altering the function of $GABA_A$, N-methyl-D-aspartate (NMDA), or $5\text{-}HT_2$ receptors.

Another intracellular signaling molecule implicated in anxiety and fear responses is the tyrosine kinase Fyn. Fyn is a member of the Src family of tyrosine kinases that can associate with and phosphorylate a variety of molecules. Inactivation of the *fyn* gene in mice results in increased anxiety-like behavior to naturally aversive stimuli in the light–dark box and novelty tests [256]. These mice also display enhanced learned fear responses in the passive-avoidance test. Fyn is highly expressed in the limbic system and has been implicated in NMDA receptor–mediated synaptic plasticity, NCAM-dependent neurite outgrowth, and myelination [257–259]. Whether any or all of these processes are involved in the enhanced anxiety exhibited in the $Fyn^{-/-}$ mice is unclear.

The NF-kB transcription factor family is linked to a number of receptors, including TNFα, and controls the expression of many genes involved in cell survival, proliferation, and regulation of inflammatory and stress responses. It has recently been shown that mice lacking the p50 subunit of NF-kB have a reduced anxiety-like phenotype [260]. These mutant mice showed reduced avoidance and autonomic arousal in the open field and EPM. In immune cells, NF-kB factors are kept inactive by association with inhibitory proteins belonging to the IkB family and activating stimuli induce the phosphorylation, polyubiquitination, and proteasome degradation of IkBs, allowing NF-kB to translocate into the nucleus and activate target genes. In contrast, it seems that either NF-kB is constitutively active in neurons [261] or normal neuronal activity is sufficient to keep a substantial amount of NF-kB in an active form. Since it is expressed during development [262], NF-kB may regulate the development of brain circuits, and consequently the reduced anxiety-like phenotype of p50 knockout mice could be due to abnormal brain development.

GR is another transcription factor (activated via the HPA axis and glucocorticoid hormones) and is well known to be involved in stress response and some anxiety disorders. As discussed later, a brief period of controllable stress experienced with general arousal and excitement can be beneficial, but chronically elevated levels of circulating corticosteroids are believed to enhance vulnerability to a variety of diseases, including affective disorders. Therefore it is not surprising that the genetic manipulation of GR results in changes in emotionality in mice. Reduced anxiety-like phenotype was found in a brain-specific GR knockout [263] and in a GR-antisense model with reduced GR expression in brain and some peripheral tissues [264], while GR overexpression in forebrain results in increased anxiety-like behavior [265]. Together, these findings indicate that a sustained increase in GR activity in brain is associated with increased anxiety-like behavior.

In addition to its role in the regulation of calcium and phosphate homeostasis and in bone formation, vitamin D is also thought to be involved in brain function. Genetic ablation of the vitamin D receptor (VDR), another nuclear receptor linked to transcription, results in increased anxiety-like behavior in a battery of behavioral tests [266].

Still another group of transcription factors associated with anxiety-like behavior is the family of cyclic adenosine monophosphate (cAMP)-responsive nuclear factors that consist of CREB, CRE modulator (CREM), and activating transcription factor 1 (ATF-1) [267]. A conditional CREB mutation that inactivates all isoforms in the brain or the disruption of the two major transcriptionally active CREB isoforms (α and δ) increases anxiety-like responses in mice in different behavioral tests, including the EPM [268]. In CREB-deficient mice, the expression of CREM isoforms is increased [269]; thus, the higher anxiety-like phenotype may be attributable to this change. Indeed, CREM-deficient mice display reduced anxiety-like behavior in the EPM test and also exhibit hyperactivity [270], indicating that CREM activity may be linked to neuronal modulation promoting anxiety.

BC1 RNA is a small non–messenger RNA common in dendritic microdomains of neurons in rodents, and it is believed to play a role in translational regulation. Mice mutant for BC1 show behavioral changes consistent with increased anxiety and reduced exploration [271]. These data indicate that an anxiety-like phenotype can be induced by disturbing gene expression beyond transcription at the translational level.

Taken together, defects in intracellular processes involving second messengers, transcription factors, and translational factors can lead to alterations in anxiety in mice. To better understand the neurobiology of anxiety, it will be critical to identify the specific mRNAs and proteins whose altered synthesis in neurons of the fear/anxiety pathway is associated with the expression of the behavioral phenotype. In any event, the common feature of these molecular changes is that they could all eventually influence morphological and/or functional plasticity in the nervous system (see further discussion on this topic below).

1.11.1 Modeling Complex Genetics of Anxiety in Mice: Oligogenic Anxiety-Like Conditions in Mice

Genetic studies on various mouse phenotypes clearly indicate that most behavioral traits are heritable and are specified by multiple genes or QTLs. For example, mapping studies have estimated that the individual anxiety-related behavioral differences in the DeFries recombinant inbred strains of mice are the result of the interaction between four to six QTLs for each behavior; the largest QTL explains no more than half of the variance attributable to the detected QTL [15, 272, 273]. However, QTLs can consist of hundreds of genes, and these studies are not designed to analyze the contribution of individual genes to anxiety. An alternative strategy to study the combined effect of two or more genes on behavior is to use double- and triple-knockout mice. A recent report analyzed anxiety-related behaviors in double 5-HTT$^{-/-}$ and BDNF$^{+/-}$ mutant mice [274]. These mice, as compared to 5-HTT$^{-/-}$, BDNF$^{+/-}$, and wild-type mice, displayed a significantly higher level of anxiety-like behavior, reduced levels of 5-HT and 5-hydroxyindole acetic acid in the hippocampus and hypothalamus, and greater increases in plasma ACTH after a stressful stimulus. These findings support the hypothesis that genetic changes in BDNF expression interact with 5-HT to modulate anxiety and stress-related behaviors.

Another double-knockout strain lacking both monoamine oxidase (MAO) A and B, two enzymes responsible for the degradation of monoamines, shows anxiety-like behavior in various tests [275]. Neither the MAO_A nor the MAO_B knockout mutants display anxiety in these tests, indicating that an interaction between the two MAO genes leads to a novel phenotype [276, 277]. Since monoamine levels are higher in the double knockouts than in the single mutants, the abnormal behavior of $MAO_{A/B}$ mutants is likely the consequence of altered monoaminergic neurotransmission.

1.12 EFFECTS OF EARLY-LIFE ENVIRONMENT ON ANXIETY

1.12.1 Early-Life Experience on Expression of Anxiety in Later Life

A large body of evidence supports the notion that early-life environmental effects alter life-long stress-coping mechanisms. Unlike human studies, which are predominantly retrospective with a large number of environmental variables, animal research has focused on the effect of "handling" and maternal care during postnatal development. Brief handling of pups results in life-long decreases in behavioral and endocrine responses to stress while animals separated from their mothers/litters for longer periods of time (i.e., for several hours) exhibit increased anxiety [278–280]. Later studies determined that the critical feature of short-term handling was the increase in maternal care [licking and grooming (LG)] following the return of pups [281]. Variability in maternal care can produce large differences in adult behavior and hormonal responsiveness to stress. Pups nursed by mothers with either a high or a low level of LG and arched-back nursing (ABN) show a decreased and increased level of anxiety-like behavior in adult life (open field, novelty-suppressed feeding, and shock-probe burying assays), respectively [281–284]. Also, offspring of high LG–ABN mothers (as well as briefly handled pups) have reduced plasma levels of ACTH and corticosterone in adulthood following stressful stimuli such as restraint stress when compared to the offspring of low LG–ABN mothers (or nonhandled pups) [285]. Furthermore, these animals show increased glucocorticoid feedback sensitivity, increased hippocampal GR mRNA expression, and decreased hypothalamic CRH mRNA levels.

Interestingly, pups born to low LG–ABN mothers but cross fostered to high LG–ABN mothers develop low anxiety-like behaviors in adulthood, but high LG–ABN pups reared by low LG–ABN mothers do not develop increased anxiety-like responses in adulthood [285]. Furthermore, the maternal behavior of female offspring from low LG–ABN mothers can be changed by cross fostering them to high LG–ABN mothers. The reverse, however, is not true because daughters of high LG–ABN mothers raised by low LG–ABN dams have high LG–ABN maternal behavior [281, 286]. Finally, offspring of low LG–ABN mothers, if cross fostered to high LG–ABN mothers, show hormonal levels similar to those observed for offspring of high LG–ABN mothers [285]. These findings suggest that environmental effects may overpower genetic predispositions, particularly in cases where such modification would be beneficial for survival.

Although experiments related to both postnatal handling and maternal behavior clearly show a nongenomic influence on anxiety-like behavior, the transmission mechanism of this effect has been difficult to elucidate. It has been hypothesized that environmental influences exert some level of control on the development of HPA and the regulation of HPA function via a number of neurotransmitter systems, including the noradrenergic, GABAergic, and glutamatergic systems [287, 288]. For example, rat pups of high LG–ABN dams show altered $GABA_A$ receptor subunit expression in the amygdala, LC, medial prefrontal cortex, and hippocampus that could contribute to their reduced anxiety-like behavior as compared to pups from low LG–ABN dams [289, 290]. In addition to the GABAergic system, other potential factors mediating the environmental effects include the glutamatergic system and neurotrophins such as BDNF. Liu et al. [291] found that adult offspring of high LG–ABN Long Evans dams show increased hippocampal synaptogenesis and better spatial learning and memory than low LG–ABN offspring and that these differences could be equalized if low LG–ABN pups were cross fostered to high LG–ABN dams. More specifically, increased LG–ABN of offspring resulted in increased hippocampal mRNA expression of NR2A and NR2B NMDA receptor subunits at postnatal day 8, a change that was sustained into adulthood. Consistent with the regulation of the BDNF gene by NMDA receptors [292], increased levels of BDNF, but not NGF or NT-3, mRNA were observed in the dorsal hippocampus of eight-day-old high LG–ABN pups [291]. Most recently, it has been reported that the maternal effect is linked to alterations in methylation and chromatin structure at the GR promoter in the offspring [291a]. It has been proposed that downregulation of hippocampal GR in the pups of low nursing mothers compromises feedback inhibition in the hypothalamic pituitary adrenal axis ultimately leading to higher anxiety states [291a]. Since GR knockout mice have reduced anxiety [263] and GR overexpression in forebrain results in increased anxiety-like behavior [265], it is possible that the maternally-induced regulation is specific for a subset of GRs and does not involve the GR pool implicated in the stress related actions of glucocorticoids.

1.12.2 Interaction of Environment with Genes in Establishing Level of Anxiety

Although the interaction of genes and environment in shaping personality is well accepted, direct experimental evidence to support this notion has been difficult to obtain in humans. Recent association studies, however, have clearly indicated that genetic and environmental factors act together, enhancing the phenotype beyond the level established by either factor alone. For example, promoter polymorphism in 5-HTT can influence anxiety-related behavior (s/s genotype represents a predisposition to neuroticism/anxiety) [9], and a recent report showed that this polymorphism moderates the influence of stressful life events on depression. Individuals with one or two copies of the s allele of the 5-HTT promoter polymorphism exhibited more depressive symptoms in relation to stressful life events than l/s individuals [293]. Although this study was focused on depression, anxiety is a common symptom in depression, and future studies may reveal evidence of an interaction between an individual's 5-HTT allelic makeup and environmental insults in anxiety disorders. This connection has already been made in primates. Rhesus monkeys have a 5-HTT polymorphism similar to that found in humans, and it was shown that although both mother-reared and nursery-reared heterozygote (l/s) animals demonstrate increased affective responding (a measure of temperament) relative to l/l homozygotes, nursery-reared but not mother-reared l/s infants exhibited lower orientation scores than their l/l counterparts [294]. Also, monkeys with deleterious early rearing experiences were differentiated by genotype in cerebrospinal fluid concentrations of the 5-HT metabolite, 5-hydroxyindoleacetic acid, while monkeys reared normally were not [295]. Another study found that separation-induced increases in ACTH levels were modulated by both rearing condition and 5-HTT polymorphism [296]. During separation, animals with l/s genotypes had higher ACTH levels than l/l animals, and peer-reared l/s animals had higher ACTH levels than all other groups, including mother-reared animals.

Rodents are more amenable to such studies, and there have been a number of reports on the effect of early-life experience and gene interaction on later-life behavior. For example, early-life handling or cross fostering of highly neophobic BALB/c mice to less neophobic C57BL/6 mice equalizes both the behavioral and the benzodiazepine receptor expression differences between these two strains as well as decreasing the ACTH release following an acute stressor of BALB/c mice in adulthood [284, 297–299]. Furthermore, the effect of the $5HT_{1A}$ receptor gene on the anxiety-like behavior may be modulated by the environment. In a recent study, Weller et al. documented that F1 $5HT_{1A}R^{+/-}$ offspring reared by $5HT_{1A}R^{-/-}$ mothers have increased ultrasonic vocalization (USV) when compared to F1 $5HT_{1A}R^{+/-}$ offspring raised by $5HT_{1A}R^{+/+}$ dams [300]. However, contrary to expectations, F1 $5HT_{1A}R^{+/-}$ offspring reared by $5HT_{1A}R^{-/-}$ mothers have decreased measures of anxiety in the EPM as adults when compared to F1 $5HT_{1A}R^{+/-}$ offspring raised by $5HT_{1A}R^{+/+}$ dams. Also, $5HT_{1A}R^{-/-}$ pups reared by either $5HT_{1A}R^{-/-}$ or $5HT_{1A}R^{+/-}$ dams produced less isolation-induced response (USV) than their $5HT_{1A}R^{+/+}$ controls [300]. Although it is difficult to consolidate these seemingly contradictory results, these experiments show that the level of anxiety associated with $5HT_{1A}R$ deficiency can be altered by environmental factors.

In addition to early environmental influences, later-life or adult environment can also influence the expression of emotionality, as demonstrated in mouse models. As discussed previously, lack of the nociceptin/orphanin FQ gene leads to an enhanced anxiety phenotype in mice [184, 185]. The strength of the behavioral expression of the phenotype is dependent, however, on environmental influences such as social interactions. Ouagazzal et al. found that homozygous mutant animals, when housed alone, performed similarly to their wild-type controls on tests of emotional reactivity. Enhanced emotionality became apparent only when the singly housed animals were introduced to group housing (five animals per cage) that induced greater levels of aggression and increased anxiety responses [301].

Taken together, these data show that both genetic and environmental factors have an important role in establishing emotionality in mammals. Often, these factors work together, enhancing the phenotype beyond the level established by either factor alone. Other times, the environmental influences can partially or fully rescue undesirable phenotypes caused by genetic predispositions or mutations, enhancing the likelihood of the organism's survival.

1.13 CONCLUSIONS: NEUROBIOLOGY OF ANXIETY DISORDERS

Combining what is known about anxiety disorders (including symptomatology, pharmacology, and biochemistry) with the genetic and molecular information gathered from the diverse knockout mouse strains that exhibit alterations in anxiety-like behavior, it becomes apparent that anxiety-related pathways and processes involve communication between neurons (including neuronal messengers and their receptors) and/or signaling within cells (Fig. 1.6 [302]). Since the manipulation of a ligand, its receptor, and a coupled intracellular signaling elicits a similar anxiety-like behavior, it is possible to cluster these molecules to pathways. Many of these pathways eventually converge onto regulation of transcription and/or translation, and one can hypothesize that anxiety-like behavior is the result of changes, at least in part, at the level of gene expression (Fig. 1.6). Indeed, the genetic manipulation of transcription (by CREB, GR, VDR, and NF-kB; see previous sections) can also result in changes in anxiety levels.

Several of these "anxiety-related pathways" can be established. For example, the "serotonergic" pathway consists of receptors controlling the release of 5-HT (5-HT$_{1A}$ and 5-HT$_{1B}$ receptors), 5-HTT, postsynaptic 5-HT receptors, and mitogen-activated protein kinase/extracellular regulated protein kinase (MAPK/ERK) signaling (Fig. 1.6). As described in this chapter, a change in any of these components can lead to altered emotional behavior. The proper function of this pathway is especially crucial during early postnatal development, and one can hypothesize that abnormal signaling via this system alters the development of neuronal networks and consequently function, manifested as abnormal fear/anxiety response. BDNF, whose deficiency has also been associated with anxiety-like behavior, is also linked to the MAPK–ERK signaling (Fig. 1.6), suggesting that the two distinct anxiety-associated traits (deficit in 5-HT$_{1A}$ and BDNF) may share downstream targets. In addition to the convergence of various pathways, the same extracellular signal can diverge to various intracellular pathways illustrated by the coupling of the 5-HT$_{1A}$ receptor to both the MAPK–ERK and NF-kB pathways [303–307] (Fig. 1.6). Such divergence obviously broadens the clusters of affected genes. Since manipulation of the p50 subunit of NF-kB (activated by cytokines) can also be linked to anxiety-like behavior, crosstalk is extensive at the signaling level and therefore within and between anxiety-related pathways. Although the function of 5-HT and BDNF pathways is altered not only as a result of mutations and genetic polymorphisms but also by the environment, another "anxiety-related" pathway consisting of CRH, ACTH, and GR is especially sensitive to environmental changes. As with the other pathways, activation of this pathway by chronic stress eventually alters gene regulation (via GR).

It is hypothesized that abnormalities in these pathways at any level lead to, via altered gene expression, changes in neuronal morphology and/or function. Indeed, a number of knockout mouse strains with an anxiety-like phenotype as well as rodents following chronic stress show altered dendritic arborization in hippocampus and amygdala [308, 309], abnormal synapse formation [126, 250, 310], and altered electrical properties of neurons [311]. These changes result in abnormal neuronal network activity characterized by a deficit in short-term plasticity (i.e., hippocampal paired pulse facilitation and inhibition) [210, 312, 313], abnormalities in long-term potentiation [250, 312], an increase in network excitability [210, 311, 314], and abnormal activation or inhibition of brain regions as measured by fMRI [74, 75, 78]. In anxiety disorders, multiple molecular pathways may be simultaneously affected in multiple brain regions, consistent with the multitude of associated symptoms. Importantly, all commonly used anxiolytic drugs [benzodiazepines, selective

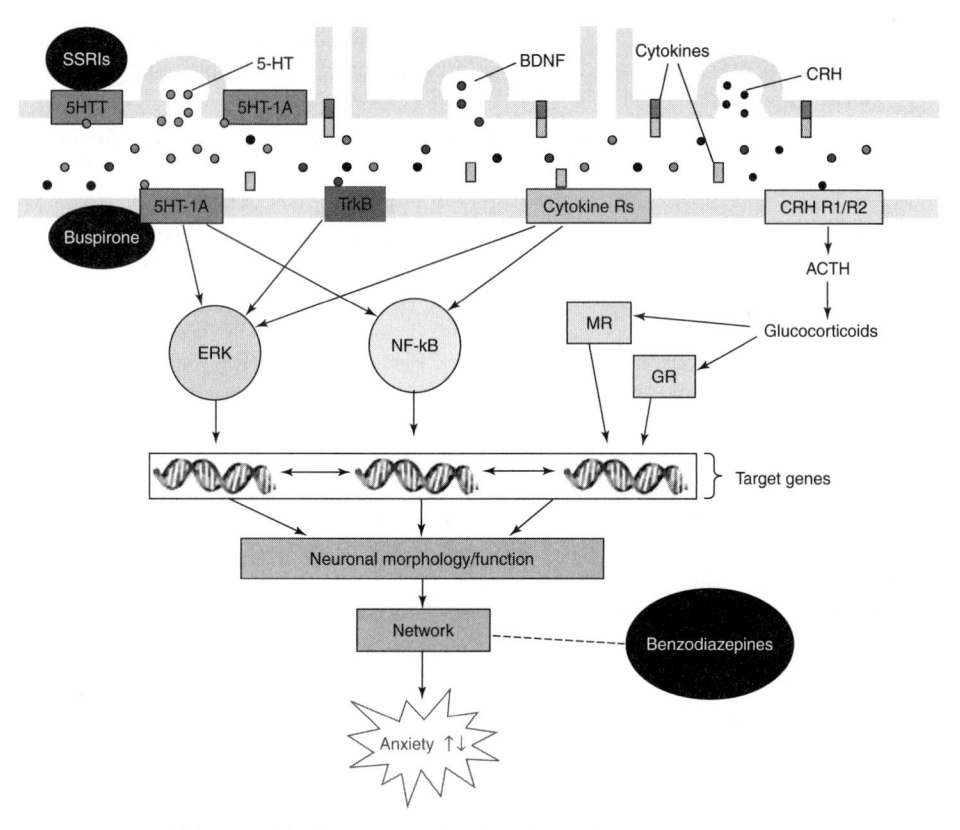

Figure 1.6 Unifying model of pathogenesis of anxiety. Pharmacological and genetic studies indicate that defects in specific substrates of neuronal communication (e.g.,5-HT, GABA, 5-HT receptors), intracellular signaling (e.g., ERK), and gene expression (GR) may be involved in anxiety-related behavior. These extracellular neuronal messengers and their associated receptors and coupled intracellular signaling form specific pathways. Abnormalities in these molecular pathways at various levels can directly modify the function/morphology of the neuronal network associated with fear, ultimately producing changes in anxiety levels. (See color insert.)

serotonin reuptake inhibitors (SSRIs), and buspirone] can be integrated into the model described above, indicating that the genetic data are consistent with the pharmacological data and that anxiolytic drugs target and modulate the molecular and cellular pathways which apparently control or establish (during development) the level of anxiety (Fig. 1.6).

REFERENCES

1. Eysenck, H. J. I. E. (1990). Biological dimensions of personality. In: *Handbook of Personality: Theory and Research*, L. A. Pervin, Ed. Guilford, New York, pp. 244–276.
2. Eysenck, H. J. (1967). *The Biological Basis of Personality*. Charles C. Thomas, Springfield, IL.
3. Costa, P. T. J., and McCrae, R. R. (1992). Normal personality assessment in clinical practice: The NEO Personality Inventory. *Psychol. Assess.* 4, 5–13.

4. Jang, K. L., McCrae, R. R., Angleitner, A., Riemann, R., and Livesley, W. J. (1998). Heritability of facet-level traits in a cross-cultural twin sample: Support for a hierarchical model of personality. *J. Pers. Soc. Psychol.* 74, 1556–1565.

5. American Psychiatric-Association (APA) (1994). *Diagnostic and Statistical Manual of Mental Disorders*, 4th edn. APA, Washington, DC.

6. Sherman, S. L., DeFries, J. C., Gottesman, I. I., Loehlin, J. C., Meyer, J. M., Pelias, M. Z., Rice, J., and Waldman, I. (1997). Behavioral genetics '97: ASHG statement. Recent developments in human behavioral genetics: Past accomplishments and future directions. *Am. J. Hum. Genet.* 60, 1265–1275.

7. Fullerton, J., Cubin, M., Tiwari, H., Wang, C., Bomhra, A., Davidson, S., Miller, S., Fairburn, C., Goodwin, G., Neale, M. C., Fiddy, S., Mott, R., Allison, D. B., and Flint, J. (2003). Linkage analysis of extremely discordant and concordant sibling pairs identifies quantitative-trait loci that influence variation in the human personality trait neuroticism. *Am. J. Hum. Genet.* 72, 879–890.

8. Neale, B. M., Sullivan, P. F., and Kendler, K. S. (2005). A genome scan of neuroticism in nicotine dependent smokers. *Am. J. Med. Genet. B Neuropsychiatr. Genet.* 132, 65–69.

9. Lesch, K. P., Bengel, D., Heils, A., Sabol, S. Z., Greenberg, B. D., Petri, S., Benjamin, J., Muller, C. R., Hamer, D. H., and Murphy, D. L. (1996). Association of anxiety-related traits with a polymorphism in the serotonin transporter gene regulatory region. *Science* 274, 1527–1531.

10. Jiang, X., Xu, K., Hoberman, J., Tian, F., Marko, A. J., Waheed, J. F., Harris, C. R., Marini, A. M., Enoch, M. A., and Lipsky, R. H. (2005). BDNF variation and mood disorders: A novel functional promoter polymorphism and Val66Met are associated with anxiety but have opposing effects. *Neuropsychopharmacology* 30, 1353–1361.

11. Lang, U. E., Hellweg, R., Kalus, P., Bajbouj, M., Lenzen, K. P., Sander, T., Kunz, D., and Gallinat, J. (2005). Association of a functional BDNF polymorphism and anxiety-related personality traits. *Psychopharmacology (Berl.)* 180, 95–99.

12. Flint, J., Corley, R., DeFries, J. C., Fulker, D. W., Gray, J. A., Miller, S., and Collins, A. C. (1995). A simple genetic basis for a complex psychological trait in laboratory mice. *Science* 269, 1432–1435.

13. Gershenfeld, H. K., Neumann, P. E., Mathis, C., Crawley, J. N., Li, X., and Paul, S. M. (1997). Mapping quantitative trait loci for open-field behavior in mice. *Behav. Genet.* 27, 201–210.

14. Gershenfeld, H. K., and Paul, S. M. (1997). Mapping quantitative trait loci for fear-like behaviors in mice. *Genomics* 46, 1–8.

15. Henderson, N. D., Turri, M. G., DeFries, J. C., and Flint, J. (2004). QTL analysis of multiple behavioral measures of anxiety in mice. *Behav. Genet.* 34, 267–293.

16. Soldz, S., and Vaillant, G. E. (1999). The Big Five personality traits and the life course: A 45-year longitudinal study. *J. Res. Pers.* 33, 208–232.

17. McAdams, D. P. (1992). The five-factor model in personality: A critical appraisal. *J. Pers.* 60, 329–361.

18. McCrae, R. R., and Costa, P. T., Jr. (1997). Personality trait structure as a human universal. *Am. Psychol.* 52, 509–516.

19. John, O. P. (1990). The "Big Five" factor taxonomy: Dimensions of personality in the natural language and in questionnaires. In: *Handbook of Personality: Theory and Research*, L. A. Pervin, Ed. Guilford, New York, pp. 66–100.

20. Benjamin, J., Li, L., Patterson, C., Greenberg, B. D., Murphy, D. L., and Hamer, D. H. (1996). Population and familial association between the D4 dopamine receptor gene and measures of novelty seeking. *Nat. Genet.* 12, 81–84.
21. Gray, J. A., and McNaughton, N. (2000). *The Neuropsychology of Anxiety.* Oxford University Press, Oxford.
22. Cloninger, C. R. (1987). A systematic method for clinical description and classification of personality variants. A proposal. *Arch. Gen. Psychiatry* 44, 573–588.
23. Loehlin, J. C., Horn, J. M., and Willerman, L. (1990). Heredity, environment, and personality change: Evidence from the Texas Adoption Project. *J. Pers.* 58, 221–243.
24. Hogg, S. (1996). A review of the validity and variability of the elevated plus-maze as an animal model of anxiety. *Pharmacol. Biochem. Behav.* 54, 21–30.
25. Bourin, M., and Hascoet, M. (2003). The mouse light/dark box test. *Eur. J. Pharmacol.* 463, 55–65.
26. Blanchard, D. C., Griebel, G., and Blanchard, R. J. (2003). The Mouse Defense Test Battery: Pharmacological and behavioral assays for anxiety and panic. *Eur. J. Pharmacol.* 463, 97–116.
27. Belzung, C. (2001). Rodent models of anxiety-like behaviors: Are they predictive for compounds acting via non-benzodiazepine mechanisms? *Curr. Opin. Investig. Drugs.* 2, 1108–1111.
28. Uys, J. D., Stein, D. J., Daniels, W. M., and Harvey, B. H. (2003). Animal models of anxiety disorders. *Curr Psychiatry Rep.* 5, 274–281.
29. Griebel, G. (1995). 5-Hydroxytryptamine-interacting drugs in animal models of anxiety disorders: More than 30 years of research. *Pharmacol. Ther.* 65, 319–395.
30. Rodgers, R. J., Cao, B. J., Dalvi, A., and Holmes, A. (1997). Animal models of anxiety: An ethological perspective. *Braz. J. Med. Biol. Res.* 30, 289–304.
31. Rodgers, R. J. (1997). Animal models of 'anxiety': Where next?. *Behav. Pharmacol.* 8, 477–496; discussion 497–504.
32. Weiss, S. M., Lightowler, S., Stanhope, K. J., Kennett, G. A., and Dourish, C. T. (2000). Measurement of anxiety in transgenic mice. *Rev. Neurosci.* 11, 59–74.
33. Lister, R. G. (1987). The use of a plus-maze to measure anxiety in the mouse. *Psychopharmacology (Berl.)* 92, 180–185.
34. Treit, D., and Fundytus, M. (1988). Thigmotaxis as a test for anxiolytic activity in rats. *Pharmacol. Biochem. Behav.* 31, 959–962.
35. Crawley, J. N. (1981). Neuropharmacologic specificity of a simple animal model for the behavioral actions of benzodiazepines. *Pharmacol. Biochem. Behav.* 15, 695–699.
36. Rodgers, R. J., Boullier, E., Chatzimichalaki, P., Cooper, G. D., and Shorten, A. (2002). Contrasting phenotypes of C57BL/6JolaHsd. 129S2/SvHsd and 129/SvEv mice in two exploration-based tests of anxiety-related behaviour. *Physiol. Behav.* 77, 301–310.
37. Gross, C., Santarelli, L., Brunner, D., Zhuang, X., and Hen, R. (2000). Altered fear circuits in 5-HT(1A) receptor KO mice. *Biol. Psychiatry* 48, 1157–1163.
38. Bailey, S. J., and Toth, M. (2004). Variability in the benzodiazepine response of serotonin 5-HT1A receptor null mice displaying anxiety-like phenotype: Evidence for genetic modifiers in the 5-HT-mediated regulation of GABA(A) receptors. *J. Neurosci.* 24, 6343–6351.
39. File, S. E. (1985). Animal models for predicting clinical efficacy of anxiolytic drugs: Social behaviour. *Neuropsychobiology* 13, 55–62.

40. Geller, I., Kulak, J. T., Jr., and Seifter, J. (1962). The effects of chlordiazepoxide and chlorpromazine on a punishment discrimination. *Psychopharmacologia* 3, 374–385.

41. Vogel, J. R., Beer, B., and Clody, D. E. (1971). A simple and reliable conflict procedure for testing anti-anxiety agents. *Psychopharmacologia* 21, 1–7.

42. Davis, M. (1990). Animal models of anxiety based on classical conditioning: The conditioned emotional response (CER) and the fear-potentiated startle effect. *Pharmacol. Ther.* 47, 147–165.

43. Bienvenu, O. J., Samuels, J. F., Costa, P. T., Reti, I. M., Eaton, W. W., and Nestadt, G. (2004). Anxiety and depressive disorders and the five-factor model of personality: A higher- and lower-order personality trait investigation in a community sample. *Depress. Anxiety* 20, 92–97.

44. Friedman, B. H., and Thayer, J. F. (1998). Autonomic balance revisited: Panic anxiety and heart rate variability. *J. Psychosom. Res.* 44, 133–151.

45. Jacob, C. P., Strobel, A., Hohenberger, K., Ringel, T., Gutknecht, L., Reif, A., Brocke, B., and Lesch, K. P. (2004). Association between allelic variation of serotonin transporter function and neuroticism in anxious cluster C personality disorders. *Am. J. Psychiatry* 161, 569–572.

46. Sen, S., Burmeister, M., and Ghosh, D. (2004). Meta-analysis of the association between a serotonin transporter promoter polymorphism (5-HTTLPR) and anxiety-related personality traits. *Am. J. Med. Genet. B Neuropsychiatr. Genet.* 127, 85–89.

47. Organization, W. H. (1992). *The ICD-10 Classification of Mental and Behavioral Disorders—Clinical Description and Diagnostic Guidelines.* World Health Organization, Geneva.

48. Slade, T., and Andrews, G. (2001). DSM-IV and ICD-10 generalized anxiety disorder: Discrepant diagnoses and associated disability. *Soc. Psychiatry Psychiatr. Epidemiol.* 36, 45–51.

49. Andrews, G., and Slade, T. (2002). The classification of anxiety disorders in ICD-10 and DSM-IV: A concordance analysis. *Psychopathology* 35, 100–106.

50. Noyes, R.H.-S.R. (2004). *The Anxiety Disorders.* Cambridge University Press, Cambridge.

51. Avgustinovich, D. F., Lipina, T. V., Bondar, N. P., Alekseyenko, O. V., and Kudryavtseva, N. N. (2000). Features of the genetically defined anxiety in mice. *Behav Genet.* 30, 101–109.

52. Trullas, R., and Skolnick, P. (1993). Differences in fear motivated behaviors among inbred mouse strains. *Psychopharmacology (Berl.)* 111, 323–331.

53. van Gaalen, M. M., and Steckler, T. (2000). Behavioural analysis of four mouse strains in an anxiety test battery. *Behav. Brain Res.* 115, 95–106.

54. Berrettini, W. H., Harris, N., Ferraro, T. N., and Vogel, W. H. (1994). Maudsley reactive and non-reactive rats differ in exploratory behavior but not in learning. *Psychiatr. Genet.* 4, 91–94.

55. Liebsch, G., Linthorst, A. C., Neumann, I. D., Reul, J. M., Holsboer, F., and Landgraf, R. (1998). Behavioral, physiological, and neuroendocrine stress responses and differential sensitivity to diazepam in two Wistar rat lines selectively bred for high- and low-anxiety-related behavior. *Neuropsychopharmacology* 19, 381–396.

56. Domino, E. F., French, J., Pohorecki, R., Galus, C. F., and Pandit, S. K. (1989). Further observations on the effects of subhypnotic doses of midazolam in normal volunteers. *Psychopharmacol. Bull.* 25, 460–465.

57. Gupta, A., Lind, S., Eklund, A., and Lennmarken, C. (1997). The effects of midazolam and flumazenil on psychomotor function. *J. Clin. Anesth.* 9, 21–25.

58. Glue, P., Wilson, S., Coupland, N., Ball, D., and Nutt, D. (1995). The relationship between benzodiazepine receptor sensitivity and neuroticism. *Anxiety Disord.* 9, 33–45.
59. Glue, P., and Nutt, D. J. (1991). Benzodiazepine receptor sensitivity in panic disorder. *Lancet* 337, 563.
60. Roy-Byrne, P. P., Cowley, D. S., Greenblatt, D. J., Shader, R. I., and Hommer, D. (1990). Reduced benzodiazepine sensitivity in panic disorder. *Arch. Gen. Psychiatry* 47, 534–538.
61. Roy-Byrne, P., Wingerson, D. K., Radant, A., Greenblatt, D. J., and Cowley, D. S. (1996). Reduced benzodiazepine sensitivity in patients with panic disorder: Comparison with patients with obsessive-compulsive disorder and normal subjects. *Am. J. Psychiatry* 153, 1444–1449.
62. Cowley, D. S., Ha, E. H., and Roy-Byrne, P. P. (1997). Determinants of pharmacologic treatment failure in panic disorder. *J. Clin. Psychiatry* 58, 555–561; quiz 562–563.
63. Pratt, J. A. (1992). The neuroanatomical basis of anxiety. *Pharmacol. Ther.* 55, 149–181.
64. Davis, M. (1992). The role of the amygdala in fear and anxiety. *Annu. Rev. Neurosci.* 15, 353–375.
65. LeDoux, J. E., Iwata, J., Cicchetti, P., and Reis, D. J. (1988). Different projections of the central amygdaloid nucleus mediate autonomic and behavioral correlates of conditioned fear. *J. Neurosci.* 8, 2517–2529.
66. LeDoux, J. E., Cicchetti, P., Xagoraris, A., and Romanski, L. M. (1990). The lateral amygdaloid nucleus: Sensory interface of the amygdala in fear conditioning. *J. Neurosci.* 10, 1062–1069.
67. Liberzon, I., Taylor, S. F., Amdur, R., Jung, T. D., Chamberlain, K. R., Minoshima, S., Koeppe, R. A., and Fig, L. M. (1999). Brain activation in PTSD in response to trauma-related stimuli. *Biol. Psychiatry* 45, 817–826.
68. Nutt, D. J., and Malizia, A. L. (2004). Structural and functional brain changes in posttraumatic stress disorder. *J. Clin. Psychiatry* 65 (Suppl. 1), 11–17.
69. Dilger, S., Straube, T., Mentzel, H. J., Fitzek, C., Reichenbach, J. R., Hecht, H., Krieschel, S., Gutberlet, I., and Miltner, W. H. (2003). Brain activation to phobia-related pictures in spider phobic humans: An event-related functional magnetic resonance imaging study. *Neurosci. Lett.* 348, 29–32.
70. Massana, G., Serra-Grabulosa, J. M., Salgado-Pineda, P., Gasto, C., Junque, C., Massana, J., Mercader, J. M., Gomez, B., Tobena, A., and Salamero, M. (2003). Amygdalar atrophy in panic disorder patients detected by volumetric magnetic resonance imaging. *Neuroimage* 19, 80–90.
71. Szeszko, P. R., Robinson, D., Alvir, J. M., Bilder, R. M., Lencz, T., Ashtari, M., Wu, H., and Bogerts, B. (1999). Orbital frontal and amygdala volume reductions in obsessive-compulsive disorder. *Arch. Gen. Psychiatry* 56, 913–919.
72. De Bellis, M. D., Casey, B. J., Dahl, R. E., Birmaher, B., Williamson, D. E., Thomas, K. M., Axelson, D. A., Frustaci, K., Boring, A. M., Hall, J., and Ryan, N. D. (2000). A pilot study of amygdala volumes in pediatric generalized anxiety disorder. *Biol. Psychiatry* 48, 51–57.
73. Thomas, K. M., Drevets, W. C., Dahl, R. E., Ryan, N. D., Birmaher, B., Eccard, C. H., Axelson, D., Whalen, P. J., and Casey, B. J. (2001). Amygdala response to fearful faces in anxious and depressed children. *Arch. Gen. Psychiatry* 58, 1057–1063.
74. Bystritsky, A., Pontillo, D., Powers, M., Sabb, F. W., Craske, M. G., and Bookheimer, S. Y. (2001). Functional MRI changes during panic anticipation and imagery exposure. *Neuroreport* 12, 3953–3957.

75. Lanius, R. A., Williamson, P. C., Hopper, J., Densmore, M., Boksman, K., Gupta, M. A., Neufeld, R. W., Gati, J. S., and Menon, R. S. (2003). Recall of emotional states in posttraumatic stress disorder: An fMRI investigation. *Biol. Psychiatry* 53, 204–210.
76. Shin, L. M., Whalen, P. J., Pitman, R. K., Bush, G., Macklin, M. L., Lasko, N. B., Orr, S. P., McInerney, S. C., and Rauch, S. L. (2001). An fMRI study of anterior cingulate function in posttraumatic stress disorder. *Biol. Psychiatry* 50, 932–942.
77. Bremner, J. D., Staib, L. H., Kaloupek, D., Southwick, S. M., Soufer, R., and Charney, D. S. (1999). Neural correlates of exposure to traumatic pictures and sound in Vietnam combat veterans with and without posttraumatic stress disorder: A positron emission tomography study. *Biol. Psychiatry* 45, 806–816.
78. Rauch, S. L., Whalen, P. J., Shin, L. M., McInerney, S. C., Macklin, M. L., Lasko, N. B., Orr, S. P., and Pitman, R. K. (2000). Exaggerated amygdala response to masked facial stimuli in posttraumatic stress disorder: A functional MRI study. *Biol. Psychiatry* 47, 769–776.
79. De Bellis, M. D., Hall, J., Boring, A. M., Frustaci, K., and Moritz, G. (2001). A pilot longitudinal study of hippocampal volumes in pediatric maltreatment-related posttraumatic stress disorder. *Biol. Psychiatry* 50, 305–309.
80. Bonne, O., Brandes, D., Gilboa, A., Gomori, J. M., Shenton, M. E., Pitman, R. K., and Shalev, A. Y. (2001). Longitudinal MRI study of hippocampal volume in trauma survivors with PTSD. *Am. J. Psychiatry* 158, 1248–1251.
81. Gilbertson, M. W., Shenton, M. E., Ciszewski, A., Kasai, K., Lasko, N. B., Orr, S. P., and Pitman, R. K. (2002). Smaller hippocampal volume predicts pathologic vulnerability to psychological trauma. *Nat. Neurosci.* 5, 1242–1247.
82. Lindauer, R. J., Vlieger, E. J., Jalink, M., Olff, M., Carlier, I. V., Majoie, C. B., den Heeten, G. J., and Gersons, B. P. (2004). Smaller hippocampal volume in Dutch police officers with posttraumatic stress disorder. *Biol. Psychiatry* 56, 356–363.
83. Wignall, E. L., Dickson, J. M., Vaughan, P., Farrow, T. F., Wilkinson, I. D., Hunter, M. D., and Woodruff, P. W. (2004). Smaller hippocampal volume in patients with recent-onset posttraumatic stress disorder. *Biol. Psychiatry* 56, 832–836.
84. Villarreal, G., and King, C. Y. (2001). Brain imaging in posttraumatic stress disorder. *Semin. Clin. Neuropsychiatry* 6, 131–145.
85. Pujol, J., Soriano-Mas, C., Alonso, P., Cardoner, N., Menchon, J. M., Deus, J., and Vallejo, J. (2004). Mapping structural brain alterations in obsessive-compulsive disorder. *Arch. Gen. Psychiatry* 61, 720–730.
86. Saxena, S., Brody, A. L., Schwartz, J. M., and Baxter, L. R. (1998). Neuroimaging and frontal-subcortical circuitry in obsessive-compulsive disorder. *Br. J. Psychiatry* Suppl., 35, 26–37.
87. LeDoux, J. E. (2000). Emotion circuits in the brain. *Annu. Rev. Neurosci.* 23, 155–184.
88. Cahill, L., and McGaugh, J. L. (1998). Mechanisms of emotional arousal and lasting declarative memory. *Trends Neurosci.* 21, 294–299.
89. Davis, M., Rainnie, D., and Cassell, M. (1994). Neurotransmission in the rat amygdala related to fear and anxiety. *Trends Neurosci.* 17, 208–214.
90. Bannerman, D. M., Grubb, M., Deacon, R. M., Yee, B. K., Feldon, J., and Rawlins, J. N. (2003). Ventral hippocampal lesions affect anxiety but not spatial learning. *Behav. Brain Res.* 139, 197–213.
91. Kjelstrup, K. G., Tuvnes, F. A., Steffenach, H. A., Murison, R., Moser, E. I., and Moser, M. B. (2002). Reduced fear expression after lesions of the ventral hippocampus. *Proc Natl Acad Sci USA* 99, 10825–10830.

92. Degroot, A., and Treit, D. (2004). Anxiety is functionally segregated within the septohippocampal system. *Brain Res.* 1001, 60–71.

93. File, S. E., Kenny, P. J., and Cheeta, S. (2000). The role of the dorsal hippocampal serotonergic and cholinergic systems in the modulation of anxiety. *Pharmacol. Biochem. Behav.* 66, 65–72.

94. Malleret, G., Hen, R., Guillou, J. L., Segu, L., and Buhot, M. C. (1999). 5-HT1B receptor knock-out mice exhibit increased exploratory activity and enhanced spatial memory performance in the Morris water maze. *J. Neurosci.* 19, 6157–6168.

95. Shah, A. A., and Treit, D. (2004). Infusions of midazolam into the medial prefrontal cortex produce anxiolytic effects in the elevated plus-maze and shock-probe burying tests. *Brain Res.* 996, 31–40.

96. Shah, A. A., and Treit, D. (2003). Excitotoxic lesions of the medial prefrontal cortex attenuate fear responses in the elevated-plus maze, social interaction and shock probe burying tests. *Brain Res.* 969, 183–194.

97. Sullivan, R. M., and Gratton, A. (2002). Behavioral effects of excitotoxic lesions of ventral medial prefrontal cortex in the rat are hemisphere-dependent. *Brain Res.* 927, 69–79.

98. Gonzalez, L. E., Rujano, M., Tucci, S., Paredes, D., Silva, E., Alba, G., and Hernandez, L. (2000). Medial prefrontal transection enhances social interaction I: Behavioral studies. *Brain Res.* 887, 7–15.

99. Sullivan, G. M., Coplan, J. D., Kent, J. M., and Gorman, J. M. (1999). The noradrenergic system in pathological anxiety: A focus on panic with relevance to generalized anxiety and phobias. *Biol. Psychiatry* 46, 1205–1218.

100. Graeff, F. G., Viana, M. B., and Mora, P. O. (1997). Dual role of 5-HT in defense and anxiety. *Neurosci. Biobehav. Rev.* 21, 791–799.

101. Schlegel, S., Steinert, H., Bockisch, A., Hahn, K., Schloesser, R., and Benkert, O. (1994). Decreased benzodiazepine receptor binding in panic disorder measured by IOMAZENIL-SPECT. A preliminary report. *Eur. Arch. Psychiatry Clin. Neurosci.* 244, 49–51.

102. Kaschka, W., Feistel, H., and Ebert, D. (1995). Reduced benzodiazepine receptor binding in panic disorders measured by iomazenil SPECT. *J. Psychiatr. Res.* 29, 427–434.

103. Tiihonen, J., Kuikka, J., Rasanen, P., Lepola, U., Koponen, H., Liuska, A., Lehmusvaara, A., Vainio, P., Kononen, M., Bergstrom, K., Yu, M., Kinnunen, I., Akerman, K., and Karhu, J. (1997). Cerebral benzodiazepine receptor binding and distribution in generalized anxiety disorder: A fractal analysis. *Mol. Psychiatry* 2, 463–471.

104. Nutt, D. J., Glue, P., Lawson, C., and Wilson, S. (1990). Flumazenil provocation of panic attacks. Evidence for altered benzodiazepine receptor sensitivity in panic disorder. *Arch. Gen. Psychiatry* 47, 917–925.

105. Sieghart, W. (2000). Unraveling the function of GABA(A) receptor subtypes. *Trends Pharmacol. Sci.* 21, 411–413.

106. Rudolph, U., Crestani, F., and Mohler, H. (2001). GABA(A) receptor subtypes: Dissecting their pharmacological functions. *Trends Pharmacol. Sci.* 22, 188–194.

107. Essrich, C., Lorez, M., Benson, J. A., Fritschy, J. M., and Luscher, B. (1998). Postsynaptic clustering of major GABAA receptor subtypes requires the gamma 2 subunit and gephyrin. *Nat. Neurosci.* 1, 563–571.

108. Smith, S. S., Gong, Q. H., Hsu, F. C., Markowitz, R. S., Ffrench-Mullen, J. M., and Li, X. (1998). GABA(A) receptor alpha4 subunit suppression prevents withdrawal properties of an endogenous steroid. *Nature* 392, 926–930.

109. Dalvi, A., and Rodgers, R. J. (1996). GABAergic influences on plus-maze behaviour in mice. *Psychopharmacology (Berl.)* 128, 380–397.

110. Belzung, C., Misslin, R., Vogel, E., Dodd, R. H., and Chapouthier, G. (1987). Anxiogenic effects of methyl-beta-carboline-3-carboxylate in a light/dark choice situation. *Pharmacol. Biochem. Behav.* 28, 29–33.

111. Sanders, S. K., and Shekhar, A. (1995). Regulation of anxiety by GABAA receptors in the rat amygdala. *Pharmacol. Biochem. Behav.* 52, 701–706.

112. Rowlett, J. K., Platt, D. M., Lelas, S., Atack, J. R., and Dawson, G. R. (2005). Different GABAA receptor subtypes mediate the anxiolytic, abuse-related, and motor effects of benzodiazepine-like drugs in primates. *Proc. Natl. Acad. Sci. USA* 102, 915–920.

113. Johnston, A. L., and File, S. E. (1986). 5-HT and anxiety: Promises and pitfalls. *Pharmacol. Biochem. Behav.* 24, 1467–1470.

114. Inoue, T., Izumi, T., Li, X. B., Huang, J. Z., Kitaichi, Y., Nakagawa, S., and Koyama, T. (2004). Biological basis of anxiety disorders and serotonergic anxiolytics. *Nihon Shinkei Seishin Yakurigaku Zasshi* 24, 125–131 (in Japanese).

115. Blier, P., Pineyro, G., el Mansari, M., Bergeron, R., and de Montigny, C. (1998). Role of somatodendritic 5-HT autoreceptors in modulating 5-HT neurotransmission. *Ann. NY Acad. Sci.* 861, 204–216.

116. Goldberg, M. E., Salama, A. I., Patel, J. B., and Malick, J. B. (1983). Novel non-benzodiazepine anxiolytics. *Neuropharmacology* 22, 1499–1504.

117. Bremner, J. D., Krystal, J. H., Southwick, S. M., and Charney, D. S. (1996). Noradrenergic mechanisms in stress and anxiety: II. Clinical studies. *Synapse* 23, 39–51.

118. Bremner, J. D., Krystal, J. H., Southwick, S. M., and Charney, D. S. (1996). Noradrenergic mechanisms in stress and anxiety: I. Preclinical studies. *Synapse* 23, 28–38.

119. Taylor, D. P., Riblet, L. A., Stanton, H. C., Eison, A. S., Eison, M. S., and Temple, D. L. Jr. (1982). Dopamine and antianxiety activity. *Pharmacol. Biochem. Behav.* 17 (Suppl. 1), 25–35.

120. Navarro, J. F., Luna, G., Garcia, F., and Pedraza, C. (2003). Effects of L-741,741, a selective dopamine receptor antagonist, on anxiety tested in the elevated plus-maze in mice. *Methods Find. Exp. Clin. Pharmacol.* 25, 45–47.

121. Millan, M. J., Brocco, M., Papp, M., Serres, F., La Rochelle, C. D., Sharp, T., Peglion, J. L., and Dekeyne, A. (2004). S32504, a novel naphtoxazine agonist at dopamine D3/D2 receptors: III. Actions in models of potential antidepressive and anxiolytic activity in comparison with ropinirole. *J. Pharmacol. Exp. Ther.* 309, 936–950.

122. Griebel, G. (1999). Is there a future for neuropeptide receptor ligands in the treatment of anxiety disorders? *Pharmacol. Ther.* 82, 1–61.

123. Steckler, T., and Holsboer, F. (1999). Corticotropin-releasing hormone receptor subtypes and emotion. *Biol. Psychiatry.* 46, 1480–1508.

124. von Bardeleben, U., and Holsboer, F. (1988). Human corticotropin releasing hormone: Clinical studies in patients with affective disorders, alcoholism, panic disorder and in normal controls. *Prog. Neuropsychopharmacol. Biol. Psychiatry* 12 (Suppl.), S165–S187.

125. Arborelius, L., Owens, M. J., Plotsky, P. M., and Nemeroff, C. B. (1999). The role of corticotropin-releasing factor in depression and anxiety disorders. *J. Endocrinol.* 160, 1–12.
126. McEwen, B. S. (2004). Protection and damage from acute and chronic stress: Allostasis and allostatic overload and relevance to the pathophysiology of psychiatric disorders. *Ann. NY Acad. Sci.* 1032, 1–7.
127. de Kloet, E. R., Oitzl, M. S., and Joels, M. (1993). Functional implications of brain corticosteroid receptor diversity. *Cell. Mol. Neurobiol.* 13, 433–455.
128. Strohle, A., and Holsboer, F. (2003). Stress responsive neurohormones in depression and anxiety. *Pharmacopsychiatry* 36 (Suppl. 3), S207–S214.
129. McEwen, B. S. (2000). The neurobiology of stress: From serendipity to clinical relevance. *Brain Res.* 886, 172–189.
130. Koob, G. F., and Heinrichs, S. C. (1999). A role for corticotropin releasing factor and urocortin in behavioral responses to stressors. *Brain Res.* 848, 141–152.
131. Sherman, J. E., and Kalin, N. H. (1987). The effects of ICV-CRH on novelty-induced behavior. *Pharmacol. Biochem. Behav.* 26, 699–703.
132. Sutton, R. E., Koob, G. F., Le Moal, M., Rivier, J., and Vale, W. (1982). Corticotropin releasing factor produces behavioural activation in rats. *Nature* 297, 331–333.
133. Berridge, C. W., and Dunn, A. J. (1989). Restraint-stress-induced changes in exploratory behavior appear to be mediated by norepinephrine-stimulated release of CRF. *J. Neurosci.* 9, 3513–3521.
134. Butler, P. D., Weiss, J. M., Stout, J. C., and Nemeroff, C. B. (1990). Corticotropin-releasing factor produces fear-enhancing and behavioral activating effects following infusion into the locus coeruleus. *J. Neurosci.* 10, 176–183.
135. Carrasco, G. A., and Van de Kar, L. D. (2003). Neuroendocrine pharmacology of stress. *Eur. J. Pharmacol.* 463, 235–272.
136. De Kloet, E. R., Sutanto, W., Rots, N., van Haarst, A., van den Berg, D., Oitzl, M., van Eekelen, A., and Voorhuis, D. (1991). Plasticity and function of brain corticosteroid receptors during aging. *Acta Endocrinol. (Copenh.)* 125 (Suppl. 1), 65–72.
137. Diorio, D., Viau, V., and Meaney, M. J. (1993). The role of the medial prefrontal cortex (cingulate gyrus) in the regulation of hypothalamic-pituitary-adrenal responses to stress. *J. Neurosci.* 13, 3839–3847.
138. Heilig, M., and Widerlov, E. (1990). Neuropeptide Y: An overview of central distribution, functional aspects, and possible involvement in neuropsychiatric illnesses. *Acta Psychiatr. Scand.* 82, 95–114.
139. Heilig, M., Soderpalm, B., Engel, J. A., and Widerlov, E. (1989). Centrally administered neuropeptide Y (NPY) produces anxiolytic-like effects in animal anxiety models. *Psychopharmacology (Berl.)* 98, 524–529.
140. Wahlestedt, C., Pich, E. M., Koob, G. F., Yee, F., and Heilig, M. (1993). Modulation of anxiety and neuropeptide Y-Y1 receptors by antisense oligodeoxynucleotides. *Science* 259, 528–531.
141. Harro, J., Vasar, E., and Bradwejn, J. (1993). CCK in animal and human research on anxiety. *Trends Pharmacol. Sci.* 14, 244–249.
142. Mosconi, M., Chiamulera, C., and Recchia, G. (1993). New anxiolytics in development. *Int. J. Clin. Pharmacol. Res.* 13, 331–344.
143. Abelson, J. L. (1995). Cholecystokinin in psychiatric research: A time for cautious excitement. *J. Psychiatr. Res.* 29, 389–396.
144. Herranz, R. (2003). Cholecystokinin antagonists: Pharmacological and therapeutic potential. *Med. Res. Rev.* 23, 559–605.

145. Saria, A. (1999). The tachykinin NK1 receptor in the brain: Pharmacology and putative functions. *Eur. J. Pharmacol.* 375, 51–60.
146. Brodin, E., Rosen, A., Schott, E., and Brodin, K. (1994). Effects of sequential removal of rats from a group cage, and of individual housing of rats, on substance P, cholecystokinin and somatostatin levels in the periaqueductal grey and limbic regions. *Neuropeptides* 26, 253–260.
147. Otsuka, M., and Yoshioka, K. (1993). Neurotransmitter functions of mammalian tachykinins. *Physiol. Rev.* 73, 229–308.
148. Nikolaus, S., Huston, J. P., and Hasenohrl, R. U. (1999). The neurokinin-1 receptor antagonist WIN51,708 attenuates the anxiolytic-like effects of ventralpallidal substance P injection. *Neuroreport* 10, 2293–2296.
149. Anisman, H., Merali, Z., Poulter, M. O., and Hayley, S. (2005). Cytokines as a precipitant of depressive illness: Animal and human studies. *Curr. Pharm. Des.* 11, 963–972.
150. Lesch, K. P. (2001). Molecular foundation of anxiety disorders. *J. Neural. Transm.* 108, 717–746.
151. Finn, D. A., Rutledge-Gorman, M. T., and Crabbe, J. C. (2003). Genetic animal models of anxiety. *Neurogenetics* 4, 109–135.
152. Jetty, P. V., Charney, D. S., and Goddard, A. W. (2001). Neurobiology of generalized anxiety disorder. *Psychiatr. Clin. North Am.* 24, 75–97.
153. Hariri, A. R., Mattay, V. S., Tessitore, A., Kolachana, B., Fera, F., Goldman, D., Egan, M. F., and Weinberger, D. R. (2002). Serotonin transporter genetic variation and the response of the human amygdala. *Science* 297, 400–403.
154. Munafo, M. R., Clark, T., and Flint, J., (2004). Does measurement instrument moderate the association between the serotonin transporter gene and anxiety-related personality traits? A meta-analysis. *Mol. Psychiatry* 10, 415–419.
155. Ansorge, M. S., Zhou, M., Lira, A., Hen, R., and Gingrich, J. A. (2004). Early life blockade of the 5-HT transporter alters emotional behavior in adult mice. *Science* 306, 879–881.
156. Neumeister, A., Bain, E., Nugent, A. C., Carson, R. E., Bonne, O., Luckenbaugh, D. A., Eckelman, W., Herscovitch, P., Charney, D. S., and Drevets, W. C. (2004). Reduced serotonin type 1A receptor binding in panic disorder. *J. Neurosci.* 24, 589–591.
157. Mann, J. J. (1999). Role of the serotonergic system in the pathogenesis of major depression and suicidal behavior. *Neuropsychopharmacology* 21, 99S–105S.
158. Lopez, J. F., Chalmers, D. T., Little, K. Y., and Watson, S. J. (1998). A.E. Bennett Research Award. Regulation of serotonin1A, glucocorticoid, and mineralocorticoid receptor in rat and human hippocampus: Implications for the neurobiology of depression. *Biol. Psychiatry* 43, 547–573.
159. Lemonde, S., Turecki, G., Bakish, D., Du, L., Hrdina, P. D., Bown, C. D., Sequeira, A., Kushwaha, N., Morris, S. J., Basak, A., Ou, X. M., and Albert, P. R. (2003). Impaired repression at a 5-hydroxytryptamine 1A receptor gene polymorphism associated with major depression and suicide. *J. Neurosci.* 23, 8788–8799.
160. Lesch, K. P., Aulakh, C. S., Wolozin, B. L., and Murphy, D. L. (1992). Serotonin (5-HT) receptor, 5-HT transporter and G protein-effector expression: Implications for depression. *Pharmacol. Toxicol.* 71 (Suppl. 1), 49–60.
161. Sen, S., Nesse, R. M., Stoltenberg, S. F., Li, S., Gleiberman, L., Chakravarti, A., Weder, A. B., and Burmeister, M. (2003). A BDNF coding variant is associated with

the NEO personality inventory domain neuroticism, a risk factor for depression. *Neuropsychopharmacology* 28, 397–401.

162. Lang, U. E., Hellweg, R., and Gallinat, J. (2004). BDNF serum concentrations in healthy volunteers are associated with depression-related personality traits. *Neuropsychopharmacology* 29, 795–798.

163. Egan, M. F., Kojima, M., Callicott, J. H., Goldberg, T. E., Kolachana, B. S., Bertolino, A., Zaitsev, E., Gold, B., Goldman, D., Dean, M., Lu, B., and Weinberger, D. R. (2003). The BDNF val66met polymorphism affects activity-dependent secretion of BDNF and human memory and hippocampal function. *Cell* 112, 257–269.

164. Kash, S. F., Tecott, L. H., Hodge, C., and Baekkeskov, S. (1999). Increased anxiety and altered responses to anxiolytics in mice deficient in the 65-kDa isoform of glutamic acid decarboxylase. *Proc. Natl. Acad. Sci. USA* 96, 1698–1703.

165. Asada, H., Kawamura, Y., Maruyama, K., Kume, H., Ding, R., Ji, F. Y., Kanbara, N., Kuzume, H., Sanbo, M., Yagi, T., and Obata, K. (1996). Mice lacking the 65 kDa isoform of glutamic acid decarboxylase (GAD65) maintain normal levels of GAD67 and GABA in their brains but are susceptible to seizures. *Biochem. Biophys. Res. Commun.* 229, 891–895.

166. Asada, H., Kawamura, Y., Maruyama, K., Kume, H., Ding, R. G., Kanbara, N., Kuzume, H., Sanbo, M., Yagi, T., and Obata, K. (1997). Cleft palate and decreased brain gamma-aminobutyric acid in mice lacking the 67-kDa isoform of glutamic acid decarboxylase. *Proc. Natl. Acad. Sci. USA* 94, 6496–6499.

167. Sherif, F., Harro, J., el-Hwuegi, A., and Oreland, L. (1994). Anxiolytic-like effect of the GABA-transaminase inhibitor vigabatrin (gamma-vinyl GABA) on rat exploratory activity. *Pharmacol. Biochem. Behav.* 49, 801–805.

168. Gogos, J. A., Morgan, M., Luine, V., Santha, M., Ogawa, S., Pfaff, D., and Karayiorgou, M. (1998). Catechol-*O*-methyltransferase-deficient mice exhibit sexually dimorphic changes in catecholamine levels and behavior. *Proc. Natl. Acad. Sci. USA* 95, 9991–9996.

169. Xu, F., Gainetdinov, R. R., Wetsel, W. C., Jones, S. R., Bohn, L. M., Miller, G. W., Wang, Y. M., and Caron, M. G. (2000). Mice lacking the norepinephrine transporter are supersensitive to psychostimulants. *Nat Neurosci.* 3, 465–471.

170. Bengel, D., Murphy, D. L., Andrews, A. M., Wichems, C. H., Feltner, D., Heils, A., Mossner, R., Westphal, H., and Lesch, K. P. (1998). Altered brain serotonin homeostasis and locomotor insensitivity to 3,4-methylenedioxymethamphetamine ("Ecstasy") in serotonin transporter-deficient mice. *Mol. Pharmacol.* 53, 649–655.

171. Murphy, D. L., Li, Q., Engel, S., Wichems, C., Andrews, A., Lesch, K. P., and Uhl, G. (2001). Genetic perspectives on the serotonin transporter. *Brain Res. Bull.* 56, 487–494.

172. Lira, A., Zhou, M., Castanon, N., Ansorge, M. S., Gordon, J. A., Francis, J. H., Bradley-Moore, M., Lira, J., Underwood, M. D., Arango, V., Kung, H. F., Hofer, M. A., Hen, R., and Gingrich, J. A. (2003). Altered depression-related behaviors and functional changes in the dorsal raphe nucleus of serotonin transporter-deficient mice. *Biol. Psychiatry* 54, 960–971.

173. Stenzel-Poore, M. P., Heinrichs, S. C., Rivest, S., Koob, G. F., and Vale, W. W. (1994). Overproduction of corticotropin-releasing factor in transgenic mice: A genetic model of anxiogenic behavior. *J. Neurosci.* 14, 2579–2584.

174. Stenzel-Poore, M. P., Duncan, J. E., Rittenberg, M. B., Bakke, A. C., and Heinrichs, S. C. (1996). CRH overproduction in transgenic mice: Behavioral and immune system modulation. *Ann. NY Acad. Sci.* 780, 36–48.

175. Dunn, A. J., and Swiergiel, A. H. (1999). Behavioral responses to stress are intact in CRF-deficient mice. *Brain Res.* 845, 14–20.

176. Muglia, L., Jacobson, L., and Majzoub, J. A. (1996). Production of corticotropin-releasing hormone-deficient mice by targeted mutation in embryonic stem cells. *Ann. NY Acad. Sci.* 780, 49–59.

177. Weninger, S. C., Dunn, A. J., Muglia, L. J., Dikkes, P., Miczek, K. A., Swiergiel, A. H., Berridge, C. W., and Majzoub, J. A. (1999). Stress-induced behaviors require the corticotropin-releasing hormone (CRH) receptor, but not CRH. *Proc. Natl. Acad. Sci. USA* 96, 8283–8288.

178. Vetter, D. E., Li, C., Zhao, L., Contarino, A., Liberman, M. C., Smith, G. W., Marchuk, Y., Koob, G. F., Heinemann, S. F., Vale, W., and Lee, K. F. (2002). Urocortin-deficient mice show hearing impairment and increased anxiety-like behavior. *Nat. Genet.* 31, 363–369.

179. Karolyi, I. J., Burrows, H. L., Ramesh, T. M., Nakajima, M., Lesh, J. S., Seong, E., Camper, S. A., and Seasholtz, A. F. (1999). Altered anxiety and weight gain in corticotropin-releasing hormone-binding protein-deficient mice. *Proc. Natl. Acad. Sci. USA* 96, 11595–11600.

180. Burrows, H. L., Nakajima, M., Lesh, J. S., Goosens, K. A., Samuelson, L. C., Inui, A., Camper, S. A., and Seasholtz, A. F. (1998). Excess corticotropin releasing hormone-binding protein in the hypothalamic-pituitary-adrenal axis in transgenic mice. *J. Clin. Invest.* 101, 1439–1447.

181. Bannon, A. W., Seda, J., Carmouche, M., Francis, J. M., Norman, M. H., Karbon, B., and McCaleb, M. L. (2000). Behavioral characterization of neuropeptide Y knockout mice. *Brain Res.* 868, 79–87.

182. Konig, M., Zimmer, A. M., Steiner, H., Holmes, P. V., Crawley, J. N., Brownstein, M. J., and Zimmer, A. (1996). Pain responses, anxiety and aggression in mice deficient in pre-proenkephalin. *Nature* 383, 535–538.

183. Good, A. J., and Westbrook, R. F. (1995). Effects of a microinjection of morphine into the amygdala on the acquisition and expression of conditioned fear and hypoalgesia in rats. *Behav. Neurosci.* 109, 631–641.

184. Koster, A., Montkowski, A., Schulz, S., Stube, E. M., Knaudt, K., Jenck, F., Moreau, J. L., Nothacker, H. P., Civelli, O., and Reinscheid, R. K. (1999). Targeted disruption of the orphanin FQ/nociceptin gene increases stress susceptibility and impairs stress adaptation in mice. *Proc. Natl. Acad. Sci. USA* 96, 10444–10449.

185. Reinscheid, R. K., and Civelli, O. (2002). The orphanin FQ/nociceptin knockout mouse: A behavioral model for stress responses. *Neuropeptides* 36, 72–76.

186. Poo, M. M. (2001). Neurotrophins as synaptic modulators. *Nat. Rev. Neurosci.* 2, 24–32.

187. Lessmann, V., Gottmann, K., and Malcangio, M. (2003). Neurotrophin secretion: Current facts and future prospects. *Prog. Neurobiol.* 69, 341–374.

188. Jones, K. R., Farinas, I., Backus, C., and Reichardt, L. F. (1994). Targeted disruption of the BDNF gene perturbs brain and sensory neuron development but not motor neuron development. *Cell* 76, 989–999.

189. MacQueen, G. M., Ramakrishnan, K., Croll, S. D., Siuciak, J. A., Yu, G., Young, L. T., and Fahnestock, M. (2001). Performance of heterozygous brain-derived neurotrophic factor knockout mice on behavioral analogues of anxiety, nociception, and depression. *Behav. Neurosci.* 115, 1145–1153.

190. Rios, M., Fan, G., Fekete, C., Kelly, J., Bates, B., Kuehn, R., Lechan, R. M., and Jaenisch, R. (2001). Conditional deletion of brain-derived neurotrophic factor in the postnatal brain leads to obesity and hyperactivity. *Mol. Endocrinol.* 15, 1748–1757.

190a. Chen, Z. Y., Jing, D., Bath, K. G., Ieraci, A., Khan, T., Siao, C. J., Herrera, D. G., Toth, M., Yang, C., McEwen, B. S., Hempstead, B. L. and Lee, F. S. (2006) Genetic variant BDNF (Val66Met) polymorphism alters anxiety-related behavior, *Science* 314, 140–143.

191. Connor, T. J., Song, C., Leonard, B. E., Merali, Z., and Anisman, H. (1998). An assessment of the effects of central interleukin-1beta, -2, -6, and tumor necrosis factor-alpha administration on some behavioural, neurochemical, endocrine and immune parameters in the rat. *Neuroscience* 84, 923–933.

192. Fiore, M., Alleva, E., Probert, L., Kollias, G., Angelucci, F., and Aloe, L. (1998). Exploratory and displacement behavior in transgenic mice expressing high levels of brain TNF-alpha. *Physiol. Behav.* 63, 571–576.

193. Golan, H., Levav, T., Mendelsohn, A., and Huleihel, M. (2004). Involvement of tumor necrosis factor alpha in hippocampal development and function. *Cereb. Cortex.* 14, 97–105.

194. Yamada, K., Iida, R., Miyamoto, Y., Saito, K., Sekikawa, K., Seishima, M., and Nabeshima, T. (2000). Neurobehavioral alterations in mice with a targeted deletion of the tumor necrosis factor-alpha gene: Implications for emotional behavior. *J. Neuroimmunol.* 111, 131–138.

195. Kustova, Y., Sei, Y., Morse, H. C. Jr., and Basile, A. S. (1998). The influence of a targeted deletion of the IFNgamma gene on emotional behaviors. *Brain Behav. Immun.* 12, 308–324.

196. Crestani, F., Lorez, M., Baer, K., Essrich, C., Benke, D., Laurent, J. P., Belzung, C., Fritschy, J. M., Luscher, B., and Mohler, H. (1999). Decreased GABAA-receptor clustering results in enhanced anxiety and a bias for threat cues. *Nat. Neurosci.* 2, 833–839.

197. Wick, M. J., Radcliffe, R. A., Bowers, B. J., Mascia, M. P., Luscher, B., Harris, R. A., and Wehner, J. M. (2000). Behavioural changes produced by transgenic overexpression of gamma2L and gamma2S subunits of the GABAA receptor. *Eur. J. Neurosci.* 12, 2634–2638.

198. McKernan, R. M., and Whiting, P. J. (1996). Which GABAA-receptor subtypes really occur in the brain? *Trends Neurosci.* 19, 139–143.

199. Kralic, J. E., O'Buckley, T. K., Khisti, R. T., Hodge, C. W., Homanics, G. E., and Morrow, A. L. (2002). GABA(A) receptor alpha-1 subunit deletion alters receptor subtype assembly, pharmacological and behavioral responses to benzodiazepines and zolpidem. *Neuropharmacology* 43, 685–694.

200. Sur, C., Wafford, K. A., Reynolds, D. S., Hadingham, K. L., Bromidge, F., Macaulay, A., Collinson, N., O'Meara, G., Howell, O., Newman, R., Myers, J., Atack, J. R., Dawson, G. R., McKernan, R. M., Whiting, P. J., and Rosahl, T. W. (2001). Loss of the major GABA(A) receptor subtype in the brain is not lethal in mice. *J. Neurosci.* 21, 3409–3418.

201. Vicini, S., Ferguson, C., Prybylowski, K., Kralic, J., Morrow, A. L., and Homanics, G. E. (2001). GABA(A) receptor alpha1 subunit deletion prevents developmental changes of inhibitory synaptic currents in cerebellar neurons. *J. Neurosci.* 21, 3009–3016.

202. Low, K., Crestani, F., Keist, R., Benke, D., Brunig, I., Benson, J. A., Fritschy, J. M., Rulicke, T., Bluethmann, H., Mohler, H., and Rudolph, U. (2000). Molecular and neuronal substrate for the selective attenuation of anxiety. *Science.* 290, 131–134.

203. Reynolds, D. S., McKernan, R. M., and Dawson, G. R. (2001). Anxiolytic-like action of diazepam: Which GABA(A) receptor subtype is involved? *Trends Pharmacol. Sci.* 22, 402–403.

204. Boehm, S. L. II, Ponomarev, I., Jennings, A. W., Whiting, P. J., Rosahl, T. W., Garrett, E. M., Blednov, Y. A., and Harris, R. A. (2004). Gamma-aminobutyric acid A receptor subunit mutant mice: New perspectives on alcohol actions. *Biochem. Pharmacol.* 68, 1581–1602.

205. Collinson, N., Kuenzi, F. M., Jarolimek, W., Maubach, K. A., Cothliff, R., Sur, C., Smith, A., Otu, F. M., Howell, O., Atack, J. R., McKernan, R. M., Seabrook, G. R., Dawson, G. R., Whiting, P. J., and Rosahl, T. W. (2002). Enhanced learning and memory and altered GABAergic synaptic transmission in mice lacking the alpha 5 subunit of the GABAA receptor. *J. Neurosci.* 22, 5572–5580.

206. Rodgers, R. J., and Johnson, N. J. (1995). Factor analysis of spatiotemporal and ethological measures in the murine elevated plus-maze test of anxiety. *Pharmacol. Biochem. Behav.* 52, 297–303.

207. Heisler, L. K., Chu, H. M., Brennan, T. J., Danao, J. A., Bajwa, P., Parsons, L. H., and Tecott, L. H. (1998). Elevated anxiety and antidepressant-like responses in serotonin 5-HT1A receptor mutant mice. *Proc. Natl. Acad. Sci. USA* 95, 15049–15054.

208. Ramboz, S., Oosting, R., Amara, D. A., Kung, H. F., Blier, P., Mendelsohn, M., Mann, J. J., Brunner, D., and Hen, R. (1998). Serotonin receptor 1A knockout: An animal model of anxiety-related disorder. *Proc. Natl. Acad. Sci. USA* 95, 14476–14481.

209. Parks, C. L., Robinson, P. S., Sibille, E., Shenk, T., and Toth, M. (1998). Increased anxiety of mice lacking the serotonin1A receptor. *Proc. Natl. Acad. Sci. USA* 95, 10734–10739.

210. Sibille, E., Pavlides, C., Benke, D., and Toth, M. (2000). Genetic inactivation of the serotonin(1A) receptor in mice results in downregulation of major GABA(A) receptor alpha subunits, reduction of GABA(A) receptor binding, and benzodiazepine-resistant anxiety. *J. Neurosci.* 20, 2758–2765.

211. He, M., Sibille, E., Benjamin, D., Toth, M., and Shippenberg, T. (2001). Differential effects of 5-HT1A receptor deletion upon basal and fluoxetine-evoked 5-HT concentrations as revealed by in vivo microdialysis. *Brain Res.* 902, 11–17.

212. Bortolozzi, A., Amargos-Bosch, M., Toth, M., Artigas, F., and Adell, A. (2004). In vivo efflux of serotonin in the dorsal raphe nucleus of 5-HT1A receptor knockout mice. *J. Neurochem.* 88, 1373–1379.

213. Parsons, L. H., Kerr, T. M., and Tecott, L. H. (2001). 5-HT(1A) receptor mutant mice exhibit enhanced tonic, stress-induced and fluoxetine-induced serotonergic neurotransmission. *J. Neurochem.* 77, 607–617.

214. Gross, C., Zhuang, X., Stark, K., Ramboz, S., Oosting, R., Kirby, L., Santarelli, L., Beck, S., and Hen, R. (2002). Serotonin1A receptor acts during development to establish normal anxiety-like behaviour in the adult. *Nature* 416, 396–400.

215. Pattij, T., Groenink, L., Hijzen, T. H., Oosting, R. S., Maes, R. A., van der Gugten, J., and Olivier, B. (2002). Autonomic changes associated with enhanced anxiety in 5-HT(1A) receptor knockout mice. *Neuropsychopharmacology* 27, 380–390.

216. Pattij, T., Hijzen, T. H., Groenink, L., Oosting, R. S., van der Gugten, J., Maes, R. A., Hen, R., and Olivier, B. (2001). Stress-induced hyperthermia in the 5-HT(1A) receptor knockout mouse is normal. *Biol. Psychiatry* 49, 569–574.

217. Boschert, U., Amara, D. A., Segu, L., and Hen, R. (1994). The mouse 5-hydroxytryptamine1B receptor is localized predominantly on axon terminals. *Neuroscience* 58, 167–182.

218. Gothert, M. (1990). Presynaptic serotonin receptors in the central nervous system. *Ann. NY Acad. Sci.* 604, 102–112.
219. Zhuang, X., Gross, C., Santarelli, L., Compan, V., Trillat, A. C., and Hen, R. (1999). Altered emotional states in knockout mice lacking 5-HT1A or 5-HT1B receptors. *Neuropsychopharmacology* 21, 52S–60S.
220. Phillips, T. J., Hen, R., and Crabbe, J. C. (1999). Complications associated with genetic background effects in research using knockout mice. *Psychopharmacology (Berl.)* 147, 5–7.
220a. Weisstaub, N. V., Zhou, M., Lira, A., Lambe, E., Gonzalez-Maeso, J., Hornung, J. P., Sibille, E., Underwood, M., Itohara, S., Dauer, W. T., Ansorge, M. S., Morelli, E., Mann, J. J., Toth, M., Aghajanian, G., Sealfon, S. C., Hen, R. and Gingrich, J. A. (2006) Cortical 5-HT2A receptor signaling modulates anxiety-like behaviors in mice, *Science* 313, 536–540.
221. Vaughan, J., Donaldson, C., Bittencourt, J., Perrin, M. H., Lewis, K., Sutton, S., Chan, R., Turnbull, A. V., Lovejoy, D., Rivier, C. et al. (1995). Urocortin, a mammalian neuropeptide related to fish urotensin I and to corticotropin-releasing factor. *Nature* 378, 287–292.
222. Moreau, J. L., Kilpatrick, G., and Jenck, F. (1997). Urocortin, a novel neuropeptide with anxiogenic-like properties. *Neuroreport* 8, 1697–1701.
223. Contarino, A., Dellu, F., Koob, G. F., Smith, G. W., Lee, K. F., Vale, W., and Gold, L. H. (1999). Reduced anxiety-like and cognitive performance in mice lacking the corticotropin-releasing factor receptor 1. *Brain Res.* 835, 1–9.
224. Smith, G. W., Aubry, J. M., Dellu, F., Contarino, A., Bilezikjian, L. M., Gold, L. H., Chen, R., Marchuk, Y., Hauser, C., Bentley, C. A., Sawchenko, P. E., Koob, G. F., Vale, W., and Lee, K. F. (1998). Corticotropin releasing factor receptor 1-deficient mice display decreased anxiety, impaired stress response, and aberrant neuroendocrine development. *Neuron* 20, 1093–1102.
225. Bale, T. L., Contarino, A., Smith, G. W., Chan, R., Gold, L. H., Sawchenko, P. E., Koob, G. F., Vale, W. W., and Lee, K. F. (2000). Mice deficient for corticotropin-releasing hormone receptor-2 display anxiety-like behaviour and are hypersensitive to stress. *Nat. Genet.* 24, 410–414.
226. Kishimoto, T., Radulovic, J., Radulovic, M., Lin, C. R., Schrick, C., Hooshmand, F., Hermanson, O., Rosenfeld, M. G., and Spiess, J. (2000). Deletion of crhr2 reveals an anxiolytic role for corticotropin-releasing hormone receptor-2. *Nat. Genet.* 24, 415–419.
227. Coste, S. C., Kesterson, R. A., Heldwein, K. A., Stevens, S. L., Heard, A. D., Hollis, J. H., Murray, S. E., Hill, J. K., Pantely, G. A., Hohimer, A. R., Hatton, D. C., Phillips, T. J., Finn, D. A., Low, M. J., Rittenberg, M. B., Stenzel, P., and Stenzel-Poore, M. P. (2000). Abnormal adaptations to stress and impaired cardiovascular function in mice lacking corticotropin-releasing hormone receptor-2. *Nat. Genet.* 24, 403–409.
228. Bale, T. L., Picetti, R., Contarino, A., Koob, G. F., Vale, W. W., and Lee, K. F. (2002). Mice deficient for both corticotropin-releasing factor receptor 1 (CRFR1) and CRFR2 have an impaired stress response and display sexually dichotomous anxiety-like behavior. *J. Neurosci.* 22, 193–199.
229. Steiner, H., Fuchs, S., and Accili, D. (1997). D3 dopamine receptor-deficient mouse: Evidence for reduced anxiety. *Physiol. Behav.* 63, 137–141.
230. Dulawa, S. C., Grandy, D. K., Low, M. J., Paulus, M. P., and Geyer, M. A. (1999). Dopamine D4 receptor-knock-out mice exhibit reduced exploration of novel stimuli. *J. Neurosci.* 19, 9550–9556.

231. Martin, M., Ledent, C., Parmentier, M., Maldonado, R., and Valverde, O. (2002). Involvement of CB1 cannabinoid receptors in emotional behaviour. *Psychopharmacology (Berl.)* 159, 379–387.

232. Haller, J., Bakos, N., Szirmay, M., Ledent, C., and Freund, T. F. (2002). The effects of genetic and pharmacological blockade of the CB1 cannabinoid receptor on anxiety. *Eur. J. Neurosci.* 16, 1395–1398.

233. Degroot, A., and Nomikos, G. G. (2004). Genetic deletion and pharmacological blockade of CB1 receptors modulates anxiety in the shock-probe burying test. *Eur. J. Neurosci.* 20, 1059–1064.

234. Lahdesmaki, J., Sallinen, J., MacDonald, E., Kobilka, B. K., Fagerholm, V., and Scheinin, M. (2002). Behavioral and neurochemical characterization of alpha(2A)-adrenergic receptor knockout mice. *Neuroscience* 113, 289–299.

235. Baldwin, H. A., and File, S. E. (1989). Caffeine-induced anxiogenesis: The role of adenosine, benzodiazepine and noradrenergic receptors. *Pharmacol. Biochem. Behav.* 32, 181–186.

236. Ledent, C., Vaugeois, J. M., Schiffmann, S. N., Pedrazzini, T., El Yacoubi, M., Vanderhaeghen, J. J., Costentin, J., Heath, J. K., Vassart, G., and Parmentier, M. (1997). Aggressiveness, hypoalgesia and high blood pressure in mice lacking the adenosine A2a receptor. *Nature* 388, 674–678.

237. Schiffmann, S. N., and Vanderhaeghen, J. J. (1993). Adenosine A2 receptors regulate the gene expression of striatopallidal and striatonigral neurons. *J. Neurosci.* 13, 1080–1087.

238. Blednov, Y. A., Stoffel, M., Chang, S. R., and Harris, R. A. (2001). GIRK2 deficient mice. Evidence for hyperactivity and reduced anxiety. *Physiol. Behav.* 74, 109–117.

239. Lesage, F., Duprat, F., Fink, M., Guillemare, E., Coppola, T., Lazdunski, M., and Hugnot, J. P. (1994). Cloning provides evidence for a family of inward rectifier and G-protein coupled K^+ channels in the brain. *FEBS Lett.* 353, 37–42.

240. Karschin, C., Dissmann, E., Stuhmer, W., and Karschin, A. (1996). IRK(1–3) and GIRK(1–4) inwardly rectifying K^+ channel mRNAs are differentially expressed in the adult rat brain. *J. Neurosci.* 16, 3559–3570.

241. Costall, B., Kelly, M. E., Naylor, R. J., and Onaivi, E. S. (1989). The actions of nicotine and cocaine in a mouse model of anxiety. *Pharmacol. Biochem. Behav.* 33, 197–203.

242. Brioni, J. D., O'Neill, A. B., Kim, D. J., and Decker, M. W. (1993). Nicotinic receptor agonists exhibit anxiolytic-like effects on the elevated plus-maze test. *Eur. J. Pharmacol.* 238, 1–8.

243. Paylor, R., Nguyen, M., Crawley, J. N., Patrick, J., Beaudet, A., and Orr-Urtreger, A. (1998). Alpha7 nicotinic receptor subunits are not necessary for hippocampal-dependent learning or sensorimotor gating: A behavioral characterization of Acra7-deficient mice. *Learn. Mem.* 5, 302–316.

244. Ross, S. A., Wong, J. Y., Clifford, J. J., Kinsella, A., Massalas, J. S., Horne, M. K., Scheffer, I. E., Kola, I., Waddington, J. L., Berkovic, S. F., and Drago, J. (2000). Phenotypic characterization of an alpha 4 neuronal nicotinic acetylcholine receptor subunit knock-out mouse. *J. Neurosci.* 20, 6431–6441.

245. Huang, E. J., and Reichardt, L. F. (2003). Trk receptors: Roles in neuronal signal transduction. *Annu. Rev. Biochem.* 72, 609–642.

246. Koponen, E., Voikar, V., Riekki, R., Saarelainen, T., Rauramaa, T., Rauvala, H., Taira, T., and Castren, E. (2004). Transgenic mice overexpressing the full-length neurotrophin receptor trkB exhibit increased activation of the trkB-PLCgamma pathway, reduced anxiety, and facilitated learning. *Mol. Cell. Neurosci.* 26, 166–181.

247. Sandi, C. (2004). Stress, cognitive impairment and cell adhesion molecules. *Nat. Rev. Neurosci.* 5, 917–930.

248. Stork, O., Welzl, H., Wotjak, C. T., Hoyer, D., Delling, M., Cremer, H., and Schachner, M. (1999). Anxiety and increased 5-HT1A receptor response in NCAM null mutant mice. *J. Neurobiol.* 40, 343–355.

249. Law, J. W., Lee, A. Y., Sun, M., Nikonenko, A. G., Chung, S. K., Dityatev, A., Schachner, M., and Morellini, F. (2003). Decreased anxiety, altered place learning, and increased CA1 basal excitatory synaptic transmission in mice with conditional ablation of the neural cell adhesion molecule L1. *J. Neurosci.* 23, 10419–10432.

250. Manabe, T., Togashi, H., Uchida, N., Suzuki, S. C., Hayakawa, Y., Yamamoto, M., Yoda, H., Miyakawa, T., Takeichi, M., and Chisaka, O. (2000). Loss of cadherin-11 adhesion receptor enhances plastic changes in hippocampal synapses and modifies behavioral responses. *Mol. Cell. Neurosci.* 15, 534–546.

251. Yamagata, M., Sanes, J. R., and Weiner, J. A. (2003). Synaptic adhesion molecules. *Curr. Opin. Cell. Biol.* 15, 621–632.

252. Chen, C., Rainnie, D. G., Greene, R. W., and Tonegawa, S. (1994). Abnormal fear response and aggressive behavior in mutant mice deficient for alpha-calcium-calmodulin kinase II. *Science* 266, 291–294.

253. Kennedy, M. B. (1997). The postsynaptic density at glutamatergic synapses. *Trends Neurosci.* 20, 264–268.

254. Braun, A. P., and Schulman, H. (1995). The multifunctional calcium/calmodulin-dependent protein kinase: From form to function. *Annu. Rev. Physiol.* 57, 417–445.

255. Bowers, B. J., Collins, A. C., Tritto, T., and Wehner, J. M. (2000). Mice lacking PKC gamma exhibit decreased anxiety. *Behav. Genet.* 30, 111–121.

256. Miyakawa, T., Yagi, T., Watanabe, S., and Niki, H. (1994). Increased fearfulness of Fyn tyrosine kinase deficient mice. *Brain Res. Mol. Brain Res.* 27, 179–182.

257. Grant, S. G. (1996). Analysis of NMDA receptor mediated synaptic plasticity using gene targeting: Roles of Fyn and FAK non-receptor tyrosine kinases. *J. Physiol. Paris* 90, 337–338.

258. Beggs, H. E., Baragona, S. C., Hemperly, J. J., and Maness, P. F. (1997). NCAM140 interacts with the focal adhesion kinase p125(fak) and the SRC-related tyrosine kinase p59(fyn). *J. Biol. Chem.* 272, 8310–8319.

259. Seiwa, C., Sugiyama, I., Yagi, T., Iguchi, T., and Asou, H. (2000). Fyn tyrosine kinase participates in the compact myelin sheath formation in the central nervous system. *Neurosci. Res.* 37, 21–31.

260. Kassed, C. A., and Herkenham, M. (2004). NF-kappaB p50-deficient mice show reduced anxiety-like behaviors in tests of exploratory drive and anxiety. *Behav. Brain Res.* 154, 577–584.

261. Kaltschmidt, C., Kaltschmidt, B., Neumann, H., Wekerle, H., and Baeuerle, P. A. (1994). Constitutive NF-kappa B activity in neurons. *Mol. Cell. Biol.* 14, 3981–3992.

262. Schmidt-Ullrich, R., Memet, S., Lilienbaum, A., Feuillard, J., Raphael, M., and Israel, A. (1996). NF-kappaB activity in transgenic mice: Developmental regulation and tissue specificity. *Development* 122, 2117–2128.

263. Tronche, F., Kellendonk, C., Kretz, O., Gass, P., Anlag, K., Orban, P. C., Bock, R., Klein, R., and Schutz, G. (1999). Disruption of the glucocorticoid receptor gene in the nervous system results in reduced anxiety. *Nat. Genet.* 23, 99–103.

264. Pepin, M. C., Pothier, F., and Barden, N. (1992). Impaired type II glucocorticoid-receptor function in mice bearing antisense RNA transgene. *Nature* 355, 725–728.

265. Wei, Q., Lu, X. Y., Liu, L., Schafer, G., Shieh, K. R., Burke, S., Robinson, T. E., Watson, S. J., Seasholtz, A. F., and Akil, H. (2004). Glucocorticoid receptor overexpression in forebrain: A mouse model of increased emotional lability. *Proc. Natl. Acad. Sci. USA* 101, 11851–11856.

266. Kalueff, A. V., Lou, Y. R., Laaksi, I., and Tuohimaa, P. (2004). Increased anxiety in mice lacking vitamin D receptor gene. *Neuroreport* 15, 1271–1274.

267. Montminy, M. (1997). Transcriptional regulation by cyclic AMP. *Annu. Rev. Biochem.* 66, 807–822.

268. Valverde, O., Mantamadiotis, T., Torrecilla, M., Ugedo, L., Pineda, J., Bleckmann, S., Gass, P., Kretz, O., Mitchell, J. M., Schutz, G., and Maldonado, R. (2004). Modulation of anxiety-like behavior and morphine dependence in CREB-deficient mice. *Neuropsychopharmacology* 29, 1122–1133.

269. Blendy, J. A., Kaestner, K. H., Schmid, W., Gass, P., and Schutz, G. (1996). Targeting of the CREB gene leads to up-regulation of a novel CREB mRNA isoform. *EMBO. J.* 15, 1098–1106.

270. Maldonado, R., Smadja, C., Mazzucchelli, C., and Sassone-Corsi, P. (1999). Altered emotional and locomotor responses in mice deficient in the transcription factor CREM. *Proc. Natl. Acad. Sci. USA* 96, 14094–14099.

271. Lewejohann, L., Skryabin, B. V., Sachser, N., Prehn, C., Heiduschka, P., Thanos, S., Jordan, U., Dell'Omo, G., Vyssotski, A. L., Pleskacheva, M. G., Lipp, H. P., Tiedge, H., Brosius, J., and Prior, H. (2004). Role of a neuronal small non-messenger RNA: Behavioural alterations in BC1 RNA-deleted mice. *Behav. Brain. Res.* 154, 273–289.

272. Turri, M. G., Henderson, N. D., DeFries, J. C., and Flint, J. (2001). Quantitative trait locus mapping in laboratory mice derived from a replicated selection experiment for open-field activity. *Genetics* 158, 1217–1226.

273. Turri, M. G., DeFries, J. C., Henderson, N. D., and Flint, J. (2004). Multivariate analysis of quantitative trait loci influencing variation in anxiety-related behavior in laboratory mice. *Mamm. Genome.* 15, 69–76.

274. Ren-Patterson, R. F., Cochran, L. W., Holmes, A., Sherrill, S., Huang, S. J., Tolliver, T., Lesch, K. P., Lu, B., and Murphy, D. L., (2005). Loss of brain-derived neurotrophic factor gene allele exacerbates brain monoamine deficiencies and increases stress abnormalities of serotonin transporter knockout mice, *J. Neurosci. Res.* 79, 756–771.

275. Chen, K., Holschneider, D. P., Wu, W., Rebrin, I., and Shih, J. C. (2004). A spontaneous point mutation produces monoamine oxidase A/B knock-out mice with greatly elevated monoamines and anxiety-like behavior. *J. Biol. Chem.* 279, 39645–39652.

276. Grimsby, J., Toth, M., Chen, K., Kumazawa, T., Klaidman, L., Adams, J. D., Karoum, F., Gal, J., and Shih, J. C. (1997). Increased stress response and beta-phenylethylamine in MAOB-deficient mice. *Nat. Genet.* 17, 206–210.

277. Cases, O., Seif, I., Grimsby, J., Gaspar, P., Chen, K., Pournin, S., Muller, U., Aguet, M., Babinet, C., Shih, J. C. et al. (1995). Aggressive behavior and altered amounts of brain serotonin and norepinephrine in mice lacking MAOA. *Science* 268, 1763–1766.

278. Meaney, M. J., Diorio, J., Francis, D., Widdowson, J., LaPlante, P., Caldji, C., Sharma, S., Seckl, J. R., and Plotsky, P. M. (1996). Early environmental regulation of forebrain glucocorticoid receptor gene expression: Implications for adrenocortical responses to stress. *Dev. Neurosci.* 18, 49–72.

279. Plotsky, P. M., and Meaney, M. J. (1993). Early, postnatal experience alters hypothalamic corticotropin-releasing factor (CRF) mRNA, median eminence CRF content and stress-induced release in adult rats. *Brain Res. Mol. Brain Res.* 18, 195–200.

280. Kalinichev, M., Easterling, K. W., Plotsky, P. M., and Holtzman, S. G. (2002). Long-lasting changes in stress-induced corticosterone response and anxiety-like behaviors as a consequence of neonatal maternal separation in Long-Evans rats. *Pharmacol. Biochem. Behav.* 73, 131–140.

281. Francis, D. D., and Meaney, M. J. (1999). Maternal care and the development of stress responses. *Curr. Opin. Neurobiol.* 9, 128–134.

282. Meaney, M. J. (2001). Maternal care, gene expression, and the transmission of individual differences in stress reactivity across generations. *Annu. Rev. Neurosci.* 24, 1161–1192.

283. Menard, J. L., Champagne, D. L., and Meaney, M. J. (2004). Variations of maternal care differentially influence "fear" reactivity and regional patterns of cFos immunoreactivity in response to the shock-probe burying test. *Neuroscience* 129, 297–308.

284. Caldji, C., Tannenbaum, B., Sharma, S., Francis, D., Plotsky, P. M., and Meaney, M. J. (1998). Maternal care during infancy regulates the development of neural systems mediating the expression of fearfulness in the rat. *Proc. Natl. Acad. Sci. USA* 95, 5335–5340.

285. Liu, D., Diorio, J., Tannenbaum, B., Caldji, C., Francis, D., Freedman, A., Sharma, S., Pearson, D., Plotsky, P. M., and Meaney, M. J. (1997). Maternal care, hippocampal glucocorticoid receptors, and hypothalamic-pituitary-adrenal responses to stress. *Science* 277, 1659–1662.

286. Champagne, F., and Meaney, M. J. (2001). Like mother, like daughter: Evidence for non-genomic transmission of parental behavior and stress responsivity. *Prog. Brain Res.* 133, 287–302.

287. Forray, M. I., and Gysling, K. (2004). Role of noradrenergic projections to the bed nucleus of the stria terminalis in the regulation of the hypothalamic-pituitary-adrenal axis. *Brain Res. Brain Res. Rev.* 47, 145–160.

288. Herman, J. P., Mueller, N. K., and Figueiredo, H. (2004). Role of GABA and glutamate circuitry in hypothalamo-pituitary-adrenocortical stress integration. *Ann. NY Acad. Sci.* 1018, 35–45.

289. Caldji, C., Diorio, J., and Meaney, M. J. (2003). Variations in maternal care alter GABA(A) receptor subunit expression in brain regions associated with fear. *Neuropsychopharmacology* 28, 1950–1959.

290. Caldji, C., Diorio, J., Anisman, H., and Meaney, M. J. (2004). Maternal behavior regulates benzodiazepine/GABAA receptor subunit expression in brain regions associated with fear in BALB/c and C57BL/6 mice. *Neuropsychopharmacology* 29, 1344–1352.

291. Liu, D., Diorio, J., Day, J. C., Francis, D. D., and Meaney, M. J. (2000). Maternal care, hippocampal synaptogenesis and cognitive development in rats. *Nat. Neurosci.* 3, 799–806.

291a. Weaver, I. C., Cervoni, N., Champagne, F. A., D'Alessio, A. C., Sharma, S., Seckl, J. R., Dymov, S., Szyf, M. and Meaney, M. J. (2004) Epigenetic programming by maternal behavior, *Nat Neurosci.* 7, 847–854.

292. Marini, A. M., Rabin, S. J., Lipsky, R. H., and Mocchetti, I. (1998). Activity-dependent release of brain-derived neurotrophic factor underlies the neuroprotective effect of N-methyl-D-aspartate. *J. Biol. Chem.* 273, 29394–29399.

293. Caspi, A., Sugden, K., Moffitt, T. E., Taylor, A., Craig, I. W., Harrington, H., McClay, J., Mill, J., Martin, J., Braithwaite, A., and Poulton, R. (2003). Influence of life stress on depression: Moderation by a polymorphism in the 5-HTT gene. *Science* 301, 386–389.

294. Champoux, M., Bennett, A., Shannon, C., Higley, J. D., Lesch, K. P., and Suomi, S. J. (2002). Serotonin transporter gene polymorphism, differential early rearing, and behavior in rhesus monkey neonates. *Mol. Psychiatry* 7, 1058–1063.
295. Bennett, A. J., Lesch, K. P., Heils, A., Long, J. C., Lorenz, J. G., Shoaf, S. E., Champoux, M., Suomi, S. J., Linnoila, M. V., and Higley, J. D. (2002). Early experience and serotonin transporter gene variation interact to influence primate CNS function. *Mol. Psychiatry* 7, 118–122.
296. Barr, C. S., Newman, T. K., Shannon, C., Parker, C., Dvoskin, R. L., Becker, M. L., Schwandt, M., Champoux, M., Lesch, K. P., Goldman, D., Suomi, S. J., and Higley, J. D. (2004). Rearing condition and rh5-HTTLPR interact to influence limbic-hypothalamic-pituitary-adrenal axis response to stress in infant macaques. *Biol. Psychiatry* 55, 733–738.
297. Crawley, J. N., Belknap, J. K., Collins, A., Crabbe, J. C., Frankel, W., Henderson, N., Hitzemann, R. J., Maxson, S. C., Miner, L. L., Silva, A. J., Wehner, J. M., Wynshaw-Boris, A., and Paylor, R. (1997). Behavioral phenotypes of inbred mouse strains: Implications and recommendations for molecular studies. *Psychopharmacology (Berl.)* 132, 107–124.
298. Anisman, H., Zaharia, M. D., Meaney, M. J., and Merali, Z. (1998). Do early life events permanently alter behavioral and hormonal responses to stressors? *Int. J. Dev. Neurosci.* 16, 149–164.
299. Zaharia, M. D., Kulczycki, J., Shanks, N., Meaney, M. J., and Anisman, H. (1996). The effects of early postnatal stimulation on Morris water-maze acquisition in adult mice: Genetic and maternal factors. *Psychopharmacology (Berl.)* 128, 227–239.
300. Weller, A., Leguisamo, A. C., Towns, L., Ramboz, S., Bagiella, E., Hofer, M., Hen, R., and Brunner, D. (2003). Maternal effects in infant and adult phenotypes of 5HT1A and 5HT1B receptor knockout mice. *Dev. Psychobiol.* 42, 194–205.
301. Ouagazzal, A. M., Moreau, J. L., Pauly Evers, M., and Jenck, F. (2003). Impact of environmental housing conditions on the emotional responses of mice deficient for nociceptin/orphanin FQ peptide precursor gene. *Behav. Brain Res.* 144, 111–117.
302. Wood, S. J., and Toth, M. (2001). Molecular pathways of anxiety revealed by knockout mice. *Mol. Neurobiol.* 23, 101–119.
303. Della Rocca, G. J., Mukhin, Y. V., Garnovskaya, M. N., Daaka, Y., Clark, G. J., Luttrell, L. M., Lefkowitz, R. J., and Raymond, J. R. (1999). Serotonin 5-HT1A receptor-mediated Erk activation requires calcium/calmodulin-dependent receptor endocytosis. *J. Biol. Chem.* 274, 4749–4753.
304. Cowen, D. S., Sowers, R. S., and Manning, D. R. (1996). Activation of a mitogen-activated protein kinase (ERK2) by the 5-hydroxytryptamine1A receptor is sensitive not only to inhibitors of phosphatidylinositol 3-kinase, but to an inhibitor of phosphatidylcholine hydrolysis. *J. Biol. Chem.* 271, 22297–22300.
305. Cowen, D. S., Molinoff, P. B., and Manning, D. R. (1997). 5-Hydroxytryptamine1A receptor-mediated increases in receptor expression and activation of nuclear factor-kappaB in transfected Chinese hamster ovary cells. *Mol. Pharmacol.* 52, 221–226.
306. Garnovskaya, M. N., van Biesen, T., Hawe, B., Casanas Ramos, S., Lefkowitz, R. J., and Raymond, J. R. (1996). Ras-dependent activation of fibroblast mitogen-activated protein kinase by 5-HT1A receptor via a G protein beta gamma-subunit-initiated pathway. *Biochemistry* 35, 13716–13722.
307. Adayev, T., Ray, I., Sondhi, R., Sobocki, T., and Banerjee, P. (2003). The G protein-coupled 5-HT1A receptor causes suppression of caspase-3 through MAPK and protein kinase Calpha. *Biochim. Biophys. Acta* 1640, 85–96.

308. Magarinos, A. M., McEwen, B. S., Flugge, G., and Fuchs, E. (1996). Chronic psychosocial stress causes apical dendritic atrophy of hippocampal CA3 pyramidal neurons in subordinate tree shrews. *J. Neurosci.* 16, 3534–3540.
309. Vyas, A., Mitra, R., Shankaranarayana Rao, B. S., and Chattarji, S. (2002). Chronic stress induces contrasting patterns of dendritic remodeling in hippocampal and amygdaloid neurons. *J. Neurosci.* 22, 6810–6818.
310. McEwen, B. S., and Magarinos, A. M. (2001). Stress and hippocampal plasticity: Implications for the pathophysiology of affective disorders. *Hum. Psychopharmacol.* 16, S7–S19.
311. Rainnie, D. G., Bergeron, R., Sajdyk, T. J., Patil, M., Gehlert, D. R., and Shekhar, A. (2004). Corticotrophin releasing factor-induced synaptic plasticity in the amygdala translates stress into emotional disorders. *J. Neurosci.* 24, 3471–3479.
312. Carter, A. R., Chen, C., Schwartz, P. M., and Segal, R. A. (2002). Brain-derived neurotrophic factor modulates cerebellar plasticity and synaptic ultrastructure. *J. Neurosci.* 22, 1316–1327.
313. Sarnyai, Z., Sibille, E. L., Pavlides, C., Fenster, R. J., McEwen, B. S., and Toth, M. (2000). Impaired hippocampal-dependent learning and functional abnormalities in the hippocampus in mice lacking serotonin(1A) receptors. *Proc. Natl. Acad. Sci. USA* 97, 14731–14736.
314. Salome, N., Salchner, P., Viltart, O., Sequeira, H., Wigger, A., Landgraf, R., and Singewald, N. (2004). Neurobiological correlates of high (HAB) versus low anxiety-related behavior (LAB): Differential Fos expression in HAB and LAB rats. *Biol. Psychiatry* 55, 715–723.

2

PHARMACOTHERAPY OF ANXIETY

JON R. NASH[1] AND DAVID J. NUTT[2]
[1]*University of Bristol, Bristol, United Kingdom and* [2]*University of Bristol, School of Medical Science, Bristol, United Kingdom*

2.1	Introduction		60
2.2	Clinical Management of Anxiety		60
2.3	Diagnosis of Anxiety Disorders		61
2.4	Anxiolytic Drugs		62
	2.4.1	Drugs Acting via Monoamine Neurotransmission	63
		2.4.1.1 Antidepressants	64
		2.4.1.2 5-HT_{1A} Receptor Agonists	70
		2.4.1.3 β Blockers	71
		2.4.1.4 Antipsychotics	71
	2.4.2	Drugs Acting via Amino Acid Neurotransmission	72
		2.4.2.1 Benzodiazepines	73
		2.4.2.2 Anticonvulsants	74
	2.4.3	Drugs with Other Mechanisms of Action	75
		2.4.3.1 Antihistamines	75
		2.4.3.2 Lithium	75
2.5	Pharmacotherapy for Anxiety Disorders		75
	2.5.1	Generalized Anxiety Disorder	77
	2.5.2	Obsessive-Compulsive Disorder	77
	2.5.3	Panic Disorder and Agoraphobia	78
	2.5.4	Post traumatic Stress Disorder	79
	2.5.5	Social Anxiety Disorder (Social Phobia)	79
	2.5.6	Specific Phobia	80
	2.5.7	Anxiety Symptoms in Depressive Disorders	80
2.6	Conclusions and Future Directions		81
References			82

Handbook of Contemporary Neuropharmacology, Edited by David R. Sibley, Israel Hanin, Michael Kuhar, and Phil Skolnick. Copyright © 2007 John Wiley & Sons, Inc.

2.1 INTRODUCTION

The medical treatment of anxiety disorders is passing through an interesting phase. The range of therapeutic options is expanding and public interest in the field is high. Longstanding controversies, such as the relative merits of psychological therapies versus medication and the safety of medical treatments of anxiety, are debated in the national media. Patients are increasingly active participants in the therapeutic process using widely available sources of medical information, while government guidelines seek to standardize prescribing practice and have provoked debate within the medical profession. The management of anxiety continues to sit uncomfortably between primary and secondary care and in many ways remains the poor relation within mental health care in most if not all countries. Nevertheless current medical practice is based on a substantial volume of research evidence and clinical experience, and it is possible to justify with confidence the treatment options put before patients.

The diagnostic concept of anxiety has undergone progressive evolution since Donald Klein described the discrimination of panic disorder from other neuroses [1]. New diagnostic categories have emerged, and although some discrepancies remain between different classifications, general agreement has been reached for the diagnostic validity of the main categories. This has allowed quantitative measurement of the prevalence and economic burden of anxiety disorders in epidemiological surveys [2, 3], and this evidence has been a key factor driving research into anxiolytic therapies.

The rapid advances of the past 15 years have also been driven by developments in a diversity of other disciplines, including preclinical and clinical pharmacology, cognitive and experimental psychology, and neuroscience (particularly neuroimaging). Research from areas such as genetics and molecular biology is only just beginning to have an impact. This chapter describes the current basis of pharmacotherapy for anxiety disorders, but with the pace of scientific discovery this is a field that is likely to undergo further change in the years ahead.

2.2 CLINICAL MANAGEMENT OF ANXIETY

Management of an anxious patient involves far more than the prescription of medication (Fig. 2.1). Establishing the diagnosis of a specific anxiety disorder is a critical part of the assessment process that may greatly influence the treatment offered. Anxiety disorders frequently present with comorbid conditions such as depression, alcohol or substance use problems, and other anxiety disorders, which must be detected and managed appropriately. A patient tends to present when anxiety causes impairment of their social, occupational, or domestic functioning, and identification of the key complaints helps in drawing up an effective management plan; for example, a patient with generalized anxiety disorder may complain that insomnia impairs his or her ability to work, and management should include strategies to improve sleep efficiency as well as treatment of the anxiety. Most anxiety disorders and any concomitant depression are associated with an increased risk of suicidal thoughts and acts of deliberate self-harm, and these should be carefully assessed and monitored during treatment.

Psychoeducation helps engagement and improves recovery. Models of anxiety disorders have been described in both the biological and psychological dimensions,

```
                    ┌─────────────────────┐
                    │ Diagnostic assessment│
                    └─────────────────────┘
                      ↙        ↓        ↘
         ┌──────────────┐ ┌──────────┐ ┌────────────────────┐
         │ Comorbidity  │ │ Primary  │ │Functional impairment│
         │Other anxiety │ │diagnosis │ │     Domestic        │
         │  disorder    │ │ of anxiety│ │    Occupational    │
         │  Depression  │ │ disorder │ │      Social         │
         │Harmful use of│ └──────────┘ └────────────────────┘
         │alcohol/drugs │      ↓
         └──────────────┘ ┌──────────┐
                          │Treatment │
                          │   plan   │
                          └──────────┘
```

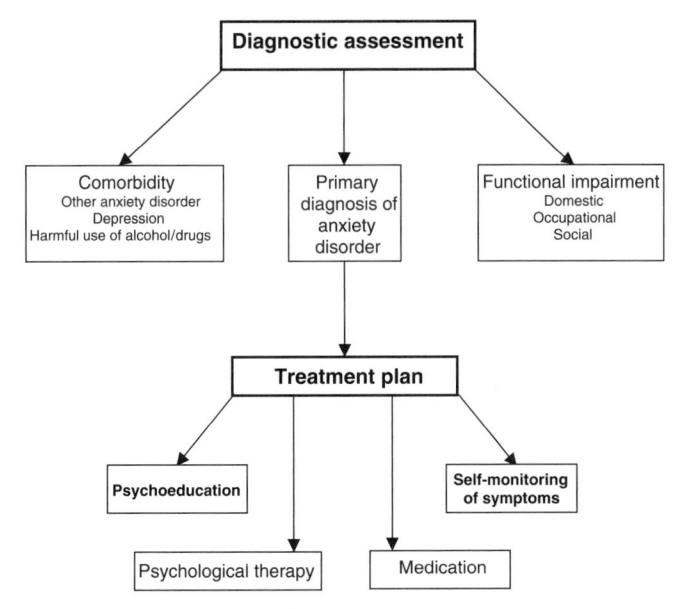

Figure 2.1 Clinical assessment of anxious patient.

and patients benefit from an explanation, tailored to their level of understanding, in each dimension. This can be reinforced by the use of educative literature [4]. Treatment efficacy is improved when patients monitor and record their symptoms [5].

A management plan is negotiated with the patient by considering any appropriate biological and psychological treatments. A combination of drug and psychological therapies can be more effective than either alone [6]. The patient may have preconceptions about specific therapies, often as a result of their anxiety; for example, a patient with panic disorder fears the effects of drugs and a patient with social anxiety baulks at the suggestion of group therapy. An open discussion of benefits and adverse effects, including long-term side effects, is likely to improve compliance. Although medications are generally well tolerated, some side effects commonly occur, and anxious patients tend to experience more than others [7]. Progress with treatment should be encouraged by regular review, particularly in the early stages.

2.3 DIAGNOSIS OF ANXIETY DISORDERS

Although every method for categorizing anxiety disorders has its shortcomings, in current clinical practice the diagnostic criteria of the American Psychiatric Association [fourth edition of the Diagnostic and Statistical Manual of Mental Disorders (DSM-IV)] is most commonly used [8]. *Anxiety disorder* is divided into syndromes with clear operational criteria. In particular, the criteria are clearly stated for a symptomatic individual to become a case, and this diagnostic threshold is defined either by the level of distress experienced by the individual or in terms of impairment of occupational, social, or domestic functioning. Patients may have symptoms from more than one diagnostic category, but it is important to elicit the primary diagnosis, as this will influence the recommended treatment. Comorbid disorders, usually a

TABLE 2.1 Diagnostic Criteria for Major Anxiety Disorders

Generalized anxiety disorder (GAD)	Excessive worry/anxiety about various matters for at least 6 months; difficulty in controlling worry; accompanying somatic symptoms (effects of chronic tension); clinically important distress or impairment of functioning
Obsessive-compulsive disorder (OCD)	Presence of obsessions (thoughts) or compulsions (behaviors); symptoms felt by patient to be unreasonable or excessive; clinically important distress or impairment of functioning
Panic disorder with/ without agoraphobia[a]	Severe fear or discomfort peaking within 10 min; characteristic physical/psychological symptoms; episodes are recurrent and some unexpected; anxiety about further attacks or consequences of attacks
Post-traumatic stress disorder (PTSD)	Severe traumatic event that threatened death or serious harm; felt intense fear, horror, or helplessness; repeated reliving experiences; phobic avoidance of trauma-related stimuli; hyperarousal; symptoms lasting >1 month and causing clinically important distress or impairment of functioning
Social anxiety disorder	Recurrent fears of social or performance situations; situations avoided or endured with distress; clinically important distress or impairment of functioning
Specific phobia	Persistent fear/avoidance of specific object or situation; phobic stimulus immediately provoking anxiety response; clinically important distress or impairment of functioning.

Source: After DSM-IV.
[a]Agoraphobia: anxiety about place/situation where panic attack is distressing or escape difficult; situation is avoided, endured with distress or companion is required.

second anxiety disorder, mood disorder, or substance use disorder, are common and must be detected. The key diagnostic criteria for the major anxiety disorders are given in Table 2.1.

2.4 ANXIOLYTIC DRUGS

The use of substances for their anxiolytic properties dates from the beginning of recorded human history. The last century saw the development of their use for medical purposes, and major progress was made in the 1990s, "the decade of anxiety," as advances in neuroscience provided a basis for the design of new treatments. There are now drugs available that are better tolerated, although not necessarily more effective, than their predecessors. Despite growing knowledge of the complex neural pathways involved in anxiety, it is notable that the actions of current drugs occur via a small number of neurotransmitter systems, with the most important being the monoaminergic neurotransmitters [serotonin (5-HT), noradrenaline, and to a lesser extent dopamine] and the amino acid neurotransmitters [chiefly γ-aminobutyric acid (GABA) but also glutamate].

2.4.1 Drugs Acting via Monoamine Neurotransmission

Interest in this field originated with the serendipitous discovery of the tricyclic antidepressants (TCAs) and monoamine oxidase inhibitors (MAOIs), when these drugs were later found to exert their anxiolytic effects via actions on monoamine systems. Recent research, rather than clarifying the role of these neurotransmitters in anxiety pathways, has tended to present an increasingly complex picture [9]. Nevertheless these advances have led to the development of "designer drugs" with selective effects on serotonergic and noradrenergic neurones. Drugs such as the selective serotonin reuptake inhibitors (SSRIs) do not exceed their predecessors in terms of anxiolytic efficacy [10], but improved tolerability has led to their adoption as first-line treatments for anxiety disorders. The historical development of drugs in this field is illustrated in Fig. 2.2.

The monoamines are relatively simple molecules that are synthesized within neurons from dietary amino acids. They facilitate transmission in neural pathways that originate in brain stem nuclei and have descending projections to the autonomic nervous system and widespread ascending projections to sites in the limbic system and cortex. In addition to the control of anxiety responses, these pathways modulate many other aspects of behavioral function, including mood, appetite, and sleep.

Among the monoamines the role of 5-HT in anxiety is best understood, but the picture is complex as increased serotonergic activity may be anxiogenic or anxiolytic depending on the site and duration of action [11]. 5-HT is released into the synapse and either binds to postsynaptic receptors or reenters the neuron via a specific transporter (Fig. 2.3). The serotonergic neuron regulates its own firing rate via the action of inhibitory autoreceptors. Anxiety disorders have been shown to be associated with various alterations in the serotonergic neuron including reduced

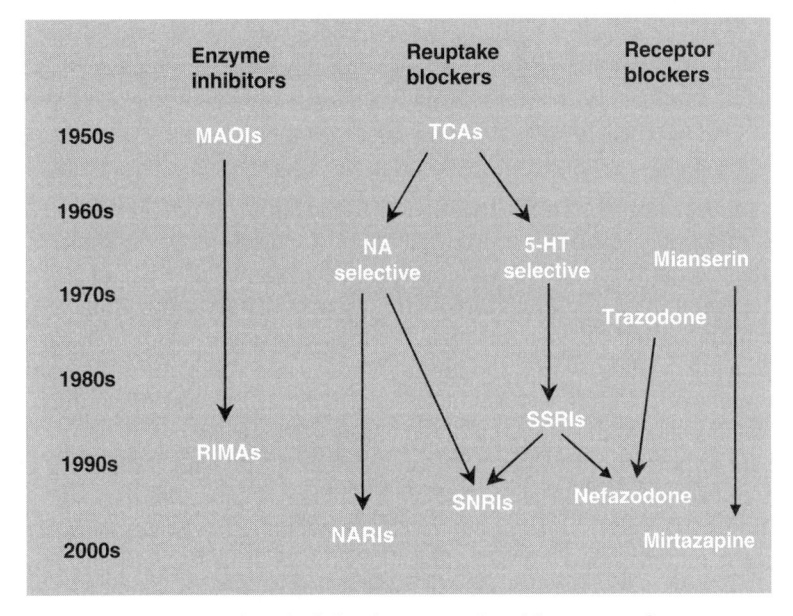

Figure 2.2 Historical development of antidepressant drugs.

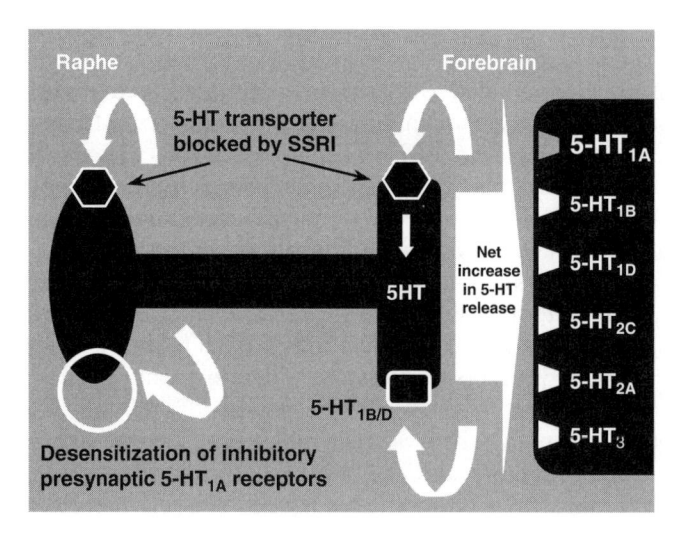

Figure 2.3 Actions of anxiolytic drugs on serotonergic neurone.

binding to presynaptic and postsynaptic 5-HT$_{1A}$ receptors [12] and possibly with a genetic variation in the 5-HT transporter [13].

Anxiolytic drugs can alter monoaminergic neurotransmission by increasing synaptic availability or by direct action on postsynaptic receptors. Mechanisms for increasing monoamine availability include promoting release by blocking inhibitory autoreceptors, decreasing reuptake by blocking transporters, and decreasing metabolism by inhibiting oxidative enzymes. Monoamines are also implicated in the pathophysiology of depression, and drugs that increase their synaptic availability tend to have antidepressant effects. These drugs have been traditionally classified as antidepressants, although they have a primary role as anxiolytics and are currently the major drug class in the field. Other anxiolytic drugs acting via monoamines are the postsynaptic serotonin receptor partial agonist buspirone, the β-adrenoceptor blockers, and drugs classed as antipsychotics, which are primarily antagonists at postsynaptic monoamine receptors.

2.4.1.1 Antidepressants. Taken together the efficacy of antidepressants covers the spectrum of anxiety disorders, although there are important differences between drugs in the group (Table 2.2). Several new antidepressants have been marketed since the SSRIs: venlafaxine and mirtazapine are discussed later; nefazodone, a serotonin reuptake inhibitor and postsynaptic 5-HT$_2$ blocker, showed promise in early studies but was recently withdrawn by its manufacturers; and reboxetine, a noradrenaline reuptake inhibitor (NARI), showed benefits in panic disorder in one published study [14] and further evidence of its anxiolytic efficacy is awaited.

There are important difference between antidepressants and other drug groups in the onset and course of their actions (Fig. 2.4). There is often an increase in anxiety on initiation of therapy, and anxiolytic effects occur later. In comparative studies improvement matches that on benzodiazepines after four weeks [15]. Withdrawal effects, particularly rebound anxiety, are less problematic with antidepressants than with benzodiazepines, although stopping treatment is associated with a significant

TABLE 2.2 The Use of Antidepressants in Anxiety Disorders

Parameter	SSRI/SNRI[a]	TCA	Mirtazapine	MAOI/RIMA[b]
Efficacy	GAD, OCD, panic disorder PTSD, social anxiety disorder	Panic disorder, OCD (GAD, PTSD)	Panic disorder, PTSD	Panic disorder, PTSD, social anxiety disorder
Tolerability	Onset worsening, side effects on initiation, few long-term effects	Onset worsening, side effects on initiation, some long-term effects	Few side effects on initiation, few long-term side effects	Significant short- and long-term side effects, special dietary requirements, moclobemide better tolerated
Safety	Relatively safe in overdose	Significant overdose toxicity	Relatively safe in overdose	Significant overdose toxicity (less with moclobemide)
Discontinuation syndrome	Well-described, more common with paroxetine and venlafaxine, uncommon with fluoxetine	Well described	Not reported	Reported

Note: For items in brackets the evidence is less strong.
[a] Serotonin and noradrenaline receptor inhibitor.
[b] Monoamine oxidase inhibitor/reversible inhibitor of monoamine oxidase.

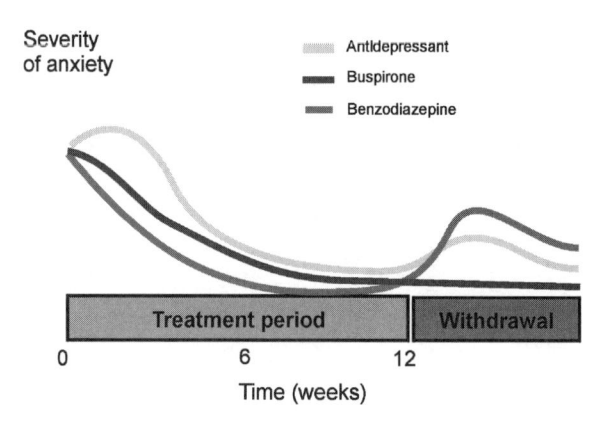

Figure 2.4 Onset and course of action of anxiolytic drugs. (See color insert.)

risk of relapse and a withdrawal (discontinuation) syndrome has been described for most of the antidepressants with short half-lives.

2.4.1.1.1 SSRIs. These drugs increase the availability of synaptic 5-HT by selectively blocking the 5-HT reuptake transporter (Fig. 2.3). In preclinical and human studies acute doses are anxiogenic [16] but chronic administration has anxiolytic effects, possibly due to downregulation of presynaptic autoreceptors [17]. There are five SSRIs widely available: citalopram, fluoxetine, fluvoxamine, paroxetine, and sertraline. Escitalopram, the S enantiomer of citalopram, has been demonstrated to be effective in several studies of anxiety disorders and has the same spectrum of efficacy as citalopram [18]. The SSRIs as a class are now widely considered to be appropriate first-line anxiolytic drugs; in particular, paroxetine, one of the most potent 5-HT reuptake blockers, has been licensed in the United Kingdom for the treatment of each of the major anxiety disorders. Efficacy has been clearly demonstrated for SSRIs in randomized controlled trials of up to six months, but in common with other antidepressants research evidence is lacking for longer term efficacy.

A major advantage of the SSRIs is their improved tolerability relative to the TCAs and benzodiazepines, which has been demonstrated in comparisons of drugs from these classes [19, 20]. Nevertheless they are not without side effects: On initiation nausea, anxiety, jitteriness, and insomnia are related to the starting dose; later sedation, asthenia, headache, sweating, and sexual dysfunction may occur. Hyponatremia is a problem most likely to be seen in the elderly. Some effects are particular to individual drugs within the class [21]. For example, paroxetine has some anticholinergic properties and can cause dry mouth, constipation, and urinary hesitancy; sertraline is more likely to cause dyspepsia and diarrhea; and fluoxetine has agonist activity at 5-HT_{2C} receptors, causing headache, agitation, and loss of appetite, possibly explaining its efficacy in bulimia [22].

Although SSRI overdose can cause seizures, coma, and cardiac abnormalities [23], these toxic effects occur only in large overdoses or in combination with other drugs. Fatality rates are very substantially lower than with TCA overdose [24, 25]. Public attention has been drawn to reports of suicidal and aggressive thoughts and behavior associated with SSRI therapy [26]. The scientific basis for this assertion is disputed, and a number of conflicting factors have been considered [27, 28]. Both anxiety disorders and related depression significantly increase the risk of suicide and successful treatment reduces this risk. However, there are periods within treatment when clinical factors can lead to an increased risk; for example, as energy levels improve, the patient may be more likely to act upon existing suicidal thoughts, and this phenomenon was observed before the advent of antidepressants. Furthermore there may be factors specific to antidepressant therapy that cause increased suicidality, such as side effects of agitation, restlessness, and increased anxiety which are possibly due to activation of postsynaptic 5-HT$_2$ receptors by increased synaptic 5-HT. These factors have been particularly highlighted as relating to the use of SSRIs but are in reality common to most antidepressants. The assessment and monitoring of suicidality are an integral part of the clinical management of any patient with anxiety or depression. It is debatable whether SSRI therapy presents a special risk in this area, and taking a broader view it appears that SSRI treatment is associated with reduced suicidality on a population level [29, 30].

A further controversy that has surfaced in the lay media is the misleading claim that SSRIs have "addictive" properties. This centers around reports of patients suffering symptoms when trying to discontinue medication. In many cases these symptoms are a recurrence of the original anxiety disorder, often as a result of suboptimal treatment, although an important difference between antidepressants and benzodiazepines is that rebound anxiety (a rapid return of the original symptoms) has not been clearly demonstrated with antidepressants. There is also a well-described transient discontinuation syndrome associated with SSRI withdrawal, that is, a reaction occurring as brain levels of the drug are falling that is not a feature of the underlying disorder [28, 31]. The most frequently occurring symptoms are dizziness, nausea, and headache (Table 2.3), with a typical duration of two to four days. The syndrome is most common with paroxetine, possibly due to its anticholinergic activity, and is very uncommon with fluoxetine due to the long half-life of its metabolites [32]. Although prominently highlighted with SSRIs, a similar syndrome has been observed with most, although not all, antidepressants. It can start as soon as 48 h after the final dose, and although most cases resolve within two to three weeks, symptoms may rarely last longer than this. Difficult cases can be managed by reinstituting the drug and withdrawing slowly, if necessary using liquid preparations, or by switching to a drug with a long half-life such as fluoxetine. Patients should be counseled about possible withdrawal problems at the start of therapy, although with careful management significant problems should not be common.

TABLE 2.3 SSRI Discontinuation Syndrome

Symptoms	**Neurological symptoms**: dizziness, tremor, vertigo, paraesthesia/shooting pains
	Psychological symptoms: anxiety, confusion, memory problems
	Somatic distress: nausea, headache, lethargy
	Hyperarousal: agitation, restlessness, insomnia, irritability
Risk factors	**Treatment factors**: longer duration of treatment, rapid discontinuation, short half-life drug, possibly increased dose
	Patient factors: possibly younger age, any psychiatric diagnosis
Therapeutic strategies	Careful assessment, reassurance, reinstitute therapy if necessary, taper slowly (over 1 month), switch to fluoxetine

SSRIs may interact with other drugs that have effects on 5-HT neurotransmission, including TCAs, buspirone, sumatriptan, and tryptophan, but particularly important is the interaction with MAOIs that can lead to a synergistic increase in synaptic 5-HT. This can result in the potentially lethal "serotonin syndrome," comprising restlessness, irritability, tremor, sweating, and hyperreflexia [33]. In clinical practice there should be a washout of two weeks between discontinuing MAOI therapy and starting SSRI; a washout of one to two weeks should follow SSRI discontinuation (five weeks for fluoxetine). The drugs have variable potential for drug interactions via hepatic cytochrome P450 enzymes (Table 2.4). Citalopram and escitalopram have the lowest potential for interactions.

Expert sources and government guidelines recommend SSRIs as first-line drug treatments of anxiety disorders [34–37]. In preparation for treatment a full discussion of potential benefits and anticipated side effects (including discontinuation effects) should be held with the patient [38]. Some patients have difficulty initiating treatment because of anxiety about side effects. In these cases the drug may be increased slowly from a low starting dose, if necessary using the syrup form of fluoxetine or paroxetine, or a benzodiazepine may be used to cover the initiaition period.

There is little research evidence to guide a decision on duration of treatment. Studies have shown continued improvement for up to 12 months, and for most disorders there is a significant relapse rate when treatment is stopped [39–41]. Guidelines suggest continuing for 12–24 months if treatment is successful, but a longer duration may be required for some patients (Table 2.5). Treatment disconti-

TABLE 2.4 SSRIs and Hepatic Cytochrome P450 Enzymes

Enzymes	Inhibitor of Enzymes
Citalopram/escitalopram	—
Fluoxetine	2D6 (potent)
	3A4 (potent)
Fluvoxamine	1A2 (potent)
	3A4 (potent)
	2D6 (moderate)
Paroxetine	2D6 (potent)
	3A4 (moderate)
Sertraline	2D6 (moderate)

TABLE 2.5 Patients Requiring Long-Term Treatment

Patient factors	Illness factors
Comorbid mood disorder	Severely disabling symptoms
Comorbid anxiety disorder	Chronic illness (> 2 years)
Physical ill-health	Recurrent episodes
Personality disorder	Incomplete response to treatment
Age > 50 years	

nuation should be carefully planned and it is sensible to slowly taper off SSRIs as a matter of routine.

2.4.1.1.2 SNRIs. Venlafaxine is a serotonin and noradrenaline reuptake inhibitor (SNRI). It shares these properties with the TCAs amitriptyline, clomipramine, and imipramine, but it is the first selective SNRI with low affinity for muscarinic, histaminic, and α-adrenergic receptors. At low doses serotonergic effects predominate, but at higher doses (above 150 mg daily) the reuptake of noradrenaline is also significantly blocked [42]. It is not yet clear whether these noradrenergic effects confer additional benefit in the treatment of anxiety disorders. Venlafaxine is available as immediate- and extended-release (XR) preparations.

There is a large evidence base for the antidepressant efficacy of venlafaxine and increasing evidence for its use in anxiety disorders, including GAD [43], OCD [44], and social anxiety disorder [45], and for anxiety symptoms associated with depression [46]. Side effects on initiation of therapy are similar to those of SSRIs with nausea being the most common, and higher doses can cause elevation of blood pressure. A discontinuation syndrome similar to that seen with SSRIs has been reported. Toxicity causes cardiac conduction problems, seizures, and coma. There is a disputed suggestion that venlafaxine overdose may be associated with a higher mortality than that of the SSRIs [47]. This has led to the U.K. government recommending restriction of its prescription to secondary care [48], which appears a perverse decision when the mortality associated with venlafaxine overdose is substantially less than with other antidepressants, such as the tricyclics, which can be prescribed without restriction [25]. Although metabolized by the hepatic cytochrome CYP2D6, venlafaxine does not inhibit this enzyme and has a low potential for drug interactions.

Other SNRIs have been in development for some time and have recently been marketed on the basis of their antidepressant efficacy. As yet their efficacy in anxiety disorders is unproven, although the SNRI duloxetine was shown to be effective for anxiety symptoms associated with depression [49].

2.4.1.1.3 TCAs. This group includes compounds with actions on a range of neurotransmitter systems. Their antidepressant efficacy is primarily mediated by inhibition of the reuptake of 5-HT and noradrenaline, although side effects such as sedation may also have clinical benefits. Their efficacy in anxiety disorders is supported by a long history of clinical experience and a solid evidence base from controlled trials. Studies support the use of clomipramine (a potent 5-HT reuptake inhibitor) in panic disorder and OCD [50, 51], of imipramine in panic disorder and GAD [52, 53], and of amitriptyline in PTSD [54]. No controlled studies support the use of TCAs in social anxiety disorder.

A meta-analysis of controlled studies suggested superior efficacy of clomipramine over SSRIs in OCD [55], but this has not been demonstrated in direct comparisons, and the use of SSRIs has superceded that of TCAs because of advantages in safety and tolerability [56]. Side effects of TCAs include anticholinergic effects (drowsiness, dry mouth, blurred vision, and constipation), antihistaminergic effects (drowsiness and weight gain), and postural hypotension caused by α_1-adrenoceptor blockade, as well as the side effects common to SSRIs. Some effects are dose related, and as the usual practice is to titrate the dose slowly upward, this often leads to patients being maintained on subtherapeutic doses. A discontinuation syndrome similar to that with SSRIs is well described, and withdrawal should be tapered. Overdose is associated with a significant mortality due to hypotension, cardiac arrhythmias, metabolic acidosis, seizures, and coma [25]. Interactions can occur with other drugs with central nervous system (CNS) effects (particularly MAOIs), and with drugs that affect hepatic metabolism.

2.4.1.1.4 Mirtazapine. Mirtazapine has a novel mechanism of action that in theory should promote anxiolytic effects, although solid evidence from studies in anxiety disorders is awaited. It increases synaptic release of 5-HT and noradrenaline via blockade of presynaptic inhibitory α_2-adrenoceptors as well as blocking postsynaptic 5-HT$_2$ and 5-HT$_3$ receptors and H$_1$ histamine receptors. Mirtazapine has good efficacy for anxiety symptoms associated with depression [57] and in controlled studies was superior to placebo in PTSD [58], equivalent to fluoxetine in panic disorder [59], and reduced social anxiety symptoms in heavy drinkers [60].

The actions of mirtazapine lead to a unique side-effect profile. Important effects are sedation, drowsiness, dry mouth, increased appetite, and weight gain. It does not cause initial worsening of anxiety. Tolerance to the sedative properties occurs after a few weeks, and paradoxically higher doses tend to be less sedating. Overdose does not cause serious toxic effects other than sedation. It has the potential for interaction with drugs that inhibit the cytochrome P450 2D6 and 3A4 isoenzymes, although reports of interactions are rare. Discontinuation symptoms have not yet been reported.

2.4.1.1.5 MAOIs. These drugs increase synaptic availability of 5-HT, noradrenaline, and dopamine by inhibiting their intracellular metabolism. The classical MAOIs phenelzine and tranylcypromine bind irreversibly to monoamine oxidase, while the newer drug moclobemide is a reversible inhibitor of monoamine oxidase A (RIMA). The long history of clinical use of MAOIs in panic disorder, PTSD, and social anxiety disorder is supported by several controlled trials [61–63], whereas the evidence for moclobemide is less conclusive. Both positive and negative studies have been published in panic disorder and social anxiety disorder, and meta-analysis suggests a lower response rate in social anxiety disorder than with SSRIs [64]. Brofaromine, a reversible MAOI, was effective in a controlled trial in social anxiety disorder but is no longer marketed.

The classical MAOIs have a significant side-effect profile, including dizziness, drowsiness, insomnia, headache, postural hypotension, and anticholinergic effects. Asthenia, weight gain, and sexual dysfunction can occur during long-term use. A hypertensive reaction (cheese reaction) may follow the ingestion of foods containing tyramine, which must therefore be removed from the diet. Overdose can be fatal due to seizures, cardiac arrhythmias, and hypotension. Interactions can occur with sympathomimetics, antihypertensives, and most psychoactive drugs, and a washout of two weeks is advised when switching from a MAOI to another antidepressant. Moclobemide is better tolerated, although at high doses (>900 mg daily) its binding becomes less reversible and dietary restrictions should be observed. The main side effects are dizziness and insomnia. Overdose toxicity is less, although fatalities have been reported.

2.4.1.2 5-HT$_{1A}$ Receptor Agonists. Buspirone is a partial agonist at postsynaptic 5-HT$_{1A}$ receptors in the limbic system but a full agonist at autoreceptors in the raphe [65]. Acute dosage inhibits 5-HT release, but this recovers with continued administration.

It has anxiolytic effects that take several weeks to emerge, although in contrast to antidepressants it does not cause worsening of symptoms at initiation (Fig. 2.4). Buspirone is effective in the treatment of GAD [66] and for anxiety symptoms in depression [67], either as monotherapy or combined with an SSRI. Response is less favorable if the patient has recently taken a benzodiazepine [68]. Evidence is lacking to support the use of buspirone in other anxiety disorders. Other drugs in this class have demonstrated anxiolytic properties in preclinical studies. Gepirone is effective for anxiety symptoms associated with depression [69] and tandospirone is licensed for use as an anxiolytic in Japan.

Buspirone is well tolerated, particularly by the elderly [70]. Common side effects include dizziness, anxiety, nausea, and headache. It does not cause sexual dysfunction and does not appear to be associated with a discontinuation syndrome. Overdose causes drowsiness but not serious toxic effects. A potential for interaction with drugs that inhibit the cytochrome P450 3A4 isoenzyme is not a significant problem in clinical practice. GAD is usually a chronic condition and buspirone is suitable for long-term treatment. Patients should be advised to expect a slow onset of benefits and reviewed regularly in the early stages of treatment.

2.4.1.3 β Blockers. The rationale for using β-adrenoceptor blockers for the treatment of anxiety is twofold: first, for the control of symptoms caused by autonomic arousal (e.g., palpitations, tremor) and, second because of the postulated but poorly understood involvement of central noradrenergic activity in anxiety pathways. There is a history of clinical use of these drugs in each of the five major anxiety disorders, but evidence is lacking from controlled clinical trials, and positive findings have often been superceded by later negative studies. Early trials were carried out with propranolol and the more cardioselective atenolol, which has mainly peripheral effects. The efficacy of atenolol in performance anxiety suggests that not all of the effects are centrally mediated [71]. Recently there has been interest in pindolol, a β Blocker that also blocks 5-HT$_{1A}$ autoreceptors and may promote serotonergic neurotransmission. Studies using pindolol to augment SSRI treatment of anxiety disorders have had mixed results [72–74].

Commonly β blockers cause side effects including bradycardia, hypotension, fatigue, and bronchospasm. Overdose can cause fatal cardiogenic shock. Because of the doubtful evidence for efficacy and poor tolerability and safety, their use in anxiety disorders is limited. They may have a circumscribed role in the prevention of performance anxiety [75].

2.4.1.4 Antipsychotics. This category contains drugs with various mechanisms of action that have clinical antipsychotic effects that are thought to be mediated via antagonism of D$_2$ dopamine receptors in the limbic system and cortex. They are loosely divided into two groups: older "classical" drugs such as haloperidol and chlorpromazine that are potent D$_2$ blockers and "atypical" antipsychotics that have a lower affinity for D$_2$ receptors but also block 5-HT$_2$ receptors. The history of clinical use of classical antipsychotics as "major tranquilizers" for anxiety disorders has little support from controlled trials [76]. Evidence is greatest in OCD for the augmentation of SSRI treatment with haloperidol [77] and the atypical drugs risperidone [78] and quetiapine [79]. Recent controlled trials have reported benefits for the atypical drug olanzapine in social anxiety disorder [80] and for olanzapine and risperidone in addition to SSRIs in PTSD [81, 82]. Open studies are reporting efficacy for atypical antipsychotics in other anxiety disorders, and it may be that their clinical use expands in the future. The atypicals have advantages in tolerability and safety over the older drugs, particularly a lower incidence of extrapyramidal movement disorders, although they may cause sedation, weight gain, and metabolic effects. Their metabolism by cytochrome P450 enzymes leads to a potential for interaction with many coprescribed drugs.

2.4.2 Drugs Acting via Amino Acid Neurotransmission

Glutamate is the major excitatory amino acid in the brain and has a key role as a neurotransmitter in memory, learning, and stress responses. Glutamate receptors are present throughout the CNS but differ widely according to their localization and function [83], and as a result have not been easy to identify as targets for pharmacological manipulation (see also Chapters 10 and 11 in Volume I of this handbook). The role of glutamate in facilitating new learning has been established for some time, and it has recently been suggested that augmenting glutamate transmission may enhance recovery from anxiety disorders by accelerating the learning of new, nonanxious responses [84].

GABA is formed by the decarboxylation of glutamate and is the major inhibitory neurotransmitter (see also Chapters 12 and 13 in Volume I of this handbook). Recent research has centerd on the role of the $GABA_A$ receptor as the mediator of the anxiolytic and sedative effects of drugs such as alcohol and the benzodiazepines [85]. This complex transmembrane receptor consists of five linked subunits in a ring structure around a central chloride ion channel (Fig. 2.5). Binding of the endogenous neurotransmitter changes the configuration of the receptor, causing an increased permeability to chloride ions and inhibiting neuronal firing. Exogenous drugs bind to different sites on the receptor and affect its function, either in a direct fashion or by modulating the effects of GABA. The structure of the receptor depends on the configuration of its protein subunits, and nearly 20 subtypes have been found in the brain, with differences in topographical distribution and between individuals. Different receptor subtypes have different sensitivity to drugs such as alcohol and

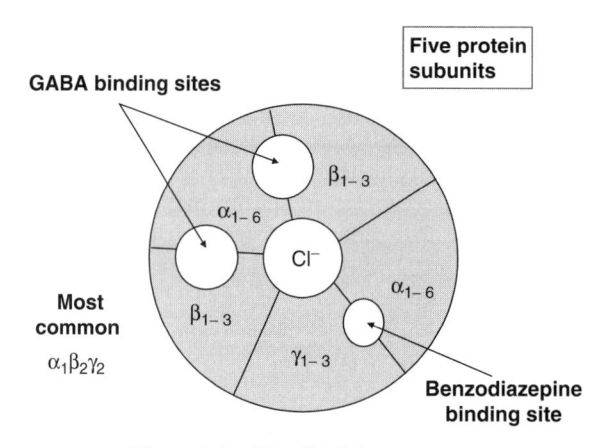

Figure 2.5 The $GABA_A$ receptor.

may explain differences in the sensitivity of individuals to these drugs. Abnormalities of the $GABA_A$ receptor have been identified in humans with anxiety disorders [86].

For most of the second half of the twentieth century the benzodiazepines were the mainstay of the treatment of anxiety. They have now been surpassed by antidepressants in terms of overall efficacy and tolerability, but despite concerns about their long-term safety, they remain an important therapeutic option. The group of anticonvulsants contains a number of drugs that act via GABA or glutamate neurotransmission and have a limited but interesting role in the treatment of particular anxiety disorders.

2.4.2.1 Benzodiazepines. The efficacy of benzodiazepines has been proven in anxiety disorders through extensive clinical experience and controlled trials [87, 88], although it is important to note that they are not effective at treating comorbid depression and there is less evidence to support their use in OCD and PTSD. Their anxiolytic effects have an immediate onset, and in contrast to other groups they do not cause a worsening of anxiety when therapy is initiated (Fig. 2.4). They are generally well tolerated, although side effects such as sedation, loss of balance, and impaired psychomotor performance may be problematic for some patients. There are reported associations with road traffic accidents [89] and with falls and fractures in the elderly [90]. They are relatively safe in overdose [91], although the risk is increased if taken in combination with alcohol or other sedative drugs.

The major controversy surrounding the use of benzodiazepines has concerned the risks of long-term treatment, specifically tolerance, abuse, dependence, and withdrawal effects. From being the most widely prescribed psychotropic drug they suffered a major backlash, although a more balanced view of their place in treatment has subsequently emerged [92] and they continue to be favored by patients and prescribers [93]. After 40 years of clinical experience there is little evidence of tolerance to the anxiolytic effects of benzodiazepines [94]. Abuse (taking in excess of the prescribed dose) is uncommon except in individuals with a history of abuse of other drugs, who may not be suitable for benzodiazepine therapy [95]. There is, however, a consensus that adverse effects on discontinuation are more common than with other anxiolytics [96]. A careful clinical assessment is indicated in this situation, as these effects may be caused by recurrence or rebound (recurrence with increased intensity) of the original anxiety symptoms.

A benzodiazepine withdrawal syndrome has been described in some patients discontinuing therapy (Table 2.6). Although potentially serious, it is generally mild and self-limiting (up to six weeks) but may accompany or provoke a recurrence of anxiety symptoms and cause great concern to the patient. As with any other treatment, the risks and benefits of benzodiazepine therapy should be carefully assessed and discussed with the patient. Monotherapy will not be first-line treatment for the majority of patients, but benzodiazepines offer a valuable option that should not be discounted.

The potential for interactions with other medications comes from two sources: the exacerbation of sedation and impaired psychomotor performance by other drugs also causing these effects and alterations in the hepatic metabolism of benzodiazepines by drugs that are either inducers or inhibitors of cytochrome P450 enzymes. The increased toxicity in combination with alcohol is mostly pharmacodynamic but may partly be due to the inhibition of metabolism of some benzodiazepines by high alcohol concentrations. Other drugs that may have additive effects on sedation include

TABLE 2.6 Benzodiazepine Withdrawal Syndrome

Symptoms	**Hyperarousal**: anxiety, irritability, insomnia, restlessness
	Neuropsychological effects: dysphoria, perceptual sensitisation, tinnitus, confusion, psychosis
	Autonomic lability: sweating, tachycardia, hypertension, tremor, dizziness
	Seizures
Risk factors	**Treatment factors**: treatment duration > 6 months/High dose/Short-acting drug/Abrupt cessation
	Patient factors: severe premorbid anxiety/Alcohol/substance use/disorder/Female/Dysfunctional personality/Panic disorder
Therapeutic strategies	Gradual tapering; switch to long-acting drug, e.g., diazepam; cover with secondary agent (anticonvulsant, antidepressant); cognitive behavioral therapy

TCAs, antihistamines, opioid analgesics, and the α_2-adrenoceptor agonists clonidine and lofexidine. Most benzodiazepines undergo oxidative metabolism in the liver that may be enhanced by enzyme inducers (e.g., carbamazepine, phenytoin) or slowed by inhibitors (sodium valproate, fluoxetine, fluvoxamine). Oxazepam, lorazepam, and temazepam are directly conjugated and are not subject to these interactions.

The specific clinical use of the numerous available benzodiazepines depends on their individual pharmacokinetic and pharmacodynamic properties. Drugs with a high affinity for the $GABA_A$ receptor (alprazolam, clonazepam, lorazepam) have high anxiolytic efficacy, and these drugs may have a particular role in panic disorder where subsensitivity of $GABA_A$ receptors has been demonstrated [97, 98]; drugs with a short duration of action (temazepam) are used as hypnotics to minimize daytime sedative effects; diazepam has a long half-life and duration of action and may be favored for long-term use or when there is a past history of withdrawal problems; oxazepam has a slow onset of action and may be less susceptible to abuse.

Guidance on the clinical indications for benzodiazepine therapy is available from various sources [35, 36, 95]. Long-term therapy is most likely to present problems with discontinuation and is usually reserved for cases that have proven resistant to treatment with antidepressants alone. Patients may benefit from a two- to four-week course of a benzodiazepine while antidepressant therapy is initiated, as this counteracts the increased anxiety caused by some drugs [99]. A benzodiazepine may be useful as a hypnotic in some cases of anxiety disorder and can be used by phobic patients on an occasional basis before exposure to a feared situation.

Benzodiazepines are additionally discussed in Chapter 3.

2.4.2.2 Anticonvulsants. There is an overlap between the clinical syndromes of anxiety and epilepsy. Panic disorder and PTSD can present with symptoms similar to temporal lobe seizures, alcohol and drug withdrawal states can cause both anxiety and seizures, and some drugs (e.g., barbiturates and benzodiazepines) act as both anticonvulsants and anxiolytics. Most anticonvulsants act via the neurotransmission of GABA or glutamate and in recent years have offered a promising field for the development of novel anxiolytic therapies [83, 100]. Although preclinical studies have demonstrated their anxiolytic properties, the evidence base in humans is less impressive and in practice they are reserved for second-line or adjunctive therapy. Drug interactions mediated via hepatic enzymes are a significant feature of this group.

Gabapentin increases GABA activity by a mechanism that is unclear. It causes dose-related sedation and dizziness. It has been shown in controlled trials to be effective in social anxiety disorder [101] and to benefit some patients with panic disorder [102]. Pregabalin is a related compound that has recently demonstrated efficacy in GAD in a phase III study [103].

Lamotrigine blocks voltage-gated sodium channels and inhibits release of glutamate. A controlled study found efficacy in PTSD [104]. Important side effects include fever and skin reactions.

The historical use of sodium valproate for anxiety is poorly supported by clinical trials. A randomized study showed efficacy in panic disorder [105] and benefit has been reported in open studies in OCD and PTSD. The major side effects are tremor, nausea, ataxia, and weight gain and there is the potential for drug interactions via inhibition of hepatic enzymes.

No satisfactory randomized controlled trials have been published demonstrating the efficacy of carbamazepine in anxiety disorders, although it has a history of use as an anxiolytic in panic disorder and PTSD. It has an unfavorable side-effect profile (nausea, dizziness, ataxia) and multiple drug interactions due to induction of liver enzymes. Levetiracetam has anxiolytic activity in preclinical studies and was helpful for patients with social anxiety in an open study [106]. Tiagabine blocks neuronal uptake of GABA and has reported benefits in panic disorder and PTSD [107]. Topiramate has complex actions on GABA and glutamate and was found to be helpful for some symptoms of PTSD [108]. Vigabatrin inhibits GABA metabolism and has been shown to block provoked panic attacks in healthy volunteers [109].

2.4.3 Drugs with Other Mechanisms of Action

2.4.3.1 Antihistamines. The longstanding use in some countries of hydroxyzine, a centrally acting H_1 histamine receptor antagonist, is supported by positive findings in controlled trials in GAD [110–112]. Hydroxyzine promotes sleep and its anxiolytic effects have an early onset. Although it causes sedation, tolerance to this effect often occurs and effects on psychomotor performance are smaller than with benzodiazepines [113]. It is well tolerated and withdrawal effects have not been reported. Although the evidence for its efficacy is not large, hydroxyzine provides an option for some patients with GAD for whom standard treatments are unsuitable.

2.4.3.2 Lithium. Lithium is effective in the treatment of mood disorders. Its mechanism of action is unclear, but is likely to be via modification of intracellular second-messenger systems. There are no controlled trials demonstrating the efficacy of lithium in anxiety disorders, but there have been case reports of its use as an augmenting agent in panic disorder and OCD. Its high toxicity and poor tolerability limit its use in anxiety in the absence of a stronger evidence base.

2.5 PHARMACOTHERAPY FOR ANXIETY DISORDERS

An overview of appropriate drug treatments for each of the major anxiety disorders as well as for depression with prominent anxiety symptoms is shown in Table 2.7.

TABLE 2.7 Pharmacotherapy for Anxiety Disorders

Disorder	First-Line Treatments	Second-Line Treatments	Other Treatments	Augmenting Agents
Generalised anxiety disorder	Venlafaxine 75–150 mg, SSRI (e.g., paroxetine 20 mg, escitalopram, 10 mg)	Imipramine 150 mg, buspirone 15–60 mg	Diazepam 5–30 mg, hydroxyzine 200–400 mg	Benzodiazepines (e.g., diazepam 5–30 mg)
Obsessive-compulsive disorder	SSRI (e.g., fluoxetine 20–60 mg, fluvoxamine 50–300 mg, paroxetine 20–60 mg, sertraline 50–200 mg)	Clomipramine 150–250 mg	—	Haloperidol 5–15 mg, quetiapine 25–600 mg, risperidone 1–3 mg
Panic disorder	SSRI ± benzodiazepine (e.g., citalopram 20–60 mg, escitalopram 5–20 mg, paroxetine 10 mg daily increasing to max 50 mg daily	Clomipramine 150 mg, imipramine 150 mg, phenelzine 30–60 mg, alprazolam 3–6 mg	Clonazepam 0.5–3 mg, diazepam 5–30 mg, lorazepam 2–6 mg Gabapentin, 500–1000 mg	Benzodiazepines (e.g., diazepam 5–30 mg), pindolol
Post traumatic stress disorder	SSRI (e.g., paroxetine 20–50 mg, sertraline 50–200 mg)	Amitriptyline 150–200 mg, mirtazapine 30–45 mg, phenelzine 30–60 mg	Carbamazepine 250–500 mg, lamotrigine 100–200 mg, venlafaxine 75–150 mg	Olanzapine 2.5–5 mg
Social anxiety disorder	SSRI (e.g., paroxetine 20–50 mg), venlafaxine 75–150 mg	Phenelzine 30–60 mg	Clonazepam 0.5–3 mg, gabapentin 500–1000 mg, moclobemide 600 mg, olanzapine 2.5–5 mg	Benzodiazepines (e.g., diazepam 5–30 mg), buspirone 20–40 mg
Specific phobia	—	SSRI (e.g., paroxetine 20 mg)	Benzodiazepines (e.g., diazepam 5–10 mg)	
Depression with concomitant anxiety	SSRI ± benzodiazepine (e.g., paroxetine 20–40 mg), mirtazapine 30–45 mgm venlafaxine 75–150 mg	Amitriptyline 75–150 mg, clomipramine 75–150 mg	—	Benzodiazepines (e.g., diazepam 5–30 mg)

Note: Doses are the suggested total daily dosage.

This overview represents the current view of the authors based on their interpretation of the published evidence and their extensive clinical experience.

2.5.1 Generalized Anxiety Disorder

GAD is a prevalent, chronic, disabling disorder that is comorbid with other anxiety or mood disorders in the majority of cases [114]. While it is a relatively new diagnostic concept, longitudinal studies have reinforced its validity [115]. The core symptoms are chronic worry and tension, and GAD frequently presents with somatic complaints such as headache, myalgia, or insomnia [116]. The diagnosis requires symptoms to be present for at least 6 months, although the duration of illness at presentation is usually much longer than this. The presence of comorbidity leads to a worse prognosis [117]. Cognitive behavioral therapy (CBT) is a structured psychological therapy usually delivered by a trained therapist on an individual basis over 10–15 weekly sessions. It aims to elicit erroneous thinking patterns that lead to anxious thoughts and to train the patient to challenge them and adopt new thinking strategies. CBT has been shown to be effective in GAD and should be considered if available [118].

Recommended drugs for GAD are antidepressants, benzodiazepines, buspirone, and hydroxyzine [114]. The use of antipsychotics is not supported by controlled trials and is discouraged due to their poor long-term tolerability. Pregabalin (related to the anticonvulsant gabapentin) was effective in preliminary trials and may be a future treatment option [103].

Recent evidence has brought about a shift in prescribing in GAD, and now the usual choice for first-line treatment will be an antidepressant. Suitable drugs include venlafaxine [43] and the SSRI paroxetine [119]. A nonsedating TCA such as imipramine could also be used if tolerated and where the risk of suicide is deemed to be low [53]. Little research is available to guide a decision on treatment duration, and a standard recommendation for anxiety disorders would be to continue therapy for at least 12 months following clinical improvement [34]. Buspirone is also appropriate for long-term therapy in the absence of comorbid depression [120].

Benzodiazepines are effective as monotherapy [53] but are rarely used as first-line therapy in this context because of their side-effect profile. They have a useful short-term role for the rapid control of anxiety symptoms or for the control of somatic symptoms such as muscle tension and insomnia, particularly in the early stages of antidepressant therapy. Hydroxyzine has a limited role but can be considered if other treatments are unsuitable [111].

2.5.2 Obsessive-Compulsive Disorder

OCD is a disabling disorder that runs a chronic or recurrent course ([121]; see also Chapter 6). It is diagnosed by the presence of obsessions (recurrent, intrusive thoughts, images, or impulses that are experienced as irrational and unpleasant) or compulsions (repetitive behaviors that are performed to reduce a feeling of unease). The symptoms are present for at least 1 h every day and cause impairment of important functions. Prevalence has been measured in various populations and is around 1–2%. Symptoms start as early as the first decade and have often been present in excess of 10 years at presentation [122]. Depression occurs in more than

50% of cases and there is significant comorbidity with other anxiety disorders, eating disorders, and tic disorders. Although classified with the anxiety disorders, OCD is distinct from the rest of this group in its epidemiological profile and neurobiology. In clinical terms OCD symptoms respond to drugs that enhance serotonergic neurotransmission but not to noradrenergic drugs and poorly to benzodiazepines.

The recommended first-line drugs for OCD are SSRIs and the TCA clomipramine [123]. The required dosage is generally higher than that required for other disorders (e.g., clomipramine 150–250 mg, paroxetine 40–60 mg) and SSRIs have advantages in safety and tolerability. Long-term treatment may be required. There is good evidence for the efficacy of CBT and there may be added benefits from combining psychological and pharmacological therapies [124]. In cases poorly responsive to SSRI treatment augmentation with the antipsychotics haloperidol, risperidone, or quetiapine has support from clinical trials, and addition of buspirone, lithium, and the serotonin precursor L-tryptophan has also been tried. In severe treatment-resistant cases the neurosurgical procedure stereotactic cingulotomy should be considered [125].

2.5.3 Panic Disorder and Agoraphobia

This is also a common, chronic, and disabling disorder with its peak incidence in young adulthood [35]. A panic attack is defined as the sudden onset of anxiety symptoms rising to a peak within 10 min. DSM-IV requires 4 of 13 defined symptoms to be present. The symptoms are physical symptoms corresponding to those caused by autonomic arousal and psychological symptoms (fear of a catastrophic event) and depersonalization/derealization (an altered perception of oneself or the world around). Panic disorder occurs when there are recurrent panic attacks, some of which are uncued or unexpected, and there is fear of having further attacks. Agoraphobia is present in around half of cases [3] and is a poor prognostic indicator. For some patients the anticipatory anxiety or agoraphobia may be considerably more disabling than the original panic attacks. Panic disorder is comorbid with episodes of depression at some stage in the majority of cases [126], with social anxiety disorder and to a lesser extent GAD and PTSD, and with alcohol dependence and personality disorder. Comorbidity results in increased severity and poor response to treatment. Panic disorder is associated with a significantly increased risk of suicide, and this is increased further by the presence of comorbid depression [127].

There is solid evidence for pharmacotherapy for panic disorder with SSRIs [128], the TCAs clomipramine and imipramine [50, 52] and the benzodiazepines alprazolam, clonazepam, lorazepam, and diazepam [129–132]. Therapy is likely to be required for a minimum of 12 months, and the favorable tolerability of SSRIs will usually lead to their choice as first line therapy. Patients with panic disorder are sensitive to drug effects, so a low initial dose may be used and titrated up or a benzodiazepine may be coadministered for the first 2–4 weeks. Stopping treatment is associated with discontinuation effects and an increased risk of relapse and should be approached with caution. CBT is an effective treatment for panic disorder, and additional benefits may be gained from combination therapy [133].

Other drugs effective in controlled studies include the antidepressants phenelzine [61], moclobemide [134], venlafaxine [135], mirtazapine [59] and reboxetine [14] and the anticonvulsants sodium valproate [105] and gabapentin [102].

2.5.4 Post traumatic Stress Disorder

This is another anxiety disorder that is common although underdiagnosed and is usually severely disabling [136]. The diagnosis is given when specific psychological and physical symptoms follow exposure to a traumatizing event that invokes fear, horror, and helplessness. Symptoms fall into three categories: reexperiencing phenomena (flashbacks, nightmares, distress when memories of trauma are triggered), persistent avoidance of triggers to memory of the trauma and general numbing, and hyperarousal (insomnia, irritability, poor concentration, hypervigilance, increased startle response). Symptoms must persist for more than one month after the trauma. PTSD is highly comorbid with depression [137] and substance use disorders and is associated with previous exposures to trauma and a previous history of anxiety disorders. PTSD carries the highest risk of suicide among the anxiety disorders [138]. Without effective treatment it generally runs a chronic, unremitting course.

The evidence base for pharmacotherapy is shallow although improving. Efficacy is established for the SSRIs paroxetine [139], fluoxetine [140], and sertraline [141] and the TCA amitriptyline [54]. Treatment is started at standard dose but may be titrated upward (e.g., paroxetine 20–50 mg). Results from long-term studies are awaited, but treatment should be continued for a minimum of 12 months. Medication is given alongside psychotherapy, usually cognitive and exposure therapies [142]. Other treatments include the antidepressants phenelzine and mirtazapine, the anticonvulsants lamotrigine, sodium valproate, carbamazepine, and tiagabine, and augmentation with the atypical antipsychotic olanzapine. The use of benzodiazepines is not advised as their efficacy is not established and withdrawal symptoms may be particularly distressing. If insomnia is problematic, then a nonbenzodiazepine hypnotic may be prescribed.

2.5.5 Social Anxiety Disorder (Social Phobia)

This disorder is characterized by anxiety symptoms in social or performance situations accompanied by a fear of embarrassment or humiliation. Situations are avoided or endured with distress. There may be a specific fear of one or two situations (most commonly public speaking) or of three or more situations in the generalized subtype. Epidemiological studies find this to be the most prevalent anxiety disorder among the general population [143]. Peak onset is around the time of adolescence and the resulting impairments can have a profound effect on social and occupational development. If untreated it tends to follow a chronic, unremitting course. Social anxiety disorder is frequently comorbid with depression, other anxiety disorders, alcohol problems, and eating disorders. It is associated with an increased rate of suicide that is significantly higher in the presence of comorbidity [144].

Drug treatment studies have focused on the generalized subtype [145]. The largest evidence base is for the SSRIs, which are accepted to be the drug treatment of choice. Treatment is started at standard dose and increased as necessary (e.g., paroxetine 20–50 mg). Duration of treatment is usually for at least 12 months, and there is benefit from combination with CBT [146]. The other class of antidepressant to be considered is the MAOIs, as phenelzine and moclobemide have controlled trial data to support their use [63]. TCAs have no proven efficacy and evidence for venlafaxine and mirtazapine is awaited. Among the benzodiazepines only clonazepam has been shown to be effective as monotherapy, possibly due to its effects on 5-HT$_{1A}$ receptors [147]. Benzodiazepines may also be used to augment SSRI treatment. Other drugs to consider are the anticonvulsant gabapentin and the antipsychotic olanzapine. The β blockers are not effective in generalized social anxiety disorder but have a role in symptomatic control in specific performance anxiety.

2.5.6 Specific Phobia

In this disorder the patient has an inappropriate or excessive fear of a particular stimulus or situation, such as animals, heights, or thunder. An anxiety reaction is consistently and rapidly evoked on exposure to the stimulus, and there is anticipatory anxiety. Population studies have found a surprisingly high prevalence and associated disability, for example a lifetime prevalence of 12% in the National Comorbidity Survey [143]. The standard treatment for specific phobia is behavioral therapy, and patients rarely require pharmacological treatment. Nevertheless there are clinical and pharmacological similarities between patients with specific phobias and those with other anxiety disorders, particularly panic disorder [148], and it might be predicted that anxiolytic medications would have beneficial effects. A small controlled study found an improvement in measures of fear and avoidance after a four-week trial of the SSRI paroxetine [149], and there is also a role for the use of a short-acting benzodiazepine to control anxiety prior to exposure to the feared stimulus. A further interesting finding with potentially wider application is that the benefits of psychological therapy for height phobia were increased by the use of D-serine, a drug that enhances N-methyl-D-aspartate (NMDA) glutamate receptor functioning [150]. This may have been due to the effects of this drug in promoting learning and "overwriting" of conditioned phobic responses.

2.5.7 Anxiety Symptoms in Depressive Disorders

The prevalence of depression in patients with anxiety disorders is high, as is the prevalence of anxiety in patients with depression [151, 152]. Among patients presenting for treatment of anxiety symptoms, a large proportion will have a primary diagnosis of depression. In these situations it is critical to offer a treatment plan that will prove effective against both anxiety and depression [153]. The presence of both disorders together causes an increase in disability, increased severity of symptoms, a higher likelihood of suicidal thoughts, and a poor response to treatment [154].

Antidepressants would be the obvious drug class to select in this patient group, and a number of controlled studies have demonstrated their efficacy. Both SSRIs and TCAs are effective, with the most evidence being for the SSRI paroxetine and the TCAs clomipramine and amitriptyline [155–157]. Comparative studies favor the SSRIs because of their better tolerability, and safety is also a factor in a group at high risk of suicide. Recent studies have demonstrated the efficacy of the new antidepressants venlafaxine [46] and mirtazapine [57] in this group, and as their tolerability matches that of the SSRIs, they should also be considered as first-line treatment. Benzodiazepines produce a rapid improvement in anxiety but are ineffective at treating depression [158] and are not suitable for long-term treatment in this context. They have a short-term role on initiation of antidepressant therapy in selected patients.

2.6 CONCLUSIONS AND FUTURE DIRECTIONS

We have demonstrated that the recent shift in clinical practice toward the use of antidepressants, particularly SSRIs, for the first-line treatment of anxiety disorders is supported by research evidence from randomized controlled trials. Although there has been some negative reporting of the use of SSRIs, the overall situation with regard to anxiety disorders remains one of underdiagnosis and undertreatment, so it should be expected that SSRI use will continue to increase. Clinical practice may be refined in future years as important gaps in the current knowledge base are filled, including the optimal duration of treatment, the identification of patients at particular risk of relapse, the benefits of combining drugs with psychotherapy, and suitable options for patients resistant to first-line treatments. Health policy in the United Kingdom appears to be shifting toward the management of anxiety disorders in primary care [37], and this may potentially lead to an increase in provision of psychological therapies and further raise the profile of anxiety disorders.

New drugs available for the treatment of depression may also prove to be effective for anxiety disorders. In the immediate future these will be drugs acting on the monoamine system. While the prime position of the SSRIs has been reinforced by evidence for the role of 5-HT in anxiety, newer antidepressants such as the SNRIs and mirtazapine have a dual action on serotonergic and noradrenergic neurotransmission. This dual action appears to confer additional benefits in the treatment of depression, but it is not yet clear whether the same is true in anxiety disorders. Further clinical studies are required to fully define the role of venlafaxine and mirtazapine, and clarification of the role of noradrenaline in anxiety is likely to occur.

Many other drug groups with actions on monoaminergic neurons have demonstrated anxiolytic properties in preclinical studies and may in the future prove to be effective treatments. The most likely candidates at present are the azapirones, which are partial agonists at $5-HT_{1A}$ receptors and have already demonstrated antidepressant and anxiolytic activity in humans [65]. Other potential candidates include the $5-HT_{2C}$ receptor antagonist and melatonin receptor agonist agomelatine [159], other $5-HT_{2C}$ antagonists [160], $5-HT_{1B}$ receptor agonists and antagonists [161] and $5-HT_4$ antagonists [162].

It is only in recent years that drugs acting via GABA neurotransmission have been supplanted as first-line treatments, and new drugs in this class with improved tolerability compared to the benzodiazepines are likely to be marketed in the near future [163]. Other GABAergic drugs already marketed for their anticonvulsant properties, such as the selective GABA reuptake inhibitor (SGRI) tiagabine, may prove to have useful efficacy in anxiety disorders [164]. Further down the line agonists that are selective for specific subunits of the $GABA_A$ receptor offer the prospect of drugs that are anxiolytic but with fewer sedative properties [165].

Overall it is remarkable that current pharmacological strategies are centerd around such a small number of brain mechanisms. Future strategies may involve glutamate neurotransmission, particularly inhibition of mGlu5 receptors [166], and neuropeptides such as corticotropin-releasing factor antagonists ([167]; see also Chapter 5) and substance P antagonists [168, 169]. A continued expansion in the range of anxiolytic therapies should be anticipated.

REFERENCES

1. Klein, D. F. (1964). Delineation of two drug-responsive anxiety syndromes. *Psychopharmacologia* 5, 397–408.
2. Kessler, R. C., McGonagle, K. A., Zhao, S., Nelson, C. B., Hughes, M., Eshleman, S., Wittchen, H.-U., and Kendler, K. S. (1994). Lifetime and 12-month prevalence of DSM-III-R psychiatric disorders in the United States: Results from the National Comorbidity Survey. *Arch. Gen. Psychiatry* 51, 8–19.
3. Wittchen, H. U., Reed, V., and Kessler, R. C. (1998). The relationship of agoraphobia and panic in a community sample of adolescents and young adults. *Arch. Gen. Psychiatry* 55, 1017–1024.
4. Dannon, P. N., Iancu, I., and Grunhaus, L. (2002). Psychoeducation in panic disorder patients: Effect of a self-information booklet in a randomized, masked-rater study. *Depress. Anxiety* 16, 71–76.
5. Febbraro, G. A., and Clum, G. A. (1998). Meta-analytic investigation of the effectiveness of self-regulatory components in the treatment of adult problem behaviors. *Clin. Psychol. Rev.* 18, 143–161.
6. Barlow, D. H., Gorman, J. M., Shear, M. K., and Woods, S. W. (2000). Cognitive-behavioral therapy, imipramine, or their combination for panic disorder: A randomized controlled trial. *JAMA* 283, 2529–2536.
7. Davies, S. J., Jackson, P. R., Ramsay, L. E., and Ghahramani, P. (2003). Drug intolerance due to nonspecific adverse effects related to psychiatric morbidity in hypertensive patients. *Arch. Intern. Med.* 163, 592–600.
8. American Psychiatric Association (APA) (1994). *Diagnostic and Statistical Manual of Mental Disorders*, 4th ed., APA, Washington, DC.
9. Argyropoulos, S. V., and Nutt, D. J. (2003). Neurochemical aspects of anxiety. In *Anxiety Disorders*, D. J. Nutt and J. C. Ballenger, Eds. Blackwell Science, Oxford, pp. 183–199.
10. Bakker, A., van Balkom, A. J., and Spinhoven, P. (2002). SSRIs vs. TCAs in the treatment of panic disorder: A meta-analysis. *Acta Psychiatr. Scand* 106, 163–167.
11. Gordon, J. A., and Hen, R. (2004). The serotonergic system and anxiety. *Neuromol. Med.* 5, 27–40.
12. Neumeister, A., Bain, E., Nugent, A. C., Carson, R. E., Bonne, O., Luckenbaugh, D. A., Eckelman, W., Herscovitch, P., Charney, D. S., and Drevets, W. C. (2004). Reduced serotonin type 1A receptor binding in panic disorder. *J. Neurosci.* 24, 589–591.
13. Gallinat, J., Strohle, A., Lang, U. E., Bajbouj, M., Kalus, P., Montag, C., Seifert, F., Wernicke, C., Rommelspacher, H., Rinneberg, H., and Schubert, F. (2005). Association of human hippocampal neurochemistry, serotonin transporter genetic variation, and anxiety. *Neuroimage* 15, 123–131.
14. Versiani, M., Cassano, G., Perugi, G., Benedetti, A., Mastalli, L., Nardi, A., and Savino, M. (2002). Reboxetine, a selective norepinephrine reuptake inhibitor, is an effective and well-tolerated treatment for panic disorder. *J. Clin. Psychiatry* 63, 31–37.
15. Rocca, P., Fonzo, V., Scotta, M., Zanalda, E., and Ravizza, L. (1997). Paroxetine efficacy in the treatment of generalized anxiety disorder. *Acta Psychiatr. Scand.* 95, 444–450.
16. Bell, C. J., and Nutt, D. J. (1998). Serotonin and panic. *Br. J. Psychiatry* 172, 465–471.
17. Blier, P. (2003). The pharmacology of putative early-onset antidepressant strategies. *Eur. Neuropsychopharmacol.* 13, 57–66.

18. Waugh, J., and Goa, K. L. (2003). Escitalopram: A review of its use in the management of major depressive and anxiety disorders. *CNS Drugs* 17, 343–362.
19. Zohar, J., and Judge, R. (1996). Paroxetine versus clomipramine in the treatment of obsessive-compulsive disorder. *Br. J. Psychiatry* 169, 468–474.
20. Kasper, S., and Resinger, E. (2001). Panic disorder: The place of benzodiazepines and selective serotonin reuptake inhibitors. *Eur. Neuropsychopharmacol.* 11, 307–321.
21. Goodnick, P. J., and Goldstein, B. J. (1998). SSRIs in affective disorders—I. Basic pharmacology. *J. Psychopharmacol.* 12(Suppl. B), S5–S20.
22. Bacaltchuk, J., and Hay, P. (2003). Antidepressants versus placebo for people with bulimia nervosa. *Cochrane Database Syst. Rev* 4, CD003391.
23. Barbey, J. T., and Roose, S. P. (1998). SSRI safety in overdose. *J. Clin. Psychiatry* 59(Suppl. 15), 42–48.
24. Mason, J., Freemantle, N., and Eccles, M. (2000). Fatal toxicity associated with antidepressant use in primary care. *Br. J. Gen. Pract.* 50, 366–370.
25. Nutt, D. J. (2005). Death by tricyclic: The real antidepressant scandal?. *J. Psychopharmacol.* 19, 123–124.
26. Healy, D. (2003). Lines of evidence on the risks of suicide with selective serotonin reuptake inhibitors. *Psychother. Psychosom.* 72, 71–79.
27. Fergusson, D., Doucette, S., Glass, K. C., Shapiro, S., Healy, D., Hebert, P., and Hutton, B. (2005). Association between suicide attempts and selective serotonin reuptake inhibitors: Systematic review of randomised controlled trials. *BMJ* 330, 396–399.
28. Nutt, D. J. (2003). Death and dependence: Current controversies over the selective serotonin reuptake inhibitors. *J. Psychopharmacol.* 17, 355–364.
29. Carlsten, A., Waern, M., Ekedahl, A., and Ranstam, J. (2001). Antidepressant medication and suicide in Sweden. *Pharmacoepidemiol. Drug Saf.* 10, 525–530.
30. Khan, A., Khan, S., Kolts, R., and Brown, W. A. (2003). Suicide rates in clinical trials of SSRIs, other antidepressants, and placebo: Analysis of FDA reports. *Am. J. Psychiatry* 160, 790–792.
31. Haddad, P. (1998). The SSRI discontinuation syndrome. *J. Psychopharmacol.* 12, 305–313.
32. Michelson, D., Fava, M., Amsterdam, J., Apter, J., Londborg, P., Tamura, R., and Tepner, R. G. (2000). Interruption of selective serotonin reuptake inhibitor treatment. Double-blind, placebo-controlled trial. *Br. J. Psychiatry* 176, 363–368.
33. Boyer, E. W., and Shannon, M. (2005). The serotonin syndrome. *N. Engl. J. Med.* 352, 1112–1120.
34. American Psychiatric Association (APA) (1998). *Practice Guidelines for the Treatment of Patients with Panic Disorder*. APA, Washington, DC.
35. Ballenger, J. C., Davidson, J. R., Lecrubier, Y., Nutt, D. J., Baldwin, D. S., den Boer, J. A., Kasper, S., and Shear, M. K. (1998). Consensus statement on panic disorder from the International Consensus Group on Depression and Anxiety. *J. Clin. Psychiatry* 59(Suppl. 8), 47–54.
36. Bandelow, B., Zohar, J., Hollander, E., Kasper, S., and Moller, H. J. (2002). World Federation of Societies of Biological Psychiatry (WFSBP) guidelines for the pharmacological treatment of anxiety, obsessive-compulsive and posttraumatic stress disorders. *World J. Biol. Psychiatry* 3, 171–199.

37. NHS National Institute for Clinical Excellence (2004). Management of anxiety (panic disorder, with or without agoraphobia, and generalised anxiety disorder) in adults in primary, secondary and community care. Available at www.nice.org.uk.
38. Bull, S. A., Hu, X. H., Hunkeler, E. M., Lee, J. Y., Ming, E. E., Markson, L. E., and Fireman, B. (2002). Discontinuation of use and switching of antidepressants: Influence of patient-physician communication. *JAMA* 288, 1403–1409.
39. Ballenger, J. C. (2004). Remission rates in patients with anxiety disorders treated with paroxetine. *J. Clin. Psychiatry* 65, 1696–1707.
40. Lecrubier, Y., and Judge, R. (1997). Long-term evaluation of paroxetine, clomipramine and placebo in panic disorder. Collaborative Paroxetine Panic Study Investigators. *Acta Psychiatr. Scand.* 95, 153–160.
41. Michelson, D., Pollack, M., Lydiard, R. B., Tamura, R., Tepner, R., and Tollefson, G. (1999). Continuing treatment of panic disorder after acute response: Randomised, placebo-controlled trial with fluoxetine. The Fluoxetine Panic Disorder Study Group. *Br. J. Psychiatry* 174, 213–218.
42. Melichar, J. K., Haida, A., Rhodes, C., Reynolds, A. H., Nutt, D. J., and Malizia, A. L. (2001). Venlafaxine occupation at the noradrenaline reuptake site: In-vivo determination in healthy volunteers. *J. Psychopharmacol.* 15, 9–12.
43. Allgulander, C., Hackett, D., and Salinas, E. (2001). Venlafaxine extended release (ER) in the treatment of generalised anxiety disorder: Twenty-four-week placebo-controlled dose-ranging study. *Br. J. Psychiatry* 179, 15–22.
44. Denys, D., van der Wee, N., van Megen, H. J., and Westenberg, H. G. (2003). A double blind comparison of venlafaxine and paroxetine in obsessive-compulsive disorder. *J. Clin. Psychopharmacol.* 23, 568–575.
45. Liebowitz, M. R., Gelenberg, A. J., and Munjack, D. (2005). Venlafaxine extended release vs placebo and paroxetine in social anxiety disorder. *Arch. Gen. Psychiatry* 62, 190–198.
46. Silverstone, P. H., and Ravindran, A. (1999). Once-daily venlafaxine extended release (XR) compared with fluoxetine in outpatients with depression and anxiety. *J. Clin. Psychiatry* 60, 22–28.
47. Buckley, N. A., and McManus, P. R. (2002). Fatal toxicity of serotoninergic and other antidepressant drugs: Analysis of United Kingdom mortality data. *BMJ* 325, 1332–1333.
48. NHS National Institute for Clinical Excellence (2004). Management of depression in primary and secondary care. Available at www.nice.org.uk.
49. Dunner, D. L., Goldstein, D. J., Mallinckrodt, C., Lu, Y., and Detke, M. J. (2003). Duloxetine in treatment of anxiety symptoms associated with depression. *Depress. Anxiety* 18, 53–61.
50. Lecrubier, Y., Bakker, A., Dunbar, G., and Judge, R. (1997). A comparison of paroxetine, clomipramine and placebo in the treatment of panic disorder. Collaborative Paroxetine Panic Study Investigators. *Acta Psychiatr. Scand.* 95, 145–152.
51. Clomipramine Collaborative Study Group (1991). Clomipramine in the treatment of patients with obsessive-compulsive disorder. *Arch. Gen. Psychiatry* 48, 730–738.
52. Cross-National Collaborative Panic Study (1992). Drug treatment of panic disorder. Comparative efficacy of alprazolam, imipramine, and placebo. *Br. J. Psychiatry* 160, 191–202.
53. Rickels, K., Downing, R., Schweizer, E., and Hassman, H. (1993). Antidepressants for the treatment of generalized anxiety disorder. A placebo-controlled comparison of imipramine, trazodone, and diazepam. *Arch. Gen. Psychiatry* 50, 884–895.

54. Davidson, J. R., Kudler, H. S., Saunders, W. B., Erickson, L., Smith, R. D., Stein, R. M., Lipper, S., Hammett, E. B., Mahorney, S. L., and Cavenar, J. O. (1993). Predicting response to amitriptyline in posttraumatic stress disorder. *Am. J. Psychiatry* 150, 1024–1029.
55. Kobak, K. A., Greist, J. H., Jefferson, J. W., Katzelnick, D. J., and Henk, H. J. (1998). Behavioral versus pharmacological treatments of obsessive compulsive disorder: A meta-analysis. *Psychopharmacology (Berl.)* 136, 205–216.
56. Zohar, J., and Westenberg, H. G. (2000). Anxiety disorders: A review of tricyclic antidepressants and selective serotonin reuptake inhibitors. *Acta Psychiatr. Scand. Suppl.* 403, 39–49.
57. Fawcett, J., and Barkin, R. L. (1998). A meta-analysis of eight randomized, double-blind, controlled clinical trials of mirtazapine for the treatment of patients with major depression and symptoms of anxiety. *J. Clin. Psychiatry* 59, 123–127.
58. Davidson, J. R., Weisler, R. H., Butterfield, M. I., Casat, C. D., Connor, K. M., Barnett, S., and van Meter, S. (2003). Mirtazapine vs. placebo in posttraumatic stress disorder: A pilot trial. *Biol. Psychiatry* 53, 188–191.
59. Ribeiro, L., Busnello, J. V., Kauer-Sant'Anna, M., Madruga, M., Quevedo, J., Busnello, and E. A., Kapczinski, F. (2001). Mirtazapine versus fluoxetine in the treatment of panic disorder. *Braz. J. Med. Biol. Res.* 34, 1303–1307.
60. Liappas, J., Paparrigopoulos, T., Tzavellas, E., and Christodoulou, G. (2003). Alcohol detoxification and social anxiety symptoms: A preliminary study of the impact of mirtazapine administration. *J. Affect. Disord.* 76, 279–284.
61. Sheehan, D. V., Ballenger, J., and Jacobsen, G. (1980). Treatment of endogenous anxiety with phobic, hysterical, and hypochondriacal symptoms. *Arch. Gen. Psychiatry* 37, 51–59.
62. Frank, J. B., Kosten, T. R., Giller, E. L., and Dan, E. (1988). A randomized clinical trial of phenelzine and imipramine for posttraumatic stress disorder. *Am. J. Psychiatry* 145, 1289–1291.
63. Versiani, M., Nardi, A. E., Mundim, F. D., Alves, A. B., Liebowitz, M. R., and Amrein, R. (1992). Pharmacotherapy of social phobia. A controlled study with moclobemide and phenelzine. *Br. J. Psychiatry* 161, 353–360.
64. van der Linden, G. J., Stein, D. J., and van Balkom, A. J. (2000). The efficacy of the selective serotonin reuptake inhibitors for social anxiety disorder (social phobia): A meta-analysis of randomized controlled trials. *Int. Clin. Psychopharmacol.* 15(Suppl. 2), S15–S23.
65. Blier, P., and Ward, N. M. (2003). Is there a role for 5-HT(1A) agonists in the treatment of depression? *Biol. Psychiatry* 53, 193–203.
66. Enkelmann, R. (1991). Alprazolam versus buspirone in the treatment of outpatients with generalized anxiety disorder. *Psychopharmacology (Berl.)* 105, 428–432.
67. Rickels, K., Amsterdam, J. D., Clary, C., Puzzuoli, G., and Schweizer, E. (1991). Buspirone in major depression: A controlled study. *J. Clin. Psychiatry* 52, 34–38.
68. DeMartinis, N., Rynn, M., Rickels, K., and Mandos, L. (2000). Prior benzodiazepine use and buspirone response in the treatment of generalized anxiety disorder. *J. Clin. Psychiatry* 61, 91–94.
69. Alpert, J. E., Franznick, D. A., Hollander, S. B., and Fava, M. (2004). Gepirone extended-release treatment of anxious depression: Evidence from a retrospective subgroup analysis in patients with major depressive disorder. *J. Clin. Psychiatry* 65, 1069–1075.

70. Bohm, C., Robinson, D. S., Gammans, R. E., Shrotriya, R. C., Alms, D. R., Leroy, A., and Placchi, M. (1990). Buspirone therapy in anxious elderly patients: A controlled clinical trial. *J. Clin. Psychopharmacol.* 10(Suppl. 3), 47S–51S.

71. Gorman, J. M., Liebowitz, M. R., Fyer, A. J., Campeas, R., and Klein, D. F. (1985). Treatment of social phobia with atenolol. *J. Clin. Psychopharmacol.* 5, 298–301.

72. Hirschmann, S., Dannon, P. N., Iancu, I., Dolberg, O. T., Zohar, J., and Grunhaus, L. (2000). Pindolol augmentation in patients with treatment-resistant panic disorder: A double-blind, placebo-controlled trial. *J. Clin. Psychopharmacol.* 20, 556–559.

73. Dannon, P. N., Sasson, Y., Hirschmann, S., Iancu, I., Grunhaus, L. J., and Zohar, J. (2000). Pindolol augmentation in treatment-resistant obsessive compulsive disorder: A double-blind placebo controlled trial. *Eur. Neuropsychopharmacol.* 10, 165–169.

74. Stein, M. B., Sareen, J., Hami, S., and Chao, J. (2001). Pindolol potentiation of paroxetine for generalized social phobia: A double-blind, placebo-controlled, crossover study. *Am. J. Psychiatry* 158, 1725–1727.

75. Elman, M. J., Sugar, J., Fiscella, R., Deutsch, T. A., Noth, J., Nyberg, M., Packo, K., and Anderson, R. J. (1998). The effect of propranolol versus placebo on resident surgical performance. *Trans. Am. Ophthalmol. Soc.* 96, 283–291.

76. El-Khayat, R., and Baldwin, D. S. (1998). Antipsychotic drugs for non-psychotic patients: Assessment of the benefit/risk ratio in generalized anxiety disorder. *J. Psychopharmacol.* 12, 323–329.

77. McDougle, C. J., Goodman, W. K., Leckman, J. F., Lee, N. C., Heninger, G. R., and Price, L. H. (1994). Haloperidol addition in fluvoxamine-refractory obsessive-compulsive disorder. A double-blind, placebo-controlled study in patients with and without tics. *Arch. Gen. Psychiatry* 51, 302–308.

78. McDougle, C. J., Epperson, C. N., Pelton, G. H., Wasylink, S., and Price, L. H. (2000). A double-blind, placebo-controlled study of risperidone addition in serotonin reuptake inhibitor-refractory obsessive-compulsive disorder. *Arch. Gen. Psychiatry* 57, 794–801.

79. Atmaca, M., Kuloglu, M., Tezcan, E., and Gecici, O. (2002). Quetiapine augmentation in patients with treatment resistant obsessive-compulsive disorder: A single-blind, placebo-controlled study. *Int. Clin. Psychopharmacol.* 17, 115–119.

80. Barnett, S. D., Kramer, M. L., Casat, C. D., Connor, K. M., and Davidson, J. R. (2002). Efficacy of olanzapine in social anxiety disorder: A pilot study. *J. Psychopharmacol.* 16, 365–368.

81. Stein, M. B., Kline, N. A., and Matloff, J. L. (2002). Adjunctive olanzapine for SSRI-resistant combat-related PTSD: A double-blind, placebo-controlled study. *Am. J. Psychiatry* 159, 1777–1779.

82. Bartzokis, G., Lu, P. H., Turner, J., Mintz, J., and Saunders, C. S. (2005). Adjunctive risperidone in the treatment of chronic combat-related posttraumatic stress disorder. *Biol. Psychiatry* 57, 474–479.

83. Kent, J. M., Mathew, S. J., and Gorman, J. M. (2002). Molecular targets in the treatment of anxiety. *Biol. Psychiatry* 52, 1008–1030.

84. Ledgerwood, L., Richardson, R., and Cranney, J. (2005). D-Cycloserine facilitates extinction of learned fear: Effects on reacquisition and generalized extinction. *Biol. Psychiatry* 57, 841–847.

85. Nutt, D. J., and Malizia, A. L. (2001). New insights into the role of the GABA(A)-benzodiazepine receptor in psychiatric disorder. *Br. J. Psychiatry* 179, 390–396.

86. Roy-Byrne, P. P. (2005). The GABA-benzodiazepine receptor complex: Structure, function, and role in anxiety. *J. Clin. Psychiatry* 66(Suppl. 2), 14–20.

87. Faravelli, C., Rosi, S., and Truglia, E. (2003). Treatments: Benzodiazepines. In *Anxiety disorders*, D. J. Nutt and J. C. Ballenger, Eds. Blackwell Science, Oxford, pp. 315–338.
88. Stevens, J. C., and Pollack, M. H. (2005). Benzodiazepines in clinical practice: Consideration of their long-term use and alternative agents. *J. Clin. Psychiatry* 66(Suppl. 2), 21–27.
89. Barbone, F., McMahon, A. D., Davey, P. G., Morris, A. D., Reid, I. C., McDevitt, D. G., and MacDonald, T. M. (1998). Association of road-traffic accidents with benzodiazepine use. *Lancet* 352, 1331–1336.
90. Wang, P. S., Bohn, R. L., Glynn, R. J., Mogun, H., and Avorn, J. (2001). Hazardous benzodiazepine regimens in the elderly: Effects of half-life, dosage, and duration on risk of hip fracture. *Am. J. Psychiatry* 158, 892–898.
91. Buckley, N. A., Dawson, A. H., Whyte, I. M., and O'Connell, D. L. (1995). Relative toxicity of benzodiazepines in overdose. *BMJ* 310, 219–221.
92. Williams, D. D., and McBride, A. (1998). Benzodiazepines: time for reassessment. *Br. J. Psychiatry* 173, 361–362.
93. Bruce, S. E., Vasile, R. G., Goisman, R. M., Salzman, C., Spencer, M., Machan, J. T., and Keller, M. B. (2003). Are benzodiazepines still the medication of choice for patients with panic disorder with or without agoraphobia?. *Am. J. Psychiatry* 160, 1432–1438.
94. Rickels, K., and Schweizer, E. (1998). Panic disorder: Long-term pharmacotherapy and discontinuation. *J. Clin. Psychopharmacol.* 18, 12S–18S.
95. Task Force Report of the American Psychiatric Association (1990). *Benzodiazepine Dependence, Toxicity and Abuse.* American Psychiatric Association, Washington, DC.
96. Schweizer, E., and Rickels, K. (1998). Benzodiazepine dependence and withdrawal: A review of the syndrome and its clinical management. *Acta Psychiatr. Scand.* 393, S95–S101.
97. Nutt, D. J., Glue, P., Lawson, C., and Wilson, S. (1990). Flumazenil provocation of panic attacks. Evidence for altered benzodiazepine receptor sensitivity in panic disorder. *Arch. Gen. Psychiatry* 47, 917–925.
98. Roy-Byrne, P. P., Cowley, D. S., Greenblatt, D. J., Shader, R. I., and Hommer, D. (1990). Reduced benzodiazepine sensitivity in panic disorder. *Arch. Gen. Psychiatry* 47, 534–538.
99. Goddard, A. W., Brouette, T., Almai, A., Jetty, P., Woods, S. W., and Charney, D. (2001). Early coadministration of clonazepam with sertraline for panic disorder. *Arch. Gen. Psychiatry* 58, 681–686.
100. van Ameringen, M., Mancini, C., Pipe, B., and Bennett, M. (2004). Antiepileptic drugs in the treatment of anxiety disorders: Role in therapy. *Drugs* 64, 2199–2220.
101. Pande, A. C., Davidson, J. R., Jefferson, J. W., Janney, C. A., Katzelnick, D. J., Weisler, R. H., Greist, J. H., and Sutherland, S. M. (1999). Treatment of social phobia with gabapentin: A placebo-controlled study. *J. Clin. Psychopharmacol.* 19, 341–348.
102. Pande, A. C., Pollack, M. H., Crockatt, J., Greiner, M., Chouinard, G., Lydiard, R. B., Taylor, C. B., Dager, S. R., and Shiovitz, T. (2000). Placebo-controlled study of gabapentin treatment of panic disorder. *J. Clin. Psychopharmacol.* 20, 467–471.
103. Pande, A. C., Crockatt, J. G., Feltner, D. E., Janney, C. A., Smith, W. T., Weisler, R., Londborg, P. D., Bielski, R. J., Zimbroff, D. L., Davidson, J. R., and Liu-Dumaw, M. (2003). Pregabalin in generalized anxiety disorder: A placebo-controlled trial. *Am. J. Psychiatry* 160, 533–540.
104. Hertzberg, M. A., Butterfield, M. I., Feldman, M. E., Beckham, J. C., Sutherland, S. M., Connor, K. M., and Davidson, J. R. (1999). A preliminary study of lamotrigine for the treatment of posttraumatic stress disorder. *Biol. Psychiatry* 45, 1226–1229.

105. Lum, M., Fontaine, R., Elie, R., and Ontiveros, A. (1991). Probable interaction of sodium divalproex with benzodiazepines. *Prog. Neuropsychopharmacol. Biol. Psychiatry* 15, 269–273.

106. Simon, N. M., Worthington, J. J., Doyle, A. C., Hoge, E. A., Kinrys, G., Fischmann, D., Link, N., and Pollack, M. H. (2004). An open-label study of levetiracetam for the treatment of social anxiety disorder. *J. Clin. Psychiatry* 65, 1219–1222.

107. Lydiard, R. B. (2003). The role of GABA in anxiety disorders. *J. Clin. Psychiatry* 64(Suppl. 3), 21–27.

108. Berlant, J., and van Kammen, D. P. (2002). Open-label topiramate as primary or adjunctive therapy in chronic civilian posttraumatic stress disorder: A preliminary report. *J. Clin. Psychiatry* 63, 15–20.

109. Zwanzger, P., Baghai, T. C., Schuele, C., Strohle, A., Padberg, F., Kathmann, N., Schwarz, M., Moller, H. J., and Rupprecht, R. (2001). Vigabatrin decreases cholecystokinin-tetrapeptide (CCK-4) induced panic in healthy volunteers. *Neuropsychopharmacology* 25, 699–703.

110. Ferreri, M., and Hantouche, E. G. (1998). Recent clinical trials of hydroxyzine in generalized anxiety disorder. *Acta Psychiatr. Scand.* 393(Suppl.), 102–108.

111. Lader, M., and Scotto, J. C. (1998). A multicentre double-blind comparison of hydroxyzine, buspirone and placebo in patients with generalized anxiety disorder. *Psychopharmacology (Berl.)* 139, 402–406.

112. Llorca, P. M., Spadone, C., Sol, O., Danniau, A., Bougerol, T., Corruble, E., Faruch, M., Macher, J. P., Sermet, E., and Servant, D. (2002). Efficacy and safety of hydroxyzine in the treatment of generalized anxiety disorder: A 3-month double-blind study. *J. Clin. Psychiatry* 63, 1020–1027.

113. de Brabander, A., and Deberdt, W. (1990). Effects of hydroxyzine on attention and memory. *Hum. Psychopharmacol.* 5, 357–362.

114. Ballenger, J. C., Davidson, J. R., Lecrubier, Y., Nutt, D. J., Borkovec, T. D., Rickels, K., Stein, D. J., and Wittchen, H. U. (2001). Consensus statement on generalized anxiety disorder from the International Consensus Group on Depression and Anxiety. *J. Clin. Psychiatry* 62(Suppl. 11), 53–58.

115. Kessler, R. C., DuPont, R. L., Berglund, P., and Wittchen, H. U. (1999). Impairment in pure and comorbid generalized anxiety disorder and major depression at 12 months in two national surveys. *Am. J. Psychiatry* 156, 1915–1923.

116. Lydiard, R. B. (2000). An overview of generalized anxiety disorder: Disease state—Appropriate therapy. *Clin. Ther.* 22(Suppl. A), 3–19.

117. Yonkers, K. A., Warshaw, M. G., Massion, A. O., and Keller, M. B. (1996). Phenomenology and course of generalised anxiety disorder. *Br. J. Psychiatry* 168, 308–313.

118. Durham, R. C., Murphy, T., Allan, T., Richard, K., Treliving, L. R., and Fenton, G. W. (1994). Cognitive therapy, analytic psychotherapy and anxiety management training for generalised anxiety disorder. *Br. J. Psychiatry* 165, 315–323.

119. Stocchi, F., Nordera, G., Jokinen, R. H., Lepola, U. M., Hewett, K., Bryson, H., Iyengar, M. K., and Paroxetine Generalized Anxiety Disorder Study Team (2003). Efficacy and tolerability of paroxetine for the long-term treatment of generalized anxiety disorder. *J. Clin. Psychiatry* 64, 250–258.

120. Rakel, R. E. (1990). Long-term buspirone therapy for chronic anxiety: A multicenter international study to determine safety. *South Med. J.* 83, 194–198.

121. Sasson, Y., Zohar, J., Chopra, M., Lustig, M., Iancu, I., and Hendler, T. (1997). Epidemiology of obsessive-compulsive disorder: A world view. *J. Clin. Psychiatry* 58(Suppl. 12), 7–10.

122. Hollander, E., Greenwald, S., Neville, D., Johnson, J., Hornig, C. D., and Weissman, M. M. (1996). Uncomplicated and comorbid obsessive-compulsive disorder in an epidemiologic sample. *Depress. Anxiety* 4, 111–119.

123. Pigott, T. A., and Seay, S. M. (1999). A review of the efficacy of selective serotonin reuptake inhibitors in obsessive-compulsive disorder. *J. Clin. Psychiatry* 60, 101–106.

124. Hohagen, F., Winkelmann, G., Rasche-Ruchle, H., Hand, I., Konig, A., Munchau, N., Hiss, H., Geiger-Kabisch, C., Kappler, C., Schramm, P., Rey, E., Aldenhoff, J., and Berger, M. (1998). Combination of behaviour therapy with fluvoxamine in comparison with behaviour therapy and placebo. Results of a multicentre study. *Br. J. Psychiatry Suppl.* 35, 71–78.

125. Jenike, M. A., Baer, L., Ballantine, T., Martuza, R. L., Tynes, S., Giriunas, I., Buttolph, M. L., and Cassem, N. H. (1991). Cingulotomy for refractory obsessive-compulsive disorder. A long-term follow-up of 33 patients. *Arch. Gen. Psychiatry* 48, 548–555.

126. Stein, M. B., Tancer, M. E., and Uhde, T. W. (1990). Major depression in patients with panic disorder: Factors associated with course and recurrence. *J. Affect. Disord.* 19, 287–296.

127. Lepine, J. P., Chignon, J. M., and Teherani, M. (1993). Suicide attempts in patients with panic disorder. *Arch. Gen. Psychiatry* 50, 144–149.

128. Boyer, W. (1995). Serotonin uptake inhibitors are superior to imipramine and alprazolam in alleviating panic attacks: A meta-analysis. *Int. Clin. Psychopharmacol.* 10, 45–49.

129. Ballenger, J. C., Burrows, G. D., DuPont, R.L., Lesser, I. M., Noyes, R., Jr., Pecknold, J. C., Rifkin, A., and Swinson, R. P. (1988). Alprazolam in panic disorder and agoraphobia: Results from a multicenter trial. I. Efficacy in short-term treatment. *Arch. Gen. Psychiatry* 45, 413–422.

130. Beauclair, L., Fontaine, R., Annable, L., Holobow, N., and Chouinard, G. (1994). Clonazepam in the treatment of panic disorder: A double-blind, placebo-controlled trial investigating the correlation between clonazepam concentrations in plasma and clinical response. *J. Clin. Psychopharmacol.* 14, 111–118.

131. Charney, D. S., and Woods, S. W. (1989). Benzodiazepine treatment of panic disorder: A comparison of alprazolam and lorazepam. *J. Clin. Psychiatry* 50, 418–423.

132. Noyes, R., Burrows, G. D., Reich, J. H., Judd, F. K., Garvey, M. J., Norman, T. R., Cook, B. L., and Marriott, P. (1996). Diazepam versus alprazolam for the treatment of panic disorder. *J. Clin. Psychiatry* 57, 349–355.

133. Oehrberg, S., Christiansen, P. E., Behnke, K., Borup, A. L., Severin, B., Soegaard, J., Calberg, H., Judge, R., Ohrstrom, J. K., and Manniche, P. M. (1995). Paroxetine in the treatment of panic disorder. A randomised, double-blind, placebo-controlled study. *Br. J. Psychiatry* 167, 374–379.

134. Tiller, J. W., Bouwer, C., and Behnke, K. (1999). Moclobemide and fluoxetine for panic disorder. International Panic Disorder Study Group. *Eur. Arch. Psychiatry Clin. Neurosci.* 249(Suppl. 1), 7–10.

135. Pollack, M. H., Worthington, J. J., III, Otto, M. W., Maki, K. M., Smoller, J. W., Manfro, G. G., Rudolph, R., and Rosenbaum, J. F. (1996). Venlafaxine for panic disorder: Results from a double-blind, placebo-controlled study. *Psychopharmacol. Bull.* 32, 667–670.

136. Ballenger, J. C., Davidson, J. R., Lecrubier, Y., Nutt, D. J., Foa, E. B., Kessler, R. C., McFarlane, A. C., and Shalev, A. Y. (2000). Consensus statement on posttraumatic stress disorder from the International Consensus Group on Depression and Anxiety. *J. Clin. Psychiatry* 61(Suppl. 5), 60–66.

137. Kessler, R. C., Sonnega, A., Bromet, E., Hughes, M., and Nelson, C. B. (1995). Posttraumatic stress disorder in the National Comorbidity Survey. *Arch. Gen. Psychiatry* 52, 1048–1060.

138. Davidson, J. R., Hughes, D., Blazer, D. G., and George, L. K. (1991). Post-traumatic stress disorder in the community: an epidemiological study. *Psychol. Med.* 21, 713–721.

139. Tucker, P., Zaninelli, R., Yehuda, R., Ruggiero, L., Dillingham, K., and Pitts, C. D. (2001). Paroxetine in the treatment of chronic posttraumatic stress disorder: Results of a placebo-controlled, flexible-dosage trial. *J. Clin. Psychiatry*. 62, 860–868.

140. Connor, K. M., Sutherland, S. M., Tupler, L. A., Malik, M. L., and Davidson, J. R. (1999). Fluoxetine in post-traumatic stress disorder. Randomised, double-blind study. *Br. J. Psychiatry* 175, 17–22.

141. Brady, K., Pearlstein, T., Asnis, G. M., Baker, D., Rothbaum, B., Sikes, C. R., and Farfel, G. M. (2000). Efficacy and safety of sertraline treatment of posttraumatic stress disorder: A randomized controlled trial. *JAMA* 283, 1837–1844.

142. Foa, E. B. (2000). Psychosocial treatment of posttraumatic stress disorder. *J. Clin. Psychiatry* 61(Suppl. 5), 43–48.

143. Magee, W. J., Eaton, W. W., Wittchen, H. U., McGonagle, K. A., and Kessler, R. C. (1996). Agoraphobia, simple phobia, and social phobia in the National Comorbidity Survey. *Arch. Gen. Psychiatry* 53, 159–168.

144. Schneier, F. R., Johnson, J., Hornig, C. D., Liebowitz, M. R., and Weissman, M. M. (1992). Social phobia. Comorbidity and morbidity in an epidemiologic sample. *Arch. Gen. Psychiatry* 49, 282–288.

145. Ballenger, J. C., Davidson, J. R., Lecrubier, Y., Nutt, D. J., Bobes, J., Beidel, D. C., Ono, Y., and Westenberg, H. G. (1998). Consensus statement on social anxiety disorder from the International Consensus Group on Depression and Anxiety. *J. Clin. Psychiatry* 59(Suppl. 17), 54–60.

146. Blomhoff, S., Haug, T. T., Hellstrom, K., Holme, I., Humble, M., Madsbu, H. P., and Wold, J. E. (2001). Randomised controlled general practice trial of sertraline, exposure therapy and combined treatment in generalised social phobia. *Br. J. Psychiatry* 179, 23–30.

147. Davidson, J. R., Potts, N., Richichi, E., Krishnan, R., Ford, S. M., Smith, R., and Wilson, W. H. (1993). Treatment of social phobia with clonazepam and placebo. *J. Clin. Psychopharmacol.* 13, 423–428.

148. Verburg, C., Griez, E., and Meijer, J. (1994). A 35% carbon dioxide challenge in simple phobias. *Acta Psychiatr. Scand.* 90, 420–423.

149. Benjamin, J., Ben-Zion, I. Z., Karbofsky, E., and Dannon, P. (2000). Double-blind placebo-controlled pilot study of paroxetine for specific phobia. *Psychopharmacology (Berl.)* 149, 194–196.

150. Ressler, K. J., Rothbaum, B. O., Tannenbaum, L., Anderson, P., Graap, K., Zimand, E., Hodges, L., and Davis, M. (2004). Cognitive enhancers as adjuncts to psychotherapy: Use of D-cycloserine in phobic individuals to facilitate extinction of fear. *Arch. Gen. Psychiatry* 61, 1136–1144.

151. Tylee, A., Gastpar, M., Lepine, J. P., and Mendlewicz, J. (1999). Identification of depressed patient types in the community and their treatment needs: Findings from the DEPRES II (Depression Research in European Society II) survey. *Int. Clin. Psychopharmacol.* 14, 153–165.

152. Kessler, R. C., Stang, P. E., Wittchen, H. U., Ustun, T. B., Roy-Burne, P. P., and Walters, E. E. (1998). Lifetime panic-depression comorbidity in the National Comorbidity Survey. *Arch. Gen. Psychiatry* 55, 801–808.

153. Nutt, D. J. (2000). Treatment of depression and concomitant anxiety. *Eur. Neuropsychopharmacol.* 10(Suppl. 4), 433–437.

154. Lepine, J. P., Gastpar, M., Mendlewicz, J., and Tylee, A. (1997). Depression in the community: the first pan-European study DEPRES (Depression Research in European Society). *Int. Clin. Psychopharmacol.* 12, 19–29.

155. Feighner, J. P., Cohn, J. B., Fabre, L. F., Jr., Fieve, R. R., Mendels, J., Shrivastava, R. K., and Dunbar, G. C. (1993). A study comparing paroxetine placebo and imipramine in depressed patients. *J. Affect Disord.* 28, 71–79.

156. Ravindran, A. V., Judge, R., Hunter, B. N., Bray, J., and Morton, N. H. (1997). A double-blind, multicenter study in primary care comparing paroxetine and clomipramine in patients with depression and associated anxiety. *J. Clin. Psychiatry* 58, 112–118.

157. Stott, P. C., Blagden, M. D., and Aitken, C. A. (1993). Depression and associated anxiety in primary care: A double-blind comparison of paroxetine and amitriptyline. *Eur. Neuropsychopharmacol.* 3, 324–325.

158. Lenox, R. H., Shipley, J. E., Peyser, J. M., Williams, J. M., and Weaver, L. A. (1984). Double-blind comparison of alprazolam versus imipramine in the inpatient treatment of major depressive illness. *Psychopharmacol. Bull.* 20, 79–82.

159. Millan, M. J., Brocco, M., Gobert, A., and Dekeyne, A. (2005). Anxiolytic properties of agomelatine, an antidepressant with melatoninergic and serotonergic properties: Role of 5-HT2C receptor blockade. *Psychopharmacology (Berl.)* 177, 448–458.

160. Campbell, B. M., and Merchant, K. M. (2003). Serotonin 2C receptors within the basolateral amygdala induce acute fear-like responses in an open-field environment. *Brain Res.* 993, 1–9.

161. Tatarczynska, E., Klodzinska, A., Stachowicz, K., and Chojnacka-Wojcik, E. (2004). Effects of a selective 5-HT1B receptor agonist and antagonists in animal models of anxiety and depression. *Behav. Pharmacol.* 15, 523–534.

162. Smriga, M., and Torii, K. (2003). L-Lysine acts like a partial serotonin receptor 4 antagonist and inhibits serotonin-mediated intestinal pathologies and anxiety in rats. *Proc. Natl. Acad. Sci. USA* 100, 15370–15375.

163. Ashton, C. H., and Young, A. H. (2003). GABA-ergic drugs: Exit stage left, enter stage right. *J. Psychopharmacol.* 17, 174–178.

164. Schaller, J. L., Thomas, J., and Rawlings, D. (2004). Low-dose tiagabine effectiveness in anxiety disorders. *Med. Gen. Med.* 17, 8.

165. Dawson, G. R., Collinson, N., and Atack, J. R. (2005). Development of subtype selective GABAA modulators. *CNS Spectr.* 10, 21–27.

166. Spooren, W., and Gasparini, F. (2004). mGlu5 receptor antagonists: A novel class of anxiolytics?. *Drug News Perspect.* 17, 251–257.

167. Ayala, A. R., Pushkas, J., Higley, J. D., Ronsaville, D., Gold, P. W., Chrousos, G. P., Pacak, K., Calis, K. A., Gerald, M., Lindell, S., Rice, K. C., and Cizza, G. (2004). Behavioral, adrenal, and sympathetic responses to long-term administration of an oral corticotropin-releasing hormone receptor antagonist in a primate stress paradigm. *J. Clin. Endocrinol. Metab.* 89, 5729–5737.

168. Argyropoulos, S. V., and Nutt, D. J. (2000). Substance P antagonists: Novel agents in the treatment of depression. *Expert Opin. Investig. Drugs* 9, 1871–1875.

169. Herpfer, I., and Lieb, K. (2005). Substance P receptor antagonists in psychiatry: Rationale for development and therapeutic potential. *CNS Drugs* 19, 275–293.

3

BENZODIAZEPINES

Hartmut Lüddens[1] and Esa R. Korpi[2]

[1]*Laboratory of Molecular Biology, University of Mainz, Mainz, Germany and*
[2]*Institute of Biomedicine/Pharmacology, Biomedicum Helsinki, University of Helsinki, Helsinki, Finland*

3.1	Introduction	93
3.2	Pharmacology of Benzodiazepine Receptor Ligands	97
	3.2.1 Therapeutic Action of BZ Receptor Ligands	97
	3.2.2 Endogenous Benzodiazepine Site Ligands	98
	3.2.3 Modulation of Single-Cell GABA Response by Benzodiazepines	99
	3.2.4 Tolerance and Dependence to BZ	100
	3.2.5 Metabolism of BZ Receptor Ligands	101
3.3	$GABA_A$/Benzodiazepine Receptors	103
	3.3.1 Subunit and Subtype Structural Diversity	103
	3.3.2 Functional Domains	105
	3.3.2.1 GABA and BZ Binding Pocket	105
	3.3.2.2 Assembly, Clustering, and Surface Expression	108
	3.3.3 Diversity of Brain Distribution	110
	3.3.4 BZ Functional Diversity as Revealed by Gene Knockout and Knockin Models	112
3.4	Structure Activity Relation of Benzodiazepines	114
3.5	Future Developments	116
	Acknowledgment	117
	References	117

3.1 INTRODUCTION

The widespread use of benzodiazepines (BZs) is largely due to their powerful anxiolytic and hypnotic properties in combination with safety even at high dosages when used alone without other central nervous system (CNS) depressant drugs or alcohol. Strictly speaking, only the 1,4- and 1,5-benzodiazepines (Figs. 3.1–3.3) belong to this class of compounds. But since the development of chlordiazepoxide (see below), a large number of chemically unrelated groups of tranquilizers have been

Handbook of Contemporary Neuropharmacology, Edited by David R. Sibley, Israel Hanin, Michael Kuhar, and Phil Skolnick. Copyright © 2007 John Wiley & Sons, Inc.

	R1	R2	R3	R7	R2'
Clonazepam	-H	=O	-H	-NO$_2$	-H
Diazepam	-CH$_3$	=O	-H	-Cl	-H
Nordiazepam	-H	=O	-H	-Cl	-H
Flurazepam	-CH$_2$CH$_2$N(C$_2$H$_5$)$_2$	=O	-H	-Cl	-F
Flunitrazepam	-CH$_3$	=O	-H	-NO$_2$	-F
Lorazepam	-H	=O	-OH	-Cl	-Cl
Quazepam	-CH$_2$CF$_3$	=S	-H	-Cl	-F
2-Oxo-quazepam	-CH$_2$CF$_3$	=O	-H	-Cl	-F

Figure 3.1 Structure of 1,4-benzodiazepines. Shown are several subtype non-selective 1,4-benzodiazepines as well as two ligands with some preference for α_1-containing GABA$_A$/BZ receptors (quazepam and 2-oxoquazepam).

	R2'
Triazolam	-Cl
Alprazolam	-H

Midazolam

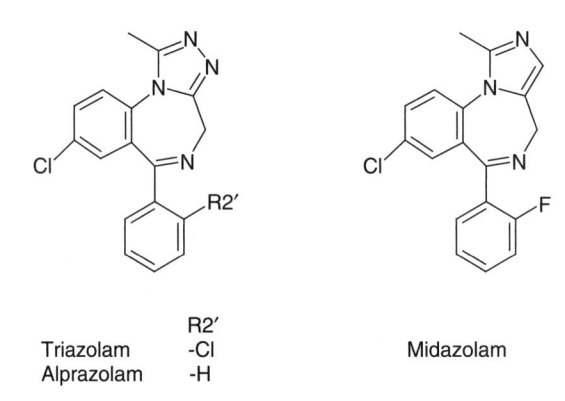

Figure 3.2 Structure of two triazolo-1,4-benzodiazepines and midazolam. All compounds shown are non-selective to various GABA$_A$/BZ-receptor subtypes.

synthesized which act with high affinity and specificity via the BZ receptor sites. Among the most important classes are the triazolopyridazines (e.g., CI 218,872; Fig. 3.4), imidazopyridines (e.g., zolpidem; Fig. 3.4), and β-carbolines (e.g., β-carboline-3-methylester; Fig. 3.4).

The first known and intensively studied synthetic tranquilizers were the barbiturates meprobamate, reserpine, and chlorpromazine. In an attempt to circumvent the molecular manipulation approach and to obtain a novel chemical type of tranquilizer, Leo H. Sternbach and colleagues, who developed the first BZ compounds, did not start from a biochemical or pharmacological point but from the viewpoint of a chemist in that

	R7
RO15-4513	-N$_3$
Flumazenil	-F

Figure 3.3 Structure of two imidazo-1,4-BZs. Whereas RO 15-4513 is a partial negative modulator on α_1-, α_2-, α_3-, and α_5-containing receptors and recognizes all GABA$_A$/BZ receptors with high affinity, flumazenil is an antagonist and binds with high affinity only to α_1-, α_2-, α_3-, and α_5-containing receptors and with a much lower affinity to α_4- and α_6-containing receptors.

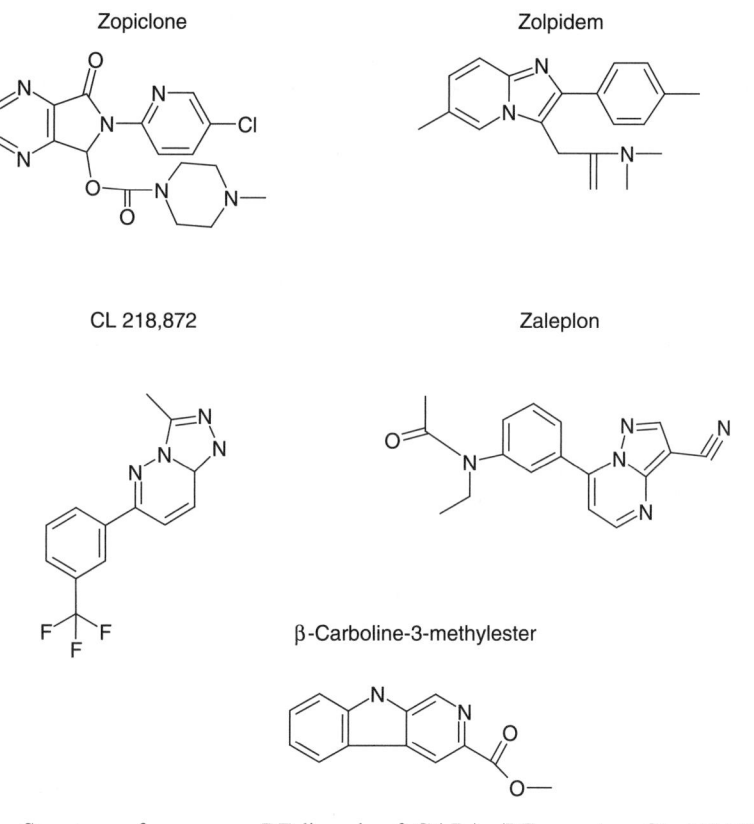

Figure 3.4 Structure of some non-BZ ligands of GABA$_A$/BZ receptor. CL 218,872 is the prototypical α_1-preferring ligand. As well, β-carboline-3-methylester is a long-known α_1-preferring ligand, but in contrast to CL 218,872, it is a full negative modulator. Zolpidem is the most selective GABA$_A$/BZ receptor ligand known binding with high affinity only to α_1-containing receptors and with moderate affinity to α_2- and α_3-containing receptors. Zaleplon and zopiclone are less selective than the former two but still do not display the full functionality of the classical 1,4-BZs.

he postulated that the structures should be more or less unexplored, be easily obtainable, and be demanding for a synthetic chemist [1]. Even more so, their discovery was not the planned synthesis of a given structure but the result of an unexpected chemical reaction. Thus, the structure of the first in this series of tranquilizers, generically named chlordiazepoxide and marketed as Librium, was only established some time after its synthesis and after it had been shown to be an efficient minor tranquilizer.

Twenty years after the first human in vivo pharmacological testing the molecular targets of BZ ligands were simultaneously described by three groups using [^{3}H]diazepam as a tool [2–4]. Since then, research into the action and function of BZ has taken advantage of the ease with which the ligands can be measured in vivo and in vitro using their tritiated forms. The novel selective labeled ligands, in conjunction with the development of molecular biology techniques, paved the ground to study the biochemical and neurobiological functions of the BZ in such detail that they are now among the best understood neuropharmacological agents.

Even before the BZ binding sites were described on a molecular level, it was speculated that γ-aminobutyric acid (GABA) plays a crucial role in the central action of BZ [5, 6]. Gradually, a picture evolved in which neuronal BZ binding sites were physically coupled to GABA type A (GABA$_A$) receptors to form the GABA$_A$/BZ receptor complex [7–9]. This model was further proven by demonstrating that affinity-purified BZ receptors contain sites for the specific GABA$_A$ agonist [^{3}H]muscimol [10]. On sodium dodecyl sulfate–polyacrylamide gel electrophoresis (SDS–PAGE) the purified protein separated into two major bands, labeled α (50 kDa) and β (57 kDa). By irreversibly photolabeling BZ receptors with [^{3}H]flunitrazepam the 50-kDa band is strongly labeled, but tissue-specific heterogeneity of the central BZ receptor was demonstrated by showing that other than the α and the β bands specifically incorporated [^{3}H]flunitrazepam [11]. Only the introduction of the molecular binding techniques finally settled the issue and started a new area in BZ ligand development and GABA$_A$/BZ receptor research.

Shortly after the discovery of BZ binding sites in the CNS, specific high-affinity [^{3}H]diazepam binding was described in various peripheral tissues and in transformed cells of neuronal origin [4, 12]. These sites are physically and pharmacologically distinct from sites present in tissues derived from the neuronal crest during ontogeny [13–15]. Though diazepam (Fig. 3.1) and most other clinically important BZs [16] bind with high affinity to both sites, other BZ ligands preferentially recognize one or the other: The 4′-chloro-substituted diazepam (RO 5-4864) and the isoquinoline Pk 11195 recognize only the "peripheral-type" site, while flumazenil (RO 15-1788, Fig. 3.3) and clonazepam (Fig. 3.1) are specific ligands for the "central-type" BZ site. The distribution of the "central-type" receptors made them likely candidates for the therapeutic action of the BZs; the peripheral sites were originally termed "acceptors" to denote a lack of physiological or pharmacological function [17]. Since then, the peripheral-type BZ receptor protein was shown to be located in the outer mitochondrial membrane [18] and to be most likely involved in cholesterol uptake and steroid exchange across that membrane [19, 20]. It is an 18-kDa protein with five transmembrane α-helical domains [see 21], clearly different from subunits of the GABA$_A$ receptor. This BZ recognition site is unlikely to be involved in the central action generally associated with BZ. Therefore, the remainder of the text will concentrate on the GABA$_A$/BZ receptors. For a more detailed discussion on the structure of GABA receptors, see Chapter 12 in volume I of this handbook.

3.2 PHARMACOLOGY OF BENZODIAZEPINE RECEPTOR LIGANDS

3.2.1 Therapeutic Action of BZ Receptor Ligands

The 1,4-BZs exhibit remarkably similar clinical profiles, demonstrating anxiolytic, sedative, myorelaxant, anticonvulsant, amnestic, and respiratory depressant properties. However, there is a separation in the doses needed to achieve these effects, though the size of the therapeutic window differs slightly between different BZs. Only when it comes to receptor subtype selective compounds can sedation be more prevalent than any of the other effects (see Fig. 3.5).

A large number of new BZ receptor ligands have been evaluated preclinically and clinically in recent years, all of them structurally different from the classical 1,4- and 1,5-BZs. These compounds include the hypnotic agents zolpidem, zaleplon, and zopiclone (Fig. 3.4). The imidazopyridine zolpidem is a highly potent sedative and hypnotic [22]. In contrast to the classical BZ it does not seem to alter sleep architecture or induce rebound insomnia after discontinuation [23, 24]. Zolpidem decreases sleep latency and increases sleep duration and reduces the number of awakenings [25]. Zolpidem has rapid metabolism with metabolic elimination $T_{1/2\beta}$ values of 1.5–3 h, and when used at normal evening doses to treat insomnia, the residual cognitive impairment effects the next morning are negligible. While zaleplon may be best indicated for the delayed onset of sleep, zolpidem and zopiclone may be better indicated for maintaining a complete night's sleep [26]. For a detailed discussion on the hypnotic properties of benzodiazepines, see Chapter 6 in volume III of this handbook.

BZs are relatively safe, even in large doses. However, especially when administered together with other sedative substances, that is, ethanol, barbiturates, or opiates, toxic effects may result. These include general apathy, muscular atonia, ataxia, and inhibition of the respiratory system. Under severe intoxication flumazenil can be given as an antidote, though care must be taken as this compound has a much shorter

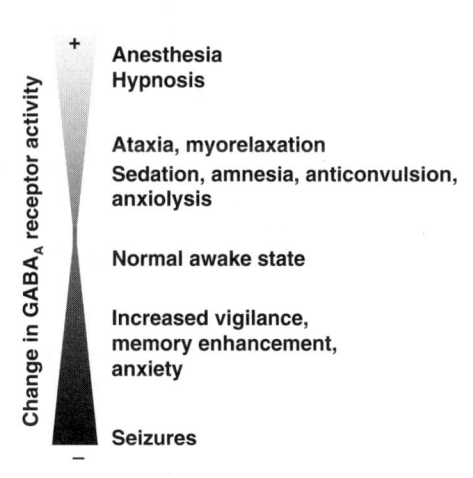

Figure 3.5 Correlation of activity at $GABA_A$ receptors with clinical effects. The intrinsic activity of BZ receptor ligands ranges on a continuum from full positive (top) to full negative modulators (bottom). Receptor-subtype-specific compounds with the less than full efficacy may avoid unwanted GABA-mediated effects.

half-life than many other BZ ligands in clinical use, which might make the repeated administration necessary.

3.2.2 Endogenous Benzodiazepine Site Ligands

Ever since the discovery of the BZ receptors, scientists have been interested in finding endogenously produced substances that would act naturally via these binding sites and would be called endozepines. Many substances have been described that interfere with BZ binding [27–29], but a definitive proof of physiological significance of any of these compounds is still missing. Without going into details of each putative compound, a few of them are still being investigated and may finally prove to be active endogenous BZ ligands, at least in certain pathophysiological conditions.

It has been clearly demonstrated that 1,4-BZs are present in the body and brain, even in postmortem brains from patients deceased 20 years before the first BZs have been synthesized [30, 31], suggesting that, for example, N-desmethyldiazepam could be formed by endogenous enzymes. These pathways have been poorly characterized in humans, and, therefore, the compounds might originate from plants or bacteria known to be able to synthesize BZs. As well, BZ ligands with negatively modulating properties may be endogenously formed from the β-carboline series of compounds [32], although some of the early compounds isolated from urine may not be present in brain or be artifacts of the isolation procedure [33, 34].

One of the most interesting cases has been the discovery of a peptide of about 100 amino acids called diazepam binding inhibitor (DBI). DBI was suggested to act as an endogenous inverse agonist at $GABA_A$/BZ receptors [35, 36]. It is a competitive inhibitor of [^{3}H]flumazenil binding to central $GABA_A$ receptors and to [^{3}H]RO 5-4864 binding to peripheral-type mitochondrial BZ receptors [37]. It is present in several different forms and mostly in brain glial cells and tumors and in peripheral tissues [38, 39]. Interestingly, DBI was found to be a member of the acyl-coenzyme A (CoA) binding protein family (ACBP [40, 41]), which have been implicated in many cellular functions including the modulation of acyl-CoA concentrations within cells and are considered products of widely conserved housekeeping genes. The gene also contains a sterol regulatory element [42], which allows DBI/ACBP to be regulated with other genes affecting lipid metabolism. DBI/ACBP has also been shown to activate steroidogenesis by facilitating cholesterol transport to the inner mitochondrial membrane, a process mediated by the peripheral-type BZ receptor [43, 44]. Thus, DBI is a ligand for the mitochondrial BZ receptor but might not be so relevant as an endogenous BZ acting on the central $GABA_A$ receptors. Since various BZ molecules have very variable affinities to the peripheral sites (see above), the behavioral and physiological actions of all these drugs cannot be mediated by these sites.

Stupor associated with hepatic encephalopathy has been treated with flumazenil [45–47], and while amelioration of the symptoms has been observed, it is apparently not so effective to become the only routine therapy [48]. Its efficacy indicates increased amounts of endogenous BZs in these patients, which has been confirmed both in patient samples and from tissues of animals with hepatic failure. The identities of the increased endogenous ligands are not yet settled, but they include BZ like structures and DBI-like peptides [49–52]. Furthermore, in acute intermittent porphyria there are increased concentrations of hemoglobin metabolites, of which hemin and protoporphyrin IX have been shown to potentiate at micromolar sensitivity the GABA responses of the $\alpha_1\beta_2\gamma_2$ GABA$_A$ receptors via flumazenil-sensitive BZ sites [53]. Interestingly, the latter compounds are also known to have even higher affinities toward the guinea pig brain peripheral-type BZ receptors [54].

The physiological relevance of the naturally produced BZs or other endogenous ligands still remains unclear, but from the experimental point of view it should be kept in mind that the recent BZ site point-mutated mouse models (see below) have not revealed clear behavioral or physiological alterations without drug challenges. This fact does not support any major role for the endogenous BZ site ligands in normal brain function, although they might be involved in pathological conditions, such as hepatic encephalopathy.

3.2.3 Modulation of Single-Cell GABA Response by Benzodiazepines

Detailed analysis of single-channel kinetics confirmed early reports [55] that BZs do not affect GABA-induced single-channel conductance or the average channel open duration [56–58] but increase channel-opening frequency by elevating the number of bursts [56, 57]. Zolpidem has little or no effect on mIPSC frequency, rise time, or amplitude but causes a significant prolongation of the miniature inhibitory postsynaptic current (mIPSC) decay [59]. The negative modulatory β-carboline DMCM (compare β-CCM in Fig. 3.4) reduces the channel-opening frequency without altering open duration or channel conductance; that is, it behaves inversely to positive modulating BZ [58]. BZ potentiation of the GABA response is discussed as originating from an increased affinity for GABA (Fig. 3.6). In this case, BZ should increase the average channel open duration as is observed with increased GABA

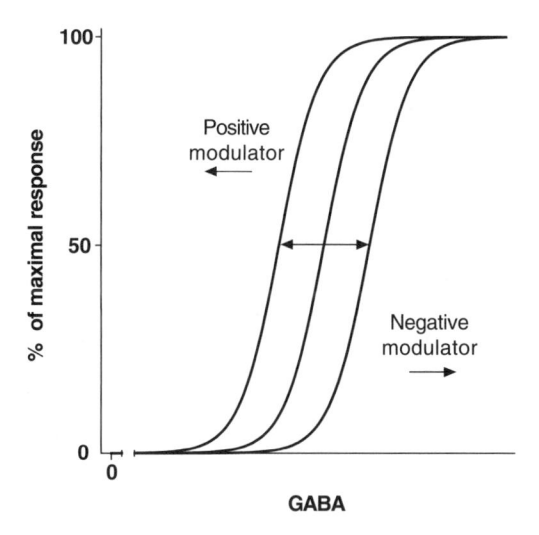

Figure 3.6 Effect of positive and negative modulators at BZ recognition site. Positive modulators shift the dose–response curve of GABA at a given GABA$_A$ receptor subtype to the left, whereas negative modulators right shift the curve. At the level of spontaneous inhibitory postsynaptic currents, the modulators mainly affect the current decay. Neither class has any effect on the maximal response of GABA or any effect in the absence of GABA, that is, the endogenous neurotransmitter controls the postsynaptic effect, unless the synaptic GABA release fails to saturate the postsynaptic receptors.

concentrations [56], but kinetic analysis [57] does not support such a mechanism [58]. The increased channel-opening frequency might be explained by an increased affinity at only one of multiple binding sites, different transitions into desensitized states, or altered coupling between binding site and channel [56].

In view of the close to saturating concentrations of GABA in the synaptic clefts of most neurons, BZ receptor ligands might exert their effects mainly by an increase in the decay time constants, thus prolonging the action of GABA [60]. In some neurons, the number of $GABA_A$ receptors in their synapses differ and BZ can increase the mIPSC amplitudes in those synapses with a high number of receptors apparently not saturated by released GABA, while no amplitude potentiation takes place in the synapses with low $GABA_A$ receptor number [61]. BZs can also act on extrasynaptic receptors (e.g., [62]), where the surrounding GABA concentrations are insufficient to cause the maximal effect, although quite a number of extrasynaptic receptors are BZ nonsensitive as they lack the γ_2 subunits [63].

The actions of BZ on $GABA_A$ receptors at single receptor and synapse levels must finally be converted to effects on activities of neuronal pathways and circuitries, which then affect widespread physiological and mental processes.

3.2.4 Tolerance and Dependence to BZ

The GABAergic system has been implicated in the mechanisms of drug abuse, in the abuse not only of BZ-positive modulators but also of other drugs of abuse, such as ethanol, opioids, cannabinoids, nicotine, and stimulants [64]. This is of no surprise, since the GABAergic system is so widespread and regulates most brain systems. Furthermore, novel mechanisms via GABAergic pathways have been proposed to be responsible for the rewarding actions of $GABA_A$ receptor–positive modulators and antagonists after intracerebral injections into different regions of ventral tegmental and caudal hypothalamic regions [65–67]. Effects of chronic use leading to tolerance and abuse to BZ compounds can be examined at the levels of $GABA_A$ receptor sensitivity, receptor subunit alterations, and counteracting adaptations in other neuronal systems.

Chronic treatment of experimental animals or neuronal cell cultures with BZ agonists have shown that the receptor binding determined by various ligands does not alter much [68, 69], suggesting that $GABA_A$ receptor subunit levels are rather stable even during continued receptor stimulation. Similar disappointing results have been obtained when receptor subunit gene transcription has been evaluated by subunit-specific oligonucleotide probes for messenger RNA (mRNA) [70], indicating that the receptor subunit synthesis remains mostly stable. In addition, subunit switches, such as a general change in dominance from γ_2 to δ subunit-containing receptors, have been excluded [70]. Still, there has been a more consistent finding of reduced GABA sensitivity after BZ treatment, especially a reduced or even abolished GABA stimulation of [^{3}H]BZ binding [68, 71], indicating that, while the binding sites are intact, they are in a state where allosteric interactions can no longer facilitate receptor function. Along this line, a similar loss of potentiation after chronic BZ treatment has been observed in the GABA actions stimulated by BZ [68]. It is possible that the reduced coupling between $GABA_A$ receptor binding site domains by chronic treatments is due to altered posttranslational processing of receptor subunits/subtypes and/or by receptor endocytosis, as it can take place rapidly within a few hours [72].

On the other hand, some research groups have been able to find defined alterations in brain regional $GABA_A$ receptor subunit expression, which might correlate with the emergence of tolerance to various BZ agonists. In frontoparietal motor and somatosensory cortex of rats, at least α_1-subunit expression decreased and that of α_3, α_5, $\beta_{2/3}$, and γ_2 subunits increased in a region-selective manner during a 14-day diazepam treatment that resulted in tolerance [73]. The suggested antipanic compound alprazolam alters the expression of brain stem α_3-, β_1-, and γ_2-subunit expression in rats [74]. A defined reduction in the hippocampal α_5-subunit expression in mice has been suggested to be mainly responsible for the tolerance development to low doses of diazepam [75], in keeping with earlier experiments showing reduced binding of the α_5-subunit-selective ligand [^{3}H]RY-80 in the hippocampal CA1 region in rats after flurazepam treatment [76]. Thus, it seems that there are several receptor-subtype-dependent mechanisms for tolerance development, partly depending on the animal species and behavioral assays used for tolerance assessment, and conditioning mechanisms, as hinted by the involvement of the hippocampal receptor subtypes. These mechanisms might thus be brain region specific. However, we also need more receptor-subtype-selective functional studies to understand the brain pathways involved in the BZ tolerance mechanisms.

The apparent diversity of the mechanisms accounting for BZ tolerance is further complicated by adaptations in other mechanisms than the $GABA_A$ receptor. Acute diazepam administration at low sedative doses induces the expression of several genes in the cerebral cortex of mice, including growth factors, such as brain-derived neurotophic factor, and transcription factors and kinases [77]. Interestingly, calcium/calmodulin-dependent protein kinase II remained upregulated at least 40 h after a single diazepam dose. All these changes were dependent on the α_1-subunit-containing receptors as they were absent in α_1(H101R) knockin mice. One of the most interesting findings has been the increased function and protein levels of α-amino-3-hydroxy-5-methylisoxazole-4-propionic acid (AMPA)–type glutamate receptors in the hippocampus during chronic treatment with flurazepam or diazepam [78–80]. Especially the GluR-A (GluR-1) subunit of AMPA-type glutamate receptors has been upregulated in certain brain regions by many other drugs of abuse, such as morphine, cocaine, and amphetamine [81–84]. This indicates that the AMPA receptor facilitation, upregulation, and/or increased cell surface targeting are not specific for BZ tolerance or withdrawal. These non-$GABA_A$ receptor adaptations might become important targets for reducing tolerance, dependence, and withdrawal phenomena to BZs and other drugs of abuse.

Most of the dependence experiments have been carried out with long-acting BZ ligands, such as diazepam and flurazepam. However, all full agonists, independent of the duration of action, possess the property of inducing tolerance and dependence. Importantly, the partial agonists so far studied usually do not induce strong tolerance or withdrawal symptoms at experimentally relevant doses [85–88]. However, as none of these has passed into clinical use, we can only refer to these reviews on these compounds.

3.2.5 Metabolism of BZ Receptor Ligands

As detailed before, the pharmacological action of all chemically related BZs in clinical use is similar with the exception of the antagonist flumazenil, though minor variations in the affinity and efficacy between the various subtypes have been reported. As these minor differences in the receptor actions between the ligands are unlikely to explain all observed clinical variances, they may be mainly or even exclusively due to differences in the absorption and metabolism of the drugs. As even the absorption is close to complete for most of the BZ receptor ligands of this chemical class, most differences can be traced back to the respective metabolic paths. After oral administration the time to peak levels detected in the plasma ranges from 30 min (~1 h for diazepam) up to 8 h. As well, the biological half-life of BZ varies greatly between a few hours (e.g., alprazolam, brotizolam) and more than 20 h (e.g., diazepam). As many BZs are extensively metabolized by the cytochrome P450 system in the gastrointestinal tract and liver and, furthermore, many of the metabolites are pharmacologically active, the duration of action of a BZ administration is often unrelated to the biotransformation of the parental compound. Two extreme examples are diazepam and flurazepam with their main and bioactive metabolites N-desmethyl-diazepam (nordiazepam) and N-desalkyl-flurazepam, respectively, which are eliminated from plasma with half-lives of 80–100 and 50 h, respectively. These differences readily explain that ultra-short-acting ligands are more suitable for the induction of sleep, longer acting ones suited for sleep maintenance and sedation, and very long acting BZ ligands for long-term treatment of anxiety, respectively.

All BZ compounds with nonfused substitutions at position 1 or 2 of the seven-membered ring, like diazepam and flurazepam, undergo a rapid modification of this substituent, resulting in the active NOR metabolites (NOR = *nitrogen ohne radikal*, German, meaning a nitrogen without any substituent). Thus, given the structural similarity of the BZ it is not surprising that quite a number of metabolic pathways converge on nordiazepam (Fig. 3.1). This compound can be metabolized to the active oxazepam by hydroxylation at position 3 of the diazepine ring before it is finally inactivated through glucuronidization at this hydroxyl position and excreted. As for compounds with a fused ring between positions 1 and 2 (midazolam, triazolam, and alprazolam; Fig. 3.2), the first step in inactivation cannot be performed and they are directly hydroxylated, glucuronidized, and excreted.

Non-BZ compounds such as the hypnotics zaleplon, zopiclone, and zolpidem (Fig. 3.4) are generally rapidly absorbed and reach their maximal concentrations within 1–2 h. Zopiclone is extensively metabolized by N demethylation, N oxidation, and decarboxylation. Its chiral center leads to stereoselective pharmacokinetics. Zolpidem is oxidized in the methyl groups and hydroxylated in the imidazolepyridine ring system [89].

Cytochrome P450 (CYP) 3A4 oxidase, located in the enterocytes of the small bowel and liver hepatocytes, is involved in the metabolism of a number of BZ receptor ligands, especially midazolam, triazolam, alprazolam, diazepam, flunitrazepam, and zopiclone [90–92]. The enzyme is inhibited by a number of other drugs, including the antidepressants fluoxetine and nefazodone, the macroglide antibiotic erythromycin, antifungal azoles, and the human immunodeficiency virus (HIV) protease inhibitor ritonavir as well as grapefruit juice. In the context of the mentioned BZ receptor ligands inhibition of CYP3A4 may lead to prolonged sedation, especially when patients are under stable drug treatment and one of the inhibitors is added. For example, midazolam plasma levels (i.e., areas under the curve) at the same dose can vary 400-fold depending on whether CYP 3A4 inhibitor (e.g., itraconazole) or inducer (e.g., rifampicin) is being coadministered [93], which produces clear effects on its clinically wanted sedative and unwanted motor-impairing actions.

3.3 GABA$_A$/BENZODIAZEPINE RECEPTORS

3.3.1 Subunit and Subtype Structural Diversity

GABA$_A$ receptors are members of the superfamily of ligand-gated ion channels which should be termed Cys loop receptors in order to exclude the structurally unrelated ionotropic glutamate receptors. They are heteropentameric ion channels, although the initial purification of bovine GABA$_A$ receptors suggested that only two proteins are involved in the formation of these Cys loop receptors [10]. Now it is common knowledge that GABA$_A$ receptors are composed of an array of polysubunits (α_{1-6}, β_{1-3}, γ_{1-3}, ϵ, δ, π, and θ), all of which are products of separate genes [94–96]. Their variety is even intensified by several splice forms, for example, α_6, β_2, and γ_2 subunits.

The ρ_{1-3} subunits mainly or exclusively present in the retina show similar structural characteristics and exhibit a high sequence identity to the above-mentioned subunits. They are picrotoxin sensitive but insensitive to bicuculline, the prototypic competitive GABA$_A$ antagonist, and to baclofen, the prototypic GABA$_B$ receptor agonist, and have thus been classified as GABA$_C$ receptor subunits [97, 98]. The classification of GABA$_A$ and GABA$_C$ receptors basing on a single pharmacological characteristic is controversial as only few features are common to all GABA$_A$ receptors. Thus, Kai Kaila proposed the terms GABA$_i$ and GABA$_m$ for GABA$_A$ + GABA$_C$ and GABA$_B$ receptors, respectively, with i standing for ionotropic and m for metabotropic (personal communication to HL).

Common features of all these subunits as well as for the glycine and nicotinic acetylcholine receptor subunits include four putative transmembrane regions and the so-called cysteine loop, located in the N-terminal extracellular domain and characterized by two cysteine residues spaced by 13 otherwise largely divergent amino acids which gave the group its name. Another hallmark of GABA$_A$ receptors is a conserved sequence in the second transmembrane region encompassing the amino acids TTVLTMTT. Though this sequence has been used to retrieve 13 of the known GABA$_A$ receptors [99], it is only partially conserved in the more recently identified subunits ϵ, π, and ρ_{1-3} and hardly recognizable in θ. In view of the fact that five of the eight amino acids are possibly lining the ion channel proper [100], the divergence of the ϵ and θ subunits warrants further investigation into the channel properties of receptors containing these subunits. However, with respect to BZ neither the ϵ nor the θ or δ subunits confer sensitivity to these ligands and the resulting receptors have not been shown to respond to these ligands. All subunits contain recognition sites for N glycosylation in the so-called large intracellular loop between transmembrane regions 3 and 4. The glycosylation adds to the theoretical molecular weight of the subunits, which ranges from 52 kDa for the unprocessed α_1 subunit, that is, still containing the 20- to 30-amino-acid-long leader sequence necessary for plasma membrane targeting, and 62 kDa for the α_4 subunit. This varies only marginally between mammalian species (e.g., between man, mouse, or rat), as the sequence identity between these species is mostly higher than 98%. Furthermore, no substantial pharmacological differences have been observed between the mentioned species. Exceptions to the rule are the non-BZ-relevant ϵ and θ subunits, which display only about 70% sequence identity between human, mouse, and rat [96].

BZ receptor–positive modulator ligands, such as diazepam, CL 218,872, and zolpidem, distinguish two GABA$_A$ receptor subtypes differing mainly in their α- and γ-subunit variants [101]. They characteristically display a high affinity to the α_1-subunit-containing receptors, but CL 218,872 and zolpidem differ from diazepam in having reduced affinity to α_2-, α_3-, and α_5-containing receptors [102, 103]. All these ligands are inactive at α_4- and α_6-subunit-containing receptors. This classification can be extended further, since some $\alpha\beta\gamma$ combinations differentiate between these ligands: zolpidem binds with poor affinity to α_5- and/or γ_3-subunit-containing receptors [104], while CL 218,872 has 10-fold higher affinity (low nanomolar) toward $\alpha_1\beta_3\gamma_3$ receptors than to any other α_1- or $\gamma_{2/3}$-subunit-containing receptors. The functional significance of this interaction has not been studied, but if existing at all in native brain, it represents only a minor pool of receptors as CL 218,872 fails to distinguish any high-affinity components in displacement analysis with rat hippocampal and cerebrocortical receptors [105]. This is but one example of the special properties that can be observed in recombinant receptors but does not seem to exist in appreciable amounts in native brain. It is important to note that the behavioral profiles of diazepam, CL 218,872, and zolpidem are quite different and their behavioral efficacy cannot be deduced from competitive ligand binding assays. Thus, CL 218,872 is a low-efficacy anxiolytic, diazepam a potent anxiolytic, and zolpidem a very potent hypnotic with little anxiolytic efficacy. These differences may be explained by their efficacies: CI 218,872 is a partial positive modulator, diazepam a wide-range full-partial positive modulator, and zolpidem an α_1-subunit-preferring full positive modulator [106]. Therefore, competitive binding assay results need to be complemented with data on the intrinsic efficacies of the compounds before making any behaviorally relevant predictions. Even in the case that both data sets are available, behavioral effects may be due to receptor populations that cannot be mimicked in vitro. This has been seen, for example, in the granule cells of the cerebellum: Though the array of subunits is restricted to α_1, α_6, β_2, β_3, and δ, only 50% of the pharmacology seen in rat brain slices could be accounted for by any of possible subunit combinations in vitro [107]. The same issue becomes important when one attempts to apply in vitro selectivity data into human brain imaging studies with the purpose of visualizing various subtypes of GABA$_A$ receptor.

Exchanging the β subunit in ternary $\alpha_i\beta_j\gamma_2$ receptors did not significantly alter the BZ binding characteristics [108, 109] for flunitrazepam, DMCM, FG8205, zolpidem, or CL 218,872 between the β_1, β_2, and β_3 isoforms in electrophysiological recordings [109]. Accordingly, Puia [110] reported for diazepam or bretazenil only a tendency toward a decreased potentiation while exchanging β_1 with the β_2 or the β_3 subunit in $\alpha_i\beta_j\gamma_2$ receptors. Sigel, however, observed a severalfold higher potentiation in $\alpha_{1/3}\beta_2\gamma_2$ receptors, as compared to $\alpha_{1/3/5}\beta_1\gamma_2$ [111]. The minor relevance of the β subunits in ternary receptors to BZ pharmacology was also seen when studied by [^{35}S]TBPS binding, although, in $\alpha_5\beta_j\gamma_{2/3}$ and to a lesser extent in $\alpha_3\beta_j\gamma_{2/3}$ receptors, the β_3 variant was required for high-affinity [^{35}S]TBPS binding [101, 104]. Interestingly, this correlates with the notion that α_5-subunit mRNA colocalizes with β_3 mRNA [112, 113]. Another study on homo-oligomeric β_3 channels reported this subunit to be sufficient for high-affinity [^{35}S]TBPS binding [114].

The receptor structures are further altered by posttranslational modifications, but the roles of these processes in function and in pharmacological specificity have not been well established. The receptor subunits show sequence similarity of about 70% within classes and about 30% between classes.

3.3.2 Functional Domains

3.3.2.1 GABA and BZ Binding Pocket.
Addition of the neurotransmitter triggers a small rotation of the extracellular domains of the receptor subunits [115], which then opens the channel pore formed by the adjoining transmembrane 2 TM2 regions of the five subunits as predicted from the data obtained with nicotinic acetylcholine receptors [116]. Using disulfide bond mapping in recombinant $GABA_A$ $\alpha_1\beta_1$ mutant receptors, Horenstein et al. [117] demonstrated that the extracellular portion of the TM2-lined pore is more flexible than the intracellular portion and that these domains of the α_1 and β_1 subunits rotate asymmetrically, since homologous residues (α_1T261C and β_1T256C) form disulfide bonds only when the receptors are activated by GABA. The resulting covalent modification keeps the channels open.

The physical pore properties of $GABA_A$ receptors are remarkably invariant among different subunit compositions (see [118]). Still, different compounds exert their action on the receptor via a range of different modes. For example, pentobarbital increases the mean duration of opening time and the mean number of openings per burst [119], but, as described before, BZ-positive modulators increase the open frequency [119] and BZ-negative modulators decrease it. Furthermore, though picrotoxinin does not directly interact with the binding site for pentobarbital, it produces the opposite effects on the receptor; that is, it reduces the mean number of openings per burst and shortens the mean open time [119]. Picrotoxinin protects the covalent modification of an α_1 V257C substitution by a sulfhydryl reagent in the intracellular portion of the TM2 region [120], possibly because of a direct steric hindrance by picrotoxinin, suggesting the direct blockade of the channel pore by ligands of this type.

The minimal structural requirement for $GABA_A$ receptors gated by GABA is a heteropentamer built from two different subunits with one peptide derived from the α class and the other from the β class of variants [121]. Thus, it was expected that both subunit classes contribute to the formation of the GABA binding pocket. Indeed, a number of amino acids on members of both classes, most of them conserved within a subunit class, have been identified as being involved in high-affinity agonist binding. The first one in this series was recognized by the F-to-L mutation at position 64 in the rat α_1 subunit in an electrophysiological assay [111, 122], later confirmed by direct photolabeling of the site with [^{3}H]muscimol [123]. Whereas the homologous residue in the α_5 variant was shown to be involved in the formation of the GABA binding pocket, the equivalent residues in the β_2 and γ_2 subunits do not affect GABA binding [122]. The two neighboring amino acids R66, corresponding to R70 in α_5, and S68 in the α_1 variant have been reported to contribute to the GABA binding domain [124, 125], as well as R120 in α_1 and its counterpart R123 in α_5 [125, 126].

[^{3}H]RO 15-4513 (Fig. 3.3) binding to BZ sites is differently modulated by GABA in various recombinant receptors. In $\alpha_1\beta_2\gamma_2$ receptors, GABA reduces its binding, which is in agreement with the classification of RO 15-4513 as a negative modulator [127]. In the $\alpha_6\beta_2\gamma_2$ receptors, GABA enhances significantly the binding. [^{3}H]RO 15-4513 binding is sensitive to diazepam in $\alpha_1\beta_2\gamma_2$ ($K_i = 16$ nM [128]) and α_6(Q100)$\beta_2\gamma_2$ ($K_i = 1.3\,\mu$M [129]) receptors but insensitive in $\alpha_6\beta_2\gamma_2$ receptors. These actions are also consistent with electrophysiological results ([130, 131], but see [132]), demonstrating that negative modulators act like positive modulators at $\alpha_6\beta_x\gamma_2$ and $\alpha_4\beta_x\gamma_2$ receptors. The observation that the intrinsic activities of flumazenil, ranging from antagonistic to partial positive modulatory, and RO 15-4513, ranging from partial negative modulatory to partial positive modulatory, depended on the amino acid replacing the H101 [133] supports the idea that the amino acid at this position affects the intramolecular transduction of an allosteric effect and not only the ligand binding domain structure.

In the years after cloning the first $GABA_A$ receptor subunit complementary DNAs (cDNAs) site-directed mutagenesis has contributed to the identification of residues on single subunits in a receptor complex involved in specificity, selectivity, and efficacy differences of BZ receptor ligands. In many cases the approach proceeded over the construction of chimeric proteins derived from two subunits with largely differing properties to finally point to a single amino acid. Another possible procedure employed the high sequence identity between subunits of a given class to directly point to amino acid candidates explaining physiological and pharmacological differences between $GABA_A$ receptors. The first approach was used to largely explain the molecular basis of the so-called BZ type I and type II receptors. An E is conserved in all α variants at the position 201 besides in α_1. Its exchange by a G leads to an increase in the affinity for the α_1-preferring compounds CL 218,872 and 2-oxoquazepam [134]. Further identified amino acids are T208 and I215 of the human α_5 subunit which confer high subtype selectivity of the partial inverse agonist L-655,708 to $\alpha_5\beta\gamma_2$ receptors in α_5(T208S, I215V)$\beta_1\gamma_2$ receptors [135], the homologous residues affecting also the affinity of zolpidem in α_1(S208T, V215I)$\beta_1\gamma_2$ receptors. However, these residues only slightly reduced the affinity of CL 218,872 binding. Still, these effects stress the importance of the whole domain between amino acid residues 201 and 215 in BZ binding [136, 137].

One of the most instrumental amino acid residues in the elucidation of BZ pharmacology is the H (in α_1, α_2, α_3, and α_5) to R (in α_4 and α_6) transition at a position corresponding to R100 in α_6. The single R-to-H substitution at positions 99 of α_4 and 100 of α_6 imparts sensitivity of these receptors to diazepam [137, 138]. Furthermore, diazepam insensitivity can be conferred to α_1 receptors by replacing the corresponding H101 with an R [138]. The point mutation only changes the affinity for diazepam but does not interfere with the affinity for GABA [139], a fact that has been utilized to dissect the behavioral pharmacological actions of classical BZs such as diazepam and at least partially attribute their diverse actions on receptors containing individual α subunits (see below). As well, diazepam-insensitive $\alpha_6\beta_2\gamma_2$ receptors can be converted to a diazepam-preferring species by four amino acid exchanges in the α_6 variant, thus reversing the rank order of potency of BZ receptor ligands in mutated as compared to wild-type receptors [137].

As briefly noted before, the same amino acid residue in the α_6 subunit has been identified as being polymorphic in rats: Alcohol-insensitive (AT) and alcohol-sensitive (ANT) rat lines were developed by selective outbreeding for differential sensitivity to the motor-impairing effects of an acutely administered moderate dose of ethanol (2 g/kg) [140]. The motor impairment was measured with a tilting plane test on a rough surface [141], which evaluates quick postural adaptations, supposedly needed cerebellar adjustment. The ANT rats are abnormally BZ agonist sensitive and have also slightly greater sensitivity to the motor-impairing actions of barbiturates, intravenous anesthetics, N-methyl-D-aspartate receptor antagonists, and neurosteroid agonists [142–145]. There are no overall differences in brain $GABA_A$ receptors between the ANT and AT rat lines [146, 147], but the binding of [^{3}H]RO 15-4513 to the cerebellum in ANT rats is about 100-fold more sensitive to diazepam and lorazepam than the binding in AT rat samples [148, 149], resulting in reduced "diazepam-insensitive" BZ binding in ANT rats. This is caused by a single nucleotide exchange in the $GABA_A$ receptor granule cell–specific α_6 subunit gene in the ANT rats leading to an R-to-Q exchange [150]. Interestingly, even if ANT rats differ from AT rats only in their cerebellar granule cell sensitivity to diazepam, in behavioral tests for the anxiolytic activity of diazepam they show heightened responses as compared to AT rats [151], suggesting that the cerebellum is also important for emotional behavior. Interestingly, the highly alcohol sensitive ANT rats consume voluntarily less alcohol than the alcohol-insensitive AT rats [152]. In proof, Saba et al. [153] have recently described a Sardinian alcohol-nonpreferring rat line to spontaneously have exactly the same mutation as the ANT rats in the α_6 subunit. However, whether these presumably α_6-subunit-mediated effects of alcohol are due to receptors containing the γ_2 subunit and have to be thus classified as $GABA_A/BZ$ receptors have still to be evaluated, especially in light of the more recent publication of the high sensitivity of $\alpha_6\beta_3\delta$ receptors against ethanol [154].

As outlined before, all $GABA_A$ receptors of the composition $\alpha_i\beta_j\gamma_k$ ($i = 1,...,6$, $j = 1,...,3$, $k = 2, 3$) are BZ sensitive. Thus, it was only a question of time before the γ_2 subunit was molecularly dissected to identify amino acids crucial in BZ pharmacology. In this line, a single amino acid residue has been identified in the γ_2 subunit, which seems to critically determine the efficacy of a given BZ receptor ligand with a $GABA_A$ receptor subtype [155]. If T142 in γ_2 is converted to serine, the channel response of the resulting $\alpha_1\beta_1\gamma_2$ receptor to 5 µM GABA is increased by flumazenil and RO 15-4513 (instead of being unaffected or decreased in the corresponding wild-type receptors), thus converting negative or neutral allosteric modulators into positive ones. The F at position 77 of the γ_2 subunit is homologous to the above-mentioned F64 in the α_1 and α_6 subunits. Whereas the latter is required for high-affinity GABA functionality, the former is involved in high-affinity binding of several BZ receptor ligands, for example, zolpidem, the β-carboline DMCM, diazepam, and CI 218,872 [136, 156]. A similar correspondence between GABA and BZ responsiveness was found for amino acids involved in the GABA recognition on the β subunit [157] and BZ binding site on the homologous α-subunit residues [158]. Both findings substantiate the claim that the BZ binding site is a "converted" agonist recognition site.

Recently, two domains in the γ_2 subunit have been identified as transducing elements for the BZ activity, one being in the region TM1, the other in the adjacent region TM2 including the following short extracellular loop [159]. Together these domains may form the structural basis for the enhancement of GABA-induced currents by BZ receptor ligands.

For some BZ site ligands, such as β-carbolines, an additional binding site on $GABA_A$ receptors independent of γ_2 subunits has been suggested [160, 161]. In addition to the function as a negative modulator on the BZ site at low micromolar concentrations, DMCM, ethyl-β-carboline-3-carboxylate (β-CCE), and propyl-β-carboline-3-carboxylate (β-CCP) at high micromolar concentrations potentiate the $GABA_A$ receptor function through a supposedly loreclezole-associated binding site in the β_2 and β_3 subunits [162]. This positive modulatory effect is independent of the α variant present in the receptor complex and is more pronounced in α_6-containing receptors due to the lack of inhibition (negative modulation) by the BZ binding site

[160, 161]. This site can be detected especially in the cerebellar granule cell layer by using [^{35}S]TBPS autoradiography, and it is decreased in the absence of α_6 subunits [163] but retained in γ_2(F77I) point-mutated mice [164], which show absence of DMCM-induced convulsions and presence of DMCM-induced motor impairment. As the effects are insensitive to flumazenil, they cannot be classified as being BZ receptor mediated though they are due to long known BZ receptor ligands.

An additional low-affinity BZ site has been suggested based on receptor assays in frog oocytes [165]. Diazepam, flunitrazepam, and midazolam but not flurazepam at micromolar concentrations produced strong enhancement of currents induced by a low GABA effective concentration (EC$_3$ sic!) in $\alpha_1\beta_2\gamma_2$ as well as $\alpha_1\beta_2$ receptors. In line with the subunit restrictions given before, nanomolar concentrations of all tested BZ agonists enhanced GABA responses in $\alpha_1\beta_2\gamma_2$ receptors, but to a lower extent than the micromolar concentrations of the active ones in γ_2-less receptors. Importantly, only the nanomolar actions were blocked by the selective antagonist flumazenil. It remains to be shown in vivo whether these effects have any functional role, the simple test being the demonstration of flumazenil-insensitive sedation or anesthesia by the above-mentioned active BZs.

3.3.2.2 Assembly, Clustering, and Surface Expression. Most but not all GABA$_A$ receptors assemble as *hetero*pentamers and require signaling sequences for the specific interaction of the subunits. One of the sequences was identified employing a natural splice variant of the α_6 subunit which is alternatively spliced in about 20% of its transcripts in rat brain, causing a 10-amino-acid deletion of the amino acids E57 up to Q66, thus including the residues F and R, positions 63/65 and 64/66 in α_6 and α_1, respectively [166]. When this spliced α_6 subunit is expressed in HEK 293 cells together with β_2 and γ_2 subunits, no binding activity of GABA or any BZ ligand is detected. Similarly, when the same subunits are expressed in *Xenopus* oocytes, no GABA-responsive channels are formed, though the transcript is translated in vitro. On a first glance, this result corroborates the idea that the GABA and/or BZ binding domains are at least partly in the extracellular region of the α subunits. Taylor et al. [167] have, however, shown that the short alternatively spliced α_6 subunit does not assemble into receptors that reach the plasma membrane, indicating that the deleted domain or a subsequent tertiary structural alteration affects membrane targeting. A stretch of 70 amino acids in the second half of the N-terminal extracellular domain was identified to be important for the homo-oligomeric assembly of the GABA$_C$ receptor ρ_1 but not the ρ_2 subunits [168]. In rat α_1 and γ_2 subunits, domains have been detected [α_1(80–100) and γ_2(91–104)] that are necessary for subunit interaction, assembly, and formation of BZ binding site [169, 170] in recombinant $\alpha_1\beta_3\gamma_2$ receptors. Another adjacent region of the γ_2 subunit [γ_2(83–93)] might be needed for interaction with β_3 subunits [170].

Recently, a glia-derived protein was identified in the CNS of the mollusk *Lymnea* [171]. This protein binds acetylcholine, shows a 15% sequence identity to the N-termini of nicotinic acetylcholine receptor subunits at domains that are suggested to be important in the formation of the agonist binding sites, and contains a cysteine loop with 12 (instead of 13) intervening amino acids. It lacks the membrane-spanning domains, thus forming soluble (i.e., non-membrane-bound), *homo*pentameric complexes [172]. This stresses the importance of the extracellular N-terminus for the assembly of subunits in this family of ligand-gated ion channels. Importantly, there are already data to suggest that at least BZ binding sites can be formed by truncated N-terminal extracellular domains in GABA$_A$ receptor α_1- and γ_2-subunit dimers, whereas [^{3}H]muscimol binding apparently requires also transmembrane domains of the α_1 subunits together with truncated β_3 subunits [170].

The altered pharmacology of native GABA$_A$ receptors and changes in the γ_2- and α_4-subunit levels in δ-subunit-deficient mice indicate that the δ subunit preferentially assembles in the forebrain with α_4 subunits, where it interferes with the coassembly of α_4 and γ_2 subunits, the γ_2 subunit being recruited into additional functional receptors in its absence. This provokes the question of how GABA$_A$ receptor subunit assembly is regulated in the normal brain. Little further is known besides that the N-terminal domains of the α subunits are obligatory for this process [167, 173], elegantly proven by the assembly of the homopentameric acetylcholine binding protein of *Lymnea* [172]. Two scenarios exist to explain these results, that is, either the concentration of δ subunit exceeds that of the γ_2 subunit or the δ subunit has a higher probability than the γ_2 subunit in assembling with α_4 and α_6 subunits. In both scenarios, δ and γ_2 subunits compete with each other during assembly into functional receptors in neurons, a process which could efficiently limit the number of receptor subtypes, that is, subunit combinations, produced and especially the number of BZ-responsive GABA$_A$ receptors. However, recombinant $\alpha_4\beta_3\gamma_2\delta$ GABA$_A$ receptors are formed in HEK 293 cells [174] where the γ_2 and δ subunits assemble into functional receptors as demonstrated by their selective electrophysiological and pharmacological properties, though at a reduced expression level. However, fibroblasts may lack molecular features such as clustering proteins [175–177] that might be needed for the selective assembly or ideal function of subunits in vivo, thus further enlarging the once-thought narrow gap between the in vitro and in vivo properties of GABA$_A$ receptors.

The γ_2 and γ_3 subunits not only confer BZ sensitivity to the resulting GABA$_A$ receptors but also are instrumental in the subcellular targeting of the receptors, that is, the clustering of the receptors and/or the synaptic versus the extrasynaptic location of the receptors. Two main players have been identified to be involved in these cellular processes, gephyrin and GABA$_A$ receptor-associated protein (GABARAP). In the following we will briefly outline their properties. Gephyrin, initially described as a 93-kDa protein copurified with glycine receptors [178], is now known to be more widely expressed in the CNS as well as peripheral tissue, even in areas devoid of the glycine receptor [179]. Mice lacking gephyrin die at day 1 after birth (P1) and exhibit a reduced number of clustered glycine receptors at their synapses but not an overall loss of glycine receptors [180]. As well, a significant reduction in the punctuate immunoreactivity toward the GABA$_A$ receptor α_2 and γ_2 subunits is observed in spinal cord sections of these mice [181]. In primary hippocampal neuronal cultures synaptically clustered GABA$_A$ receptors are reduced but their intracellular pool is increased. Together with results from γ_2 knockout mice, which exhibit a loss of clustered GABA$_A$ receptors [182, 183], these data provide evidence for a dominant role for gephyrin and probably the $\gamma_{2/3}$ subunits in GABA$_A$/BZ receptor clustering. The pool of GABA$_A$ receptors clustered extrasynaptically, as detected by $\beta_{2/3}$- and γ_2-specific antibodies in wild-type hippocampal neurons, is reduced during development, but even after 30 days in culture it amounts to 50% of all clusters [184]. This leaves open the question on the mode of specific targeting of these clusters or the precise subunit composition of extrasynaptic versus synaptic clusters.

Employing the yeast two-hybrid system, a ubiquitously expressed protein was identified to interact with a part of the large intracellular loop of the γ_2 subunit [185]. In spite of its distribution pattern it was called GABARAP. It exhibits sequence similarity with light chain 3 of microtubule-associated proteins and a putative tubulin binding motif, which apparently directly interact with microtubules and tubulin, respectively [186]. Recombinant $\alpha_1\beta_2\gamma_{2L}$ receptors expressed together with GABARAP have variable GABA sensitivity and channel kinetics depending on whether the receptors are in clusters or diffusely distributed on the cell membrane [175]. Using again the technique of yeast two-hybrid screening, Kanematsu et al. [187] found an inositol 1,4,5-trisphosphate binding protein, called p130, that may bind to GABARAP and inhibit the binding of γ_2 subunit to GABARAP. The p130 knockout mice show reduced sensitivity to diazepam in both behavioral and hippocampal electrophysiological experiments, whereas GABA-induced receptor currents are unaltered. The roles of the GABARAP and p130 are still unresolved, especially as the GABARAP-deficient mouse line appears to have no defects in $GABA_A$ receptor membrane targeting [188].

Insertion of proteins into the plasma membrane and the half time of surface expression represent a highly regulated process. Thus, it is not really astonishing that there are proteins regulating these processes. In this line the ubiquitin-like protein Plic-1 has been found to interact with several α and β subunits of the $GABA_A$ receptor [189]. This protein seems to be important for facilitation of $GABA_A$ receptor surface expression and intracellular stabilization of subunits. Recently, it was shown that $GABA_A$ receptors are constitutively internalized by clathrin-dependent endocytosis [190], which could be traced to the interaction of β and γ_2 subunits with the adaptin complex AP2. This interaction may be functionally important in vivo as the blockade of endocytosis increased the amplitude of GABA-induced miniature inhibitory postsynaptic currents in hippocampal neurons by two. The internalization of the $\alpha_1\beta_2$ and $\alpha_1\beta_2\gamma_2$ receptors in HEK 293 cells is strongly modulated by phosphorylation/dephosphorylation reactions [191], but the modulations might not be $GABA_A$ receptor specific. Especially, the role of protein kinase C–mediated phosphorylation of receptor interacting proteins needs to be assessed. The functional and pharmacological regulation of receptor surface expression, subunit stabilization, and internalization thus remain to be studied, but the present scarce data already suggest that these mechanisms may also vary between different $GABA_A$ receptor subtypes [192].

Whether the factors described here contribute to the mentioned discrepancy between the observed in vitro and in vivo effects of BZ receptor ligands will be a major focus of BZ research. Further, they might be important for the receptor regulation during tolerance development. Even more so, the results may even point to future pharmacological targets to treat disorders currently medicated with BZ receptor ligands.

3.3.3 Diversity of Brain Distribution

Early autoradiographic experiments have shown $GABA_A$ receptor–associated GABA site labeling using [^{3}H]muscimol as a ligand [193]. More thorough examination, however, has raised the suspicion that the high-affinity binding of GABA site ligands does not distribute as widely in the CNS as BZ site or channel site ligands labeled by [^{3}H]BZ and [^{35}S]TBPS, respectively. The GABA binding site as seen with [^{3}H]muscimol is concentrated especially to the cerebellar granule cell layer and thalamus, whereas the diencephalon and colliculi are hardly labeled contrasting with the labeling patterns by [^{3}H]BZ and [^{35}S]TBPS. Thus, [^{3}H]muscimol autoradiographies indicate that GABA site labeling reveals only a fraction of all GABA$_A$ receptors, though it is the prototypic agonist acting on all GABA$_A$ receptor subtypes in functional assays at high nanomolar–low micromolar concentrations. High-affinity [^{3}H]muscimol binding to rat brain sections was proposed to be associated with δ-containing receptors [194, 195]. This was corroborated by the findings that [^{3}H]muscimol binding to GABA sites is reduced in cerebellar sections from α$_6$ knockout mice [163] exhibiting a reduced number of α$_6$- and/or δ-subunit-containing receptors [196] and that in δ-deficient mice [197] the high-affinity [^{3}H]muscimol binding is reduced in both the cerebellum and forebrain [145]. In contrast, [^{3}H]RO 15-4513 binding to BZ sites of the cerebellum and forebrain is increased in $δ^{-/-}$ animals, which was, at least partly, due to an increase in diazepam-insensitive receptors. Concurrently the amount of the γ$_2$ subunit, as determined by Western blotting, is increased and that of α$_4$ decreased in $δ^{-/-}$ animals, while the level of the α$_1$ subunit remains unchanged [145], indicating augmented assembly of γ$_2$ subunits with α$_6$ and α$_4$ subunits in the absence of the δ subunit. This points to an increased expression of BZ receptors as a compensation to the decrease of high-affinity GABA recognition sites [128, 198, 199].

As stated before, GABA$_A$ receptors responsive to BZ receptor ligands require any α variant together with any β subunit and either γ$_2$ or γ$_3$. In these configurations the β subunits are known to contribute little to the differences in the BZ ligand–mediated effects and the γ$_3$ subunit is rare (see below). Therefore, mainly the α subunits determine the pharmacological and physiological responses of GABA$_A$ receptors to BZ receptor ligands. Thus, the following description focuses on the α$_1$ variant distribution in the CNS, especially as the γ$_2$ subunit is found in nearly all brain regions, though to different intensities [200].

The α$_1$ subunit appears to be the most abundant subunit in the CNS, missing only in a few regions and often colocalizing with the β$_2$ subunit [112, 113, 201–203]. Strong α$_2$- and α$_3$-subunit expression seems to inversely correlate with α$_1$ expression. These two subunits as well as α$_3$ and α$_5$ are abundant in the hippocampus [113, 202]. The α$_3$β$_1$γ$_2$-subunit combination is reported for serotonergic neurons of the raphe nuclei and cholinergic neurons of the basal forebrain [204–206]. Some subunits dominate during embryonic development, for example, α$_2$, α$_3$, and α$_5$ [202, 207, 208], but are reduced or even absent in defined regions in the adult brain [209]. The time-delimited presence of specific subunits during ontogenesis in defined brain regions appears to be essential for normal development [210, 211]. Other neurons, for example, the cerebellar Purkinje cells, maintain their subunit composition of α$_1$β$_{2/3}$γ$_2$ throughout all pre- and postnatal stages [202]. It is also possible that more than one α subunit is in a pentameric complex [212, 213].

The α$_5$ subunit, concentrated in the adult hippocampus and olfactory bulb [113, 214], is part of a receptor with negligible affinity for BZ receptor ligands such as the imidazopyridine zolpidem [103, 215] (see Fig. 3.4). Major amounts of the α$_4$ subunit are found in the hippocampus and thalamus and often colocalize with the δ subunit [198]. The α$_6$ subunit, also found to colocalize with the δ subunit, appears to be almost exclusively restricted to the cerebellar granule cells [128] with some traces found in the dorsal cochlear nucleus [216, 217], a brain area developmentally derived from cerebellar precursors.

The β$_1$ mRNA signals are strongest in the hippocampus, less pronounced in the claustrum and parts of the stria terminale, and weak in the amygdala and hypothalamus [113, 218, 219], whereas the β_2 subunit shows more widespread distribution that seems to be inversely correlated to the β_1 and β_3 concentrations, for example, in the hypothalamus and in parts of the hippocampus [113, 218, 219]. Here the β_3 subunit is strong, mainly in CA1 and CA2, but as well in the olfactory bulb, cortex, caudate putamen, nucleus accumbens, and hypothalamus. Like for the α variants, studies on the distribution of the β_1, β_2, and β_3 subunits during pre- and postnatal ontogeny indicate an independent regulation of their expression in different brain regions that suggests a role during development [202, 209, 220]. A line of proof is a mouse line devoid of the chromosomal region encoding α_5 and β_3 that bears a neonatally lethal cleft palate [221]. Introduction of a transgene coding for the β_3 subunit rescued these mice [211], thus proving not only the responsibility of β_3 for the cleft palate but also the role of the β_3 variant in development, in this specific case outside the CNS. These observations provoke the question of whether BZ can cause congenital malformations. Indeed, there have been early reports to this end [222, 223], which, however, could not be substantiated in more recent studies [224, 225].

The ubiquitous presence of the γ_2 subunit and hence the BZ receptor is contrasted by the restricted distribution of the γ_1 and γ_3 variants. Messenger RNA encoding the γ_1 subunit is limited to regions of the amygdala, septum, and hypothalamus [226]; the γ_3 subunit is largely present in the olfactory bulb, cortex, basal nuclei, and medial geniculate of the thalamus [99, 113, 227].

Immunoprecipitation studies with an α_6 antibody suggested that between 10 and 40% α_6 subunit is combined with the α_1 subunit [212, 228]. Caruncho and Costa [228a], however, concluded from double immunolabelings of freeze-fracture replicas that these two subunits do not colocalize within the same receptor complex. Based on mRNA and protein colocalization, further subunit combinations containing more than one α variant have been suggested, such as $\alpha_1\alpha_3\beta_{2/3}\gamma_2$ [203, 213, 229]. However, immunoprecipitation studies might include incompletely assembled receptors as well as receptors not inserted into the outer cell membrane [192]. As well some receptor pools might be underestimated in such studies because they are not readily solubilized by conventional detergent treatments [230].

In addition to the differences between [^{3}H]BZ and [^{3}H]muscimol binding distribution, there exists a large discrepancy between the high-affinity [^{3}H]GABA site ligand binding to brain sections, membrane homogenates, or recombinant receptor preparations on one side and the low-affinity binding of these ligands suggested from allosteric actions in functional assays employing electrophysiological methods and [^{35}S]TBPS and [^{3}H]BZ binding assays on the other side. Whereas the former is uniformly in the range of tens of nanomolar [104], the latter varies from high nanomolar to the micromolar range [101, 118, 231]. As this discrepancy holds true for single-receptor preparations, it cannot be due to receptor heterogeneity but rather must be an intrinsic receptor property. One likely explanation is the interconversion between a low-affinity and a high-affinity state, which, however, still awaits a definite biochemical proof.

3.3.4 BZ Functional Diversity as Revealed by Gene Knockout and Knockin Models

The most dramatic increase in knowledge about the functional diversity of BZ receptor ligands has been obtained in the past years by the use of knockout models and even more pronounced by mouse knockin models for $GABA_A$/BZ receptors.

These studies revealed that the deficiency of some subunits such as the $GABA_A$ receptor γ_2 and the before-mentioned β_3 subunit cannot be compensated for in the developing brain. Mouse lines devoid of these subunits are severely compromised [210, 232], and thus absence of these subunits is incompatible with life, at least during development.

The α_5-subunit gene, the expression of which is largely restricted to the hippocampus but as well present in parts of the cortex and more widespread in prenatal development, has been disrupted in mice and their behavior has been analyzed. They show enhanced platform learning in the Morris water maze and normal behavior and normal sensitivity to BZ agonists in the elevated-plus maze test of anxiety [233]. It is thus possible that inhibition of α_5-subunit-containing receptors might help in improving cognitive functions, though the basic function of this subunit can obviously not be to curtail learning ability. A more philosophical aspect is the idea that forgetting is as essential for life as learning. Interestingly, as mentioned above, reduction of the expression of this subunit in the hippocampus seems to correlate with tolerance development to prolonged BZ treatment in animal models [75, 76].

The lack of γ_3, α_6, and δ subunits, and even in view of the data cited above, the lack of the α_5 variant does not produce any strong behavioral or physiological phenotype [197, 233–237]. Even more surprisingly, the homozygotic loss of α_1 or β_2 subunits resulting in a 50% reduction of all $GABA_A$ receptors [238] is associated with neither lethal or strong behavioral effects, indicating functional compensation. However, though a general increase in other α-subunit expressions would be expected in these mice, the contrary was found: The α_6-subunit-dependent BZ-positive modulator-insensitive [^{3}H]RO 15-4513 binding is reduced by about 30%, suggesting that proper assembly or membrane targeting of the α_6 subunits needs the presence of α_1 subunits [238]. More recent experiments on the α_1 knockout mice have revealed clear compensations, especially by increased α_2 and α_3 subunits in the forebrain [239].

The proposal that the α_6 subunit plays a significant role in the action of alcohol [240] warranted an analysis of the behavior of α_6-subunit-deficient mice behavior in response to sedative compounds [235, 236]. Two independently generated α_6 knockout lines lack the subunit-specific [^{3}H]RO 15-4513 binding in the cerebellar granule cell layer but neither exhibit any immediately apparent motor learning or coordination deficits nor is their alcohol and anesthetic sensitivity different from that of wild-type animals [241]. However, their motor function is more readily affected by diazepam than that of the wild-type mice [242]. A potassium leak current carried via the Task-1 channel is increased in $\alpha_6^{-/-}$ mice, most likely needed to counteract the loss of inhibition in the cerebellar granule cells [243]. Analogous phenomena similar to this may occur in all other $GABA_A$ knockout mice, obscuring the biological significance of the subunits and hindering the interpretation of the lack of apparent behavioral consequences.

To overcome these obstacles, Rudolph, Möhler, and co-workers as well as Rosahl, Whiting, and co-workers utilized a gene knockin approach that alters the diazepam-sensitive sites in α_1-, α_2-, α_3-, and α_5-subunit-containing receptors into insensitive ones by exchanging the H to R at the position N-terminal to the cysteine loop that is crucial for diazepam sensitivity [138]. These mouse models produced information on the behavioral roles of $GABA_A$ receptor subtypes. Initially, this approach was thought to provide the final answers to the $GABA_A$ receptor subtype-specific actions of BZ receptor ligands. In the first round of experiments two groups independently reported that in α_1(H101R) mutant mice diazepam is no longer sedative and amnestic, partially lost its anticonvulsant effects, but retained normal anxiolytic properties [244, 245]. However, α_1(H101R) mice react normally to diazepam with respect to sleep-related parameters [246]; most like hypnotic sleep-related effects most likely involve other GABA$_A$ receptor subtypes.

The α_2(H101R) mice, that is, mice with a BZ-insensitive α_2 variant, did not display clear anxiolytic responses to diazepam, while their sedative responses to BZs were normal [247]. This is not surprising in view of the involvement of a number of brain regions in anxiety-related behavior, including the amygdala, a structure with high α_2 content, mammilary bodies, and dorsal hippocampus (see [113, 248]). More recent data, however, put into question the involvement of solely the α_2 subunit in the anxiolytic effects of BZ receptor ligands. Along this line, α_3-containing receptors may mediate anxiolytic effects of novel subtype-selective BZ ligands [249, 250]. Interestingly, the α_3(H126R) mice showed no deficits in the actions of diazepam [251], though the α_3 subunit is strategically expressed in important monoaminergic nuclei [203] believed to be involved in the regulation of emotional behavior. As well, even α_5-containing receptors cannot be totally excluded to be involved in anxiety behavior [252]. Further experiments with these models will be important to exclude compensatory alterations in the GABAergic or other systems which may occur in spite of the absence of any proven endogenous BZ receptor ligands (see above) and in the absence of any overt physiological changes in GABA sensitivity of the mutated α variants. As well, the roles of these subtypes in behaviors such as tolerance and dependence to BZs need to be clarified. The muscle-relaxing effects of BZ receptor ligands seem to be largely mediated by the α_2 subunit as in the BZ-insensitive α_2 variant mice the myorelaxant action of diazepam was almost completely abolished [251].

As well, the role of the α_5 variant in the action of BZ receptor ligands did not become as clear as hoped for when mice carrying the H-to-R mutation were analyzed [253]: Diazepam no longer exerted the full muscle-relaxing effect seen with high doses of BZ ligands, but the sedative, anticonvulsant, and anxiolytic effects of diazepam were unaffected in these mutant mice. Surprisingly, the point mutation resulted in a selective reduction of α_5-containing GABA$_A$ receptors in hippocampal pyramidal cells resulting in an overall loss of 20% of the α_5 protein, which in itself did not change the above-mentioned effects but changed the response in a trace fear-conditioning task in which a tone associated with an electric shock was separated by an empty time interval independent of any external BZ. Though these results can be taken as a hint for the involvement of the α_5 subunit in some type(s) of associative learning, the role of BZ receptor ligands is still open for discussion. The same mutant mice did not develop any tolerance to the α_1-mediated sedative effects of diazepam which was interpreted as a regulatory crosstalk between two GABA$_A$ receptor subtypes [75].

3.4 STRUCTURE ACTIVITY RELATION OF BENZODIAZEPINES

In a strict sense all BZ receptor ligands are GABA$_A$R subtype selective as none of these ligands recognizes all native or heterologously expressed ligand-gated ion channels of this type, simply because, contrary to previous beliefs, not all GABA$_A$R are BZ receptors. Slightly more relevant to the pharmacology of BZ receptor ligands is the observation that not a single ligand in clinical use binds to all BZ receptors with similar affinity, simply because no BZ receptor ligand recognizes $GABA_A$/BZ receptors containing the α_4 or α_6 subunits, resulting in the term "diazepam-insensitive" (DI) BZ receptors for $\alpha_{4/6}\beta_j\gamma_2$ receptors. However, these receptors bind the azido derivative of flumazenil, RO 15-4513, with high affinity that is identical to all receptors of the configuration $\alpha_i\beta_j\gamma_2$ ($i = 1,...,4, 6; j = 1, 2,...,3$) and this ligand binds to α_5-containing BZ receptors with an even 10-fold higher affinity. Still, this selectivity does not play any role in clinical practice, whereas compounds which selectively recognize any given receptor of the types $\alpha_i\beta_j\gamma_2$ ($i = 1, 2, 3, 5$ with any $j = 1, 2, 3$) would be highly desirable.

Two different strategies have been employed to probe the structural requirements of BZ receptor ligands with specific receptor subtypes. One might be called the "molecular path," in which putative subtype-selective compounds are tested on an array of recombinant receptor subunit combinations with biochemical and/or electrophysiological methods. The second one assumes that certain aspects of pharmacological BZ receptor ligand effects are mediated through defined receptor subpopulations and might be called the "behavioral path." A third possible route has not yet been taken and presumably it will take some time before it will lead to a successful end in the field of the BZ receptor ligands. It takes advantage of structural data of the receptor to fit appropriate molecules directly into the pharmacophore. Especially the latter but also the first route is hampered by the continuum of effect size of these BZ receptor ligands from full negative modulators up to full positive modulators, though, on the other hand, this range of effect size has facilitated the development of so-called functional selective compounds, in which the given compound binds to some or all receptor subtypes but the efficacy is, at best, zero on one type and 100% on the other.

As far back as 1993, intrinsic efficacy differences were supported to mediate the differing effects of BZ receptor ligands [254], although the molecular diversity of $GABA_A$/BZ receptors was traced to the existence of several α variants already in 1989 [108]. A fuller appreciation to its now-known extent came in the following years [103, 128, 198], although BZ type I over BZ type II preferring compounds like CL 218,872, quazepam, and 2-oxo-quazepam were identified over 20 years ago [255–258]. The first subtype-specific structure–activity analysis was made under the assumption that in the cerebellum [^{3}H]flunitrazepam binding represents a single receptor population [259], an assumption we now know to be essentially but not totally correct as only 90% of all diazepam-sensitive receptors in this brain region contain the α_1 variant and thus represent the BZ type I receptors. Zolpidem is now the most subtype-selective BZ receptor ligand in clinical use. It displays a 12- to 25-fold higher affinity to α_1-containing receptors as to α_2- and α_3-containing receptors, paired with negligible affinity to all other α variant receptors [103, 260]. Recently, a zolpidem derivative was shown to be even more α_1 selective than zolpidem: This compound only recognizes the most abundant $\alpha_1\beta_j\gamma_2$ receptors [261] but still displays anxiolytic-like properties.

It took a few more years before the first molecular modeling approaches were performed in the search for α-subunit-preferring compounds with a single receptor population [262, 263], in this specific case, the α_6-containing and thus one of the two theoretically possible diazepam-insensitive receptors. By analyzing close to 50 BZs

[263], the authors concluded that the ester substituent and substitutions at position 6 besides the obvious position 7 of imidazo-[1,4]benzodiazepines (compare Fig. 3.3) have a marked influence on the ratio of affinity for diazepam-sensitive to diazepam-insensitive receptor subtypes. However, no ligand was identified that had a substantially higher affinity to α_6-containing receptors or a ratio of affinities substantially in favor of α_6-containing receptors.

More comprehensive pharmacophore models were proposed in the following years and included not only the α_6-containing receptors but also $\alpha_{1/2/3}$- and especially α_5-containing GABA$_A$/BZ receptors. For the latter it had been observed that imidazobenzodiazepines are generally α_5 receptor selective [104, 264]. A lipophilic pocket present in the general pharmacophore of all GABA$_A$/BZ receptors [265] seems to be smaller in α_1-containing receptors than that present in α_5-containing receptors [264]. This may account for the high affinity of zolpidem to α_1 receptors as it may lead to a strong lipophilic–lipophilic interaction only possible in the restricted space. Thus, increasing the size of the substituent at position R7 in Figure 3.3 increased the selectivity for α_5-containing receptors and finally resulted in the development of RY-80, a high-affinity, high-selectivity ligand for α_5 receptors [266]. A similar strategy yielded the α_5-selective ligand L-655,708 that exhibits an affinity in the same order of magnitude [267]. By exchanging two amino acids in α_1 into the corresponding residues of α_5 (α_1S205T,V212I) the binding selectivity of α_5 against L-655,708 was transferred to α_1-containing receptors [135]. Both ligands as well as a number of other ligands identified as α_5 selective [268] are negative modulators at the BZ recognition site. A good candidate for a positive modulator on this receptor subtype is still missing, if at all desirable in view of the fact that negative modulators at this site are developed as putative "cognition enhancers," thus leading to the speculation that positive modulators should lead to learning deficits.

In recent years a number of compounds have been published that are selective for the other members beside α_5 of the former BZ type II receptor group, that is, α_2 and/ or α_3 receptors [250, 269]. However, in most instances the compounds are not selective for the latter receptors in the sense that they bind with a high enough difference in affinity to produce a subtype-selective effect but they more pronouncedly differ in their efficacies exerted on α_1, α_2, α_3, and α_5 receptors. One of these compounds is a negative modulator and anxiogenic in vivo at doses that minimize the occupancy at other than α_3 receptor subtypes, again suggesting that the α_3 receptor subtype may play a role in anxiety.

3.5 FUTURE DEVELOPMENTS

The existing mechanisms to extrinsically regulate the BZ-modulated GABAergic system are widespread and of tremendous clinical importance, although they represent only a substructure of the GABA$_A$ system, which again is only a part of all inhibitory processes in the CNS. Nonetheless, the entire clinical or scientific potential of the BZ-dependent inhibition has probably not been exhaustively explored, mainly due to the large heterogeneity of the GABA$_A$/BZ receptor system. We are still awaiting $\alpha_i\beta_x\gamma_2$ ($i = 2,\ldots,6$) receptor subtype–specific drugs to come into clinical practice. Even less is known of BZ receptors containing the γ_3 instead of the γ_2 variant. There is no reason to believe that a minor receptor population is of minor importance [270, 271]. As well, the old story of partial versus full modulators, at both sides of the scale, that is, positive and negative modulators, has not completely unfolded [272]. It is most likely that the use of these "fine-tuning" substances could finally benefit patients. In the extreme, this could lead to a drug only suitable for the treatment of a minor population of affected persons, regardless of whether diagnosed with anxiety-related diseases, epilepsy, insomnia, or drug-related problems. Another open question is the differential activation of synaptic versus extrasynaptic receptors, though it is open to discussion whether this can be achieved at all with any BZ ligand.

As reviewed elsewhere, genetic variations of the $GABA_A$ receptor subunit may affect the susceptibility to many neuropsychiatric diseases [88]. When we better understand the underlying, perhaps neuronal cell population–specific, pathophysiological mechanisms, we may be able to find a stronger rationale for developing improved BZ ligand–based therapeutics.

ACKNOWLEDGMENT

This work was supported by the Academy of Finland (ERK) and the Deutsche Forschungsgemeinschaft (HL).

REFERENCES

1. Sternbach, L. H. (1978). The benzodiazepine story. In *Progress in Drug Research*, J. Ernst, Ed. Birkhäuser Verlag, Basel, pp. 229–266.
2. Bosmann, H. B., Case, K. R., and DiStefano, P. (1977). Diazepam receptor characterization: Specific binding of a benzodiazepine to macromolecules in various areas of rat brain. *FEBS Lett.* 82(2), 368–372.
3. Möhler, H., and Okada, T. (1977). Benzodiazepine receptors: Demonstration in the central nervous system. *Science* 198, 849–851.
4. Squires, R. F., and Braestrup, C. (1977). Benzodiazepine receptors in the rat brain. *Nature* 266, 732–734.
5. Costa, E., et al. (1975). New concepts on the mechanism of action of benzodiazepines. *Life Sci.* 17, 167–186.
6. Haefely, W., et al. (1975). Possible involvement of GABA in the central actions of benzodiazepines. In *Mechanism of Action of Benzodiazepines*. E. Costa, and P. Greengard, Eds. Raven, New York, pp. 131–151.
7. Gavish, M., and Snyder, S. H. (1980). Benzodiazepine recognition sites on GABA receptors. *Nature* 287, 651–652.
8. Karobath, M., Sperk, G., and Schonbeck, G. (1978). Evidence for an endogenous factor interfering with ^{3}H-diazepam binding to rat brain membranes. *Eur. J. Pharmacol.* 49, 323–326.
9. Tallman, J. F., Thomas, J. W., and Gallager, D. W. (1978). GABAergic modulation of benzodiazepine binding site sensitivity. *Nature* 288, 609–610.
10. Sigel, E., et al. (1983). A γ-aminobutyric acid/benzodiazepine receptor complex of bovine cerebral cortex. *J. Biol. Chem.* 258(11), 6965–6971.
11. Sieghart, W., and Karobath, M. (1980). Molecular heterogeneity of benzodiazepine receptors. *Nature* 286, 285–287.
12. Syapin, P. J., and Skolnick, P. (1979). Characterization of benzodiazepine binding sites in cultured cells of neuronal origin. *J. Neurochem.* 32, 1047–1051.

13. Marangos, P. J., et al. (1982). Characterization of peripheral-type benzodiazepine binding sites in brain using [^{3}H]Ro 5-4864. *Mol. Pharmacol.* 22, 26–32.

14. Paul, S., Marangos, P., and Skolnick, P. (1981). The benzodiazepine-GABA-chloride-ionophore receptor complex: Common site of minor tranquilizer action. *Biol. Psychiatry* 16, 213–229.

15. Schoemaker, H., et al. (1983). Specific, high-affinity binding sites for [^{3}H]Ro 5-4864 in rat brain and kidney. *J. Pharmacol. Exp. Ther.* 225, 61–69.

16. Lueddens, H. W., and Skolnick, P. (1987). "Peripheral"-type benzodiazepine receptors in the kidney: Regulation of radioligand binding by anions and DIDS. *Eur. J. Pharmacol.* 133(2), 205–214.

17. Richards, J. G., and Möhler, H. (1984). Benzodiazepine receptors. *Neuropharmacology* 23(2B), 233–242.

18. Anholt, R. R., et al. (1986). The peripheral-type benzodiazepine receptor. Localization to the mitochondrial outer membrane. *J. Biol. Chem.* 261(2), 576–583.

19. Papadopoulos, V., et al. (1990). The peripheral-type benzodiazepine receptor is functionally linked to Leydig cell steroidogenesis. *J. Biol. Chem.* 265(7), 3772–3779.

20. Papadopoulos, V., Nowzari, F. B., and Krueger, K. E. (1991). Hormone-stimulated steroidogenesis is coupled to mitochondrial benzodiazepine receptors. Tropic hormone action on steroid biosynthesis is inhibited by flunitrazepam. *J. Biol. Chem.* 266(6), 3682–3687.

21. Lacapere, J. J., and Papadopoulos, V. (2003). Peripheral-type benzodiazepine receptor: Structure and function of a cholesterol-binding protein in steroid and bile acid biosynthesis. *Steroids* 68(7/8), 569–585.

22. Salva, P., and Costa, J. (1995). Clinical pharmacokinetics and pharmacodynamics of zolpidem. Therapeutic implications. *Clin. Pharmacokinet.* 29(3), 142–153.

23. Besset, A., et al. (1995). Effects of zolpidem on the architecture and cyclical structure of sleep in poor sleepers. *Drugs Exp. Clin. Res.* 21(4), 161–169.

24. Terzano, M. G., and Parrino, L. (1995). Effect of hypnotic drugs on sleep architecture. *Pol. J. Pharmacol.* 46(5), 487–490.

25. Roth, T., Roehrs, T., and Vogel, G. (1995). Zolpidem in the treatment of transient insomnia: A double-blind, randomized comparison with placebo. *Sleep* 18(4), 246–251.

26. Drover, D. R. (2004). Comparative pharmacokinetics and pharmacodynamics of short-acting hypnosedatives: Zaleplon, zolpidem and zopiclone. *Clin. Pharmacokinet.* 43(4), 227–238.

27. Skolnick, P., et al. (1979). CNS benzodiazepine receptors: Physiological studies and putative endogenous ligands. *Pharmacol. Biochem. Behav.* 10(5), 815–823.

28. Haefely, W. (1988). Endogenous ligands of the benzodiazepine receptor. *Pharmacopsychiatry* 21(1), 43–46.

29. Davis, L. G., Manning, R. W., and Dawson, W. E. (1984). Putative endogenous ligands to the benzodiazepine receptor: What can they tell us? *Drug Dev. Res.* 4(1), 31–37.

30. Sangameswaran, L., and de Blas, A. L. (1985). Demonstration of benzodiazepine-like molecules in the mammalian brain with a monoclonal antibody to benzodiazepines. *Proc. Natl. Acad. Sci. USA* 82(16), 5560–5564.

31. Sangameswaran, L., et al. (1986). Purification of a benzodiazepine from bovine brain and detection of benzodiazepine-like immunoreactivity in human brain. *Proc. Natl. Acad. Sci. USA* 83(23), 9236–9240.

32. Pena, C., et al. (1986). Isolation and identification in bovine cerebral cortex of N-butyl β-carboline-3-carboxylate, a potent benzodiazepine binding inhibitor. *Proc. Natl. Acad. Sci. USA* 83(13), 4952–4956.
33. Braestrup, C., Nielsen, M., and Olsen, C. E. (1980). Urinary and brain β-carboline-3-carboxylates as potent inhibitors of brain benzodiazepine receptors. *Proc. Natl. Acad. Sci. USA* 77(4), 2288–2292.
34. Nielsen, M., and Braestrup, C. (1980). Ethyl β-carboline-3-carboxylate shows differential benzodiazepine receptor interaction. *Nature* 286, 606–607.
35. Guidotti, A., et al. (1983). Isolation, characterization, and purification to homogeneity of an endogenous polypeptide with agonistic action on benzodiazepine receptors. *Proc. Natl. Acad. Sci. USA* 80(11), 3531–3535.
36. Alho, H., et al. (1987). Studies of a brain polypeptide functioning as a putative endogenous ligand to benzodiazepine recognition sites in rats selectively bred for alcohol related behavior. *Alcohol Alcohol Suppl.* 1, 637–641.
37. Costa, E., and Guidotti, A. (1991). Diazepam binding inhibitor (DBI): A peptide with multiple biological actions. *Life Sci.* 49(5), 325–344.
38. Alho, H., Varga, V., and Krueger, K. E. (1994). Expression of mitochondrial benzodiazepine receptor and its putative endogenous ligand diazepam binding inhibitor in cultured primary astrocytes and C-6 cells: Relation to cell growth. *Cell Growth Differ.* 5(9), 1005–1014.
39. Alho, H., et al. (1995). Increased expression of diazepam binding inhibitor in human brain tumors. *Cell Growth Differ.* 6(3), 309–314.
40. Mogensen, I. B., et al. (1987). A novel acyl-CoA-binding protein from bovine liver. Effect on fatty acid synthesis. *Biochem. J.* 241(1), 189–192.
41. Knudsen, J., and Nielsen, M. (1990). Diazepam-binding inhibitor: A neuropeptide and/or an acyl-CoA ester binding protein? *Biochem. J.* 265(3), 927–929.
42. Swinnen, J. V., et al. (1998). Identification of diazepam-binding inhibitor/acyl-CoA-binding protein as a sterol regulatory element-binding protein-responsive gene. *J. Biol. Chem.* 273(32), 19938–19944.
43. Papadopoulos, V., et al. (1991). Diazepam binding inhibitor and its processing products stimulate mitochondrial steroid biosynthesis via an interaction with mitochondrial benzodiazepine receptors. *Endocrinology* 129(3), 1481–1488.
44. Papadopoulos, V., Berkovich, A., and Krueger, K. E. (1991). The role of diazepam binding inhibitor and its processing products at mitochondrial benzodiazepine receptors: Regulation of steroid biosynthesis. *Neuropharmacology* 30(12B), 1417–1423.
45. Meier, R., and Gyr, K. (1988). Treatment of hepatic encephalopathy (HE) with the benzodiazepine antagonist flumazenil: A pilot study. *Eur. J. Anaesthesiol. Suppl.* 2(139), 139–146.
46. Grimm, G., et al. (1988). Improvement of hepatic encephalopathy treated with flumazenil. *Lancet* 2(8625), 1392–1394.
47. Goulenok, C., et al. (2002). Flumazenil vs. placebo in hepatic encephalopathy in patients with cirrhosis: A meta-analysis. *Aliment. Pharmacol. Ther.* 16(3), 361–372.
48. Als-Nielsen, B., Gluud, L. L., and Gluud, C. (2004). Benzodiazepine receptor antagonists for hepatic encephalopathy. *Cochrane Database Syst. Rev.* 2004(2), CD002798.
49. Olasmaa, M., et al. (1990). Endogenous benzodiazepine receptor ligands in human and animal hepatic encephalopathy. *J. Neurochem.* 55(6), 2015–2023.

50. Rothstein, J. D., et al. (1989). Cerebrospinal fluid content of diazepam binding inhibitor in chronic hepatic encephalopathy. *Ann. Neurol.* 26(1), 57–62.
51. Butterworth, R. F., et al. (1991). Increased brain content of the endogenous benzodiazepine receptor ligand, octadecaneuropeptide (ODN), following portacaval anastomosis in the rat. *Peptides* 12(1), 119–125.
52. Basile, A. S., et al. (1990). The GABA$_A$ receptor complex in hepatic encephalopathy. Autoradiographic evidence for the presence of elevated levels of a benzodiazepine receptor ligand. *Neuropsychopharmacology* 3(1), 61–71.
53. Ruscito, B. J., and Harrison, N. L. (2003). Hemoglobin metabolites mimic benzodiazepines and are possible mediators of hepatic encephalopathy. *Blood* 102(4), 1525–1528.
54. Verma, A., Nye, J. S., and Snyder, S. H. (1987). Porphyrins are endogenous ligands for the mitochondrial (peripheral-type) benzodiazepine receptor. *Proc. Natl. Acad. Sci. USA* 84(8), 2256–2260.
55. Study, R. E., and Barker, J. L. (1981). Diazepam and ($-$)-pentobarbital: Fluctuation analysis reveals different mechanisms for potentiation of γ-aminobutyric acid responses in cultured central neurons. *Proc. Natl. Acad. Sci. USA* 78, 7180–7184.
56. MacDonald, R. L., and Olsen, R. W. (1994). GABA$_A$ Receptor channels. *Annu. Rev. Neurosci.* 17, 569–602.
57. MacDonald, R. L., and Twyman, R. E. (1992). Kinetic properties and regulation of GABA$_A$ receptor channels. *Ion Channels* 3, 315–343.
58. Rogers, C. J., Twyman, R. E., and Macdonald, R. L. (1994). Benzodiazepine and β-carboline regulation of single GABA$_A$ receptor channels of mouse spinal neurones in culture. *J. Physiol. London* 475(1), 69–82.
59. Belelli, D., et al. (2005). Extrasynaptic GABA$_A$ receptors of thalamocortical neurons: A molecular target for hypnotics. *J. Neurosci.* 25(50), 11513–11520.
60. Cope, D. W., Hughes, S. W., and Crunelli, V. (2005). GABA$_A$ receptor-mediated tonic inhibition in thalamic neurons. *J. Neurosci.* 25(50), 11553–11563.
61. Nusser, Z., Cull-Candy, S., and Farrant, M. (1997). Differences in synaptic GABA(A) receptor number underlie variation in GABA mini amplitude. *Neuron* 19(3), 697–709.
62. Lindquist, C. E., Ebert, B., and Birnir, B. (2003). Extrasynaptic GABA$_A$ channels activated by THIP are modulated by diazepam in CA1 pyramidal neurons in the rat brain hippocampal slice. *Mol. Cell Neurosci.* 24(1), 250–257.
63. Farrant, M., and Nusser, Z. (2005). Variations on an inhibitory theme: Phasic and tonic activation of GABA$_A$ receptors. *Nat. Rev. Neurosci.* 6(3), 215–229.
64. Koob, G. F., and Le Moal, M. (2006). *Neurobiology of Addiction*. Elsevier, London.
65. Ikemoto, S. (2005). The supramammillary nucleus mediates primary reinforcement via GABA$_A$ receptors. *Neuropsychopharmacology* 30(6), 1088–1095.
66. Laviolette, S. R., and van der Kooy, D. (2001). GABA$_A$ receptors in the ventral tegmental area control bidirectional reward signalling between dopaminergic and non-dopaminergic neural motivational systems. *Eur. J. Neurosci.* 13(5), 1009–1015.
67. Laviolette, S. R., and van der Kooy, D. (2004). GABA$_A$ receptors signal bidirectional reward transmission from the ventral tegmental area to the tegmental pedunculopontine nucleus as a function of opiate state. *Eur. J. Neurosci.* 20(8), 2179–2187.
68. Hutchinson, M. A., Smith, P. F., and Darlington, C. L. (1996). The behavioural and neuronal effects of the chronic administration of benzodiazepine anxiolytic and hypnotic drugs. *Prog. Neurobiol.* 49(1), 73–97.

69. Bateson, A. N. (2002). Basic pharmacologic mechanisms involved in benzodiazepine tolerance and withdrawal. *Curr. Pharm. Des.* 8(1), 5–21.
70. Pratt, J. A., Brett, R. R., and Laurie, D. J. (1998). Benzodiazepine dependence: From neural circuits to gene expression. *Pharmacol. Biochem. Behav.* 59(4), 925–934.
71. Gallager, D. W., et al. (1984). Chronic benzodiazepine treatment decreases postsynaptic GABA sensitivity. *Nature* 308(5954), 74–77.
72. Holt, R. A., Bateson, A. N., and Martin, I. L. (1999). Decreased GABA enhancement of benzodiazepine binding after a single dose of diazepam. *J. Neurochem.* 72(5), 2219–2222.
73. Pesold, C., et al. (1997). Tolerance to diazepam and changes in $GABA_A$ receptor subunit expression in rat neocortical areas. *Neuroscience* 79(2), 477–487.
74. Tanay, V. M., et al. (2001). Common effects of chronically administered antipanic drugs on brainstem $GABA_A$ receptor subunit gene expression. *Mol. Psychiatry* 6(4), 404–412.
75. van Rijnsoever, C., et al. (2004). Requirement of α5-$GABA_A$ receptors for the development of tolerance to the sedative action of diazepam in mice. *J. Neurosci.* 24(30), 6785–6790.
76. Li, M., Szabo, A., and Rosenberg, H. C. (2000). Down-regulation of benzodiazepine binding to α5 subunit-containing γ-aminobutyric $acid_A$ receptors in tolerant rat brain indicates particular involvement of the hippocampal CA1 region. *J. Pharmacol. Exp. Ther.* 295(2), 689–696.
77. Huopaniemi, L., et al. (2004). Diazepam-induced adaptive plasticity revealed by α1 $GABA_A$ receptor-specific expression profiling. *J. Neurochem.* 88(5), 1059–1067.
78. Izzo, E., et al. (2001). Glutamic acid decarboxylase and glutamate receptor changes during tolerance and dependence to benzodiazepines. *Proc. Natl. Acad. Sci. USA* 98(6), 3483–3488.
79. van Sickle, B. J., Xiang, K., and Tietz, E. I. (2004). Transient plasticity of hippocampal CA1 neuron glutamate receptors contributes to benzodiazepine withdrawal-anxiety. *Neuropsychopharmacology* 29(11), 1994–2006.
80. van Sickle, B. J., and Tietz, E. I. (2002). Selective enhancement of AMPA receptor-mediated function in hippocampal CA1 neurons from chronic benzodiazepine-treated rats. *Neuropharmacology* 43(1), 11–27.
81. Fitzgerald, L. W., et al. (1996). Drugs of abuse and stress increase the expression of GluR1 and NMDAR1 glutamate receptor subunits in the rat ventral tegmental area: Common adaptations among cross-sensitizing agents. *J. Neurosci.* 16(1), 274–282.
82. Lu, W., and Wolf, M. E. (1999). Repeated amphetamine administration alters AMPA receptor subunit expression in rat nucleus accumbens and medial prefrontal cortex. *Synapse* 32(2), 119–131.
83. Zhang, X. F., et al. (1997). Increased responsiveness of ventral tegmental area dopamine neurons to glutamate after repeated administration of cocaine or amphetamine is transient and selectively involves AMPA receptors. *J. Pharmacol. Exp. Ther.* 281(2), 699–706.
84. Carlezon, W. A., Jr., and Nestler, E. J. (2002). Elevated levels of GluR1 in the midbrain: A trigger for sensitization to drugs of abuse. *Trends Neurosci.* 25(12), 610–615.
85. Haefely, W., Martin, J. R., and Schoch, P. (1990). Novel anxiolytics that act as partial agonists at benzodiazepine receptors. *Trends Pharmacol. Sci.* 11, 452–456.
86. Doble, A., and Martin, I. L. (1992). Multiple benzodiazepine receptors: No reason for anxiety. *Trends Pharmacol. Sci.* 13(2), 76–81.

87. Costa, E., and Guidotti, A. (1996). Benzodiazepines on trial: A research strategy for their rehabilitation. *Trends Pharmacol. Sci.* 17(5), 192–200.
88. Korpi, E. R., and Sinkkonen, S. T. (2006). $GABA_A$ receptor subtypes as targets for neuropsychiatric drug development. *Pharmacol. Ther.* 109, 12–32.
89. Chouinard, G., Lefko-Singh, K., and Teboul, E. (1999). Metabolism of anxiolytics and hypnotics: Benzodiazepines, buspirone, zoplicone, and zolpidem. *Cell. Mol. Neurobiol.* 19(4), 533–552.
90. Dresser, G. K., Spence, J. D., and Bailey, D. G. (2000). Pharmacokinetic-pharmacodynamic consequences and clinical relevance of cytochrome P450 3A4 inhibition. *Clin. Pharmacokinet.* 38(1), 41–57.
91. Hesse, L. M., et al. (2001). CYP3A4 is the major CYP isoform mediating the in vitro hydroxylation and demethylation of flunitrazepam. *Drug Metab. Dispos.* 29(2), 133–140.
92. Tanaka, E. (1999). Clinically significant pharmacokinetic drug interactions with benzodiazepines. *J. Clin. Pharm. Ther.* 24(5), 347–355.
93. Backman, J. T., et al. (1998). The area under the plasma concentration-time curve for oral midazolam is 400-fold larger during treatment with itraconazole than with rifampicin. *Eur. J. Clin. Pharmacol.* 54(1), 53–58.
94. Barnard, E.A., et al. (1998). International union of pharmacology. XV. Subtypes of γ-aminobutyric acid$_A$ receptors: Classification on the basis of subunit structure and receptor function. *Pharmacol. Rev.* 50(2), 291–313.
95. Bonnert, T. P., et al. (1999). θ, a novel γ-aminobutyric acid type$_A$ receptor subunit. *Proc. Natl. Acad. Sci. USA* 96(17), 9891–9896.
96. Sinkkonen, S. T., et al. (2000). $GABA_A$ receptor ε and θ subunits display unusual structural variation between species and are enriched in the rat locus ceruleus. *J. Neurosci.* 20(10), 3588–3595.
97. Johnston, G. A., et al. (1975). Cis- and trans-4-aminocrotonic acid as GABA analogues of restricted conformation. *J. Neurochem.* 24(1), 157–160.
98. Nistri, A., and Sivilotti, L. (1985). An unusual effect of γ-aminobutyric acid on synaptic transmission of frog tectal neurones in vitro. *Br. J. Pharmacol.* 85(4), 917–921.
99. Herb, A., et al. (1992). The third γ subunit of the γ-aminobutyric acid type A receptor family. *Proc. Natl. Acad. Sci. USA* 89(12), 1433–1437.
100. Xu, M., and Akabas, M. H. (1996). Identification of channel-lining residues in the M2 membrane-spanning segment of the $GABA_A$ receptor α1 subunit. *J. Gen. Physiol.* 107(2), 195–205.
101. Lüddens, H., and Korpi, E. R. (1995). GABA antagonists differentiate between recombinant $GABA_A$/benzodiazepine receptor subtypes. *J. Neurosci.* 15(10), 6957–6962.
102. Pritchett, D. B., et al. (1989). Importance of a novel $GABA_A$ receptor subunit for benzodiazepine pharmacology. *Nature* 338(6216), 582–585.
103. Pritchett, D. B., and Seeburg, P. H. (1990). γ-Aminobutyric acid$_A$ receptor α$_5$-subunit creates novel type II benzodiazepine receptor pharmacology. *J. Neurochem.* 54(5), 1802–1804.
104. Lüddens, H., Seeburg, P. H., and Korpi, E.R. (1994). Impact of β and γ variants on ligand-binding properties of γ-aminobutyric acid type A receptors. *Mol. Pharmacol.* 45(5), 810–814.
105. Korpi, E. R., Gründer, G., and Lüddens, H. (2002). Drug interactions in $GABA_A$ receptors. *Prog. Neurobiol.* 67(2), 113–159.

106. Korpi, E. R., and Lüddens, H. (1997). Furosemide interactions with brain GABA$_A$ receptors. *Br. J. Pharmacol.* 120, 741–748.

107. Hevers, W., and Lüddens, H. (2002). Pharmacological heterogeneity of γ-aminobutyric acid receptors during development suggests distinct classes of rat cerebellar granule cells in situ. *Neuropharmacology* 42(1), 34–47.

108. Pritchett, D. B., Lüddens, H., and Seeburg, P. H. (1989). Type I and type II GABA$_A$-benzodiazepine receptors produced in transfected cells. *Science* 245(4924), 1389–1392.

109. Hadingham, K. L., et al. (1993). Role of the β subunit in determining the pharmacology of human γ-aminobutyric acid type A receptors. *Mol. Pharmacol.* 44(6), 1211–1218; correction (1994) 46(1), 211.

110. Puia, G., et al. (1992). Molecular mechanisms of the partial allosteric modulatory effects of bretazenil at γ-aminobutyric acid type A receptor. *Proc. Natl. Acad. Sci. USA* 89(8), 3620–3624.

111. Sigel, E., et al. (1990). The effect of subunit composition of rat brain GABA$_A$ receptors on channel function. *Neuron* 5(5), 703–711.

112. Laurie, D. J., Seeburg, P. H., and Wisden, W. (1992). The distribution of 13 GABA$_A$ receptor subunit mRNAs in the rat brain. II. Olfactory bulb and cerebellum. *J. Neurosci.* 12(3), 1063–1076.

113. Wisden, W., et al. (1992). The distribution of 13 GABA$_A$ receptor subunit mRNAs in the rat brain. I. Telencephalon, diencephalon, mesencephalon. *J. Neurosci.* 12(3), 1040–1062.

114. Slany, A., et al. (1995). Rat β3 subunits expressed in human embryonic kidney 293 cells form high affinity [^{35}S]t-butylbicyclophosphorothionate binding sites modulated by several allosteric ligands of γ-aminobutyric acid type A receptors. *Mol. Pharmacol.* 48(3), 385–391.

115. Unwin, N. (1995). Acetylcholine receptor channel imaged in the open state. *Nature* 373, 37–43.

116. Unwin, N. (1993). Nicotinic acetylcholine receptor at 9 Å resolution. *J. Mol. Biol.* 229(4), 1101–1124.

117. Horenstein, J., et al. (2001). Protein mobility and GABA-induced conformational changes in GABA$_A$ receptor pore-lining M2 segment. *Nat. Neurosci.* 4(5), 477–485.

118. Hevers, W., and Lüddens, H. (1998). The diversity of GABA$_A$ receptors. Pharmacological and electrophysiological properties of GABA$_A$ channel subtypes. *Mol. Neurobiol.* 18(1), 35–86.

119. Twyman, R. E., Rogers, C. J., and Macdonald, R. L. (1989). Pentobarbital and picrotoxin have reciprocal actions on single GABA$_A$ receptor channels. *Neurosci. Lett.* 96(1), 89–95.

120. Xu, M., Covey, D. F., and Akabas, M. H. (1995). Interaction of picrotoxin with GABA$_A$ receptor channel-lining residues probed in cysteine mutants. *Biophys. J.* 69(5), 1858–1867.

121. Schofield, P. R., et al. (1987). Sequence and functional expression of the GABA$_A$ receptor shows a ligand-gated receptor super-family. *Nature* 328(6127), 221–227.

122. Sigel, E., et al. (1992). Point mutations affecting antagonist affinity and agonist dependent gating of GABA$_A$ receptor channels. *EMBO J.* 11(6), 2017–2023.

123. Smith, G. B., and Olsen, R. W. (1994). Identification of a [^{3}H]muscimol photoaffinity substrate in the bovine γ-aminobutyric acid$_A$ receptor α subunit. *J. Biol. Chem.* 269(32), 20380–20387.

124. Boileau, A. J., et al. (1999). Mapping the agonist binding site of the GABA$_A$ receptor: Evidence for a β-strand. *J. Neurosci.* 19(12), 4847–4854.

125. Hartvig, L., et al. (2000). Two conserved arginines in the extracellular *N*-terminal domain of the GABA$_A$ receptor α5 subunit are crucial for receptor function. *J. Neurosci.* 75(4), 1746–1753.

126. Westh-Hansen, S. E., et al. (1999). Arginine residue 120 of the human GABA$_A$ receptor α1, subunit is essential for GABA binding and chloride ion current gating. *Neuroreport* 10(11), 2417–2421.

127. Bonetti, E. P., et al. (1989). Ro 15-4513: Partial inverse agonism at the BZR and interactions with ethanol. *Pharmacol. Biochem. Behav.* 31(3), 733–749.

128. Lüddens, H., et al. (1990). Cerebellar GABA$_A$ receptor selective for a behavioural alcohol antagonist. *Nature* 346(6285), 648–651.

129. Korpi, E. R., and Seeburg, P. H. (1993). Natural mutation of GABA$_A$ receptor α6 subunit alters benzodiazepine affinity but not allosteric GABA effects. *Eur. J. Pharmacol.* 247(1), 23–27.

130. Wafford, K. A., et al. (1993). Functional comparison of the role of γ subunits in recombinant human γ-aminobutyric acid$_A$/benzodiazepine receptors. *Mol. Pharmacol.* 44(2), 437–442.

131. Knoflach, F., et al. (1996). Pharmacological modulation of the diazepam-insensitive recombinant γ-aminobutyric acid$_A$ receptors α4β2γ2 and α6β2γ2. *Mol. Pharmacol.* 50(5), 1253–1261.

132. Kleingoor, C., et al. (1991). Inverse but not full benzodiazepine agonists modulate recombinant α6β2γ2 GABA$_A$ receptors in transfected human embryonic kidney cells. *Neurosci. Lett.* 130(2), 169–172.

133. Dunn, S. M., et al. (1999). Mutagenesis of the rat α1 subunit of the γ-aminobutyric acid$_A$ receptor reveals the importance of residue 101 in determining the allosteric effects of benzodiazepine site ligands. *Mol. Pharmacol.* 56(4), 768–774.

134. Pritchett, D. B., and Seeburg, P. H. (1991). γ-Aminobutyric acid type A receptor point mutation increases the affinity of compounds for the benzodiazepine site. *Proc. Natl. Acad. Sci. USA* 88(4), 1421–1425.

135. Casula, M. A., et al. (2001). Identification of amino acid residues responsible for the α5 subunit binding selectivity of L-655,708, a benzodiazepine binding site ligand at the GABA$_A$ receptors. *J. Neurochem.* 77(2), 445–451.

136. Buhr, A., Baur, R., and Sigel, E. (1997). Subtle changes in residue 77 of the γ subunit of α1β2γ2 GABA$_A$ receptors drastically alter the affinity for ligands of the benzodiazepine binding site. *J. Biol. Chem.* 272(18), 11799–11804.

137. Wieland, H. A., and Lüddens, H. (1994). Four amino acid exchanges convert a diazepam-insensitive, inverse agonist-preferring GABA$_A$ receptor into a diazepam-preferring GABA$_A$ receptor. *J. Med. Chem.* 37(26), 4576–4580.

138. Wieland, H., Lüddens, H., and Seeburg, P. H. (1992). A single histidine in GABA$_A$ receptors is essential for benzodiazepine agonist binding. *J. Biol. Chem.* 267(3), 1426–1429.

139. Kleingoor, C., et al. (1993). Current potentiation by diazepam but not GABA sensitivity is determined by a single histidine residue. *Neuroreport* 4(2), 187–190.

140. Eriksson, K., and Rusi, M. (1981). Finnish selection studies on alcohol-related behaviors: General outline, NIAAA Research Monograph 6. In *Development Animal Models as Pharmacogenetic Tools.* G. E. McClearn, R. A. Deitrich, and G. Erwin, Ed. U.S. Government Printing Office, Washington, DC, pp. 87–117.

141. Arvola, A., Sammalisto, L., and Wallgren, H. (1958). A test for level of alcohol intoxication in the rat. *Q. J. Stud. Alcohol* 19(4), 563–572.

142. Hellevuo, K., Kiianmaa, K., and Korpi, E. R. (1989). Effect of GABAergic drugs on motor impairment from ethanol, barbital and lorazepam in rat lines selected for differential sensitivity to ethanol. *Pharmacol. Biochem. Behav.* 34, 399–404.

143. Yildirim, Y., et al. (1997). Propofol induced ataxia hypnosis in rat lines selected for differential alcohol sensitivity. *Pharmacol. Toxicol.* 80(1), 44–48.

144. Toropainen, M., et al. (1997). Behavioral sensitivity and ethanol potentiation of the N-methyl-D-aspartate receptor antagonist MK-801 in a rat line selected for high ethanol sensitivity. *Alcohol Clin. Exp. Res.* 21(4), 666–671.

145. Korpi, E. R., et al. (2001). Increased behavioral neurosteroid sensitivity in a rat line selectively bred for high alcohol sensitivity. *Eur. J. Pharmacol.* 421(1), 31–38.

146. Malminen, O., and Korpi, E. R. (1988). GABA/benzodiazepine receptor/chloride ionophore complex in brains of rat lines selectively bred for differences in ethanol-induced motor impairment. *Alcohol* 5(3), 239–249; 5(6), 523.

147. Uusi-Oukari, M., and Korpi, E. R. (1992). Functional properties of $GABA_A$ receptors in two rat lines selected for high and low alcohol sensitivity. *Alcohol* 9(3), 261–269.

148. Uusi-Oukari, M., and Korpi, E. R. (1990). Diazepam sensitivity of an imidazobenzodiazepine, [^{3}H]Ro 15-4513, in cerebellar membranes from two rat lines developed for high and low alcohol sensitivity. *J. Neurochem.* 54, 1980–1987.

149. Uusi-Oukari, M., and Korpi, E. R. (1991). Specific alterations in the cerebellar $GABA_A$ receptors of an alcohol-sensitive ANT rat line. *Alcohol Clin. Exp. Res.* 15(2), 241–248.

150. Korpi, E. R., et al. (1993). Benzodiazepine-induced motor impairment linked to point mutation in cerebellar $GABA_A$ receptor. *Nature* 361(6410), 356–359.

151. Vekovischeva, O. Y., et al. (1999). Cerebellar $GABA_A$ receptors and anxiolytic action of diazepam. *Brain Res.* 837(1/2), 184–187.

152. Sarviharju, M., and Korpi, E. R. (1993). Ethanol sensitivity and consumption in F2 hybrid crosses of ANT and AT rats. *Alcohol* 10(5), 415–418.

153. Saba, L., et al. (2001). The R100Q mutation of the $GABA_A$ α6 receptor subunit may contribute to voluntary aversion to ethanol in the sNP rat line. *Brain Res. Mol. Brain Res.* 87(2), 263–270.

154. Wallner, M., Hanchar, H. J., and Olsen, R. W. (2003). Ethanol enhances α4β3δ and α6β3δ γ-aminobutyric acid type A receptors at low concentrations known to affect humans. *Proc. Natl. Acad. Sci. USA* 100(25), 15218–15223.

155. Mihic, S. J., et al. (1994). A single amino acid of the human γ-aminobutyric acid type A receptor γ2 subunit determines benzodiazepine efficacy. *J. Biol. Chem.* 269(52), 32768–32773.

156. Wingrove, P. B., et al. (1997). Key amino acids in the γ subunit of the γ-aminobutyric $acid_A$ receptor that determine ligand binding and modulation at the benzodiazepine site. *Mol. Pharmacol.* 52(5), 874–881.

157. Amin, J., and Weiss, D. S. (1993). $GABA_A$ receptor needs two homologous domains of the β-subunit for activation by GABA but not by pentobarbital. *Nature* 366(6455), 565–569.

158. Amin, J., Brooks Kayal, A., and Weiss, D. S. (1997). Two tyrosine residues on the α subunit are crucial for benzodiazepine binding and allosteric modulation of γ-aminobutyric $acid_A$ receptors. *Mol. Pharmacol.* 51(5), 833–841.

159. Jones-Davis, D. M., et al. (2005). Structural determinants of benzodiazepine allosteric regulation of $GABA_A$ receptor currents. *J. Neurosci.* 25(35), 8056–8065.

160. Stevenson, A., et al. (1995). β-Carboline γ-aminobutyric acid$_A$ receptor inverse agonists modulate γ-aminobutyric acid via the loreclezole binding site as well as the benzodiazepine site. *Mol. Pharmacol.* 48(6), 965–969.
161. Saxena, N. C., and Macdonald, R. L. (1996). Properties of putative cerebellar γ-aminobutyric acid$_A$ receptor isoforms. *Mol. Pharmacol.* 49(3), 567–579.
162. Wingrove, P. B., et al. (1994). The modulatory action of loreclezole at the γ-aminobutyric acid type A receptor is determined by a single amino acid in the β$_2$ and β$_3$ subunit. *Proc. Natl. Acad. Sci. USA* 91(10), 4569–4573.
163. Mäkelä, R., et al. (1997). Cerebellar γ-aminobutyric acid type a receptors: Pharmacological subtypes revealed by mutant mouse lines. *Mol. Pharmacol.* 52(3), 380–388.
164. Leppa, E., et al. (2005). Agonistic effects of the β-carboline DMCM revealed in GABA$_A$ receptor γ2 subunit F77I point-mutated mice. *Neuropharmacology* 48(4), 469–478.
165. Walters, R. J., et al. (2000). Benzodiazepines act an GABA$_A$ receptors via two distinct and separable mechanisms. *Nat. Neurosci.* 3(12), 1274–1281.
166. Korpi, E. R., et al. (1994). Small *N*-terminal deletion by splicing in cerebellar α6 subunit abolishes GABA$_A$ receptor function. *J. Neurochem.* 63(3), 1167–1170.
167. Taylor, P. M., et al. (2000). Identification of residues within GABA$_A$ receptor α subunits that mediate specific assembly with receptor β subunits. *J. Neurosci.* 20(4), 1297–1306.
168. Enz, R., and Cutting, G. R. (1999). Identification of 70 amino acids important for GABA$_C$ receptor ρ1 sub-unit assembly. *Brain Res.* 846(2), 177–185.
169. Klausberger, T., et al. (2000). GABA$_A$ receptor assembly. Identification and structure of γ2 sequences forming the intersubunit contacts with α1 and β3 subunits. *J. Biol. Chem.* 275(12), 8921–8928.
170. Klausberger, T., et al. (2001). Alternate use of distinct intersubunit contacts controls GABA$_A$ receptor assembly and stoichiometry. *J. Neurosci.* 21(23), 9124–9133.
171. Smit, A.B., et al. (2001). A glia-derived acetylcholine-binding protein that modulates synaptic transmission. *Nature* 411(6835), 261–268.
172. Brejc, K., et al. (2001). Crystal structure of an ACh-binding protein reveals the ligand-binding domain of nicotinic receptors. *Nature* 411(6835), 269–276.
173. Tretter, V., et al. (1997). Stoichiometry and assembly of a recombinant GABA$_A$ receptor subtype. *J. Neurosci.* 17(8), 2728–2737.
174. Hevers, W., Korpi, E. R., and Lüddens, H. (2000). Assembly of functional α6β3γ2δ GABA$_A$ receptors in vitro. *Neuroreport* 11(18), 4103–4106.
175. Chen, L., et al. (2000). The γ-aminobutyric acid type A (GABA$_A$) receptor-associated protein (GABARAP) promotes GABA$_A$ receptor clustering and modulates the channel kinetics. *Proc. Natl. Acad. Sci. USA* 97(21), 11557–11562.
176. Kneussel, M., and Betz, H. (2000). Receptors, gephyrin and gephyrin-associated proteins: Novel insights into the assembly of inhibitory postsynaptic membrane specializations. *J. Physiol.* 525(Pt. 1), 1–9.
177. Everitt, A. B., et al. (2004). Conductance of recombinant GABA channels is increased in cells co-expressing GABA$_A$ A receptor-associated protein. *J. Biol. Chem.* 279(21), 21701–21706.
178. Pfeiffer, F., Graham, D., and Betz, H. (1982). Purification by affinity chromatography of the glycine receptor of rat spinal cord. *J. Biol. Chem.* 257(16), 9389–9393.
179. Prior, P., et al. (1992). Primary structure and alternative splice variants of gephyrin, a putative glycine receptor-tubulin linker protein. *Neuron* 8(6), 1161–1170.

180. Feng, G., et al. (1998). Dual requirement for gephyrin in glycine receptor clustering and molybdoenzyme activity. *Science* 282(5392), 1321–1324.
181. Kneussel, M., et al. (1999). Loss of postsynaptic $GABA_A$ receptor clustering in gephyrin-deficient mice. *J. Neurosci.* 19(21), 9289–9297.
182. Craig, A. M., et al. (1996). Clustering of gephyrin at GABAergic but not glutamatergic synapses in cultured rat hippocampal neurons. *J. Neurosci.* 16(10), 3166–3177.
183. Essrich, C., et al. (1998). Postsynaptic clustering of major $GABA_A$ receptor subtypes requires the γ2 subunit and gephyrin. *Nat. Neurosci.* 1(7), 563–571.
184. Scotti, A. L., and Reuter, H. (2001). Synaptic and extrasynaptic γ-aminobutyric acid type A receptor clusters in rat hippocampal cultures during development. *Proc. Natl. Acad. Sci. USA* 98(6), 3489–3494.
185. Wang, H., et al. (1999). $GABA_A$-receptor-associated protein links $GABA_A$ receptors and the cytoskeleton. *Nature* 397(6714), 69–72.
186. Wang, H., and Olsen, R. W. (2000). Binding of the $GABA_A$ receptor-associated protein (GABARAP) to microtubules and microfilaments suggests involvement of the cytoskeleton in GABARAP-$GABA_A$ receptor interaction. *J. Neurochem.* 75(2), 644–655.
187. Kanematsu, T., et al. (2002). Role of the PLC-related, catalytically inactive protein p130 in $GABA_A$ receptor function. *EMBO J.* 21(5), 1004–1011.
188. O'Sullivan, G. A., et al. (2005). GABARAP is not essential for GABA receptor targeting to the synapse. *Eur. J. Neurosci.* 22(10), 2644–2648.
189. Bedford, F. K., et al. (2001). $GABA_A$ receptor cell surface number and subunit stability are regulated by the ubiquitin-like protein Plic-1. *Nat. Neurosci.* 4(9), 908–916.
190. Kittler, J. T., et al. (2000). Analysis of $GABA_A$ receptor assembly in mammalian cell lines and hippocampal neurons using γ2 subunit green fluorescent protein chimeras. *Mol. Cell. Neurosci.* 16(4), 440–452.
191. Cinar, H., and Barnes, E. M., 2001. Clathrin-independent endocytosis of $GABA_A$ receptors in HEK 293 cells. *Biochemistry* 40(46), 14030–14036.
192. Connolly, C. N., et al. (1996). Assembly and cell surface expression of heteromeric and homomeric γ-aminobutyric acid type A receptors. *J. Biol. Chem.* 271(1), 89–96.
193. Olsen, R. W., McCabe, R. T., and Wamsley, J. K. (1990). $GABA_A$ receptor subtypes: Autoradiographic comparison of GABA, benzodiazepine, and convulsant binding sites in the rat central nervous system. *J. Chem. Neuroanat.* 3(1), 59–76.
194. Shivers, B. D., et al. (1989). Two novel $GABA_A$ receptor subunits exist in distinct neuronal subpopulations. *Neuron* 3(3), 327–337.
195. Quirk, K., et al. (1995). Characterisation of δ-subunit containing $GABA_A$ receptors from rat brain. *Eur. J. Pharmacol. Mol. Pharmacol. Section* 290(3), 175–181.
196. Uusi-Oukari, M., et al. (2000). Long-range interactions in neuronal gene expression: Evidence from gene targeting in the $GABA_A$ receptor β2-α6-α1-γ2 subunit gene cluster. *Mol. Cell. Neurosci.* 16(1), 34–41.
197. Mihalek, R. M., et al. (1999). Attenuated sensitivity to neuroactive steroids in γ-aminobutyrate type A receptor δ subunit knockout mice. *Proc. Natl. Acad. Sci. USA* 96(22), 12905–12910.
198. Wisden, W., et al. (1991). Cloning, pharmacological characteristics and expression pattern of the rat $GABA_A$ receptor $α_4$ subunit. *FEBS Lett.* 289(2), 227–230.
199. Benke, D., Michel, C., and Mohler, H. (1997). $GABA_A$ receptors containing the α4 subunit: Prevalence, distribution, pharmacology, and subunit architecture in situ. *J. Neurochem.* 69(2), 806–814.

200. Gutierrez, A., Khan, Z. U., and De Blas, A. L. (1994). Immunocytochemical localization of γ2 short and γ2 long subunits of the GABA$_A$ receptor in the rat brain. *J. Neurosci.* 14(11 Pt. 2), 7168–7179.
201. Benke, D., et al. (1991). Immunochemical identification of the α1- and α3-subunits of the GABA$_A$-receptor in rat brain. *J. Recept. Res.* 11(1/4), 407–424.
202. Laurie, D. J., Wisden, W., and Seeburg, P. H. (1992). The distribution of thirteen GABA$_A$ receptor subunit mRNAs in the rat brain. III. Embryonic and postnatal development. *J. Neurosci.* 12(11), 4151–4172.
203. Fritschy, J. M., et al. (1992). Five subtypes of type A γ-aminobutyric acid receptors identified in neurons by double and triple immunofluorescence staining with subunit-specific antibodies. *Proc. Natl. Acad. Sci. USA* 89(15), 6726–6730.
204. Benke, D., et al. (1994). Distribution, prevalence, and drug binding profile of γ-aminobutyric acid type A receptor subtypes differing in the β-subunit variant. *J. Biol. Chem.* 269(43), 27100–27107.
205. Gao, B., et al. (1993). Neuron-specific expression of GABA$_A$ receptor subtypes: Differential association of the α1- and α3-subunits with serotonergic and GABAergic neurons. *Neuroscience* 54(4), 881–892.
206. Gao, B., and Fritschy, J. M. (1995). Cerebellar granule cells in vitro recapitulate the in vivo pattern of GABA$_A$-receptor subunit expression. *Dev. Brain Res.* 88(1), 1–16.
207. Poulter, M. O., et al. (1992). Differential and transient expression of GABA$_A$ receptor α-subunit mRNAs in the developing rat CNS. *J. Neurosci.* 12(8), 2888–2900.
208. Poulter, M. O., et al. (1993). Co-existent expression of GABA$_A$ receptor β2, β3 and γ2 subunit messenger RNAs during embryogenesis and early postnatal development of the rat central nervous system. *Neuroscience* 53(4), 1019–1033.
209. Fritschy, J. M., et al. (1994). Switch in the expression of rat GABA$_A$-receptor subtypes during postnatal development: An immunohistochemical study. *J. Neurosci.* 14(9), 5302–5324.
210. Günther, U., et al. (1995). Benzodiazepine-insensitive mice generated by targeted disruption of the γ2 subunit gene of γ-aminobutyric acid type A receptors. *Proc. Natl. Acad. Sci. USA* 92(17), 7749–7753.
211. Culiat, C. T., et al. (1995). Deficiency of the β3 subunit of the type A γ-aminobutyric acid receptor causes cleft palate in mice. *Nat. Genet.* 11(3), 344–346.
212. Lüddens, H., Killisch, I., and Seeburg, P. H. (1991). More than one alpha variant may exist in a GABA$_A$/benzodiazepine receptor complex. *J. Recept. Res.* 11(1–4), 535–551.
213. Benke, D., et al. (2004). Analysis of the presence and abundance of GABA$_A$ receptors containing two different types of α subunits in murine brain using point-mutated α subunits. *J. Biol. Chem.* 279(42), 43654–43660.
214. Fritschy, J. M., and Möhler, H. (1995). GABA$_A$-receptor heterogeneity in the adult rat brain: Differential regional and cellular distribution of seven major subunits. *J. Comp. Neurol.* 359(1), 154–194.
215. Arbilla, S., et al. (1986). High affinity [^{3}H]zolpidem binding in the rat brain: An imidazopyridine with agonist properties at central benzodiazepine receptors. *Eur. J. Pharmacol.* 130(3), 257–263.
216. Varecka, L., et al. (1994). GABA$_A$/benzodiazepine receptor α6 subunit mRNA in granule cells of the cerebellar cortex and cochlear nuclei: Expression in developing and mutant mice. *J. Comp. Neurol.* 339(3), 341–352.
217. Bahn, S., Jones, A., and Wisden, W. (1997). Directing gene expression to cerebellar granule cells using γ-aminobutyric acid type A receptor α6 subunit transgenes. *Proc. Natl. Acad. Sci. USA* 94(17), 9417–9421.

218. Zhang, J. H., Sato, M., and Tohyama, M. (1991). Region-specific expression of the mRNAs encoding β subunits (β1, β2, and β3) of GABA$_A$ receptor in the rat brain. *J. Comp. Neurol.* 303(4), 637–657.

219. Lolait, S. J., et al. (1989). Pharmacological characterization and region-specific expression in brain of the β2- and β3-subunits of the rat GABA$_A$ receptor. *FEBS Lett.* 258(1), 17–21.

220. Zdilar, D., et al. (1992). Differential expression of GABA$_A$/benzodiazepine receptor β1, β2, and β3 subunit mRNAs in the developing mouse cerebellum. *J. Comp. Neurol.* 326(4), 580–594.

221. Culiat, C. T., et al. (1993). Concordance between isolated cleft palate in mice and alterations within a region including the gene encoding the β3-subunit of the type A γ-aminobutyric acid receptor. *Proc. Natl. Acad. Sci. USA* 90(11), 5105–5109.

222. Takeno, S., Nakagawa, M., and Sakai, T. (1990). Teratogenic effects of nitrazepam in rats. *Res. Commun. Chem. Pathol. Pharmacol.* 69(1), 59–70.

223. Laegreid, L., et al. (1989). Teratogenic effects of benzodiazepine use during pregnancy. *J. Pediatr.* 114(1), 126–131.

224. Lin, A. E., et al. (2004). Clonazepam use in pregnancy and the risk of malformations. *Birth Defects Res. A Clin. Mol. Teratol.* 70(8), 534–536.

225. Eros, E., et al. (2002). A population-based case-control teratologic study of nitrazepam, medazepam, tofisopam, alprazolam and clonazepam treatment during pregnancy. *Eur. J. Obstet. Gynecol. Reprod. Biol.* 101(2), 147–154.

226. Quirk, K., et al. (1994). γ-Aminobutyric acid type A receptors in the rat brain can contain both γ2 and γ3 subunits, but γ1 does not exist in combination with another γ subunit. *Mol. Pharmacol.* 45(6), 1061–1070.

227. Knoflach, F., et al. (1991). The γ3-subunit of the GABA$_A$-receptor confers sensitivity to benzodiazepine receptor ligands. *FEBS Lett.* 293(1/2), 191–194.

228. Pollard, S., Thompson, C. L., and Stephenson, F. A. (1995). Quantitative characterization of α6 and α1 subunit-containing native γ-aminobutyric acidA receptors of adult rat cerebellum demonstrates two α subunits per receptor oligomer. *J. Biol. Chem.* 270(36), 21285–21290.

228a. Caruncho, H. J., and Costa, E. (1994). Double-immunolabelling analysis of GABA$_A$ receptor subunits in label-fracture replicas of cultured rat cerebellar granule cells. *Recept. Channel* 2, 143–153.

229. De Blas, A. L. (1996). Brain GABA$_A$ receptors studied with subunit-specific antibodies. *Mol. Neurobiol.* 12(1), 55–71.

230. Sigel, E., and Kannenberg, K. (1996). GABA$_A$-receptor subtypes. *Trends Neurosci.* 19(9), 386.

231. Böhme, I., Rabe, H., and Lüddens, H. (2004). Four amino acids in the α subunits determine the GABA sensitivities of GABA$_A$ receptor subtypes. *J. Biol. Chem.* 279(34), 35193–35200.

232. Homanics, G. E., et al. (1997). Mice devoid of γ-aminobutyrate type A receptor β3 subunit have epilepsy, cleft palate, and hypersensitive behavior. *Proc. Natl. Acad. Sci. USA* 94(8), 4143–4148.

233. Collinson, N., et al. (2001). Role of the α5 subunit of the GABA$_A$ receptor in learning and memory. *Behav. Pharmacol.* 12(Suppl.1), S22.

234. Culiat, C. T., et al. (1994). Phenotypic consequences of deletion of the γ3, α5, or β3 subunit of the type A γ-aminobutyric acid receptor in mice. *Proc. Natl. Acad. Sci. USA* 91(7), 2815–2818.

235. Jones, A., et al. (1997). Ligand-gated ion channel subunit partnerships: $GABA_A$ receptor α6 subunit gene inactivation inhibits δ subunit expression. *J. Neurosci.* 17(4), 1350–1362.
236. Homanics, G. E., et al. (1997). Gene knockout of the α6 subunit of the γ–aminobutyric acid type A receptor: Lack of effect on responses to ethanol, pentobarbital, and general anesthetics. *Mol. Pharmacol.* 51(4), 588–596.
237. Homanics, G. E., et al. (1999). Normal electrophysiological and behavioral responses to ethanol in mice lacking the long splice variant of the γ2 subunit of the γ-aminobutyrate type A receptor. *Neuropharmacology* 38(2), 253–265.
238. Sur, C., et al. (2001). Loss of the major $GABA_A$ receptor subtype in the brain is not lethal in mice. *J. Neurosci.* 21(10), 3409–3418.
239. Kralic, J. E., et al. (2002). Molecular and pharmacological characterization of $GABA_A$ receptor α1 subunit knockout mice. *J. Pharmacol. Exp. Ther.* 302(3), 1037–1045.
240. Korpi, E. R., et al. (1994). Role of $GABA_A$ receptors in the actions of alcohol and alcoholism: Recent advances. *Alcohol Alcoholism* 29, 115–129.
241. Homanics, G. E., et al. (1998). Ethanol tolerance and withdrawal responses in $GABA_A$ receptor α6 subunit null allele mice and in inbred C57BL/6J and strain 129/SvJ mice. *Alcohol Clin. Exp. Res.* 22(1), 259–265.
242. Korpi, E. R., et al. (1999). Cerebellar granule-cell-specific $GABA_A$ receptors attenuate benzodiazepine-induced ataxia: Evidence from α6-subunit-deficient mice. *Eur. J. Neurosci.* 11(1), 233–240.
243. Brickley, S. G., et al. (2001). Adaptive regulation of neuronal excitability by a voltage-independent potassium conductance. *Nature* 409, 88–92.
244. Rudolph, U., et al. (1999). Benzodiazepine actions mediated by specific γ-aminobutyric $acid_A$ receptor subtypes. *Nature* 401, 796–800.
245. McKernan, R. M., et al. (2000). Sedative but not anxiolytic properties of benzodiazepines are mediated by the $GABA_A$ receptor α1 subtype. *Nat. Neurosci.* 3(6), 587–592.
246. Tobler, I., et al. (2001). Diazepam-induced changes in sleep: Role of the α1 $GABA_A$ receptor subtype. *Proc. Natl. Acad. Sci. USA* 98(11), 6464–6469.
247. Löw, K., et al. (2000). Molecular and neuronal substrate for the selective attenuation of anxiety. *Science* 290(5489), 131–134.
248. Millan, M. J. (2003). The neurobiology and control of anxious states. *Prog. Neurobiol.* 70, 83–244.
249. Dias, R., et al. (2005). Evidence for a significant role of α3-containing $GABA_A$ receptors in mediating the anxiolytic effects of benzodiazepines. *J. Neurosci.* 25(46), 10682–10688.
250. Atack, J. R., et al. (2005). Anxiogenic properties of an inverse agonist selective for α3 subunit-containing $GABA_A$ receptors. *Br. J. Pharmacol.* 144(3), 357–366.
251. Crestani, F., et al. (2001). Molecular targets for the myorelaxant action of diazepam. *Mol. Pharmacol.* 59(3), 442–445.
252. Navarro, J. F., Buron, E., and Martin-Lopez, M. (2002). Anxiogenic-like activity of L-655,708, a selective ligand for the benzodiazepine site of $GABA_A$ receptors which contain the α5 subunit, in the elevated plus-maze test. *Prog. Neuropsychopharmacol. Biol. Psychiatry* 26(7/8), 1389–1392.
253. Crestani, F., et al. (2002). Trace fear conditioning involves hippocampal α5 $GABA_A$ receptors. *Proc. Natl. Acad. USA* 99(13), 8980–8985.
254. Haefely, W. E., et al. (1993). The multiplicity of actions of benzodiazepine receptor ligands. *Can. J. Psychiatry* 38(Suppl. 4), S102–S108.

255. Squires, R. F., et al. (1979). Some properties of brain specific benzodiazepine receptors: New evidence for multiple receptors. *Pharmacol. Biochem. Behav.* 10, 825–830.
256. Sieghart, W., et al. (1983). Several new benzodiazepines selectively interact with a benzodiazepine receptor subtype. *Neurosci. Lett.* 38(1), 73–78.
257. Iorio, L. C., Barnett, A., and Billard, W. (1984). Selective affinity of 1-*N*-trifluoroethyl benzodiazepines for cerebellar type 1 receptor sites. *Life Sci.* 35(1), 105–113.
258. Billard, W., et al. (1988). Selective affinity of the benzodiazepines quazepam and 2-oxo-quazepam for BZ1 binding site and demonstration of 3H-2-oxo-quazepam as a BZ1 selective radioligand. *Life Sci.* 42(2), 179–187.
259. Sieghart, W., and Schuster, A. (1984). Affinity of various ligands for benzodiazepine receptors in rat cerebellum and hippocampus. *Biochem. Pharmacol.* 33(24), 4033–4038.
260. Dämgen, K., and Lüddens, H. (1999). Zaleplon displays a selectivity to recombinant $GABA_A$ receptors different from zolpidem, zopiclone and benzodiazepines. *Neurosci. Res. Comm.* 25(3), 139–148.
261. Selleri, S., et al. (2005). A novel selective $GABA_A$ α1 receptor agonist displaying sedative and anxiolytic-like properties in rodents. *J. Med. Chem.* 49(21), 6756–6760.
262. Korpi, E. R., Uusi-Oukari, M., and Wegelius, K. (1992). Substrate specificity of diazepam-insensitive cerebellar [^{3}H]Ro 15-4513 binding sites. *Eur. J. Pharmacol.* 213, 323–329.
263. Wong, G., et al. (1993). Synthetic and computer-assisted analysis of the structural requirements for selective, high-affinity ligand binding to diazepam-insensitive benzodiazepine receptors. *J. Med. Chem.* 36(13), 1820–1830.
264. Liu, R. Y., et al. (1996). Synthesis and pharmacological properties of novel 8-substituted imidazobenzodiazepines: High-affinity, selective probes for α5-containing $GABA_A$ receptors. *J. Med. Chem.* 39(9), 1928–1934.
265. Zhang, W., et al. (1995). Development of a comprehensive pharmacophore model for the benzodiazepine receptor. *Drug Des. Discov.* 12(3), 193–248.
266. Skolnick, P., et al. (1997). [^{3}H]RY 80: A high affinity, selective ligand for γ–aminobutyric acid$_A$ receptors containing alpha–5 subunits. *J. Pharmacol. Exp. Therap.* 283(2), 488–493.
267. Quirk, K., et al. (1996). [^{3}H]L-655,708, a novel ligand selective for the benzodiazepine site of $GABA_A$ receptors which contain the α5 subunit. *Neuropharmacology* 35(9/10), 1331–1335.
268. van Niel, M. B., et al. (2005). A new pyridazine series of $GABA_A$ α5 ligands. *J. Med. Chem.* 48(19), 6004–6011.
269. Collins, I., et al. (2002). 3-Heteroaryl-2-pyridones: Benzodiazepine site ligands with functional delectivity for α2/α3-subtypes of human $GABA_A$ receptor-ion channels. *J. Med. Chem.* 45(9), 1887–1900.
270. Rudolph, U., Crestani, F., and Möhler, H. (2001). $GABA_A$ receptor subtypes: Dissecting their pharmacological functions. *Trends Pharmacol. Sci.* 22(4), 188–194.
271. Vicini, S., and Ortinski, P. (2004). Genetic manipulations of $GABA_A$ receptor in mice make inhibition exciting. *Pharmacol. Ther.* 103(2), 109–120.
272. Haefely, W., et al. (1992). Partial agonists of benzodiazepine receptors for the treatment of epilepsy, sleep, and anxiety disorders. *Adv. Biochem. Psychopharmacol.* 47(379), 379–394.

4

NEUROACTIVE STEROIDS IN ANXIETY AND STRESS

DEBORAH A. FINN[1] AND ROBERT H. PURDY[2]

[1]*Oregon Health and Science University and Department of Veterans Affairs, Portland, Oregon*
and [2]*The Scripps Research Institute, La Jolla, California*

4.1	Introduction		134
4.2	Neuroactive Steroid Chemistry and Pharmacology		135
	4.2.1	Brain and Peripheral Sources of Neuroactive Steroids	135
	4.2.2	Actions on $GABA_A$ Receptors and Other Ligand-Gated Ion Channels	137
	4.2.3	Enantiomeric Selectivity of Neuroactive Steroids	141
	4.2.4	Behavioral Effects	142
4.3	Effects of Neurosteroids in Animal Models of Anxiety and Stress		142
	4.3.1	Elevated-Plus Maze	143
	4.3.2	Geller–Seifter and Vogel Conflict Tests	145
	4.3.3	Light–Dark Box	146
	4.3.4	Acoustic Startle and Fear-Potentiated Startle	147
	4.3.5	Mirrored Chamber	147
	4.3.6	Open-Field Activity	148
	4.3.7	Defensive Burying Behavior	149
	4.3.8	Separation-Induced Ultrasonic Vocalizations	150
	4.3.9	Modified Forced-Swim Test	150
	4.3.10	Mild Mental Stress Models and Social Isolation	151
4.4	Neuroactive Steroid Interactions with Stress-Induced Behaviors		152
	4.4.1	HPA Axis and Stress	153
	4.4.2	Anxiety-Related Disorders	154
	4.4.3	Depression	156
	4.4.4	Acute and Chronic Effects of Alcohol	157
	4.4.5	Stress-Induced Drug Reinstatement	159
4.5	Conclusions and Outlook		160
Acknowledgments			161
References			161

Handbook of Contemporary Neuropharmacology, Edited by David R. Sibley, Israel Hanin, Michael Kuhar, and Phil Skolnick. Copyright © 2007 John Wiley & Sons, Inc.

4.1 INTRODUCTION

Rapid membrane effects of certain specific metabolites of steroid hormones provide a mechanism by which these metabolites can influence brain function and behavior in addition to the classical genomic actions of the parent steroid hormones. It was over 60 years ago that the pioneering studies of Hans Selye [1] reported the sedative–anesthetic activity of the hormones progesterone and deoxycorticosterone, where among 75 steroids tested by systemic (i.p.) administration in rodents, 5β-pregnanedione was the most active. This led to the introduction of hydroxydione sodium (21-hydroxy-5β-pregnane-3,20-dione succinate, sodium salt) as the first steroidal anesthetic in 1955 [2]. However, it was Margarethe Holzbauer and her colleagues, during the 1969–1985 period, who isolated and identified pregnenolone, progesterone, allopregnanolone (3α,5α-THP), epiallopregnanolone (3β,5α-THP), allopregnanedione (5α-dihydroprogesterone, or 5α-DHP), 20α-dihydroprogesterone, and allopregnanediol (5α-pregnane-3α,20α-diol) from ovarian venous blood of the rat and measured the ovarian content and secretion rates of these steroids during proestrus [3]. Their work was seminal but is often forgotten. Holzbauer and colleagues [4] further demonstrated the *in vivo* secretion of pregnenolone, progesterone, and 3α,5α-THP by the adrenal gland of the rat in quantities similar to those secreted by the ovary during estrus. Their laboratory later provided an outdated organic extract of adrenal venous blood that was found to contain similar amounts of allotetrahydrodeoxycorticosterone (3α, 21-dihydroxy-5α-pregnan-20-one; alloTHDOC) and 3α,5α-THP by radioimmunoassay (RIA) after separation of the steroid fraction by high-performance liquid chromatography (HPLC; R. Purdy, unpublished).

Two decades ago, γ-aminobutyric acid A (GABA$_A$) receptors were found to be sensitive to modulation by steroids, providing the first hint at a mechanism underlying the reported rapid (on the order of seconds) onset of action of these steroids. Subsequent to the initial demonstration by Harrison and Simmonds [5] that alphaxalone (3α-hydroxy-5α-pregnan-11,20-dione, a metabolite of 11-dehydrocorticosterone found in patients with congenital adrenal hyperplasia exhibiting 21- hydroxylase deficiency [6]) potentiated GABA-gated chloride currents, evidence has accumulated that alphaxalone and structurally related steroid derivatives have rapid membrane actions via an interaction with ligand-gated ion channels [7–11]. This evidence has given rise to the term *neuroactive steroids*, to distinguish them from *neurosteroids*, which are synthesized *de novo* from cholesterol in nervous tissue [12]. Behaviorally, GABA agonist neuroactive steroids are now recognized to possess especially potent anesthetic, hypnotic, anxiolytic, and anticonvulsant properties [13].

An understanding of the physiological role of neuroactive steroids is essential for their acceptance as modulators of stress and anxiety. It is apparent that these endogenously occurring steroids can reach levels in the rat brain that are capable of modulating GABA$_A$ receptors. 3α,5α-THP and alloTHDOC have been measured in brain and plasma, where their levels have been shown to fluctuate in response to stress in rats [14], and during the estrous and menstrual cycles of rats and humans, respectively [8]. Brain and plasma levels of 3α,5α-THP temporally follow those of progesterone in the female rat (i.e., peak brain levels are observed during estrus in the rat and dramatically increase during pregnancy). Both 3α,5α-THP and alloTHDOC are detectable in the normal male rat brain, but the levels are low under most circumstances. However, exposure of male rats to stressors such as ambient temperature swim, footshock, or CO_2 inhalation resulted in a rapid 4- to 20-fold increase in brain levels of 3α,5α-THP and alloTHDOC [14, 15] to the equivalent of 10–30 nM. Similar concentrations are observed in female rats during estrus, while concentrations can increase to approximately 100 nM during pregnancy [8, 16, 17], documenting that basal 3α,5α-THP levels are higher in females than in males. These concentrations achieved *in vivo* are within the range of concentrations previously shown to potentiate the *in vitro* action of GABA at $GABA_A$ receptors, suggesting that fluctuations in endogenous 3α,5α-THP levels in rodents and both 3α,5α-THP and 3α,5β-THP levels in humans may be physiologically relevant. Evidence in support of this idea has been reviewed recently [18].

4.2 NEUROACTIVE STEROID CHEMISTRY AND PHARMACOLOGY

4.2.1 Brain and Peripheral Sources of Neuroactive Steroids

The term *neurosteroid* was introduced by Baulieu [19] to designate a steroid hormone derivative found in brain at concentrations that were independent of its plasma concentration, and the story of their discovery and function has been recently reviewed [12]. Endogenous concentrations of the progesterone metabolite 3α,5α-THP have been detected in brain, plasma, and adrenals of male and female rats and in female rat ovaries [4, 8, 15, 20–23]. Brain 3α,5α-THP levels have been detected in rat, mouse, dog, monkey, and human [8, 15, 22–28]. Compared with 3α,5α-THP, the 5β-reduced epimer is present in the rat in much lower abundance, if at all [27]. In addition, brain 3α, 5α-THP concentration is detectable at lower levels in adrenalectomized animals and is higher than plasma 3α,5α-THP levels in intact animals [15, 22, 23].

A number of studies have established that the enzymes identified in classic steroidogenic tissues are likewise found in the nervous system [29]. Thus, the endogenous concentration of neuroactive steroids in the brain most likely reflects a combination of neuroactive compounds produced there *de novo* as well as steroids metabolized to neuroactive compounds in the brain but derived from circulating precursors. For this reason, it has recently been proposed that the definition of the term neurosteroid be broadened to include both sources of neuroactive steroids [29]. It also is noteworthy that all neurosteroids identified to date have been found to have neuroactive effects in some behavioral assay. The most recent study identified the major neurosteroid in the amphibian brain as 7α-hydroxypregnenolone and subsequently determined that this neurosteroid acts as a neuronal activator to stimulate locomotor activity of breeding newts [30]. A schematic of the biosynthetic pathway of neuroactive steroid formation from cholesterol is depicted in Fig. 4.1.

Many methods have been used to quantify steroidal compounds. These include RIA, gas chromatography–mass spectrometry (GC/MS), HPLC, and liquid chromatography–mass spectrometry (LC/MS). While these techniques are successful in the analysis of steroids, it has been difficult to achieve quantitative analysis of small samples of neurosteroids because of their low concentrations in nervous tissues. Highly specific analytical methods are required to analyze small quantities of neurosteroids and their sulfates. Only with extremely sensitive methods of analysis is it possible to discover whether neurosteroids are synthesized in nervous tissues in quantities sufficient to affect neuronal activity and whether these neurosteroids are distributed uniformly in brain.

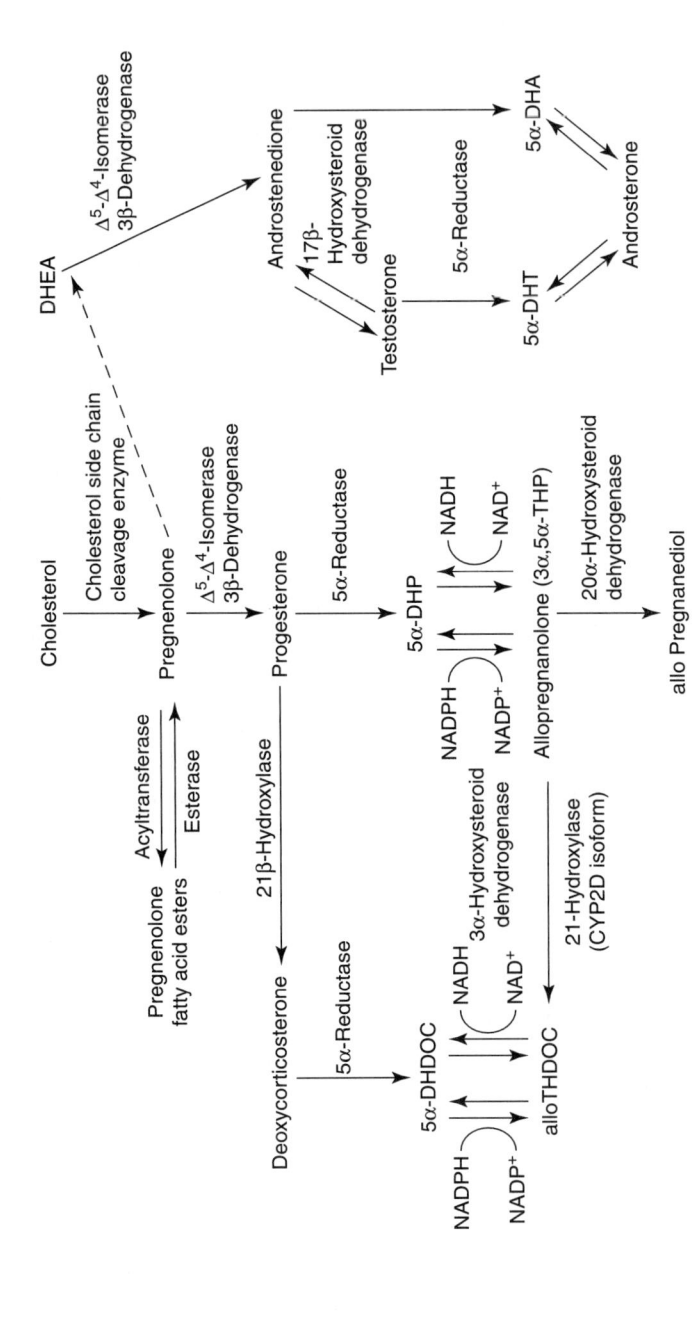

Figure 4.1 Biosynthesis of select neurosteroids. Depicted is the biosynthetic pathway for the neurosteroids 3α,5α-THP, alloTHDOC, allopregnanediol, and androsterone, which are potent positive modulators of GABA$_A$ receptors. The fatty acid esters of pregnenolone, which are storage forms of pregnenolone in brain, are shown. The broken line indicates that 17-OH pregnenolone is omitted from the diagram in the formation of DHEA from pregnenolone. Note also that brain cytochrome P450 (CYP2D) isoforms have been shown recently to exhibit 21-hydroxylase activity in the brain, which can convert progesterone, DHP, or 3α,5α-THP to their respective deoxycorticosterone derivatives[37]. Abbreviations: DHEA, dehydroepiandrosterone; DHDOC, dihydrodeoxycorticosterone; DHP, dihydroprogesterone; THDOC, tetrahydrodeoxycorticosterone; DHT, dihydrotestosterone; DHA, dihydroandrostenedione. (Modified from Finn et al. [241]).

In the initial identification of dehydroepiandrosterone sulfate (DHEAS) [31] and pregnenolone sulfate (PREGS) [32] in the rat brain, a conjugated steroid fraction from brain extracts was prepared by chromatography on a column of Sephadex LH-20 and termed the *sulfate fraction*. This was free from unconjugated steroids, steroidal esters of fatty acids (lipoidal steroids), and steroidal glucosiduronates. This sulfate fraction was then hydrolyzed by solvolysis in ethyl acetate for 12–16 h at 37°C, and the hydrolyzed products were purified on a column of Lipidex 5000. The purified steroids were converted to their trimethylsilyl ethers and characterized by GC/MS as DHEA and PREG. On the basis that the levels of DHEA and PREG separately measured from the hydrolyzed sulfate fraction from brain extracts by RIA were markedly elevated compared to corresponding levels in blood and were found in extracts of brain tissue from rats previously adrenalectomized and orchiectomized, DHEAS and PREGS were described as neurosteroids. A considerable body of electrophysiological, pharmacological, and physiological work has subsequently been carried out on these two presumed neurosteroid sulfates [33]. Meanwhile, Prasad et al. [34], demonstrated that when extracts of brain were heated and treated with triethylamine or various reducing agents such as ferrous sulfate, larger amounts of DHEA and PREG could be measured by GC/MS, compared to simple extraction without such treatments. They suggested that there might be steroidal hydroperoxides or peroxides in brain that had not yet been characterized.

Recently, two laboratories have independently cast grave doubts on the existence of significant amounts of DHEAS and PREGS in the adult rat brain. Using a nonexchangeable internal standard of [3α,11,11-^{2}H$_3$] allopregnanolone sulfate and a tracer amount of [1,2,6,7-^{3}H$_4$] DHEA sulfate, Liu et al. [35] were unable to find detectable amounts of DHEAS, PREGS, and any of the four pregnenolone sulfates in nonhydrolyzed extracts of the adult Sprague–Dawley male and female rats using LC/microelectrospray MS (LC/micro-ESI–MS). Shimada et al. [36] also have found only low amounts, 0.53 ± 0.28 ng/g, of PREGS in nonhydrolyzed extracts from adult Wistar rat brain using a unique derivatization procedure followed by LC/micro-ES–MS. This compares to the value of about 20 ng/g brain of PREGS originally reported using solvolysis and measurement by RIA [32]. At present, there are no reports of other PREG-containing compounds that could account for this 20-ng/g brain level. Thus, the nature of the majority of PREG-containing compound(s) in the sulfate fraction from extracts of the rodent brain remains a mystery. It would require low microgram amounts of such a compound to be identified (after purification) using the most sensitive microprocedure of high-resolution proton magnetic resonance instrumentation.

4.2.2 Actions on GABA$_A$ Receptors and Other Ligand-Gated Ion Channels

After alphaxalone was found to potentiate GABA-gated chloride currents [5], the progesterone metabolite 3α,5α-THP and the deoxycorticosterone metabolite alloTHDOC were determined to be potent positive modulators of GABA$_A$ receptors. The relationship between plasma levels of corticosterone and alloTHDOC, measured by RIA in various stages of immobilization stress in adult male Sprague–Dawley rats, is illustrated in Fig. 4.2. It also has been demonstrated that alloTHDOC can be formed in brain and in the periphery from 3α,5α-THP through 21- hydroxylase activity [37] of cytochrome P450 (CYP2D) isoforms (Fig. 4.1). Therefore, we do not know at

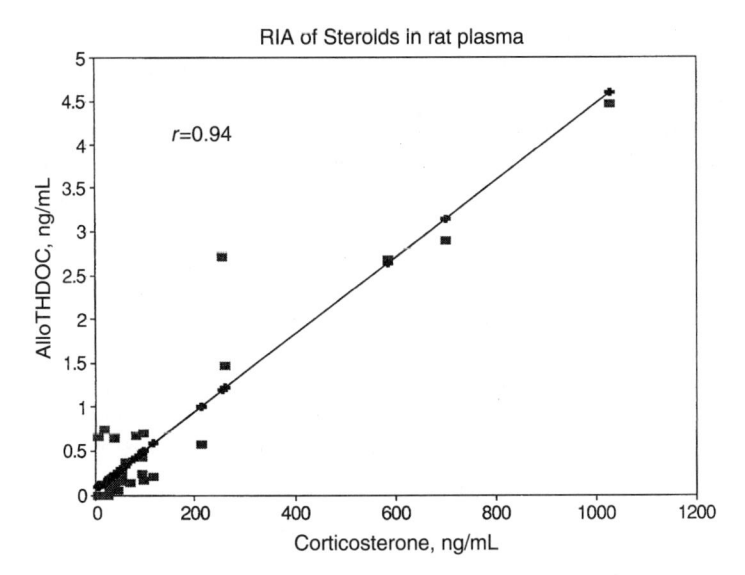

Figure 4.2 The relationship between plasma levels of alloTHDOC and corticosterone in adult male Sprague–Dawley rats before and at various times during 30 min of immobilization stress. The rectangles are the values measured by RIA. The crosses are the values for the calculated regression line for $r = 0.94$. (Data from R. H. Purdy and N. Hagino, unpublished.)

present if the levels of alloTHDOC in brain are the result of synthesis from deoxycorticosterone (DOC) or allopregnanolone or both.

The above 3α-hydroxysteroids enhanced GABA-stimulated chloride flux in rat brain synaptoneurosomes at nanomolar concentrations [38] and interacted with known modulatory sites on $GABA_A$ receptors in a noncompetitive manner [39, 40]. These pregnane neurosteroids have a saturated steroid A ring (see Fig. 4.3 for the steroid four-ring structures of the four epimeric pregnanolones formed in primates).

Notably, the interaction of pregnane neurosteroids with $GABA_A$ receptors was stereospecific, in that the two key features necessary for activity were a 5α- or 5β-reduced steroid A ring and a 3α-OH group. The 3β analogues (i.e., 3β-hydroxy, 5α- or 5β-reduced pregnanes; epiallopregnanolone and epipregnanolone, respectively; Fig. 4.3) were devoid of activity or exhibited a partial inverse agonist profile. Progesterone, estradiol, corticosterone, 5α-dihydrotestosterone, and cholesterol were inactive *in vitro*. In the case of alloTHDOC, the 5β isomer (i.e., 5β-THDOC) had a partial agonist pharmacological profile [41]. Metabolism of 3α,5α-THP to allopregnanediol also yielded a steroid with efficacy as a partial agonist [42]. Among all the endogenously occurring steroids examined, 3α,5α-THP was the most potent, followed by its 5β stereoisomer (pregnanolone or 3α,5β-THP) and alloTHDOC [40]. Importantly, the positive modulatory effect of neurosteroids at $GABA_A$ receptors was relatively specific, in that these steroids did not interact with any other known neurotransmitter receptor in the nanomolar-to-low-micromolar concentration range.

Electrophysiological studies revealed that GABAergic steroids facilitated the open state of the GABA-gated channel (frequency and duration, nanomolar concentrations) and could directly activate $GABA_A$ receptors in the absence of GABA at higher (micromolar) concentrations [43]. For a more detailed description of the

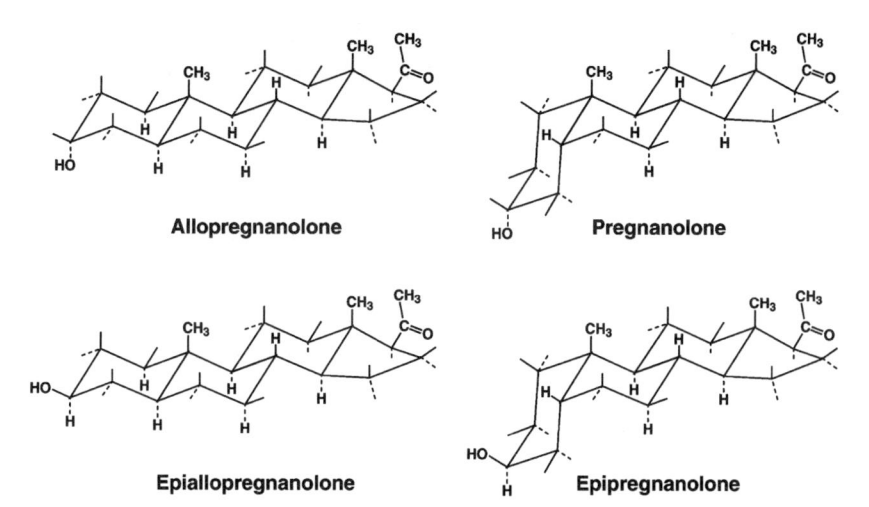

Figure 4.3 Structures of four epimeric pregnanolones. In the two allo (5α) steroids, the 3-hydroxyl group is axial in allopregnanolone (3α) and equatorial in epiallopregnanolone (3β), whereas in the 5β steroids the reverse is the case, with the 3-hydroxyl group being equatorial in pregnanolone (3α) and axial (3β) in epipregnanolone.

perturbation of GABA-gated ion channel kinetics by neurosteroids, the reader is referred to several excellent reports [44–46]. In general, the stereospecificity and enantioselectivity required for neuroactive steroid modulation of GABA$_A$ receptors are features that would be consistent with a specific steroid binding site on GABA$_A$ receptors [46–49]. However, use of recombinant subunit expression studies in conjunction with site-directed mutagenesis has not defined a steroid binding pocket on GABA$_A$ receptors. Thus, the molecular mechanism(s) underlying the perturbation of GABA$_A$ receptor function by neuroactive steroids remains to be determined.

Steroids with GABA-negative actions also have been reported (e.g., PREGS and DHEAS). Whereas PREGS and DHEAS antagonized GABA-gated chloride uptake and conductance in a noncompetitive manner [50, 51], PREGS also markedly reduced glycine-activated chloride currents [52] and enhanced N-methyl-D-aspartate (NMDA)–gated currents and elevations in intracellular calcium (Ca^{2+}) [53, 54]. Recent work also demonstrated that the C$_{3,5}$ reduction of cortisol, which is a primary regulator of the stress response in humans, generated compounds with negative modulatory activity at GABA$_A$ receptors [55]. Notably, 3α,5β-cortisol inhibited muscimol-stimulated chloride uptake with an median inhibitory concentration (IC$_{50}$) of 13 μM, whereas a 10 μM concentration of cortisol, 11-deoxycortisol, 5α-dihydrocortisol, 3α,5α-cortisol, and 3α,5β-11-deoxycortisol exhibited weak negative modulatory activity on muscimol-stimulated chloride uptake. Therefore, cortisol metabolism may produce steroids with GABA-negative action.

A possible role for pregnane 3-sulfate steroids in the modulation of NMDA receptor function also has been described. Although pregnanolone (3α,5β-THP; 50 μM) failed to alter NMDA induced cation influx through the NMDA receptor, its 3-position sulfate derivative dose dependently inhibited this NMDA receptor current in chick spinal cord neurons with an EC$_{50}$ of 62 μM [56], and it suppressed NMDA-mediated increases in intracellular Ca^{2+} in rat hippocampal neurons with an IC$_{50}$ of

37 μM [57]. Similarly, 100 μM concentrations of either 3α,5α-THP-sulfate or epipregnanolone-sulfate antagonized NMDA receptor cation conductance by 25 and 50%, respectively [58]. Pregnane 3-sulfates were found to modulate NMDA receptor function in a non-competitive fashion [56, 57], and their inhibitory interaction with this receptor likely involved a specific and separate binding site from positive modulators such as PREGS and related steroids [58–60]. Notably, sulfated and nonsulfated pregnane neurosteroids also had opposing effects on $GABA_A$ receptor function [61]. Thus, even though sulfation of steroids is a major enzymatic reaction of metabolism, secretion, and homeostasis of steroids in the periphery, it may have a role greater than merely facilitating secretion because it also can change the pharmacological activity of steroids in the CNS [29]. While the role of sulfation in the modulation of excitatory and inhibitory ion channels by neurosteroids has yet to be demonstrated *in vivo*, it is possible that the addition and removal of the sulfate group could be a critical control point for neurosteroid modulation of neurotransmitter receptors [62].

In addition to the potent modulation of $GABA_A$ receptor function by pregnane steroids, evidence also indicates that these steroids can interact with other ionotropic receptor systems at micromolar concentrations. Progesterone, 5α-DHP, and 3α,5α-THP inhibited $^{86}Rb^+$ efflux through neuronal nicotinic acetylcholine (nACh) receptors derived from mouse thalamus with apparent K_i values of 38, 5.3, and 17.5 μM, respectively [63]. In most cases, neurosteroid antagonism of nACh receptors *in vitro* was observed at concentrations between 10 and 100 μM—levels that are three- to five-fold greater than those estimated to be present in mammalian brain [64]. The inhibition of nACh receptors by progesterone occurred in a noncompetitive manner, did not require the presence of cognate ligand, and was likely dependent on the receptor subunit combinations expressed [65–67]. The attachment of the side chain with a β orientation at the 17 position of the neurosteroid imparted greater inhibitory potency at nACh receptors, whereas, in contrast to $GABA_A$ receptors, the orientation of the hydroxyl group at the 3 position had little impact upon neurosteroid efficacy [68]. Although the sensitivity of various nACh receptor subunit combinations to neurosteroids has yet to be examined, it appears unlikely that a physiologically relevant concentration of pregnane steroids could alter nACh receptor activity.

Progesterone dose dependently inhibited serotonin-evoked currents through serotonin type 3 (5-HT_3) receptors from rat nodose ganglion with an EC_{50} of 31 μM, whereas its A-ring-reduced metabolite 3α,5α-THP (50 μM) exhibited no observable effect on this measure [69]. In contrast, *in vitro* studies suggest that pregnane steroids are functional antagonists at 5-HT_3 receptors. 3α,5α-THP (10 μM) attenuated serotonin-mediated current by 30–35% in HEK 293 cells [70], while alloTHDOC and alphaxalone inhibited 5-HT-induced [^{14}C]-guanidinium influx in N1E-115 cells with IC_{50} values of 19 and 44 μM, respectively [71]. Similar to neurosteroid interactions at nACh receptors, the substituent at the 3 position of the steroid A ring had little consequence for the antagonist profile of pregnane neurosteroids at 5-HT_3 receptors [70]. The degree of stereospecificity in neurosteroid modulation of 5-HT_3 receptors remains ambiguous, especially when considering a recent finding that the potency of neurosteroids in inhibiting 5-HT_3 receptor–mediated current was correlated with their lipophilicity [71], thereby suggesting a mechanism involving disruption of lipids adjacent to the receptor.

T-type (low-voltage-activated) Ca^{2+} channels, which act over a range of membrane potentials near the resting potential of most cells and are thought to play an important role in controlling cellular excitability [72–75], can be blocked by micromolar concentrations of 3α,5α-THP and alphaxalone [76]. The authors also demonstrated that the 5α-reduced neuroactive steroids were potent peripheral analgesic agents [76]. Notably, structural modifications that eliminated the blocking effect on T-type Ca^{2+} channels but maintained $GABA_A$ receptor potentiation resulted in a complete loss of peripheral analgesic effects. Taken in conjunction with data indicating that $GABA_A$ receptors play a role in centrally mediated effects of neuroactive steroids [77], it is likely that the peripheral analgesic action of 5α-reduced neuroactive steroids is mediated primarily by T channels and only to a smaller extent by $GABA_A$ receptors.

Recent reports documenting neurosteroid interactions with metabotropic sigma 1 (σ_1) receptors are noteworthy. Importantly, the pregnane neurosteroids 3α,5α-THP and epipregnanolone were devoid of σ_1 receptor activity [78]. In contrast, progesterone has been identified as one of the most potent neurosteroid inhibitors of agonist binding to the σ_1 receptor [78, 79]. Furthermore, blockade of progesterone's conversion to its pregnane metabolites via a 5α-reductase inhibitor (finasteride) resulted in attenuated agonist binding to the σ_1 receptor, presumably due to augmented levels of progesterone [80]. Clearly, pregnane neurosteroids play little if any physiological role in modulating σ_1 receptor function.

Therefore, 3α,5α-THP, alloTHDOC, and 3α,5β-THP, the three most potent pregnane neurosteroids characterized to date, have nanomolar potencies at $GABA_A$ receptors, and consequently, these actions undoubtedly have physiological significance [18]. Interactions of pregnane neurosteroids at nACh, $5-HT_3$, and NMDA receptors occur within the range 10–100 μM and are unlikely to have physiological relevance, even under challenge conditions (i.e., stress or pregnancy).

4.2.3 Enantiomeric Selectivity of Neuroactive Steroids

Studies of the binding and electrophysiological activity of neuroactive steroids have demonstrated that the effect of GABAergic steroids does not result from steroid binding at the benzodiazepine, barbiturate, picrotoxin, or GABA sites of these receptor complexes. These results have led to the concept of unique binding sites for a group of neuroactive steroids on $GABA_A$ receptor complexes [10, 61, 81, 82]. Although there is no current demonstration of the effective binding of a radioactive steroid ligand to such sites, a significant correlation has been obtained between physiological and behavioral effects and *in vitro* structure-activity relationships of GABAergic steroids [83].

Specificity in the interaction of neuroactive steroids with neurotransmitter systems is most convincingly demonstrated by the results of Covey et al. [47] with non–naturally occurring enantiomers of both positive and negative modulators of GABAergic neurotransmission. Allopregnanolone (3α,5α-THP) and pregnanolone (3α,5β-THP) occur naturally in one entiomerically pure form, as illustrated in Fig 4.3. The mirror images of these compounds, known as ent steroids, are shown in Fig 4.4. and were prepared by total synthesis. Here the optically active centers at carbon atoms 3, 5, 8, 9, 10, 13, 14, and 17 are opposite to the configurations in the natural steroids (originally isolated from human pregnancy urine). High entioselectivity was

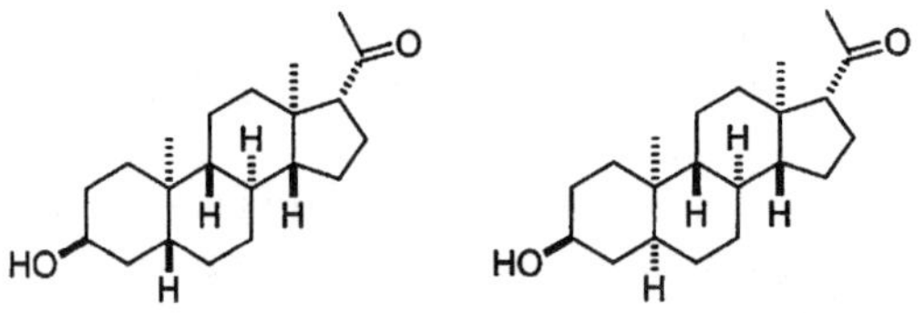

Figure 4.4 Enantiomeric structures of *ent*-allopregnanolone and *ent*-pregnanolone. These synthetic compounds are both much less potent positive modulators of $GABA_A$ receptors when compared to their natural enantiomers shown in Fig. 4.3. [47].

found for 3α,5α-THP when compared to *ent*-3α,5α-THP. However, the entioselectivity for 3α,5β-THP was markedly lower than that for 3α,5α-THP, consistent with different binding sites for 3α-hydroxy-5α- and 3α-hydroxy-5β-pregnanes. This difference was confirmed by the use of the first specific inhibitor of 3α,5α-THP, 3α-hydroxy-5α-androst-16-ene-17-phenyl, which only weakly affects the *in vitro* and *in vivo* activity of 3α,5β-THP [84].

4.2.4 Behavioral Effects

Neurosteroids that are positive modulators of $GABA_A$ receptors possess anesthetic [85], hypnotic [86], anticonvulsant [17, 87–93], and anxiolytic [93–100] properties [13]. While 3α,5β-THP was equipotent with 3α,5α-THP as an anxiolytic [95, 98, 101], it was much less potent as an anticonvulsant [101]. The 3β-stereoisomer of 3α,5α-THP was inactive in all tests. The effects of pregnane neurosteroids on cognitive function also have been extensively evaluated on conditioned learning and spatial learning tasks [102]. Regardless of the paradigm utilized (e.g., win-shift foraging paradigm, Morris water maze, Y-maze discrimination task), 3α,5α-THP, 3α,5β-THP, and epipregnanolone exhibited a behavioral profile associated with working (spatial) memory deficits [102–105]. Collectively, these behavioral responses closely follow the anticipated patterns based on *in vitro* evidence and suggest that GABAergic steroids modify the functioning of central $GABA_A$ receptors *in vivo*. Therefore, if the findings with exogenous administration of 3α,5α-THP are indicative of $GABA_A$ receptor sensitivity to endogenous 3α,5α-THP concentration, then endogenous neurosteroids may participate in the physiological control of central nervous system (CNS) excitability.

4.3 EFFECTS OF NEUROSTEROIDS IN ANIMAL MODELS OF ANXIETY AND STRESS

Rodent models of human generalized anxiety symptoms take advantage of a variety of behaviors within the natural behavioral repertoire of rodents that have been interpreted to be "anxiety-like." While these tasks are based on putative parallels between human and rodent symptoms of anxiety, it is not known whether a rodent experiences "anxiety" in the same way as humans. With this in mind, different behavioral principles seem to underlie various animal models of anxiety such that paradigms can be based on spontaneous exploration, a learned response, conflict behavior, or a combination of these ideas. Most of these tasks utilize approach–avoidance behaviors in rodents that can provide a good indication of a rodent's response to conflict in the natural environment. A number of detailed reviews are available on this topic [106–111]. Here, we will briefly describe tasks that have been well validated in terms of their specificity for anxiety-like behaviors and the ability to demonstrate anxiolytic effects with a variety of GABAergic neuroactive steroids. The paradigms described below are good choices for testing hypotheses related to the modulatory effect of neuroactive steroids on anxiety-related behavior. However, these tests also can be influenced by factors unrelated to anxiety. It is therefore recommended that any animal model be tested on more than one anxiety test, so that different sensory and motor modalities can be examined. Alternatively, anti-anxiety effects in multiple tasks that measure both increases and decreases in responding can control for motor effects.

4.3.1 Elevated-Plus Maze

One of the most well-validated animal models of anxiety is the elevated-plus maze task [112–115], as it is able to detect both anxiolytic and anxiogenic agents in rodents [113]. This task is based on a rodent's natural avoidance of open, elevated alleys that was described almost 50 years ago [116]. Thus, the test sets up a conflict for the rodent between its tendency to explore a novel environment and its tendency to avoid the aversive properties of an open, elevated environment. Typically, mice and rats perform similarly on the elevated-plus maze, although performance on this task can be influenced by light level [117].

The apparatus consists of two open and two enclosed horizontal perpendicular arms of the same size and shape that are at right angles to each other. These four arms extend from a central platform (approximately 5×5 cm), forming the shape of a plus, and are elevated approximately 50 cm above the floor. The two open arms are simple runways with a minimal lip that allows the animal to see the edge without falling off the arm. The enclosed arms are closed runways with high walls that can be opaque. Typically, an animal is placed on the central platform (i.e., at the junction of the four arms) and allowed to explore freely for 5 min. During the 5-min test period, the number of entries into the open and closed arms as well as the amount of time spent in the open and closed arms is measured. Ideally, for an arm entry to be measured, all four paws should be within the arm. If the task is videotaped, additional anxiety-related behaviors can be quantified (see below) [107, 118]. However, the most commonly reported index of anxiety with this task is the percentage of open-arm entries or open-arm time, which is a proportion of the total number of entries or total time of the test, multiplied by 100. Normally, mice prefer the closed arms of the elevated-plus maze. Anxiolytic drugs typically increase the proportion of open-arm entries and the time spent on the open arm [93, 112, 118–122], whereas anxiogenic drugs or treatments decrease the percentage of open-arm entries or time [113, 123].

Comprehensive profiling of behavior also can be achieved by performing detailed videotaped analysis of untreated rodents on the elevated-plus maze, yielding a catalog of readily identifiable behaviors that have been referred to as *risk assessment* [107]. Examples include rearing, head dipping, stretched attend postures, closed-arm returns (i.e., doubling back in, rather than leaving, a closed arm), and several non exploratory behaviors [118]. "Protected" versus "unprotected" forms of these behaviors can be differentiated based on wall contact. This distinction is based on recent evidence that the most important feature producing open-arm avoidance is the absence of thigmotactic cues (i.e., walls), rather than the height of the maze [123]. Thus, this ethological approach provides multidimensionality to the analysis of elevated-plus maze behavior [107].

An important consideration for interpretation of elevated-plus maze data is that any treatment that affects motor behavior may influence the percentage of open-arm entries or time spent in the open arms. This is due to the fact that the paradigm requires the animal to locomote for a period of 5 min. However, the total number of entries as well as number of entries into the closed arms will give an indication of whether the treatment is influencing activity per se, and closed-arm entries are the most validated measure of activity [106, 124]. In this case, independent paradigms that specifically analyze locomotor behavior are recommended.

Consistent with a GABA-agonist pharmacological profile, the neurosteroids $3\alpha,5\alpha$-THP and $3\alpha,5\beta$-THP exhibit significant anxiolytic effects on the elevated plus-maze following systemic (1–20 mg/kg, i.p.) [93, 98, 100, 125] or intracerebroventricular (1.25–10 µg, i.c.v.) [95] administration. Both steroids significantly increased the proportion of open-arm entries and open-arm time. A similar anxiolytic effect was observed following administration of alloTHDOC (5–20 mg/kg, i.p.) [100]. Detailed behavioral analyses demonstrated that the anxiolytic effects of alloTHDOC, $3\alpha,5\alpha$-THP, and $3\alpha,5\beta$-THP did not reliably decrease measures of risk assessment and were not associated with a change in activity level, in contrast to the anxiolytic profile of a 1-mg/kg dose of diazepam [100]. However, in one study, a decrease in total entries, taken as an index of sedation, was observed following administration of a 10 µg (i.c.v.) dose of $3\alpha,5\alpha$-THP [95]. Systemic administration of allopregnanediol, a partial agonist at $GABA_A$ receptors, produced anxiolytic effects within a dose range of 10–40 mg/kg, i.p. [126]. Both systemic and i.c.v. administration of the 3β-stereoisomer of $3\alpha,5\alpha$-THP ($3\beta,5\alpha$-THP) had no effect on elevated-plus maze behavior or locomotor activity [95, 100], consistent with reports of its inability to potentiate GABA-gated currents. Therefore, GABA agonist neurosteroids produce anxiolytic effects in the rodent elevated-plus maze, and their anxiolytic profile can be partially distinguished from that of a well-characterized benzodiazepine (i.e., diazepam).

Recent findings in progesterone receptor (PR) knockout mice indicate that the anxiolytic effect of progesterone was due to its conversion to $3\alpha,5\alpha$-THP [127]. With this mouse model, a targeted null mutation of the PR gene eliminated the function of both PR-A and PR-B subtypes of the PR. Administration of progesterone (50 and 75 mg/kg) or $3\alpha,5\alpha$-THP (2 and 5 mg/kg) to PR knockout and wild-type mice significantly increased open-arm entries and time. Notably, the anxiolytic effect of progesterone was blocked by pretreatment with finasteride (50 mg/kg), a 5α-reductase inhibitor that prevents the conversion of progesterone to $3\alpha,5\alpha$-THP, in both genotypes [127]. Finasteride pretreatment did not alter $3\alpha,5\alpha$-THP's anxiolytic effect in either genotype. These results indicate that the anxiolytic action of progesterone does not require PRs, but does require its conversion to $3\alpha,5\alpha$-THP.

In contrast, neurosteroids that are noncompetitive antagonists of $GABA_A$ receptors have mixed effects on anxiety-related behavior. For example, systemic administration of DHEA and DHEAS exhibited anxiolytic effects on the elevated-plus maze [128], whereas pregnenolone had anxiogenic properties [129]. PREGS had a biphasic effect on elevated-plus maze behavior, exhibiting anxiolytic effects at low doses and anxiogenic effects at increasing doses [129]. Although data for DHEAS and PREGS are limited, it is possible that the mixed effects of these GABA antagonist steroids reflect confounding effects on activity level or the reduced ability of sulfated steroids to cross the blood–brain barrier.

Recent findings indicate that microinjection of GABA agonist neuroactive steroids or agents that increase neurosteroid levels into the hippocampus can produce anxiolytic effects. Specifically, microinjection of 2.5 and 5-μg doses of pregnanolone (3α,5β-THP) into the dorsal hippocampus of male rats significantly increased the proportion of time spent in the open arms of the elevated-plus maze [130]. Similar behavioral effects were seen when the hippocampus was microinjected with agonists of peripheral mitochondrial benzodiazepine receptors, which led to an increase of brain 3α,5α-THP [131].

With regard to the neurobiology of stress and anxiety, the role of the hippocampus has been described as a "comparator system" that can detect whether a threat is familiar or novel, thus requiring either a conditioned automatic response or higher order processing, respectively [132]. The septum, posterior cingulate, and thalamic nuclei also have been implicated in this role [133]. Overall, the hippocampus is important in traumatic memory consolidation and, with the entorhinal cortex, in contextual fear–conditioned behaviors. Projections from the hippocampus to the bed nucleus of the stria terminalis (BNST) and from the BNST to hypothalamic and brain stem sites may be involved in the expression of contextual fear conditioning (see Section 4.3.4).

4.3.2 Geller–Seifter and Vogel Conflict Tests

Both of these paradigms are conflict tests that utilize operant responding for a food reward [134] or a water reward [135], with electric shock as the aversive component in both tasks. The number of lever presses for either the food or water reward, in conjunction with a mild shock that is delivered on a fixed-ratio schedule, is the variable of interest. Anxiolytic drugs typically increase the number of lever presses, or the number of shocks that are acceptable, for the food or water reward. Although weeks of training on the lever-press task are required, these paradigms have the advantage that once stable performance baselines are established, the same animal can be used repeatedly to examine drug effects by comparing these data with its baseline (i.e., it is its own control). These tasks also have the advantage of an additional internal control, unpunished responding, that gives an indication of nonspecific drug effects. While both the Geller–Seifter and Vogel paradigms have been used primarily in rats, there are data on neurosteroid effects in mice as well.

Early work in Sprague–Dawley rats and Swiss Webster mice demonstrated that both alloTHDOC (10, 15, and 20 mg/kg, i.p.) and 3α,5α-THP (20 mg/kg, i.p.) had anxiolytic effects in the Vogel and Geller–Seifter conflict tests, respectively [94, 97]. Both steroids significantly increased punished responding without significantly influencing unpunished responding. However, a trend for sedation was found following the highest dose of alloTHDOC. Subsequent studies have confirmed these initial findings and demonstrated that systemic administration of 3α,5α-THP [98, 99], 3α,5β-THP [98], and alphaxalone [96] significantly enhanced punished drinking, consistent with their positive modulatory effects at $GABA_A$ receptors.

Another study compared the anxiolytic potential of four pregnanediols, differing only in the stereochemical orientation (α or β) of the steroid A ring and the 20-OH group [126]. The effects of these pregnanediols were examined in the Vogel test following i.c.v. administration and compared to those of their 20-ketone analogs (i.e., 3α,5α-THP and 3α,5β-THP). All four pregnanediols significantly enhanced punished drinking at doses ranging from 10 to 60 μg, whereas 3α,5α-THP and 3α,5β-THP enhanced punished responding when administered at 2.5- and 5-μg doses, respectively [126]. Doses of 3β,5α-THP up to 100 μg were inactive in the Vogel test, consistent with this steroid's lack of activity at $GABA_A$ receptors. These results suggest that some endogenously occurring pregnanediol metabolites (e.g., Fig. 4.3) also may influence physiological processes related to anxiety via an action at $GABA_A$ receptors, in addition to the actions of their parent steroids 3α,5α-THP and 3α,5β-THP.

As discussed in chapters on the neurobiology of stress and anxiety disorders, the amygdala plays a pivotal role in the assessment of and response to danger. The amygdala has extensive connections to the cortex and locus ceruleus and projections to the striatum, hypothalamus, midbrain, and brain stem. Thus, it can exert control over locomotor, neuroendocrine, autonomic, and respiratory responses. In addition, the amygdala also is seen as the common pathway and processor of "fear" [136]. Recent work demonstrated that infusion of 3α,5α-THP (8 μg per side) into the central nucleus of the amygdala (CeA) of male and ovariectomized (OVX) female rats produced a significant anxiolytic effect, measured by a significant increase in punished responding in the modified Geller Seifter conflict test [137]. Likewise, bilateral infusion of 3α,5α-THP (8 μg per side) into the CeA significantly increased open-arm time and open-arm entries on the elevated plus maze, compared to vehicle-infused controls. Bilateral infusion of the noncompetitive $GABA_A$ receptor steroid antagonists PREGS (0.0018 μg side) or DHEAS (2–8 μg per side) into the CeA had no effect on punished or unpunished responding, nor did i.c.v. administration of these two steroids at doses ranging from 1 to 20 μg [137]. Collectively, these findings suggest that the CeA is a key region involved in the mechanisms underlying the anxiolytic effects of 3α,5α-THP.

4.3.3 Light–Dark Box

Conceptually similar to the elevated-plus maze, the light–dark exploration task is based on the conflict between a rodent's tendency to explore a novel environment and the aversive properties of a brightly lit open field [138, 139]. The apparatus is an acrylic box divided by a panel into a large open area (28 cm long × 28 cm wide) and a slightly smaller enclosed area that is painted black (28 cm long × 19 cm wide). The open area is illuminated to 355 lux, whereas the light level in the dark chamber is low (2 lux). Typically, the animal is placed in the center of the light area, facing away from the entrance to the dark chamber, and behavior is recorded for 5–10 min. The number of transitions between the light and dark chambers, the time spent in both chambers, as well as the latency to enter the dark chamber, can be quantified by photocell array or manually. A chamber crossing is defined as all four paws of the mouse inside the chamber. The number of transitions and the time spent in the light chamber are the most commonly used variables. Anxiolytic drugs increase the number of transitions as well as the amount of time spent in the light chamber, relative to the dark chamber, which are believed to be indicators of the animal's willingness to explore the brightly lit open area [94, 139].

Interpretation of the light–dark box data can be confounded by effects of treatments on locomotor activity, particularly when the number of transitions is the only variable that is utilized. This appears to be more of a problem with anxiogenic drugs or treatments, as low levels of general activity have been shown to produce false positives [140]. Thus, it is recommended that independent testing for locomotor function be conducted in new classes of drugs in order to detect stimulant or sedative properties that could confound interpretation of the light–dark transition measure.

Early work found that alloTHDOC (7.5–15 mg/kg, i.p.) significantly increased the number of light–dark transitions in Swiss Webster mice [94]. There was no decrease in generalized locomotion, although a trend for sedation was found following administration of a 30-mg/kg dose of alloTHDOC. Subsequent studies in Swiss Webster mice documented dose-dependent anxiolytic effects of alloTHDOC (20 and 40 mg/kg, i.p.) and 3α,5α-THP (10–40 mg/kg, i.p.) with the light–dark box and that the 3β stereoisomer of 3α,5α-THP was inactive in this task [97, 98].

4.3.4 Acoustic Startle and Fear-Potentiated Startle

It was over 50 years ago that conditioned fear could be revealed by the magnitude of the startle response to an auditory stimulus [141]. This fear-potentiated startle paradigm involves pairing a neutral stimulus (e.g., light) with a footshock prior to the auditory stimulus [136, 142]. During testing, startle is elicited by the auditory stimulus alone (normal acoustic startle) or the auditory stimulus in the presence of the footshock-paired neutral stimulus (potentiated startle). The fear-potentiated startle effect only occurs following prior light–shock pairings, and not when lights and shocks have been presented in an unpaired or random fashion [143]. Presenting the conditioned stimulus repeatedly without further light/shock pairings will extinguish the prior fear conditioning (i.e., enhanced startle response) [144]. Notably, anxiolytic drugs reduce fear potentiated startle, whereas drugs that induce anxiety in people will increase potentiated startle in rodents [136].

Intracerebroventricular administration of corticotropin-releasing factor (CRF) can increase the amplitude of the acoustic startle response [145–147], whereas CRF peptide antagonists exhibit anxiolytic effects in the fear-potentiated startle paradigm [137, 147, 148]. Recently, it was reported that CRF-potentiated startle was significantly reduced in OVX female rats treated acutely or chronically with progesterone as well as in lactating female rats (high progesterone levels) [149]. Administration of 3α,5α-THP (10 mg/kg, i.p.) had a similar effect, suggesting that the effect of progesterone to reduce CRF-potentiated startle might be due to its metabolism to 3α,5α-THP. However, neither chronic progesterone nor 3α,5α-THP attenuated fear-potentiated startle [149]. Taken in conjunction with work indicating that the BNST, but not the CeA, is required for the elevation of startle after CRF infusion [150], the disparity in the effects of progesterone and 3α,5α-THP on CRF- versus fear-potentiated startle may reflect differential sensitivity of these brain regions to the steroids.

4.3.5 Mirrored Chamber

The chamber-of-mirrors procedure was first described in 1990 [151] as a measure of anxiety in rodents. This test generates an approach–avoidance conflict behavior which is based on early work [152] indicating that several vertebrate species demonstrate behavioral responses to mirrors such as aggressive threats and approach–avoidance behavior. The chamber consists of a mirrored cube 30 cm on a side which is open on one side and placed inside the center of an opaque Plexiglas box (40 × 40 × 30.5 cm). Thus, a 5-cm corridor completely surrounds the five-sided mirrored chamber. A sixth mirror is placed against the container wall opposite the single open side of the mirrored chamber. With the exception of the initial report in which mice were tested for 30 min [151], mice are placed in the corridor outside the mirrored chamber. Latency to enter the mirrored chamber, number of entries, time per entry, and total time in the mirrored chamber are recorded for a period of 5–10 min [153–156]. In this assay, a mouse avoids entering the mirrored chamber, whereas it will enter readily if the walls of the chamber are not mirrored [151]. However, a recent study in three inbred strains of mice in which the mirrors in the chamber were replaced with white or gray tiles suggested that a brightness or position effect in the chamber also could explain the avoidance behavior in certain genotypes [156]. Nonetheless, the mirrored-chamber procedure has been validated in terms of being responsive to a wide spectrum of anxiolytic agents at doses that do not affect locomotor activity [151, 153–155]. Recently, a modified version of the mirrored chamber was validated in the mouse to detect both anxiolytic and anxiogenic agents [157].

Neurosteroids also exhibited anxiolytic effects, measured by the behavior of mice in the mirrored test of anxiety [155]. Administration of progesterone (1–10 mg/kg) or its reduced metabolite 3α,5α-THP (0.5 and 1 mg/kg) produced a dose-dependent anxiolytic response, measured by increased number of entries and total time spent in the mirrored chamber as well as by decreased latency to enter the chamber. Consistent with the GABA agonist profile of 3α,5α-THP, the anxiolytic effect was blocked by coadministration of picrotoxin, a $GABA_A$ receptor chloride channel antagonist. In contrast, administration of a neurosteroid with GABA antagonist properties (DHEAS, 1 and 2 mg/kg) produced an anxiogenic response, measured by a decrease in the number of entries and total time spent in the mirrored chamber as well as an increase in the latency to enter the chamber. Therefore, both anxiolytic and anxiogenic effects of neurosteroids have been demonstrated that are consistent with their activity at $GABA_A$ receptors.

4.3.6 Open-Field Activity

Open-field activity is the oldest and simplest measure of rodent emotional behavior [158, 159]. Briefly, spontaneous exploratory locomotion, proximity to the walls and central arena, and number of fecal boli deposited are quantified in a brightly lit novel open field for a period of 5–10 min. Whereas fully automated systems are widely used, the scoring also can be performed manually. Thigmotaxis is measured by comparing activity in the center with activity in the perimeter of the open field. An animal exhibiting high perimeter and low center activity would be interpreted as possessing high levels of anxiety. However, an important distinction is that open-field activity is not a specific measure of anxiety or as specific a measure of anxiolytic drug response, compared to other tasks described in this section. Nonetheless, open-field activity does provide a useful measure of normal versus abnormal exploratory behavior. With this *proviso* in mind, early work documented that systemic administration of 3α,5α-THP and alloTHDOC (20 mg/kg, i.p.)

significantly increased activity in the open-field test, whereas the 3β epimer of 3α, 5α-THP was inactive [97].

4.3.7 Defensive Burying Behavior

Defensive burying refers to rodent behavior of displacing bedding material to remove or avoid aversive (unfamiliar and/or harmful) objects from their habitat. Together with flight, freezing, and fighting, defensive burying is part of the behavioral repertoire of unconditioned defensive reactions in an animal [160]. The shock-prod defensive burying procedure was first described in 1978 by Pinel and Treit [161]. Using a familiar test chamber, the animal is confronted with a wire-wrapped prod (or probe) that is inserted through a small hole in one of the test chamber walls so that the prod is approximately 2 cm above the bedding. Following the first contact with the electrified prod (in which the animal receives an electric shock), the animal's behavior is either observed or videotaped for a test session of 10–15 min. Typically, rodents will cover the shock source with cage litter or bedding. The latency and time to the first prod contact (shock) and the latency time to initiate burying behavior are recorded. The most commonly used measures of this defensive behavior have been the frequency and duration of time spent on prod-directed burying behavior as well as the height of the bedding material around the shock prod. In general, anxiolytic drugs suppress conditioned defensive burying, as measured by a reduction in the mean duration of burying behavior [160].

As with other animal models of anxiety-related behaviors, an ethological analysis of several concurrent and competitive behavioral indices of fear/anxiety, avoidance, reactivity, and exploration can provide a better understanding of the full defensive behavioral repertoire in rodents [160]. The following behavioral categories can be distinguished: ambulation, rearing, immobility, burying, grooming, prod-explore (i.e., oriented toward prod in a stretch/attend-like posture), and eating/drinking. One benefit of this ethological analysis stems from the fact that there is considerable variation across individual animals and studies in the mean time that animals engage in burying, which also represents only a small portion (between 3 and 30%) of the behaviors exhibited during the 10–15-min test. Thus, in addition to measuring defensive burying, one can quantify other avoidance/defensive behaviors (i.e., decreased prod exploration, increased freezing/immobility) as well as general exploratory and other behaviors (i.e., ambulation, rearing, grooming, and consummatory activities). While this paradigm has the advantage of requiring much less ambulatory locomotor activity than other tasks, it does have the potential confound that treatments producing behavioral sedation may produce false positives on this task (i.e., decreased defensive burying due to sedation). This task also has been well characterized for rats but not for mice.

The GABAergic neuroactive steroids 3α,5α-THP (0.25–1.0 mg/kg) and 3α,5β-THP suppressed burying behavior in this task, consistent with their anxiolytic profile [125, 162]. Progesterone (1–4 mg/kg) also was effective, whereas PREGS (1–4 mg/kg) was not [162]. Additional studies determined that microinjection of 3α,5β-THP into the dorsal hippocampus or the lateral septum significantly decreased burying behavior [130]. These microinjection studies are consistent with data indicating that the posterior parts of the septal region, the dorsal hippocampus, the caudal shell of the nucleus accumbens, and the dorsal raphe nuclei are critical parts of the neural circuitry underlying defensive burying [160].

4.3.8 Separation-Induced Ultrasonic Vocalizations

The rat pup ultrasonic vocalization procedure has been shown to detect a wide range of anxiolytic and anxiogenic compounds [163]. In rat pups, vocalizations in the frequency range of 35–45 kHz are produced in the first two postnatal weeks and are associated with social isolation. Most investigators count the number of calls using a microphone sensitive to high-frequency sounds connected to a signal detection device, such as a bat detector, that transduces the sounds into the audible range. However, it also is recommended that nonvocal variables such as changes in ambient and body temperature, locomotion, and coordination should be monitored to determine whether the effects of a treatment are specific for vocal behavior [163]. Variations of this procedure have been referred to as maternal separation, early deprivation, or social isolation [164].

Initial studies determined that benzodiazepine agonists (such as diazepam and chlordiazepoxide) decreased the number of ultrasonic vocalizations in isolated rat pups at doses lower than those that produced muscle relaxation and sedation [165]. The GABAergic neurosteroids $3\alpha,5\alpha$-THP and alloTHDOC also significantly decreased the number of ultrasonic vocalizations in isolated rat pups [166–169]. Repeated administration of alloTHDOC to infant rats during postnatal days 2–10 prior to recurring separation from their mothers significantly attenuated the increase in anxiety-related behavior that was evident in rats administered vehicle, when the animals were tested on the elevated-plus maze as adults [168]. In the study by Patchev et al. [168], repeated maternal separation also produced neuroendocrine alterations related to dysregulation of the hypothalamic–pituitary–adrenal (HPA) axis in adult rats, and these endocrine responses were significantly reduced in the animals administered repeated alloTHDOC as infants. In contrast, a study that utilized a slightly different maternal separation procedure did not observe a difference in anxiety related behavior in adult rats that had been repeatedly separated from their mothers as infants versus non-isolated controls [169]. However, as adults, non-isolated controls treated daily with $3\alpha,5\alpha$-THP during postnatal days 2–6 exhibited less anxiety-like behavior than all other groups, including isolated rats treated with $3\alpha,5\alpha$-THP. Postnatal treatment with $3\alpha,5\alpha$-THP also eliminated the sex difference in anxiety-related behavior that was apparent in non-injected adult rats. In general, these studies suggest that chronic treatment with the GABAergic neurosteroids alloTHDOC and $3\alpha,5\alpha$-THP may offset the behavioral and neuroendocrine changes that occur as a result of adverse early-life events.

4.3.9 Modified Forced-Swim Test

The forced-swim test is considered an animal model of depression, rather than of anxiety. Since many of the core symptoms of depression are difficult to measure in laboratory animals, many of the available animal models of depression are based on the actions of known antidepressants or on the responses to stress [170]. The forced-swim test was initially developed in the rat [171] and later in the mouse [172]. In this model, rodents are forced to swim in a confined environment. The animals initially swim around and attempt to escape and eventually assume an immobile position. On subsequent tests, the latency to immobility is decreased [170, 173]. The immobility is thought to reflect either a failure of persistence in escape-directed behavior (i.e., behavioral despair) or the development of passive behavior that disengages the animal from active forms of coping with stressful stimuli. A drug or treatment that produces an increase in immobility would be considered to produce depressive-like behavior, whereas a drug that increases escape-directed behavior (i.e., decreased immobility) would be considered to have an antidepressant effect. However, one drawback of the Porsolt forced-swim test is that it is not sensitive to the selective serotonin reuptake inhibitor (SSRI) class of antidepressant compounds.

In an effort to enhance the sensitivity of the forced-swim test in rodents so that it could be SSRI responsive, several simple procedural modifications were made [173]. Increasing the water depth to 30 cm produced less immobility time because animals could not contact the cylinder bottom with their paws. Rating the predominant behavior over 5-s intervals allowed the distinction of the following behaviors: climbing, horizontal swimming, and immobility. With regard to the putative antidepressant effects of neurosteroids, systemic (0.5, 1 or 2 mg/kg, i.p.) or i.c.v. (1 or 2 μg per mouse) administration of 3α,5α-THP dose dependently reduced the duration of immobility in the modified Porsolt forced-swim test [174, 175]. This antidepressant-like effect of 3α,5α-THP was potentiated by pretreatment with the GABA$_A$ receptor agonist muscimol [174] or ethanol [175], whereas it was blocked by pretreatment with the GABA$_A$ receptor antagonist bicuculline. Administration of progesterone (2 mg/kg) to OVX female rats also was effective at producing effects in the forced-swim test that were similar to that of the tricyclic antidepressants [176]. The ability of progesterone to decrease immobility by increasing climbing behavior was comparable to that observed during days 14 and 17 of pregnancy. Thus, physiological states in which progesterone levels are high can produce antidepressant-like effects, presumably due to progesterone's reduction to 3α,5α-THP.

Chronic ethanol withdrawal, which has been reported to decrease endogenous 3α,5α-THP levels (see Section 4.4.4), produced an increase in immobility on the modified forced-swim test [175]. Notably, subthreshold doses of 3α,5α-THP (0.25 or 0.5 μg per mouse) reversed the depressive-like symptoms associated with ethanol withdrawal. Recent findings also indicated that withdrawal from daily progesterone injections significantly increased immobility in the modified forced-swim test in female DBA/2 mice (E. H. Beckley and D. A. Finn, unpublished results). There was a further increase in immobility when the metabolism of progesterone was blocked with administration of finasteride, suggesting that withdrawal from progesterone or progesterone metabolites produced an increase in depressive-like behavior. These findings are consistent with recent work suggesting that some symptoms of progesterone withdrawal are due to withdrawal from 3α,5α-THP [177, 178]. Although speculative at this point, these findings are consistent with an inverse relationship between fluctuations in endogenous 3α,5α-THP levels and depressive-like symptoms (i.e., ↑ 3α,5α-THP, ↓ depression; ↓ 3α,5α-THP, ↑ depression).

4.3.10 Mild Mental Stress Models and Social Isolation

As described in Section 4.1, acute exposure of male rodents to a variety of stressors rapidly increased brain 3α,5α-THP and alloTHDOC to the equivalent of 10–30 nM concentrations [14, 15]. Recent work also demonstrated that immobilizing rats on their backs for 20 min produced a significant increase in brain 3α,5α-THP levels as well as in levels of the precursor steroids pregnenolone, progesterone, and 5α-DHP [179]. Notably, when the vocalizations of the rats were recorded during the period of immobilization and subsequently played for 1 h to a group of unrestrained rats (referred to as mild mental stress or "din stress" by the authors), there was a slight but significant increase in brain 3α,5α-THP, 5α-DHP, progesterone, and pregnenolone levels in 66% of the rats [179]. Thus, acute exposure to physical stressors or stressors encompassing a psychological component can increase the synthesis of GABAergic neuroactive steroids to levels that should facilitate GABAergic neurotransmission in the brain.

In contrast, long-term social isolation after weaning significantly decreased brain 3α,5α-THP and alloTHDOC levels in male rodents [180–182]. There is conflicting evidence on the specific point(s) in the neurosteroid biosynthetic pathway where social isolation might be altering GABAergic neurosteroid levels. Whereas one study demonstrated that social isolation also decreased brain pregnenolone and progesterone levels [181], a second study provided evidence that the effect of social isolation occurred at a point downstream from progesterone [182]. In the study by Dong et al. [182], social isolation did not alter progesterone levels, but it significantly decreased the expression and protein levels of the enzyme 5α-reductase (see Fig. 4.1 for biosynthetic pathway). Nonetheless, the decreases in GABAergic neurosteroid levels were associated with an increase in anxiety-like behavior, measured by a significant decrease in percentage of open-arm time on the elevated-plus maze and a significant decrease in punished responding in the Vogel conflict test [181]. Social isolation also produced a decrease in biochemical and electrophysiological measures of $GABA_A$ receptor function [181] as well as decreased sensitivity to the hypnotic effect of GABAergic compounds [180, 183]. Thus, the period of exposure to stress may produce opposite effects on endogenous neuroactive steroid levels in the brain.

4.4 NEUROACTIVE STEROID INTERACTIONS WITH STRESS-INDUCED BEHAVIORS

From the results summarized in Section 4.3, it is apparent that GABA agonist neurosteroids have anxiolytic properties. However, their role as endogenous modulators of anxiety is less clear. For example, systemic administration of progesterone has anxiolytic effects, measured by elevated-plus maze behavior, via its metabolism to 3α,5α-THP, since inhibiting the enzymatic conversion of progesterone to 3α,5α-THP blocked the anxiolytic effect of progesterone [184]. Likewise, results from a recent study suggest that the ability of progesterone to attenuate CRF- enhanced acoustic startle response might be due to progesterone's metabolism to 3α,5α-THP, since administration of 3α,5α-THP had a similar effect, whereas use of a progestin that was not metabolized to 3α,5α-THP (i.e., medroxy-progesterone) did not [149]. While the putative modulatory role of brain versus peripheral-derived 3α,5α-THP on anxiety-related behavior is not clear, recent work has examined the effect of ligands that stimulate biosynthesis of 3α,5α-THP in adrenalectomized–gonadectomized (ADX–GDX) and intact animals [131, 185]. These ligands, which activate peripheral benzodiazepine receptors, significantly increased brain levels of 3α,5α-THP to a greater extent in the intact versus ADX–GDX rats, yet the increase in brain 3α,5αTHP also was associated with a marked anti-conflict effect in the Vogel test. Thus, it is possible that peripheral sources of 3α,5αTHP may have a greater impact in modulating anxiety-related behavior than brain-derived 3α,5αTHP.

4.4.1 HPA Axis and Stress

Acute stress of many types results in the release of CRF, adrenocorticotropic hormone (ACTH), and cortisol in humans and corticosterone in rodents (see Fig. 4.5) [186]. Corticosteroids bind to mineralocorticoid receptors (MRs) and glucocorticoid receptors (GRs), which are colocalized in brain regions important in the regulation of anxiety, such as the hippocampus, septum, and amygdala. A recent report indicated that increased corticosterone levels in rodents were highly correlated with measures of risk assessment [187]. Several animal models of anxiety have demonstrated that both MR and GR can modulate specific aspects of anxiety, as antagonists for both receptor subtypes have been shown to have anxiolytic effects [186].

GRs are found in higher concentrations in regions involved in feedback regulation of the hormonal stress response. GRs have a 10-fold lower affinity for corticosterone than MRs, becoming occupied only during stress and at the circadian peak, whereas

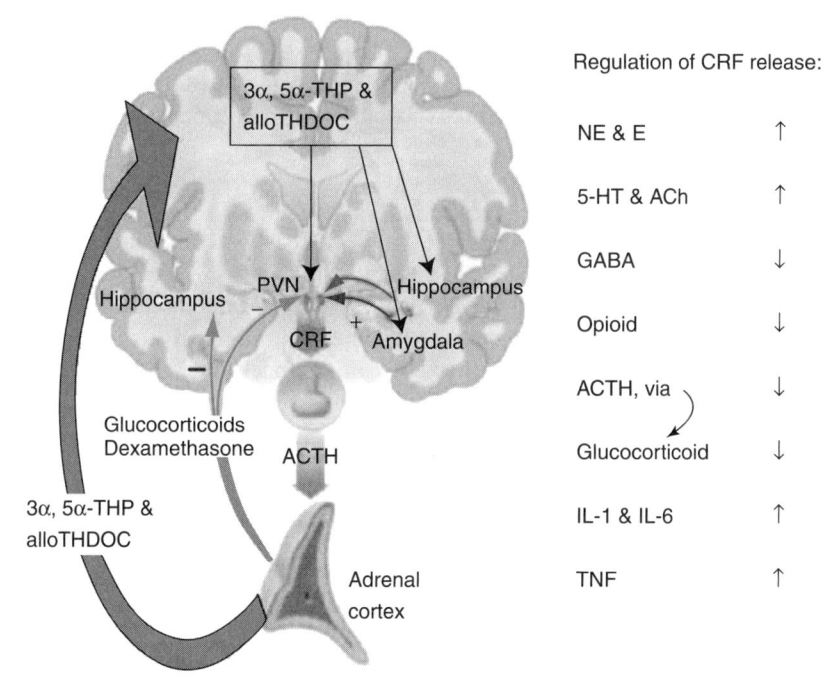

Figure 4.5 Various points of control for regulation of the HPA axis by neurosteroids, neurotransmitters, ACTH, glucocorticoids, and the immune system[186, 222, 224, 284–286]. A variety of stressors activate the HPA axis, which is typically observed as an increase in glucocorticoids from the adrenal cortex. Stress also produces an increase in levels of the GABAergic neurosteroids 3α,5α-THP and alloTHDOC in the brain via the circulation and *de novo* synthesis. (Adapted from Nestler et al. [170].) (See color insert.)

MR is almost completely occupied under basal conditions. Since it is believed that GR action is mainly regulated by hormone level, with MR action being influenced by receptor density, endogenous corticosteroids can play an important role in the maintenance of homeostatic equilibrium via its two receptors [188, 189]. High corticosteroid levels, such as those elicited by exposure to an acute stressor, decrease the number of GRs, which in turn results in increased corticosterone secretion and feedback resistance.

One of the many neurotransmitters that can modulate HPA axis activity is the GABAergic system, as the GABAergic innervation of CRF-producing cells of the hypothalamic paraventricular nucleus (PVN) has been shown to be particularly important for the control of HPA axis activity [190]. For example, GABAergic function in the PVN was increased after ADX and was normalized when corticosteroid levels were restored [191]. A series of elegant studies recently determined that corticosterone can modulate GABAergic function in PVN neurons within hours in a mode different from that of neurosteroids (i.e., presynaptic vs. postsynaptic effect) [192]. Restraint stress was found to decrease GABAergic inhibition by 50%, suggesting that the corticosterone-induced changes in GABAergic function in the PVN also occur with natural fluctuations in this hormone level due to stress exposure.

Adding another level of complexity to regulation of the HPA axis, acute stressors and activation of the HPA axis also can increase levels of the GABAergic neurosteroids 3α,5α-THP and alloTHDOC (see Figs. 4.2 and 4.5 and Section 4.1). One possibility is that a stress-induced increase in GABAergic neurosteroids could participate in the adaptation to the stress response. Consistent with this idea, administration of 3α,5αTHP reduced anxiety that was induced by CRF [193] in addition to exerting actions within the hypothalamus to dampen the activity of the HPA axis [193, 194].

4.4.2 Anxiety-Related Disorders

Alterations in HPA axis function are suggested in posttraumatic stress disorder (PTSD), as shown by a decrease in cortisol levels and increased suppression of cortisol levels with the GR agonist dexamethasone (dexamethasone suppression test, DST), suggesting enhanced sensitivity to cortisol feedback [195, 196]. Patients with PTSD also had a blunted ACTH response to CRF versus control subjects, suggesting hypersecretion of CRF [197]. Consistent with this observation, patients with combat-related PTSD had elevated levels of CRF in the cerebrospinal fluid (CSF) [198]. However, more recent work suggested that women with PTSD do not differ from traumatized subjects or non-traumatized controls in basal cortisol levels [199]. When the subjects were challenged with a dose of ACTH that had been reported to elicit cortisol responses equivalent to that seen following extreme naturalistic stressors, the cortisol responses were significantly increased in the patients with PTSD versus other subjects. An independent study determined that, following a CRF challenge dose, cortisol levels determined hourly in CSF over a 6 h period were significantly elevated in patients with PTSD compared to matched control subjects [200]. Whereas baseline DHEA levels did not differ between the patients in the study by Rasmusson et al. [199], the increase in DHEA in response to the ACTH challenge was significantly greater in the PTSD patients. The authors hypothesized that the anti-glucocorticoid properties of DHEA might antagonize glucocorticoid negative feedback within the brain and pituitary, which would ultimately result in an increase in the adrenal capacity for cortisol release due to a facilitation of CRF or ACTH release.

CSF levels of CRF have also been shown to be elevated in patients with obsessive compulsive disorder [201], but not panic disorder [202]. However, an additional study demonstrating no difference in baseline CSF levels of CRF between control subjects and patients with generalized anxiety disorder, panic disorder, or obsessive-compulsive disorder [203] suggests that these patients did not exhibit tonic hypersecretion of CRF. Therefore, evidence for dysfunction of CRF or HPA systems in anxiety disorders has been inconsistent [204].

A recent study by Strohle and colleagues in patients with panic disorder [205] demonstrated that panic attacks induced by sodium lactate and cholecystokinin tetrapeptide were accompanied by marked decreases in circulating levels of 3α, 5α-THP and 3α,5β-THP, with concomitant increases in the neuroactive steroid antagonist 3β,5α-THP. Similar changes were not observed in control subjects. Baseline 3α,5α-THP levels in these patients were increased [206], particularly in the early follicular phase of the menstrual cycle [207]. It is possible that during an induced panic attack patients with panic disorder fail to maintain compensatory increased 3α,5α-THP levels. Therefore, neuroactive steroids may play a role in the pathophysiology of panic disorders.

Early work suggested that examination stress produced a significant increase in the density of peripheral benzodiazepine receptors (PBRs), compared to unstressed controls [208]. Although PBRs play a role in the translocation of cholesterol from the outer to the inner mitochondrial membrane [209], which represents the rate-limiting step for the synthesis of neuroactive steroids (see Fig. 4.1) [210], the physiological consequence of the increased PBR with regard to neuroactive steroid biosynthesis was not known. More recent work determined that PhD examination stress increased heart rate, blood pressure, plasma 3α,5α-THP, and cortisol levels and the density of PBR when compared with baseline levels [211]. The increase in plasma cortisol was not correlated with the increase in PBR density, suggesting that the acute stress–induced increase in cortisol levels did not depend on rapid biosynthesis. Notably, the increase in plasma 3α,5α-THP was significantly positively correlated with increased PBR density. Although no causal relationship can be drawn from these findings, it is possible that use of synthetic PBR agonists to enhance the synthesis of 3α,5α-THP could be useful in the treatment of anxiety disorders [211].

A number of studies in which various animal models of anxiety were utilized demonstrated that injection of CRF into the locus ceruleus, paraventricular nucleus of the hypothalamus, BNST, and CeA produced signs and symptoms that were identical to animals in response to stress as well as those observed in patients with anxiety disorders [137, 148, 212–215]. Notably, central CRF systems, in addition to those that participate in the control of the HPA axis, contribute to affective behavior regulation [216]. In male rats, alfaxalone, the 11-keto derivative of 3α,5α-THP, was shown to attenuate the anxiogenic behavioral effects of CRF and swim stress without reducing the CRF-induced increases in plasma ACTH [217]. Alfaxalone also inhibited the startle enhancing effects of CRF in male rats without disrupting CRF-stimulated locomotor activity [218]. At doses of 5 and 10 μg i.c.v., 3α, 5α-THP counteracted the anxiogenic action of 5 μg CRF in male rats and prevented the adrenalectomy-induced upregulation of CRF gene expression [193]. Both progesterone and 3α,5α-THP attenuated CRF-enhanced acoustic startle, whereas the progestin medroxyprogesterone acetate enhanced CRF-induced startle [149]. Thus, CRF appears to play a significant role in anxiety-related and stress-related states that can be attenuated by GABAergic neuroactive steroids. Collectively, the data also suggest that agents acting at CRF receptors may have therapeutic value in anxiety disorders. Indeed, the development of CRF receptor antagonists as novel anxiolytics is being actively pursued (see chapter 5) [215].

For a more detailed discussion of neuroactive steroids in psychopathology and menstrual cycle–linked CNS disorders, the reader is referred to the reviews by Dubrovsky [219], and Backstrom et al., [220] and chapter 21 in volume I of this handbook.

4.4.3 Depression

Evidence suggests that stressful life events can produce hyperactivity of the HPA axis and can increase vulnerability to depression [170, 221–225]. In general, patients with major depressive disorder exhibit elevated plasma cortisol and CRF levels, with approximately 50% of patients displaying an impaired suppression of cortisol secretion after dexamethasone administration (DST test) [225]. Patients with stress-associated disorders such as depression appear to escape from glucocorticoid negative feedback, resulting in a persistent activation of the HPA axis.

Protracted social isolation in rodents produces behavioral symptoms also found in depression, in addition to producing a significant decrease in cortical 3α,5α-THP levels and a decrease in expression of the biosynthetic enzyme 5α-reductase [182]. Taken in conjunction with the finding that 3α,5α-THP has antidepressant properties [174], manipulation of neuroactive steroid biosynthesis may have therapeutic benefits. Studies in patients with unipolar depression found a 60% decrease in 3α,5α-THP content in CSF or plasma, compared to values in normal subjects [226–228]. Treatment with fluoxetine, a broad-spectrum antidepressant that inhibits serotonin reuptake, for 8–10 weeks normalized the levels of 3α,5α-THP in the depressed patients. Improvement in symptomatology and the increase in 3α,5α-THP concentrations in CSF were significantly, positively correlated in the study by Uzunova et al. [227]. It was subsequently determined that fluoxetine altered 3α,5α-THP biosynthesis by increasing the affinity of 5α-DHP for the enzyme 3α-hydroxysteroid dehydrogenase (see Fig. 4.1) [229]. Data in rats indicate that the effect of fluoxetine on 3α,5α-THP biosynthesis was rapid; significant increases in brain 3α,5α-THP levels were observed between 15 and 120 min post injection of fluoxetine [230]. This ability of fluoxetine to shift the activity of the 3α-hydroxysteroid dehydrogenase enzyme toward the reductive direction (i.e., toward the formation of 3α,5α-THP from 5α-DHP) provides evidence for a possible role of neuroactive steroids in successful antidepressant therapy.

There are massive levels of progesterone ($\sim 5 \times 10^{-7}$ M) in maternal plasma during human pregnancy near term. These levels are much greater (5- to 50-fold) than those that occur in most other pregnant mammals, including non-human primates [231]. It is therefore not surprising that the combined levels of 3α,5α-THP and 3α.5β-THP approach 15 ng/mL or $\sim 5 \times 10^{-8}$ M near term (Fig. 4.6), although there are wide individual variations. There is only a very limited transfer of progesterone from maternal plasma into the fetus, but it does enter the

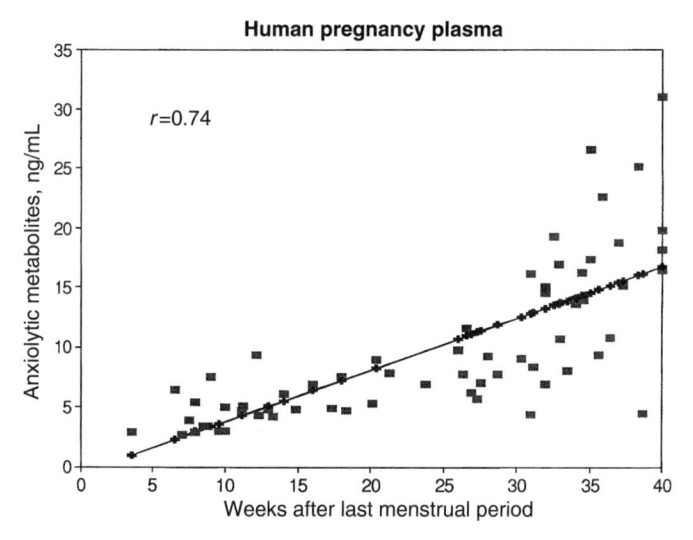

Figure 4.6 Combined levels of anxiolytic metabolites of progesterone, allopregnanolone, and pregnanolone, measured in 11 normal women during pregnancy. The weeks of gestation were established from last menstrual period. The levels of the anxiolytic metabolites were measured in duplicate by specific RIA after extraction of serum and separation of the individual neuroactive steroids as described by Purdy et al. [21] and Schmidt et al. [287]. (Data from R. Purdy and D. Castracane, unpublished.)

fetal circulation from the placental syncytiotrophoblast where it is synthesized and then converted in the fetus to 3α,5α-THP and its sulfate [232].

The etiology of depression in childbearing women is poorly understood, but it has been suggested that the very large changes in progesterone and its anxiolytic metabolites in the postpartum period may predispose some women to depression [233, 234]. These dramatic postpartum changes are illustrated in Fig. 4.7 as the dramatic logarithmic decrease in concentrations of progesterone, 3α,5α-THP, and 3α,5β-THP in the maternal plasma of three normal women. A more detailed time profile of pregnanolone isomers in the postpartum period has been provided by Hill et al. [235]. Gilbert Evans et al. [236] have found a significant reduction in the concentrations of 3α,5α-THP plus 3α,5β-THP in pregnant women with a history of postpartum depression at 36–38 weeks, regardless of their current state of depression. Their results suggest that depression history was associated with an underlying dysregulation of these neuroactive steroids.

4.4.4 Acute and Chronic Effects of Alcohol

Acute and chronic administration of alcohol also activates the HPA axis, measured by an increase in plasma corticosterone in rodents [237–241]. Elegant work by the Rivier laboratory demonstrated that i.p. or intragastric administration of alcohol produced a rapid, significant increase in plasma ACTH levels [242] and neuronal activity in the cell bodies of the PVN of the hypothalamus that express CRF and vasopressin [238, 239]. Since available *in vivo* evidence had not consistently

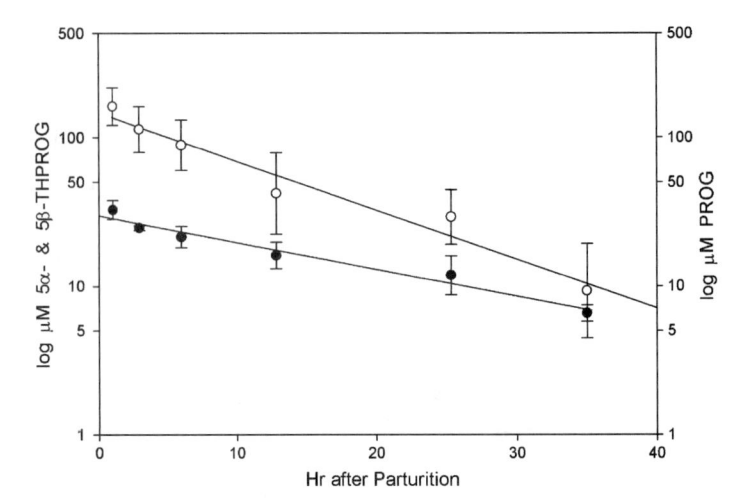

Figure 4.7 Logarithm of sum of micromolar concentrations (± standard error of the mean) of progesterone (PROG, open circles) and sum of its two anxiolytic metabolites (closed circles), allopregnanolone (5α-THPROG) and pregnanolone (5β-THPROG), obtained in the plasma from three women up to 36 h after parturition. The anxiolytic metabolites were measured by RIA as described in Fig. 4.6. Progesterone was measured by RIA in duplicate using a standard kit from ICN (Costa Mesa, CA). (Data from R.H. Purdy and D. Castracane, unpublished.)

demonstrated whether acute administration of alcohol influenced pituitary activity, independent of CRF and vasopressin, the mechanism by which ethanol stimulated the HPA axis was uncertain. However, recent findings shed some light on the specific sites of action of ethanol on the activity of the HPA axis. Specifically, i.c.v. and i.p. administration of alcohol increased the expression of proopiomelanocortin (POMC) in the anterior pituitary with a time course that corresponded to ACTH release [243]; these responses were completely abolished by immunoneutralization of CRF and vasopressin. This finding provides strong evidence that the stimulatory effect of acute alcohol administration on the HPA axis requires the release of endogenous CRF and vasopressin, rather than a direct pituitary influence of alcohol on the corticotropes.

Acute administration of anesthetics, including ethanol, also has been shown to increase plasma levels of progesterone, the parent steroid of 3α,5α-THP, in male rats [244]. This initial finding was recently extended with the demonstration that acute injection of ethanol doses ranging from 1 to 4 g/kg significantly increased cortical 3α,5α-THP levels to pharmacologically active concentrations in rats and mice [245–247]. Acute alcohol intoxication also increased plasma 3α,5α-THP levels in male and female adolescent humans [248, 249]. Due to the fact that the pharmacological profile of ethanol is similar to that of 3α,5α-THP, it has been suggested that certain behavioral effects of ethanol and 3α,5α-THP might share a GABAergic mechanism [250, 251]. Taken in conjunction with the demonstration that manipulating endogenous 3α,5α-THP levels altered specific behavioral and physiological effects of ethanol (i.e., ↑ 3α,5α-THP, ↑ ethanol effect; ↓ 3α,5α-THP, ↓ ethanol effect) [246, 252], these data suggest that an ethanol-induced increase in endogenous 3α, 5α-THP levels might potentiate or prolong certain behavioral effects of ethanol via its action at $GABA_A$ receptors. Since additional studies demonstrated that the endocrine response to acutely administered alcohol was principally due to steroid biosynthesis in adrenal and gonadal tissue [253–255], it is possible that endogenous $3\alpha,5\alpha$-THP levels might play a role in the modulation of the excitability of the HPA axis in response to stress (see Fig. 4.5) and in the modulation of cortical $3\alpha,5\alpha$-THP concentration after ethanol injection.

Electrophysiological recordings from CA1 pyramidal neurons determined that the action of ethanol on $GABA_A$ receptor–mediated inhibitory postsynaptic current amplitude was biphasic [256]. Initially, there was a rapid, direct effect of ethanol on $GABA_A$ receptor activity, followed by an indirect effect that was believed to be mediated by the synthesis of $3\alpha,5\alpha$-THP. Furthermore, it has been clearly demonstrated by these electrophysiological methods that ethanol increases GABAergic transmission at both presynaptic and postsynaptic sites in rat central amygdala neurons [257], as well as altering glutamatergic transmission in this tissue [258]. This poses the possibility of neuroactive steroid action at both of these sites of neurotransmission within the amygdala.

4.4.5 Stress-Induced Drug Reinstatement

Drug relapse is a major problem in the treatment of drug addiction in humans [259]. Early work in monkeys and rodents used a reinstatement procedure as an animal model of drug relapse [260–263]. In the reinstatement model, laboratory animals initially are trained to lever press for access to drugs in operant chambers, which produces robust self-administration behavior. The drug-reinforced responding is extinguished when saline is substituted for the drug solution or when the infusion pump is disconnected (i.e., the animal stops pressing the lever and responding to the stimuli previously associated with drug delivery). During reinstatement tests, animals are given access to the levers, but the drug remains unavailable, making it possible to test for the ability of various events to reinitiate drug-seeking behavior. The results from a number of laboratories have determined that the following events are extremely effective in promoting operant-reinforced responding on the lever previously associated with drug: reexposure to the drug (i.e., priming injection), acute exposure to stressful stimuli (e.g., footshock), and environmental stimuli (e.g., cues) previously associated with drug self-administration [264–268].

In the 1990s, many studies demonstrated that exposure to intermittent footshock was at least as effective as priming injections of cocaine, heroin, or nicotine and even more effective than priming injections of alcohol in promoting high levels of responding in tests of reinstatement over a range of footshock durations (10–60 min) [269–273]. Administration of CRF (0.3 and 1 µg, i.c.v.) potently reinstated heroin-seeking behavior, whereas the CRF antagonist α-helical CRF_{9-41} (3 and 10 µg, i.c.v.) attenuated stress-induced but not heroin-induced reinstatement [274]. Additional studies determined that ADX and corticosterone replacement did not alter footshock-induced reinstatement to alcohol [275], whereas the nonselective CRF antagonist D-Phe-CRF_{12-41} (0.3 and 1 µg, i.c.v.) and the nonpeptide CRF_1 receptor antagonist CP-154,526 (15–30 mg/kg, subcutaneous) significantly decreased reinstatement of alcohol-, heroin-, and cocaine-seeking behavior that was induced by intermittent footshock [275, 276]. These data suggest that extra hypothalamic CRF systems are involved in stress-induced drug reinstatement behavior.

With regard to neurosteroid effects on drug reinstatement, a single study has demonstrated that priming injections of 3α,5α-THP (3 and 7.5 mg/kg, i.p.) dose dependently reinstated previously extinguished responding for ethanol but not for sucrose [277]. In contrast, conditioned stimuli reinstated previously extinguished ethanol- and sucrose-seeking behavior, suggesting that the mechanisms that subserve cue-induced reinstatement do not depend on the nature of the positive reinforcer tested. However, the fact that 3α,5α-THP selectively promoted responding for ethanol after a period of abstinence suggests that $GABA_A$ receptor modulation may contribute to the processes involved in reinstatement of ethanol-seeking behavior.

Notably, several neuroactive steroids also modulate ethanol self-administration behavior. The initial study determined that 3α,5α-THP significantly increased ethanol-reinforced operant responding in male rats [278] by enhancing responses during the initial run of a 30-min operant session. A subsequent study determined that 3α,5α-THP selectively enhanced ethanol-reinforced operant responding when a sucrose solution was concurrently available [279], suggesting specificity for 3α,5α-THP in modulating ethanol self-administration in male rats. Consistent with these findings, 3α,5α-THP dose dependently increased ethanol preference drinking during the first hour of 2-h limited-access sessions in male mice [280, 280a]. In contrast to the results with 3α,5α-THP, epipregnanolone and a novel neuroactive steroid with a 3α-carboxyl group (3α,5β-20-oxo-pregnane-3-carboxylic acid, termed PCA) dose dependently reduced operant ethanol self-administration in male rats [281]. The opposite effect of epipregnanolone and PCA on ethanol self-administration may be related to different inhibitory actions of these compounds on either $GABA_A$ or NMDA receptors, respectively [282, 283]. Thus, dual modulation of inhibitory and excitatory neurotransmitter systems by certain neuroactive steroids may provide a novel therapeutic potential for modifying the reinforcing effects of addictive drugs.

4.5 CONCLUSIONS AND OUTLOOK

There has been an exponential increase in basic science and clinical investigations of neuroactive steroids in the last two decades. Methodological advances in the specificity, sensitivity, and accuracy of measurement of nonconjugated neuroactive steroids are still continuing. The chemical nature of the "sulfate-like" esters of PREG and DHEA in brain has yet to be elucidated, even though these esters are predominant in mammalian blood. Since anesthetic neuroactive steroids such as alfaxalone were introduced five decades ago, there has been a continuing interest in the development of other synthetic neuroactive steroids for the clinical treatment of neurological disorders, including stress and anxiety. Additionally, neuroactive steroids have been linked to pathogenesis in menstrual cycle–linked disorders of the CNS.

Several thousand synthetic steroids have been assayed for their interactions as allosteric modulators of neurotransmitter systems. New compounds with unusual properties continue to be reported. Yet, in our opinion, universal recognition of the neurophysiological and neuropharmacological importance of neuroactive steroids awaits definitive demonstration of their clinical importance and therapeutic advantage.

ACKNOWLEDGMENTS

This is publication number 17678-NP from The Scripps Research Institute. This work was supported by U.S. National Institutes of Health grants AA06420, AA12439, and AA10760 from the National Institute on Alcohol Abuse and Alcoholism and by the U.S. Department of Veterans Affairs (DAF). The immobilization experiment described in Fig. 4.2 was performed in the laboratory of Nobuyoshi Hagino at the University of Texas Health Sciences Center, San Antonio, TX. The samples of plasma from pregnant women used to generate the data shown in Figs. 4.6 and 4.7 were generously provided by V. Daniel Castracane at Texas University Health Sciences Center, Amarillo, TX. The radioimmunoassays used to generate the data in Figs. 4.2, 4.6 and 4.7 were performed by Perry Moore at the Southwest Foundation for Biomedical Research, San Antonio, TX, under a contract from the National Institute of Mental Health. We gratefully acknowledge the editorial contributions of Elizabeth Gordon, Michael Arends, Mellany Santos, Eric Zorrilla, Dewleen Baker, and Mathew Ford and helpful conversations with collaborators John Crabbe and Tamara Phillips as well as invaluable assistance from members of the Finn Laboratory on various aspects of this work.

REFERENCES

1. Selye, H. (1942). Correlations between the chemical structure and the pharmacological actions of the steroids. *Endocrinology* 30, 437–453.
2. Laubach, G. D., Pan, S. Y., and Rudel, H. W. (1955). Steroid anesthetic agent. *Science* 122, 78.
3. Holzbauer, M. (1976). Physiological aspects of steroids with anaesthetic properties. *Med. Biol.* 54, 227–242.
4. Holzbauer, M., Birmingham, M. K., De Nicola, A. F., et al. (1985). In vivo secretion of 3α-hydroxy-5α-pregnan-20-one, a potent anaesthetic steroid, by the adrenal gland of the rat. *J. Steroid Biochem.* 22, 97–102.
5. Harrison, N. L., and Simmonds, M. A. (1984). Modulation of the GABA receptor complex by a steroid anaesthetic. *Brain Res.* 323, 287–292.
6. Merke, D. P., Bornstein, S. R., Avila, N. A., et al. (2002). Future directions in the study and management of congenital adrenal hyperplasia due to 21-hydroxylase deficiency. *Ann. Intern. Med.* 136, 320–334.
7. McEwen, B. S. (1991). Non-genomic and genomic effects of steroids on neural activity. *Trends Pharmacol. Sci.* 12, 141–147.
8. Paul, S. M., and Purdy, R. H. (1992). Neuroactive steroids. *FASEB J.* 6, 2311–2322.
9. Brann, D. W., Hendry, L. B., and Mahesh, V. B. (1995). Emerging diversities in the mechanism of action of steroid hormones. *J. Steroid Biochem. Mol. Biol.* 52, 113–133.
10. Lambert, J. J., Belelli, D., Hill-Venning, C., et al. (1995). Neurosteroids and $GABA_A$ receptor function. *Trends Pharmacol. Sci.* 16, 295–303.
11. Rupprecht, R., and Holsboer, F. (1999). Neuroactive steroids: Mechanisms of action and neuropsychopharmacological perspectives. *Trends Neurosci.* 22, 410–416.
12. Baulieu, E. E., Robel, P., and Schumacher, M. (2001). Neurosteroids: Beginning of the story. *Int. Rev. Neurobiol.* 46, 1–32.

13. Gasior, M., Carter, R. B., and Witkin, J. M. (1999). Neuroactive steroids: Potential therapeutic use in neurological and psychiatric disorders. *Trends Pharmacol. Sci.* 20, 107–112.
14. Barbaccia, M. L., Serra, M., Purdy, R. H., et al. (2001). Stress and neuroactive steroids. *Int. Rev. Neurobiol.* 46, 243–272.
15. Purdy, R. H., Morrow, A. L., Moore, P. H. Jr., et al. (1991). Stress-induced elevations of γ-aminobutyric acid type A receptor-active steroids in the rat brain. *Proc. Natl. Acad. Sci. USA* 88, 4553–4557.
16. Concas, A., Mostallino, M. C., Porcu, P., et al. (1998). Role of brain allopregnanolone in the plasticity of gamma-aminobutyric acid type A receptor in rat brain during pregnancy and after delivery. *Proc. Natl. Acad. Sci. USA* 95, 13284–13289.
17. Finn, D. A., and Gee, K. W. (1994). The estrus cycle, sensitivity to convulsants and the anticonvulsant effect of a neuroactive steroid. *J. Pharmacol. Exp. Ther.* 271, 164–170.
18. Belelli, D., and Lambert, J. J. (2005). Neurosteroids: Endogenous regulators of the $GABA_A$ receptor. *Nat. Rev. Neurosci.* 6, 565–575.
19. Baulieu, E. E. (1981). Steroid hormones in the brain: Several mechanisms? In: *Steroid Hormone Regulation of the Brain.* Series title: *Wenner-Gren Center International Symposium,* Vol. 34, K. Fuxe, J. A. Gustafsson, and L. Wetterberg, Eds., Pergamon, Oxford, pp. 3–14.
20. Ichikawa, S., Sawada, T., Nakamura, Y., et al. (1974). Ovarian secretion of pregnane compounds during the estrous cycle and pregnancy in rats. *Endocrinology* 94, 1615–1620.
21. Purdy, R. H., Moore, P. H. Jr., Rao, P. N., et al. (1990). Radioimmunoassay of 3α-hydroxy-5α-pregnan-20-one in rat and human plasma. *Steroids* 55, 290–296.
22. Corpechot, C., Young, J., Calvel, M., et al. (1993). Neurosteroids: 3α-Hydroxy-5α-pregnan-20-one and its precursors in the brain, plasma and steroidogenic glands of male and female rats. *Endocrinology* 133, 1003–1009.
23. Cheney, D. L., Uzunov, D., Costa, E., et al. (1995). Gas chromatographic-mass fragmentographic quantitation of 3α-hydroxy-5α-pregnan-20-one (allopregnanolone) and its precursors in blood and brain of adrenalectomized and castrated rats. *J. Neurosci.* 15, 4641–4650.
24. Karavolas, H. J., Bertics, P. J., Hidges, D., et al. (1984). Progesterone processing by neuroendocrine structures. In *Metabolism of Hormonal Steroids in the Neuroendocrine Structures,* F. Celotti, F. Naftolin, and L. Martini Eds. Raven, New York pp. 149–170.
25. Korneyev, A., Guidotti, A., and Costa, E. (1993). Regional and interspecies differences in brain progesterone metabolism. *J. Neurochem.* 61, 2041–2047.
26. Mathur, C., Prasad, V. V., Raji, V. S., et al. (1993). Steroids and their conjugates in the mammalian brain. *Proc. Natl. Acad. Sci. USA* 90, 85–88.
27. Mellon, S. (1994). Neurosteroids: Biochemistry, modes of action, and clinical relevance. *J. Clin. Endo. Metab.* 78, 1003–1008.
28. Bixo, M., Andersson, A., Winblad, B., et al. (1997). Progesterone, 5α-pregnane-3,20-dione and 3α-hydroxy-5α-pregnane-20-one in specific regions of the human female brain in different endocrine states. *Brain Res.* 764, 173–178.
29. Mellon, S. H., and Vaudry, H. (2001). Biosynthesis of neurosteroids and regulation of their synthesis. *Int. Rev. Neurobiol.* 46, 33–78.
30. Matsunaga, M., Ukena, K., Baulieu, E. -E., and Tsutsui, K. (2004). 7α-Hydroxypregnenolone acts as a neuronal activator to stimulate locomotor activity of breeding newts by means of the dopamine system. *Proc. Natl. Acad. Sci. USA* 101, 17282–17287.

31. Corpechot, C., Robel, P., Axelson, M., et al. (1991). Characterization and measurement of dehydroepiandrosterone sulfate in rat brain. *Proc. Natl. Acad. Sci. USA* 78, 4704–4707.

32. Corpechot, C., Synguelakis, M., Talha, S., et al. (1983). Pregnenolone and its sulfate ester in the rat brain. *Brain Res.* 270, 119–125.

33. Vallee, M., Mayo, W., Koob, G. F., et al. (2003). Neuroactive steroids: New biomarkers of cognitive aging. *J. Steroid Biochem. Mol. Biol.* 85, 329–335.

34. Prasad, V. V. K., Vegesna, S. R., Welch, M., et al. (1994). Precursors of the neurosteroids. *Proc. Natl. Acad. Sci. USA* 91, 3220–3223.

35. Liu, S., Sjovall, J., and Griffiths, W. J. (2003). Neurosteroids in rat brain: Extraction, isolation, and analysis by nanoscale liquid chromatography-electrospray mass spectrometry. *Anal. Chem.* 75, 5835–5846.

36. Shimada, K., Higashi, T., and Mitamura, K. (2002). Development of analyses of biological steroids using chromatography: Special reference to Vitamin D compounds and neurosteroids. *Chromatography* 24, 1–6.

37. Kishimoto, W., Hiroi, T., Shiraishi, M., et al. (2004). Cytochrome P450 2D catalyze steroid 21-hydroxylation in the brain. *Endocrinology* 145, 699–705.

38. Morrow, A. L., Suzdak, P. D., and Paul, S. M. (1987). Steroid hormone metabolites potentiate GABA receptor-mediated chloride ion flux with nanomolar potency. *Eur. J. Pharmacol.* 142, 483–485.

39. Gee, K. W., Bolger, M. B., Brinton, R. E., et al. (1988). Steroid modulation of the chloride ionophore in rat brain: Structure-activity requirements, regional dependence and mechanism of action. *J. Pharmacol. Exp. Ther.* 246, 803–812.

40. Belelli, D., Lan, N. C., and Gee, K. W. (1990). Anticonvulsant steroids and the GABA/benzodiazepine receptor-chloride ionophore complex. *Neurosci. Biobehav. Rev.* 14, 315–322.

41. Xue, B. G., Whittemore, E. R., Park, C. H., et al. (1997). Partial agonism by 3α, 21-dihydroxy-5β-pregnan-20-one at the γ-aminobutyric$_A$ receptor neurosteroid site. *J. Pharmacol. Exp. Ther.* 281, 1095–1101.

42. Belelli, D., and Gee, K. W. (1989). 5α-Pregnan-3α, 20α-diol behaves like a partial agonist in the modulation of GABA-stimulated chloride ion uptake by synaptoneurosomes. *Eur. J. Pharmacol.* 167, 173–176.

43. Lambert, J. J., Belelli, D., Peden, D. R., et al. (2003). Neurosteroid modulation of GABA$_A$ receptors. *Prog. Neurobiol.* 71, 67–80.

44. Twyman, R. E., and MacDonald, R. L. (1992). Neurosteroid regulation of GABA$_A$ receptor single-channel kinetic properties of mouse spinal cord neurons in culture. *J. Physiol.* 456, 215–245.

45. Zhu, W. J., and Vicini, S. (1997). Neurosteroid prolongs GABA$_A$ channel deactivation by altering kinetics of desensitized states. *J. Neurosci.* 17, 4022–4031.

46. Lambert, J. J., Belelli, D., Harney, S. C., et al. (2001). Modulation of native and recombinant GABA$_A$ receptors by endogenous and synthetic neuroactive steroids. *Brain Res. Rev* 37, 68–80.

47. Covey, D. F., Evers, A. S., Mennerick, S., et al. (2001). Recent developments in structure-activity relationships for steroid modulators of GABA$_A$ receptors. *Brain Res. Rev.* 37, 91–97.

48. Hamilton, N. M. (2002). Interaction of steroids with the GABA$_A$ receptor. *Curr. Top Med. Chem.* 2, 887–902.

49. Akk, G., Bracamontes, J. R., Covey, D. F., et al. (2004). Neuroactive steroids have multiple actions to potentiate GABA$_A$ receptors. *J. Physiol.* 558, 59–74.

50. Majewska, M. D., and Schwartz, R. D. (1987). Pregnenolone-sulfate: An endogenous antagonist of the γ-aminobutyric acid receptor complex in brain? *Brain Res.* 404, 355–360.
51. Majewska, M. D., Demirgoren, S., Spivak, C. E., et al. (1990). The neurosteroid dehydroepiandrosterone sulfate is an allosteric antagonist of the $GABA_A$ receptor. *Brain Res.* 526, 143–146.
52. Wu, F. S., Gibbs, T. T., and Farb, D. H. (1990). Inverse modulation of γ-aminobutyric acid- and glycine-induced currents by progesterone. *Mol. Pharmacol.* 37, 597–602.
53. Wu, F. S., Gibbs, T. T., and Farb, D. H. (1991). Pregnenolone sulfate: A positive allosteric modulator at the N-methyl-D-aspartate receptor. *Mol. Pharmacol.* 40, 333–336.
54. Irwin, R. P., Maragakis, N. J., Rogawski, M. A., et al. (1992). Pregnenolone sulfate augments NMDA receptor mediated increases in intracellular Ca^{2+} in cultured rat hippocampal neurons. *Neurosci. Lett.* 141, 30–34.
55. Penland, S. N., and Morrow, A. L. (2004). 3α, 5β-Reduced cortisol exhibits antagonist properties on cerebral cortical $GABA_A$ receptors. *Eur. J. Pharmacol.* 506, 129–132.
56. Park-Chung, M., Wu, F. S., and Farb, D. H. (1994). 3α-Hydroxy-5β-pregnan-20-one sulfate: A negative modulator of the NMDA-induced current in cultured neurons. *Mol. Pharmacol.* 46, 146–150.
57. Irwin, R. P., Lin, S. Z., Rogawski, M. A., et al. (1994). Steroid potentiation and inhibition of N-methyl-D-aspartate receptor-mediated intracellular Ca^{++} responses: Structure-activity studies. *J. Pharmacol. Exp. Ther.* 271, 677–682.
58. Park-Chung, M., Wu, F. S., Purdy, R. H., et al. (1997). Distinct sites for inverse modulation of N-methyl-D-aspartate receptors by sulfated steroids. *Mol. Pharmacol.* 52, 1113–1123.
59. Yaghoubi, N., Malayev, A., Russek, S. J., et al. (1998). Neurosteroid modulation of recombinant ionotropic glutamate receptors. *Brain Res.* 803, 153–160.
60. Weaver, C. E., Land, M. B., Purdy, R. H., et al. (2000). Geometry and charge determine pharmacological effects of steroids on N-methyl-D-aspartate receptor-induced Ca^{2+} accumulation and cell death. *J. Pharmacol. Exp. Ther.* 293, 747–754.
61. Park-Chung, M., Malayev, A., Purdy, R. H., et al. (1999). Sulfated and unsulfated steroids modulate γ-aminobutyric acid$_A$ receptor function through distinct sites. *Brain Res.* 83, 72–87.
62. Gibbs, T. T., and Farb, D. H. (2000). Dueling enigmas: Neurosteroids and sigma receptors in the limelight. *Science STKE [Electronic Resource]: Signal Transduction Knowledge Environment* 60 (Nov. 28), 1–4.
63. Bullock, A. E., Clark, A. L., Grady, S. R., et al. (1997). Neurosteroids modulate nicotinic receptor function in mouse striatal and thalamic synaptosomes. *J. Neurochem.* 68, 2412–2423.
64. Pereira, E. F., Hilmas, C., Santos, M. D., et al. (2002). Unconventional ligands and modulators of nicotinic receptors. *J. Neurobiol.* 53, 479–500.
65. Bertrand, D., Valera, S., Bertrand, S., et al. (1991). Steroids inhibit nicotinic acetylcholine receptors. *Neuroreport* 2, 277–280.
66. Ke, L., and Lukas, R. J. (1996). Effects of steroid exposure on ligand binding and functional activities of diverse nicotinic acetylcholine receptor subtypes. *J. Neurochem.* 67, 1100–1112.
67. Valera, S., Ballivet, M., and Bertrand, D. (1992). Progesterone modulates a neuronal nicotinic acetylcholine receptor. *Proc. Natl. Acad. Sci. USA* 89, 9949–9953.
68. Paradiso, K., Sabey, K., Evers, A. S., et al. (2000). Steroid inhibition of rat neuronal nicotinic α4β2 receptors expressed in HEK 293 cells. *Mol. Pharmacol.* 58, 341–351.

69. Wu, F. S., Lai, C. P., and Liu, B. C. (2000). Non-competitive inhibition of 5-HT$_3$ receptor-mediated currents by progesterone in rat nodose ganglion neurons. *Neurosci. Lett.* 278, 37–40.

70. Wetzel, C. H., Hermann, B., Behl, C., et al. (1998). Functional antagonism of gonadal steroids at the 5-hydroxytryptamine type 3 receptor. *Mol. Endocrinol.* 12, 1441–1451.

71. Barann, M., Gothert, M., Bruss, M., et al. (1999). Inhibition by steroids of [^{14}C]-guanidinium flux through the voltage-gated sodium channel and the cation channel of the 5-HT$_3$ receptor of N1E-115 neuroblastoma cells. *Naunyn-Schmiedeberg's Arch. Pharmacol.* 360, 234–241.

72. Carbone, E., and Lux, H. D. (1984). A low-voltage activated, fully inactivating Ca channel in vertebrate sensory neurones. *Nature* 310, 501–502.

73. Huguenard, J. R. (1996). Low-threshold calcium currents in central nervous system neurons. *Annu. Rev. Physiol.* 58, 329–348.

74. Ertel, S. I., Ertel, E. A., and Clozel, J. P. (1997). T-type Ca^{2+} channels and pharmacological blockade: Potential pathophysiological relevance. *Cardiovasc. Drugs Ther.* 11, 723–739.

75. Perez-Reyes, E. (2003). Molecular physiology of low-voltage-activated T-type calcium channels. *Physiol. Rev.* 83, 117–161.

76. Pathirathna, S., Brimelow, B. C., Jagodic, M. M., et al. (2005). New evidence that both T-type calcium channels and GABA$_A$ channels are responsible for the potent peripheral analgesic effects of 5α-reduced neuroactive steroids. *Pain* 114, 429–443.

77. Nadeson, R., and Goodchild, C. S. (2000). Antinociceptive properties of neurosteroids. II. Experiments with Saffan and its components alphaxalone and alphadolone to reveal separation of anaesthetic and antinociceptive effects and the involvement of spinal cord GABA$_A$ receptors. *Pain* 88, 31–39.

78. Maurice, T., Urani, A., Phan, V. L., et al. (2001). The interaction between neuroactive steroids and the σ$_1$ receptor function: Behavioral consequences and therapeutic opportunities. *Brain Res. Rev.* 37, 116–132.

79. Su, T. P., London, E. D., and Jaffe, J. H. (1988). Steroid binding at sigma receptors suggests a link between endocrine, nervous, and immune systems. *Science* 240, 219–221.

80. Maurice, T., Phan, V. L., Urani, A., et al. (1999). Neuroactive neurosteroids as endogenous effectors for the sigma$_1$ (σ$_1$) receptor: Pharmacological evidence and therapeutic opportunities. *Jpn. J. Pharmacol.* 81, 125–155.

81. Gee, K. W., McCauley, L. D., and Lan, N. C. (1995). A putative receptor for neurosteroids on the GABA$_A$ receptor complex: The pharmacological properties and therapeutic potential of epalons. *Crit. Rev. Neurobiol.* 9, 207–227.

82. Olsen, R. W., and Sapp, D. W. (1995). Neuroactive steroid modulation of GABA$_A$ receptors. *Adv. Biochem. Psychopharmacol.* 48, 57–74.

83. Hawkinson, J. E., Kimbrough, C. L., Belelli, D., et al. (1994). Correlation of neuroactive steroid modulation of [^{35}S]t-butylbicyclophosphorothionate and [^{3}H]flunitrazepam binding and γ-aminobutyric acid$_A$ receptor function. *Mol. Pharmacol.* 46, 977–985.

84. Mennerick, S., He, Y., Jiang, X., et al. (2004). Selective antagonism of 5alpha-reduced neurosteroid effects at GABA(A) receptors. *Mol. Pharmacol.* 65, 1191–1197.

85. Mok, W. M., Herschkowitz, S., and Krieger, N. R. (1991). In vivo studies identify 5α-pregnan-3α-ol-20-one as an active anesthetic agent. *J. Neurochem.* 57, 1296–1301.

86. Mendelson, W. B., Martin, J. V., Perlis, M., et al. (1987). Sleep induction by an adrenal steroid in the rat. *Psychopharmacology* 93, 226–229.

87. Belelli, D., Bolger, M. B., and Gee, K. W. (1989). Anticonvulsant profile of the progesterone metabolite 5α-pregnan-3α-ol-20-one. *Eur. J. Pharmacol.* 166, 325–329.
88. Kokate, T. G., Svensson, B. E., and Rogawski, M. A. (1994). Anticonvulsant activity of neurosteroids: Correlation with γ-aminobutyric acid-evoked chloride current potentiation. *J. Pharmacol. Exp. Ther.* 270, 1223–1229.
89. Kokate, T. G., Cohen, A. L., Karp, E., et al. (1996). Neuroactive steroids protect against pilocarpine- and kainic acid-induced limbic seizures and status epilepticus in mice. *Neuropharmacology* 35, 1049–1056.
90. Devaud, L. L., Purdy, R. H., and Morrow, A. L. (1995). The neurosteroid, 3α-hydroxy-5α-pregnan-20-one, protects against bicuculline-induced seizures during ethanol withdrawal in rats. *Alcohol. Clin. Exp. Res.* 19, 350–355.
91. Devaud, L. L., Purdy, R. H., Finn, D. A., et al. (1996). Sensitization of γ-aminobutyric acid$_A$ receptors to neuroactive steroids in rats during ethanol withdrawal. *J. Pharmacol. Exp. Ther.* 278, 510–517.
92. Finn, D. A., Roberts, A. J., and Crabbe, J. C. (1995). Neuroactive steroid sensitivity in Withdrawal Seizure Prone and -Resistant mice. *Alcohol Clin. Exp. Res.* 19, 410–415.
93. Finn, D. A., Roberts, A. J., Lotrich, F., et al. (1997). Genetic differences in behavioral sensitivity to a neuroactive steroid. *J. Pharmacol. Exp. Ther.* 280, 820–828.
94. Crawley, J. N., Glowa, J. R., Majewska, M. D., et al. (1986). Anxiolytic activity of an endogenous adrenal steroid. *Brain Res.* 398, 382–385.
95. Bitran, D., Hilvers, R. J., and Kellogg, C. K. (1991). Anxiolytic effects of 3α-hydroxy-5α[β]-pregnan-20-one: Endogenous metabolites that are active at the GABA$_A$ receptor. *Brain Res.* 561, 157–161.
96. Britton, K. T., Page, M., Baldwin, H., et al. (1991). Anxiolytic activity of steroid anesthetic alphaxalone. *J. Pharmacol. Exp. Ther.* 258, 124–129.
97. Wieland, S., Lan, N. C., Mirasedeghi, S., et al. (1991). Anxiolytic activity of the progesterone metabolite 5α-pregnan-3α-ol-20-one. *Brain Res.* 565, 263–268.
98. Wieland, S., Belluzzi, J. D., Stein, L., et al. (1995). Comparative behavioral characterization of the neuroactive steroids 3α-OH,5α-pregnan-20-one and 3α-OH,5β-pregnan-20-one in rodents. *Psychopharmacology* 118, 65–71.
99. Brot, M. D., Akwa, Y., Purdy, R. H., et al. (1997). The anxiolytic-like effects of the neurosteroid allopregnanolone: Interactions with GABA$_A$ receptors. *Eur. J. Pharmacol.* 325, 1–7.
100. Rodgers, R. J., and Johnson, N. J. T. (1998). Behaviorally selective effects of neuroactive steroids on plus-maze anxiety in mice. *Pharmacol. Biochem. Behav.* 59, 221–232.
101. Melchior, C. L., and Allen, P. M. (1992). Interaction of pregnenolone and pregnenolone sulfate with ethanol and pentobarbital. *Pharmacol. Biochem. Behav.* 42, 605–611.
102. Vallee, M., Mayo, W., Koob, G. F., et al. (2001). Neurosteroids in learning and memory processes. *Int. Rev. Neurobiol.* 46, 273–320.
103. Melchior, C. L., and Ritzmann, R. F. (1996). Neurosteroids block the memory-impairing effects of ethanol in mice. *Pharmacol. Biochem. Behav.* 53, 51–56.
104. Ladurelle, N., Eychenne, B., Denton, D., et al. (2000). Prolonged intracerebroventricular infusion of neurosteroids affects cognitive performances in the mouse. *Brain Res.* 858, 371–379.
105. Matthews, D. B., Morrow, A. L., Tokunaga, S., et al. (2002). Acute ethanol administration and acute allopregnanolone administration impair spatial memory in the Morris water task. *Alcohol Clin. Exp. Res.* 26, 1747–1751.

106. File, S. E., Lippa, A. S., Beer, B., et al. (1997). Animal tests of anxiety. In J. N. Crawley, C. R. Gerfen, R. McKay, M. A. Rogawski, D. R. Sibley, and P. Skolnick Eds. *Current Protocols in Neuroscience*. Wiley, New York, pp. 8.3.1–8.3.22.

107. Rodgers, R. J., Cao, B. J., Dalvi, A., et al. (1997). Animal models of anxiety: An ethological perspective. *Braz. J. Med. Biol. Res.* 30, 289–304.

108. Martin, P. (1998). Animal models sensitive to anti-anxiety agents. *Acta. Psychiatr. Scand. Suppl.* 393, 74–80.

109. Koob, G. F., Henrichs, S. C., and Britton, K. (1998). Animal models of anxiety disorders In: Schatzberg, A. F. and Nemeroff, C. B. Eds., *Textbook of Pharmacology*, 2nd ed., American Psychiatric Press, Washington DC, pp. 133–144.

110. Crawley, J. N. (1999). Evaluating anxiety in rodents. In: *Handbook of Molecular-Genetic Techniques for Brain and Behavior Research*, Series title: *Techniques in the Behavioral and Neural Sciences*, Vol. 13, W.E. Crusio, R.T. Gerlai, Eds., Elsevier Science BV, Amsterdam, pp. 667–673.

111. Finn, D. A., Rutledge-Gorman, M. T., and Crabbe, J. C. (2003). Genetic animal models of anxiety. *Neurogenetics* 4, 109–135.

112. Pellow, S., Chopin, P., File, S. E., et al. (1985). Validation of open:closed arm entries in an elevated plus-maze as a measure of anxiety in the rat. *J. Neurosci. Methods* 14, 149–167.

113. Lister, R. G. (1987). The use of a plus-maze to measure anxiety in the mouse. *Psychopharmacology* 92, 180–185.

114. Trullas, R., and Skolnick, P. (1993). Differences in fear motivated behaviors among inbred mouse strains. *Psychopharmacology* 111, 323–331.

115. Cole, J. C., and Rodgers, R. J. (1994). Ethological evaluation of the effects of acute and chronic buspirone treatment in the murine elevated plus-maze test: Comparison with haloperidol. *Psychopharmacology* 114, 288–296.

116. Montgomery, K. C. (1955). The relation between fear induced by novel stimulation and exploratory behavior. *J. Comp. Physiol. Psychol.* 48, 254–260.

117. Lamberty, Y., and Gower, A. J. (1996). Arm width and brightness modulation of spontaneous behaviour of two strains of mice tested in the elevated plus-maze. *Physiol. Behav.* 59, 439–444.

118. Rodgers, R. J., Cole, J. C., Cobain, M. R., et al. (1992). Anxiogenic-like effects of fluprazine and eltoprazine in the mouse elevated plus maze: Profile comparisons with 8-OH-DPAT, CGS 12066B, TFMPP and mCPP. *Behav. Pharmacol.* 3, 621–634.

119. Handley, S. L., and Mithani, S. (1984). Effects of alpha-adrenoceptor agonists and antagonists in a maze exploration model of "fear"-motivated behaviour. *Naunyn Schemiedeberg's Arch. Pharmacol.* 327, 1–5.

120. Handley, S. L., and McBlane, J. W. (1993). An assessment of the elevated X-maze for studying anxiety and anxiety-modulating drugs. *J. Pharmacol. Toxicol. Methods* 29, 129–138.

121. Treit, D. (1985). The inhibitory effect of diazepam on defensive burying: Anxiolytic vs. analgesic effects. *Pharmacol. Biochem. Behav.* 22, 47–52.

122. Dawson, G. R., and Tricklebank, M. D. (1995). Use of the elevated plus maze in the search for novel anxiolytic agents. *Trends Pharmacol. Sci.* 16, 33–36.

123. Treit, D., Menard, J., and Royan, C. (1993). Anxiogenic stimuli in the elevated plus-maze. *Pharmacol. Biochem. Behav.* 44, 463–469.

124. Fernandes, C., and File, S. E. (1996). The influence of open arm ledges and maze experience in the elevated plus-maze. *Pharmacol. Biochem. Behav.* 54, 31–40.

125. Gomez, C., Saldivar-Gonzalez, A., Delgado, G., et al. (2002). Rapid anxiolytic activity of progesterone and pregnanolone in male rats. *Pharmacol. Biochem. Behav.* 72, 543–550.
126. Carboni, E., Wieland, S., Lan, N. C., et al. (1996). Anxiolytic properties of endogenously occurring pregnanediols in two rodent models of anxiety. *Psychopharmacology* 126, 173–178.
127. Reddy, D. S., O'Malley, B. W., and Rogawski, M. A. (2005). Anxiolytic activity of progesterone in progesterone receptor knockout mice. *Neuropharmacology* 48, 14–24.
128. Melchior, C. L., and Ritzmann, R. F. (1994a). Dehydroepiandrosterone is an anxiolytic in mice on the plus maze. *Pharmacol. Biochem. Behav.* 47, 437–441.
129. Melchior, C. L., and Ritzmann, R. F. (1994b). Pregnenolone and pregnenolone sulfate, alone and with ethanol, in mice on the plus-maze. *Pharmacol. Biochem. Behav.* 48, 893–897.
130. Bitran, D., Dugan, M., Renda, P., et al. (1999). Anxiolytic effects of the neuroactive steroid pregnanolone (3α-OH-5β-pregnan-20-one) after microinjection in the dorsal hippocampus and lateral septum. *Brain Res.* 850, 217–224.
131. Bitran, D., Foley, M., Audette, D., et al. (2000). Activation of peripheral mitochondrial benzodiazepine receptors in the hippocampus stimulates allopregnanolone synthesis and produces anxiolytic-like effects in the rat. *Psychopharmacology* 151, 64–71.
132. Gray, J. A. (1982). Precis of the neuropsychology of anxiety: An enquiry into the functions of the septo-hippocampal system. *Behav. Brain Sci.* 5, 469–534.
133. Gabriel, M. (1993). Discriminative avoidance learning: A model system In: *Neurobiology of Cingulate Cortex and Limbic Thalamus: A Comprehensive Handbook.* B. A. Vogt and M. Gabriel, Eds., Birkhauser, Boston, pp. 478–523.
134. Geller, I., and Seifter, J. (1960). The effects of meprobamate, barbiturates, d-amphetamine and promazine on experimentally induced conflict in the rat. *Psychopharmacologia* 1, 482–491.
135. Vogel, J. R., Beer, B., and Clody, D. E. (1971). A simple and reliable conflict procedure for testing anti-anxiety agents. *Psychopharmacologia* 21, 1–7.
136. Davis, M. (1992). The role of the amygdala in fear-potentiated startle: Implications for animal models of anxiety. *Trends Pharmacol. Sci.* 13, 35–41.
137. Akwa, Y., Purdy, R. H., Koob, G. F., et al. (1999). The amygdala mediates the anxiolytic-like effect of the neurosteroid allopregnanolone in rat. *Behav. Brain Res.* 106, 119–125.
138. Crawley, J., and Goodwin, F. K. (1980). Preliminary report of a simple animal behavior model for the anxiolytic effects of benzodiazepines. *Pharmacol. Biochem. Behav.* 13, 167–170.
139. Crawley, J. N. (1981). Neuropharmacologic specificity of a simple animal model for the behavioral actions of benzodiazepines. *Pharmacol. Biochem. Behav.* 15, 695–699.
140. Crawley, J. N., Skolnick, P., and Paul, S. M. (1984). Absence of intrinsic actions of benzodiazepine antagonists on an exploratory model of anxiety in the mouse. *Neuropharmacology* 23, 531–537.
141. Brown, J. S., Kalish, H. I., and Farber, I. E. (1951). Conditioned fear as revealed by magnitude of startle response to an auditory stimulus. *J. Exp. Psychol.* 41, 317–328.
142. Lang, P. J., Davis, M., and Ohman, A. (2000). Fear and anxiety: Animal models and human cognitive psychophysiology. *J. Affect. Disord.* 61, 137–159.
143. Davis, M., and Astrachan, D. I. (1978). Conditioned fear and startle magnitude: Effects of different footshock or backshock intensities used in training. *J. Exp. Psychol.: Anim. Behav. Process* 4, 95–103.

144. Falls, W. A., Miserendino, M. J. D., and Davis, M. (1992). Extinction of fear-potentiated startle: Blockade by infusion of an NMDA antagonist into the amygdala. *J. Neurosci.* 12, 854–863.

145. Swerdlow, N. R., Geyer, M. A., Vale, W. W., et al. (1986). Corticotropin-releasing factor potentiates acoustic startle in rats: Blockade by chlordiazepoxide. *Psychopharmacology* 88, 147–152.

146. Liang, K. C., Melia, K. R., Miserendino, M. J., et al. (1992). Corticotropin-releasing factor: Long-lasting facilitation of the acoustic startle reflex. *J. Neurosci.* 12, 2303–2312.

147. Koob, G. F., and Heinrichs, S. C. (1999). A role for corticotropin releasing factor and urocortin in behavioral responses to stressors. *Brain Res.* 848, 141–152.

148. Steckler, T., and Holsboer, F. (1999). Corticotropin-releasing hormone receptor subtypes and emotion. *Biol. Psychiatry* 46, 1480–1508.

149. Toufexis, D. J., Davis, C., Hammond, A., et al. (2004). Progesterone attenuates corticotropin-releasing factor-enhanced but not fear-potentiated startle via the activity of its neuroactive metabolite, allopregnanolone. *J. Neurosci.* 24, 10280–10287.

150. Lee, Y., and Davis, M. Role of the hippocampus, the bed nucleus of the stria terminalis, and the amygdala in the excitatory effect of corticotropin-releasing hormone on the acoustic startle reflex. *J. Neurosci.* 17, 6434–6446.

151. Toubas, P. L., Abla, K. A., Cao, W., et al. (1990). Latency to enter a mirrored chamber: A novel behavioral assay for anxiolytic agents. *Pharmacol. Biochem. Behav.* 35, 121–126.

152. Gallup, G. G. Jr. (1968). Mirror-image stimulation. *Psychol. Bull.* 70, 782–793.

153. Cao, W., Burkholder, T., Wilkins, L., et al. (1993). A genetic comparison of behavioral actions of ethanol and nicotine in the mirrored chamber. *Pharmacol. Biochem. Behav.* 45, 803–809.

154. Seale, T. W., Niekrasz, I., and Garrett, K. M. (1996). Anxiolysis by ethanol, diazepam and buspirone in a novel murine behavioral assay. *Neuroreport* 7, 1803–1808.

155. Reddy, D. S., and Kulkarni, S. K. (1997). Differential anxiolytic effects of neurosteroids in the mirrored chamber behavior test in mice. *Brain Res.* 752, 61–71.

156. Lamberty, Y. (1998). The mirror chamber test for testing anxiolytics: Is there a mirror-induced stimulation? *Physiol. Behav.* 64, 703–705.

157. Kliethermes, C. L., Finn, D. A., and Crabbe, J. C. (2003). Validation of a modified mirrored chamber sensitive to anxiolytics and anxiogenics in mice. *Psychopharmacology* 169, 190–197.

158. Hall, C. S. (1936). Emotional behavior in the rat: III. The relationship between emotionality and ambulatory activity. *J. Comp. Psychol.* 22, 345–352.

159. Henderson, N. D. (1967). Prior treatment effects on open field behaviour of mice: A genetic analysis. *Anim. Behav.* 15, 364–376.

160. De Boer, S. F., and Koolhaas, J. M. (2003). Defensive burying in rodents: Ethology, neurobiology and psychopharmacology. *Eur. J. Pharmacol.* 463, 145–161.

161. Pinel, J. P., and Treit, D. (1978). Burying as a defensive response in rats. *J. Comp. Physiol. Psychol.* 92, 708–712.

162. Picazo, O., and Fernandez-Guasti, A. (1995). Anti-anxiety effects of progesterone and some of its reduced metabolites: An evaluation using the burying behavior test. *Brain Res.* 680, 135–141.

163. Winslow, J. T., and Insel, T. R. (1991). The infant rat separation paradigm: A novel test for novel anxiolytics. *Trends Pharmacol. Sci.* 12, 402–404.

164. Lehmann, J., and Feldon, J. (2000). Long-term biobehavioral effects of maternal separation in the rat: Consistent or confusing? *Rev. Neurosci.* 11, 383–408.
165. Gardner, C. R. (1985). Distress vocalization in rat pups: A simple screening method for anxiolytic drugs. *J. Pharmacol. Methods* 14, 181–187.
166. Zimmerberg, B., Brunelli, S. A., and Hofer, M. A. (1994). Reduction of rat pup ultrasonic vocalizations by the neuroactive steroid allopregnanolone. *Pharmacol. Biochem. Behav.* 47, 735–738.
167. Zimmerberg, B., Rackow, S. H., and George-Friedman, K. P. (1999). Sex-dependent behavioral effects of the neurosteroid allopregnanolone (3α, 5α-THP) in neonatal and adult rats after postnatal stress. *Pharmacol. Biochem. Behav.* 64, 717–724.
168. Patchev, V. K., Montkowski, A., Rouskova, D., et al. (1997). Neonatal treatment of rats with the neuroactive steroid tetrahydrodeoxycorticosterone (THDOC) abolishes the behavioral and neuroendocrine consequences of adverse early life events. *J. Clin. Invest.* 99, 962–966.
169. Zimmerberg, B., and Kajunski, E. W. (2004). Sexually dimorphic effects of postnatal allopregnanolone on the development of anxiety behavior after early deprivation. *Pharmacol. Biochem. Behav.* 78, 465–471.
170. Nestler, E. J., Barrot, M., DiLeone, R. J., et al. (2002). Neurobiology of depression. *Neuron* 34, 13–25.
171. Porsolt, R. D., LePichon, M., and Jalfre, M. (1977). Depression: A new animal model sensitive to antidepressant treatments. *Nature* 266, 730–732.
172. Porsolt, R. D. (2000). Animal models of depression: Utility for transgenic research. *Rev. Neurosci.* 11, 53–58.
173. Cryan, J. F., Markou, A., and Lucki, I. (2002). Assessing antidepressant activity in rodents: Recent developments and future needs. *Trends Pharmacol. Sci.* 23, 238–245.
174. Khisti, R. T., Chopde, C. T., and Jain, S. P. (2000). Antidepressant-like effect of the neurosteroid 3α-hydroxy-5α-pregnan-20-one in mice forced swim test. *Pharmacol. Biochem. Behav.* 67, 137–143.
175. Hirani, K., Khisti, R. T., and Chopde, C. T. (2002). Behavioral action of ethanol in Porsolt's forced swim test: Modulation by 3α-hydroxy-5α-pregnan-20-one. *Neuropharmacology* 43, 1339–1350.
176. Molina-Hernandez, M., and Tellez-Alcantara, N. P. (2001). Antidepressant-like actions of pregnancy, and progesterone in Wistar rats forced to swim. *Psychoneuroendocrinology* 26, 479–491.
177. Smith, S. S., Gong, Q. H., Li, X., et al. (1998a). Withdrawal from 3alpha-OH-5alpha-pregnan-20-one using a pseudopregnancy model alters the kinetics of hippocampal $GABA_A$-gated current and increases the $GABA_A$ receptor alpha4 subunit in association with increased anxiety. *J. Neurosci.* 18, 5275–5284.
178. Smith, S. S., Gong, Q. H., Hsu, F. C., et al. (1998b). GABA(A) receptor alpha4 subunit suppression prevents withdrawal properties of an endogenous steroid. *Nature* 392, 926–930.
179. Higashi, T., Takido, N., and Shimada, K. (2005). Studies on neurosteroids XVII. Analysis of stress-induced changes in neurosteroid levels in rat brains using liquid chromatography-electron capture atmospheric pressure chemical ionization-mass spectrometry. *Steroids* 70, 1–11.
180. Matsumoto, K., Uzunova, V., Pinna, G., et al. (1999). Permissive role of brain allopregnanolone content in the regulation of pentobarbital-induced righting reflex loss. *Neuropharmacology* 38, 955–963.

181. Serra, M., Pisu, M. G., Littera, M., et al. (2000). Social isolation-induced decreases in both the abundance of neuroactive steroids and GABA$_A$ receptor function in rat brain. *J. Neurochem* 75, 732–740.

182. Dong, E., Matsumoto, K., Uzunova, V., et al. (2001). Brain 5α-dihydroprogesterone and allopregnanolone synthesis in a mouse model of protracted social isolation. *Proc. Natl. Acad. Sci. USA* 98, 2849–2854.

183. Pinna, G., Uzunova, V., Matsumoto, K., et al. (2000). Brain allopregnanolone regulates the potency of the GABA$_A$ receptor agonist muscimol. *Neuropharmacology* 39, 440–448.

184. Bitran, D., Shiekh, M., and McLeod, M. (1995). Anxiolytic effect of progesterone is mediated by the neurosteroid allopregnanolone at brain GABA$_A$ receptors. *J. Neuroendocrinol* 7, 171–177.

185. Serra, M., Madau, P., Chessa, M. F., et al. (1999). 2-Phenyl-imidazo[1,2-a]pyridine derivatives as ligands for peripheral benzodiazepine receptors: Stimulation of neurosteroid synthesis and anticonflict action in rats. *Br. J. Pharmacol.* 127, 177–187.

186. Korte, S. M. (2001). Corticosteroids in relation to fear, anxiety and psychopathology. *Neurosci. Biobehav. Rev.* 25, 117–142.

187. Rodgers, R. J., Haller, J., Holmes, A., et al. (1999). Corticosterone response to the plus-maze: High correlation with risk assessment in rats and mice. *Physiol. Behav.* 68, 47–53.

188. De Kloet, E. R. (1991). Brain corticosteroid receptor balance and homeostatic control. *Front. Neuroendocrinol.* 12, 95–164.

189. Sapolsky, R. M. (1996). Stress, glucocorticoids, and damage to the nervous system: The current state of confusion. *Stress* 1, 1–19.

190. Cole, R. L., and Sawchenko, P. E. (2002). Neurotransmitter regulation of cellular activation and neuropeptide gene expression in the paraventricular nucleus of the hypothalamus. *J. Neurosci.* 22, 959–969.

191. Verkuyl, J. M., and Joels, M. (2003). Effect of adrenalectomy on miniature inhibitory postsynaptic currents in the paraventricular nucleus of the hypothalamus. *J. Neurophysiol.* 89, 237–245.

192. Verkuyl, J. M., Karst, H., and Joels, M. (2005). GABAergic transmission in the rat paraventricular nucleus of the hypothalamus is suppressed by corticosterone and stress. *Eur. J. Neurosci.* 21, 113–121.

193. Patchev, V. K., Shoaib, M., Holsboer, F., et al. (1994). The neurosteroid tetrahydroprogesterone counteracts corticotropin-releasing hormone-induced anxiety and alters the release and gene expression of corticotropin-releasing hormone in the rat hypothalamus. *Neuroscience* 62, 265–271.

194. Patchev, V. K., Hassan, A. H., Holsboer, D. F., et al. (1996). The neurosteroid tetrahydroprogesterone attenuates the endocrine response to stress and exerts glucocorticoid-like effects on vasopressin gene transcription in the rat hypothalamus. *Neuropsychopharmacology* 15, 533–540.

195. Yehuda, R., Southwick, S. M., Krystal, J. H., et al. (1993). Enhanced suppression of cortisol following dexamethasone administration in posttraumatic stress disorder. *Am. J. Psychiatry* 150, 83–86.

196. Yehuda, R., Levengood, R. A., Schmeidler, J., et al. (1996). Increased pituitary activation following metyrapone administration in post-traumatic stress disorder. *Psychoneuroendocrinology* 21, 1–16.

197. Smith, M. A., Davidson, J., Ritchie, J. C., et al. (1989). The corticotropin-releasing hormone test in patients with posttraumatic stress disorder. *Biol. Psychiatry* 26, 349–355.

198. Bremner, J. D., Southwick, S. M., Darnell, A., et al. (1996). Chronic PTSD in Vietnam combat veterans: Course of illness and substance abuse. *Am. J. Psychiatry* 153, 369–375.

199. Rasmusson, A. M., Vasek, J., Lipschitz, D. S., et al. (2004). An increased capacity for adrenal DHEA release is associated with decreased avoidance and negative mood symptoms in women with PTSD. *Neuropsychopharmacology* 29, 1546–1557.

200. Baker, D. G., Ekhator, N. N., Kasckow, J. W., et al. (2005). Higher levels of basal serial CSF cortisol in combat veterans with posttraumatic stress disorder. *Am. J. Psychiatry* 162, 992–994.

201. Altemus, M., Swedo, S. E., Leonard, H. L., et al. (1994). Changes in cerebrospinal fluid neurochemistry during treatment of obsessive-compulsive disorder with clomipramine. *Arch. Gen. Psychiatry* 51, 794–803.

202. Jolkkonen, J., Lepola, U., Bissette, G., et al. (1993). CSF corticotropin-releasing factor is not affected in panic disorder. *Biol. Psychiatry* 33, 136–138.

203. Fossey, M. D., Lydiard, R. B., Ballenger, J. C., et al. (1996). Cerebrospinal fluid corticotropin-releasing factor concentrations in patients with anxiety disorders and normal comparison subjects. *Biol. Psychiatry* 39, 703–707.

204. Charney, D. S., and Bremner, J. D. (1999). The neurobiology of anxiety disorders. In: *Neurobiology of Mental Illness*, D. S. Charney and E. J. Nestler, Eds., Oxford University Press, New York, pp. 494–517.

205. Strohle, A., Romeo, E., di Michele, F., et al. (2003). Induced panic attacks shift gamma-aminobutyric acid type A receptor modulatory neuroactive steroid composition in patients with panic disorder: Preliminary results. *Arch. Gen. Psychiatry* 60, 161–168.

206. Strohle, A., Romeo, E., di Michele, F., et al. (2002). GABA(A) receptor-modulating neuroactive steroid composition in patients with panic disorder before and during paroxetine treatment. *Am. J. Psychiatry* 159, 145–147.

207. Brambilla, F., Biggio, G., Pisu, M. G., et al. (2003). Neurosteroid secretion in panic disorder. *Psychiatry Res* 118, 107–116.

208. Karp, L., Weizman, A., Tyano, S., et al. (1989). Examination stress, platelet peripheral benzodiazepine binding sites, and plasma hormone levels. *Life Sci.* 44, 1077–1082.

209. Krueger, K. E., and Papadopoulos, V. (1990). Peripheral-type benzodiazepine receptors mediate translocation of cholesterol from outer to inner mitochondrial membranes in adrenocortical cells. *J. Biol. Chem.* 265, 15015–15022.

210. Krueger, K. E., and Papadopoulos, V. (1992). Mitochondrial benzodiazepine receptors and the regulation of steroid biosynthesis. *Annu. Rev. Pharmacol. Toxicol.* 32, 211–237.

211. Droogleever Fortuyn, H. A., van Broekhoven, F., Span, P. N., et al. (2004). Effects of PhD examination stress on allopregnanolone and cortisol plasma levels and peripheral benzodiazepine receptor density. *Psychoneuroendocrinology* 29, 1341–1344.

212. Sutton, R. E., Koob, G. F., Le Moal, M., et al. (1982). Corticotropin releasing factor produces behavioural activation in rats. *Nature* 297, 331–333.

213. Butler, P. D., Weiss, J. M., Stout, J. C., et al. (1990). Corticotropin-releasing factor produces fear-enhancing and behavioral activating effects following infusion into the locus coeruleus. *J. Neurosci.* 10, 176–183.

214. Dunn, A. J., and Berridge, C. W. (1990). Physiological and behavioral responses to corticotropin-releasing factor administration: Is CRF a mediator of anxiety or stress responses? *Brain Res. Rev.* 15, 71–100.

215. Griebel, G. (1999). Is there a future for neuropeptide receptor ligands in the treatment of anxiety disorders? *Pharmacol. Ther.* 82, 1–61.

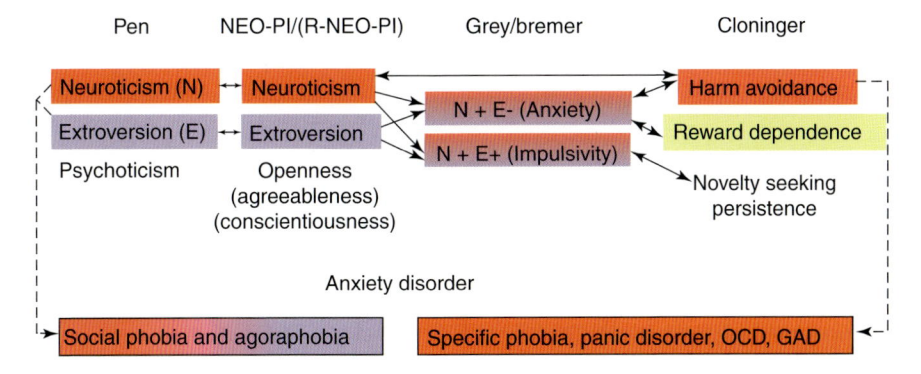

Figure 1.1 Psychological traits and models. According to various models, personality consists of three to five fundamental traits. Arrows indicate corresponding traits in the various models. Traits are highly variable in individuals, but most individuals fall in between the extremes of a trait. Behavior outside of this range can be considered abnormal. For example, higher than normal level of neuroticism (in the PEN model) or harm avoidance (in the Cloninger model) is characteristic for anxiety disorders.

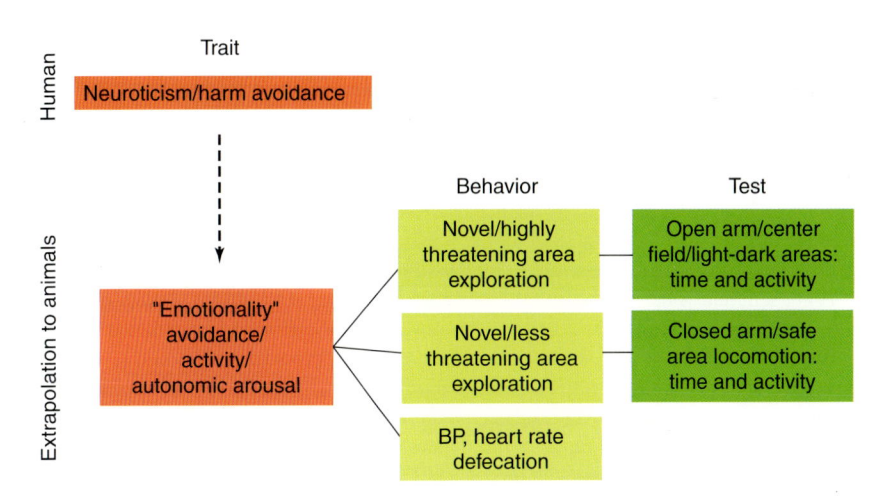

Figure 1.2 Measures of "emotionality" in rodents. The human trait of neuroticism is extrapolated to the measures of emotionality in rodents: avoidance, activity, and autonomic arousal (AvAcAa). AvAcAa can be quantified in well-established behavioral models. Exploration of a low and a moderate to highly threatening environment provides measures of avoidance and activity, while physiological functions provide measurements of autonomic arousal.

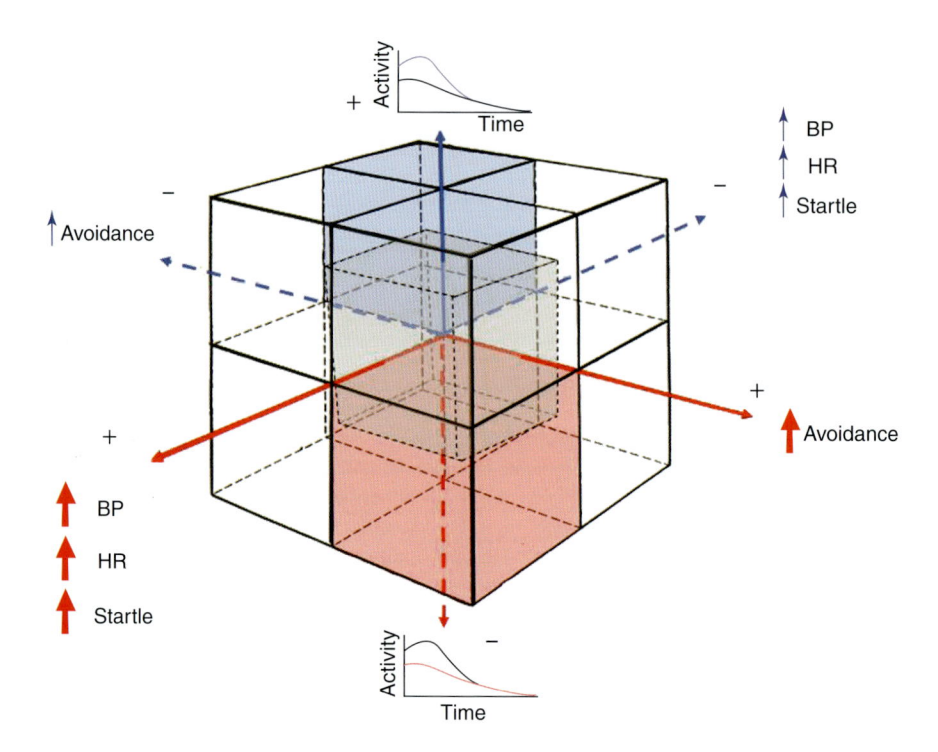

Figure 1.3 The three dimensions (AvAcAa) of emotionality in rodents in three-dimensional representation. Avoidance (Av) is plotted on the *x* axis, the positive spectrum representing increased levels of avoidance in stress-inducing environments or following stress-inducing stimuli and the negative spectrum representing attenuation of avoidance or even increased risk-taking behavior. Activity (Ac) as a response to stress and fear is plotted on the *y* axis, with the positive spectrum corresponding to increased levels of activity in a moderate to highly stressful environment. Following habituation, the activity is not different. Decreased activity in such an environment would be plotted in the negative spectrum of the *y* axis. Finally, the *z* axis is used for autonomic arousal (Aa) elicited by fearful or stressful stimuli, including increased heart rate, increased blood pressure, heightened levels of muscle tension (as measured by the startle response), defecation, and urination. A positive or negative deviation from the normal level of autonomic arousal can be represented by the positive and negative spectra of this axis, respectively. The normal range of these measures in a population is represented by the grey cube. Increased anxiety-like behavior can be conceptualized as increased avoidance, reduced activity, and increased arousal beyond the normal range of variations, denoted by the red area of the cube. Reduced anxiety-like behavior or increased novelty-seeking/risk-taking behavior is characterized by attenuation of avoidance, increased activity, and reduced autonomic arousal, highlighted by the blue area of the cube.

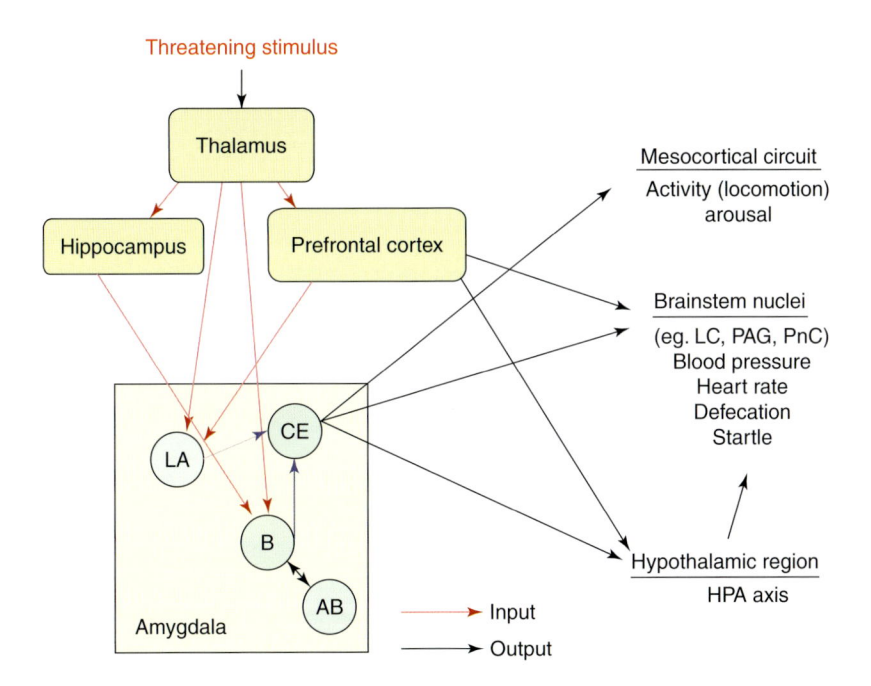

Figure 1.4 Brain regions involved in processing fear, stress, and emotionality in animals. Threatening stimuli are received and processed by brain regions such as the thalamus, hippocampus, prefrontal cortex (PFC), and amygdala. The amygdala sends projections to a number of target regions. These include brain stem nuclei such as the locus ceruleus (LC), periaqueductal gray (PAG), and pontine nucleus caudalis (PnC), which mediate various forms of autonomic arousal. The amygdala is also connected to the mesocortical circuit that mediates arousal and activity (as measured by locomotion in mice) and the hypothalamic region which controls glucocorticoid levels through the hypothalamic–pituitary-adrenal (HPA) axis. The PFC, which is involved in executive functions such as attention, also sends projections directly to the brain stem and the hypothalamus.

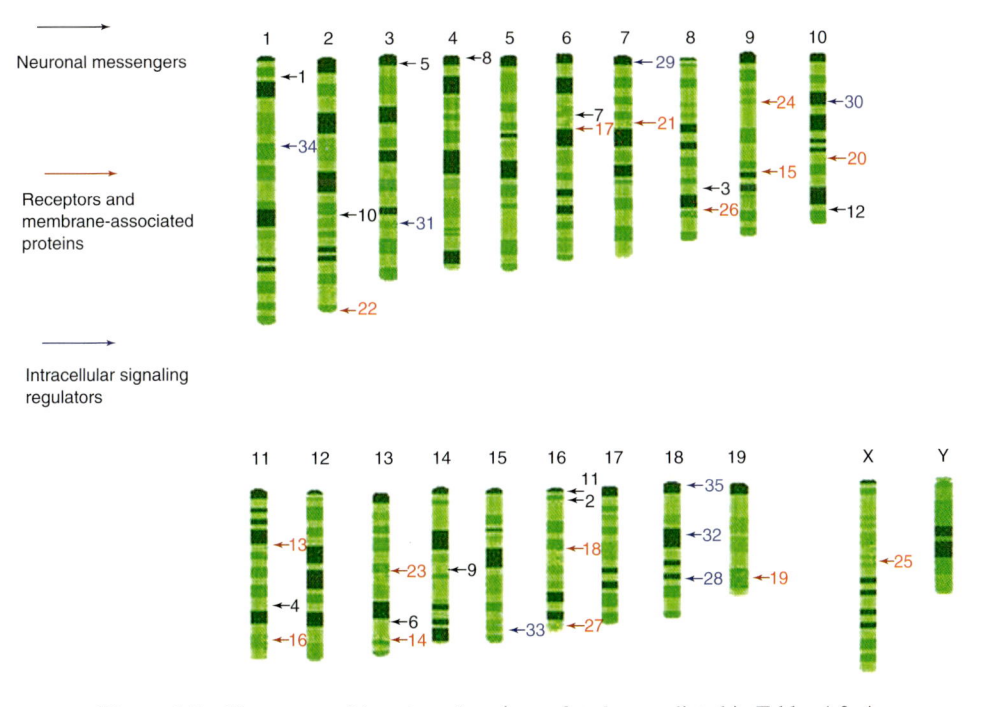

Figure 1.5 Chromosomal location of anxiety-related genes listed in Tables 1.2–4.

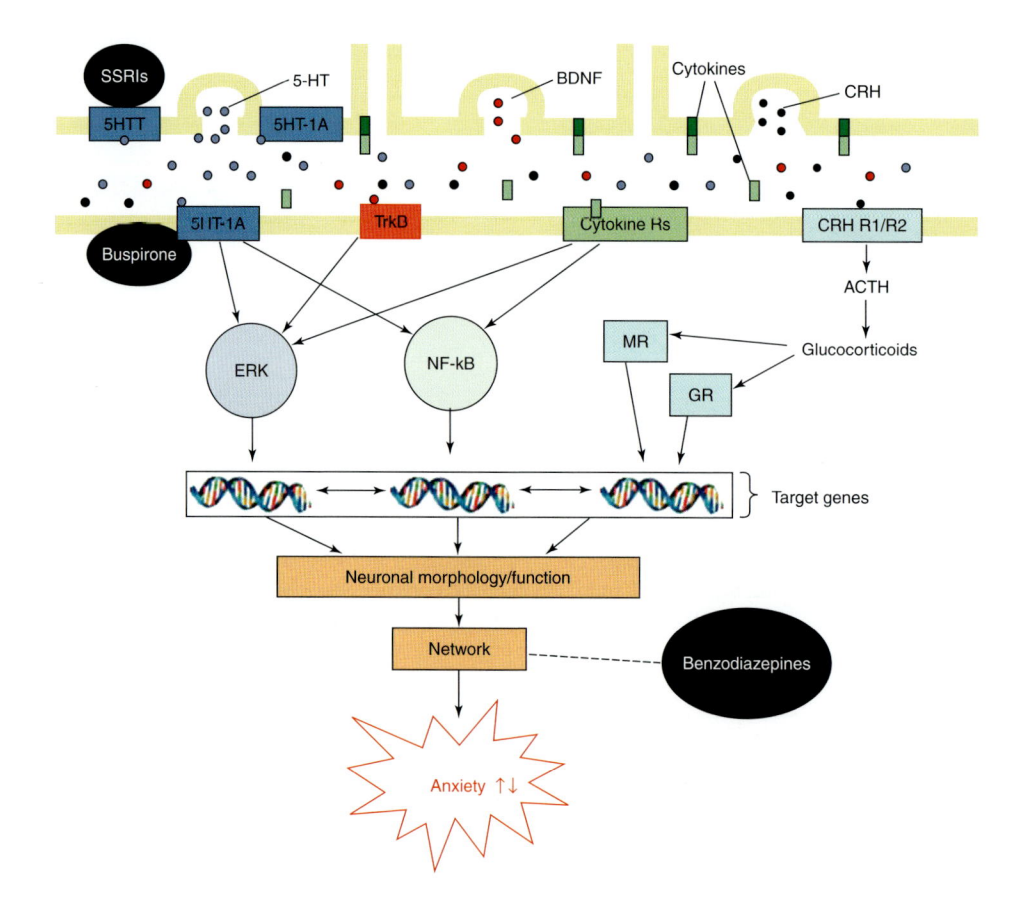

Figure 1.6 Unifying model of pathogenesis of anxiety. Pharmacological and genetic studies indicate that defects in specific substrates of neuronal communication (e.g., 5-HT, GABA, 5-HT receptors), intracellular signaling (e.g., ERK), and gene expression (GR) may be involved in anxiety-related behavior. These extracellular neuronal messengers and their associated receptors and coupled intracellular signaling form specific pathways. Abnormalities in these molecular pathways at various levels can directly modify the function/morphology of the neuronal network associated with fear, ultimately producing changes in anxiety levels.

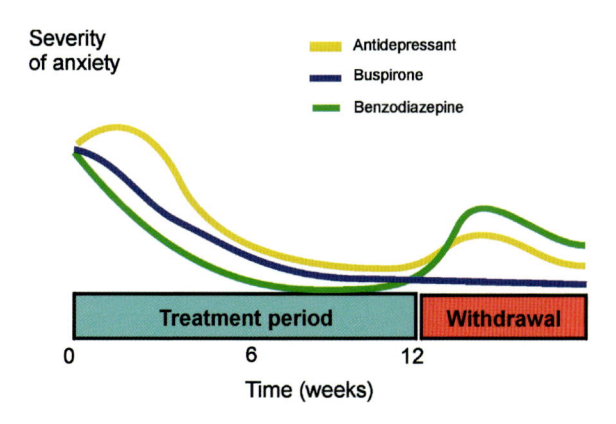

Figure 2.4 Onset and course of action of anxiolytic drugs.

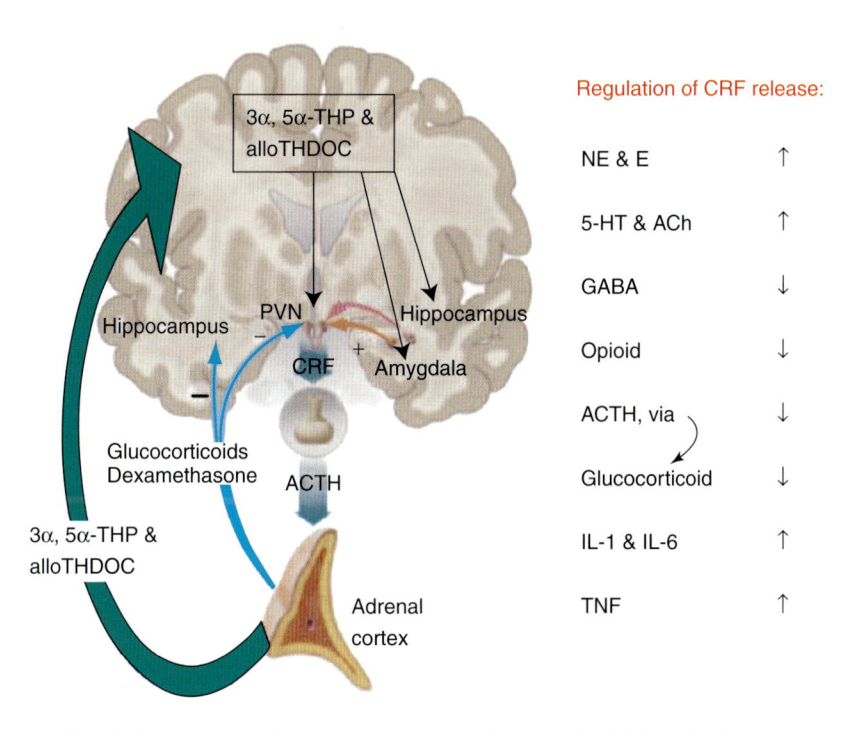

Figure 4.5 Various points of control for regulation of the HPA axis by neurosteroids, neurotransmitters, ACTH, glucocorticoids, and the immune system [186, 222, 224, 284–286]. A variety of stressors activate the HPA axis, which is typically observed as an increase in glucocorticoids from the adrenal cortex. Stress also produces an increase in levels of the GABAergic neurosteroids 3α,5α-THP and alloTHDOC in the brain via the circulation and *de novo* synthesis. (Adapted from Nestler et al. [170].)

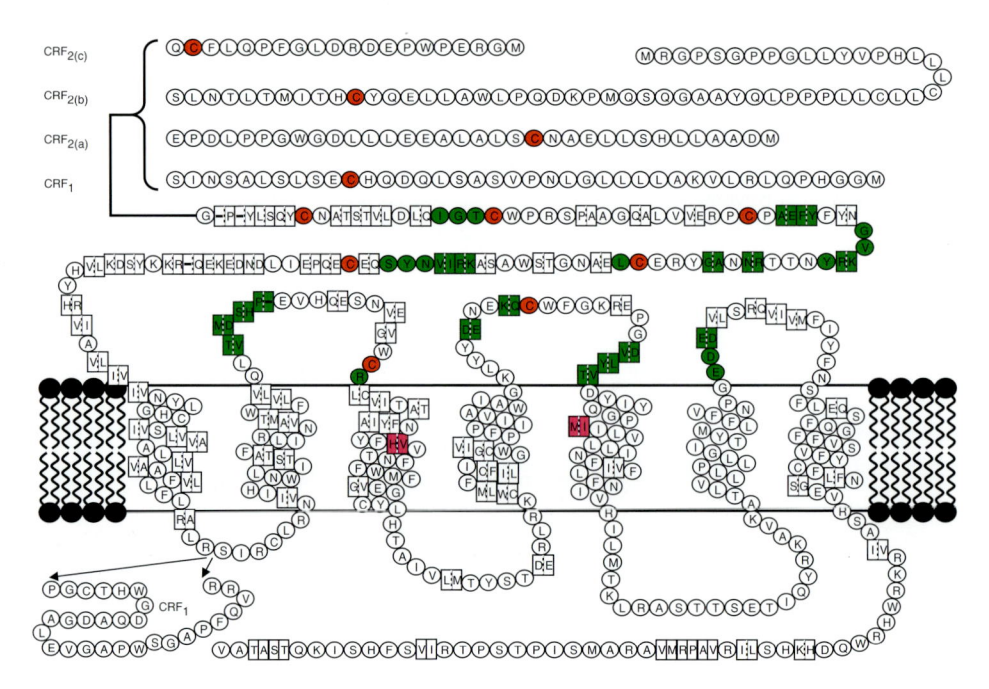

Figure 5.1 Topographical representation of human CRF receptor subtypes and isoforms. The three splice variants of the N domain of the CRF_2 receptor are illustrated. Within the remainder of the receptor, conserved residues between CRF_1 and CRF_2 receptors are in circles, whereas differing residues are indicated by squares (CRF_1 receptor residue on the left-hand side, CRF_2 receptor on the right-hand side). Residues shaded red are cysteines conserved throughout the CRF and class B receptor families. Residues shaded green have been implicated in peptide ligand binding [130–139] whereas residues shaded pink have been implicated in nonpeptide antagonist binding [130]. The position of transmembrane helices have been predicted based on amino acid sequence hydropathy analysis—the precise position of the helices is not presently known. (Figure adapted from *Celltransmissions* with permission from Sigma-Aldrich [196].)

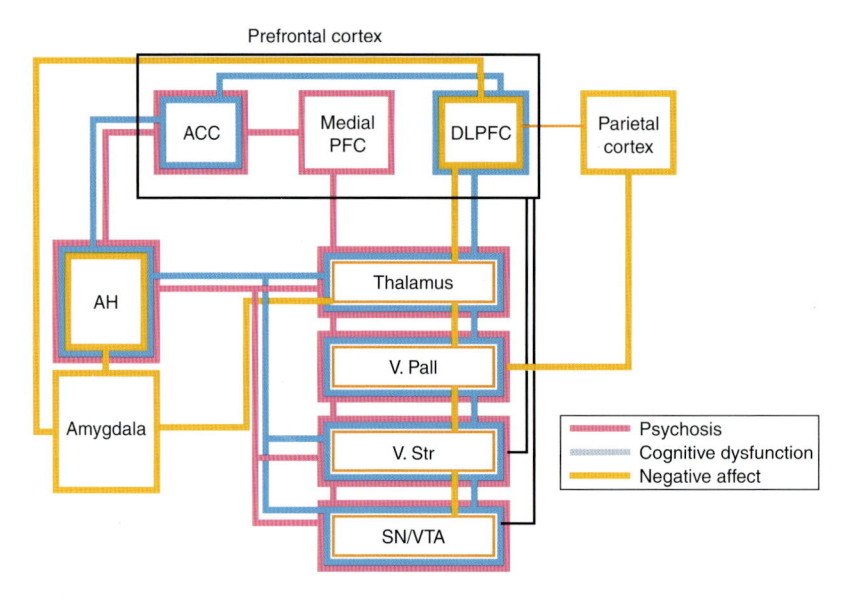

Figure 7.1 Schematic of hypothetical neural systems underlying the three symptom domains: psychosis, cognitive dysfunction, and negative affect. AH = anterior hippocampus; ACC = anterior cingulate; PFC = prefrontal cortex; DLPFC = dorsolateral prefrontal cortex; V. Pall = ventral pallidum; V Str. = ventral stiatum; SN/VTA = substantia nigra/ventral tegmental area.

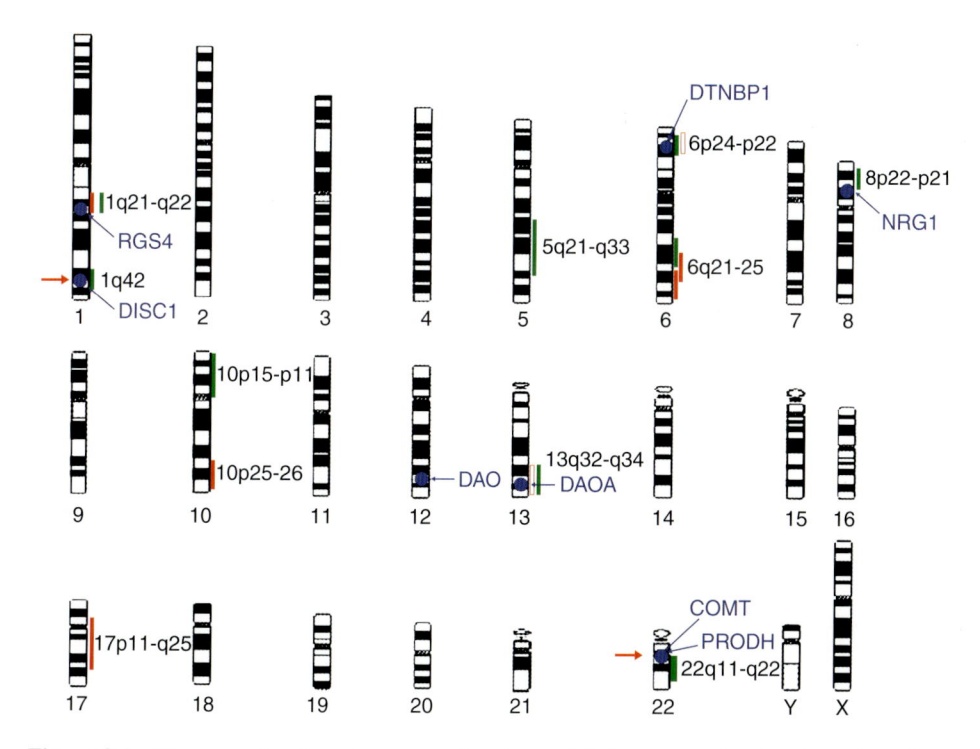

Figure 9.1 Ideogram showing chromosomal regions of linkage to schizophrenia and candidate genes that may be associated. Vertical bars denote regions where evidence for linkage has been found in more than one study (green) and where linkage has reached genomewide significance (red) according to the criteria of Lander and Kruglyak [19]. Arrows (red) identify regions where chromosomal abnormalities are involved with schizophrenia. The chromosomal positions of the major candidate genes discussed in this chapter are also displayed.

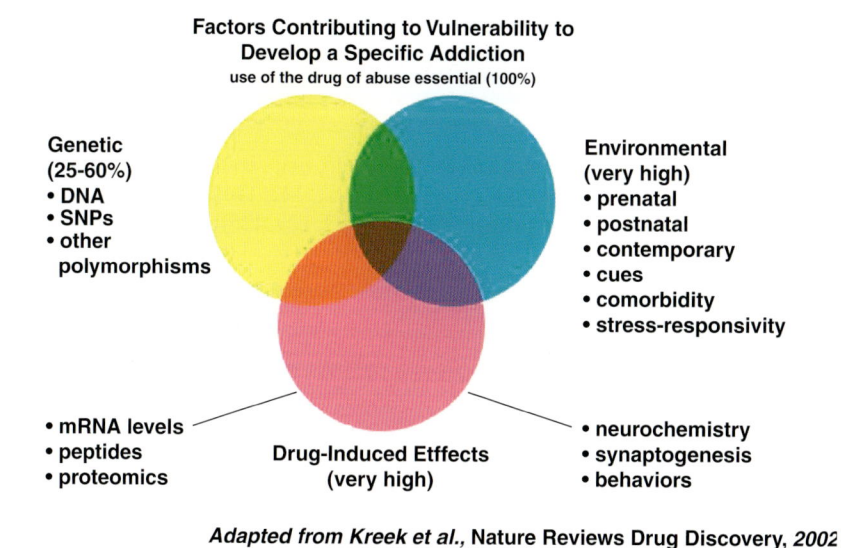

Figure 13.2 Factors contributing to vulnerability to develop a specific addiction. (Adapted from Kreek et al., *Nature Reviews Drug Discovery*, 2002.)

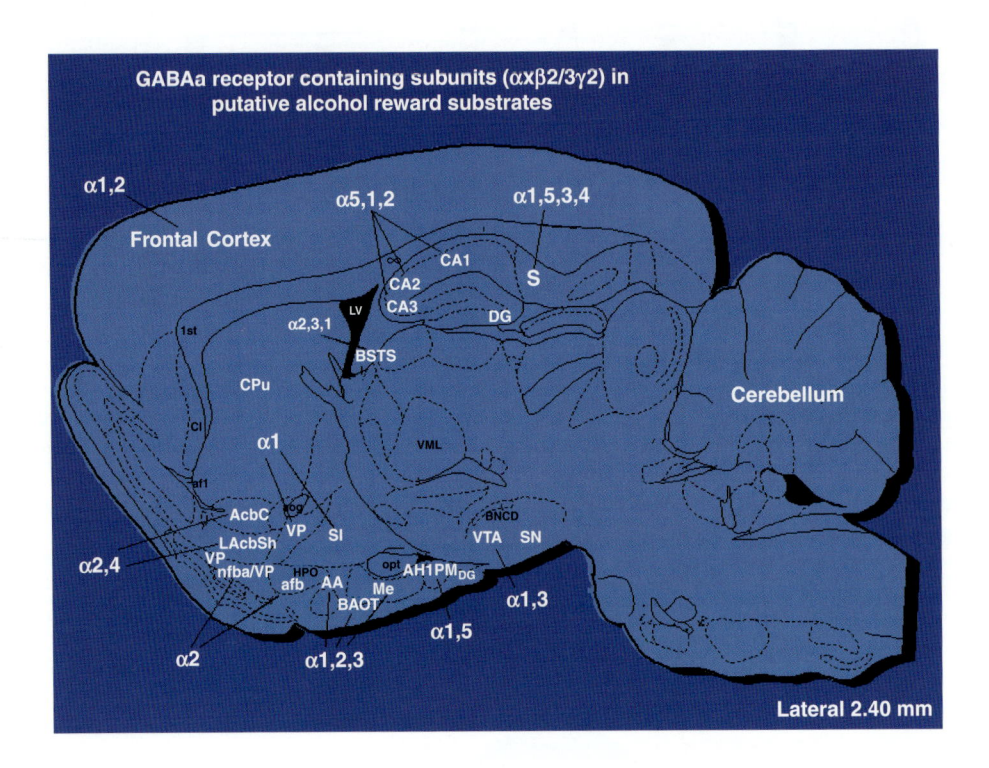

Figure 14.13 Distribution of $GABA_A$ receptor containing subunits (e.g., $\alpha x\beta 2/3\gamma 2$) in putative alcohol reward substrates based on in vitro immunocytochemistry [141, 142, 146], in situ hybridization [143, 146, 213, 214], and in vivo neurobehavioral [18, 19, 30, 37, 123, 125] studies.

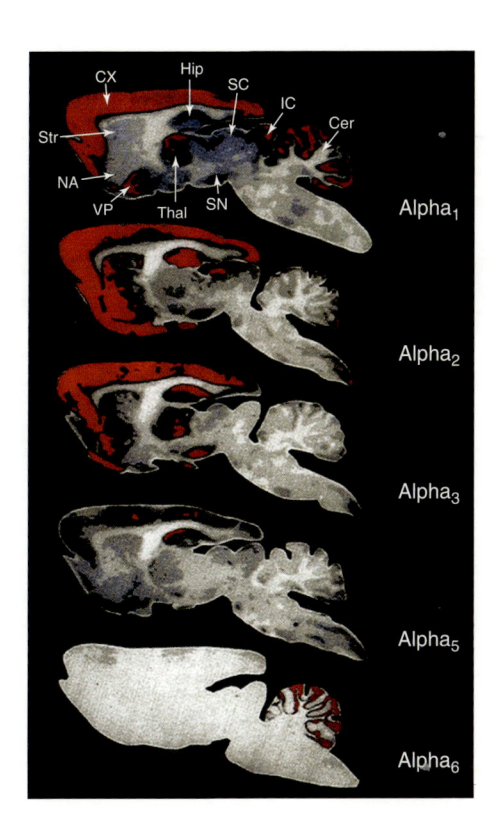

Figure 14.15 Distribution of $GABA_A$ receptor containing subunits α_1-$\alpha_6\beta_2\gamma_2$ in rat CNS based on immunocytochemistry studies by Turner and colleagues [142].

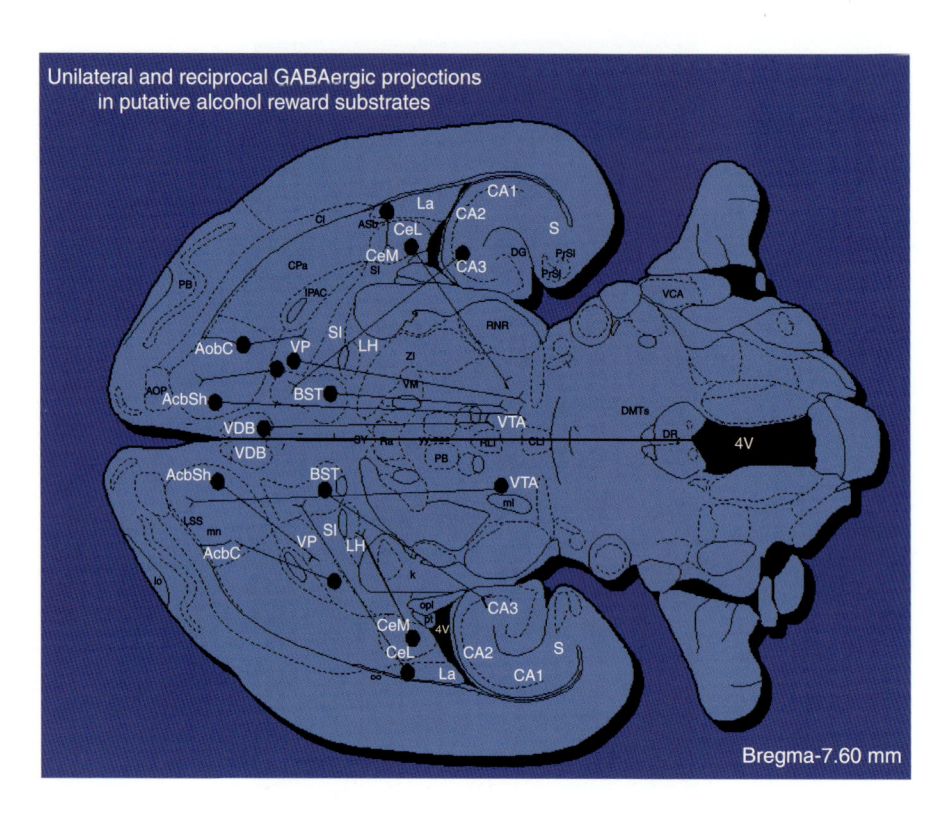

Figure 14.16 Illustration of both unilateral and reciprocal GABAergic projections in putative alcohol reward substrates based on histological mapping studies [64, 87, 88, 94, 95, 215–217].

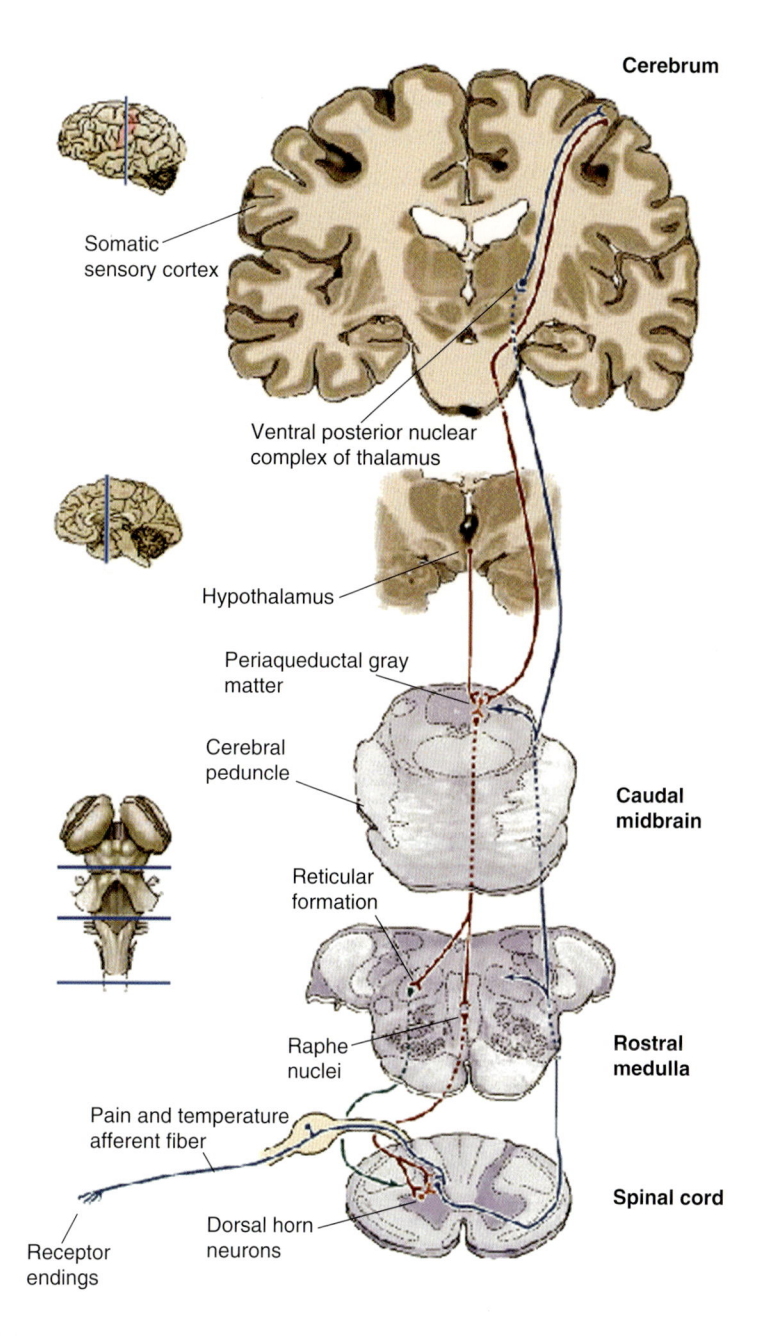

Figure 20.1 Ascending spinothalamic tract. Major pathways for pain (and temperature) sensation. (a) Spinothalamic system. (b) Trigeminal pain and temperature system, which carries information about these sensations from the face. (Reproduced with permission from D. Purues et al. (2001). *NeuroScience*. Sinauer, Sunderland, MA, Fig. 10.3).

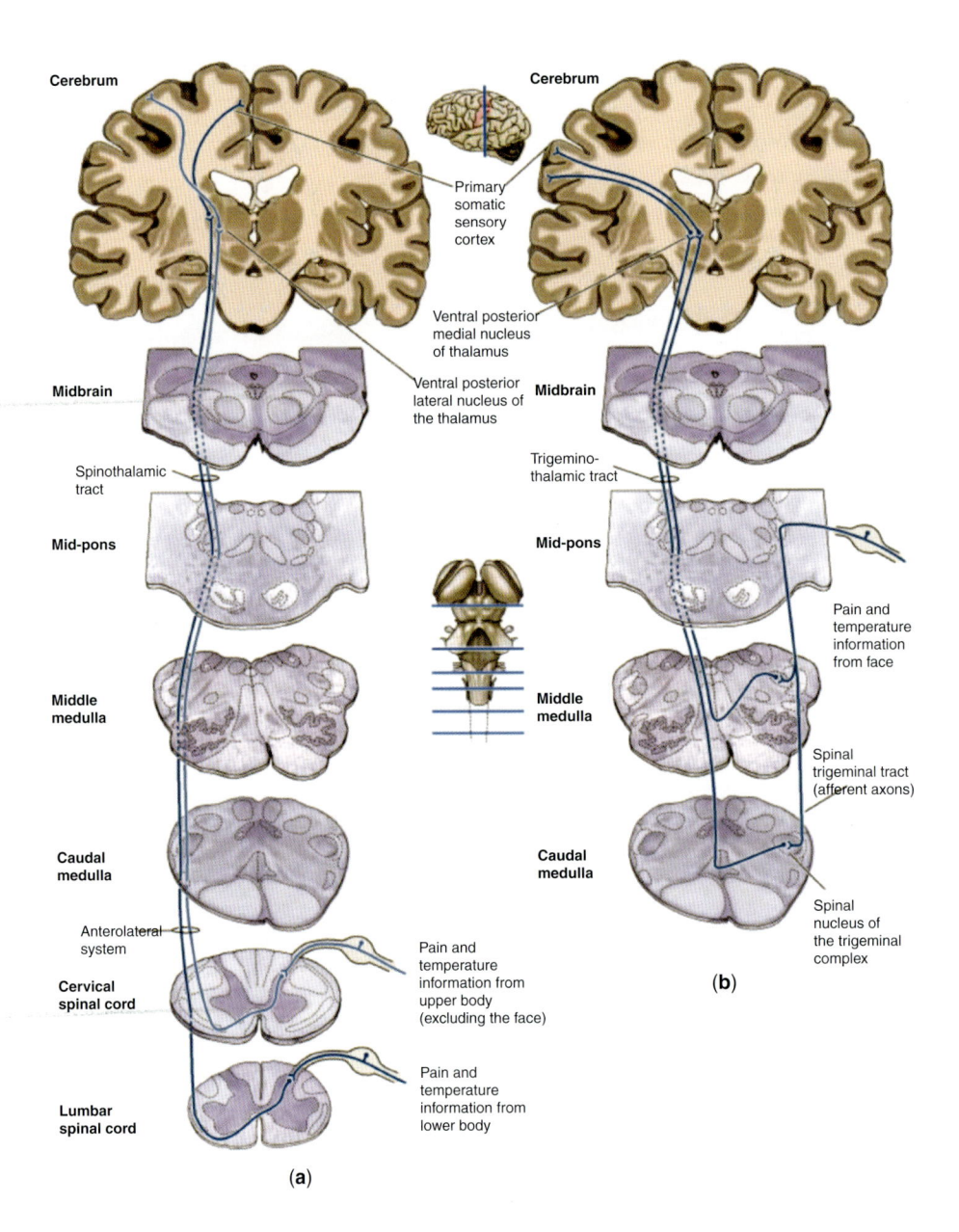

Figure 20.3 Descending pain modulatory pathways. The descending systems that modulate the transmission of ascending pain signals. These modulatory systems originate in the somatic sensory cortex, the hypothalamus, the periaqueductal gray matter of the midbrain, the raphe nuclei, and other nuclei of the rostral ventral medulla. Complex modulatory effects occur at each of these sites, as well as in the dorsal horn. (Reproduced with permission from D. Purues et al. (2001). *NeuroScience*. Sinauer, Sunderland, MA, Fig. 10.5).

216. Heinrichs, S. C., and Koob, G. F. (2004). Corticotropin-releasing factor in brain: A role in activation, arousal, and affect regulation. *J. Pharmacol. Exp. Ther.* 311, 427–440.

217. Britton, K. T., McLeod, S., Koob, G. F., et al. (1992). Pregnane steroid alphaxalone attenuates anxiogenic behavioral effects of corticotropin releasing factor and stress. *Pharmacol. Biochem. Behav.* 41, 399–403.

218. Swerdlow, N. R., and Britton, K. T. (1994). Alphaxalone, a steroid anesthetic, inhibits the startle-enhancing effects of corticotropin releasing factor, but not strychnine. *Psychopharmacology* 115, 141–146.

219. Dubrovsky, B. O. (2005). Steroids, neuroactive steroids and neurosteroids in psychopathology. *Prog. Neuropsychopharmacol. Biol. Psychiatry* 29, 169–192.

220. Backstrom, T., Andersson, A., Andree, L., et al. (2003). Pathogenesis in menstrual cycle-linked CNS disorders. In *Steroids and the Nervous System*, Series title: *Annals of the New York Academy of Sciences*, Vol. 1007, G. C. Panzica and R. C. Melcangi, Eds. New York Academy of Sciences, New York, pp. 42–53.

221. Arborelius, L., Owens, M. J., Plotsky, P. M., et al. (1999). The role of corticotropin-releasing factor in depression and anxiety disorders. *J. Endocrinol.* 160, 1–12.

222. Makino, S., Hashimoto, K., and Gold, P. W. (2002). Multiple feedback mechanisms activating corticotropin-releasing hormone system in the brain during stress. *Pharmacol. Biochem. Behav.* 73, 147–158.

223. Reul, J. M. H. M., and Holsboer, F. (2002). Corticotropin-releasing factor receptors 1 and 2 in anxiety and depression. *Curr. Opin. Pharmacol.* 2, 23–33.

224. Tsigos, C., and Chrousos, G. P. (2002). Hypothalamic-pituitary-adrenal axis, neuroendocrine factors and stress. *J. Psychosom. Res.* 53, 865–871.

225. Claes, S. J. (2004). Corticotropin-releasing hormone (CRH) in psychiatry: From stress to psychopathology. *Ann. Med.* 36, 50–61.

226. Romeo, E., Strohle, A., Spalletta, G., et al. (1998). Effects of antidepressant treatment on neuroactive steroids in major depression. *Am. J. Psychiatry.* 155, 910–913.

227. Uzunova, V., Sheline, Y., Davis, J. M., et al. (1998). Increase in the cerebrospinal fluid content of neurosteroids in patients with unipolar major depression who are receiving fluoxetine or fluvoxamine. *Proc. Natl. Acad. Sci. USA,* 95, 3239–3244.

228. Strohle, A., Pasini, A., Romeo, E., et al. (2000). Fluoxetine decreases concentrations of 3α,5α-tetrahydrodeoxycorticosterone (THDOC) in major depression. *J. Psychiatr. Res.* 34, 183–186.

229. Griffin, L. D., and Mellon, S. H. (1999). Selective serotonin reuptake inhibitors directly alter activity of neurosteroidogenic enzymes. *Proc. Natl. Acad. Sci. USA,* 96, 13512–13517.

230. Uzunov, D. P., Cooper, T. B., Costa, E., et al. (1996). Fluoxetine-elicited changes in brain neurosteroid cotent measured by negative ion mass fragmentography. *Proc. Natl. Acad. Sci. USA,* 93, 12599–12604.

231. Pepe, G. J., and Albrecht, E. D. (1995). Actions of placental and fetal adrenal steroid hormones in primate pregnancy. *Endocr. Rev.* 16, 608–648.

232. Dombroski, R. A., Casey, M. L., and MacDonald, P. C. (1997). 5-α-Dihydroprogesterone formation in human placenta from 5α-pregnan-3β/α-ol-20-ones and 5-pregnan-3β-yl-20-one sulfate. *J. Steroid Biochem. Mol. Biol.* 63, 155–163.

233. Epperson, C. N. (1999). Postpartum major depression: Detection and treatment. *Am. Fam. Physician* 59, 2247–2254, 2259–2260.

234. Nappi, R. E., Petraglia, F., Luisi, S., et al. (2001). Serum allopregnanolone in women with postpartum "blues". *Obstet. Gynecol.* 97, 77–80.

235. Hill, M., Bicikova, M., Parizek, A., et al. (2001). Neuroactive steroids, their precursors and polar conjugates during parturition and postpartum in maternal blood: 2. Time profiles of pregnanolone isomers. *J. Steroid Biochem. Mol. Biol.* 78, 51–57.

236. Gilbert Evans, S. E., Ross, L. E., Sellers, E. M., et al. (2005). 3alpha-reduced neuroactive steroids and their precursors during pregnancy and the postpartum period. *Gynecol. Endocrinol.* 21, 268–279.

237. Rivier, C. (1993). Female rats release more corticosterone than males in response to alcohol: Influence of circulating sex steroids and possible consequences for blood alcohol levels. *Alcohol. Clin. Exp. Res.* 17, 854–859.

238. Ogilvie, K., Lee, S., and Rivier, C. (1997). Effect of three different modes of alcohol administration on the activity of the rat hypothalamic-pituitary-adrenal axis. *Alcohol. Clin. Exp. Res.* 21, 467–476.

239. Ogilvie, K., Lee, S., and Rivier, C. (1998). Divergence in the expression of molecular markers of neuronal activation in the parvocellular paraventricular nucleus of the hypothalamus evoked by alcohol administration via different routes. *J. Neurosci.* 18, 4344–4352.

240. Finn, D. A., Gallaher, E. J., and Crabbe, J. C. (2000). Differential change in neuroactive steroid sensitivity during ethanol withdrawal. *J. Pharmacol. Exp. Ther.* 292, 394–405.

241. Finn, D. A., Sinnott, R. S., Ford, M. M., et al. (2004b). Sex differences in the effect of ethanol injection and consumption on brain allopregnanolone levels in C57BL/6 mice. *Neuroscience* 123, 813–819.

242. Rivier, C. (1996). Alcohol stimulates ACTH secretion in the rat: Mechanisms of action and interactions with other stimuli. *Alcohol. Clin. Exp. Res.* 20, 240–254.

243. Lee, S., Selvage, D., Hansen, K., et al. (2004). Site of action of acute alcohol administration in stimulating the rat hypothalamic-pituitary-adrenal axis: Comparison between the effect of systemic and intracerebroventricular injection of this drug on pituitary and hypothalamic responses. *Endocrinology* 145, 4470–4479.

244. Korneyev, A., Costa, E., and Guidotti, A. (1993a). During anesthetic-induced activation of the hypothalamic pituitary adrenal axis, blood-borne steroids fail to contribute to the anesthetic effect. *Neuroendocrinology* 57, 559–565.

245. Barbaccia, M. L., Affricano, D., Trabucchi, M., et al. (1999). Ethanol markedly increases "GABAergic" neurosteroids in alcohol-preferring rats. *Eur. J. Pharmacol.* 384, R1–R2.

246. VanDoren, M. J., Matthews, D. B., Janis, G. C., et al. (2000). Neuroactive steroid 3α-hydroxy-5α-pregnan-20-one modulates electrophysiological and behavioral actions of ethanol. *J. Neurosci.* 20, 1982–1989.

247. Finn, D. A., Ford, M. M., Wiren, K. W., et al. (2004a). The role of pregnane neurosteroids in ethanol withdrawal: Behavioral genetic approaches. *Pharmacol. Ther.* 101, 91–112.

248. Torres, J. M., and Ortega, E. (2003). Alcohol intoxication increases allopregnanolone levels in female adolescent humans. *Neuropsychopharmacology* 28, 1207–1209.

249. Torres, J. M., and Ortega, E. (2004). Alcohol intoxication increases allopregnanolone levels in male adolescent humans. *Psychopharmacology* 172, 352–355.

250. Grobin, A. C., Matthews, D. B., Devaud, L. L., et al. (1998). The role of $GABA_A$ receptors in the acute and chronic effects of ethanol. *Psychopharmacology* 139, 2–19.

251. Morrow, A. L., VanDoren, M. J., Penland, S. N., et al. (2001). The role of GABAergic neuroactive steroids in ethanol action, tolerance and dependence. *Brain Res. Rev.* 37, 98–109.

252. Dazzi, L., Serra, M., Seu, E., et al. (2002). Progesterone enhances ethanol-induced modulation of mesocortical dopamine neurons: Antagonism by finasteride. *J. Neurochem.* 83, 1103–1109.

253. Budec, M., Koko, V., Milovanovic, T., et al. (2002). Acute ethanol treatment increases level of progesterone in ovariectomized rats. *Alcohol* 26, 173–178.

254. Khisti, R. T., VanDoren, M. J., O'Buckley, T., et al. (2003). Neuroactive steroid 3α-hydroxy-5α-pregnan-20-one modulates ethanol-induced loss of righting reflex in rats. *Brain Res.* 980, 255–265.

255. O'Dell, L. E., Alomary, A. A., Vallee, M., et al. (2004). Ethanol-induced increases in neuroactive steroids in the rat brain and plasma are absent in adrenalectomized and gonadectomized rats. *Eur. J. Pharmacol.* 484, 241–247.

256. Sanna, E., Talani, G., Busonero, F., et al. (2004). Brain steroidogenesis mediates ethanol modulation of $GABA_A$ receptor activity in rat hippocampus. *J. Neurosci.* 24, 6521–6530.

257. Roberto, M., Madamba, S. G., Moore, S. D., et al. (2003). Ethanol increases GABAergic transmission at both pre- and postsynaptic sites in rat central amygdala neurons. *Proc. Natl. Acad. Sci. USA* 100, 2053–2058.

258. Roberto, M., Schweitzer, P., Madamba, S. G., et al. (2004). Acute and chronic ethanol alter glutamatergic transmission in rat central amygdala: An in vitro and in vivo analysis. *J. Neurosci.* 24, 1594–1603.

259. O'Brien, C. P. (1997). A range of research-based pharmacotherapies for addiction. *Science* 278, 66–70.

260. Stretch, R., Gerber, G. J., and Wood, S. M. (1971). Factors affecting behavior maintained by response-contingent intravenous infusions of amphetamine in squirrel monkeys. *Can. J. Physiol. Pharmacol.* 49, 581–589.

261. Davis, W. M., and Smith, S. G. (1976). Role of conditioned reinforcers in the initiation, maintenance and extinction of drug-seeking behavior. *Pavlov. J. Biol. Sci.* 11, 222–236.

262. de Wit, H., and Stewart, J. (1981). Reinstatement of cocaine-reinforced responding in the rat. *Psychopharmacology* 75, 134–143.

263. de Wit, H., and Stewart, J. (1983). Drug reinstatement of heroin-reinforced responding in the rat. *Psychopharmacology* 79, 29–31.

264. Stewart, J. (2000). Pathways to relapse: The neurobiology of drug- and stress-induced relapse to drug-taking. *J. Psychiatry Neurosci.* 25, 125–136.

265. Sarnyai, Z., Shaham, Y., and Heinrichs, S. C. (2001). The role of corticotropin-releasing factor in drug addiction. *Pharmacol. Rev.* 53, 209–243.

266. Shalev, U., Grimm, J. W., and Shaham, Y. (2002). Neurobiology of relapse to heroin and cocaine seeking: A review. *Pharmacol. Rev.* 54, 1–42.

267. Shaham, Y., Erb, S., and Stewart, J. (2000). Stress-induced relapse to heroin and cocaine seeking in rats: A review. *Brain Res. Rev.* 33, 13–33.

268. Shaham, Y., Shalev, U., Lu, L., et al. (2003). The reinstatement model of drug relapse: History, methodology and major findings. *Psychopharmacology* 168, 3–20.

269. Shaham, Y., and Stewart, J. (1995). Stress reinstates heroin-seeking in drug-free animals: An effect mimicking heroin, not withdrawal. *Psychopharmacology* 119, 334–341.

270. Erb, S., Shaham, Y., and Stewart, J. (1996). Stress reinstates cocaine-seeking behavior after prolonged extinction and a drug-free period. *Psychopharmacology* 128, 408–412.

271. Shaham, Y., Adamson, L. K., Grocki, S., et al. (1997a). Reinstatement and spontaneous recovery of nicotine-seeking in rats. *Psychopharmacology* 130, 396–403.
272. Le, A. D., Quan, B., Juzytch, W., et al. (1998). Reinstatement of alcohol-seeking by priming injections of alcohol and exposure to stress in rats. *Psychopharmacology* 135, 169–174.
273. Buczek, Y., Le, A. D., Wang, A., et al. (1999). Stress reinstates nicotine seeking but not sucrose solution seeking in rats. *Psychopharmacology* 144, 183–188.
274. Shaham, Y., Funk, D., Erb, S., et al. (1997b). Corticotropin-releasing factor, but not corticosterone, is involved in the stress-induced relapse to heroin-seeking in rats. *J. Neurosci.* 17, 2605–2614.
275. Le, A. D., Harding, S., Juzytsch, W., et al. (2000). The role of corticotropin-releasing factor in stress-induced relapse to alcohol-seeking behavior in rats. *Psychopharmacology* 150, 317–324.
276. Shaham, Y., Erb, S., Leung, S., et al. (1998). CP-154,426, a selective, non-peptide antagonist of the corticotropin-releasing factor 1 receptor attenuates stress-induced relapse to drug seeking in cocaine- and heroin-trained rats. *Psychopharmacology* 137, 184–190.
277. Nie, H., and Janak, P. H. (2003). Comparison of reinstatement of ethanol- and sucrose-seeking by conditioned stimuli and priming injections of allopregnanolone after extinction in rats. *Psychopharmacology* 168, 222–228.
278. Janak, P. H., Redfern, J. E., and Samson, H. H. (1998). The reinforcing effects of ethanol are altered by the endogenous neurosteroid, allopregnanolone. *Alcohol. Clin. Exp. Res.* 22, 1106–1112.
279. Janak, P. H., and Gill, M. T. (2003). Comparison of the effects of allopregnanolone with direct GABAergic agonists on ethanol self-administration with and without concurrently available sucrose. *Alcohol* 30, 1–7.
280. Sinnott, R. S., Phillips, T. J., and Finn, D. A. (2002). Alteration of voluntary ethanol and saccharin consumption by the neurosteroid allopregnanolone in mice. *Psychopharmacology* 162, 438–447.
280a. Ford, M. M., Nickel, J. D., Phillips, T. J., et al. (2005). Neurosteroid modulators of $GABA_A$ receptors differentially modulate ethanol intake patterns in male C57BL/6Jmice. *Alcohol. Clin. Exp. Res.* 29, 1630–1640.
281. O'Dell, L. E., Purdy, R. H., Covey, D. F., et al. (2005). Epipregnanolone and a novel synthetic neuroactive steroid reduce alcohol self-administration in rats. *Pharmacol. Biochem. Behav.* 81, 543–550.
282. Wang, M., He, Y., Eisenman, L. N., et al. (2002). 3β-Hydroxypregnane steroids are pregnenolone sulfate-like $GABA_A$ receptor antagonists. *J. Neurosci.* 22, 3366–3375.
283. Mennerick, S., Zeng, C. M., Benz, A., et al. (2001). Effects on gamma-aminobutyric acid $(GABA)_A$ receptors of a neuroactive steroid that negatively modulates glutamate neurotransmission and augments GABA neurotransmission. *Mol. Pharmacol.* 60, 732–741.
284. Johnson, E. O., Kamilaris, T. C., Chrousos, G. P., and Gold, P. W. (1992). Mechanisms of stress: A dynamic overview of hormonal and behavioral homeostasis. *Neurosci. Biobehav. Rev.* 16, 115–130.
285. Herman, J. P., and Cullinan, W. E. (1997). Neurocircuitry of stress: Central control of the hypothalamo-pituitary-adrenocortical axis. *Trends Neurosci.* 20, 78–84.
286. Holsboer, F. (1999). The rationale for corticotropin-releasing hormone receptor (CRH-R) antagonists to treat depression and anxiety. *J. Psychiatr. Res.* 33, 181–214.
287. Schmidt, P. J., Purdy, R. H., Moore, P. H., Jr., et al. (1994). Circulating levels of anxiolytic steroids in the luteal phase in women with premenstrual syndrome and in control subjects. *J. Clin. Endocrinol. Metab.* 79, 1256–1260.

5

EMERGING ANXIOLYTICS: CORTICOTROPIN-RELEASING FACTOR RECEPTOR ANTAGONISTS

DIMITRI E. GRIGORIADIS AND SAMUEL R. J. HOARE
Neurocrine Biosciences, San Diego, California

5.1	Introduction	177
5.2	CRF Receptor/Ligand Family	179
	5.2.1 Ligands for CRF Receptor Family	180
	5.2.2 Subtypes and Distribution of CRF Receptor	181
5.3	Peptide Ligand Pharmacology of CRF_1 and CRF_2 Receptors	185
	5.3.1 Mechanisms of Peptide Ligand Binding to CRF_1 and CRF_2 Receptors	190
5.4	Nonpeptide Ligands for CRF_1 Receptors	195
	5.4.1 Mechanism of Nonpeptide Ligand Interaction with CRF_1 Receptor	195
5.5	Potential for Therapeutic Intervention in Anxiety and Depression	196
5.6	Conclusions	198
	References	199

5.1 INTRODUCTION

The corticotropin-releasing factor (CRF) system is widely accepted as the primary mediator of an organism's response to stress. CRF is one of a number of neurohormones synthesized in discrete hypothalamic nuclei where in response to a stressor is secreted into the portal vasculature where it acts directly at the pituitary. At the pituitary, and more specifically at the anterior pituitary, CRF binds to cognate receptors resulting in the release of the proopiomelanocortin-derived peptide adrenocorticotropic hormone (ACTH). This in turn acts at the adrenal gland to secrete glucocorticoids, and these steroids feed back at the level of the hypothalamus and the anterior pituitary to attenuate the release of CRF and ACTH, respectively. This hormone loop is known as the hypothalamic–pituitary–adrenal (HPA) axis and is tightly regulated in mediating the stress response. In addition to its endocrine effects, CRF is widely distributed, synthesized, and secreted from extrahypothalamic

Handbook of Contemporary Neuropharmacology, Edited by David R. Sibley, Israel Hanin, Michael Kuhar, and Phil Skolnick. Copyright © 2007 John Wiley & Sons, Inc.

sites within the central nervous system (CNS) acting on higher centers of the brain where it mediates the appropriate response of the organism to various physical and psychological stressors.

Although the modern concept that hypothalamic secretions were the key mediators of the stress response dates back to the works of Sir Geoffrey Harris and Hans Selye in the early 1950s [1, 2], it was the independent determination from the experiments of Guillemin and Rosenberg [3] and Saffran and Schally [4] that provided the first direct evidence of a hypothalamic factor (CRF) that was responsible, under stressful situations, for regulating the production of ACTH. The identity of this specific factor, however, was not discovered until 30 years later when Vale and colleagues [5] reported the isolation, characterization, synthesis, and in vitro and in vivo biological activities of CRF from sheep hypothalamus. Once this peptide was characterized, evidence began to accumulate that this stress hormone may play a major role in human affective disorders. Nemeroff and colleagues made one of the first observations implicating this system in depression by demonstrating that the cerebrospinal fluid (CSF) of depressed patients contained elevated levels of the CRF peptide itself, suggesting a hypersecretion of this hormone in the brain during this disease [6]. At the same time, two groups independently demonstrated that in depressed individuals the ACTH response to systemic administration of CRF was blunted, suggesting a downregulation of the system [7–9], and a positive correlation was observed between CSF concentrations of CRF and the degree of post–dexamethasone suppression of plasma cortisol [10]. These data taken together indicated the tight control of a system whereby elevated levels of CRF in the CNS could cause the downregulation or desensitization of the receptors at the pituitary, thereby causing a blunting of the ACTH response upon exogenous administration of CRF. Further corroboration of this hypothesis was presented by the findings that in suicide victims CRF receptor binding sites were significantly decreased in postmortem frontal cortical tissue, again consistent with the mechanism of elevated levels of CRF in brain causing a homologous downregulation of CRF receptors [11].

Examination of CRF in detail presented further evidence that this system plays a key role in the manifestation of anxiety and depression. Levels of CRF in the CNS of depressed individuals who had undergone successful treatment paradigms were found to be altered in a direction consistent with the hypothesis that elevated levels of CRF were manifesting the disease symptomatology. For example, when CRF was measured in the CSF of depressed individuals before and after successful electroshock convulsive therapy (ECT), the elevated levels of CRF in the CSF was found to decrease following ECT and corresponded to patient improvement in mood [12]. Another study, performed on 24 patients suffering from major depression and treated for six to eight weeks with antidepressants, interestingly found that although no differences in the CSF levels of CRF were observed between pre- and posttreatment, despite clinical improvement, those patients who did not relapse in the following six months had a significant reduction in CSF concentrations of CRF while those that relapsed did not. These findings suggest that the hyperactivity of CRF in the CNS may predispose patients to relapse following treatment and are consistent with the findings of a higher risk of relapse in patients that exhibit elevated levels of cortisol following concomitant administration of the CRF/dexamethasone suppression test [13]. Furthermore, while the simple measurement of CRF peptide in the brain may not accurately reflect the hyperactivity of the system in these disorders, clinical studies to date are in agreement that CRF levels in the CSF generally decrease in parallel with clinical recovery regardless of the treatment paradigm used [14, 15].

More than a decade later, the receptors for this neurohormone were identified and cloned from a variety of species, including human. The ability to look biochemically at the cloned human receptor accelerated the identification and characterization of nonpeptide small molecules that could block these receptors and paved the way for the development of novel therapeutics for disorders associated with a dysregulated stress axis, including anxiety and depression. This chapter provides a brief overview of the CRF system, including the known ligands and receptor subtypes, and details the different interactions between the ligands (both peptide and nonpeptide) and these receptors. With the relatively recent discovery of nonpeptide antagonists for the CRF system, the similarities and differences between the receptor/ligand interactions will be examined and the preliminary evidence and potential for their utility as anxiolytics and antidepressants will be presented.

5.2 CRF RECEPTOR/LIGAND FAMILY

Since the discovery of ovine CRF from the sheep hypothalamus, other functional CRF peptides have been identified from many species, including rat [16], human [17], goat [18], cow [19], pig [20], suckerfish (urotensin-I, isolated from the urophysis extract of the sucker (teleost) fish *Catostomus commersoni* [21, 22]), and xenopus (sauvagine isolated from a skin extract of the South American tree frog *Phyllomedusa sauvegei* [23, 24]). All of these peptides demonstrated the ability to cause the secretion of ACTH from primary cultures of rat anterior pituitary cells [25]. Initially, urotensin-I was thought to subserve the role of CRF in the fish; however, the discovery of two independent CRF genes in this species [26] prompted many laboratories to begin searching for the presence of other CRF-like molecules in mammals. In 1995, with the aid of immunocytochemical methodologies, a urotensin-like molecule was isolated from the Edinger–Westphal nucleus of the rat brain which had high homology (63% sequence identity) to urotensin-I [27]. This new peptide, termed urocortin, was cloned, synthesized, and found to stimulate the secretion of ACTH both in vitro and in vivo. The human homolog of urocortin was subsequently identified by the cloning of its messenger RNA (mRNA) from a human genomic brain library and localized to human chromosome 2 [28]. These initial findings became the basis for the discovery of a family of mammalian urocortin peptides which, as will be described below, have distinct distributions and pharmacological profiles but whose precise relevance to human physiology or pathophysiology is not yet completely understood.

CRF and its related peptides mediate their actions through high-affinity binding sites in various peripheral and central tissues. In addition, a high-affinity soluble binding site exists, the CRF binding protein, which is expressed predominantly in the brain and pituitary and is presumed to modulate the activity of CRF itself [29]. Both the natural peptides and the close analog peptides have been radiolabeled and used in radioligand binding and receptor autoradiographic studies of the distribution of CRF receptors and their role(s) in physiological processes. There have been numerous publications that have described the radioligand binding characteristics of CRF receptors using those available radioligands in a variety of tissues (for a review see [30–33]). The receptors for CRF exist as two distinct subtypes encoded by separate genes and have been termed CRF_1 and CRF_2. Both receptors belong to the class B family of G-protein-coupled receptors (GPCRs), which includes receptors for secretin, vasoactive intestinal peptide (VIP), calcitonin, and glucagon, among others. CRF_1 receptors positively regulate the accumulation of cyclic adenosine monophosphate (cAMP) in response to CRF in both heterologously expressed systems and native tissues from brain and periphery and are therefore coupled to G_s as the major signal transduction mechanism [34, 35]. The CRF_2 receptor has also been shown to couple through G_s and stimulate the production of cAMP, but thus far only in heterologously expressed cell lines containing the human, rat, or mouse forms [36–38].

5.2.1 Ligands for CRF Receptor Family

Since the discovery of ovine CRF, many peptides from multiple species have been discovered that play similar functional roles as described above. In addition to urocortin 1 (UCN1), two other mammalian peptides have been identified from the mouse and human termed urocortin 2 (UCN2) and urocortin 3 (UCN3) [39, 40]. In the human, these same peptides have been identified as stresscopin (SCP) and stresscopin-related peptide (SRP) [41]. The species homology between mouse and human is 76% for SRP/UCN2 and 90% for SCP/UCN3 and these peptides share approximately 30–40% homology with rat/human (r/h) CRF and urocortin. (for a review see [42]). While UCN1 has equal affinity for both CRF receptor subtypes, UCN2 and UCN3 are selective for the CRF_2 receptor subtype and have little or no affinity for the CRF binding protein (described in detail below).

CRF and the related urocortins have been localized to a variety of tissues within the body. The literature is replete with articles detailing the localization and distribution of CRF and the urocortins both from the mRNA and the protein levels. While a full description is beyond the scope of this chapter, briefly, within the CNS, CRF is widely distributed with the highest levels evident in the hypothalamus, amygdala, cortical regions, and cerebellum (reviewed in [31, 43–47]). In general, the distributions of CRF and the urocortins are remarkably nonoverlapping with one exception and a common localization to hypothalamic structures. UCN1 demonstrates the highest levels of expression in regions such as the Edinger–Westphal nucleus, substantia nigra, lateral superior olive, dorsal raphe nucleus, and hypothalamus [27, 48–50]. UCN2 is also discretely localized to hypothalamic nuclei, specifically the paraventricular, supraoptic, and arcuate nuclei as well as in the brain stem [40]. UCN3 is primarily localized to the hypothalamus and more specifically in the preoptic and paraventricular nuclei. It is also highly expressed in medial amygdala, lateral septum (indicating an association with the CRF_2 receptor), and bed nucleus of the stria terminalis [51]. In addition, these peptides have been localized in a variety of peripheral tissues, including the skin and skeletal muscle [52], human heart and kidney [53], and the colon, suggesting a role for stress-induced gastrointestinal (GI) function [54–56].

To date, there are no known endogenous physiological antagonists for the CRF receptor system, however; various truncations of agonist peptides, with deletions of the first 8–11 N-terminal amino acids, have resulted in potent peptide antagonists, both selective and nonselective with respect to their affinities at the CRF_1 and CRF_2

receptor subtypes. These peptides have shed new light not only on understanding the physiology of the CRF system but also for the elucidation of the discrete interactions of the peptide/ligand complex. As with the agonist peptides either deletions of the C-terminal amino acids or simple deamidation of the carboxy terminus renders these peptides essentially inactive at CRF receptors, suggesting that at some level the binding requirements for these ligands have some similarities between the two receptor subtypes. Deletions of the agonist peptides or modifications in the N-terminus, however, have successfully identified potent and functional receptor antagonists that are both selective and nonselective for the CRF receptor subtypes. Peptides such as α-helical CRF(9–41) [57], d-PheCRF(12-41) [58], and astressin [59] were synthesized and found to be potent functional antagonists at both the CRF_1 and CRF_2 receptor subtypes. Antisauvagine-30 [60], an N terminally truncated form of sauvagine, and the more recent cyclized astressin-2B [61] are two peptides that have approximately 400- to 500-fold selectivity for the CRF_2 receptor over the CRF_1 receptor, and these peptides have been recently used to begin dissecting out specific roles of the CRF_2 receptor subtype in a variety of in vivo studies [62, 63]. As will be discussed below, the peptide interactions with the receptors lie largely with the extracellular N-terminal domain of the receptors, and it is precisely the composition of the N-terminus of the peptides that confers agonist activity. This point is illustrated elegantly by the recent studies examining the interactions of the peptide antagonist astressin and the expressed soluble form of the N-terminus of the CRF_1 receptor [64].

5.2.2 Subtypes and Distribution of CRF Receptor

The current understanding of the subfamily of CRF receptors encompasses two receptor subtypes termed CRF_1 and CRF_2 receptors, with the CRF_2 receptor existing in three identified splice variant isoforms ($CRF_{2(a)}$, $CRF_{2(b)}$, and $CRF_{2(c)}$). Prior to the cloning and elucidation of the subtypes of CRF receptors, the labeled agonists $[^{125}I]r/hCRF$ and $[^{125}I]ovine(o)$ CRF were used to elucidate the binding characteristics and anatomical distribution of CRF receptors in the brain, and many publications exist describing the binding characteristics of these prototypical labeled compounds (for review see [30–33]). Indeed, early drug discovery efforts utilized these ligands in native brain homogenate preparations (typically rat frontal cortex or cerebellar tissues) to identify nonpeptide molecules as potential antagonists. Fortunately, these early pharmacological characterizations and drug discovery efforts were largely unaffected by the discovery of a second family member (the CRF_2 receptor) by virtue of the fact that the prototypical endogenous peptides $[^{125}I]r/hCRF$ and $[^{125}I]oCRF$ have lower affinity for the CRF_2 receptor subtype (10–100 nM), making them essentially in vitro selective tools for the CRF_1 receptor under the conditions in which they were being used. The subsequent radiolabeling of the amphibian peptide sauvagine (from frog skin, *P. sauvagei* [23]), which has high affinity for both the CRF_1 and CRF_2 receptor subtypes, allowed for the first time the discrimination of CRF_1 and CRF_2 receptor pharmacology and distribution [65].

The CRF_1 receptor was first cloned from a human corticotropic tumor and characterized as a 415-amino-acid receptor belonging to the class B subfamily of GPCRs with a characteristically large N-terminus, linked to seven putative transmembrane domains terminating with an intracellular C-terminal tail and reported along with an alternatively spliced form of which included a 29-amino-acid insert in the first intracellular loop (Fig. 5.1) [66]. This was shortly followed by the cloning of the rat form of this receptor by the same group [67]. Following the cloning and characterization of the CRF_1 receptor the second subtype of this family was identified and termed the CRF_2 receptor [37] and was also subsequently identified from a variety of species [36–38]. This subtype had approximately 71% identity with the CRF_1 receptor and was shown to exist as three independent splice variants differing from each other only at the extreme N-terminal end (see Fig. 5.1). The chromosomal mapping of the human CRF_2 gene has also been determined and has been localized to chromosome 7p21–p15 [68]. As with any rapidly expanding family of proteins, consistency of molecular nomenclature is difficult to maintain. The literature unfortunately contains a number of different designations for this family of receptors, including CRF-RA [67] and PC-CRF [36, 69] for the CRF_1 receptor; $CRF_{2\alpha}$ [37] for the $CRF_{2(a)}$ receptor; CRF-RB [67], $CRF_{2\beta}$ [37], and HM-CRF [36] for the $CRF_{2(b)}$ receptor; and $CRF_{2\gamma}$ [70] for the $CRF_{2(c)}$ receptor. In an attempt to maintain some consistency with other GPCR families of receptors, a nomenclature for these subtypes has recently been proposed according to the International Union of Basic and Clinical Pharmacology (IUPHAR) convention for the naming of receptors, and these receptors should be referred to hereafter as CRF_1, $CRF_{2(a)}$, $CRF_{2(b)}$, and $CRF_{2(c)}$ receptors [71].

Compared to the CRF_1 receptor, the $CRF_{2(a)}$ receptor is a 411-amino-acid protein with the typical glycosylation sites in the N-terminal domain, The $CRF_{2(b)}$ receptor, which has been cloned from rat, mouse, and human, contains 431 amino acids and differs from the 411-amino-acid $CRF_{2(a)}$ isoform in that the first 34 amino acids in the N-terminal extracellular domain are replaced by a unique sequence 54 amino acids in length [37, 72]. The $CRF_{2(c)}$ receptor has thus far only been identified in the amygdala of the human brain [70]. This splice variant uses yet a different 5′ alternative exon for its amino terminus and replaces the first 34-amino-acid sequence of the $CRF_{2(a)}$ receptor with a unique 20-amino-acid sequence (see Fig. 5.1). Very recently a soluble splice variant of the mouse $CRF_{2(a)}$ receptor has been identified and characterized. This soluble protein appears to localize in the same discrete anatomical brain regions of the mouse brain and may represent yet another mechanism through which this system can modulate the activity of its endogenous agonists [73].

There have also been a number of splice variants for the CRF_1 receptor reported in the literature; however, the physiological significance of these variants still remains to be determined. Besides the first 29-amino-acid variant first described in the initial pituitary tumor library described above, a second splice variant for the CRF_1 receptor ($CRF_{1\gamma}$) derived from human hypothalamus has been reported where a large portion of the N-terminal domain is deleted. This protein, however, has lower affinity for agonists and appears to be weakly functional when expressed in mammalian cell lines [74]. Finally, a third splice variant identified from human pregnant myometrium ($CRF_{1\delta}$) contains a deletion of 14 amino acids in the C-terminus of the seventh transmembrane domain. On heterologous expression of this receptor, it was found that while binding of agonist ligands was largely unaffected, this receptor could not couple through G proteins and was therefore functionally inactive [75]. While these receptor splice variants offer insight into the structure and functional conformations of the CRF_1 receptor, their in vivo

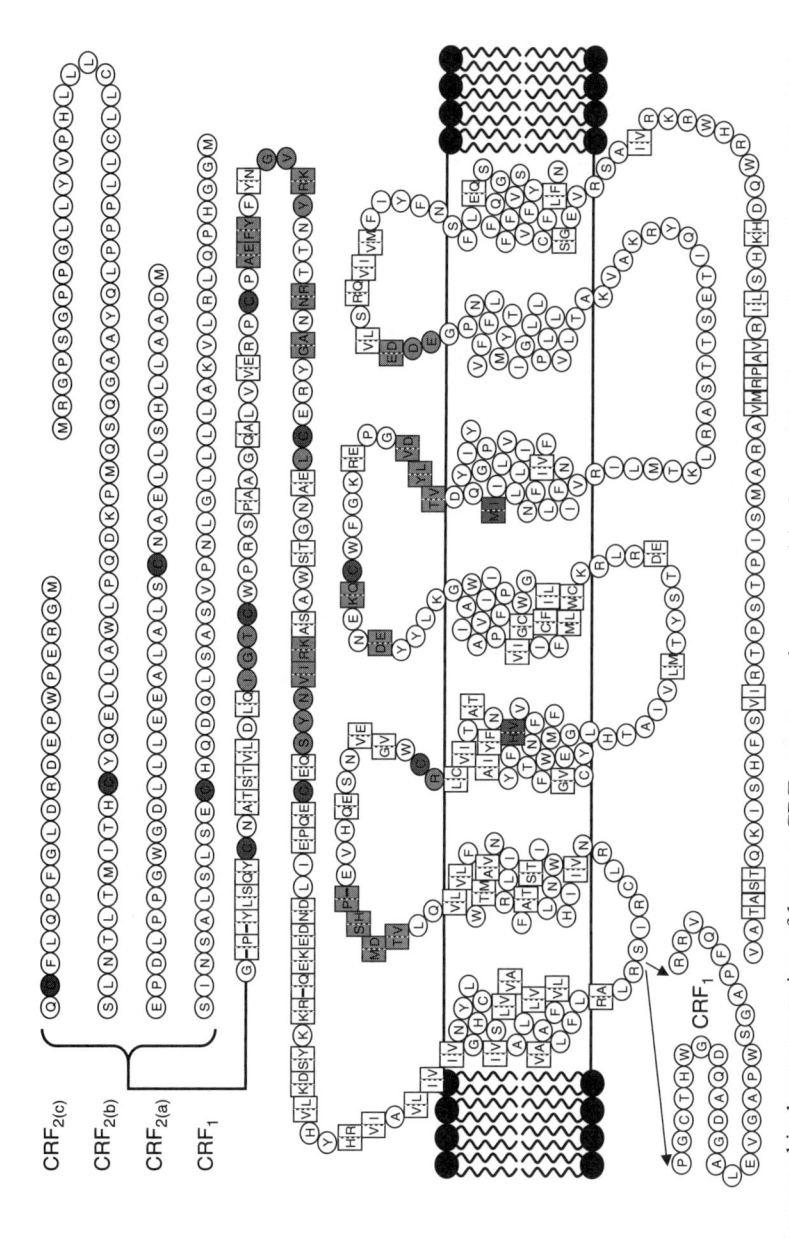

Figure 5.1 Topographical representation of human CRF receptor subtypes and isoforms. The three splice variants of the N domain of the CRF$_2$ receptor are illustrated. Within the remainder of the receptor, conserved residues between CRF$_1$ and CRF$_2$ receptors are in circles, whereas differing residues are indicated by squares (CRF$_1$ receptor residue on the left-hand side, CRF$_2$ receptor on the right-hand side). Residues shaded red are cysteines conserved throughout the CRF and class B receptor families. Residues shaded green have been implicated in peptide ligand binding [130–139] whereas residues shaded pink have been implicated in nonpeptide antagonist binding [130]. The position of transmembrane helices have been predicted based on amino acid sequence hydropathy analysis—the precise position of the helices is not presently known. (Figure adapted from *Celltransmissions* with permission from Sigma-Aldrich [196].) (See color insert.)

physiological relevance will have to await further mRNA and protein expression determinations in native tissues.

Many studies have described in great detail the anatomical distribution of the CRF receptor subtypes and isoforms in a variety of species using both receptor autoradiographic studies with [^{125}I]sauvagine or [^{125}I]oCRF and in situ hybridization studies using probes that are both subtype specific and isoform selective (reviewed in great detail in [76–80]). The highest density of CRF_1 receptors exists in the pituitary gland, where CRF_1 expression clustered on corticotropes related to its effects on the release of ACTH from the anterior lobe of the pituitary [77]. High levels of CRF_1 receptors have been localized in brain to the cerebral cortical areas, amygdala, and hippocampus in rodents and also in hypothalamus and amygdala in nonhuman primates (for review see [77, 80]). There are also a number of peripheral sites to which CRF receptors have been localized, including adrenals, and throughout the immune and reproductive systems where levels of CRF_1 mRNA have been localized in the testis and ovary [81–83]. A major peripheral site of high expression for this receptor is the GI tract [84–86]. Localization studies have suggested a distinct functional role for this protein in gut function and motility and compliment the reported actions of CRF and related endogenous peptides that have been examined in detail [63, 87, 88] and mimic the effects of stress on gastric and colonic motility [89, 90]. In fact, the concept of stress-induced pathophysiology in the gut and the role of the CRF receptors in mediating this pathology is currently generating a great deal of interest for drug discovery. The potential utility of CRF receptor antagonists for GI stress disorders such as irritable bowel syndrome have been recently reviewed [91–94].

The localization and distribution of the CRF_2 receptor are quite different and more varied within the CNS and across species than the CRF_1 receptor. Unlike the similarities in CNS distribution of the CRF_1 receptor between species, the CRF_2 receptor exhibits more species differences in the localization of receptor subtypes between rodent, nonhuman primate, and human tissues. Within the rat brain, $CRF_{2(a)}$ receptor expression is generally confined to subcortical structures, including the lateral septal region, the bed nucleus of the stria terminalis, the amygdaloid area, and the olfactory bulb [77], whereas in higher order species such as human and nonhuman primates the $CRF_{2(a)}$ receptor is distributed in high densities across the cortical regions as well as the brain structures described in rodents [77]. While the role of the CRF_2 receptor in anxiety disorders still requires some clarification, some recent studies have begun to demonstrate that at least the $CRF_{2(a)}$ receptor may well facilitate the manifestation of anxiety. The lateral septum, by virtue of widespread reciprocal connections throughout the brain, is implicated in a variety of physiological processes playing a central role in classical limbic circuitry and thus potentially integrating a variety of emotional conditions including fear and aggression. In fact, it has recently been demonstrated that acute antagonism of the CRF_2 receptor in the lateral septum using the nonselective peptide antagonists produced a specific reduction in stress-induced behavior. This effect was not produced by the administration of selective CRF_1 receptor antagonists into this brain region [95]. In addition, it has been shown that selective peptide antagonists for the CRF_2 receptor administered intracerebroventricularly in mice were able to attenuate CRF or UCN2-induced increases in acoustic startle, suggesting in this model that the CRF_2 receptor may participate in the progression of the anxiety response [96]. In addition, CRF_2 receptor knockout studies have demonstrated that mice lacking the

CRF$_2$ receptor gene exhibit anxiety-like effects as well as a hypersensitivity to stress, further suggesting a role for this subtype in the overall response to stress [97]. Key to the understanding of the role of this receptor in anxiety or depression, of course, will be the development of selective nonpeptide receptor antagonists and their evaluation in primate models of disease. With these tools, a solid understanding of the role of this receptor subtype can be defined and the CRF$_{2(a)}$ receptor may yet represent an additional target for the development of novel anxiolytics.

The CRF$_{2(b)}$ splice form is localized primarily on nonneuronal elements, such as the choroid plexus of the ventricular system and cerebral arterioles. In the periphery, CRF$_{2(b)}$ mRNA is expressed at high levels in both cardiac and skeletal muscle with lower levels evident in both lung and intestine [77, 98]. Most recently the CRF$_{2(b)}$ receptor has been localized in the human cardiovascular system where the ligands UCN2 and UCN3 have been shown to cause vasodilation [99, 100]. Interestingly, these effects, if shown to be able to counteract the pressor effects of centrally mediated CRF$_1$ receptor effects of CRF and urocortin, may define a tight regulation of stress-induced cardiovascular changes [100]. The CRF$_{2(c)}$ isoform has yet to be identified in the rodent; however, reverse transcriptase polymerase chain reaction (RT-PCR) analysis of human brain mRNA demonstrated expression in septum, amygdala, hippocampus, and frontal cortex [70]. A full characterization of the CRF$_{2(c)}$ subtype and the role it may play in physiology or pathophysiology still remains to be determined. As with the CRF$_1$ receptor, the CRF$_2$ receptor is also highly expressed and localized to the GI tract [56, 84] and there have been recent reports demonstrating clear efficacy of the selective CRF$_2$ agonists UCN2 and UCN3 on GI motility and pain responses [101], further suggesting that this receptor subtype may be involved in the manifestation of stress- or anxiety-induced pathophysiology.

5.3 PEPTIDE LIGAND PHARMACOLOGY OF CRF$_1$ AND CRF$_2$ RECEPTORS

As defined above, the CRF receptor and ligand system is unusual in that the receptors are activated by multiple endogenous ligands (CRF, UCN1, UCN2, and UCN3 [42, 71, 102]). The receptors have been shown to couple to multiple G proteins and intracellular signaling pathways [103, 104] (reviewed in [105, 106]), but in general the most common signaling pathway is stimulation of cAMP production through activation of the G$_s$ G protein. Peptide selectivity for the receptors has been assessed by measuring stimulation of cAMP accumulation. For the mammalian receptors overexpressed in cultured cell systems, CRF itself is moderately selective for CRF$_1$ over CRF$_2$ receptors [36, 37, 41, 65, 107–110], UCN1 is nonselective for the two subtypes [39–41, 108], and UCN2 and UCN3 are selective for the CRF$_2$ over the CRF$_1$ receptor [39–41, 109]. Interestingly, these peptides do not demonstrate any appreciable differences in activation potency when assessed at the three splice variants of the CRF$_2$ receptor (CRF$_{2(a)}$, CRF$_{2(b)}$, and CRF$_{2(c)}$) [70, 111]. A similar CRF$_1$/CRF$_2$ receptor selectivity profile has been demonstrated for receptors expressed endogenously (i.e., at normal physiological levels) in tissues and receptor-expressing cell lines [39, 41, 112–115]. For example, the pharmacological rank-order profile of peptide agonists at CRF$_1$ receptors in the AtT20 mouse corticotrope tumor cell line and CRF$_{2(b)}$ receptors in A7r5 rat smooth muscle cells is similar to that in

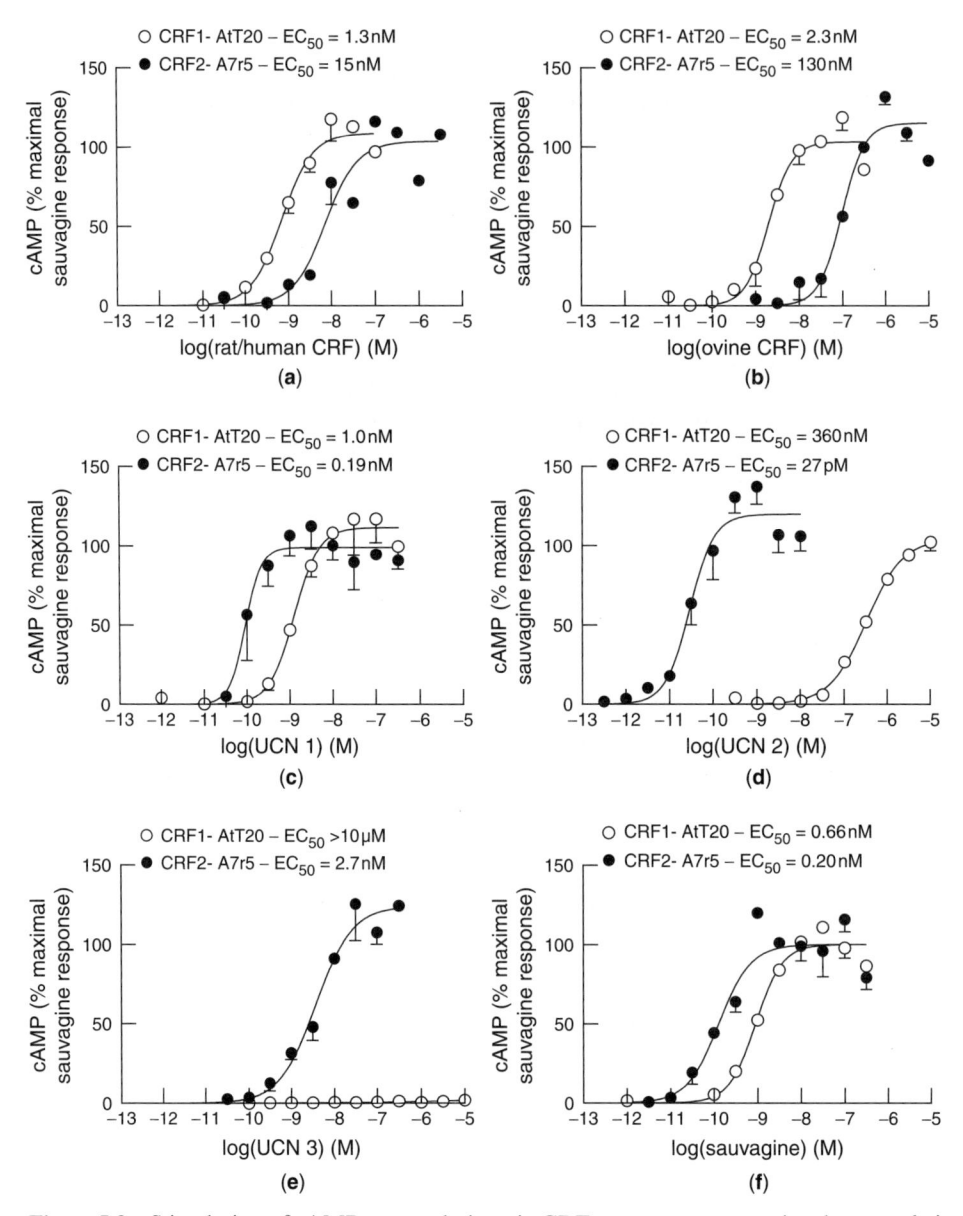

Figure 5.2 Stimulation of cAMP accumulation via CRF receptors expressed endogenously in model cell lines by CRF-related peptides. cAMP accumulation was measured in the mouse AtT20 corticotrope cell line, which expresses CRF_1, and the rat A7r5 aortic smooth muscle cell line, expressing $CRF_{2(b)}$. EC_{50} values are the mean of three experiments. (Data compiled from [116].)

heterologously expressed receptor systems (Fig. 5.2) [116]. This validation is important because receptor overexpression can distort pharmacological behavior of agonist ligands, for example resulting in enhancement of agonist potency [reduction of median effective concentration (EC_{50})] or enhancement of efficacy (enhanced E_{max}).

As described above, synthetic peptide antagonists have been developed, by N-terminal truncation and amino acid substitution of the endogenous peptide agonists [57, 59–61, 109, 117, 118]. N-terminal truncation of CRF [57, 109], UCN1 [119], UCN2 [109], and sauvagine [60, 61] results in a loss of receptor activation but retention of detectable receptor binding. Certain critical amino acid substitutions of these truncated peptides increase affinity for one or both CRF receptors [57, 59–61]. For example, the nonselective antagonist astressin is a CRF(12–41) fragment with substitutions designed to enhance affinity (L-Phe^{11} to D-Phe^{11}) and a lactam between residues 30 and 33 that stabilizes α-helical structure in the C-terminal portion of the peptide [61]. The extent of α helicity correlates well with the antagonist potency [57, 117]. Recently even shorter C-terminal analogs of astressin (12 amino acids, residues 30–41) have been reported that possess comparable potency to the parent peptide [118]. N-terminal truncation of sauvagine together with certain substitutions yielded the CRF_2-selective antagonists antisauvagine-30 [60] and astressin$_2$-B [61]. In addition to the truncated forms of agonists that yield antagonists, numerous peptide chimeras have also been developed by combining sequence fragments of the different endogenous peptides. Examples include cortagine, an agonist selective for the CRF_1 receptor over the CRF_2 receptor [110].

Peptide ligand binding to CRF_1 and CRF_2 receptors has been measured using radiolabeled peptides. Both receptor subtypes are readily labeled by [^{125}I]sauvagine [65, 116, 120, 121], an agonist, and [^{125}I]astressin [121, 122], an antagonist. Other radioligands include radiolabeled UCN1 [122–124] for CRF_1 and CRF_2 receptors, [^{125}I]oCRF for selectively labeling CRF_1 [30, 124, 125], and [^{125}I]antisauvagine-30 for selectively labeling CRF_2 [126]. Ligand binding affinity for G-protein-coupled receptors is dependent on the conformational state of the receptor. In general, agonists bind with higher affinity to the G-protein-coupled state (RG state) than the uncoupled receptor (R state), whereas antagonist binding does not discriminate between these states [127, 128]. Taking this differential binding pharmacology into account can be important for identifying receptor subtypes in tissues and for understanding ligand binding mechanisms (see below). For CRF receptors the RG state can be selectively labeled using a radiolabeled agonist [30, 65, 116, 120, 121, 124, 125] such as [^{125}I]sauvagine [116, 121]. The R state can be generated using guanosine triphosphate (GTP) or its nonhydrolyzable analogs (such as GTPγS). These guanine nucleotides bind the α subunit of heterotrimeric G proteins, leading to the breakdown of the receptor–G protein complex [129]. The resulting R state of CRF receptors can be labeled by the antagonist [^{125}I]astressin [116, 121, 122]. For the CRF_1 receptor, peptide agonists bind with much higher affinity to the RG state than to the R state (Fig. 5.3, Table 5.1) and vary from 77-fold for UCN1 to 690-fold for oCRF [121]. This finding suggests uncoupling the G protein from its receptor substantially reduces binding of peptide agonists to the CRF_1 receptor, implying agonism results at least in part from ligand discriminating the RG state over the R state. By contrast, peptide agonist binding to the CRF_2 receptor is much less sensitive to the conformational state of the receptor with a change of 1.2-fold higher affinity for RG for UCN1 to a 6.5-fold difference for UCN2 (Fig. 5.3, Table 5.1 [116]). This finding suggests that for the CRF_2 receptor uncoupling receptor from G protein does not strongly affect peptide agonist binding, a hypothesis supported by the only slight reduction of [^{125}I]sauvagine binding produced by GTPγS (Fig. 5.3i) [65, 116, 120, 126]. Peptide antagonist affinity for both receptors was unaffected by

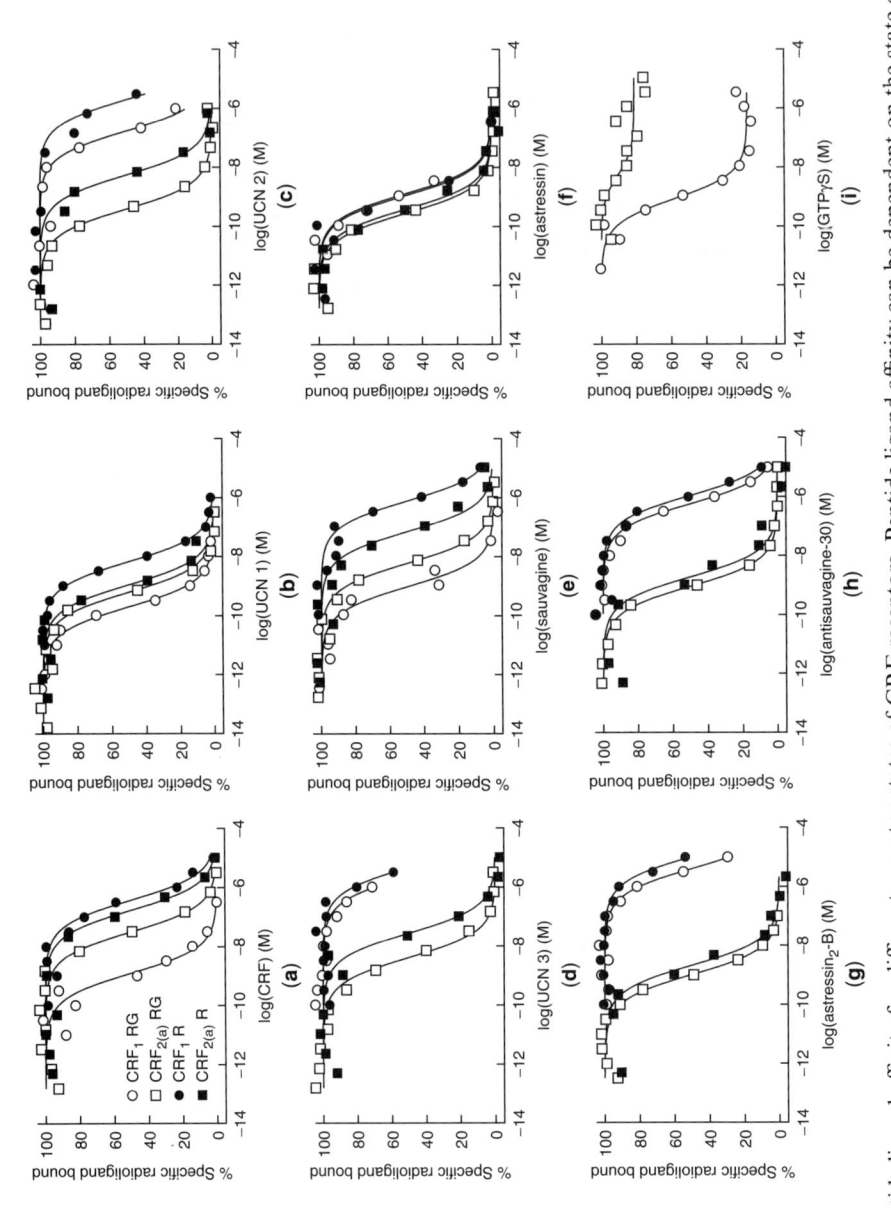

Figure 5.3 Peptide ligand affinity for different receptor states of CRF receptors. Peptide ligand affinity can be dependent on the state of the receptor. Peptide affinity for the G-protein-coupled state (RG state) of the human CRF_1 and $CRF_{2(a)}$ receptors can be measured by competition against a radiolabeled peptide agonist ([^{125}I]sauvagine). Peptide affinity for the receptor uncoupled from G protein (R state) was measured in competition versus a radiolabeled antagonist peptide ([^{125}I]astressin) in the presence of GTPγS. This guanine nucleotide binds the α subunit of heterotrimeric G proteins, leading to the breakdown of the receptor–G protein complex. Data for the human CRF_1 receptor are for this receptor in membranes prepared from LtK$^-$ mouse fibroblasts [121]. Data for the human $CRF_{2(a)}$ receptor are for this receptor in Chinese hamster ovary cell membranes. (Data compiled from [116, 121].)

TABLE 5.1 Peptide Ligand Affinity (nM) for R and RG States of Human CRF_1 and $CRF_{2(a)}$ Receptors[a,b]

Peptide Ligand	RG State		R State	
	CRF_1 K_i (nM)	CRF_2 K_i (nM)	CRF_1 K_i (nM)	CRF_2 K_i (nM)
r/hCRF	0.30	19	270	38
oCRF	0.29	150	200	320
hUCN1	0.039	0.27	3.0	0.33
hUCN2	130	0.17	640	1.1
hUCN3	>1000	1.3	>1000	6.6
Sauvagine	0.45	2.6	230	11
Astressin	0.43	0.15	0.67	0.11
Antisauvagine-30	150	0.29	340	0.40
Astressin$_2$-B	950	0.49	4200	0.57

[a]*Source:* Data compiled from [116, 121].
[b]Peptide ligand affinity for G-protein-coupled (RG) receptor state was measured in competition versus a radiolabeled agonist peptide ($[^{125}I]$sauvagine) for human CRF_1 or $CRF_{2(a)}$ receptors expressed in mammalian cells (L+k$^-$ cells [121] and CHO cells, respectively [116]). Peptide affinity for the receptor uncoupled from G protein (R state) was measured in competition versus a radiolabeled antagonist peptide ($[^{125}I]$astressin) in the presence of GTPγS. This guanine nucleotide binds the α subunit of heterotrimeric G proteins, leading to the breakdown of the receptor–G protein complex.

the conformational state of the receptor (Figs. 5.3f–h, Table 5.1 [108, 116, 121, 122, 124, 126]), implying antagonism results from a lack of discrimination between RG and R states.

Peptide ligand selectivity for binding one CRF receptor over the other has historically been determined using radiolabeled agonists [65, 108, 116, 120, 121, 123], particularly $[^{125}I]$sauvagine. Under these conditions, affinity estimates for receptors are likely those for the RG state of CRF_1 and CRF_2 receptors. Selectivity in binding the RG state approximately correlates with selectivity in functional cAMP accumulation experiments: in the binding assays, r/hCRF is selective for CRF_1 over CRF_2 (63-fold for cloned human CRF_1 and $CRF_{2(a)}$ receptors; Table 5.1, Fig. 5.3a); oCRF is more CRF_1 selective (520-fold, Table 5.1); UCN1 and sauvagine are nonselective (Table 5.1, Figs. 5.3b,e); UCN2 and UCN3 are strongly CRF_2 selective (760-fold and >770-fold, respectively, Table 5.1, Figs. 5.3c,d); astressin is a nonselective antagonist (Table 5.1, Fig. 5.3f); and astressin$_2$-B and antisauvagine-30 are CRF_2-selective antagonists (510-fold and 1900-fold, respectively, Table 5.1, Figs. 5.3g,h) [39, 60, 108, 109, 116, 121, 122]. This selectivity profile has been demonstrated for CRF receptors expressed endogenously in tissues (e.g., cerebellum for CRF_1 [121] and olfactory bulb for CRF_2 [116]). A different selectivity profile is manifest for the uncoupled R state of the receptor. In this conformation, CRF peptides are no longer selective (Table 5.1, Fig. 5.3a) and UCN1 and sauvagine are slightly selective for CRF_2 over CRF_1 receptors (9.0-fold and 21-fold, respectively, Table 5.1, Figs. 5.3b,e) [116]. Therefore, in identifying the receptor subtype in tissues it is important to consider the nature of the conformational state labeled by the specific radioligand used. The use of agonist radioligands is recommended, enabling comparison with a wealth of historical data.

5.3.1 Mechanisms of Peptide Ligand Binding to CRF_1 and CRF_2 Receptors

The molecular mechanisms of peptide ligand binding to CRF receptors have been investigated using point-mutated receptors [130–139], chimeric receptors [116, 130–134, 138, 140, 141], receptor fragments [64, 119, 139, 140, 142–146], receptor–ligand crosslinking [136, 147], and nuclear magnetic resonance (NMR) chemical shift perturbation [139]. These studies have indicated a low-resolution binding orientation termed the "two-domain" model, also demonstrated for other class B GPCRs. In this mechanism, the carboxyl terminal portion of the peptides interacts with the N-terminal domain (N-domain) of the receptors, and the amino terminal portion of the peptide binds the receptors' juxtamembrane domain (J domain, comprising the transmembrane helices and intervening loops). Binding determinants in both receptor domains have been identified using receptor mutants and chimeric receptors (Fig. 5.1). Peptide ligands interact with both N- and J-domain fragments expressed in isolation (Fig. 5.4). The carboxyl terminal fragments of CRF and sauvagine

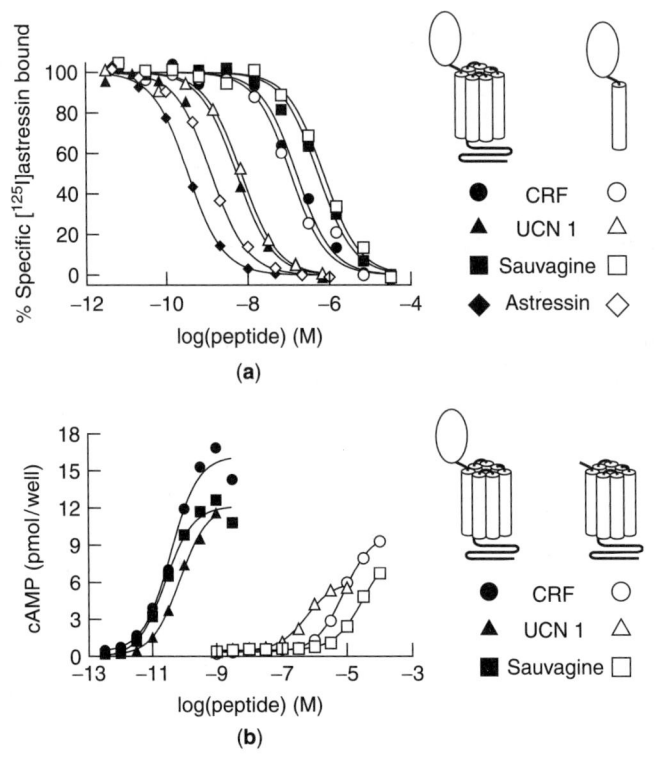

Figure 5.4 Interaction of peptide ligands with (a) N domain and (b) J domain of CRF_1 receptor. (a) Peptide ligand interaction with the N domain was measured by inhibition of [^{125}I]astressin binding to the N domain fused to the single-membrane-spanning α helix of the activinII-B receptor [140, 146]. Peptide affinity for the whole receptor was measured by inhibition of [^{125}I]astressin binding in the presence of GTPγS to uncouple receptor from G protein. (b) Peptide ligand interaction with the J domain was measured by stimulation of cAMP accumulation via a J-domain fragment [146]. Note that peptide potency on the J domain is dramatically reduced compared with the whole receptor. The peptides did not affect cAMP accumulation in nontransfected cells [146]. (Data compiled from [146].)

(astressin and antisauvagine-30, respectively) bind with high affinity to N-domain fragments of CRF_1 and CRF_2 receptors [64, 140, 144–146] (Fig. 5.4a). Modifying the carboxyl terminal residue of CRF by deamidation eliminates detectable binding to the N-domain fragment of the CRF_1 receptor but does not affect interaction with the J-domain fragment [146]. Tethering the N-terminal 16 amino acids of CRF to the J domain of the CRF_1 receptor results in receptor activation [143]. Receptor–ligand crosslinking, utilizing the CRF_1 receptor and peptides with photoactivatable side chains, indicated residue 16 of sauvagine crosslinks L257 in the second extracellular loop [136]; the extreme N-terminus and residue 12 of UCN1 bind the second extracellular loop; and residues 35 and 40 of UCN1 bind the C-terminal region of the N domain [147].

The molecular mechanism has been evaluated to a higher resolution for the interaction of astressin with the N domain, utilizing structural data for peptide and the N domain [139]. NMR, circular dichroism, and other analytical studies of CRF-related peptide structure indicate transient-to-stable formation of α helix within the C-terminal region [57, 59, 117, 118, 148, 149], depending on the experimental conditions and peptide studied. An NMR structure of a soluble N domain of the mouse $CRF_{2(b)}$ receptor was recently reported [139]. A central core contains a salt-bridge sandwiched between aromatic side chains surrounded by conserved residues. Two antiparallel β sheets are interconnected by the core. Loop regions of poorly resolved structure are adjacent to the structured core region. The tertiary structure is stabilized by three disulfide bonds (C45–C70, C60–C103, and C84–C118 for the mouse CRF_2 receptor). These three cysteines are conserved within CRF receptors and other class B GPCRs [64, 139, 144, 150]. NMR chemical-shift perturbation within the N domain upon binding astressin [139] indicates residues in and around the structured core are direct or indirect binding determinants (I67, G68, T69, G90, I91, K92, N94, A99, Y100, E102, R112, V113, N114, Y115, and S116). These residues are highly conserved within CRF receptor subtypes and species variants, suggesting a common molecular mechanism of peptide ligand binding to the N domain [139]. Mutation of I67 and R112 of the $CRF_{2(b)}$ receptor reduces affinity of astressin 120- and 6.5-fold, respectively [139]. Mutation of residues analogous to K92 and A99 of the $CRF_{2(b)}$ receptor in the CRF_1 receptor also reduces peptide ligand affinity [132]. These data can be rationalized by a molecular model of astressin interaction with the $CRF_{2(b)}$ N domain, in which the carboxyl terminal portion of astressin binds as an α helix to a broad, slightly concave surface within the structured core region [139]. Proposed interactions between an astressin and the mouse $CRF_{2(b)}$ receptor include electrostatic interaction between E39 and R112 and between K35 and E119 and hydrophobic interaction between L37 and Y115 and between I41 and P120 [139].

Less is known about the molecular interactions of the amino-terminal portion of the peptide and the J domain of the receptor. The solution structure of the amino-terminal portion of the peptide is not well characterized, and nothing is presently known of the receptor-bound structure of this region of the peptide. In addition the structure of the J domain of CRF receptors has not been determined. The transmembrane helices of this region have been modeled by homology using the crystal structure of bovine rhodopsin as a template, but the predictive utility of these models might be limited owing to the very low amino acid sequence homology between CRF receptors (class B GPCRs) and rhodopsin (a class A GPCR) [139]. The only obvious common feature between class A and B GPCRs is the potential disulfide bond between transmembrane type 3 (TM3) and extracellular loop 2, although evolutionary trace analysis has suggested a small number of other common hydrophobic amino acid residues within the transmembrane domains [151, 152]. Peptide binding determinants within the J domain are located within the predicted extracellular loops and toward the predicted extracellular ends of transmembrane helices (Fig. 5.1). These results suggest the amino-terminal portion of peptide ligand binds to the extracellular face of the J domain of CRF receptors, an arrangement that has also been suggested for other class B GPCRs [150]. Interestingly, circumstantial evidence suggests N terminally truncated CRF and sauvagine analogs can interact with the J domain of the receptors. Astressin, a 12–41 residue analog of CRF, blocks activation of a CRF_1 J-domain fragment by CRF, albeit at high concentrations [146]. Additionally, this peptide binds with 10-fold higher affinity to the whole CRF_1 receptor than an N-domain receptor, suggesting additional binding determinants within the J domain [146]. Shorter C-terminal CRF analogs (residues 30–41, peptides 19 and 20 of [118]) bind with similar affinity to the whole receptor and the N domain, suggesting residues within the 12–29 region of astressin bind the J domain of the CRF_1 receptor [153]. Finally, analysis of chimeric CRF_1/CRF_2 receptors indicated that the J domain acts as a selectivity determinant for CRF_2-selective antisauvagine-30 and astressin$_2$-B (11–40 analogs of sauvagine), suggesting these peptides interact with the J domain of the CRF_2 receptor [116]. Taken together these findings suggest peptide antagonists can bind the J domain of CRF_1 and CRF_2 receptors, possibly through interactions with amino-terminal residues of the peptides.

The J domain of the CRF_1 receptor is involved in ligand binding and conformational changes of the receptor that lead to receptor activation and desensitization. Peptide agonists stimulate cAMP accumulation via a J-domain fragment (Fig. 5.4b) [146] and the amino-terminal portion of CRF activates a J-domain fragment when tethered to this receptor [143]. In addition, full-length peptide agonist binding to the CRF_1 receptor is markedly reduced by GTPγS, whereas residue 12–41 analogs of CRF (e.g., astressin) are unaffected (see above). This finding suggests interactions of residues within the 1–11 sequence with the J domain are sensitive to G-protein coupling to the receptor. Peptides that appear to only bind the N domain (peptides 19 and 20 in [118]) do not activate the CRF_1 receptor, suggesting ligand interaction with the N domain is not required for receptor activation. These short fragments also fail to affect CRF_1 receptor internalization, whereas full-length CRF robustly stimulates internalization [153]. This result provides circumstantial evidence that ligand interaction with the J domain but not the N domain stimulates CRF_1 receptor internalization. Interestingly, astressin also stimulates CRF_1 receptor internalization, an unusual effect of an antagonist ligand [153]. This effect is mediated through receptor interaction of the 12–29 region of the peptide [153], likely through binding the J domain (see above). The receptor conformation mediating astressin-induced receptor internalization appears distinct from that for CRF; the latter ligand promotes receptor phosphorylation and arrestin recruitment to the receptor, whereas the former ligand does not [153].

The strength of peptide agonist interaction for each of the N and J domains has been quantified for the CRF_1 receptor using N- and J-domain fragments. UCN1 binds with high affinity (approximately 5 nM) to the CRF_1 N domain expressed in isolation as a membrane-proximal protein (expressed as a fusion with the single membrane-spanning α helix of the activinII-B receptor) [64, 140, 146]. CRF and sauvagine bind with lower affinity to the N domain (approximately 50 and 500 nM, respectively [64, 140, 146]). Similar data were obtained with a soluble CRF_1 N-domain fragment [64, 119, 144, 145]. Peptide ligand affinity for the membrane-anchored N-domain fragment has been compared with that for the whole CRF_1 receptor, enabling quantification of the contribution of the N domain to overall ligand affinity. In this comparison the G-protein-uncoupled (R) state of the full-length CRF_1 receptor was used, since the N domain on the extracellular membrane surface is incapable of coupling to G protein on the intracellular membrane surface. For the CRF_1 receptor these experiments demonstrated that peptide agonist affinity for the N domain is only slightly stronger (less than twofold) on the full-length, G-protein-uncoupled CRF_1 receptor than on the membrane-anchored N domain fragment, indicating the N domain contributes almost all the ligand binding energy at the R state [140, 144, 145]. Direct peptide binding to the J domain of the CRF_1 receptor is extremely weak—on the isolated J-domain fragment, peptide agonist EC_{50} for stimulating cAMP production was four to six orders of magnitude higher than EC_{50} for the whole receptor (Fig. 5.4b) [146]. Taken together these findings suggest a sequential mass action binding model for agonist peptides [146] in which peptide first binds the N domain of the CRF_1 receptor with moderate to high affinity (depending on the peptide agonist) (Fig. 5.5a). This interaction provides an "affinity trap" that enormously increases the local concentration of peptide in the vicinity of the J domain, allowing the weak J domain interaction to occur (Fig. 5.5a). This concentrating effect of N-domain binding enables significant ligand interaction to occur with the J domain at physiological levels of ligand. Ligand interaction with the J domain promotes receptor activation and stimulation of G-protein coupling leading to intracellular signaling (Fig. 5.5a). Reciprocally, G-protein coupling to the CRF_1 receptor increases the affinity of peptide agonists by 49- to 690-fold [121], likely through increasing peptide affinity for the J domain [146]. Taken together, these findings suggest a quantitative model for the CRF_1 receptor in which (1) peptide agonists bind with moderate to high affinity for the N domain (100 nM for CRF); (2) peptide binding to the J domain weakly stabilizes binding at the R state of the receptor (<2-fold for CRF); and (3) peptide binding to the J domain is strongly stabilized by G-protein coupling to the receptor (>100-fold for CRF).

Similar techniques have been applied to estimate peptide agonist affinity for the CRF_2 receptor. UCN1 and UCN2 bind with high affinity to a membrane-anchored $CRF_{2(b)}$ receptor N domain (5.4 and 16 nM, respectively), whereas UCN3, CRF, and sauvagine are less potent (>200, 79, and >200 nM, respectively) [145]. Similar data were obtained with a soluble $CRF_{2(b)}$ receptor fragment [145]. Peptide agonist affinity for the whole $CRF_{2(b)}$ receptor (R state) was significantly higher than affinity for the isolated J domain (from 2.9-fold for CRF to 33-fold for UCN2) [145], suggesting an appreciable contribution of the J domain to peptide agonist affinity at the R state (in contrast to the CRF_1 receptor for which the J domain contributed minimally to peptide agonist affinity at the R state). G-protein coupling to the $CRF_{2(a)}$ or $CRF_{2(b)}$ receptor only weakly stabilizes peptide agonist binding (e.g., 1.2- to 6.5-fold for $CRF_{2(a)}$). Within the context of the two-domain model, these results imply that, first, peptide agonists bind with moderate to high affinity to the N domain of the CRF_2 receptor (16 nM for UCN2); second, binding is moderately stabilized through peptide interaction with the J domain of the R state (33-fold for UCN2); and third,

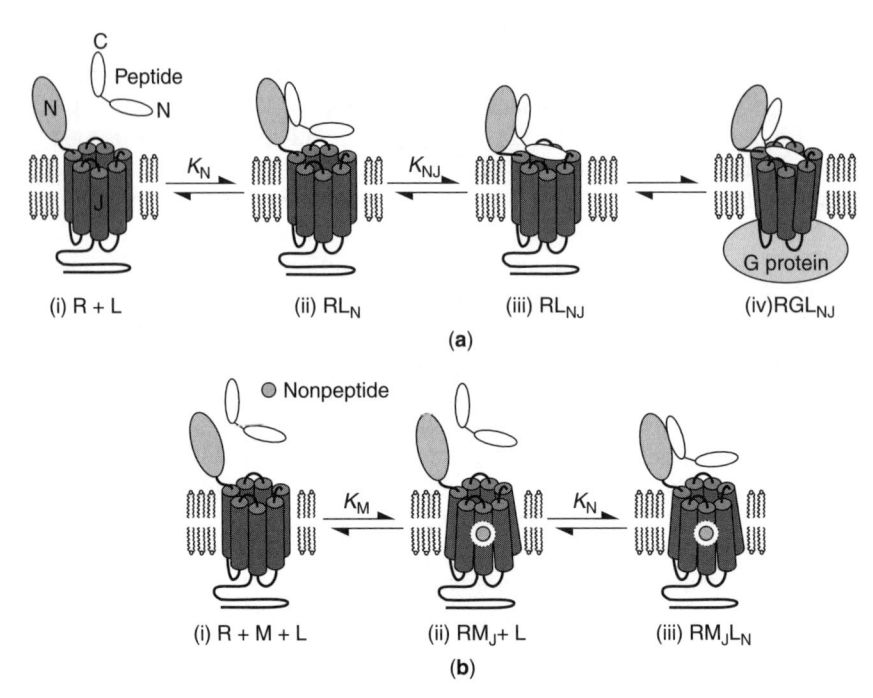

194   EMERGING ANXIOLYTICS: CORTICOTROPIN-RELEASING FACTOR

Figure 5.5 Binding models of peptide and nonpeptide ligand interaction with CRF receptors. (See [146] for a detailed description of these models.) (a) Binding model of peptide ligand interaction with CRF_1 and CRF_2 receptors. (i) The C-terminal region of the peptide (L) binds the N domain of the receptor (R) forming RL_N. (ii) This interaction enormously increases the local concentration of the N-terminal peptide region in the vicinity of the J domain, allowing (iii) their weak interaction to occur, forming RL_{NJ}. (iv) J-domain peptide binding increases receptor interaction with G protein, and reciprocally G-protein binding enhances J-domain affinity for peptide ligand. (b) Nonpeptide binding and antagonism model for CRF_1 receptor. (i) Nonpeptide ligand (M, small circle) binds within the J domain, forming RM_J. (ii) This interaction causes a change within the CRF_1 receptor that impedes peptide binding to its sites on the J domain. By blocking peptide–J domain interaction, the nonpeptide antagonist blocks peptide-stimulated receptor signaling because peptide–J domain interaction is required for G-protein activation. (iii) Nonpeptide ligand binding to the J domain does not prevent peptide interaction with the N domain, so the RM_JL_N complex can form. (Reproduced with permission from *Drug Discovery Today* [150].)

G-protein coupling to the receptor weakly enhances peptide agonist binding (6.5-fold for UCN2). Compared with the CRF_1 receptor (see above), the J domain appears to provide more binding energy for the CRF_2 receptor (at the R state), whereas G-protein coupling stabilizes binding less. The molecular basis of this difference between the two receptors remains to be determined.

Finally the strength of peptide antagonist interaction for N and J domains has been assessed. For both CRF_1 and $CRF_{2(b)}$ receptors astressin binds with high affinity to N-domain fragments (approximately 1 nM). Surprisingly, astressin affinity for the whole receptor is an order-of-magnitude higher for both CRF_1 and $CRF_{2(b)}$ receptors [145, 146], suggesting astressin binding is appreciably stabilized through interaction with the J domain. In addition, the J domain is a selectivity determinant of the CRF_2-selective antagonists antisauvagine-30 and astressin$_2$-B, shown using chimeric CRF_1/CRF_2 receptors [116]. Peptide antagonist binding is unaffected by receptor–G protein interaction [116, 121, 122]. These findings suggest peptide antagonists bind with high affinity to the N domain, with binding moderately stabilized through interaction with the J domain and with G-protein binding to the receptor having no effect.

5.4 NONPEPTIDE LIGANDS FOR CRF_1 RECEPTORS

Antagonism of central CRF_1 receptors has been rationalized as a potential next-generation treatment for anxiety and depression [154–157]. Since peptide antagonists generally possess poor pharmacokinetics (poor oral bioavailability, rapid clearance, and minimal brain penetration) and lack CRF_1 receptor selectivity, attempts have been made to develop small, orally bioavailable, brain-penetrating, CRF_1-selective nonpeptide antagonists. Numerous low-molecular-weight ligands have been developed that potently bind and antagonize the CRF_1 receptor (examples in Fig. 5.6; reviewed in detail in [156, 158, 159]). The large majority of these ligands comprise a central heterocyclic core (examples include the monocyclic SSR125543A [160, 161], the bicyclic antalarmin [162], and tricyclic NBI 35965 [163, 164]; Fig. 5.6), a "top" alkyl or branched alkyl side chain, and a "bottom" substituted aromatic ring. Regardless of the core composition, there is an essential requirement for a hydrogen bond acceptor, separated from the bottom aromatic group by a one-atom linker (e.g., SSR125543A) or by a two-atom linker (e.g., antalarmin) (see Fig. 5.6). Most, if not all, known nonpeptide antagonists display considerable selectivity for the CRF_1 receptor over the CRF_2 receptor (for a comprehensive review on structures see [156, 157]). This selectivity, combined with reasonable pharmacokinetics, has rendered compounds such as these exceptionally useful for evaluating the physiological and potential therapeutic roles of the CRF_1 receptor in animal models and, as described below, has been initially examined in an open label phase IIA clinical trial in major depressive disorder [165].

5.4.1 Mechanism of Nonpeptide Ligand Interaction with CRF_1 Receptor

The mechanism of nonpeptide ligand binding to the CRF_1 receptor has been investigated using receptor fragments [143, 146], receptor chimeras and mutagenesis [130], and quantitative analysis of ligand binding data [163, 166]. Nonpeptide antagonists bind the J domain, predominantly if not exclusively: Nonpeptide radioligand affinity for a J-domain fragment is not significantly different from that for the whole receptor and nonpeptide antagonist fully blocks peptide-stimulated cAMP accumulation via the J-domain fragment [146]. Constitutive activation of a J-domain fragment tethered to the N-terminal region of CRF is blocked by the nonpeptide antagonist antalarmin [143]. CRF_1/CRF_2 receptor chimeras identified TM3 and TM5 as selectivity determinants for selective nonpeptide antagonist with the CRF_1 receptor [130]. Exchange of two residues of the CRF_1 receptor for the corresponding residues of the CRF_2 receptor resulted in reduced nonpeptide ligand binding (H199 V in TM3 and M276I in TM5; Fig. 5.1) [130].

Nonpeptide antagonist likely binds regions within the J domain that are distinct from those for peptide ligand. The two mutations of the CRF_1 receptor implicated in nonpeptide ligand binding did not affect peptide ligand binding [130]. In addition these determinants are within the predicted transmembrane bundle (Fig. 5.1), whereas peptide ligand binding determinants have been identified principally in the extracellular loop regions of the J domain (Fig. 5.1). In addition, nonpeptide versus peptide ligand binding data display diagnostic features implying nonpeptide ligand allosterically regulates peptide ligand binding, and vice versa: Nonpeptide ligands modulate peptide radioligand dissociation from the CRF_1 receptor, and peptide ligands accelerate nonpeptide radioligand dissociation [163]. In addition peptide ligands only partially inhibit nonpeptide radioligand binding at equilibrium [163, 166]. An interesting difference was observed between the allosteric effect at G-protein-coupled and G-protein-uncoupled CRF_1 receptor states. At the R state, the allosteric effect between peptide and nonpeptide ligand binding was slight. NBI 35965 binding to the receptor reduced sauvagine affinity by only 3.0-fold. In other words, sauvagine affinity for the NBI 35965–bound receptor was 690 nM compared with 230 nM for the free receptor). In contrast, at the RG state NBI 35965 binding reduced sauvagine affinity by 180-fold.

All of these observations can be explained by the model presented in Fig 5.5b and have been described in detail [146]. In this model, nonpeptide ligand binds to sites within the transmembrane region of the J domain, distinct from the sites bound by peptide ligand (Fig. 5.5b). Nonpeptide ligand binding to this region produces a change in the receptor that impedes peptide binding to its sites on the J domain. This allosteric effect blocks peptide-stimulated signaling, since J domain interaction is required for peptide agonism (see above). However, this allosteric effect does not affect peptide binding to the N domain of the receptor (Fig. 5.5b). This model can explain why the allosteric effect is greater at the RG state than at the R state. At the RG state the J domain contributes much more binding energy for peptide ligand interaction, so blocking this interaction with nonpeptide ligand substantially reduces peptide binding affinity. At the R state the J domain contributes much less peptide binding energy, so blocking this interaction only marginally reduces peptide binding. Overall this binding model retrospectively rationalizes nonpeptide-versus-peptide binding data, explains the antagonist action of the compounds, and could be prospectively useful in the future development of nonpeptide ligands.

5.5 POTENTIAL FOR THERAPEUTIC INTERVENTION IN ANXIETY AND DEPRESSION

During the course of examining the role of the CRF system in disorders such as anxiety and depression, a number of preclinical studies have suggested that that anxiety-related disorders such as generalized anxiety disorder or panic disorder, while independent syndromes, share some clinical and biological characteristics with major depression. In addition to the circumstantial evidence presented above from clinical studies monitoring the regulation of the CRF system in various disease and treatment paradigms, there have been a great many experimental studies performed in animal models supporting the role of this system in the manifestation of anxiety- or depression-like behaviors. It is not surprising that the human disorders of anxiety and depression are difficult to model in animals. However, animal models have been widely used focusing on specific symptoms involving fear and/or fearful responses in animals that are correlated to the inappropriate responses to mildly stressful stimuli exhibited in human anxiety. For example, the findings that CRF itself has central, behavioral and arousal properties that are characteristic of other anxiogenic compounds have been well documented preclinically and relate directly to the hyperarousal that defines anxiety disorders [167, 168]. In panic disorder, a role for CRF has been suggested by the observations again of a blunted ACTH response in these patients compared to normal individuals [169, 170]. The blunted ACTH response in panic disorder patients to exogenous CRF most likely reflects processes occurring above the level of the hypothalamus and related to a central hypersecretion of CRF. In a recent preclinical study, CRF-induced deficits in prepulse inhibition (PPI) in rats were reversed by pharmacological blockade with CRF receptor antagonists. The CRF-induced deficit in animals is similar to the disruption of PPI observed in patients with panic disorder where the CRF system may also be overactive [171]. Thus, by modeling some of the physiological characteristics of a disorder, it is possible to examine the mechanisms that may underlie a specific pathophysiology. There have been a number of excellent reviews detailing the myriad animal models that have been used to dissect the precise effects and regulation of CRF in stress-related behaviors [156, 172–175].

The majority, if not all, of the small-molecule CRF receptor antagonists that have been described are primarily selective for the CRF_1 receptor subtype. The few molecules that have appeared in the literature claiming CRF_2 selectivity have been at best weak inhibitors of function at the CRF_2 receptor subtype. The efforts to further develop these compounds have focused on improving their physicochemical and pharmacokinetic properties to maximize in vivo efficacy. Nonpeptide small molecules have demonstrated efficacy in a variety of rodent models of anxiety, including changes in exploratory behavior, a measure of innate fearfulness [160, 176, 177] social interaction (anxiety) stressful situations [177–181], conditioned fear responses [182–184], and acoustic startle responses [96, 185, 186]. In addition to the rodent studies, these molecules have also demonstrated efficacy in many nonhuman primate models of anxiety. For example, both antalarmin and DMP-904 (Fig. 5.6) reduced stereotypic fear responses and decreased measures of anxiety in the human intruder stress paradigm in rhesus monkey while, in addition, significantly attenuating HPA activation and the stress-induced increase in CSF CRF [187, 188]. Chronic oral administration of antalarmin in male rhesus monkeys was also demonstrated to attenuate the stress associated with social separation in these animals [189]. Finally, CRF_1 receptor antagonists have been demonstrated to block the stress-induced visceral hyperalgesia and colonic motility in rats [190], suggesting that these molecules may also have utility in stress- or anxiety-related GI disorders [91, 94]. A thorough evaluation of the current CRF_1 receptor antagonist small molecules and their potential utility in anxiety disorders has recently been published [191].

Despite the heroic efforts expended by the pharmaceutical industry in discovering novel chemical structures that interact with the CRF receptor system, there has only been one single clinical study published in the literature describing the effects of a CRF_1 receptor antagonist in depression. In this open label non-placebo-controlled phase IIA study conducted at the Max Planck Institute of Psychiatry, Munich, the pyrazolopyrimidine R121919 (NBI 30775) was found to be well tolerated in 20 patients following a 30-day, dose escalation paradigm up to 80 mg. This compound demonstrated a significant reduction in both the Hamilton depression and anxiety

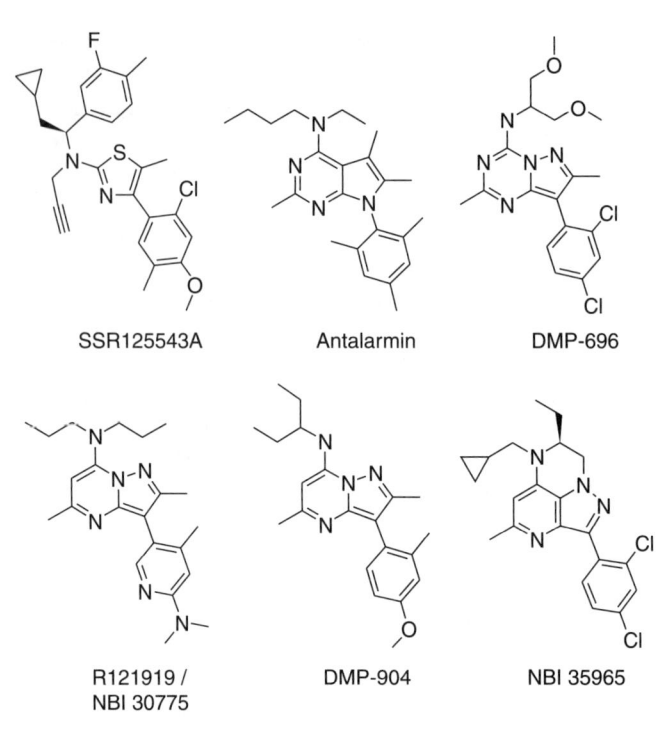

Figure 5.6 Chemical structure of nonpeptide antagonists for CRF_1 receptor. Detailed reviews of CRF_1 nonpeptide ligands can be found in [156, 158, 159].

scales HAM-D and HAM-A across the treatment period without affecting either basal HPA activity or significant blunting of an exogenously administered CRF-induced ACTH response [165]. Furthermore, this molecule was found to improve sleep-EEG patterns in both human and rat [192, 193] and in a very recent study demonstrated that this treatment did not affect weight gain or plasma leptin levels in this group of depressed individuals [194]. Although in this small open label trial the compound did not demonstrate any untoward effects in the patient population [165, 194, 195], this particular compound caused some reversible liver enzyme elevations that precluded further clinical development. Nevertheless, this initial study has provided significant support for the use of CRF_1 receptor antagonists in the treatment of depression- or anxiety-related disorders. More importantly, this study suggested that it would be possible to separate the central efficacy of CRF_1 receptor blockade from the potential peripheral side effects of rendering the HPA axis unresponsive [195].

5.6 CONCLUSIONS

The discovery of selective CRF_1 receptor antagonists has completed the first steps required in the development of novel therapeutics for stress-related disease. These newly characterized tools have in turn led to the refinement and expansion of the initial hypotheses and have identified a tangible goal of producing selective molecules that will target specific CRF-mediated behavior and physiology. While a preclinical "proof of principle" has been established whereby blockade of this system has demonstrated clear and precise functional benefits, the definitive studies in human disease have not yet been possible. Nonetheless, with the importance of this system in physiology and pathophysiology and the global efforts of academic and pharmaceutical researchers, there is little doubt that safe and selective molecules for this family of receptors will soon become available and eventually lead to some exciting novel therapeutic opportunities for neuropsychiatric and stress-related diseases. The CRF system is positioned to offer an alternative treatment option, and should the hypothesis that the cause of these disorders is manifested through an underlying overactivity of the stress system be confirmed, CRF receptor antagonists may well be the beginning of the next generation of antidepressant therapies with a novel mechanism of action.

REFERENCES

1. Harris, G. W. (1949). The relationship of the nervous system to the neurohypophysis and the adenohypophysis. *J. Endocrinol.* 6(2, Suppl.), xvii–xix.
2. Selye, H. (1950). *Stress*. Acta Medical, Montreal, Quebec, Canada.
3. Guillemin, R., and Rosenberg, B. (1955). Humoral hypothalamic control of anterior pituitary: A study with combined tissue cultures. *Endocrinology* 57, 599–607.
4. Saffran, M., Schally, A. V., and Benfey, B. G. (1955). Stimulation of the release of corticotrophin from the adenohypophysis by a neurohypophysial factor. *Endocrinology* 57, 439–444.
5. Vale, W., Spiess, J., Rivier, C., and Rivier, J. (1981). Characterization of a 41-residue ovine hypothalamic peptide that stimulates secretion of corticotropin and beta-endorphin. *Science* 213(4514), 1394–1397.
6. Nemeroff, C. B., Widerlov, E., Bissette, G., Walleus, H., Karlsson, I., Eklund, K., Kilts, C. D., Loosen, P. T., and Vale, W. (1984). Elevated concentrations of CSF corticotropin-releasing factor-like immunoreactivity in depressed patients. *Science* 226(4680), 1342–1344.
7. Gold, P. W., Chrousos, G., Kellner, C., Post, R., Roy, A., Augerinos, P., Schulte, H., Oldfield, E., and Loriaux, D. L. (1984). Psychiatric implications of basic and clinical studies with corticotropin-releasing factor. *Am. J. Psychiatry* 141(5), 619–627.
8. Holsboer, F., Muller, O. A., Doerr, H. G., Sippell, W. G., Stalla, G. K., Gerken, A., Steiger, A., Boll, E., and Benkert, O. (1984). ACTH and multisteroid responses to corticotropin-releasing factor in depressive illness: Relationship to multisteroid responses after ACTH stimulation and dexamethasone suppression. *Psychoneuroendocrinology* 9(2), 147–160.
9. Holsboer, F., Von Bardeleben, U., Gerken, A., Stalla, G. K., and Muller, O. A. (1984). Blunted corticotropin and normal cortisol response to human corticotropin-releasing factor in depression [letter]. *N. Engl. J. Med.* 311(17), 1127.
10. Roy, A., Pickar, D., Paul, S., Doran, A., Chrousos, G. P., and Gold, P. W. (1987). CSF corticotropin-releasing hormone in depressed patients and normal control subjects. *Am. J. Psychiatry* 144(5), 641–645.
11. Nemeroff, C. B., Owens, M. J., Bissette, G., Andorn, A. C., and Stanley, M. (1988). Reduced corticotropin releasing factor binding sites in the frontal cortex of suicide victims. *Arch. Gen. Psychiatry* 45(6), 577–579.

12. Nemeroff, C. B., Bissette, G., Akil, H., and Fink, M. (1991). Neuropeptide concentrations in the cerebrospinal fluid of depressed patients treated with electroconvulsive therapy. Corticotrophin-releasing factor, beta-endorphin and somatostatin. *Br. J. Psychiatry* 158, 59–63.

13. Zobel, A. W., Nickel, T., Sonntag, A., Uhr, M., Holsboer, F., and Ising, M. (2001). Cortisol response in the combined dexamethasone/CRH test as predictor of relapse in patients with remitted depression. A prospective study. *J. Psychiatr. Res.* 35(2), 83–94.

14. De Bellis, M. D., Gold, P. W., Geracioti, T. D., Jr., Listwak, S. J., and Kling, M. A. (1993). Association of fluoxetine treatment with reductions in CSF concentrations of corticotropin-releasing hormone and arginine vasopressin in patients with major depression. *Am. J. Psychiatry* 150(4), 656–657.

15. Heuser, I., Bissette, G., Dettling, M., Schweiger, U., Gotthardt, U., Schmider, J., Lammers, C. H., Nemeroff, C. B., and Holsboer, F. (1998). Cerebrospinal fluid concentrations of corticotropin-releasing hormone, vasopressin, and somatostatin in depressed patients and healthy controls: Response to amitriptyline treatment. *Depress. Anxiety* 8(2), 71–79.

16. Rivier, J., Spiess, J., and Vale, W. (1983). Characterization of rat hypothalamic corticotropin-releasing factor. *Proc. Natl. Acad. Sci. USA* 80(15), 4851–4855.

17. Shibahara, S., Morimoto, Y., Furutani, Y., Notake, M., Takahashi, H., Shimizu, S., Horikawa, S., and Numa, S. (1983). Isolation and sequence analysis of the human corticotropin-releasing factor precursor gene. *EMBO J.* 2(5), 775–779.

18. Ling, N., Esch, F., Bohlen, P., Baird, A. and Guillemin, R., (1984). Isolation and characterization of caprine corticotropin-releasing factor. *Biochem. Biophys. Res. Commun.* 122(3), 1218–1224.

19. Esch, F., Ling, N., Bohlen, P., Baird, A., Benoit, R., and Guillemin, R. (1984). Isolation and characterization of the bovine hypothalamic corticotropin-releasing factor. *Biochem. Biophys Res. Commun.* 122(3), 899–905.

20. Patthy, M., Horvath, J., Mason-Garcia, M., Szoke, B., Schlesinger, D. H., and Schally, A. V. (1985). Isolation and amino acid sequence of corticotropin-releasing factor from pig hypothalami. *Proc. Natl. Acad. Sci. USA* 82(24), 8762–8766.

21. Lederis, K., Letter, A., McMaster, D., Moore, G., and Schlesinger, D. (1982). Complete amino acid sequence of urotensin I, a hypotensive and corticotropin-releasing neuropeptide from *Catostomus*. *Science* 218(4568), 162–165.

22. Okawara, Y., Morley, S. D., Burzio, L. O., Zwiers, H., Lederis, K., and Richter, D. (1988). Cloning and sequence analysis of cDNA for corticotropin-releasing factor precursor from the teleost fish *Catostomus commersoni*. *Proc. Natl. Acad. Sci. USA* 85(22), 8439–8443.

23. Erspamer, V., Erspamer, G. F., Improta, G., Negri, L., and De Castiglione, R. (1980). Sauvagine, a new polypeptide from *Phyllomedusa sauvagei* skin. Occurrence in various *Phyllomedusa* species and pharmacological actions on rat blood pressure and diuresis. *Naunyn Schmiedebergs Arch. Pharmacol.* 312(3), 265–270.

24. Montecucchi, P. C., and Henschen, A. (1981). Amino acid composition and sequence analysis of sauvagine, a new active peptide from the skin of *Phyllomedusa sauvagei*. *Int. J. Pept. Protein Res.* 18, 113–120.

25. Rivier, C., Rivier, J., Lederis, K., and Vale, W. (1983). In vitro and in vivo ACTH-releasing activity of ovine CRF, sauvagine and urotensin I. *Regul. Pept.* 5(2), 139–143.

26. Morley, S. D., Schonrock, C., Richter, D., Okawara, Y., and Lederis, K. (1991). Corticotropin-releasing factor (CRF) gene family in the brain of the teleost fish *Catostomus commersoni* (white sucker): Molecular analysis predicts distinct precursors for two CRFs and one urotensin I peptide. *Mol. Mar. Biol. Biotechnol.* 1(1), 48–57.
27. Vaughan, J., Donaldson, C., Bittencourt, J., Perrin, M. H., Lewis, K., Sutton, S., Chan, R., Turnbull, A. V., Lovejoy, D., Rivier, C., et al. (1995). Urocortin, a mammalian neuropeptide related to fish urotensin I and to corticotropin-releasing factor [see comments]. *Nature* 378(6554), 287–292.
28. Donaldson, C. J., Sutton, S. W., Perrin, M. H., Corrigan, A. Z., Lewis, K. A., Rivier, J. E., Vaughan, J. M., and Vale, W. W. (1996). Cloning and characterization of human urocortin. *Endocrinology* 137(5), 2167–2170; erratum 137(9); 3896.
29. Kemp, C. F., Woods, R. J., and Lowry, P. J. (1998). The corticotrophin-releasing factor-binding protein: An act of several parts. *Peptides* 19(6), 1119–1128.
30. De Souza, E. B. (1987). Corticotropin-releasing factor receptors in the rat central nervous system: Characterization and regional distribution. *J. Neurosci.* 7(1), 88–100.
31. De Souza, E. B., and Nemeroff, C. B. (1990). *Corticotropin-Releasing Factor, Basic and Clinical Studies of a Neuropeptide.* CRC Press, Boca Raton, FL.
32. Owens, M. J., and Nemeroff, C. B. (1991). Physiology and pharmacology of corticotropin-releasing factor. *Pharmacol. Rev.* 43(4), 425–473.
33. Grigoriadis, D. E., Heroux, J. A., and De Souza, E. B. (1993). Characterization and regulation of corticotropin-releasing factor receptors in the central nervous, endocrine and immune systems. In *Corticotropin Releasing Factor*, D. J. Chadwick, J. Marsh, and K. Ackrill, Eds. Wiley, Chichester, West Sussex, pp. 85–101.
34. Battaglia, G., Webster, E. L., and De Souza, E. B. (1987). Characterization of corticotropin-releasing factor receptor-mediated adenylate cyclase activity in the rat central nervous system. *Synapse* 1(6), 572–581.
35. Webster, E. L., Battaglia, G., and De Souza, E. B. (1989). Functional corticotropin-releasing factor (CRF) receptors in mouse spleen: Evidence from adenylate cyclase studies. *Peptides* 10(2), 395–401.
36. Kishimoto, T., Pearse, R. V., II, Lin, C. R., and Rosenfeld, M. G. (1995). A sauvagine/corticotropin-releasing factor receptor expressed in heart and skeletal muscle. *Proc. Natl. Acad. Sci. USA* 92(4), 1108–1112.
37. Lovenberg, T. W., Liaw, C. W., Grigoriadis, D. E., Clevenger, W., Chalmers, D. T., De Souza, E. B., and Oltersdorf, T. (1995). Cloning and characterization of a functionally distinct corticotropin-releasing factor receptor subtype from rat brain. *Proc. Natl. Acad. Sci. USA* 92(3), 836–840; erratum 92(12), 5759.
38. Perrin, M., Donaldson, C., Chen, R., Blount, A., Berggren, T., Bilezikjian, L., Sawchenko, P., and Vale, W. (1995). Identification of a second corticotropin-releasing factor receptor gene and characterization of a cDNA expressed in heart. *Proc. Natl. Acad. Sci. USA* 92(7), 2969–2973.
39. Lewis, K., Li, C., Perrin, M. H., Blount, A., Kunitake, K., Donaldson, C., Vaughan, J., Reyes, T. M., Gulyas, J., Fischer, W., Bilezikjian, L., Rivier, J., Sawchenko, P. E., and Vale, W. W. (2001). Identification of urocortin III, an additional member of the corticotropin-releasing factor (CRF) family with high affinity for the CRF2 receptor. *Proc. Natl. Acad. Sci. USA* 98(13), 7570–7575.
40. Reyes, T. M., Lewis, K., Perrin, M. H., Kunitake, K. S., Vaughan, J., Arias, C. A., Hogenesch, J. B., Gulyas, J., Rivier, J., Vale, W. W., and Sawchenko, P. E. (2001).

Urocortin II: A member of the corticotropin-releasing factor (CRF) neuropeptide family that is selectively bound by type 2 CRF receptors. *Proc. Natl. Acad. Sci. USA* 98(5), 2843–2848.

41. Hsu, S. Y., and Hsueh, A. J. (2001). Human stresscopin and stresscopin-related peptide are selective ligands for the type 2 corticotropin-releasing hormone receptor. *Nat. Med.* 7(5), 605–611.

42. Dautzenberg, F. M., and Hauger, R. L. (2002). The CRF peptide family and their receptors: Yet more partners discovered. *Trends Pharmacol. Sci.* 23(2), 71–77.

43. Elde, R., Seybold, V., Sorenson, R. L., Cummings, S., Holets, V., Onstott, D., Sasek, C., Schmechel, D. E., and Oertel, W. H. (1984). Peptidergic regulation in neuroendocrine and autonomic systems. *Peptides* 5(Suppl. 1), 101–107.

44. De Souza, E. B., Insel, T. R., Perrin, M. H., Rivier, J., Vale, W. W., and Kuhar, M. J. (1985). Corticotropin-releasing factor receptors are widely distributed within the rat central nervous system: An autoradiographic study. *J. Neurosci.* 5(12), 3189–3203.

45. Petrusz, P., Merchenthaler, I., Maderdrut, J. L., and Heitz, P. U. (1985). Central and peripheral distribution of corticotropin-releasing factor. *Fed. Proc.* 44(1, Pt. 2), 229–235.

46. Emeric-Sauval, E. (1986). Corticotropin-releasing factor (CRF)—A review. *Psychoneuroendocrinology* 11(3), 277–294.

47. De Souza, E. B., and Grigoriadis, D. E. (2002). Corticotropin-releasing factor: Physiology, pharmacology and role in central nervous system disorders. In *Neuropsychopharmacology: The Fifth Generation of Progress*, K. L. Davis, D. Charney, J. T. Coyle, and C. B. Nemeroff, Eds. Lippincott Williams & Wilkins, Philadelphia, PA, pp. 91–107.

48. Kozicz, T., Yanaihara, H., and Arimura, A. (1998). Distribution of urocortin-like immunoreactivity in the central nervous system of the rat. *J. Comp. Neurol.* 391(1), 1–10.

49. Takahashi, K., Totsune, K., Sone, M., Murakami, O., Satoh, F., Arihara, Z., Sasano, H., Iino, K., and Mouri, T. (1998). Regional distribution of urocortin-like immunoreactivity and expression of urocortin mRNA in the human brain. *Peptides* 19(4), 643–647.

50. Yamamoto, H., Maeda, T., Fujimura, M., and Fujimiya, M. (1998). Urocortin-like immunoreactivity in the substantia nigra, ventral tegmental area and Edinger-Westphal nucleus of rat. *Neurosci. Lett.* 243(1–3), 21–24.

51. Li, C., Vaughan, J., Sawchenko, P. E., and Vale, W. W. (2002). Urocortin III-immunoreactive projections in rat brain: Partial overlap with sites of type 2 corticotrophin-releasing factor receptor expression. *J. Neurosci.* 22(3), 991–1001.

52. Chen, A., Blount, A., Vaughan, J., Brar, B., and Vale, W. (2004). Urocortin II gene is highly expressed in mouse skin and skeletal muscle tissues: Localization, basal expression in corticotropin-releasing factor receptor (CRFR) 1- and CRFR2-null mice, and regulation by glucocorticoids. *Endocrinology* 145(5), 2445–2457.

53. Takahashi, K., Totsune, K., Murakami, O., Saruta, M., Nakabayashi, M., Suzuki, T., Sasano, H., and Shibahara, S. (2004). Expression of urocortin III/stresscopin in human heart and kidney. *J. Clin. Endocrinol. Metab.* 89(4), 1897–1903.

54. Muramatsu, Y., Fukushima, K., Iino, K., Totsune, K., Takahashi, K., Suzuki, T., Hirasawa, G., Takeyama, J., Ito, M., Nose, M., Tashiro, A., Hongo, M., Oki, Y., Nagura, H., and Sasano, H. (2000). Urocortin and corticotropin-releasing factor receptor expression in the human colonic mucosa. *Peptides* 21(12), 1799–1809.

55. Kozicz, T., and Arimura, A. (2002). Distribution of urocortin in the rat's gastrointestinal tract and its colocalization with tyrosine hydroxylase. *Peptides* 23(3), 515–521.
56. Chatzaki, E., Charalampopoulos, I., Leontidis, C., Mouzas, I. A., Tzardi, M., Tsatsanis, C., Margioris, A. N., and Gravanis, A. (2003). Urocortin in human gastric mucosa: Relationship to inflammatory activity. *J. Clin. Endocrinol. Metab.* 88(1), 478–483.
57. Rivier, J., Rivier, C., and Vale, W. (1984). Synthetic competitive antagonists of corticotropin-releasing factor: Effect on ACTH secretion in the rat. *Science* 224(4651), 889–891.
58. Hernandez, J. F., Kornreich, W., Rivier, C., Miranda, A., Yamamoto, G., Andrews, J., Tache, Y., Vale, W., and Rivier, J. (1993). Synthesis and relative potencies of new constrained CRF antagonists. *J. Med. Chem.* 36(20), 2860–2867.
59. Miranda, A., Koerber, S. C., Gulyas, J., Lahrichi, S. L., Craig, A. G., Corrigan, A., Hagler, A., Rivier, C., Vale, W., and Rivier, J. (1994). Conformationally restricted competitive antagonists of human/rat corticotropin-releasing factor. *J. Med. Chem.* 37(10), 1450–1459.
60. Ruhmann, A., Bonk, I., Lin, C. R., Rosenfeld, M. G., and Spiess, J. (1998). Structural requirements for peptidic antagonists of the corticotropin-releasing factor receptor (CRFR): Development of CRFR2beta-selective antisauvagine-30. *Proc. Natl. Acad. Sci. USA* 95(26), 15264–15269.
61. Rivier, J., Gulyas, J., Kirby, D., Low, W., Perrin, M. H., Kunitake, K., Digruccio, M., Vaughan, J., Reubi, J. C., Waser, B., Koerber, S. C., Martinez, V., Wang, L., Tache, Y., and Vale, W. (2002). Potent and long-acting corticotropin releasing factor (CRF) receptor 2 selective peptide competitive antagonists. *J. Med. Chem.* 45(21), 4737–4747.
62. Gardiner, S., March, J., Kemp, P., Davenport, A., Wiley, K., and Bennett, T. (2005). Regional hemodynamic actions of selective CRF2 receptor ligands in conscious rats. *J. Pharmacol. Exp. Ther.* 312, 53–60.
63. Martinez, V., Wang, L., Rivier, J., Grigoriadis, D., and Tache, Y. (2004). Central CRF, urocortins and stress increase colonic transit via CRF1 receptors while activation of CRF2 receptors delays gastric transit in mice. *J. Physiol.* 556(1), 221–234. Erratum published in *J. Physiol.* 556(3), 1013.
64. Perrin, M. H., Fischer, W. H., Kunitake, K. S., Craig, A. G., Koerber, S. C., Cervini, L. A., Rivier, J. E., Groppe, J. C., Greenwald, J., Moller Nielsen, S., and Vale, W. W. (2001). Expression, purification, and characterization of a soluble form of the first extracellular domain of the human type 1 corticotropin releasing factor receptor. *J. Biol. Chem.* 276(34), 31528–31534.
65. Grigoriadis, D. E., Liu, X. J., Vaughn, J., Palmer, S. F., True, C. D., Vale, W. W., Ling, N., and De Souza, E. B. (1996). 125I-Tyro-sauvagine: A novel high affinity radioligand for the pharmacological and biochemical study of human corticotropin-releasing factor 2 alpha receptors. *Mol. Pharmacol.* 50(3), 679–686.
66. Chen, R., Lewis, K. A., Perrin, M. H., and Vale, W. W. (1993). Expression cloning of a human corticotropin-releasing-factor receptor. *Proc. Natl. Acad. Sci. USA* 90(19), 8967–8971.
67. Perrin, M. H., Donaldson, C. J., Chen, R., Lewis, K. A., and Vale, W. W. (1993). Cloning and functional expression of a rat brain corticotropin releasing factor (CRF) receptor. *Endocrinology* 133(6), 3058–3061.
68. Meyer, A. H., Ullmer, C., Schmuck, K., Morel, C., Wishart, W., Lubbert, H., and Engels, P. (1997). Localization of the human CRF2 receptor to 7p21–p15 by radiation hybrid mapping and FISH analysis. *Genomics* 40(1), 189–190.

69. Chang, C. P., Pearse, R. V. D., O'Connell, S., and Rosenfeld, M. G. (1993). Identification of a seven transmembrane helix receptor for corticotropin-releasing factor and sauvagine in mammalian brain. *Neuron* 11(6), 1187–1195.
70. Kostich, W. A., Chen, A., Sperle, K., and Largent, B. L. (1998). Molecular identification and analysis of a novel human corticotropin-releasing factor (CRF) receptor: The CRF2gamma receptor. *Mol. Endocrinol.* 12(8), 1077–1085.
71. Hauger, R. L., Grigoriadis, D. E., Dallman, M. F., Plotsky, P. M., Vale, W. W., and Dautzenberg, F. M. (2003). International Union of Pharmacology. XXXVI. Current status of the nomenclature for receptors for corticotropin-releasing factor and their ligands. *Pharmacol. Rev.* 55(1), 21–26.
72. Valdenaire, O., Giller, T., Breu, V., Gottowik, J., and Kilpatrick, G. (1997). A new functional isoform of the human CRF2 receptor for corticotropin-releasing factor. *Biochim. Biophys. Acta.* 1352(2), 129–132.
73. Chen, A. M., Perrin, M. H., Digruccio, M. R., Vaughan, J. M., Brar, B. K., Arias, C. M., Lewis, K. A., Rivier, J. E., Sawchenko, P. E., and Vale, W. W. (2005). A soluble mouse brain splice variant of type 2{alpha} corticotropin-releasing factor (CRF) receptor binds ligands and modulates their activity. *Proc. Natl. Acad. Sci. USA* 102(7), 2620–2625.
74. Ross, P. C., Kostas, C. M., and Ramabhadran, T. V. (1994). A variant of the human corticotropin-releasing factor (CRF) receptor: Cloning, expression and pharmacology. *Biochem. Biophys. Res. Commun.* 205(3), 1836–1842.
75. Grammatopoulos, D. K., Dai, Y., Randeva, H. S., Levine, M. A., Karteris, E., Easton, A. J., and Hillhouse, E. W. (1999). A novel spliced variant of the type 1 corticotropin-releasing hormone receptor with a deletion in the seventh transmembrane domain present in the human pregnant term myometrium and fetal membranes. *Mol. Endocrinol.* 13(12), 2189–2202.
76. Sawchenko, P. E., Imaki, T., Potter, E., Kovacs, K., Imaki, J., and Vale, W. (1993). The functional neuroanatomy of corticotropin-releasing factor. *Ciba Found Symp* 172, 5–21.
77. Chalmers, D. T., Lovenberg, T. W., and De Souza, E. B. (1995). Localization of novel corticotropin-releasing factor receptor (CRF2) mRNA expression to specific subcortical nuclei in rat brain: Comparison with CRF1 receptor mRNA expression. *J. Neurosci.* 15(10), 6340–6350.
78. Chalmers, D. T., Lovenberg, T. W., Grigoriadis, D. E., Behan, D. P., and De Souza, E. B. (1996). Corticotrophin-releasing factor receptors: From molecular biology to drug design. *Trends Pharmacol. Sci.* 17(4), 166–172.
79. Perrin, M. H., and Vale, W. W. (1999). Corticotropin releasing factor receptors and their ligand family. *Ann. NY Acad. Sci.* 885, 312–328.
80. Sanchez, M. M., Young, L. J., Plotsky, P. M., and Insel, T. R. (1999). Autoradiographic and in situ hybridization localization of corticotropin-releasing factor 1 and 2 receptors in nonhuman primate brain. *J. Comp. Neurol.* 408(3), 365–377.
81. Mastorakos, G., Webster, E. L., Friedman, T. C., and Chrousos, G. P. (1993). Immunoreactive corticotropin-releasing hormone and its binding sites in the rat ovary. *J. Clin. Invest.* 92(2), 961–968.
82. Vita, N., Laurent, P., Lefort, S., Chalon, P., Lelias, J. M., Kaghad, M., Le Fur, G., Caput, D., and Ferrara, P. (1993). Primary structure and functional expression of mouse pituitary and human brain corticotrophin releasing factor receptors. *FEBS Lett.* 335(1), 1–5.

83. Palchaudhuri, M. R., Wille, S., Mevenkamp, G., Spiess, J., Fuchs, E., and Dautzenberg, F. M. (1998). Corticotropin-releasing factor receptor type 1 from Tupaia belangeri—Cloning, functional expression and tissue distribution. *Eur. J. Biochem.* 258(1), 78–84.

84. Chatzaki, E., Crowe, P. D., Wang, L., Million, M., Tache, Y., and Grigoriadis, D. E. (2004). CRF receptor type 1 and 2 expression and anatomical distribution in the rat colon. *J. Neurochem.* 90(2), 309–316.

85. Chatzaki, E., Murphy, B. J., Wang, L., Million, M., Ohning, G. V., Crowe, P. D., Petroski, R., Tache, Y., and Grigoriadis, D. E. (2004). Differential profile of CRF receptor distribution in the rat stomach and duodenum assessed by newly developed CRF receptor antibodies. *J. Neurochem.* 88(1), 1–11.

86. Yuan, P. Q., Wu, S. V., and Tache, Y. (2004). CRF receptor type 1 and 2 (CRF1 and CRF2) in rat colon: Expression and CRF2 downregulation by endotoxin. *Digestive Diseases Week, AGA*, New Orleans, May 15–20.

87. Kanamoto, K., Urdanda, A., Rivier, J., and Tache, Y. (2002). Intravenous urocortin II induced gastroprotection and gastric hyperemia in anesthetized rats: Role of CRF receptor 2. *Gastroenterology* 122, A–13.

88. Saunders, P., Million, M., Miampamba, M., Wang, L., Czimmer, J., and Tache, Y. (2003). Urocortin II (Ucn II) suppresses CRF-induced activation of rat colonic motor function and myenteric neurons. *Gastroenterology* 124, A–139.

89. Tache, Y., Martinez, V., Wang, L., and Million, M. (2004). CRF1 receptor signaling pathways are involved in stress-related alterations of colonic function and viscerosensitivity: Implications for irritable bowel syndrome. *Br. J. Pharmacol.* 141(8), 1321–1330.

90. Tache, Y., and Perdue, M. H. (2004). Role of peripheral CRF signalling pathways in stress-related alterations of gut motility and mucosal function. *Neurogastroenterol. Motil.* 16(Suppl. 1), 137–142.

91. Heinrichs, S. C., and Tache, Y. (2001). Therapeutic potential of CRF receptor antagonists: A gut-brain perspective. *Exp. Opin. Investig. Drugs.* 10(4), 647–659.

92. Tache, Y., Martinez, V., Million, M., and Wang, L. (2001). Stress and the gastrointestinal tract III. Stress-related alterations of gut motor function: Role of brain corticotropin-releasing factor receptors. *Am. J. Physiol. Gastrointest. Liver Physiol.* 280(2), G173–177.

93. Tache, Y., Martinez, V., Million, M., and Maillot, C. (2002). Role of corticotropin-releasing factor subtype 1 in stress-related functional colonic alterations: Implications in irritable bowel syndrome. *Eur. J. Surg.* 128, 16–22.

94. Tache, Y. (2004). Corticotropin releasing factor receptor antagonists: Potential future therapy in gastroenterology? *Gut* 53(7), 919–921.

95. Bakshi, V. P., Smith-Roe, S., Newman, S. M., Grigoriadis, D. E., and Kalin, N. H. (2002). Reduction of stress-induced behavior by antagonism of corticotropin-releasing hormone 2 (CRH2) receptors in lateral septum or CRH1 receptors in amygdala. *J. Neurosci.* 22(7), 2926–2935.

96. Risbrough, V. B., Hauger, R. L., Pelleymounter, M. A., and Geyer, M. A. (2003). Role of corticotropin releasing factor (CRF) receptors 1 and 2 in CRF-potentiated acoustic startle in mice. *Psychopharmacology (Berl.)* 170(2), 178–187.

97. Bale, T. L., Contarino, A., Smith, G. W., Chan, R., Gold, L. H., Sawchenko, P. E., Koob, G. F., Vale, W. W., and Lee, K. F. (2000). Mice deficient for corticotropin-releasing hormone receptor-2 display anxiety-like behaviour and are hypersensitive to stress. *Nat. Genet.* 24(4), 410–414.

98. Lovenberg, T. W., Chalmers, D. T., Liu, C., and De Souza, E. B. (1995). CRF2 alpha and CRF2 beta receptor mRNAs are differentially distributed between the rat central nervous system and peripheral tissues. *Endocrinology* 136(9), 4139–4142.

99. Hashimoto, K., Nishiyama, M., Tanaka, Y., Noguchi, T., Asaba, K., Hossein, P. N., Nishioka, T., and Makino, S. (2004). Urocortins and corticotropin releasing factor type 2 receptors in the hypothalamus and the cardiovascular system. *Peptides* 25(10), 1711–1721.

100. Wiley, K. E., and Davenport, A. P. (2004). CRF2 receptors are highly expressed in the human cardiovascular system and their cognate ligands urocortins 2 and 3 are potent vasodilators. *Br. J. Pharmacol.* 143(4), 508–514.

101. Martinez, V., Wang, L., Million, M., Rivier, J., and Tache, Y. (2004). Urocortins and the regulation of gastrointestinal motor function and visceral pain. *Peptides* 25(10), 1733–1744.

102. Bale, T. L., and Vale, W. W. (2004). CRF and CRF Receptors: Role in stress responsivity and other behaviors. *Annu. Rev. Pharmacol. Toxicol.* 44, 525–557.

103. Grammatopoulos, D. K., Randeva, H. S., Levine, M. A., Katsanou, E. S., and Hillhouse, E. W. (2000). Urocortin, but not corticotropin-releasing hormone (CRH), activates the mitogen-activated protein kinase signal transduction pathway in human pregnant myometrium: An effect mediated via R1alpha and R2beta CRH receptor subtypes and stimulation of Gq-proteins. *Mol. Endocrinol.* 14(12), 2076–2091.

104. Karteris, E., Grammatopoulos, D., Randeva, H., and Hillhouse, E. W. (2000). Signal transduction characteristics of the corticotropin-releasing hormone receptors in the feto-placental unit. *J. Clin. Endocrinol. Metab.* 85(5), 1989–1996.

105. Hillhouse, E. W., Randeva, H., Ladds, G., and Grammatopoulos, D. (2002). Corticotropin-releasing hormone receptors. *Biochem. Soc. Trans.* 30(4), 428–432.

106. Blank, T., Nijholt, I., Grammatopoulos, D. K., Randeva, H. S., Hillhouse, E. W., and Spiess, J. (2003). Corticotropin-releasing factor receptors couple to multiple G-proteins to activate diverse intracellular signaling pathways in mouse hippocampus: Role in neuronal excitability and associative learning. *J. Neurosci.* 23(2), 700–707.

107. Liaw, C. W., Lovenberg, T. W., Barry, G., Oltersdorf, T., Grigoriadis, D. E., and De Souza, E. B. (1996). Cloning and characterization of the human corticotropin-releasing factor-2 receptor complementary deoxyribonucleic acid. *Endocrinology* 137(1), 72–77.

108. Dautzenberg, F. M., Py-Lang, G., Higelin, J., Fischer, C., Wright, M. B., and Huber, G. (2001). Different binding modes of amphibian and human corticotropin-releasing factor type 1 and type 2 receptors: Evidence for evolutionary differences. *J. Pharmacol. Exp. Ther.* 296(1), 113–120.

109. Brauns, O., Brauns, S., Zimmermann, B., Jahn, O., and Spiess, J. (2002). Differential responsiveness of CRF receptor subtypes to N-terminal truncation of peptidic ligands. *Peptides* 23(5), 881–888.

110. Tezval, H., Jahn, O., Todorovic, C., Sasse, A., Eckart, K., and Spiess, J. (2004). Cortagine, a specific agonist of corticotropin-releasing factor receptor subtype 1, is anxiogenic and antidepressive in the mouse model. *Proc. Natl. Acad. Sci. USA* 101(25), 9468–9473.

111. Ardati, A., Goetschy, V., Gottowick, J., Henriot, S., Valdenaire, O., Deuschle, U., and Kilpatrick, G. J. (1999). Human CRF2 alpha and beta splice variants: Pharmacological characterization using radioligand binding and a luciferase gene expression assay. *Neuropharmacology* 38(3), 441–448.

112. Olianas, M. C., and Onali, P. (1990). Presence of corticotropin-releasing factor-stimulated adenylate cyclase activity in rat retina. *J. Neurochem.* 54(6), 1967–1971.
113. Hauger, R. L., Dautzenberg, F. M., Flaccus, A., Liepold, T., and Spiess, J. (1997). Regulation of corticotropin-releasing factor receptor function in human Y-79 retinoblastoma cells: Rapid and reversible homologous desensitization but prolonged recovery. *J. Neurochem.* 68(6), 2308–2316.
114. Wang, W., Ji, P., Riopelle, R. J., and Dow, K. E. (2002). Functional expression of corticotropin-releasing hormone (CRH) receptor 1 in cultured rat microglia. *J. Neurochem.* 80(2), 287–294.
115. Kageyama, K., and Suda, T. (2003). Urocortin-related peptides increase interleukin-6 output via cyclic adenosine 5′-monophosphate-dependent pathways in A7r5 aortic smooth muscle cells. *Endocrinology* 144(6), 2234–2241.
116. Hoare, S. R., Sullivan, S. K., Fan, J., Khongsaly, K., and Grigoriadis, D. E. (2005). Peptide ligand binding properties of the corticotropin-releasing factor (CRF) type 2 receptor: Pharmacology of endogenously expressed receptors, G-protein-coupling sensitivity and determinants of CRF2 receptor selectivity. *Peptides* 26(3), 457–470.
117. Brauns, O., Brauns, S., Jenke, M., Zimmermann, B., and Dautzenberg, F. M. (2002). Secondary structure of antisauvagine analogues is important for CRF receptor antagonism: Development of antagonists with increased potency and receptor selectivity. *Peptides* 23(10), 1817–1827.
118. Yamada, Y., Mizutani, K., Mizusawa, Y., Hantani, Y., Tanaka, M., Tanaka, Y., Tomimoto, M., Sugawara, M., Imai, N., Yamada, H., Okajima, N., and Haruta, J. (2004). New class of corticotropin-releasing factor (CRF) antagonists: Small peptides having high binding affinity for CRF receptor. *J. Med. Chem.* 47(5), 1075–1078.
119. Klose, J., Fechner, K., Beyermann, M., Krause, E., Wendt, N., Bienert, M., Rudolph, R., and Rothemund, S. (2005). Impact of N-terminal domains for corticotropin-releasing factor (CRF) receptor-ligand interactions. *Biochemistry* 44(5), 1614–1623.
120. Rominger, D. H., Rominger, C. M., Fitzgerald, L. W., Grzanna, R., Largent, B. L., and Zaczek, R. (1998). Characterization of [125I]sauvagine binding to CRH2 receptors: Membrane homogenate and autoradiographic studies. *J. Pharmacol. Exp. Ther.* 286(1), 459–468.
121. Hoare, S. R., Sullivan, S. K., Pahuja, A., Ling, N., Crowe, P. D., and Grigoriadis, D. E. (2003). Conformational states of the corticotropin releasing factor 1 (CRF1) receptor: Detection, and pharmacological evaluation by peptide ligands. *Peptides* 24(12), 1881–1897.
122. Perrin, M. H., Sutton, S. W., Cervini, L. A., Rivier, J. E., and Vale, W. W. (1999). Comparison of an agonist, urocortin, and an antagonist, astressin, as radioligands for characterization of corticotropin-releasing factor receptors. *J. Pharmacol. Exp. Ther.* 288(2), 729–734.
123. Gottowik, J., Goetschy, V., Henriot, S., Kitas, E., Fluhman, B., Clerc, R. G., Moreau, J. L., Monsma, F. J., and Kilpatrick, G. J. (1997). Labelling of CRF1 and CRF2 receptors using the novel radioligand, [3H]-urocortin. *Neuropharmacology* 36(10), 1439–1446.
124. Ruhmann, A., Bonk, I., and Kopke, A. K. (1999). High-affinity binding of urocortin and astressin but not CRF to G protein-uncoupled CRFR1. *Peptides* 20(11), 1311–1319.
125. Perrin, M. H., Haas, Y., Rivier, J. E., and Vale, W. W. (1986). Corticotropin-releasing factor binding to the anterior pituitary receptor is modulated by divalent cations and guanyl nucleotides. *Endocrinology* 118(3), 1171–1179.

126. Higelin, J., Py-Lang, G., Paternoster, C., Ellis, G. J., Patel, A., and Dautzenberg, F. M. (2001). 125I-Antisauvagine-30: A novel and specific high-affinity radioligand for the characterization of corticotropin-releasing factor type 2 receptors. *Neuropharmacology* 40(1), 114–122.

127. De Lean, A., Stadel, J. M., and Lefkowitz, R. J. (1980). A ternary complex model explains the agonist-specific binding properties of the adenylate cyclase-coupled beta-adrenergic receptor. *J. Biol. Chem.* 255(15), 7108–7117.

128. Samama, P., Cotecchia, S., Costa, T., and Lefkowitz, R. J. (1993). A mutation-induced activated state of the beta 2-adrenergic receptor. Extending the ternary complex model. *J. Biol. Chem.* 268(7), 4625–4636.

129. Gilman, A. G. (1987). G proteins: Transducers of receptor-generated signals. *Annu. Rev. Biochem.* 56, 615–649.

130. Liaw, C. W., Grigoriadis, D. E., Lorang, M. T., De Souza, E. B., and Maki, R. A. (1997). Localization of agonist- and antagonist-binding domains of human corticotropin-releasing factor receptors. *Mol. Endocrinol.* 11(13), 2048–2053.

131. Liaw, C. W., Grigoriadis, D. E., Lovenberg, T. W., De Souza, E. B., and Maki, R. A. (1997). Localization of ligand-binding domains of human corticotropin-releasing factor receptor: A chimeric receptor approach. *Mol. Endocrinol.* 11(7), 980–985.

132. Dautzenberg, F. M., Wille, S., Lohmann, R., and Spiess, J. (1998). Mapping of the ligand-selective domain of the *Xenopus laevis* corticotropin-releasing factor receptor 1: Implications for the ligand-binding site. *Proc. Natl. Acad. Sci. USA* 95(9), 4941–4946.

133. Dautzenberg, F. M., Kilpatrick, G. J., Wille, S., and Hauger, R. L. (1999). The ligand-selective domains of corticotropin-releasing factor type 1 and type 2 receptor reside in different extracellular domains: Generation of chimeric receptors with a novel ligand-selective profile. *J. Neurochem.* 73(2), 821–829.

134. Sydow, S., Flaccus, A., Fischer, A., and Spiess, J. (1999). The role of the fourth extracellular domain of the rat corticotropin-releasing factor receptor type 1 in ligand binding. *Eur. J. Biochem.* 259(1/2), 55–62.

135. Wille, S., Sydow, S., Palchaudhuri, M. R., Spiess, J., and Dautzenberg, F. M. (1999). Identification of amino acids in the N-terminal domain of corticotropin-releasing factor receptor 1 that are important determinants of high-affinity ligand binding. *J. Neurochem.* 72(1), 388–395.

136. Assil-Kishawi, I., and Abou-Samra, A. B. (2002). Sauvagine crosslinks to the second extracellular loop of the corticotropin-releasing factor type 1 receptor. *J. Biol. Chem.* 227(36), 32558–32561.

137. Dautzenberg, F. M., Higelin, J., Brauns, O., Butscha, B., and Hauger, R. L. (2002). Five amino acids of the *Xenopus laevis* CRF (corticotropin-releasing factor) type 2 receptor mediate differential binding of CRF ligands in comparison with its human counterpart. *Mol. Pharmacol.* 61(5), 1132–1139.

138. Dautzenberg, F. M., and Wille, S. (2004). Binding differences of human and amphibian corticotropin-releasing factor type 1 (CRF(1)) receptors: Identification of amino acids mediating high-affinity astressin binding and functional antagonism. *Regul. Pept.* 118(3), 165–173.

139. Grace, C. R., Perrin, M. H., Digruccio, M. R., Miller, C. L., Rivier, J. E., Vale, W. W., and Riek, R. (2004). NMR structure and peptide hormone binding site of the first extracellular domain of a type B1 G protein-coupled receptor. *Proc. Natl. Acad. Sci. USA* 101(35), 12836–12841.

140. Perrin, M. H., Sutton, S., Bain, D. L., Berggren, W. T., and Vale, W. W. (1998). The first extracellular domain of corticotropin releasing factor-R1 contains major binding determinants for urocortin and astressin. *Endocrinology* 139(2), 566–570.

141. Assil, I. Q., Qi, L. J., Arai, M., Shomali, M., and Abou-Samra, A. B. (2001). Juxtamembrane region of the amino terminus of the corticotropin releasing factor receptor type 1 is important for ligand interaction. *Biochemistry* 40(5), 1187–1195.

142. Sydow, S., Radulovic, J., Dautzenberg, F. M., and Spiess, J. (1997). Structure-function relationship of different domains of the rat corticotropin-releasing factor receptor. *Mol. Brain Res.* 52(2), 182–193.

143. Nielsen, S. M., Nielsen, L. Z., Hjorth, S. A., Perrin, M. H., and Vale, W. W. (2000). Constitutive activation of tethered-peptide/corticotropin-releasing factor receptor chimeras. *Proc. Natl. Acad. Sci. USA* 97(18), 10277–10281.

144. Hofmann, B. A., Sydow, S., Jahn, O., Van Werven, L., Liepold, T., Eckart, K., and Spiess, J. (2001). Functional and protein chemical characterization of the N-terminal domain of the rat corticotropin-releasing factor receptor 1. *Protein Sci.* 10(10), 2050–2062.

145. Perrin, M. H., Digruccio, M. R., Koerber, S. C., Rivier, J. E., Kunitake, K. S., Bain, D. L., Fischer, W. H., and Vale, W. W. (2003). A soluble form of the first extracellular domain of mouse type 2beta corticotropin-releasing factor receptor reveals differential ligand specificity. *J. Biol. Chem.* 278(18), 15595–15600.

146. Hoare, S. R., Sullivan, S. K., Schwarz, D. A., Ling, N., Vale, W. W., Crowe, P. D., and Grigoriadis, D. E. (2004). Ligand affinity for amino-terminal and juxtamembrane domains of the corticotropin releasing factor type I receptor: Regulation by G-protein and nonpeptide antagonists. *Biochemistry* 43(13), 3996–4011.

147. Kratke, O., Wiesner, B., Holleran, B., Escher, E., Bienert, M., and Beyermann, M. (2004). FRET studies and photoaffinity labeling of the corticotropin releasing factor receptor type one (CRF1R) using Bpa-urocortin-I analogues. Paper presented at the International Symposium on Peptide Receptors: From gene to therapy, Montreal, Canada, July 31–August 4.

148. Lau, S. H., Rivier, J., Vale, W., Kaiser, E. T., and Kezdy, F. J. (1983). Surface properties of an amphiphilic peptide hormone and of its analog: Corticotropin-releasing factor and sauvagine. *Proc. Natl. Acad. Sci. USA* 80(23), 7070–7074.

149. Romier, C., Bernassau, J. M., Cambillau, C., and Darbon, H. (1993). Solution structure of human corticotropin releasing factor by 1H NMR and distance geometry with restrained molecular dynamics. *Prot. Eng.* 6(2), 149–156.

150. Hoare, S. R. J. (2005). Mechanisms of peptide and nonpeptide ligand binding to Class B G-protein coupled receptors. *Drug Discov. Today* 10(6), 417–427.

151. Gloriam, D. E., Schioth, H. B., and Fredriksson, R. (2005). Nine new human rhodopsin family G-protein coupled receptors: Identification, sequence characterisation and evolutionary relationship. *Biochim. Biophys. Acta* 1722(3), 235–246.

152. Schioth, H. B., and Fredriksson, R. (2005). The GRAFS classification system of G-protein coupled receptors in comparative perspective. *Gen. Comp. Endocrinol.* 142(1/2), 94–101.

153. Perry, S. J., Junger, S., Kohout, T. A., Hoare, S. R., Struthers, R. S., Grigoriadis, D. E., and Maki, R. A. (2005). Distinct conformations of the corticotropin releasing factor type 1 receptor adopted following agonist and antagonist binding are differentially regulated. *J. Biol. Chem.* 280(12), 11560–11568.

154. Holsboer, F. (1999). The rationale for corticotropin-releasing hormone receptor (CRH-R) antagonists to treat depression and anxiety. *J. Psychiatr. Res.* 33(3), 181–214.

155. Grigoriadis, D. E., Haddach, M., Ling, N., and Saunders, J. (2001). The CRF receptor: Structure, function and potential for therapeutic intervention. *Curr. Med. Chem. Central Nervous System Agents* 1, 63–97.

156. Kehne, J., and De Lombaert, S. (2002). Non-peptidic CRF1 receptor antagonists for the treatment of anxiety, depression and stress disorders. *Curr. Drug. Target. CNS Neurol. Disord.* 1(5), 467–493.

157. Saunders, J., and Williams, J. (2003). Antagonists of the corticotropin releasing factor receptor. *Prog. Med. Chem.* 41, 195–247.

158. McCarthy, J. R., Heinrichs, S. C., and Grigoriadis, D. E. (1999). Recent advances with the CRF1 receptor: Design of small molecule inhibitors, receptor subtypes and clinical indications. *Curr. Pharm. Des.* 5(5), 289–315.

159. Gilligan, P. J., Robertson, D. W., and Zaczek, R. (2000). Corticotropin releasing factor (CRF) receptor modulators: Progress and opportunities for new therapeutic agents. *J. Med. Chem.* 43(9), 1641–1660.

160. Griebel, G., Simiand, J., Steinberg, R., Jung, M., Gully, D., Roger, P., Geslin, M., Scatton, B., Maffrand, J. P., and Soubrie, P. (2002). 4-(2-Chloro-4-methoxy-5-methylphenyl)-*N*-[(1*S*)-2-cyclopropyl-1-(3-fluoro-4-methylphenyl)ethyl]5-methyl-*N*-(2-propynyl)-1,3-thiazol-2-amine hydrochloride (SSR125543A), a potent and selective corticotrophin-releasing factor(1) receptor antagonist. II. Characterization in rodent models of stress-related disorders. *J. Pharmacol. Exp. Ther.* 301(1), 333–345.

161. Gully, D., Geslin, M., Serva, L., Fontaine, E., Roger, P., Lair, C., Darre, V., Marcy, C., Rouby, P. E., Simiand, J., Guitard, J., Gout, G., Steinberg, R., Rodier, D., Griebel, G., Soubrie, P., Pascal, M., Pruss, R., Scatton, B., Maffrand, J. P., and Le Fur, G. (2002). 4-(2-Chloro-4-methoxy-5-methylphenyl)-*N*-[(1*S*)-2-cyclopropyl-1-(3-fluoro-4-methylphenyl)ethyl]5-methyl-*N*-(2-propynyl)-1,3-thiazol-2-amine hydrochloride (SSR125543A): A potent and selective corticotrophin-releasing factor(1) receptor antagonist. I. Biochemical and pharmacological characterization. *J. Pharmacol. Exp. Ther.* 301(1), 322–332.

162. Webster, E. L., Lewis, D. B., Torpy, D. J., Zachman, E. K., Rice, K. C., and Chrousos, G. P. (1996). In vivo and in vitro characterization of antalarmin, a nonpeptide corticotropin-releasing hormone (CRH) receptor antagonist: Suppression of pituitary ACTH release and peripheral inflammation. *Endocrinology* 137(12), 5747–5750.

163. Hoare, S. R., Sullivan, S. K., Ling, N., Crowe, P. D., and Grigoriadis, D. E. (2003). Mechanism of corticotropin-releasing factor type I receptor regulation by nonpeptide antagonists. *Mol. Pharmacol.* 63(3), 751–765.

164. Gross, R. S., Guo, Z., Dyck, B., Coon, T., Huang, C. Q., Lowe, R. F., Marinkovic, D., Moorjani, M., Nelson, J., Zamani-Kord, S., Grigoriadis, D. E., Hoare, S. R., Crowe, P. D., Bu, J. H., Haddach, M., McCarthy, J., Saunders, J., Sullivan, R., Chen, T. and Williams, J. P. (2005). Design and synthesis of tricyclic corticotropin-releasing factor-1 antagonists. *J. Med. Chem.* 48(18), 5780-5793.

165. Zobel, A. W., Nickel, T., Kunzel, H. E., Ackl, N., Sonntag, A., Ising, M., and Holsboer, F. (2000). Effects of the high-affinity corticotropin-releasing hormone receptor 1 antagonist R121919 in major depression: The first 20 patients treated. *J. Psychiatr. Res.* 34(3), 171–181.

166. Zhang, G., Huang, N., Li, Y. W., Qi, X., Marshall, A. P., Yan, X. X., Hill, G., Rominger, C., Prakash, S. R., Bakthavatchalam, R., Rominger, D. H., Gilligan, P. J.,

and Zaczek, R. (2003). Pharmacological characterization of a novel nonpeptide antagonist radioligand, (+/−)-N-[2-methyl-4-methoxyphenyl]-1-(1-(methoxymethyl) propyl)-6-methyl-1H-1,2,3-triazolo[4,5-c]pyridin-4-amine ([3H]SN003) for corticotropin-releasing factor1 receptors. *J. Pharmacol. Exp. Ther.* 305(1), 57–69.

167. Koob, G. F., Thatcher-Briton, K., Tazi, A., and Le Moal, M. (1988). Behavioral pharmacology of stress: Focus on CNS corticotropin-releasing factor. *Adv. Exp. Med. Biol.* 245, 25–34.

168. Koob, G. F., Cole, B. J., Swerdlow, N. R., Le Moal, M., and Britton, K. T. (1990). Stress, performance, and arousal: Focus on CRF. *NIDA Res. Monogr.* 97, 163–176.

169. Roy-Byrne, P. P., Uhde, T. W., Gold, P. W., Rubinow, D. R., and Post, R. M. (1985). Neuroendocrine abnormalities in panic disorder. *Psychopharmacol. Bull.* 21(3), 546–550.

170. Roy-Byrne, P. P., Uhde, T. W., Post, R. M., Gallucci, W., Chrousos, G. P., and Gold, P. W. (1986). The corticotropin-releasing hormone stimulation test in patients with panic disorder. *Am. J. Psychiatry* 143(7), 896–899.

171. Risbrough, V. B., Hauger, R. L., Roberts, A. L., Vale, W. W., and Geyer, M. A. (2004). Corticotropin-releasing factor receptors CRF1 and CRF2 exert both additive and opposing influences on defensive startle behavior. *J. Neurosci.* 24(29), 6545–6552.

172. Arborelius, L., Owens, M. J., Plotsky, P. M., and Nemeroff, C. B. (1999). The role of corticotropin-releasing factor in depression and anxiety disorders. *J. Endocrinol.* 160(1), 1–12.

173. Sanchez, M. M., Ladd, C. O., and Plotsky, P. M. (2001). Early adverse experience as a developmental risk factor for later psychopathology: Evidence from rodent and primate models. *Dev. Psychopathol.* 13(3), 419–449.

174. Bakshi, V. P., and Kalin, N. H. (2002). Animal models and endophenotypes of anxiety and stress disorders. In *Neuropsychopharmacology*, K. L. Davis, D. Charney, J. T. Coyle, and C. B. Nemeroff, Eds. Lippincott Williams & Wilkins, Philadelphia, PA, pp. 883–900.

175. Heinrichs, S. C., and Koob, G. F. (2004). Corticotropin-releasing factor in brain: A role in activation, arousal, and affect regulation. *J. Pharmacol. Exp. Ther.* 311(2), 427–440.

176. Griebel, G., Perrault, G., and Sanger, D. J. (1998). Characterization of the behavioral profile of the non-peptide CRF receptor antagonist CP-154,526 in anxiety models in rodents. Comparison with diazepam and buspirone. *Psychopharmacology (Berl.)* 138(1), 55–66.

177. Millan, M. J., Brocco, M., Gobert, A., Dorey, G., Casara, P., and Dekeyne, A. (2001). Anxiolytic properties of the selective, non-peptidergic CRF(1) antagonists, CP154,526 and DMP695: A comparison to other classes of anxiolytic agent. *Neuropsychopharmacology* 25(4), 585–600.

178. Harro, J., Tonissaar, M., and Eller, M. (2001). The effects of CRA 1000, a non-peptide antagonist of corticotropin-releasing factor receptor type 1, on adaptive behaviour in the rat. *Neuropeptides* 35(2), 100–109.

179. Maciag, C. M., Dent, G., Gilligan, P., He, L., Dowling, K., Ko, T., Levine, S., and Smith, M. A. (2002). Effects of a non-peptide CRF antagonist (DMP696) on the behavioral and endocrine sequelae of maternal separation. *Neuropsychopharmacology* 26(5), 574–582.

180. Overstreet, D. H., and Griebel, G. (2004). Antidepressant-like effects of CRF(1) receptor antagonist SSR125543 in an animal model of depression. *Eur. J. Pharmacol.* 497(1), 49–53.

181. Overstreet, D. H., Keeney, A., and Hogg, S. (2004). Antidepressant effects of citalopram and CRF receptor antagonist CP-154,526 in a rat model of depression. *Eur. J. Pharmacol.* 492(2/3), 195–201.

182. Hikichi, T., Akiyoshi, J., Yamamoto, Y., Tsutsumi, T., Isogawa, K., and Nagayama, H. (2000). Suppression of conditioned fear by administration of CRF receptor antagonist CP-154,526. *Pharmacopsychiatry* 33(5), 189–193.

183. Kikusui, T., Takeuchi, Y., and Mori, Y. (2000). Involvement of corticotropin-releasing factor in the retrieval process of fear-conditioned ultrasonic vocalization in rats. *Physiol. Behav.* 71(3/4), 323–328.

184. Ho, S. P., Takahashi, L. K., Livanov, V., Spencer, K., Lesher, T., Maciag, C., Smith, M. A., Rohrbach, K. W., Hartig, P. R., and Arneric, S. P. (2001). Attenuation of fear conditioning by antisense inhibition of brain corticotropin releasing factor-2 receptor. *Brain Res. Mol. Brain Res.* 89(1/2), 29–40.

185. Schulz, D. W., Mansbach, R. S., Sprouse, J., Braselton, J. P., Collins, J., Corman, M., Dunaiskis, A., Faraci, S., Schmidt, A. W., Seeger, T., Seymour, P., Tingley, F. D., III, Winston, E. N., Chen, Y. L., and Heym, J. (1996). CP-154,526: A potent and selective nonpeptide antagonist of corticotropin releasing factor receptors. *Proc. Natl. Acad. Sci. USA* 93(19), 10477–10482.

186. Chen, Y. L., Mansbach, R. S., Winter, S. M., Brooks, E., Collins, J., Corman, M. L., Dunaiskis, A. R., Faraci, W. S., Gallaschun, R. J., Schmidt, A., and Schulz, D. W. (1997). Synthesis and oral efficacy of a 4-(butylethylamino)pyrrolo[2,3-d]pyrimidine: A centrally active corticotropin-releasing factor1 receptor antagonist. *J. Med. Chem.* 40(11), 1749–1754.

187. Habib, K. E., Weld, K. P., Rice, K. C., Pushkas, J., Champoux, M., Listwak, S., Webster, E. L., Atkinson, A. J., Schulkin, J., Contoreggi, C., Chrousos, G. P., McCann, S. M., Suomi, S. J., Higley, J. D., and Gold, P. W. (2000). Oral administration of a corticotropin-releasing hormone receptor antagonist significantly attenuates behavioral, neuroendocrine, and autonomic responses to stress in primates. *Proc. Natl. Acad. Sci. USA* 97(11), 6079–6084.

188. He, L., Gilligan, P. J., Zaczek, R., Fitzgerald, L. W., Mcelroy, J., Shen, H. S., Saye, J. A., Kalin, N. H., Shelton, S., Christ, D., Trainor, G., and Hartig, P. (2000). 4-(1,3-Dimethoxyprop-2-ylamino)-2,7-dimethyl-8-(2, 4-dichlorophenyl)pyrazolo[1,5-a]-1,3,5-triazine: A potent, orally bioavailable CRF(1) receptor antagonist. *J. Med. Chem.* 43(3), 449–456.

189. Ayala, A. R., Pushkas, J., Higley, J. D., Ronsaville, D., Gold, P. W., Chrousos, G. P., Pacak, K., Calis, K. A., Gerald, M., Lindell, S., Rice, K. C., and Cizza, G. (2004). Behavioral, adrenal, and sympathetic responses to long-term administration of an oral corticotropin-releasing hormone receptor antagonist in a primate stress paradigm. *J. Clin. Endocrinol. Metab.* 89(11), 5729–5737.

190. Million, M., Grigoriadis, D. E., Sullivan, S., Crowe, P. D., Mcroberts, J. A., Zhou, H., Saunders, P. R., Maillot, C., Mayer, E. A., and Tache, Y. (2003). A novel water-soluble selective CRF(1) receptor antagonist, NBI 35965, blunts stress-induced visceral hyperalgesia and colonic motor function in rats. *Brain Res.* 985(1), 32–42.

191. Zorrilla, E. P., and Koob, G. F. (2004). The therapeutic potential of CRF(1) antagonists for anxiety. *Exp. Opin. Investig. Drugs* 13(7), 799–828.

192. Lancel, M., Muller-Preuss, P., Wigger, A., Landgraf, R., and Holsboer, F. (2002). The CRH1 receptor antagonist R121919 attenuates stress-elicited sleep disturbances in rats, particularly in those with high innate anxiety. *J. Psychiatr. Res.* 36(4), 197.

193. Held, K., Kunzel, H., Ising, M., Schmid, D. A., Zobel, A., Murck, H., Holsboer, F., and Steiger, A. (2004). Treatment with the CRH1-receptor-antagonist R121919 improves sleep-EEG in patients with depression. *J. Psychiatr. Res.* 38(2), 129–136.
194. Kunzel, H. E., Ising, M., Zobel, A. W., Nickel, T., Ackl, N., Sonntag, A., Holsboer, F., and Uhr, M. (2005). Treatment with a CRH-1-receptor antagonist (R121919) does not affect weight or plasma leptin concentration in patients with major depression. *J. Psychiatr. Res.* 39(2), 173–177.
195. Kunzel, H. E., Zobel, A. W., Nickel, T., Ackl, N., Uhr, M., Sonntag, A., Ising, M., and Holsboer, F. (2003). Treatment of depression with the CRH-1-receptor antagonist R121919: Endocrine changes and side effects. *J. Psychiatr. Res.* 37(6), 525–533.
196. Grigoriadis, D. E. (2003). Corticotropin releasing factor receptor antagonists: Potential novel therapies for human disease. *Celltransmissions* 19(4), 3–10.

6

NEUROBIOLOGY AND PHARMACOTHERAPY OF OBSESSIVE-COMPULSIVE DISORDER

JUDITH L. RAPOPORT AND GALE INOFF-GERMAIN
National Institute of Mental Health, National Institutes of Health, Bethesda, Maryland

6.1	Introduction		216
6.2	Neurobiology		216
	6.2.1	Brain Imaging Studies of OCD	217
		6.2.1.1 Structural Studies	217
		6.2.1.2 Functional Imaging Studies	219
		6.2.1.3 Magnetic Resonance Spectroscopy	220
		6.2.1.4 Neuropharmacological Implications of Brain Imaging Studies in OCD	220
	6.2.2	Genetic Studies	222
		6.2.2.1 Overview	222
		6.2.2.2 Serotonin	222
		6.2.2.3 Dopamine	223
		6.2.2.4 Glutamate	223
		6.2.2.5 Neurotransmitter Metabolism	223
		6.2.2.6 Developmental Genes	223
	6.2.3	Animal Models of OCD	224
6.3	Clinical Psychopharmacology		225
	6.3.1	Effective Monotherapies: Controlled Trials	225
	6.3.2	Augmenting Agents	225
	6.3.3	Miscellaneous Pharmacological Trials of Interest	234
	6.3.4	Induction of Obsessive-Compulsive Symptoms	234
	6.3.5	Immunomodulatory Treatments	235
6.4	Experimental Nonpharmacological Treatments		235
	6.4.1	Neurosurgery	235
	6.4.2	Transcranial Magnetic Stimulation	236
	6.4.3	Deep Brain Stimulation	236
6.5	Summary		237
	References		238

Handbook of Contemporary Neuropharmacology, Edited by David R. Sibley, Israel Hanin, Michael Kuhar, and Phil Skolnick. Copyright © 2007 John Wiley & Sons, Inc.

6.1 INTRODUCTION

Obsessive-compulsive disorder (OCD) is an anxiety disorder characterized by the presence of unwanted, senseless, intrusive, and distressing thoughts, urges, and images (obsessions) and/or repetitive behaviors (compulsions). These are generally recognized as senseless by the patient. The disorder is relatively common, affecting 2–3% of the population [1, 2]. The content of these thoughts and behaviors is often related to fear of danger to self or others; contamination concerns are particularly frequent. At least half of OCD patients have their onset before the age of 15 [3], and there is evidence (reviewed below) that early-onset patients differ somewhat in comorbidity and underlying neurobiology.

The majority (over 70%) of OCD patients have other comorbid disorders [3, 4]. The pattern of comorbidity is of great interest, as early-onset patients differ in that movement disorders such as Tourette's disorder (TD) or chronic motor tics are strongly comorbid, as is attention-deficit hyperactivity disorder (ADHD) [5, 6]. Comorbid patterns are rather nonspecific for adult-onset OCD cases but include both bipolar disorder and schizophrenia. A subgroup of childhood-onset cases is believed to have onset of OCD in relation to infection with group A β-hemolytic streptococcus, presenting a parallel condition to that of Sydenham's chorea [7, 8].

While OCD is classified as an anxiety disorder in the fourth edition of the *Diagnostic and Statistical Manual of Mental Disorders* (DSM-IV), it is given a separate chapter here as the clinical phenomenology, drug treatment response, family studies, and brain imaging data support a separate neurobiological classification for this disorder and a distinct neuropharmacological profile as well. OCD is considered a major cause of disability worldwide [9]; in spite of this, most treatment research is relatively recent with the bulk carried out in the past two decades.

This chapter presents a selective review on the neurobiology, genetics, and neuropharmacology of OCD. For a more general recent clinically oriented review of the diagnosis and treatment of this fascinating syndrome, see Jenike (2004) [10]. As is evident from this chapter, there have been significant advances in the past two decades, but there remain major opportunities for more specific understanding of this complex and probably heterogeneous illness and its treatment.

6.2 NEUROBIOLOGY

Despite the considerable interest and surge of recent work in this area, the biological basis for OCD is unknown. Clinical phenomenology has provided some important clues to the underlying neurobiology of this disorder. For example, there are striking comorbid clinical associations between OCD or OCD-like phenomena and known brain disorders, typically those involving the motor system, which led to the hypothesis that OCD is a basal ganglia disorder. These observations are not new. In his original 1885 description of basal ganglia syndromes, Gilles de la Tourette described children with senseless rituals and tormenting obsessive thoughts associated with the tics and other movements of the syndrome that bears his name. Osler, in his 1894 monograph *On Chorea and Choreiform Affections*, describes cases with chorea and classical obsessions and compulsions [11]. The initial model of OCD [12–14] formulated a frontal-striatal circuit that is dysregulated in OCD. Research on the motor system involving the planning of complex actions has proved to be particularly pertinent to OCD and most productive for clinical and brain imaging studies over time. The group of childhood-onset cases that appear to have onset of OCD in relation to group A β-hemolytic streptococcus infection provides another example of a Sydenham's chorea-like movement disorder associated with OCD and suggest a possible autoimmune subgroup [7, 15]. In spite of research implicating abnormal activity in cortical-subcortical circuitry, it is still not clear which aspects of these abnormalities are correlates and which are underlying causes of OCD. As the imaging literature has expanded, the proposed circuitry of OCD has become more complex, as discussed more fully below (and see Figs. 6.1 and 6.2 below).

6.2.1 Brain Imaging Studies of OCD

6.2.1.1 Structural Studies. Brain imaging studies have been the most important source of data concerning underlying brain abnormalities in OCD. Initial anatomic neuroimaging studies using computerized tomography (CT) and anatomic brain magnetic resonance imaging (MRI) found increased ventricular volumes in a pediatric sample [16] and smaller caudate volumes in male adolescents with childhood-onset OCD [17]. MRI studies have generally found enlarged ventricular volumes, but basal ganglia volumes have been variously reported as both increased and decreased [18, 19]. Increased thalamic volumes have also been found in drug-naive patients [20]. The most convincing lesion studies involving OCD are by far the reports of OCD onset in relation to basal ganglia lesions secondary to stroke (e.g., [21]). The variability in these volumetric findings may reflect heterogeneity in the OCD population, possibly due to differences between childhood- and later-onset populations. The latter group has been most consistent with respect to basal ganglia and orbital frontal cortex (OFC) reduction [19, 22].

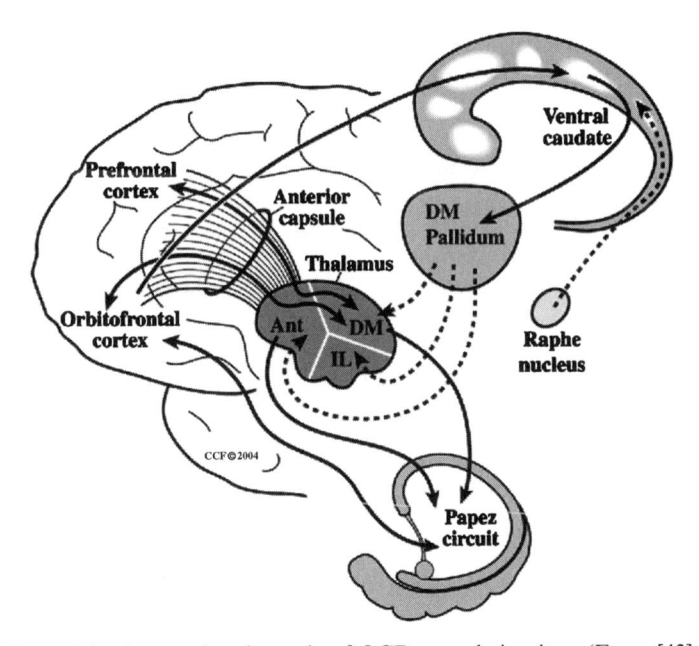

Figure 6.1 Anatomic schematic of OCD neural circuitry. (From [43].)

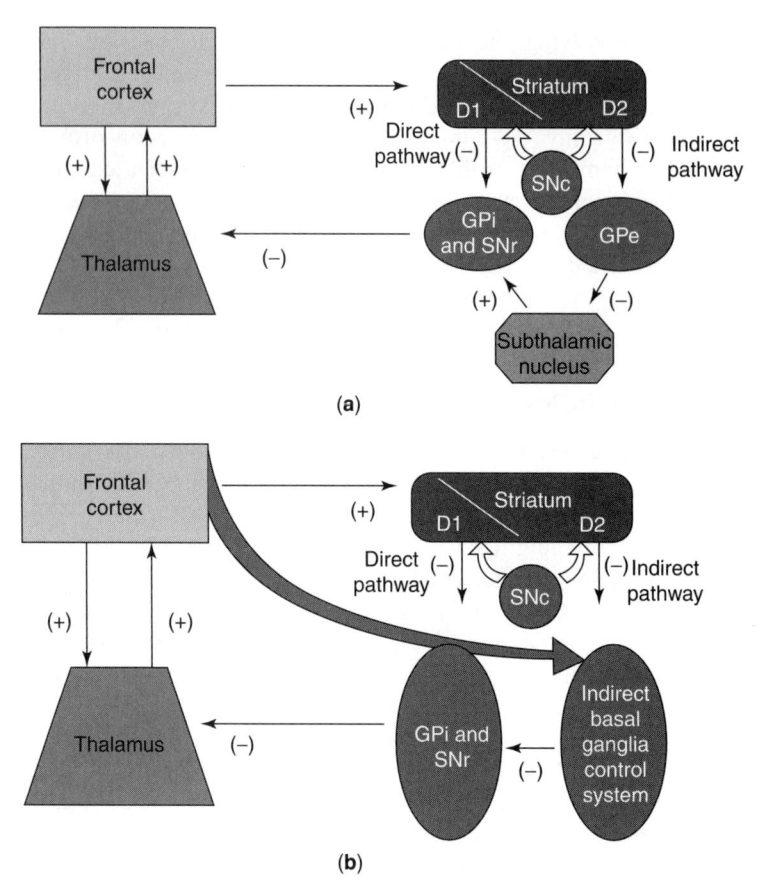

Figure 6.2 (a) Classic conception of direct and indirect frontal-basal ganglia-thalamocortical pathways. GPi and SNr, globus pallidus interna/substantia nigra, pars reticulata complex; GPe, globus pallidus externa. The frontal-subcortical circuit originates in the frontal cortex, which projects to striatum. The direct pathway projects from striatum to the GPi/SNr complex (the main output station of the basal ganglia), which projects to the thalamus, which has reciprocal, excitatory projections to and from the cortical site of origin. This pathway contains two excitatory and two inhibitory projections, making it a net positive-feedback loop. The indirect pathway also originates in the frontal cortex and projects to the striatum but then projects to the GPe, then to the subthalamic nucleus, then back to GPi/SNr, before returning to the thalamus and, finally, back to the frontal cortex. This indirect circuit has three inhibitory connections, making it a net negative-feedback loop. (b) Current conceptualization of prefrontal-basal ganglia-thalamocortical circuitry. Recent anatomic studies have called into question previous views of basal ganglia circuitry. Here, we refer to an indirect basal ganglia control system that consists of the GPe and the subthalamic nucleus. Connections within these structures are more complex than previously thought. The prefrontal cortex has excitatory projections to indirect pathway structures. In addition, the GPe directly projects to the GPi/SNr complex. Nevertheless, the net effect of activity in the indirect circuit still appears to be inhibition of the thalamus, thereby decreasing thalamocortical drive. The frontal-subcortical circuits originating in the lateral prefrontal cortex, orbitofrontal cortex, and anterior cingulate gyrus all pass through subcompartments of the medial dorsal nucleus of the thalamus. (From [18].)

6.2.1.2 Functional Imaging Studies. It is beyond the scope of this chapter to provide a thorough review of functional imaging studies in OCD. These studies have been particularly impressive in the degree of agreement across studies and methods and in their implications for treatment mechanisms. Functional methods have included both positron emission tomography (PET) and single photon emission computed tomography (SPECT) measuring cerebral blood flow (CBF) or metabolism and functional MRI (fMRI) measuring regional blood flow. Several functional studies have compared patients and controls in the resting state; others have scanned patients during symptom provocation or before and after treatment. While no finding is universally replicated, PET studies have generally shown elevated metabolism or regional cerebral blood flow (rCBF) in the OFC, anterior cingulate cortex, and basal ganglia [23]; these increases generally correlate with OCD symptoms.

Neuroimaging studies involving symptom provocation found strong correlations between OCD symptom expression and brain activation in the same regions found to be overactive, namely the OFC, anterior cingulate, and thalamus [24]. A recent SPECT study found greater responsivity of basal ganglia to symptom provocation in responders to sertraline [25]. Specifically, increases were seen in the OFC in the right caudate nucleus, left anterior cingulate (AC), and bilateral OFC. When the study was repeated with fMRI, again the right caudate, bilateral OFC, AC, and right caudate showed increased blood flow. Taken together, these studies link the expression of OCD symptoms with activation of the OFC, basal ganglia, thalamus, and limbic and paralimbic structures predominantly in the right hemisphere. In keeping with these findings, functional neuroimaging studies indicate that OCD patients show a different activation pattern [mesial temporal rather than striatal activation during learning of an implicit (procedural) sequence learning task], suggesting an alternate compensatory pathway for these subjects due presumably to striatal dysfunction. Further, these abnormalities appear specific to OCD [26].

Functional neuroimaging studies of OCD patients before and after treatment generally show decreases in the OFC or in the caudate nuclei in responders to treatment, since reductions in the caudate were seen both with fluoxetine and cognitive behavior therapy (CBT) [27]. Significant decreases were found in bilateral caudate glucose metabolism in responders to CBT compared with nonresponders [28]. These findings were not found in patients with depression, and so these appear to be disease-specific relationships. Another comprehensive examination of neural correlates of response to paroxetine in major depression, OCD, or concurrent OCD and depression also showed some diagnosis-specific differences. Treatment-related decreases in the OFC, thalamus, and ventrolateral prefrontal cortex (VLPFC) were noted for OCD responders; responders with major depression exhibited relative decreases in a large frontal area encompassing the VLPFC and medial, inferior, and dorsolateral frontal cortex. Thus, the drug-induced changes differed with respect to diagnosis and (not shown) paroxetine response versus nonresponse [29]. Perhaps most impressive has been the consistent finding that *elevated* OFC metabolism or blood flow predicts *greater* clinical response to treatment with a serotonin reuptake inhibitor (SRI). This finding has held across several functional imaging modalities and across several different SRIs.

Finally, abnormalities in the serotonin and dopamine transporter availability in unmediated OCD patients [30–33], as shown by SPECT, indicate both serotonergic and dopaminergic dysfunction in patients with OCD (although a PET study found no difference in serotonin transporter availability in OCD [33]). These important findings are being explored with higher resolution studies. They are of particular interest because of the consistent evidence, reviewed below, that low doses of dopamine antagonists potentiate the effect of selective serotonin reuptake inhibitors (SSRIs), suggesting that overactivity of the dopamine system is part of the pathophysiology of OCD.

6.2.1.3 Magnetic Resonance Spectroscopy. Most magnetic resonance spectroscopy (MRS) studies of OCD have been conducted by Rosenberg and colleagues, who found significantly increased caudate glutamatergic concentration in pediatric OCD patients compared to healthy controls [34] and also found striking decreases in glutamate concentration in the caudate in 11 children with OCD after treatment with paroxetine [35]. These findings are consistent with PET studies of adult patients indicating increased blood flow and metabolism in treatment-naive OCD patients. However, this drop in glutamate concentration appeared specific to SSRI treatment as it did not hold up for a group of OCD children responding to CBT [36]. It is notable that only caudate and not occipital glutamate concentration decreased, suggesting a localized effect of the drug. These studies, while intriguing, were done without sufficient resolution to distinguish glutamine and glutamate, and thus further understanding of these findings awaits replication with higher field strength machines.

Thus, taken together, and independent of imaging modality or type of treatment used, neuropharmacological hypotheses of OCD pathophysiology have supported the initial models put forward by Rapoport and Wise [37], Modell [12], Insel [37, 38], and Baxter [39] implicating cortical–striatal–thalamic–cortical (CSTC) loops. All of these models build on the discrete, parallel, neuroanatomic circuits connecting the prefrontal cortex, basal ganglia, and thalamus [40], although Saxena and colleagues [18] have summarized the more complex connections now documented within these structures and recent anatomic studies in primates. For example, there is a direct (excitatory) project from prefrontal cortex to the indirect (inhibitory) pathway structures. In light of the unique pattern of relationships between OCD and movement disorders, it is particularly interesting that the cortical–striatal connections provide a common substrate for both thoughts and planned movements. The excitatory projections in these circuits predominantly use glutamate as a neurotransmitter, while inhibitory ones mainly employ γ-aminobutyric acid (GABA). Several peptide transmitters also have roles within these pathways [41]. Other neurotransmitters (serotonin, dopamine, acetylcholine) modify the activity of projections between these structures. The net effect of the current model for OCD, in any case, is of an imbalance between direct and indirect pathways that leads to net overactivity of frontal–subcortical circuits.

6.2.1.4 Neuropharmacological Implications of Brain Imaging Studies in OCD. The imaging studies are almost all in agreement about the importance of the OFC, anterior cingulate, and ventral striatum. As mentioned, most consistent evidence relates OFC activity and treatment response. However, while the studies summarized above provide intriguing information about the pathways mediating OCD thoughts and behaviors, none has addressed the question of whether these findings are correlates of illness or trait markers. In fact, the normalization of caudate metabolism/blood flow with treatment and the normalization of caudate glutamate (Glx) elevation with drug treatment support imaging results as being largely state rather than trait markers. These results, together with the absence of family studies, make these findings generally ambiguous with respect to the usefulness of imaging measures as intermediate phenotypes for genetic studies.

The major neuropharmacological implications of the model is that there is increased signaling from OFC to subcortical structures (i.e., ventromedial caudate and medial dorsal thalamus). This leaves numerous possible anatomic mediators for this effect, and the imaging data do not support any single pathway. There are strong data indicating that serotonergic systems modulate OCD symptoms, as reviewed in Section 6.3.

Inhibitors of the serotonin (5-HT) transporter [5-HT reuptake inhibitors (5-HT-RIs)] produce at least some clinical benefit in most patients with OCD. Dopamine systems are also suggested by the demonstration that dopamine-blocking agents may potentiate the response to SSRI drugs [42] and, as reviewed below, for some patients this mechanism seems to have particular importance. Other neurotransmitter systems have been implicated on the basis of either the circuitry described above or brain imaging studies and include glutamate, GABA, substance P, and cholinergic and (on the basis of symptom exacerbation by naloxone, an opiate antagonist) endogenous opioid mechanisms.

Perhaps the selective regional (caudate) change in glutamate in blood flow following SSRI treatment provides the most novel treatment-related information. Initial studies in adult OCD showed that the increased metabolic rates associated with OCD symptom severity decreased after SSRI treatment [27]. However, as the major excitatory neurotransmitter system in the circuitry subsuming OCD is glutamatergic and the majority of axon terminals in the caudate nucleus are glutamatergic, stimulating 5-HT, that is, via $5-HT_{2A}$ receptors, would be expected to decrease glutamatergic efferents from the prefrontal cortex to the caudate nucleus with resulting decreased caudate glutamate concentrations. To date, there have been no studies of glutamatergic agents as monotherapies for OCD that might address this model. Future imaging studies can further extend this model (e.g., through blood flow or metabolic studies of the effects of D_2-blocking augmenting agents).

As seen in Figure 6.1, three general circuits have been assumed based on clinical, imaging, and lesion studies [43]. The first is an orbitofrontal–dorsomedial thalamic loop by way of the internal capsule. This is likely to be glutamatergic [12]. The second involves the frontal cortex–ventral caudate, dorsomedial pallidum and the intralaminar, anterior and dorsomedial thalamic nuclei. While there are multiple neurotransmitters involved in these circuits, including substance P and GABA, there are also serotonergic projections to this component from the dorsal raphe to the ventral striatum. These projections are speculated to be inhibitory. Finally, the third component includes the limbic structures and accounts for the strong anxiety component of OCD; this circuit has strong projections from the anterior cingulate cortex.

Figure 6.2 is an update to our understanding of the circuitry of the basal ganglia–thalamic–frontal loops [18]. It is included because the close association between various movement disorders, basal ganglia lesions, and OCD provides one of the unique and important leads to understanding this illness. Since the original basal ganglia models were postulated, there have been some changes to how the model of basal ganglia circuitry is viewed, most prominently the direct connection between the frontal cortex and the internal pallidum (GPe).

While it is unlikely that one neurotransmitter system will explain the basis for this complex and heterogeneous disorder, efforts have centered largely on the role of the neurotransmitter serotonin. The serotonin hypothesis of OCD that this disorder is in some way due to 5-HT dysfunction, stems from drug treatment studies [44, 45]. As reviewed below, over two decades of work has documented the efficacy and relative (to placebo and to noradrenergic antidepressant drugs) specificity of the anti-OCD effect of 5-HT uptake inhibitors [46]. However, peripheral markers of 5-HT function have not consistently indicated an abnormality in untreated patients with OCD, and exacerbation of OCD by oral administration of the 5-HT agonist m-CPP has not been consistently found [47]. Some evidence for the serotonin hypothesis has been from the genetic studies reviewed below.

Perhaps the most direct relevance of imaging studies for neuropharmacology comes from the rather consistent data on regional change in MRS or functional imaging patterns with treatment. For example, a pattern found in pre- and posttreatment studies with pediatric OCD was consistent paroxetine-induced normalization in regional (i.e., reduction in caudate but not occipital) Glx levels that correlate with treatment response [34].

6.2.2 Genetic Studies

6.2.2.1 Overview. A systematic approach to understanding the genetics of OCD would include twin, family, segregation, linkage, and association studies. Twin studies indicate concordance for OCD symptoms ranging from 26 to 87% with widely varying phenotypic definitions and sample sizes [48]. Family studies support a genetic component for OCD, particularly for populations with early age at onset. The presence of tics in probands may also predict greater familiality, as summarized by Grados et al. [49]. The findings appear complex, and heterogeneity by phenotype and by gender appears probable [50].

Genetic studies have been based on localization from linkage and from known pharmacological response. It is particularly encouraging that a 9p linkage site has recently been replicated [51, 52]. Because of the selective response of OCD to SRIs, the serotonin system has been the source for putative candidate genes. Cytogenetic studies, the studies of physical duplication, deletion, or disruption of chromosomes, are unexplored in OCD. One exception is the study of the 22q11 deletion, also known as velocardial facial syndrome (VCFS), a 3-MB microdeletion best recognized for its medical complications and association with psychosis [53]. However, OCD has also been associated with this same deletion in several studies, particularly for early-onset OCD [54, 55]. Segregation and linkage studies will not be reviewed here, but we will touch on candidate genes, which were targeted because they were involved in the metabolism of CNS neurotransmitters. Only studies with at least one independent replication are mentioned.

6.2.2.2 Serotonin. The serotonin transporter SLC6A4 on chromosome 17 is a target of SRIs. These drugs increase serotonin in the synapse by decreasing the transporter action. A functional gene 44-bp insertion/deletion polymorphism (*s* and *l* variants) within a gene promoter region (*5-HTTLPR*) has been identified and primarily *l* variants have been implicated [56], but there have been several nonreplications. This gene is highly evolutionarily conserved and regulates the entire serotonergic system. Both the serotonin transporter and some serotonin receptor subtypes such as 5-HT$_{2A}$ and 5-HT$_{2C}$ are highly expressed in the ventral striatum where they could influence the CSTC in OCD [57]. The gene has shown signals for multiple diagnoses, including ADHD, autism, bipolar disorder, and TD. The *ss* genotype is associated with poorer therapeutic response during treatment with antidepressant serotonin transporter (SERT) antagonists, the SSRIs. The 5-HT$_{1D}$ *beta* receptor gene has variants of the coding region which have been studied with preferential transmission of variant G861C (C-to-G) substitution preferentially transmitted to affecteds [58, 59] with other partial replications [60].

6.2.2.3 Dopamine. Both animal and human imaging studies have underlined the involvement of the dopaminergic system in repetitive behaviors [61, 62]. The association with movement disorders and basal ganglia disease and the well-documented efficacy of the D$_2$-blocking agent haloperidol as an augmenting agent all implicate the dopamine system in OCD. For a recent review, see [63]. There is evidence that the dopamine transporter density in the basal ganglia differs in unmedicated OCD patients in comparison to normal controls [30], suggesting further that the dopamineric neurotransmitter system is involved in the pathophysiology of OCD. The *DRD4* gene codes for a receptor with several functional polymorphisms in the form of variable numbers of tandem repeats (VNTR) identified within a particular intracellular peptide segment. The 7 repeat has been linked to ADHD, but several studies have found this association with OCD (although the specific allelic associations have been inconsistent [64–67]).

6.2.2.4 Glutamate. Several lines of evidence suggest that OCD could be a consequence of glutamatergic dysfunction. Brain imaging profiles (reviewed above) using a variety of neuroimaging techniques demonstrate alterations in the OFC, basal ganglia, and thalamus which normalize with treatment [68, 69]. These regions are linked in circuits within which glutamate is the primary excitatory neurotransmitter [70–72]. Moreover, a transgenic mouse model (see below) suggests aggravation of TD/OCD-like behavior with glutamatergic drugs [73]. Positive associations have been reported for NMDA receptors (GRIN2B) [72] and for GRIK2 (a kainate receptor) recently also associated with autism [71].

6.2.2.5 Neurotransmitter Metabolism. The X chromosome *MAOA* gene encodes monoamine oxidase A which is found in serotonergic and catecholaminergic brain neurons. (There are, however, no controlled studies indicating efficacy of MAO inhibitor drugs in OCD.) A polymorphism MAOA Eco/Rv was found to be significantly more frequent in OCD females in two studies [74, 75]. The enzyme catechol-*O*-methyl transferase (COMT) is the major degradation enzyme for catecholamine neurotransmitters. A Val–Met substitution polymorphism in codon 158 results in low enzymatic activity [76]. COMT's location in the 22q11 region associates it with VCFS, and, as mentioned above, children with VCFS frequently manifest anxiety and OCD [54].

6.2.2.6 Developmental Genes. There have been isolated reports of genes related to neurodevelopment. Hoxb8, a member of the mammalian homeobox-containing group of transcription factors, is of interest as disruption shows excessive grooming in mice [77, 78]. The developmental gene brain-derived neurotrophic factor (BDNF) was found to show significant association with OCD [79]. This is an interesting, if nonspecific, finding which bears replication.

Although genetic studies of OCD have been productive in yielding several replicated significant associations, none yet leads to new insight with respect to the neuropharmacology of OCD. One exception may be the finding of association with the mu opioid receptor [80] (see discussion of new clinical agents in Section 6.3).

6.2.3 Animal Models of OCD

Animal models are of interest in OCD for several reasons. Many OCD habits such as grooming, checking, and avoidance of fecal contamination have led to ethological models for this disorder. This implies the notion of highly conserved neural circuitry for such behavior. Unfortunately, efforts to elucidate the neural circuitry subserving OCD have been hampered by the lack of good animal models and, while some appealing "semiclinical" models (such as canine acral lick) have been published [81], other models have provided contradictory evidence [82–84]. Unlike movement disorders, many of the behaviors that are seen in OCD are inherently unique to humans (e.g., the belief that the thoughts or behaviors are senseless).

One proposed model is schedule-induced polydipsia (SIP). Food-deprived rats drink excessively when exposed to an intermittent feeding schedule, and SIP may be a displacement behavior in response to stress [85]. SSRIs reduce SIP and displacement behaviors after 14–21 days of treatment, suggesting a parallel with treatment of OCD in humans [86]. This parallel may be deceiving, however, as other antianxiety agents may increase SIP [87]. Some animal models are intriguing, such as the quinpirole (an agonist of D_2-like dopamine receptors) rat model in which repetitive cleaning behaviors are partially ameliorated by clomipramine [84]; this model focuses interest on the role of dopamine in the disorder [88]. In spite of appealing face validity (e.g., [89]), a variety of neurotransmitter systems are implicated [90]. A transgenic mouse model of comorbid TD and OCD was created by expressing a neuropotentiating cholera toxin transgene in a subset of dopamine D_1 receptors expressing neurons thought to induce cortical and amygdala glutamate output [91, 92]. It is anticipated that future models using the serotonin transporter and other putative genes will be fruitful.

To date, however, the best animal models have been inspired by the known brain circuitry of OCD. A series of studies from France has addressed regional control within the basal ganglia in primates that mediate some stereotypic and ticlike movements which might be seen as relevant to TD or possibly OCD [93, 94]. These studies utilized microinjections of bicuculline, a GABA antagonist, into various territories of the external globus pallidus (GPe). The regions were selected based on the known striato-pallidal projections to sensorimotor, associative, and limbic regions. The authors hypothesized that while sensorimotor territory injections would induce reversible abnormal movements, injections into the associative and limbic territories of the GPe would produce behavioral disorders. In fact, the bicuculline microinjections induced stereotypy when performed in the limbic part of the GPe (and ADHD-type behaviors when performed in the associative part); this is of particular interest when taken together with the modified view of the prefrontal–basal ganglia circuitry (see Fig. 6.2b) in which direct frontal GPe connectivity is now included in the model.

6.3 CLINICAL PSYCHOPHARMACOLOGY

This section focuses on selective studies addressing the major neuropharmacological issues in OCD, but excellent more general treatment reviews are available [95].

6.3.1 Effective Monotherapies: Controlled Trials

The past two decades have seen highly consistent findings that drugs that inhibit reuptake of serotonin either nonselectively (clomipramine) or selectively provide significant benefit for OCD. The major controlled trials are summarized in Table 6.1. Where pediatric trials have also been carried out, these are included. The selective effect of the SSRIs is particularly important here, as one or two double-blind comparisons with selective noradrenergic uptake inhibitors (e.g., desipramine [96]) show no efficacy of the noradrenergic medication. The well-documented efficacy of SSRIs for OCD has transformed the treatment of the disorder which earlier was treated predominantly with psychotherapy. It further differentiates OCD from depression and other anxiety disorders which may respond well to other agents predominantly affecting NE metabolism.

Table 6.1 contains representative high-quality studies documenting the efficacy for the serotonin uptake inhibitors in OCD. While clomipramine had a slightly more troublesome side-effect profile (including dry mouth, constipation, and some EKG changes), there is some consensus that it is more effective than the more selective serotonin uptake inhibiting agents. It is beyond the scope of this chapter to review the adverse effects of each of the drugs presented here. While the SSRIs are the best tolerated medications for OCD, some subjects, particularly children, have significant side effects, such as agitation, nausea, and in a small percent of cases an increased risk of suicidal ideation [115, 116]. However, generally the effect size for SRIs in OCD is substantial, and the suicidal thoughts occur early in treatment and can be handled with careful monitoring during this period.

It is also beyond the scope of this chapter to review behavioral treatment of OCD, but the reader should be aware that many find cognitive behavior therapy to be as important or more so than drug treatment for this condition [117, 118].

6.3.2 Augmenting Agents

Because the majority of patients classified as "responders" have only partial response to monotherapy with serotonin drugs, it is significant that a small but important group of controlled trials has shown benefit from the addition of another agent. These are considered augmenting agents as their effect appears to be only in conjunction with a SRI. Benefit has been shown most consistently for typical and atypical antipsychotic agents. Pharmacological augmentation strategies for treatment-resistant OCD are also well covered in a recent review [119]. Table 6.2 shows controlled trials for augmenting agents in OCD.

Table 6.2 contains a selective list of high-quality placebo-controlled studies that document the efficacy of typical and atypical antipsychotics as augmenting agents added to selective or nonselective SRIs. A single, as yet unpublished controlled trial also documented the efficacy of clonazepam as an augmenting agent [128], but the typical and atypical antipsychotics remain the only group of medications for which

TABLE 6.1 Serotonin Uptake Inhibitor Efficacy in OCD

Study	N	Design and Dose	Results	Comments
Clomipramine				
Adults: Katz et al., 1990 [97]	263	10 wks; 100–300 mg/d	>50% of CMI group (vs. <5% for placebo) became subclinical, based on NIMH-OC ($p<0.001$)	Efficacy shown in acute trial and maintained in a 1-yr DB extension
Children: DeVeaugh-Geiss et al., 1992 [98]	60	8 wks; max. daily dose: 3 mg/kg or 200 mg, whichever less	Mean CY-BOCS reduction: 37% (vs. 8% for placebo) ($p<0.05$)	Side effects typical of tricyclic antidepressants; efficacy maintained in 1-yr OL extension
Fluoxetine				
Adults: Montgomery et al., 1993 [99]	214	8 wks; fixed dose: 20, 40, 60 mg/d	40 and 60 mg were superior; response rates (Y-BOCS and CGI): 40 mg: 47%; 60 mg: 48%; 26%, 20%, 36%) ($p<0.05$)	16-wk controlled extension offered for responders; response maintained; nonresponders improved in OL extension on 60 mg
Adults: Tollefson et al., 1994 [100]; Tollefson et al., 1994 [101]	355	13 wks; fixed dose: 20, 40, 60 mg/d	All doses superior to placebo; response rates (Y-BOCS): 32–35% for all doses (vs. 8% for placebo) ($p<0.001$)	13 wks was minimum to see effects of 20 mg; in OL extension, responders maintained acute trial gains and 60 mg yielded added benefit; late-emergent adverse events: asthenia (11%), rhinitis (10%), flu syndrome (10%), abnormal dreams (9%)
Children: Geller et al., 2001 [102]	103	13 wks; max. dose: 60 mg/d	Response rates (CY-BOCS): 49% (vs. 25% for placebo) ($p=0.03$)	20–60 mg/d effective and well tolerated; side effects and drop-out rates similar for drug and placebo
Fluvoxamine				
Adults: Goodman et al., 1997 [103]	320	10 wks; max. dose: 300 mg/d	Response rates (CGI): 43% (vs. 11% for placebo) (p not provided)	Of all on fluvoxamine, mean Y-BOCS at wk 10 still in moderate range; of responders, mean decreased to mild range
Adults: Hollander et al., 2003 [104]	253	12 wks; 100–300 mg/d of CR fluvoxamine	Response rates (CGI-I): 44% (vs. 23% for placebo) ($p=0.002$)	Excluded from study if history of nonresponse to SRIs; response seen at wk 2; CR allows for more aggressive dosing

Children: Riddle et al., 2001 [105]	120	10 wks; 50–200 mg/d	Based on CY-BOCS, significant differences seen as early as wk 1 ($p = 0.007$); response rates (CY-BOCS): 42% (vs. 26% for placebo) ($p = 0.06$)	Rapid onset of action
Sertraline				
Adults: Greist et al., 1995 [106]; Greist et al., 1995 [107]	324	12 wks; fixed dose: 50, 100, 200 mg/d	Pooled sertraline group better than placebo, based on Y-BOCS ($p = 0.006$) and CGI-I ($p = 0.01$); response rates (CGI-I): 39% (vs. 30% for placebo)	Larger placebo effect than usual; those completing 3 mos of sertraline continued to improve during 40-wk extension
Adults: Koran et al., 2002 [108]	223	649 pts in 16-wk, flexible dose, SB trial; responders got additional 36 wks SB; 223 responders at 52 wks got 28 wks of 50–200 mg/d DB	During DB, sertraline better than placebo on 2 of 3 primary outcomes: dropout due to relapse/poor response (9% vs. 24%) ($p = 0.006$) and acute exacerbation of symptoms (12% vs. 35%) ($p = 0.001$)	Long-term treatment generally well tolerated; efficacy sustained among prior responders
Children: March et al., 1998 [109]	187	12 wks; up to 200 mg/d at 4 wks, then maintained for 8 more wks	Response rates (CGI-I): 42% (vs. 26% for placebo) ($p = 0.02$)	Short-term safety and effectiveness shown; efficacy differences seen at wk 3 and persisted
Paroxetine				
Adults: Hollander et al., 2003 [110]	348	12 wks; fixed dose: 20, 40, 60 mg/d	40 and 60 mg/d effective ($p < 0.05$); mean CY-BOCS reduction: 40 mg: 25%, 60 mg: 29% (vs. placebo: 13%, 20 mg: 16%)	Long-term effectiveness shown (263 acute trial responders enrolled in 6-mo, flexible dose, OL trial; 105 responders to that OL trial randomized to 6 mo, fixed dose, DB trial); some mild discontinuation symptoms if abruptly stop

(*continued*)

TABLE 6.1 (Continued)

Study	N	Design and Dose	Results	Comments
Adults: Kamijima et al., 2004 [111]	191	12 wks; 20–50 mg/d	Response rates (Y-BOCS): 50% (vs. 24% for placebo) ($p = 0.0003$)	Effective and generally well tolerated; those not adequately responding to suggested dose of 40 mg/d may benefit from 50 mg/d
Adults: Zohar & Judge, 1996 [112]	406	12 wks; paroxetine: 20–60 mg/d; CMI: 50–250 mg/d	Response rates (Y-BOCS): 55% for paroxetine ($p = 0.001$) and 55% for CMI ($p = 0.005$) (vs. 35% for placebo)	Paroxetine more effective than placebo and comparable to CMI; paroxetine better tolerated than CMI, based on some measures; more anticholinergic adverse events for CMI (53%) than paroxetine (28%), 12% for placebo
Children: Geller et al., 2004 [113]	207	10 wks; 10–50 mg/d	Response rates (CY-BOCS): 65% (vs. 41% for placebo) ($p = 0.002$)	Effective and generally well tolerated; especially gradual titration and tapering suggested due to nonlinear pharmacokinetics
Citalopram				
Adults: Montgomery et al., 2001 [114]	401	12 wks; fixed dose: 20, 40, 60 mg/d	Response rates (Y-BOCS): 20 mg: 57%, 40 mg: 52%, 60 mg: 65% (vs. 37% for placebo) ($p < 0.05$)	All three doses more effective than placebo; need larger sample to see effects of different doses; suggest starting at 20 mg, although 60 mg may be useful if need rapid response

Note: Unless noted, studies are multicenter, randomized, double-blind, placebo-controlled, acute trials with parallel design. Information on extension trials, if conducted, is provided under Comments. CGI: Clinical Global Impressions; CGI-I: Clinical Global Impressions-Improvement scores; CMI: clomipramine; DB: double blind; SB: single blind; NIMH-OC: National Institute of Mental Health Global Obsessive-Compulsive Rating Scale; OL: open label; Y-BOCS: Yale-Brown Obsessive-Compulsive Scale; CY-BOCS: Children's Yale-Brown Obsessive-Compulsive Scale; CR: controlled release.

TABLE 6.2 Controlled Trials of Augmenting Agents in Adults with OCD: Typical and Atypical Antipsychotics

Study	N	Design and Dose	Results	Comments
Haloperidol				
McDougle et al., 1994 [120]	34	OCD pts (with or without a secondary chronic tic d/o) refractory to 8 wks of fluvoxamine (max of 300 mg/d given for over 7 wks) given 4 wks haloperidol or placebo addition; haloperidol dose: 2 mg/d for 3 days, increased by 2 mg every 3 days, to a max of 10 mg/d	Based on Y-BOCS and CGI, 11/17 (65%) responded (vs. 0/17 for placebo) ($p < 0.0002$); of those with comorbid chronic tics, 8/8 responded [vs. 3 (33%) of 9 without tics or family history of tics] ($p = 0.007$)	Support for role of dopamine dysregulation in some OCD patients, particularly those with tic disorder; little or no benefit if no tic disorder; risk of tardive dyskinesia
Risperidone				
McDougle et al., 2000 [42]	36	Patients with primary OCD treated for 6 wks with risperidone ($N = 20$) or placebo ($N = 16$) addition to their SRI; risperidone started at 1 mg/d for 1 wk, with dosage increased 1 mg every week until max of 6 mg/d, as tolerated	Of study completers and based on CGI, 9/18 (50%) responded (vs. 0/15 for placebo) ($p < 0.005$)	Patients with or without comorbid tic disorder or schizotypal personality disorder may benefit; mild transient sedation; risk of tardive dyskinesia
Hollander et al., 2003 [121]	16	Patients treated for 8 wks with risperidone or placebo addition; risperidone initiated at 0.5 mg/d and gradually increased by 0.5 mg/d every 7 days over first 6 wks until max of 3 mg/d or experienced therapeutic effects or side effects	Based on Y-BOCS and CGI, 4/10 (40%) responded (vs. 0/6 for placebo) ($p = 0.12$)	Small sample but consistent with literature indicating 30–50% benefit from atypical antipsychotic addition

(*continued*)

TABLE 6.2 (*Continued*)

Study	N	Design and Dose	Results	Comments
Erzegovesi et al., 2005 [122]	39	After 12 wks of OL fluvoxamine monotherapy (max of 300 mg/d; initial study $N = 45$), both responders and nonresponders (total $N = 39$) randomly assigned to 6-wk DB addition of low-dose (0.5 mg) risperidone or placebo; fluvoxamine dose maintained	Significant interaction of "add-on treatment" × "response" × "time" ($p = 0.001$); based on Y-BOCS and CGI, during DB phase, 5 (50%) on risperidone and 2 (20%) on placebo became responders	Low dose effective; add-on treatment effective *only* in fluvoxamine-resistant subgroup; fluvoxamine-responder group had poorer effect of addition than did placebo group
Olanzapine				
Bystritsky et al., 2004 [123]	26	Treatment-refractory patients without significant comorbidity treated for 6 wks with olanzapine (started at 2.5 mg, increased to 5 mg/d for days 4–7, then 5–20 mg/day) or placebo, while continuing their SRI at stable dose	Based on Y-BOCS, 6/13 (46%) responded (vs. 0/13 for placebo) ($p = 0.01$), with mean Y-BOCS decreasing 16% in olanzapine addition group	Effect on OCD symptoms appears not to be due to antipsychotic or mood-stabilizing effects; no extrapyramidal side effects; of olanzapine patients, two (15%) discontinued: one due to lack of effect and sedation, one due to weight gain
Shapira et al., 2004 [124]	44	Partial or nonresponders to 8-wk OL fluoxetine trial (40 mg in almost all pts) treated with 6 wks olanzapine (5–10 mg) or placebo addition to fluoxetine	Groups similar; based on Y-BOCS, both groups improved over time	May have needed longer prior monotherapy

Quetiapine

Denys et al., 2004 [125]	40	Patients without significant comorbidity treated for 8 wks of up to 300 mg/d quetiapine or placebo, in addition to their SRI; quetiapine initiated at dose of 50 mg/d and increased at fixed schedule (wks 1–2: 100 mg/d; wks 3–6: 200 mg/d; wks 7–8: 300 mg/d)	Based on Y-BOCS and CGI, 8/20 (40%) responded [vs. 2/20 (10%) for placebo ($p = 0.03$)]	Effective, especially for severe obsessions; response seen within 4–6 wks; most common side effects: somnolence, dry mouth, weight gain, dizziness

Buspirone (Anxiolytic)

Grady et al., 1993 [126]	14	Crossover design, 4 wks each, placebo and buspirone addition to ongoing fluoxetine; buspirone dosage increased over 2 wks; all had stable dose of 60 mg/d for final 2 wks of active treatment	No significant effect of drug; only one patient had clinically meaningful response to buspirone (vs. 0 for placebo)	Parallels earlier study by same group showing lack of improvement for buspirone added to CMI; one patient withdrew after a seizure
McDougle et al., 1993 [127]	33	OCD patients refractory to 8 wks of fluvoxamine (up to 300 mg/d) given 6 wks buspirone ($N = 19$; initially 15 mg/d in 3 divided doses, then increased by 15 mg every other day to a max of 60 mg/d in 3 divided doses) or placebo ($N = 14$) addition to fluvoxamine continued at the same dose	No differences: based on Y-BOCS and CGI, 2/19 (11%) responded [vs. 2/14 (14%) for placebo]	Negative study

(*continued*)

TABLE 6.2 (Continued)

Study	N	Design and Dose	Results	Comments
Clonazepam (Anxiolytic)				
Pigott et al., 1992 [128]	18	2–6 mg/d added to ongoing CMI or fluoxetine (other information not available)	Added benefit demonstrated on 1 of 3 OCD rating scales	Benzodiazepine with preferential effects on serotonergic system; especially helpful if anxiety prominent; improvement seen in hours to days; typically started at 0.5 mg once or twice daily, with max of 5 mg/d when used as an antiobsessional
Desipramine (TCA)				
Barr et al., 1997 [129]	33	Desipramine or placebo added for 6 or 10 wks to SSRI treatment; desipramine daily dose adjusted weekly to obtain plasma level > 125 ng/mL if tolerated; mean final plasma level was 148.3 ng/mL (SD = 82.0)	Based on Y-BOCS, there was no drug-by-time interaction at wk 6 ($p = 0.07$) or wk 10 ($p = 0.45$)	Desipramine's relatively specific inhibition of norepinephrine reuptake was not an effective addition [30 patients completed 6 wks; 25 of these enrolled in extension; 23 (10 on desipramine, 13 on placebo) completed 10 wks]
Nortriptyline (TCA)				
Noorbala et al., 1998 [130]	30	DB nortriptyline (50 mg/d) or placebo added to 150 mg/d CMI for 8 wks	Based on Y-BOCS, both improved; but active addition showed advantage by wk 4 ($p = 0.007$); by wk 8, $p < 0.0001$	Rapid onset of action; (sample mostly female)

Lithium

McDougle et al., 1991 [131]	30	Two trials: 2-wk ($N=20$) and 4-wk ($N=10$) augmentation of ongoing fluvoxamine (200–300 mg/d); lithium initially given at 900 mg/d in 3 divided doses; dosages then adjusted to keep serum levels between 0.5 and 1.2 mmol/L	Significant change in Y-BOCS and CGI in trial 1 ($p<0.05$) but not in trial 2; based on Y-BOCS and CGI, 2/11 (18%) and 0/5 of patients having 2 wks or 4 wks, respectively, of lithium addition were responders (vs. 0/9 and 0/5 for placebo)	Generally not effective; some OL treatment also given subsequently; even 4 wks was not effective for most

Pindolol

Dannon et al., 2000 [132]	16	6 wks of pindolol ($N=8$; 2.5 mg t.i.d.) vs. placebo ($N=6$) addition to paroxetine (up to 60 mg/d)	Based on Y-BOCS, pindolol was superior to placebo ($p<0.01$) after wk 4	Results based on $N=14$ as two placebo patients dropped out

Inositol

Fux et al., 1999 [133]	10	Crossover design with 18 g/d inositol or placebo for 6 wks each, in addition to ongoing SRI (dosage range was 40–60 mg/d for fluoxetine; 200–250 mg/d for fluvoxamine; 150–225 mg/d for CMI)	Both groups improved ($p<0.000$); no significant group differences	No added effects from inositol (putative site of action intracellular; SRIs synaptic)

Note: Unless noted, studies are double blind and placebo controlled with SRI-refractory OCD patients. CGI: Clinical Global Impressions; DB: double blind; OL: open label; SRI: serotonin reuptake inhibitor; SSRI: selective serotonin reuptake inhibitor; TCA: tricyclic antidepressant; Y-BOCS: Yale-Brown Obsessive-Compulsive Scale.

there are really well-documented augmenting effects for the treatment of OCD. Increased clarity regarding criteria for defining treatment resistance and nonresponse would be useful in studies of augmenting agents and treatment in general [134].

6.3.3 Miscellaneous Pharmacological Trials of Interest

Tables 6.1 and 6.2 do not include unblinded trials or double-blind comparisons of active agents that do not also include a placebo. However, there is an intriguing list of agents for which either convincing case series or small controlled trials suggest other pharmacotherapies. Some small open studies indicate that tramadol (a mu opioid agonist) may be efficacious for OCD [135, 136]. Also, anecdotal evidence and a recent small short-term placebo-controlled, double-blind study [137, 138] suggest that oral morphine sulfate may be of benefit in treatment-resistant OCD, although, among other questions, it is unclear how often the drug should be administered. While clonazepam is widely used as an anxiolytic in OCD, a recent double-blind placebo-controlled study showed no evidence for its usefulness as monotherapy [139]. One early study examined clonazepam as an augmenting agent (see Table 6.2); an early crossover study provided initial support for its usefulness as monotherapy [140]). Other studies suggest that venlafaxine, a serotonin–norepinephrine reuptake inhibitor might be effective as monotherapy or augmenting agent [119, 141, 142]; see [143] for a review. A small study of nicotine patches given to nonsmoking OCD patients found significant improvement compared to placebo [144]; this most probably reflects a nonspecific anxiolytic effect of nicotine. Lastly, in light of evidence of hyperactivity of glutamatergic circuits in OCD, an interesting new direction involves riluzole, an antiglutamatergic agent that currently is under open-label study in adults (also, for a related published case report, see [145]).

6.3.4 Induction of Obsessive-Compulsive Symptoms

Evidence is particularly impressive that antipsychotics may augment SRI treatment of OCD. In contrast to this effect is the growing number of case reports documenting the provocation or worsening of OCD with both typical and atypical antipsychotics [146]. There has been some impression that this effect is more salient with clozapine. Speculatively, the 5-HT_2 antagonist effect of the atypical antipsychotics may disinhibit dopamine neurons, producing increased output from the orbitofrontal/cingulate cortex and thus precipitating or exacerbating OCD based on the model circuitry shown above [147]. It also has been speculated that the D_2 and 5-HT_2 receptor occupancy of atypical antipsychotics at low doses may actually antagonize the SSRI effects. Management suggestions have therefore included a trial of increased dose of the atypical agent before discontinuation [148]. Following an analysis of the effects of the nonselective 5-HT receptor agonist mCPP, which worsened OCD symptoms, a small double-blind study found that sumatriptan, a 5-HT_{1D} receptor agonist, also worsened OCD symptoms [149]. Finally, a preliminary study indicated that the mu opioid antagonist naloxone exacerbates OCD symptoms [150], although, paradoxically, another mu opioid antagonist, naltrexone, showed some efficacy in treating compulsive self-injurious behavior [151].

6.3.5 Immunomodulatory Treatments

Based on the observation that some childhood-onset OCD patients had onset apparently in relationship to infection with group A β-hemolytic streptococcus (GABHS), a subgroup of children were proposed who were hypothesized to have an autoimmune-based form of the disorder. As a partial test of this model, two treatments were examined. In the first, a controlled treatment trial of intravenous immunoglobulin (IVIG; 1 g/kg/day on two consecutive days) was carried out. The second was an open trial of plasmapheresis consisting of four to five single volume exchanges over a two-week period. These extremely interesting findings have not yet been replicated. A single trial of penicillin prophylaxis was negative [152]. In spite of growing evidence linking GABHS infection and onset of OCD [153], there remains only a single controlled trial documenting the efficacy of immunomodulatory treatment [154, 155].

6.4 EXPERIMENTAL NONPHARMACOLOGICAL TREATMENTS

In spite of the major advances in drug treatment of OCD over the past two decades, at least 10% of the OCD population remains severely affected. This amounts to hundreds of thousands of patients with a debilitating disease without effective treatment. Recent developments in techniques for direct brain manipulation have been applied both to neurological and psychiatric disorders. Given the close connection between OCD and a variety of movement disorders, it is of great interest that selected neurosurgical lesions such as subcaudate tractotomy and deep brain stimulation (DBS) have been effective in the treatment of Parkinson's and other movement disorders. Selective reviews are given below with special focus on the implications for the circuitry and potential neuropharmacology of OCD.

6.4.1 Neurosurgery

The data on neurosurgical lesion treatment for OCD consist of open trials of small numbers of patients with intractable OCD and typically high rates of comorbid Axis I disorders. Response rates across centers vary from about 20 to 60% with varying diagnostic methods and surgical procedures across centers. No randomized double-blind trials have been reported [156]. Various lesions interrupting the CSTC loops have included: anterior capsulotomy, subcaudate tractotomy, limbic leucotomy, and anterior cingulotomy. These are summarized in Table 6.3 and, as seen, interrupt the major pathways in circuits shown in Figure 6.1.

The focus of neurosurgical lesions for OCD is principally to interrupt frontal–basal ganglia and frontal–limbic connections. Reports of success in OCD patients have followed open trials of anterior capsulotomy, a lesion that aims to target connections between dorsomedial thalamus and orbital and medial prefrontal cortex. The newer technique of gamma knife capsulotomy has, at least in theory, enabled controlled trials because of the noninvasive nature of a sham lesion. (The sites of neurosurgical lesions are also the focus for trials of DBS, which, similarly, lends itself more easily to controlled trials.) It is beyond the scope of this chapter to review these studies in greater detail in the absence of any controlled trials documenting efficacy.

However, it is important to note that the circuitry involved is the same as that implicated by brain imaging studies (see above).

6.4.2 Transcranial Magnetic Stimulation

Transcranial magnetic stimulation [TMS, or repetitive transcranial magnetic stimulation (rTMS)] has been proposed as therapeutic for various psychiatric disorders, mainly depression, although stimulation characteristics remain in dispute [158]. In OCD, TMS studies have been used to explore abnormal responsivity of brain circuits, with preliminary findings of decreased neuronal inhibition and a reduced cortical silent period in the primary motor area for TD and OCD [159, 160]. While preliminary, these studies provide suggestive complementary evidence of abnormalities in cortical motor circuitry. However, to date, TMS does not appear to be therapeutically useful in OCD, although this view is based on small sample studies [161, 162] and only a single controlled trial [161].

6.4.3 Deep Brain Stimulation

The realization that chronic high-frequency stimulation resulted in clinical benefits analogous to those of neurosurgical lesioning transformed the use of functional neurosurgery for the treatment of movement disorders (primarily tremor and Parkinson's disease). The use of the more flexible and reversible DBS techniques, instead of irreversible surgical ablations and tract lesions, has been expanded to the treatment of chronic pain and psychiatric disorders, particularly intractable depression and OCD [163]. The site of stimulation overlaps somewhat with the sites of surgical lesions described in Table 6.3 and Figures 6.1 and 6.2, although there is an impressive case report of ventral caudate stimulation [164]. Thalamic and basal ganglia stimulation are most frequently used for movement disorders [165]. DBS has largely replaced pallidotomy in the treatment of Parkinson's disease.

The clinical applications have preceded the scientific understanding of the mechanisms of action of DBS, and it has been puzzling how stimulation initially thought to activate neurons could have therapeutic outcomes similar to those from lesioning of target structures. Basic work is still going on to address such fundamental topics as the volume of tissue influenced by DBS, the effects on neurotransmitter systems, and functional imaging of DBS, but several alternate hypotheses on the physiological changes induced by stimulation remain. From a neuropharmacological standpoint, it would appear that DBS affects glutamate, dopamine, and GABA systems [165]. To date, only a small number of studies have been published on DBS for OCD. Nuttin et al. [166] reported on the effects of stimulation of the internal capsule of four patients with OCD at a site described as identical to that used in capsulotomy. Beneficial effects were described in three of the four patients. The same group reported on long-term follow-up in six patients [167]. This latter study was of special interest as it included double-blind evaluation with and without the stimulation on. Three of the six were considered responders to chronic stimulation. There also has been a report of a single case with dramatic improvement [168]. Most recent is a study [169] of four cases with a short-term, blinded, off–on design and long-term, open follow-up; one patient improved dramatically during blinded and open treatment and a second showed moderate benefit during open follow-up. DBS

TABLE 6.3 Summary of Procedures for Modern Neurosurgery for Psychiatric Disorders

Procedure	Target	Rationale	Current Indications
Anterior cingulotomy	Anterior cingulum	Disconnect Papez circuit	Affective disorders, OCD, anxiety disorders
Subcaudate tractotomy	Frontobasal white matter	Disconnect frontolimbic connections	Affective disorders, OCD, anxiety disorders
Limbic leukotomy	Anterior cingulum and frontobasal white matter	Cingulotomy + subcaudate tractotomy	OCD, affective disorders
Capsulotomy	Anterior limb of internal capsule	Disconnect frontolimbic and caudate-putaminal connections	OCD, anxiety disorders, panic disorder

Source: From [157].

continues to be of interest as a probe of putative circuitry, as reports of improvement of obsessive-compulsive symptoms in patients with Parkinson's disorder, for example, suggest that subthalamic nucleus stimulation may also prove helpful [170]. For the moment, however, most work involves the placement of probes in the same area where subcaudate tractotomy is carried out, with some electrodes in part of the ventral striatum. It is clear that this is a very early stage of treatment development, but these small careful trials will be of importance in elucidating the circuitry of OCD with possible discovery of numerous possible etiologic sites for the disorder within the same circuitry.

6.5 SUMMARY

The advances of the last two decades have revolutionized our understanding and treatment of OCD. The disorder is now readily diagnosed by health care professionals, and appropriate treatments—drug treatment and behavior therapy—are available. Remarkably, the brain imaging studies have served to differentiate OCD from other anxiety disorders, and there is surprising agreement on the functional and some aspects of the anatomic abnormalities. Less successful have been the candidate gene studies, although the agreement of two independent linkage studies on a 9p locus is important. Also surprising is the degree to which there is some agreement on the gene for the D_4 receptor and 5-HT transporter in OCD. Efforts to subgroup the phenotype in terms of symptom profile have not been particularly successful, and considerably more work needs to be done, perhaps using other more neurobiological measures as alternate endophenotypes. Before this can be done, however, the conflicting data about whether brain imaging results reflect state or trait markers need to be resolved. To this end, twin and family imaging studies are needed for these and other biological measures. Such studies are ongoing at several sites.

REFERENCES

1. Karno, M., et al. (1988). The epidemiology of obsessive-compulsive disorder in five US communities. *Arch. Gen. Psychiatry* 45, 1094–1099.
2. Robins, L. N., et al. (1984). Lifetime prevalence of specific psychiatric disorders in three sites. *Arch. Gen. Psychiatry* 41(10), 949–958.
3. Rapoport, J. (1989). *Obsessive-Compulsive Disorder in Children and Adolescents*. American Psychiatric Press, Washington, DC.
4. Swinson, R. A. M., Rachman, S., and Richter, M. Eds. (1988). *Obsessive-Compulsive Disorder: Theory, Research, and Treatment*. Guilford Press, New York.
5. Pauls, D. L., et al. (1986). Gilles de la Tourette's syndrome and obsessive-compulsive disorder: Evidence supporting a genetic relationship. *Arch. Gen. Psychiatry* 43, 1180–1182.
6. Swedo, S. E. and Leonard, H. L. (1994). Childhood movement disorders and obsessive compulsive disorder. *J. Clin. Psychiatry* 55(Suppl), 32–37.
7. Swedo, S. E., Leonard, H. L., and Rapoport, J. L. (2004). The pediatric autoimmune neuropsychiatric disorders associated with streptococcal infection (PANDAS) subgroup: Separating fact from fiction. *Pediatrics* 113(4), 907–911.
8. Swedo, S. E., et al. (1997). Identification of children with pediatric autoimmune neuropsychiatric disorders associated with streptococcal infections by a marker associated with rheumatic fever [see comments]. *Am. J. Psychiatry* 15, 110–112.
9. DuPont, R. L., et al. (1995). Economic costs of obsessive-compulsive disorder. *Med. Interface* 8(4), 102–109.
10. Jenike, M. A. (2004). Clinical practice. Obsessive-compulsive disorder. *N. Engl. J. Med.* 350(3), 259–265.
11. Osler, W. (1894). *On Chorea and Choreiform Affections*. Blakiston & Sons, Philadelphia.
12. Modell, J. G., et al. (1989). Neurophysiologic dysfunction in basal ganglia/limbic striatal and thalamocortical circuits as a pathogenetic mechanism of obsessive-compulsive disorder [see comments]. *J. Neuropsychiatry Clin. Neurosci.* 1, 27–36.
13. Rapoport, J. L. (1991). Basal ganglia dysfunction as a proposed cause of obsessive-compulsive disorder. In *Psychopathology and the Brain*, B. J. Carroll and J. E. Barrett, Eds. Raven, New York, pp. 77–95.
14. Rapoport, J. L. (1989). The biology of obsessions and compulsions. *Sci. Am.* 260(3), 82–89.
15. Swedo, S. E., et al. (1989). High prevalence of obsessive-compulsive symptoms in patients with Sydenham's chorea. *Am. J. Psychiatry* 146(2), 246–249.
16. Behar, D., et al. (1984). Computerized tomography and neuropsychological test measures in adolescents with obsessive-compulsive disorder. *Am. J. Psychiatry* 141, 363–369.
17. Luxenberg, J., Swedo, S. E., and Flament, M. (1988). Neuroanatomical abnormalities in obsessive-compulsive disorder determined with quantitative X-ray computed tomography. *Am. J. Psychiatry* 145, 1089–1093.
18. Saxena, S., Bota, R. G., and Brody, A. L. (2001). Brain-behavior relationships in obsessive-compulsive disorder. *Semin. Clin. Neuropsychiatry* 6(2), 82–101.
19. Pujol, J., et al. (2004). Mapping structural brain alterations in obsessive-compulsive disorder. *Arch. Gen. Psychiatry* 61(7), 720–730.

20. Jenike, M. A., et al. (1966). Cerebral structural abnormalities in obsessive-compulsive disorder: A quantitative morphometric magnetic resonance imaging study. *Arch. Gen. Psychiatry* 53, 625–632.
21. Chacko, R., Corbin, M., and Harper, R. (2000). Acquired obsessive-compulsive disorder associated with basal ganglia lesions. *J. Neuropsychiatry Clin. Neurosci.* 12, 269–272.
22. Szeszko, P. R., et al. (2004). Brain structural abnormalities in psychotropic drug-naive pediatric patients with obsessive-compulsive disorder. *Am. J. Psychiatry* 161(6), 1049–1056.
23. Whiteside, S., Port, J., and Abramowitz, J. (2004). A meta-analysis of functional neuroimaging in obsessive-compulsive disorder. *Psychiatry Res.: Neuroimaging* 132, 69–79.
24. Rauch, S. L., et al. (1994). Regional cerebral blood flow measured during symptom provocation in obsessive-compulsive disorder using oxygen 15-labeled carbon dioxide and positron emission tomography [see comments]. *Arch. Gen. Psychiatry* 51, 62–70.
25. Hendler, T., et al. (2003). Brain reactivity to specific symptom provocation indicates prospective therapeutic outcome in OCD. *Psychiatry Res.* 124(2), 87–103.
26. Martis, B., et al. (2004). Functional magnetic resonance imaging evidence for a lack of striatal dysfunction during implicit sequence learning in individuals with animal phobia. *Am. J. Psychiatry* 161(1), 67–71.
27. Baxter, L. R., et al. (1992). Caudate glucose metabolic rate changes with both drug and behavior therapy for obsessive-compulsive disorder. *Arch. Gen. Psychiatry* 49(9), 681–689.
28. Schwartz, J. M., et al. (1996). Systematic changes in cerebral glucose metabolic rate after successful behavior modification treatment of obsessive-compulsive disorder. *Arch. Gen. Psychiatry* 53(2), 109–113.
29. Kilts, C. (2003). In vivo neuroimaging correlates of the efficacy of paroxetine in the treatment of mood and anxiety disorders. *Psychopharmacol. Bull.* 37(Suppl 1), 19–28.
30. Kim, C. H., et al. (2003). Dopamine transporter density of basal ganglia assessed with [123I]IPT SPET in obsessive-compulsive disorder. *Eur. J. Nucl. Med. Mol. Imaging* 30(12), 1637–1643.
31. Pogarell, O., et al. (2003). Elevated brain serotonin transporter availability in patients with obsessive-compulsive disorder. *Biol. Psychiatry* 54(12), 1406–1413.
32. van der Wee, N. J., et al. (2004). Enhanced dopamine transporter density in psychotropic-naive patients with obsessive-compulsive disorder shown by [123I]{beta}-CIT SPECT. *Am. J. Psychiatry* 161(12), 2201–2206.
33. Simpson, H. B., et al. (2003). Serotonin transporters in obsessive-compulsive disorder: A positron emission tomography study with [(11)C]McN 5652. *Biol. Psychiatry* 54(12), 1414–1421.
34. Rosenberg, D. R., MacMillan, S. N., and Moore, G. J. (2001). Brain anatomy and chemistry may predict treatment response in paediatric obsessive-compulsive disorder. *Int. J. Neuropsychopharmacol.* 4(2), 179–190.
35. Rosenberg, D. R., et al. (2000). Decrease in caudate glutamatergic concentrations in pediatric obsessive-compulsive disorder patients taking paroxetine. *J. Am. Acad. Child Adolesc. Psychiatry* 39(9), 1096–1103.
36. Benazon, N. R., Moore, G. J., and Rosenberg, D. R. (2003). Neurochemical analyses in pediatric obsessive-compulsive disorder in patients treated with cognitive-behavioral therapy. *J. Am. Acad. Child Adolesc. Psychiatry* 42(11), 1279–1285.

37. Rapoport, J., and Wise, S. (1988). Obsessive-compulsive disorder: Evidence for basal ganglia dysfunction. *Psychol. Bull.* 24, 380–384.
38. Insel, T. R. (1992). Toward a neuroanatomy of obsessive-compulsive disorder. *Arch. Gen. Psychiatry* 49, 739–744.
39. Baxter, L. R. Jr., et al. (1996). Brain mediation of obsessive-compulsive disorder symptoms: Evidence from functional brain imaging studies in the human and nonhuman primate. *Sem. Clin. Neuropsychiatry* 1, 32–47.
40. Alexander, G., DeLong, M., and Strick, P. (1986). Parallel organization of functionally segregated circuits linking basal ganglia and cortex. *Annu. Rev. Neurosci.* 9, 357–381.
41. Graybiel, A. M. (1990). Neurotransmitters and neuromodulators in the basal ganglia. *Trends Neurosci.* 13, 244–254.
42. McDougle, C. J., et al. (2000). A double-blind, placebo-controlled study of risperidone addition in serotonin reuptake inhibitor-refractory obsessive-compulsive disorder. *Arch. Gen. Psychiatry* 57(8), 794–801.
43. Kopell, B. J., Greenberg, B. D., and Rezai, A. R. (2004). Deep brain stimulation for psychiatric disorders. *J. Clin. Neurophysiology* 21, 51–67.
44. Flament, M. F., and Bisserbe, J. C. (1997). Pharmacologic treatment of obsessive-compulsive disorder: Comparative studies. *J. Clin. Psychiatry* 58(Suppl 12), 18–22.
45. Thoren, P., et al. (1980). Clomipramine treatment of obsessive-compulsive disorder. I. A controlled clinical trial. *Arch. Gen. Psychiatry* 37, 1281–1285.
46. Stahl, S. (1977). *Essential Psychopharmacology: Neuroscientific Basis and Practical Applications.* Cambridge University Press, Cambridge, England.
47. Micallef, J., and Blin, O. (2001). Neurobiology and clinical pharmacology of obsessive-compulsive disorder. *Clin. Neuropharmacol.* 24(4), 191–207.
48. Jonnal, A. H., et al. (2000). Obsessive and compulsive symptoms in a general population sample of female twins. *Am. J. Med. Genet.* 96(6), 791–796.
49. Grados, M. A., Walkup, J., and Walford, S. (2003). Genetics of obsessive-compulsive disorders: New findings and challenges. *Brain Dev.* 25(Suppl 1), S55–61.
50. Lochner, C., et al. (2004). Gender in obsessive-compulsive disorder: Clinical and genetic findings. *Eur. Neuropsychopharmacol.* 14(2), 105–113.
51. Hanna, G. L., et al. (2002). Genome-wide linkage analysis of families with obsessive-compulsive disorder ascertained through pediatric probands. *Am. J. Med. Genet.* 114(5), 541–552.
52. Willour, V. L., et al. (2004). Replication study supports evidence for linkage to 9p24 in obsessive-compulsive disorder. *Am. J. Hum. Genet.* 75(3), 508–513.
53. Murphy, K. C. (2002). Schizophrenia and velo-cardio-facial syndrome. *Lancet* 359(9304), 426–430.
54. Pulver, A. E., et al. (1994). Psychotic illness in patients diagnosed with velo-cardio-facial syndrome and their relatives. *J. Nerv. Ment. Dis.* 182(8), 476–478.
55. Gothelf, D., et al. (2004). Obsessive-compulsive disorder in patients with velocardiofacial (22q11 deletion) syndrome. *Am. J. Med. Genet.* 126B(1), 99–105.
56. Bengel, D., et al. (1999). Association of the serotonin transporter promoter regulatory region polymorphism and obsessive-compulsive disorder. *Mol. Psychiatry* 4(5), 463–466.
57. Hoyer, D., et al. (1986). Serotonin receptors in the human brain. I. Characterization and autoradiographic localization of 5-HT1A recognition sites. Apparent absence of 5-HT1B recognition sites. *Brain Res.* 376(1), 85–96.

58. Mundo, E., et al. (2002). 5HT1Dbeta receptor gene implicated in the pathogenesis of obsessive-compulsive disorder: Further evidence from a family-based association study. *Mol. Psychiatry* 7(7), 805–809.

59. Mundo, E., et al. (2000). Is the 5-HT(1Dbeta) receptor gene implicated in the pathogenesis of obsessive-compulsive disorder?. *Am. J. Psychiatry* 157(7), 1160–1161.

60. Camarena, B., et al. (2004). A family based association study of the 5-HT-1Dbeta receptor gene in obsessive-compulsive disorder. *Int. J. Neuropsychopharmacol.* 7(1), 49–53.

61. Graybiel, A. M., Canales, J. J., and Capper-Loup, C. (2000). Levodopa-induced dyskinesias and dopamine-dependent stereotypies: A new hypothesis. *Trends Neurosci.* 23(10 Suppl), S71–77.

62. Canales, J. J., et al. (2002). Shifts in striatal responsivity evoked by chronic stimulation of dopamine and glutamate systems. *Brain* 125(Pt 10), 2353–2363.

63. Denys, D., Zohar, J., and Westenberg, H. G. (2004). The role of dopamine in obsessive-compulsive disorder: Preclinical and clinical evidence. *J. Clin. Psychiatry* 65(Suppl 1), 11–17.

64. Cruz, C., et al. (1997). Increased prevalence of the seven-repeat variant of the dopamine D4 receptor gene in patients with obsessive-compulsive disorder with tics. *Neurosci. Lett.* 231(1), 1–4.

65. Nicolini, H., et al. (1998). [Dopamine D2 and D4 receptor genes distinguish the clinical presence of tics in obsessive-compulsive disorder]. *Gac. Med. Mex.* 134(5), 521–527.

66. Billett, E. A., Richter, M. A., and Kennedy, J. L. (1998). Genetics of obsessive-compulsive disorder. In *Obsessive-Compulsive Disorder: Theory, Research, and Treatment*, R. P. Swinson, et al., Eds. Guilford Press, New York, pp. 181–206.

67. Millet, B., et al. (2003). Association between the dopamine receptor D4 (DRD4) gene and obsessive-compulsive disorder. *Am. J. Med. Genet.* 116B(1), 55–59.

68. Carlsson, M. L. (2000). On the role of cortical glutamate in obsessive-compulsive disorder and attention-deficit hyperactivity disorder, two phenomenologically antithetical conditions. *Acta. Psychiatr. Scand.* 102(6), 401–413.

69. Carlsson, M. L. (2001). On the role of prefrontal cortex glutamate for the antithetical phenomenology of obsessive compulsive disorder and attention deficit hyperactivity disorder. *Prog. Neuropsychopharmacol. Biol. Psychiatry* 25(1), 5–26.

70. Bronstein, Y., and Cummings, J. (2001). Neurochemistry of frontal subcortical circuits. In *Frontal-Subcortical Circuits in Psychiatric and Neurological Disorders*, D. Lichter and J. Cummings, Eds. Guilford, New York, pp. 59–91.

71. Delorme, R., et al. (2004). Frequency and transmission of glutamate receptors GRIK2 and GRIK3 polymorphisms in patients with obsessive compulsive disorder. *Neuroreport* 15(4), 699–702.

72. Arnold, P. D., et al. (2004). Association of a glutamate (NMDA) subunit receptor gene (GRIN2B) with obsessive-compulsive disorder: A preliminary study. *Psychopharmacology (Berl.)* 174(4), 530–538.

73. McGrath, M. J., et al. (2000). Glutamatergic drugs exacerbate symptomatic behavior in a transgenic model of comorbid Tourette's syndrome and obsessive-compulsive disorder. *Brain Res.* 877(1), 23–30.

74. Camarena, B., et al. (2001). Additional evidence that genetic variation of MAO-A gene supports a gender subtype in obsessive-compulsive disorder. *Am. J. Med. Genet.* 105(3), 279–282.

75. Camarena, B., et al. (1998). A higher frequency of a low activity-related allele of the MAO-A gene in females with obsessive-compulsive disorder. *Psychiatr. Genet.* 8(4), 255–257.
76. Lachman, H. M., et al. (1996). Human catechol-O-methyltransferase pharmacogenetics: Description of a functional polymorphism and its potential application to neuropsychiatric disorders. *Pharmacogenetics* 6(3), 243–250.
77. Greer, J. M., and Capecchi, M. R. (2002). Hoxb8 is required for normal grooming behavior in mice. *Neuron* 33(1), 23–34.
78. Graybiel, A. M., and Saka, E. (2002). A genetic basis for obsessive grooming. *Neuron* 33(1), 1–2.
79. Hall, D., et al. (2003). Sequence variants of the brain-derived neurotrophic factor (BDNF) gene are strongly associated with obsessive-compulsive disorder. *Am. J. Hum. Genet.* 73(2), 370–376.
80. Urraca, N., et al. (2004). Mu opioid receptor gene as a candidate for the study of obsessive compulsive disorder with and without tics. *Am. J. Med. Genet.* 127B(1), 94–96.
81. Rapoport, J. L., Ryland, D. H., and Kriete, M. (1992). Drug treatment of canine acral lick: An animal model of obsessive compulsive disorder. *Arch. Gen. Psychiatry* 49, 517–521.
82. Yadin, E., Friedman, E., and Bridger, W. H. (1991). Spontaneous alternation behavior: An animal model for obsessive-compulsive disorder. *Pharmacol. Biochem. Behav.* 40, 311–315.
83. Wynchank, D., and Berk, M. (1998). Fluoxetine treatment of acral lick dermatitis in dogs: A placebo-controlled randomized double blind trial. *Depress. Anxiety* 8(1), 21–23.
84. Szechtman, H., Sulis, W., and Eilam, D. (1998). Quinpirole induces compulsive checking behavior in rats: A potential animal model of obsessive-compulsive disorder (OCD). *Behav. Neurosci.* 112(6), 1475–1485.
85. Falk, I. L. (1977). The origin and functions of adjunctive behavior. *Animal Learning Behav.* 5, 325–335.
86. Smith, C. P., et al. (1997). Anti-obsessional and antidepressant profile of besipirdine. *CNS Drug Rev.* 3, 1–23.
87. Sanger, D., and Corfield-Summer, P. K. (1979). Schedule induced drinking and thirst: A pharmacological analysis. *Pharmacol. Biochem. Behav.* 10, 471–474.
88. Szechtman, H., Culver, K., and Eilam, D. (1999). Role of dopamine systems in obsessive-compulsive disorder (OCD): Implications from a novel psychostimulant-induced animal model. *Pol. J. Pharmacol.* 51(1), 55–61.
89. Garner, J. P., et al. (2004). Barbering (fur and whisker trimming) by laboratory mice as a model of human trichotillomania and obsessive-compulsive spectrum disorders. *Comp. Med.* 54(2), 216–224.
90. van Kuyck, K., et al. (2003). Effects of electrical stimulation or lesion in nucleus accumbens on the behaviour of rats in a T-maze after administration of 8-OH-DPAT or vehicle. *Behav. Brain Res.* 140(1–2), 165–173.
91. McGrath, M., Campbell, K. M., and Veldman, M. B. (1999). Anxiety in a transgenic mouse model of cortical-limbic neuro-potentiated compulsive behavior. *Behav. Pharmacol.* 10, 435–443.
92. Nordstrom, E. J., and Burton, F. H. (2002). A transgenic model of comorbid Tourette's syndrome and obsessive-compulsive disorder circuitry. *Mol. Psychiatry* 7(6), 617–625, 524.

93. Grabli, D., et al. (2004). Behavioural disorders induced by external globus pallidus dysfunction in primates: I. Behavioural study. *Brain* 127(Pt 9), 2039–2054.

94. Francois, C., et al. (2004). Behavioural disorders induced by external globus pallidus dysfunction in primates: II. Anatomical study. *Brain* 127(Pt 9), 2055–2070.

95. Dougherty, D. D., Rauch, S. L., and Jenike, M. A. (2004). Pharmacotherapy for obsessive-compulsive disorder. *J. Clin. Psychol.* 60(11), 1195–1202.

96. Flament, M. F. (1993). [Pharmacologic treatment of obsessive compulsive disorder in the child and adolescent]. *Encephale* 19(2), 75–81.

97. Katz, R. J., DeVeaugh-Geiss, J., and Landau, P. (1990). Clomipramine in obsessive-compulsive disorder. *Biol. Psychiatry* 28(5), 401–414.

98. DeVeaugh-Geiss, J., et al. (1992). Clomipramine hydrochloride in childhood and adolescent obsessive–compulsive disorder—a multicenter trial. *J. Am. Acad. Child Adolesc. Psychiatry* 31(1), 45–49.

99. Montgomery, S. A., et al. (1993). A double-blind, placebo-controlled study of fluoxetine in patients with DSM-III-R obsessive-compulsive disorder. The Lilly European OCD Study Group. *Eur. Neuropsychopharmacol.* 3(2), 143–152.

100. Tollefson, G. D., et al. (1994). A multicenter investigation of fixed-dose fluoxetine in the treatment of obsessive-compulsive disorder. *Arch. Gen. Psychiatry* 51(7), 559–567.

101. Tollefson, G. D., et al., (1994). Continuation treatment of OCD: Double-blind and open-label experience with fluoxetine. *J. Clin. Psychiatry* 55(Suppl), 69–76; discussion 77–78.

102. Geller, D. A., et al. (2001). Fluoxetine treatment for obsessive-compulsive disorder in children and adolescents: A placebo-controlled clinical trial. *J. Am. Acad. Child Adolesc. Psychiatry* 40(7), 773–779.

103. Goodman, W. K., et al. (1997). Fluvoxamine in the treatment of obsessive-compulsive disorder and related conditions. *J. Clin. Psychiatry* 58(Suppl 5), 32–49.

104. Hollander, E., et al. (2003). A double-blind, placebo-controlled study of the efficacy and safety of controlled-release fluvoxamine in patients with obsessive-compulsive disorder. *J. Clin. Psychiatry* 64(6), 640–647.

105. Riddle, M. A., et al. (2001). Fluvoxamine for children and adolescents with obsessive-compulsive disorder: A randomized, controlled, multicenter trial. *J. Am. Acad. Child Adolesc. Psychiatry* 40(2), 222–229.

106. Greist, J., et al. (1995). Double-blind parallel comparison of three dosages of sertraline and placebo in outpatients with obsessive-compulsive disorder. *Arch. Gen. Psychiatry* 52(4), 289–295.

107. Greist, J. H., et al. (1995). A 1 year double-blind placebo-controlled fixed dose study of sertraline in the treatment of obsessive-compulsive disorder. *Int. Clin. Psychopharmacol.* 10(2), 57–65.

108. Koran, L. M., et al. (2002). Efficacy of sertraline in the long-term treatment of obsessive-compulsive disorder. *Am. J. Psychiatry* 159(1), 88–95.

109. March, J. S., et al. (1998). Sertraline in children and adolescents with obsessive-compulsive disorder: A multicenter randomized controlled trial. *JAMA* 280(20), 1752–1756.

110. Hollander, E., et al. (2003). Acute and long-term treatment and prevention of relapse of obsessive-compulsive disorder with paroxetine. *J. Clin. Psychiatry* 64(9), 1113–1121.

111. Kamijima, K., et al. (2003). Paroxetine in the treatment of obsessive-compulsive disorder: Randomized, double-blind, placebo-controlled study in Japanese patients. *Psychiatry Clin. Neurosci.* 58(4), 427–433.

112. Zohar, J., and Judge, R. (1996). Paroxetine versus clomipramine in the treatment of obsessive-compulsive disorder. OCD Paroxetine Study Investigators. *Br. J. Psychiatry* 169(4), 468–474.
113. Geller, D. A., et al. (2004). Paroxetine treatment in children and adolescents with obsessive-compulsive disorder: A randomized, multicenter, double-blind, placebo-controlled trial. *J. Am. Acad. Child Adolesc. Psychiatry* 43(11), 1387–1396.
114. Montgomery, S. A., et al. (2001). Citalopram 20 mg, 40 mg and 60 mg are all effective and well tolerated compared with placebo in obsessive-compulsive disorder. *Int. Clin. Psychopharmacol.* 16(2), 75–86.
115. Healy, D., and Whitaker, C. (2003). Antidepressants and suicide: Risk-benefit conundrums. *J. Psychiatry Neurosci.* 28(5), 331–337.
116. Wong, I. C., et al. (2004). Use of selective serotonin reuptake inhibitors in children and adolescents. *Drug Saf.* 27(13), 991–1000.
117. March, J. S. (2004). Review: Clomipramine is more effective than SSRIs for paediatric obsessive compulsive disorder. *Evid. Based Ment. Health* 7(2), 50.
118. Foa, E. B., et al. (2005). Randomized, placebo-controlled trial of exposure and ritual prevention, clomipramine, and their combination in the treatment of obsessive-compulsive disorder. *Am. J. Psychiatry* 162(1), 151–161.
119. Walsh, K. H., and McDougle, C. J. (2004). Pharmacological augmentation strategies for treatment-resistant obsessive-compulsive disorder. *Expert Opin. Pharmacother.* 5(10), 2059–2067.
120. McDougle, C. J., et al. (1994). Haloperidol addition in fluvoxamine-refractory obsessive-compulsive disorder. A double-blind, placebo-controlled study in patients with and without tics. *Arch. Gen. Psychiatry* 51(4), 302–308.
121. Hollander, E., et al. (2003). Risperidone augmentation in treatment-resistant obsessive-compulsive disorder: A double-blind, placebo-controlled study. *Int. J. Neuropsychopharmacol.* 6(4), 397–401.
122. Erzegovesi, S., et al. (2005). Low-dose risperidone augmentation of fluvoxamine treatment in obsessive-compulsive disorder: A double-blind, placebo-controlled study. *Eur. Neuropsychopharmacol.* 15(1), 69–74.
123. Bystritsky, A., et al. (2004). Augmentation of serotonin reuptake inhibitors in refractory obsessive-compulsive disorder using adjunctive olanzapine: A placebo-controlled trial. *J. Clin. Psychiatry* 65(4), 565–568.
124. Shapira, N. A., et al. (2004). A double-blind, placebo-controlled trial of olanzapine addition in fluoxetine-refractory obsessive-compulsive disorder. *Biol. Psychiatry* 55(5), 553–555.
125. Denys, D., et al. (2004). A double-blind, randomized, placebo-controlled trial of quetiapine addition in patients with obsessive-compulsive disorder refractory to serotonin reuptake inhibitors. *J. Clin. Psychiatry* 65(8), 1040–1048.
126. Grady, T. A., et al. (1993). Double-blind study of adjuvant buspirone for fluoxetine-treated patients with obsessive-compulsive disorder. *Am. J. Psychiatry* 150(5), 819–821.
127. McDougle, C. J., et al. (1993). The efficacy of fluvoxamine in obsessive-compulsive disorder: Effects of comorbid chronic tic disorder. *J. Clin. Psychopharmacol.* 13(5), 354–358.
128. Pigott, T., et al., (1992). A controlled trial of clonazepam augmentation in OCD patients treated with clomipramine or fluoxetine. Presented at the American Psychiatric Association Annual Meeting, Washington, DC, May 2–7.

129. Barr, L. C., et al. (1997). Addition of desipramine to serotonin reuptake inhibitors in treatment-resistant obsessive-compulsive disorder. *Am. J. Psychiatry* 154(9), 1293–1295.

130. Noorbala, A. A., et al. (1998). Combination of clomipramine and nortriptyline in the treatment of obsessive-compulsive disorder: A double-blind, placebo-controlled trial. *J. Clin. Pharm. Ther.* 23(2), 155–159.

131. McDougle, C. J., et al. (1991). A controlled trial of lithium augmentation in fluvoxamine-refractory obsessive-compulsive disorder: Lack of efficacy. *J. Clin. Psychopharmacol.* 11(3), 175–184.

132. Dannon, P. N., et al. (2000). Pindolol augmentation in treatment-resistant obsessive compulsive disorder: A double-blind placebo controlled trial. *Eur. Neuropsychopharmacol.* 10(3), 165–169.

133. Fux, M., Benjamin, J., and Belmaker, R. H. (1999). Inositol versus placebo augmentation of serotonin reuptake inhibitors in the treatment of obsessive-compulsive disorder: A double-blind cross-over study. *Int. J. Neuropsychopharmcol.* 2(3), 193–195.

134. Pallanti, S., Hollander, E., and Goodman, W. K. (2004). A qualitative analysis of nonresponse: Management of treatment-refractory obsessive-compulsive disorder. *J. Clin. Psychiatry* 65(Suppl 14), 6–10.

135. Shapira, N., et al. (1997). Open-label pilot study of tramadol hydrochloride in treatment-refractory obsessive-compulsive disorder. *Depress. Anxiety* 6, 170–173.

136. Goldsmith, T. B., Shapira, N. A., and Keck, P. E., Jr. (1999). Rapid remission of OCD with tramadol hydrochloride. *Am. J. Psychiatry* 156(4), 660–661.

137. Franz, B., Bullock, K. D., and Elliot, M. A. (2001). Oral morphine in treatment resistant OCD. Presented at the Fifth International Obsessive-Compulsive Disorder Conference, Sardinia, Italy, March 29–April 1.

138. Koran, L. M., et al. (2005). Double-blind treatment with oral morphine in treatment-resistant obsessive compulsive disorder. *J. Clin. Psychiatry* 66(3), 353–359.

139. Hollander, E., Kaplan, A., and Stahl, S. (2003). A double-blind placebo-controlled trial of clonazepam in obsessive-compulsive disorder. *World J. Biol. Psychiatry* 4, 30–34.

140. Hewlett, W. A., Vinogradov, S., and Agras, W. S. (1992). Clomipramine, clonazepam, and clonidine treatment of obsessive-compulsive disorder. *J. Clin. Psychopharmacol.* 12(6), 420–430.

141. Denys, D., et al. (2003). A double blind comparison of venlafaxine and paroxetine in obsessive-compulsive disorder. *J. Clin. Psychopharmacol.* 23(6), 568–575.

142. Hollander, E., et al. (2003). Venlafaxine in treatment-resistant obsessive-compulsive disorder. *J. Clin. Psychiatry* 64(5), 546–550.

143. Phelps, N. J., and Cates, M. E. (2005). The role of venlafaxine in the treatment of obsessive-compulsive disorder. *Ann. Pharmacother.* 39, 136–140.

144. Salin-Pascual, R. J. (2003). Changes in compulsion and anxiety symptoms with nicotine transdermal patches in non-smoking obsessive-compulsive disorder patients. *Rev. Invest. Clin.* 55, 650–654.

145. Coric, V., et al. (2003). Beneficial effects of the antiglutamatergic agent riluzole in a patient diagnosed with obsessive-compulsive disorder and major depressive disorder. *Psychopharmacology (Berl.)* 167(2), 219–220.

146. Lykouras, L., et al. (2003). Obsessive-compulsive symptoms induced by atypical antipsychotics. A review of the reported cases. *Prog. Neuropsychopharmacol. Biol. Psychiatry* 27(3), 333–346.

147. Graybiel, A. M., and Rauch, S. L. (2000). Toward a neurobiology of obsessive-compulsive disorder. *Neuron* 28(2), 343–347.
148. Sareen, J., et al. (2004). Do antipsychotics ameliorate or exacerbate obsessive compulsive disorder symptoms? A systematic review. *J. Affect Disord.* 82(2), 167–174.
149. Koran, L. M., Pallanti, S., and Quercioli, L. (2001). Sumatriptan, 5-HT(1D) receptors and obsessive-compulsive disorder. *Eur. Neuropsychopharmacol.* 11(2), 169–172.
150. Insel, T. R., and Pickar, D. (1983). Naloxone administration in obsessive-compulsive disorder: Report of two cases. *Am. J. Psychiatry* 140(9), 1219–1220.
151. Carrion, V. G. (1995). Naltrexone for the treatment of trichotillomania: A case report. *J. Clin. Psychopharmacol.* 15(6), 444–445.
152. Garvey, M. A., et al. (1999). A pilot study of penicillin prophylaxis for neuropsychiatric exacerbations triggered by streptococcal infections. *Biol. Psychiatry* 45(12), 1564–1571.
153. Luo, F., et al. (2004). Prospective longitudinal study of children with tic disorders and/or obsessive-compulsive disorder: Relationship of symptom exacerbations to newly acquired streptococcal infections. *Pediatrics* 113(6), 578–585.
154. Singer, H. S. (1999). PANDAS and immunomodulatory therapy. *Lancet* 354(9185), 1137–1138.
155. Snider, L. A., and Swedo, S. E. (2003). Post-streptococcal autoimmune disorders of the central nervous system. *Curr. Opin. Neurol.* 16(3), 359–365.
156. Greenberg, B. D., et al. (2003). Neurosurgery for intractable obsessive-compulsive disorder and depression: Critical issues. *Neurosurg. Clin. N. Am.* 14(2), 199–212.
157. Binder, D. K., and Iskandar, B. K. (2000). Modern neurosurgery for psychiatric disorders. *Neurosurgery* 47(1), 9–21; discussion 21–23.
158. George, M. S., et al. (2003). Transcranial magnetic stimulation. *Neurosurg. Clin. N. Am.* 14(2), 283–301.
159. Greenberg, B. D., et al. (1998). Decreased neuronal inhibition in cerebral cortex in obsessive-compulsive disorder on transcranial magnetic stimulation [letter]. *Lancet* 352(9131), 881–882.
160. Gilbert, D. L., et al. (2004). Association of cortical disinhibition with tic, ADHD, and OCD severity in Tourette syndrome. *Mov. Disord.* 19(4), 416–425.
161. Alonso, P., et al. (2001). Right prefrontal repetitive transcranial magnetic stimulation in obsessive-compulsive disorder: A double-blind, placebo-controlled study. *Am. J. Psychiatry* 158(7), 1143–1145.
162. Martin, J. L., et al. (2003). Transcranial magnetic stimulation for the treatment of obsessive-compulsive disorder. *Cochrane Database Syst. Rev.* 2003(3), CD003387.
163. Gabriels, L., et al. (2003). Deep brain stimulation for treatment-refractory obsessive-compulsive disorder: Psychopathological and neuropsychological outcome in three cases. *Acta. Psychiatr. Scand.* 107(4), 275–282.
164. Aouizerate, B., et al. (2004). Deep brain stimulation of the ventral caudate nucleus in the treatment of obsessive-compulsive disorder and major depression. Case report. *J. Neurosurg.* 101(4), 682–686.
165. McIntyre, C. C., et al. (2004). How does deep brain stimulation work? Present understanding and future questions. *J. Clin. Neurophysiol.* 21(1), 40–50.
166. Nuttin, B., et al. (1999). Electrical stimulation in anterior limbs of internal capsules in patients with obsessive-compulsive disorder. *Lancet* 354(9189), 1526.
167. Nuttin, B. J., et al. (2003). Long-term electrical capsular stimulation in patients with obsessive-compulsive disorder. *Neurosurgery* 52(6), 1263–1272; discussion 1272–1274.

168. Anderson, D., and Ahmed, A. (2003). Treatment of patients with intractable obsessive-compulsive disorder with anterior capsular stimulation. Case report. *J. Neurosurg.* 98(5), 1104–1108.
169. Abelson, J. L., et al. (2005). Deep brain stimulation for refractory obsessive-compulsive disorder. *Biol. Psychiatry* 57(5), 510–516.
170. Mallet, L., et al. (2002). Compulsions, Parkinson's disease, and stimulation. *Lancet* 360(9342), 1302–1304.

PART II

Schizophrenia and Psychosis

7

PHENOMENOLOGY AND CLINICAL SCIENCE OF SCHIZOPHRENIA

SUBROTO GHOSE AND CAROL TAMMINGA
University of Texas Southwestern Medical Center, Dallas, Texas

7.1	Introduction		252
7.2	Clinical Phenomenology and Treatment		252
	7.2.1	Psychosis	253
		7.2.1.1 Phenomenology	253
		7.2.1.2 Treatment	254
	7.2.2	Cognitive Dysfunction	254
		7.2.2.1 Phenomenology	254
		7.2.2.2 Treatment	254
	7.2.3	Negative Affect	255
		7.2.3.1 Phenomenology	255
		7.2.3.2 Treatment	255
7.3	Biological Mechanisms		256
	7.3.1	Human Brain Imaging	256
		7.3.1.1 Magnetic Resonance Imaging	256
		7.3.1.2 Magnetic Resonance Spectroscopic Imaging	256
		7.3.1.3 Functional Brain Imaging: fMRI and PET	257
	7.3.2	Human Post Mortem	260
		7.3.2.1 Structural	260
		7.3.2.2 Neurochemical	260
	7.3.3	Genetics and Phenotypes	262
7.4	Animal Models		263
	7.4.1	Cognitive Deficit Model	263
		7.4.1.1 Working Memory Deficits	263
		7.4.1.2 Declarative Memory Deficits	263
		7.4.1.3 Attention Deficits	263
	7.4.2	Genetic Models	264
	7.4.3	Psychosis Model	264
	7.4.4	Neurodevelopmental Model	265
		7.4.4.1 Disruption of Neurogenesis	265
		7.4.4.2 Lesion Models	265
7.5	Conclusion: How Far Have We Come and What are the Remaining Questions?		265
References			266

Handbook of Contemporary Neuropharmacology, Edited by David R. Sibley, Israel Hanin, Michael Kuhar, and Phil Skolnick. Copyright © 2007 John Wiley & Sons, Inc.

7.1 INTRODUCTION

Schizophrenia is a chronic psychotic illness with an unknown pathophysiology and etiology. It is the prototypical psychotic illness because of its pervasive and chronic manifestations and its human impact. Because the symptoms have their onset in early adult years and frequently run unabated throughout life, its medical need is high. Treatments are palliative, and partially effective.

The causes and mechanisms of illness will undoubtedly be complex. Neither a single brain region nor a single neurochemical alteration seems likely but several. Brain systems are thought to underlie the symptoms of the illness; some evidence suggests that the limbic system is the substrate for psychotic symptoms, the prefrontal neocortex for cognitive symptoms, and the frontoparietal cortex for the affective symptoms. A genetic vulnerability with environmental determinants of etiology is the theoretical construct guiding research.

Research into the biological basis of schizophrenia has become more informative as the tools and understanding in neuroscience itself have become more sophisticated. It has only been recent that tools for human brain research have been sensitive and reliable enough to contribute. But now, human brain imaging techniques, postmortem tissue analysis, and genetic tools are the main sources of data informing schizophrenia biology. Animal models for aspects of the illness are based on growing knowledge about the brain in schizophrenia and its genetic underpinnings. Advances in the understanding of the biology of schizophrenia are necessary to support new drug development and modify the course of illness.

7.2 CLINICAL PHENOMENOLOGY AND TREATMENT

Schizophrenia is characterized by a constellation of symptoms that include psychosis, cognitive deficits, and negative symptoms [1–7]. The course of schizophrenia is lifelong. The illness may have a precipitous onset in the late teens and early adult years followed by an episodic course sometimes with satisfactory recovery between episodes. Often other patterns of illness occur with an insidious onset, partial recovery, or a remarkable lack of recovery between episodes [8, 9]. In most affected individuals, a profound deterioration in psychosocial function occurs within the first few years of the illness [10] and then settles at a low, flatter plateau. Surprisingly, symptoms can improve in later life after 50 years of age. The Vermont study found considerable heterogeneity in outcome in later life, including frank late improvers [11, 12]. These data are consistent with several other outcome studies in Europe and the United States which report frequent good outcome in later years for individuals with schizophrenia [8, 9, 13, 14] even though divergent descriptions exist [15]. It is not known if this is due to the later years being less demanding or if the normal aging process is therapeutic in the illness. Nonetheless, the disease course of schizophrenia can be easily distinguished from traditional neurodegenerative disorders where the course is progressively downhill, such as Parkinson's disease or Alzheimer's dementia, and from traditional neurodevelopmental disorders, such as mental retardation, where the course is low and steady from early years.

The prevalence of 1% in the general population, 9% in siblings of an affected individual, 12% in offspring, and 40–50% in identical twins [16] speaks to a genetic influence, but one that does not inevitably result in schizophrenia. Schizophrenia can also occur without any family history. Several epidemiological factors have been associated with a predisposition to schizophrenia, including prenatal maternal illness during the second trimester, perinatal birth complications, and winter births [17, 18]. Each risk factor confers a modest risk alone with genetics being the strongest risk factor. Environmental factors contribute to risk, such as adolescent use of cannabis in genetically susceptible individuals [19]. Possibly when they occur together, these risks may be multiplicative. Moreover, the risk factors as a group suggest the importance of early life events in the onset of an illness whose florid symptoms appear much later in life.

Several meta-analyses have demonstrated the clustering of symptoms into at least three distinct symptom domains in schizophrenia: (1) *positive symptoms*, including hallucinations, delusions, thought disorder, and paranoia; (2) *cognitive dysfunction*, especially in attention, working memory, and executive function; and (3) *negative symptoms* such as anhedonia, social isolation, and thought poverty [1–7].

When clinical symptoms are related to imaging findings, specific brain areas are found to be differentially involved in symptom manifestations in schizophrenia. Whether these regionally specific changes are a cause or effect of the disorder is not known, but they do suggest the presence of distinct neuroanatomical substrates, possibly distinct cerebral systems, for the different symptom clusters. Accordingly, we will address these clusters as distinct entities—psychosis, cognitive dysfunction, and negative affect.

7.2.1 Psychosis

7.2.1.1 Phenomenology. Psychosis reflects a loss of touch with reality and distortion of mental functions [20]. These include delusions (distortions in thought content), hallucinations (distortion in perception), disorganized speech (distortions in language and thought process), and disorganized behavior (distortion in self-monitoring of behavior). Delusions are among the most common of the schizophrenia symptoms. They are experiences that persons with schizophrenia believe in fervently although they have no basis in fact. Common examples are delusions of persecution, in which they feel that they are being plotted against, spied on, or intentionally victimized. They may also exhibit paranoia. Other delusions may include those such as grandiosity and religiosity. Bizarre delusions are those that are clearly implausible. Hallucinations may occur in any sensory modality with auditory hallucinations being the most common. These are usually perceived as voices distinct from their own thoughts and often occur as two or more voices conversing with one another or voices maintaining a running commentary on the person's thoughts or behaviors. Disorganized thinking is another key symptom and is evaluated on the basis of the individual's speech. Schizophrenics may rapidly switch from one topic to another lacking a logical connection (loose association), making it difficult to follow their train of thought. A single, unimportant word to the listener may become the focus or topic of the next sentence. The subjects, however, believe that they make perfectly good sense. In severe disorganization, the person may be incomprehensible. Disorganized behavior may manifest in any goal-directed behavior leading to difficulty performing routine daily activities such as preparing a meal or taking a shower. The person may appear disheveled, dress peculiarly, or display inappropriate behavior.

7.2.1.2 Treatment. Antipsychotic drugs have vastly improved the lives of those afflicted with schizophrenia, although they still suffer considerable residual symptom burden and life-long psychosocial impairments. The conventional antipsychotics (butyrophenones, phenothiazines, and thioxanthenes) with potent antidopaminergic activity were used successfully to treat psychosis for 50 years, albeit with acute and chronic motor side effects. In 1990, newer drugs were introduced with higher antiserotonergic potency accompanying the dopamine receptor blockade. These drugs were less likely to cause motor side effects and dysphoria but have their own serious side effects. The metabolic syndrome (weight gain, hyperlipidemia, diabetes, hypertension) is a side effect of concern with many of the new antipsychotics. Clozapine remains the only antipsychotic with demonstrably greater antipsychotic efficacy; the mechanism of its better effect is still not known.

7.2.2 Cognitive Dysfunction

7.2.2.1 Phenomenology. The core symptoms of schizophrenia are of a cognitive nature. The particularly prominent cognitive deficits are working memory defects, attentional dysfunction, verbal and visual learning and memory, processing speed, and social learning [21–26]. No cognitive domains are entirely spared, and deficits in performance are highly intercorrelated within persons [27]. However, schizophrenic subjects in many of the studies show a particular profile of deficits that rules out the lack of motivation as a factor in performance. Neuropsychological characteristics of schizophrenia have not served to localize disease pathophysiology. For example, in schizophrenic persons, memory deficits for recurring digit occur that are consistent with temporohippocampal dysfunction [21]. Functions that are ascribed to frontal cortex are abnormal (e.g., verbal fluency, spatial performance, pattern recognition), and long-term memory is affected. Besides, persons with schizophrenia also perform tasks poorly that require sustained attention or vigilance characteristically associated with the anterior cingulate [28]. Deficits in memory possibly involving the hippocampus occur, including explicit memory, verbal memory, and working memory [29, 30]. Deficits in working memory may explain a part of the disorganization and functional deterioration observed in the illness, since the ability to hold information "on-line" is critical for organizing future thoughts and actions in the context of the recent past [31]. These characteristics of cognition in schizophrenia suggest broad cortical dysfunction.

7.2.2.2 Treatment. Existing treatments of schizophrenia have generally been unsuccessful in treating cognitive deficits in schizophrenia. There is controversy over whether second-generation antipsychotics improve cognition more than classical antipsychotics [32–34]. The MATRICS program was developed to identify potential molecular targets to treat cognitive deficits in schizophrenia [35]. Those targets judged to be most promising include a D_1 dopamine agonist [36], an α_7 nicotinic agonist [37], muscarinic agonists [38], serotonin 5-HT_{1A} and 5-HT_{2A} [39] ligands, noradrenergic agonists, [40] and modulators of the glutamate-sensitive N-methyl-D-aspartate (NMDA)–gated ionophore [41]. The metabotropic glutamate receptors mGluR 2, 3, and 5 modulate NMDA receptor function and may also provide a means to enhance cognition [42]. These drugs to improve cognition in schizophrenia are proposed as co-treatments and not as alternatives to current antipsychotics. Thus they will be tested in volunteers whose positive symptoms are optimally treated and stable. For example, some current strategies being tested include atomoxatine, a norepinephrine (NE) reuptake inhibitor that increases norepinephrine and dopamine levels in the frontal cortex, and M_1 muscarinic agonists (*N*-desmethyl clozapine, a derivative of clozapine with M_1 agonist properties).

7.2.3 Negative Affect

7.2.3.1 Phenomenology. In general, negative symptoms reflect a diminution or loss of normal functions [20]. Affective flattening, alogia, and avolition are prominent features of schizophrenia. Affective flattening is common in schizophrenia and is characterized by the person's face appearing immobile and unresponsive. The range of emotional expressiveness is diminished. Alogia, the poverty of speech, is manifested by short, empty replies. This is due not to unwillingness to speak but rather to diminution of thoughts resulting in decreased fluency and productivity of speech. Avolition is characterized by an inability to initiate and persist in goal-directed activities. The person may sit for long periods of time without showing any interest in participating in work or social activities. These subjects also have poor eye contact and reduced body language. One caveat to keep in mind is that negative symptomatology may be secondary to other factors. For this reason, it is useful to divide negative symptomatology into primary negative symptoms (or deficit symptoms) and secondary symptoms. Primary negative symptoms are the manifestations of schizophrenia and may be complicated by secondary negative symptoms that may occur because of depression, paranoia, or medication side effects. Certain antipsychotics produce extrapyramidal side effects such as bradykinesia that may mimic affective flattening. Comorbid depression can be distinguished by the presence of other symptoms of depression not found in schizophrenia. Paranoia can cause subjects to stay in a room and not talk to people, which can be mistaken as social isolation.

7.2.3.2 Treatment. Specific treatments are not available for primary negative symptoms. Antipsychotic drugs can diminish negative symptoms—an effect that may be secondary to the reduction of acute psychosis. Some studies suggest that the second-generation drugs are effective for secondary negative symptoms but they have shown no efficacy for the deficit symptoms [43]. In a longitudinal study, clozapine was found to be ineffective in treating deficit symptoms [44]. Initial promise of glutamatergic agents such as D-cycloserine [45, 46] has not been replicated in the latest larger multicenter study [47].

The clustering of symptoms and differential response of each symptom domain to medication are consistent with the concept of specific neural substrates for each cluster. While we have an understanding of the pharmacology of receptors targeted by antipsychotic medications, we do not know the cerebral mechanisms of actions of these drugs. It is probable that modulation of receptors at the cellular level can result in functional changes at the neural network level.

Systems biology concepts [48] are beginning to be applied to schizophrenia. Systems neuroscience, the study of the function of neural circuits, is concerned with the functional organization and processing of information in cellular networks, thereby linking molecular and cellular biology to behaviors such as cognitive, motivational, perceptual, and motor processes. In schizophrenia, specific neural networks may underlie each of the symptom domains. The degree of dysfunction in neural systems may vary and predominantly affected systems may have greater impact on the clinical presentation. The notion is that there are abnormal networks, not just an abnormal protein, in schizophrenia. This neural system–based approach provides a plausible and scientifically sound framework in which to conceptualize the pathophysiology of schizophrenia. We expand on this concept in the next section.

7.3 BIOLOGICAL MECHANISMS

7.3.1 Human Brain Imaging

Advances made in neuroimaging modalities allow regional in vivo observations of brain structure, chemistry, and function in persons with schizophrenia.

7.3.1.1 Magnetic Resonance Imaging. Magnetic resonance imaging (MRI) provides structural images of the brain with excellent cross-sectional anatomical detail and strong grey/white matter contrast. MRI studies report a reduction in overall brain size, an increase in ventricular size, and variable cortical wasting in schizophrenia [49–52]. These reports confirm and extend older literature using the computerized axial tomography (CAT) examination of schizophrenia that demonstrated ventricular enlargement [52]. More recently, MRI studies have reported a volume reduction in medial temporal cortical structures (hippocampus, amygdala, and parahippocampal gyrus) [53–57], thalamus [58], and striatum [59, 60]. New analytic techniques for shape analysis show regional shape differences of hippocampus [61] and thalamus [58] in schizophrenia. The volume of the superior temporal gyrus may be reduced in schizophrenia, a change that correlates with the presence of hallucinations [55, 62] and with regional electroencephalographic (EEG) changes [63]. Reduced volume [64–66] and cortical thinning [67] of the cingulate have been described. Frontal lobe abnormalities have been debated with studies showing reduction in volume [68, 69] or no change [70, 71]. The suspicion that a portion of these findings could be caused by antipsychotic treatment was raised by the results of a recent study showing haloperidol-associated increases in ventricular size and decreases in neocortical mass in first-break schizophrenia over the first three months of treatment in a study where second-generation drug treatment produced none of these alterations [72]. The extent to which the overall volume of a brain structure reflects any internal pathology, especially if the pathology is subtle, is necessarily limited. Also, while positive MRI data identify a brain area for further study, negative results do not rule out areas as pathological.

7.3.1.2 Magnetic Resonance Spectroscopic Imaging. Magnetic resonance spectroscopy (MRS) imaging allows measurement of chemical concentrations. Each metabolite is identified by its unique position on a frequency spectrum of multiple peaks; the area under each peak provides a measure of the concentration of the metabolite. Proton MRS (^{1}H MRS) studies show decreases in *N*-acetyl aspartate (NAA) in the prefrontal cortex [73–75] and temporal lobe [76–80] while others show insignificant trends or no difference [81, 82]. Similarly, reductions of NAA are seen in the anterior cingulate [83] but not in all studies [84]. NAA, found exclusively in neurons, has been speculated to reflect neuronal integrity. Phosphorous MRS (^{31}P MRS) data reflect the integrity of neuronal cell membranes. Decreased phosphomonoester resonance (precursors of membrane phospholipids) and increased phosphodiester resonances (breakdown products) in the prefrontal and temporal cortices in schizophrenia are postulated to reflect an increased turnover of membranes, possibly due to abnormalities in synaptic pruning [75, 85].

7.3.1.3 Functional Brain Imaging: fMRI and PET.
Functional MRI with BOLD (blood-oxygen-level dependent) provides dynamic physiological information and includes the BOLD technique. This technique indirectly measures changes in regional blood flow (rCBF) which reflects regional activity. Positron emission tomography (PET) imaging involves the use of a radioactive tracer to measure rCBF metabolic activity, using O-15 water or F-18 FDG (fluorodeoxyglucose), or to quantify receptors using specific radioligands.

Early PET studies with FDG reported a relative hypometabolism in frontal cortex, a finding consistent with even earlier single-photon-emission computerized tomography (SPECT) blood flow studies [86, 87]. Subsequent PET/FDG studies in schizophrenia produced inconsistent detection of frontal cortex hypometabolism, with some studies continuing to find it [88], others reporting no change in the measure [89], and still others finding frontal hypermetabolism [90]. However, a recent meta-analysis suggests that hypofrontality at rest is found in schizophrenia [91]. Still, there exists two potential confounds. First is antipsychotioc drug treatment since neuroleptics are known to reduce neuronal activity in the frontal cortex. Second, deficit symptoms in schizophrenia are associated with reduced frontal cortex activation and could serve to confound observations. Studies have certainly confirmed frontal cortex alterations in schizophrenia with variable, complex, and still incompletely understood characteristics.

7.3.1.3.1 Psychosis Neural Network.
Some investigators have suggested altered functional connections between brain regions as the cause of abnormal rCBF patterns seen in schizophrenia [89, 92, 93]. We and others have found evidence for limbic abnormalities in schizophrenia both at rest [89] and with cognitive challenge [94–96]. FDG PET scans at rest showed glucose utilization (rCMRglu) differences between normal and positive-symptom schizophrenia groups in the anterior cingulate cortex (ACC) and the hippocampus (HC) [89]. A follow-up study of similar design tested the regional associations of positive symptoms and showed that as long as patient volunteers were medication free, there was a significant association between rCMRglu in the limbic cortex (ACC plus HC) and the magnitude of positive symptoms in the illness; this correlation was not obtained when patients were medicated or with other symptom domains [97]. These studies allow us to speculate that it is the limbic cortex which is associated with the positive symptoms of the illness, while the PFC may support negative and/or cognitive symptoms. Blood flow changes in the anterior cingulate and adjacent medial frontal cortex also correlate with induction of positive symptoms with the NMDA antagonist ketamine [98]. PET scanning in hallucinating schizophrenic persons is associated with activations in several brain regions, including the medial prefrontal cortex, left superior temporal gyrus (STG), right medial temporal gyrus (MTG), left hippocampus/parahippocampal region, thalamus, putamen, and cingulate [99, 100].

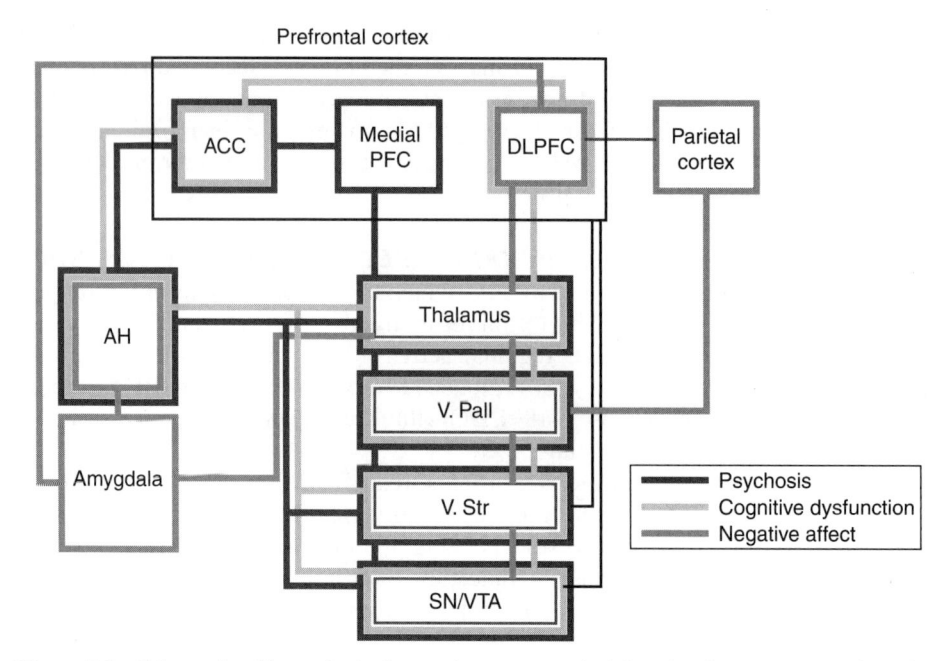

258 PHENOMENOLOGY AND CLINICAL SCIENCE OF SCHIZOPHRENIA

Figure 7.1 Schematic of hypothetical neural systems underlying the three symptom domains: psychosis, cognitive dysfunction, and negative affect. AH = anterior hippocampus; ACC = anterior cingulate; PFC = prefrontal cortex; DLPFC = dorsolateral prefrontal cortex; V. Pall = ventral pallidum; V Str. = ventral stiatum; SN/VTA = substantia nigra/ventral tegmental area. (See color insert.)

These studies provide clues to the anatomic structures that may be involved in a "psychosis neural circuit". Limbic regions, in particular, are frequently implicated in these in vivo studies. Taking these data along with anatomic considerations, we postulate that a neural system for the psychosis cluster in schizophrenia consists of the anterior hippocampus, anterior cingulate, medial PFC (BA 32), thalamus, ventral pallidum striatum, and SN/VTA (see Fig. 7.1). We postulate that the core pathology lies in the hippocampus, resulting in hippocampal dysfunction affecting other regions in the network (e.g., the ACC and medial PFC).

7.3.1.3.2 Negative Affect Neural Network. Brain activation patterns associated with negative symptoms have been studied. Hypoactivation of the frontal lobe is seen with increased negative symptoms in schizophrenia [68, 101–104]. Decrease in rCBF is observed in the prefrontal and parietal cortex among patients exhibiting negative symptoms [89, 105–107]. It is interesting to note that the DLPFC and parietal cortex have dense reciprocal interconnections [108]. Another study in predominantly negative-symptom patients implicates the medial prefrontal, dorsolateral, and prefrontal cortices [109]. Lower activity was also noted in the thalamus [89], in particular the mediodorsal nucleus of the thalamus [110]. The amygdala, a key component in the circuit of emotion, is implicated in emotional processing in schizophrenia [111]. The neural system we propose for the negative-symptom cluster includes the DLPFC, parietal cortex, amygdala/anterior hippocampus, thalamus, ventral pallidum, striatum, and SN/VTA. Of interest, deficit-symptom persons with schizophrenia exhibit greater impairment in cognitive performance [112, 113] that may reflect overlapping systems.

7.3.1.3.3 Cognitive Deficit Neural Network. In studies of verbal fluency [114] and semantic processing [115], network analysis reveals a functional disconnection between the anterior cingulate and prefrontal regions of schizophrenic subjects. Frontal lobe functional connectivity is abnormal in the schizophrenic subjects even though they had significantly activated the regions and their behavior on the tasks was not impaired. These findings suggest that the abnormalities seen in the frontal lobes of schizophrenics may be due to a problem of integration across regions and not a single regional abnormality. Functional MRI studies using cognitively demanding tasks, such as working memory tasks, produce diverse results. Manoach et al. [116, 117] used the Sternberg item recognition working memory paradigm, which required the subjects to remember either two or five digits. Unlike many PET studies of working memory, they found an increase instead of a decrease in prefrontal rCBF in the schizophrenic volunteers as compared to the normal controls. Callicott et al. [118] using the N-back task and Stevens et al. [119] using the word and tone serial position task found decreases of rCBF in inferior frontal regions of schizophrenic subjects. The task performance of the schizophrenic subjects was significantly worse on the N-back and word serial position task but was matched on the tone task. Research has shown that although rCBF increases in prefrontal regions with greater working memory demands, if working memory capacity is exceeded, the activation decreases [120]. Manoach suggests that the discrepant findings in schizophrenia may be explained by an overload of working memory in schizophrenic subjects for some tasks. In separate studies, disorganization was associated with flow in anterior cingulate and mediodorsal thalamus [106] while apomorphine, a dopamine agonist that has antipsychotic properties, normalizes anterior cingulate blood flow of schizophrenic persons during verbal fluency task performance [121]. We propose that a neural system for cognitive deficits involves the DLPFC, anterior hippocampus, anterior cingulate, thalamus, ventral pallidum, striatum, and SN/VTA (Fig. 7.1).

7.3.1.3.4 Neuroreceptor Imaging. Neuroreceptor PET and SPECT imaging allow direct assessments of receptor density and estimations of neurotransmitter release in the living brain. Human brain imaging ligand studies suggest abnormalities in D_1 receptor density in the frontal cortex of persons with schizophrenia [122, 123] leading to speculation that an agonist at the D_1 receptor may be therapeutic in treating cognitive dysfunctions in schizophrenia [124]. Imaging studies with D_2 dopamine receptor ligands reported increases in D_2 family receptors in neuroleptic-naive and neuroleptic-free schizophrenia [125], and a later report suggested its presence in psychotic nonschizophrenics [126]; however, subsequent studies using various other D_2 ligands and replications with the initial ligand have been unable to replicate this finding [127–130]. All schizophrenic individuals do not have increased D_2 family receptors in the striatum, but an alteration in D_2 density may be characteristic of a subgroup of schizophrenic patients, perhaps those with a long duration of illness or other special clinical characteristics [131]. The question remains whether D_2 family receptors are elevated in a subgroup of schizophrenic patients or reflect a confound of medication effect in the initial report. More recently, Laruelle et al. [132] measured dopamine release into the synapse using SPECT or PET imaging with low-affinity dopamine receptor ligands. They report that persons with schizophrenia have an increased release of dopamine in the striatum during the acute phases of their illness in response to amphetamine challenge compared to healthy controls [133]. A significant correlation was seen with dopamine release in the striatum and psychosis but not negative symptoms. Increased release seems not secondary to chronic antipsychotic treatment, since augmented release also occurs in first-episode patients and some family members [134]. This increase in dopaminergic tone in the striatum appears, at least in part, to be under glutamatergic regulation [135, 136]. Imaging glutamate receptors is of keen interest but is hampered by the difficulty in synthesis of such ligands, although efforts are underway [137].

Functional imaging studies have provided the most direct data on neural substrates associated with the symptom clusters while neuroreceptor imaging studies allow in vivo determination of specific receptor abnormalities and indirect measures of neurotransmitter release in specific brain regions. These studies in schizophrenic volunteers can provide in vivo data on molecular abnormalities in specific neural systems. In this section, we have proposed neural systems that may underlie each of the symptom clusters.

7.3.2 Human Post Mortem

7.3.2.1 Structural. Schizophrenia lacks identifiable neuropathological lesions such as occur in Parkinson's disease or Alzheimer's dementia. The pathology is subtle. Numerous studies utilizing a variety of techniques cite decreases in cortical thickness, abnormalities of cell size, cell number and packing density, area, neuronal organization, gross structure, and neurochemistry [138–140]. These data, however, have not been consistently replicated across laboratories, making it difficult to build a consistent story across all of the findings. This may be due to differences in patient populations, stage of illness, and medication status, although possible confounds of tissue artifact, agonal state, chronic drug treatment, lifelong-altered mental state, and relevant demographic factors must always be considered in evaluating postmortem brain tissue studies.

7.3.2.2 Neurochemical. Neurochemical studies began in schizophrenia at a time when scientists were anticipating a single protein defect. While no single defect has been found, investigators interpret studies in a broader systems context. Nonetheless, findings are often still organized by neurotransmitter system.

Studies of biochemical markers of the dopamine system in schizophrenia were stimulated by the early pharmacological observation that blockade of dopamine receptors in the brain reduces psychotic symptoms [141]. The hypothesis derived from this observation that dysfunction of the dopaminergic central nervous system (CNS) either in whole or in part accounts for psychosis in schizophrenia has been explored in all body fluids and in various conditions of rest and stimulation over the last half century [142, 143], with little real support except for the recent imaging studies that show higher occupancy of D_2 receptors by dopamine (DA) in patients with schizophrenia [144] and changes in DA release in acute illness phases [134].

More recently, because of its ubiquitous and prominent location in the CNS and because the antiglutamatergic drugs phencyclidine (PCP) and ketamine cause a schizophrenic-like reaction in humans, the glutamate system has become a focus of study. Several studies have examined ionotropic glutamate receptor subtypes [145]. Most studies have focused on the mesial temporal lobe and, in general, report abnormalities in α-amino-3-hydroxy-5-methylisoxazole-4-propionic acid (AMPA), kainate (KA), and NMDA receptor expression at the messenger RNA (mRNA), protein, and ligand binding level. In the prefrontal cortex, results are inconsistent, although recent studies report AMPA abnormalities [146, 147]. Changes are also reported in ionotropic receptor [148] and PSD 95 expression [149] in the thalamus. Few studies have examined the metabotropic glutamate receptors (mGluRs) in schizophrenia. Group II (mGluR2 and 3) receptors are implicated in animal [150] and human [151] studies. N-acetylaspartylglutamate (NAAG), an endogenous agonist of mGluR3 [152, 153], and its metabolic enzyme [154, 155] are abnormal in schizophrenia. Additionally, mGluR3 may be a risk gene for schizophrenia [156].

Evidence of γ-aminobutyric acid (GABAergic) involvement is found in reduced expression of presynaptic markers in subpopulations of interneurons in the frontal cortex and the hippocampal formation [157, 158]. GABAergic neurons can be defined by the presence of one of three calcium binding proteins, namely parvalbumin, calretinin, and calbindin. The most characteristic morphological types of neurons that express parvalbumin are the large basket and chandelier cells [159]. GAD 67 and GAT1 are decreased in the parvalbumin-expressing prefrontal interneurons [160].

The affinity of newer antipsychotic drugs for serotonergic receptors has raised speculation over the role of this neurotransmitter system in the treatment and perhaps in the pathophysiology of the illness. Years ago, serotonin was hypothesized to be central to the pathophysiology of schizophrenia, because of the psychotomimetic actions of serotonergic drugs, such as lysergic acid diethylamide (LSD) [161]. Postmortem studies have failed to find consistent change in measures of the serotonin system in schizophrenia, including in receptors (in vivo and postmortem) or in metabolites [162]. Since serotonin has been shown to modify dopamine release in striatum [163, 164], the augmented antipsychotic action of the new drugs may be mediated through modulation of dopamine release into the synapse. Indeed, drugs without any dopamine receptor affinity but with only 5-HT$_{2A}$ receptor antagonism do behave as antipsychotic drugs in animal models and show antipsychotic activity in humans [165]. Since the serotonin system has diverse receptors and functions, it is not surprising that this aspect is not yet fully explicated.

Cholinergic neurotransmission, integral to cognition and memory, may be dysfunctional in schizophrenia. Clinically, it is well known that schizophrenic patients have a much higher incidence of cigarette smoking [166]. Although "control" smokers exhibit an upregulation in nicotinic receptors [167, 168], decreased levels of nicotinic and muscarinic receptors are reported in the hippocampus frontal cortex, thalamus, and striatum in schizophrenia [169].

Molecular abnormalities are found in a number of anatomic regions and in several neurotransmitter systems in the neuropathology of schizophrenia. Abnormalities in molecular targets should be examined in terms of pathways (not only neurotransmitter pathways) affecting circuit function. Additionally, identification of primary pathology from epiphenomenon is essential. For example, neurotransmitter systems are dynamic and disruption of one system would lead to compensatory mechanisms in other relevant pathways. In general, a strategy to follow once a positive finding is made would be to confirm the finding is real and not an artifact, replicate the finding in another cohort, and determine if the molecular abnormality is part of the primary pathology. Converging data from in vivo human studies, post mortem human studies and animal model studies would provide clues to the primary pathology.

7.3.3 Genetics and Phenotypes

Schizophrenia is heritable but does not follow a simple pattern. Multiple susceptibility genes, each of small effect, are believed to exist for schizophrenia. Replicated linkages to several chromosomal regions have been made, including to 8p, 22q, 2, 3, 5q, 6p, 11q, 13q, and 20p, and there are several genes within these regions that have been associated with the illness, including neuregulin (*NRG*1) [170], dysbindin (*DTNBP*1) [171], *G72* [172], D-amino-acid oxidase (*DAAO*), regulator of G-protein signaling 4 (*RGS*4) [173], proline dehydrogenase (*ProDII*) [174], catecol-*O*-methyl transferase (*COMT*) [175, 176] and metabotropic glutamate receptor 3 (*mGluR3*) [156]. Each of these genes codes for a protein that has been speculatively linked with a purported illness mechanism [177, 178], but no clear disease pathophysiology has yet emerged. The goal of confirming a susceptibility gene for schizophrenia is to acquire molecular information about disease mechanisms, which could potentially lead to a broader understanding of the illness and be a basis for novel treatment development.

Investigators argue that an important impediment in understanding the neurobiology of schizophrenia is disease heterogeneity. This may account for the lack of firm knowledge of disease pathophysiology that is the biggest impediment to progress in therapeutics. Therefore, investigators have been attempting to define more homogeneous phenotypes of schizophrenia in persons with the illness and in family members ("endophenotypes") to test these genetically [17]. The features most often used to develop phenotypes in the illness are neurocognitive characteristics, eye movements [179–181], prepulse inhibition (PPI) [182, 183], evoked potential [184], and in vivo brain imaging features (reviewed in Gottesman and Gould [185]). These are spontaneous behaviors of the brain occurring in response to external cues that have a known neural anatomy, and hence may be more direct reflections of neural pathology [186]. The ability of some probands (60–70%) with schizophrenia to follow a smooth pendulum movement with their eyes is deficient [187]. Instead of describing smooth movements following a pendulum stimulus, some show jerky and irregular (delayed and catch-up movements) tracking patterns. Also, antisaccade eye movements (those directed away from a stimulus) are also abnormal in persons with the illness [187, 188]. PPI is a normal phenomenon evident across all sensory modalities, where a small initial ("pre") stimulus decreases the electrophysiological response to a second higher intensity stimulus. In schizophrenia, many probands show abnormal PPI, as do unaffected family members. The neural systems influencing both oculomotor movements and PPI have been well described in the animal and are believed to be highly conserved in the human [189, 190]. P50 is an electrophysiological measure produced when two equal auditory stimuli are presented 500 ms apart and their evoked potential is measured. Healthy persons show a reduced response (in amplitude) to the second signal whereas persons with schizophrenia (estimated at 80%) show less or no suppression.

These data will help identify candidate genes and allow rational selection of molecular targets for further investigation. Although genetic involvement in schizophrenia is certain, genetic makeup alone does not predict schizophrenia. Also schizophrenia typically does not manifest until the second or third decade of life, implying an interaction between genotype and other factors prior to onset of the illness. It is possible that as the brain matures (e.g., during adolescence) neural networks in the brain are developing and becoming established, a time when molecular abnormalities may become apparent.

7.4 ANIMAL MODELS

Schizophrenia, as we know it, is a uniquely human disorder; therefore creating an exact or full animal model of this illness may not be possible. It is, however, possible to create models to study aspects of disease etiology or pathophysiological mechanisms and to create models for target symptom areas. Approaches include genetic manipulations, pharmacological and environmental manipulations, and discrete anatomic lesions. These animal models produce symptoms that qualify as belonging to one or more of the three symptom clusters.

7.4.1 Cognitive Deficit Model

7.4.1.1 Working Memory Deficits. The limited cognitive capacity of animals limits the design of cognitive tasks. Olton and Samuelson [191] devised a classic task for assessing memory in the rodent, the radial arm maze. Delayed alternation problems capitalize on the rats' tendency to choose alternative maze arms or locations when rats are reexposed to an apparatus, the most common version is the T maze. Delayed nonmatching to sample tasks require a rat to remember a stimulus over a delay in which that stimulus is no longer present. Nonhuman primate working memory models include spatial delayed response, delayed match to sample, and attentional set-shifting tasks [192].

7.4.1.2 Declarative Memory Deficits. Explicit or declarative memory is abnormal in schizophrenia [193–195]. This is hippocampal dependent and has been examined in animal models. The role of the hippocampus in learning and memory tasks that encourage animals to compare and contrast odor items as they learn about them and to encode both direct and indirect relations among odors has been described [196]. Transitive inference (TI), a task of the ability to infer a relationship between items that have not been presented together, is abnormal in schizophrenia [197] and can be tested in rodents [198].

7.4.1.3 Attention Deficits. The continuous performance test (CPT) developed by Rosvold et al [199] is a paradigm used to test attention in schizophrenia. Subjects continually monitor the location of a brief visual target in one of five spatial locations that occur randomly [200], providing a measure of visuospatial attention. An analogous test for use in rodents is the five-choice serial reaction time task [201]. This test has been used to examine effects of drugs and neuroanatomical lesions on various aspects of attentional performance, including selective attention, vigilance, and executive control [202, 203].

7.4.1.3.1 Social Interactions. Social withdrawal is a significant feature in schizophrenia. Dyadic encounters have often been used to investigate social behavior in rats [204, 205]. Social recognition is assessed by quantifying the duration of social investigation during subsequent exposures to the same individual. Reexposure is characterized by a shorter investigation time. This foreshortened time is taken to represent the social recognition. Social cognition is a particular aspect of learning and memory that is selectively impaired in schizophrenia [206]. In rats, ketamine disrupts social learning, an effect that can be reversed by antipsychotic treatment [207]. The prairie vole provides another model to study social interactions. These rodents are highly social, form selective, enduring pair bonds with one mate [208, 209], and are amenable to experimental manipulation.

7.4.2 Genetic Models

A number of mutant mice for several neuroreceptors have been developed, including those for NMDA receptor subunits [210], mGluR1 [211], mGluR5 [212], dopamine receptor subtypes [213], and adrenergic α_{2A} receptors [214]. Of these, the most interesting mutant mice are those deficient in NMDA glutamate receptors generated by targeted mutation of the crucial NR1 subunit gene [210]. NR1 knockout mice display increase in activity and stereotypies that were attenuated by antipsychotic treatment. They also exhibit negative symptoms evidenced by the decrease in social interactions. These behaviors are similar to those observed in the PCP or MK-801 treated animals. Mutants for the transcription factors NPAS1 and NPAS3 have been reported to result in PPI deficits, impaired social recognition, and locomotor abnormalities [215].

7.4.3 Psychosis Model

Pharmacological models designed to perturb a particular neurotransmitter system have been described. These models induce "psychosis" but not exclusively:

1. *Glutamatergic Models* NMDA receptor antagonists, such as PCP and ketamine, induce psychotic symptoms in healthy humans [216–219] and exacerbate psychotic symptoms in patients with schizophrenia [220]. It is also found to disrupt PPI, an effect that can be reversed by atypical antipsychosis [221, 222]. In rodents, PCP administration induces behavioral activation observed as hyperlocomotion and stereotypies (positive symptoms) [223–229], impaired performance on learning and memory processes (cognitive deficit cluster) [230], and diminished social interactions (negative-symptom cluster) [229–231]. These effects can be reversed by mGluR2/3 agonists [150, 232].

2. *Dopamine Agonist Models* Hyperactivity of the mesolimbic dopaminergic system and hypoactivity in the frontal cortex have been postulated as producing positive and negative symptoms, respectively, in schizophrenia [233]. Similar to the effects of NMDA antagonists, amphetamine induces psychotic reactions in normal individuals and exacerbates symptoms in schizophrenic patients [234, 235]. Negative symptomatology, however, is not reproduced by amphetamine administration [236].

3. *Cannabinoid Model* Administration of Δ^9-tetrahydrocannabinol (Δ^9-THC), the major active component in cannabis, transiently increases positive and negative symptoms and cognitive deficits in healthy human volunteers and subjects with schizoiphrenia [237]. The *val/met* functional polymorphism in the *COMT* gene influences the development of psychosis in adolescent marijuana users [19]. Carriers of the *val158* allele, but not the *met* carriers, were much more likely to develop symptoms of psychosis. This suggests an interaction between genetic predisposition and environmental factors. In rats, Δ^9-THC influences cognitive and behavioral functions in rats [238–241].

7.4.4 Neurodevelopmental Model

7.4.4.1 Disruption of Neurogenesis. This model aims to disrupt normal cell division and maturation at specific gestational time points in an attempt to reproduce abnormalities found in schizophrenia. Prenatal injection of the mitotic inhibitor methylazoxymethanol (MAM) at day E17 produces behavioral changes mimicking the positive and negative symptoms of the disorder. Aberrant cell migration in the hippocampus and a disrupted laminar pattern in the neocortex associated with deficits in working memory [242] and other specific cognitive deficits [243] are observed in these animals. Another approach is the irradiation of monkeys in midgestation which produces cortical abnormalities reminiscent of schizophrenia [244]. Behavioral tests have not yet been reported for these monkeys.

7.4.4.2 Lesion Models. Neonatal ventral hippocampal lesions in rats have been proposed as an animal model [245]. This lesion interferes with development of the hippocampus and its associated connections with other brain regions such as the prefrontal cortex. These animals exhibit some behavioral and molecular changes observed in schizophrenia [246–248]. Lesions in other brain structures like the medial prefrontal cortex [249] have been described.

Animal models in schizophrenia have been criticized as not being definitive. While it may not be possible to reproduce the full syndrome in animals, it does not mean that animal models are not useful or informative about the discrete characteristics they demonstrate. It would be ideal if each symptom cluster and associated neural circuit could be examined separately. Each circuit, however, is not discrete and overlap is present, allowing one circuit to influence the others. Using a number of different animal models targeting specific proteins, pathways, anatomic regions, or circuits and examining the converging data will provide the most useful data.

7.5 CONCLUSION: HOW FAR HAVE WE COME AND WHAT ARE THE REMAINING QUESTIONS?

Schizophrenia is a complex disease most likely associated with multiple etiologies. Clinically, the illness can be identified by its typical presentation, but researchers endeavor to distinguish subgroups within the diagnosis "schizophrenia" in an effort to identify unique pathophysiological mechanisms. The phenotypes of schizophrenia, defined by symptoms, psychological, electrophysiological, biochemical, or physiological (i.e., rCBF) characteristics, are being proposed. The sorting of these phenotypes into biologically meaningful groups is ongoing. In brain imaging studies, distinct anatomic substrates for the three symptom clusters (psychosis, cognitive dysfunction, and negative affect) suggest the presence of specific neural networks for each cluster. It is possible that endophenotypes identified by electrophysiological or neurocognitive means also share neural network dysfunction.

A shift in conceptual framework from defects in specific proteins to defects in neural networks may represent a biologically relevant mechanism useful in investigating the pathophysiology of schizophrenia. This will require identification of relevant neural systems and an understanding of the dynamics of the systems. Then such systems could be used as a model to test function—what are the effects of disrupting one part of a network? Are there compensatory mechanisms that come into play? Are there regions that are crucial to the functioning of the system? How can we modulate the system in the diseased state to make it more efficient? The system's neuroscience approach in schizophrenia is at its very early stages of conceptualization. As an initial formulation, we propose neural networks for each of the symptom domains (Fig. 7.1). This formulation proposes that the core pathology in the hippocampus influences function of networks involving distinct cortical regions and subcortical structures.

Whether the symptom domains are manifestations of a single disease pathophysiology perturbing the neural networks or are each a partially independent disease construct remains unknown. However, heterogeneity is more often presumed about the illness, certainly with respect to etiology. An integral part of determining function of affected neural systems is understanding the molecular composition of the connections in the network. The primary molecular lesion of schizophrenia or of any one of its subgroups has not yet been identified. Whether productive leads will derive from clinical pharmacology, genetics, imaging, or phenotyping or perhaps from all is a speculation. It is the kind of discovery that will be used to target novel drug discovery. Without known molecular targets, therapeutics can advance only by serendipity, chance, or modifications of existing treatments. Hope for identifying the pivotal molecular targets for schizophrenia rests on the application of modern concepts and techniques to clearly diagnosed and characterized populations of persons with schizophrenia. There are therapeutic implications to heterogeneity: Does one treatment exist for schizophrenia or are there several symptom or syndrome-specific treatments for the illness? This question remains open, but taking clues from other illness, one would guess that several treatments will emerge.

REFERENCES

1. Liddle, P. F. (1987). The symptoms of chronic schizophrenia: A re-examination of the positive-negative dichotomy. *Br. J. Psychiatry* 151, 145–151.
2. Carpenter, Jr., W. T., and Buchanan, R. W. (1989). Domains of psychopathology relevant to the study of etiology and treatment in schizophrenia. In *Schizophrenia: Scientific Progress*, S. C. Schulz and C. A. Tamminga, Eds. Oxford University Press, New York, NY, pp. 13–22.
3. Kay, S. R., and Sevy, S. (1991). Pyramidical model of schizophrenia. *Schizophr. Bull.* 16, 537–545.

4. Arndt, S., Alliger, R. J., and Andreasen, N. C. (1991). The distinction of positive and negative symptoms. The failure of a two-dimensional model. *Br. J. Psychiatry* 158, 317–322.

5. Lenzenweger, M. F., Dworkin, R. H., and Wethington, E. (1991). Examining the underlying structure of schizophrenic phenomenology: Evidence for a three-process model. *Schizophr. Bull.* 17, 515–524.

6. Barnes, T. R., and Liddle, P. F. (1990). Evidence for the validity of negative symptoms. *Pharmacopsychiatry* 24, 43–72.

7. Andreasen, N. C., Arndt, S., Alliger, R. J., Miller, D., and Flaum, M. (1995). Symptoms of schizophrenia. Methods, meanings, and mechanisms. *Arch. Gen. Psychiatry* 52, 341–351.

8. Ciompi, L., and Muller, C. (1976). Lifestyle and age of schizophrenics. A catamnestic long-term study into old age. [German]. *Monographien aus dem Gesamtgebiete der Psychiatrie. Psychiatry Series* 1, 12–42.

9. Bleuler, M. (1978). *The Schizophrenic Disorders: Long-Term Patient and Family Studies.* Yale University Press, New Haven, CT.

10. Lieberman, J. A. (1999). Pathophysiologic mechanisms in the pathogenesis and clinical course of schizophrenia. *J. Clin. Psychiatry* 60(Suppl. 12), 9–12.

11. Harding, C. M., Brooks, G. W., Ashikaga, T., Strauss, J. S., and Breier, A. (1987). The Vermont longitudinal study of persons with severe mental illness, I: Methodology, study sample, and overall status 32 years later. *Am. J. Psychiatry* 144, 718–726.

12. Harding, C. M., Brooks, G. W., Ashikaga, T., Strauss, J. S., and Breier, A. (1987). The Vermont longitudinal study of persons with severe mental illness, II: Long-term outcome of subjects who retrospectively met DSM-III criteria for schizophrenia. *Am. J. Psychiatry* 144, 727–735.

13. Huber, G., Gross, G., and Schuttler, R. (1979). Schizophrenie: Verlaufs und socialpsychiatrische langzeit unter suchungen an den 1945 bis 1959 in Bonn hospitalisierten schizophrenen Kranken. *Monographien aus dem Gesamtgebiete der Psychiatrie* Bd 21.

14. Tsuang, M. T., Woolson, R. F., and Fleming, J. A. (1979). Long-term outcome of major psychoses. I. Schizophrenia and affective disorders compared with psychiatrically symptom-free surgical conditions. *Arch. Gen. Psychiatry* 36, 1295–1301.

15. Harvey, P. D., Bertisch, H., Friedman, J. I., Marcus, S., Parrella, M., White, L., et al. (2003). The course of functional decline in geriatric patients with schizophrenia: Cognitive-functional and clinical symptoms as determinants of change. *Am. J. Geriatr. Psychiatry* 11, 610–619.

16. Matthysse, S. W., and Kidd, K. K. (1976). Estimating the genetic contribution to schizophrenia. *Am. J. Psychiatry* 133, 185–191.

17. Mednick, S. A., and Cannon, T. D. (1991). Fetal development, birth and the syndromes of adult schizophrenia. In *Fetal Neural Development and Adult Schizophrenia*, S. A. Mednick, T. D. Cannon, C. E. Barr, and M. Lyon Eds. Cambridge University Press, New York.

18. O'Callaghan, E., Sham, P., Takei, N., Glover, G., and Murray, R. M. (1991). Schizophrenia after prenatal exposure to 1957 A2 influenza epidemic. *Lancet* 337, 1248–1250.

19. Caspi, A., Moffitt, T. E., Cannon, M., McClay, J., Murray, R., Harrington, H., Taylor, A., Arseneault, L., Williams, B., Braithwaite, A., Poulton, R., and Craig, I. W. (2005). Moderation of the effect of adolescent-onset cannabis use on adult psychosis by a functional polymorphism in the catechol-*O*-methyltransferase gene: Longitudinal evidence of a gene X environment interaction. *Biol. Psychiatry* 57, 1117–1127.

20. American Psychiatric Association (APA) (1994). *Diagnostic and Statistical Manual of Mental Disorders*, 4th ed. APA, Arlington, VA.
21. Gruzelier, J., Seymour, K., Wilson, L., Jolley, A., and Hirsch, S. (1988). Impairments on neuropsychologic tests of temporohippocampal and frontohippocampal functions and word fluency in remitting schizophrenia and affective disorders. *Arch. Gen. Psychiatry* 45, 623–629.
22. Goldberg, T. E., Ragland, J. D., Torrey, E. F., Gold, J. M., Bigelow, L. B., and Weinberger, D. R. (1990). Neuropsychological assessment of monozygotic twins discordant for schizophrenia. *Arch. Gen. Psychiatry* 47, 1066–1072.
23. Braff, D. L., Heaton, R., Kuck, J., Cullum, M., Moranville, J., Grant, I. et al. (1991). The generalized pattern of neuropsychological deficits in outpatients with chronic schizophrenia with heterogeneous Wisconsin Card Sorting Test results. *Arch. Gen. Psychiatry* 48, 891–898.
24. Gur, R. C., Saykin, A. J., and Gur, R. E. (1991). Neuropsychological study of schizophrenia. *Schizophr. Res.* 1, 153–162.
25. Liddle, P. F., and Morris, D. L. (1991). Schizophrenic syndromes and frontal lobe performance. *Br. J. Psychiatry* 158, 340–345.
26. Gold, J., Goldberg, T., and Weinberger, D. (1992). Prefrontal function and schizophrenic symptoms. *Neuropsychiatry Neuropsychol. Behav. Neurol.* 5, 253–261.
27. Sullivan, E. V., Shear, P. K., Zipursky, R. B., Sagar, H. J., and Pfefferbaum, A. (1994). A deficit profile of executive, memory, and motor functions in schizophrenia. *Biol. Psychiatry* 36, 641–653.
28. Nuechterlein, K. H., Dawson, M. E., Gitlin, M., Ventura, J., Goldstein, M. J., Snyder, K. S., et al. (1992). Developmental processes in schizophrenic disorders: Longitudinal studies of vulnerability and stress. *Schizophr. Bull.* 18, 387–425.
29. Saykin, A. J., Gur, R. C., Gur, R. E., Mozley, P. D., Mozley, L. H., Resnick, S. M., et al. (1991). Neuropsychological function in schizophrenia. Selective impairment in memory and learning. *Arch. Gen. Psychiatry* 48, 618–624.
30. Gold, J. M., Hermann, B. P., Randolph, C., Wyler, A. R., Goldberg, T. E., and Weinberger, D. R. (1994). Schizophrenia and temporal lobe epilepsy. A neuropsychological analysis. *Arch. Gen. Psychiatry* 51, 265–272.
31. Goldman-Rakic, P. S. (1994). Working memory dysfunction in schizophrenia. *J. Neuropsychiatry Clin. Neurosci.* 6, 348–357.
32. Meltzer, H. Y., and McGurk, S. R. (1999). The effects of clozapine, risperidone, and olanzapine on cognitive function in schizophrenia. *Schizophr. Bull.* 25, 233–255.
33. Meltzer, H. Y., and Sumiyoshi, T. (2003). Atypical antipsychotic drugs improve cognition in schizophrenia. *Biol. Psychiatry* 53, 265–267.
34. Green, M. F., Marder, S. R., Glynn, S. M., McGurk, S.R., Wirshing, W. C., Wirshing, D. A., Liberman, R. P., and Mintz, J. (2002). The neurocognitive effects of low-dose haloperidol: A two-year comparison with risperidone. *Biol. Psychiatry* 51, 972–978.
35. Geyer, M. A., and Tamminga, C. A. (2004). Measurement and treatment research to improve cognition in schizophrenia: Neuropharmacological aspects. *Psychopharm. (Berl.)* 174, 1–2.
36. Goldman-Rakic, P. S., Castner, S. A., Svensson, T. H., Siever, L. J., and Williams, G. V. (2004). Targeting the dopamine D_1 receptor in schizophrenia: Insights for cognitive dysfunction. *Psychopharm. (Berl.)* 174, 3–16.
37. Martin, L. F., Kem, W. R., and Freedman, R. (2004). Alpha-7 nicotinic receptor agonists: Potential new candidates for the treatment of schizophrenia. *Psychopharm. (Berl.)* 174, 55–64.

38. Friedman, J. I. (2004). Cholinergic targets for cognitive enhancement in schizophrenia: Focus on cholinesterase inhibitors and muscarinic agonists. *Psychopharm. (Berl.)* 174, 45–53.
39. Roth, B. L., Hanizavareh, S. M., Blum, A. E. (2004). Serotonin receptors represent highly favorable molecular targets for cognitive enhancement in schizophrenia and other disorders. *Psychopharm. (Berl.)* 174, 17–24.
40. Arnsten, A. F. T. (2004). Adrenergic targets for the treatment of cognitive deficits in schizophrenia. *Psychopharm. (Berl.)* 174, 25–31.
41. Coyle, J. T., and Tsai, G. (2004). The NMDA receptor glycine modulatory site: A therapeutic target for improving cognition and reducing negative symptoms in schizophrenia. *Psychopharm. (Berl.)* 174, 32–38.
42. Moghhadam, B. T. (2004). Targeting metabotropic glutamate receptors for treatment of the cognitive symptoms of schizophrenia. *Psychopharm. (Berl.)* 174, 39–44.
43. Arango, C., Buchanan, R. W., Kirkpatrick, B., and Carpenter, W. T. (2004). The deficit syndrome in schizophrenia: Implications for the treatment of negative symptoms. *Eur. Psychiatry* 19, 21–26.
44. Buchanan, R. W., Breier, A., Kirkpatrick, B., Ball, P., and Carpenter, W. T. (1998). Positive and negative symptom response to clozapine in schizophrenic patients with and without the deficit syndrome. *Am. J. Psychiatry* 155, 751–760.
45. Goff, D. C., Bottiglieri, T., Arning, E., Shih, V., Freudenreich, O., Evins, A. E., Henderson, D. C., Baer, L., and Coyle, J. (2004). Folate, homocysteine, and negative symptoms in schizophrenia. *Am. J. Psychiatry* 161, 1705–1708.
46. Heresco-Levy, U., Javitt, D. C., Ebstein, R., Vass, A., Lichtenberg, P., Bar, G., Catinari, S., and Ermilov, M. (2005). D-Serine efficacy as add-on pharmacotherapy to risperidone and olanzapine for treatment-refractory schizophrenia. *Biol. Psychiatry* 57, 577–585.
47. Carpenter, W. T., Buchanan, R. W., Javitt, D. C., Marder, S. R., Schooler, N. R., Heresco-Levy, U., Kirkpatrick, B., and McMahon, R. P. (2005). Testing two efficacy hypotheses for the treatment of negative symptoms. Abstract 115515, presented at the International Congress of Schizophrenia Research, Savannah, GA.
48. Kitano, H. (2002). Computational systems biology. *Nature* 420, 206–210.
49. Shelton, R. C. and Weinberger, D. R. (1987). Brain morphology in schizophrenia. In *Psychopharmacology: The Third Generation of Progress*, H. Y. Meltzer, Ed. Raven, New York, pp. 773–781.
50. Gur, R. E., and Pearlson, G. D. (1993). Neuroimaging in schizophrenia research. *Schizophr. Bull.* 19, 337–353.
51. Shenton, M. E., Dickey, C. C., Frumin, M., and McCarley, R. W. (2001). A review of MRI findings in schizophrenia. *Schizophr. Res.* 49, 1–52.
52. Johnstone, E. C., Crow, T. J., Frith, C. D., Husband, J., and Kreel, L. (1976). Cerebral ventricular size and cognitive impairment in chronic schizophrenia. *Lancet* 2, 924–926.
53. Lawrie, S. M., Whalley, H. C., Abukmeil, S. S., Kestelman, J. N., Miller, P., Best, J. J., Owens, D. G., and Johnstone, E. C. (2002). Temporal lobe volume changes in people at high risk of schizophrenia with psychotic symptoms. *Br. J. Psychiatry* 181, 138–143.
54. Suddath, R. L., Christison, G. W., Torrey, E. F., Casanova, M. F., and Weinberger, D. R. (1990). Anatomical abnormalities in the brains of monozygotic twins discordant for schizophrenia. *N. Engl. J. Med.* 322, 789–794.
55. Barta, P. E., Pearlson, G. D., Powers, R. E., Richards, S. S., and Tune, L. E. (1990). Auditory hallucinations and smaller superior temporal gyral volume in schizophrenia. *Am. J. Psychiatry* 147, 1457–1462.

56. Bogerts, B., Ashtari, M., Degreef, G., Alvir, J. M., Bilder, R. M., and Lieberman, J. A. (1990). Reduced temporal limbic structure volumes on magnetic resonance images in first episode schizophrenia. *Psychiatry Res.* 35, 1–13.

57. Breier, A., Buchanan, R. W., Elkashef, A., Munson, R. C., Kirkpatrick, B., and Gellad, F. (1992). Brain morphology and schizophrenia. A magnetic resonance imaging study of limbic, prefrontal cortex, and caudate structures. *Arch. Gen. Psychiatry* 49, 921–926.

58. Csernansky, J. G., Schindler, M. K., Splinter, N. R., Wang, L., Gado, M., Selemon, L. D., Rastogi-Cruz, D., Posener, J. A., Thompson, P. A., and Miller, M. I. (2004). Abnormalities of thalamic volume and shape in schizophrenia. *Am. J. Psychiatry* 161, 896–902.

59. Shihabuddin, L., Buchsbaum, M. S., Hazlett, E. A., Haznedar, M. M., Harvey, P. D., Newman, A., Schnur, D. B., Spiegel-Cohen, J., Wei, T., Machac, J., Knesaurek, K., Vallabhajosula, S., Biren, M. A., Ciaravolo, T. M., and Luu-Hsia, C. (1998). Dorsal striatal size, shape, and metabolic rate in never-medicated and previously medicated schizophrenics performing a verbal learning task. *Arch. Gen. Psychiatry* 55, 235–243.

60. Shihabuddin, L., Buchsbaum, M. S., Hazlett, E. A., Silverman, J., New, A., Brickman, A. M., Mitropoulou, V., Nunn, M., Fleischman, M. B., Tang, C., and Siever, L. J. (2001). Striatal size and relative glucose metabolic rate in schizotypal personality disorder and schizophrenia. *Arch. Gen. Psychiatry* 58, 877–884.

61. Csernansky, J. G., Joshi, S., Wang, L., Haller, J. W., Gado, M. Miller, J. P., et al. (1998). Hippocampal morphometry in schizophrenia by high dimensional brain mapping. *Proc. Natl. Acad. Sci. USA* 95, 11406–11411.

62. Shenton, M. E., Kikinis, R., Jolesz, F. A., Pollak, S. D., LeMay, M. Wible, C. G., et al. (1992). Abnormalities of the left temporal lobe and thought disorder in schizophrenia. A quantitative magnetic resonance imaging study. *N. Engl. J. Med.* 327, 604–612.

63. McCarley, R. W., Shenton, M. E., O'Donnell, B. F., Faux, S. F., Kikinis, R., Nestor, P. G., et al. (1993). Auditory P300 abnormalities and left posterior superior temporal gyrus volume reduction in schizophrenia. *Arch. Gen. Psychiatry* 50, 190–197.

64. Goldstein, J. M., Goodman, J. M., Seidman, L. J., Kennedy, D. N., Makris, N., Lee, H., Tourville, J., Caviness, V. S., Jr., Faraone, S. V., and Tsuang, M. T. (1999). Cortical abnormalities in schizophrenia identified by structural magnetic resonance imaging. *Arch. Gen. Psychiatry* 56, 537–547.

65. Sigmundsson, T., Suckling, J., Maier, M., Williams, S., Bullmore, E., Greenwood, K., Fukuda, R., Ron, M., and Toone, B. (2001). Structural abnormalities in frontal, temporal, and limbic regions and interconnecting white matter tracts in schizophrenic patients with prominent negative symptoms. *Am. J. Psychiatry* 158, 234–243.

66. Szeszko, P. R., Bilder, R. M., Lencz, T., Ashtari, M., Goldman, R. S., Reiter, G., Wu, H., and Lieberman, J. A. (2000). Reduced anterior cingulate gyrus volume correlates with executive dysfunction in men with first-episode schizophrenia. *Schizophr. Res.* 43, 97–108.

67. Narr, K. L., Toga, A. W., Szeszko, P., Thompson, P. M., Woods, R. P., Robinson, D., Sevy, S., Wang, Y., Schrock, K., and Bilder, R. M. (2005). Cortical thinning in cingulate and occipital cortices in first episode schizophrenia. *Biol. Psychiatry* 58(1), 32–40.

68. Andreasen, N. C., Flashman, L., Flaum, M., Arndt, S., Swayze, V., II, O'Leary, D. S., Ehrhardt, J. C., and Yuh, W. T. (1994). Regional brain abnormalities in schizophrenia measured with magnetic resonance imaging. *JAMA* 272, 1763–1769.

69. Schlaepfer, T. E., Harris, G. J., Tien, A. Y., Peng, L. W., Lee, S., Federman, E. B., Chase, G. A., Barta, P. E., and Pearlson, G. D. (1994). Decreased regional cortical gray matter volume in schizophrenia. *Am. J. Psychiatry* 151, 842–848.

70. Andreasen, N. C., Ehrhardt, J. C., Swayze, V. W., II, Alliger, R. J., Yuh, W. T., Cohen, G., and Ziebell, S. (1990). Magnetic resonance imaging of the brain in schizophrenia. The pathophysiologic significance of structural abnormalities. *Arch. Gen. Psychiatry* 47, 35–44.

71. Turetsky, B., Cowell, P. E., Gur, R. C., Grossman, R. I., Shtasel, D. L., and Gur, R. E. (1995). Frontal and temporal lobe brain volumes in schizophrenia. Relationship to symptoms and clinical subtype. *Arch. Gen. Psychiatry* 52, 1061–1070.

72. Lieberman, J. A., Tollefson, G. D., Charles, C., Zipursky, R., Sharma, T., Kahn, R. S., Keefe, R. S., Green, A. I., Gur, R. E., McEvoy, J., Perkins, D., Hamer, R. M., Gu, H., and Tohen, M. (HGDH Study Group) (2005). Antipsychotic drug effects on brain morphology in first-episode psychosis. *Arch Gen Psychiatry* 62, 361–370.

73. Bertolino, A., Knable, M. B., Saunders, R. C., Callicott, J. H., Kolachana, B., Mattay, V. S., Bachevalier, J., Frank, J. A., Egan, M., and Weinberger, D. R. (1999). The relationship between dorsolateral prefrontal *N*-acetylaspartate measures and striatal dopamine activity in schizophrenia. *Biol. Psychiatry* 45, 660–667.

74. Deicken, R. F., Johnson, C., and Pegues, M. (2000). Proton magnetic resonance spectroscopy of the human brain in schizophrenia. *Rev. Neurosci.* 11(2/3), 147–158.

75. Keshavan, M. S., Stanley, J. A., and Pettegrew, J. W. (2000). Magnetic resonance spectroscopy in schizophrenia: Methodological issues and findings—part II. *Biol. Psychiatry* 48, 369–380.

76. Nasrallah, H. A., Skinner, T. E., Schmalbrock, P., and Robitaille, P. M. (1994). Proton magnetic resonance spectroscopy (1H MRS) of the hippocampal formation in schizophrenia: A pilot study. *Br. J. Psychiatry* 165, 481–485.

77. Maier, M., Ron, M. A., Barker, G. J., and Tofts, P. S. (1995). Proton magnetic resonance spectroscopy: An in vivo method of estimating hippocampal neuronal depletion in schizophrenia. *Psychol. Med.* 25(6), 1201–1209.

78. Bertolino, A., Nawroz, S., Mattay, V. S., Barnett, A. S., Duyn, J. H., Moonen, C. T., Frank, J. A., Tedeschi, G., and Weinberger, D. R. (1996). Regionally specific pattern of neurochemical pathology in schizophrenia as assessed by multislice proton magnetic resonance spectroscopic imaging. *Am. J. Psychiatry* 153, 1554–1563.

79. Yurgelun-Todd, D. A., Renshaw, P. F., Gruber, S. A., Ed, M., Waternaux, C., and Cohen, B. M. (1996). Proton magnetic resonance spectroscopy of the temporal lobes in schizophrenics and normal controls. *Schizophr. Res.* 19, 55–59.

80. Deicken, R. F., Pegues, M., and Amend, D. (1999). Reduced hippocampal *N*-acetylaspartate without volume loss in schizophrenia. *Schizophr. Res.* 37, 217–223.

81. Kegeles, L. S., Shungu, D. C., Anjilvel, S., Chan, S., Ellis, S. P., Xanthopoulos, E., Malaspina, D., Gorman, J. M., Mann, J. J., Laruelle, M., and Kaufmann, C. A. (2000). Hippocampal pathology in schizophrenia: Magnetic resonance imaging and spectroscopy studies. *Psychiatry Res.* 98, 163–175.

82. Bartha, R., al-Semaan, Y. M., Williamson, P. C., Drost, D. J., Malla, A. K., Carr, T. J., Densmore, M., Canaran, G., and Neufeld, R. W. (1999). A short echo proton magnetic resonance spectroscopy study of the left mesial-temporal lobe in first-onset schizophrenic patients. *Biol. Psychiatry* 45, 1403–1411.

83. Deicken, R. F., Zhou, L., Schuff, N., and Weiner, M. W. (1997). Proton magnetic resonance spectroscopy of the anterior cingulate region in schizophrenia. *Schizophr. Res.* 27, 65–71.

84. Bertolino, A., Callicott, J. H., Elman, I., Mattay, V. S., Tedeschi, G., Frank, J. A., Breier, A., and Weinberger, D. R. (1998). Regionally specific neuronal pathology in untreated patients with schizophrenia: A proton magnetic resonance spectroscopic imaging study. *Biol. Psychiatry* 43, 641–648.

85. Reddy, R., and Keshavan, M. S. (2003). Phosphorus magnetic resonance spectroscopy: Its utility in examining the membrane hypothesis of schizophrenia. *Prostaglandins Leukot. Essent. Fatty Acids* 69, 401–415.

86. Ingvar, D. H., and Franzen, G. (1974). Abnormalities of cerebral blood flow distribution in patients with chronic schizophrenia. *Acta Psychiatr. Scand.* 50, 425–462.

87. Buchsbaum, M. S., Ingvar, D. H., Kessler, R., Waters, R. N., Cappelletti, J., van Kammen, D. P., et al. (1982). Cerebral glucography with positron tomography. *Arch. Gen. Psychiatry* 39, 251–259.

88. Buchsbaum, M. S., DeLisi, L. E., Holcomb, H. H., Cappelletti, J., King, A. C., Johnson, J., et al. (1984). Anteroposterior gradients in cerebral glucose use in schizophrenia and affective disorders. *Arch. Gen. Psychiatry* 41, 1159–1166.

89. Tamminga, C. A., Thaker, G. K., Buchanan, R., Kirkpatrick, B., Alphs, L. D., Chase, T. N., et al. (1992). Limbic system abnormalities identified in schizophrenia using positron emission tomography with fluorodeoxyglucose and neocortical alterations with deficit syndrome. *Arch. Gen. Psychiatry* 49, 522–530.

90. Cleghorn, J. M., Kaplan, R. D., Nahmias, C., Garnett, E. S., Szechtman, H., and Szechtman, B. (1989). Inferior parietal region implicated in neurocognitive impairment in schizophrenia. *Arch. Gen. Psychiatry* 46, 758–760.

91. Hill, K., Mann, L., Laws, K. R., Stephenson, C. M., Nimmo-Smith, I., and McKenna, P. J. (2004). Hypofrontality in schizophrenia: A meta-analysis of functional imaging studies. *Acta Psychiatr. Scand.* 110, 243–256.

92. Weinberger, D. R., Berman, K. F., Suddath, R., and Torrey, E. F. (1992). Evidence of dysfunction of a prefrontal-limbic network in schizophrenia: A magnetic resonance imaging and regional cerebral blood flow study of discordant monozygotic twins. *Am. J. Psychiatry* 149, 890–897.

93. Frith, C. D., Friston, K. J., Herold, S., Silbersweig, D., Fletcher, P., Cahill, C., et al. (1995). Regional brain activity in chronic schizophrenic patients during the performance of a verbal fluency task. *Br. J. Psychiatry* 167, 343–349.

94. Spence, S. A., Brooks, D. J., Hirsch, S. R., Liddle, P. F., Meehan, J., and Grasby, P. M. (1997). A PET study of voluntary movement in schizophrenic patients experiencing passivity phenomena (delusions of alien control). *Brain* 120(P. 11), 1997–2011.

95. Heckers, S., Rauch, S. L., Goff, D., Savage, C. R., Schacter, D. L. F. A. J., and Alpert, N. M. (1998). Impaired recruitment of the hippocampus during conscious recollection in schizophrenia. *Nature* 1, 318–323.

96. Artiges, E., Salame, P., Recasens, C., Poline, J. B., Attar-Levy, D., De La, R. A., et al. (2000). Working memory control in patients with schizophrenia: A PET study during a random number generation task. *Am. J. Psychiatry* 157, 1517–1519.

97. Tamminga, C. A., Vogel, M., Gao, X., Lahti, A. C., and Holcomb, H. H. (2000). The limbic cortex in schizophrenia: Focus on the anterior cingulate. *Brain Res. Brain Res. Rev.* 31, 364–370.

98. Lahti, A. C., Holcomb, H. H., Medoff, D. R., and Tamminga, C. A. (1995). Ketamine activates psychosis and alters limbic blood flow in schizophrenia. *Neuroreport* 6, 869–872.

99. Silbersweig, D. A., Stern, E., Frith, C., Cahill, C., Holmes, A., Grootoonk, S., et al. (1995). A functional neuroanatomy of hallucinations in schizophrenia. *Nature* 378, 176–179.

100. Copolov, D. L., Seal, M. L., Maruff, P., Ulusoy, R., Wong, M. T., Tochon-Danguy, H. J., and Egan, G. F. (2003). Cortical activation associated with the experience of auditory hallucinations and perception of human speech in schizophrenia: A PET correlation study. *Psychiatry Res.* 122, 139–152.

101. Volkow, N. D., Wolf, A. P., Van Gelder, P., Brodie, J. D., Overall, J. E., Cancro, R., and Gomez-Mont, F. (1987). Phenomenological correlates of metabolic activity in 18 patients with chronic schizophrenia. *Am. J. Psychiatry* 144, 151–158.

102. Andreasen, N. C., Rezai, K., Alliger, R., Swayze, V. W., II, Flaum, M., Kirchner, P., Cohen, G., and O'Leary, D. S. (1992). Hypofrontality in neuroleptic-naive patients and in patients with chronic schizophrenia. Assessment with xenon 133 single-photon emission computed tomography and the Tower of London. *Arch. Gen. Psychiatry* 49, 943–958.

103. Wolkin, A., Sanfilipo, M., Wolf, A. P., Angrist, B., Brodie, J. D., and Rotrosen, J. (1992). Negative symptoms and hypofrontality in chronic schizophrenia. *Arch. Gen. Psychiatry* 49, 959–965.

104. Schroeder, J., Buchsbaum, M. S., Siegel, B. V., Geider, F. J., Haier, R. J., Lohr, J., Wu, J., and Potkin, S. G. (1994). Patterns of cortical activity in schizophrenia. *Psychol. Med.* 24, 947–955.

105. Friston, K. J. (1992). The dorsolateral prefrontal cortex, schizophrenia and PET. *J. Neural. Transm. Suppl.* 37, 79–93.

106. Liddle, P. F., Friston, K. J., Frith, C. D., Hirsch, S. R., Jones, T., and Frackowiak, R. S. (1992). Patterns of cerebral blood flow in schizophrenia. *Br. J. Psychiatry* 160, 179–186.

107. Lahti, A. C., Holcomb, H. H., Medoff, D. R., Weiler, M. A., Tamminga, C. A., and Carpenter, W. T., Jr. (2001). Abnormal patterns of regional cerebral blood flow in schizophrenia with primary negative symptoms during an effortful auditory recognition task. *Am. J. Psychiatry* 158, 1797–1808.

108. Schwartz, M. L., and Goldman-Rakic, P. S. (1984). Callosal and intrahemispheric connectivity of the prefrontal association cortex in rhesus monkey: Relation between intraparietal and principal sulcal cortex. *J. Comp. Neurol.* 226, 403–420.

109. Potkin, S. G., Alva, G., Fleming, K., Anand, R., Keator, D., Carreon, D., Doo, M., Jin, Y., Wu, J. C., and Fallon, J. H. (2002). A PET study of the pathophysiology of negative symptoms in schizophrenia. *Am. J. Psychiatry* 159, 227–237.

110. Hazlett, E. A., Buchsbaum, M. S., Kemether, E., Bloom, R., Platholi, J., Brickman, A. M., Shihabuddin, L., Tang, C., and Byne, W. (2004). Abnormal glucose metabolism in the mediodorsal nucleus of the thalamus in schizophrenia. *Am. J. Psychiatry* 161, 305–314.

111. Gur, R. E., McGrath, C., Chan, R. M., Schroeder, L., Turner, T., Turetsky, B. I., Kohler, C., Alsop, D., Maldjian, J., Ragland, J. D., and Gur, R. C. (2002). An fMRI study of facial emotion processing in patients with schizophrenia. *Am. J. Psychiatry* 159, 1992–1999.

112. Buchanan, R. W., Strauss, M. E., Breier, A., Kirkpatrick, B., and Carpenter, W. T., Jr. (1997). Attentional impairments in deficit and nondeficit forms of schizophrenia. *Am. J. Psychiatry* 154, 363–370.

113. Buchanan, R. W., Strauss, M. E., Kirkpatrick, B., Holstein, C., Breier, A., and Carpenter, W. T., Jr. (1994). Neuropsychological impairments in deficit vs nondeficit forms of schizophrenia. *Arch. Gen. Psychiatry* 51, 804–811.

114. Spence, S. A., Liddle, P. F., Stefan, M. D., Hellewell, J. S., Sharma, T., Friston, K. J., et al. (2000). Functional anatomy of verbal fluency in people with schizophrenia and those at genetic risk. Focal dysfunction and distributed disconnectivity reappraised. *Br. J. Psychiatry* 176, 52–60.

115. Jennings, J. M., McIntosh, A. R., Kapur, S., Zipursky, R. B., and Houle, S. (1998). Functional network differences in schizophrenia: A rCBF study of semantic processing. *Neuroreport* 9, 1697–1700.

116. Manoach, D. S., Press, D. Z., Thangaraj, V., Searl, M. M., Goff, D. C., Halpern, E., et al. (1999). Schizophrenic subjects activate dorsolateral prefrontal cortex during a working memory task, as measured by fMRI. *Biol. Psychiatry* 45, 1128–1137.

117. Manoach, D. S., Gollub, R. L., Benson, E. S., Searl, M. M., Goff, D. C., Halpern, E., et al. (2000). Schizophrenic subjects show aberrant fMRI activation of dorsolateral prefrontal cortex and basal ganglia during working memory performance. *Biol. Psychiatry* 48, 99–109.

118. Callicott, J. H., Ramsey, N. F., Tallent, K., Bertolino, A., Knable, M. B., Coppola, R., et al. (1998). Functional magnetic resonance imaging brain mapping in psychiatry: Methodological issues illustrated in a study of working memory in schizophrenia. *Neuropsychopharmacology* 18, 186–196.

119. Stevens, A. A., Goldman-Rakic, P. S., Gore, J. C., Fulbright, R. K., and Wexler, B. E. (1998). Cortical dysfunction in schizophrenia during auditory word and tone working memory demonstrated by functional magnetic resonance imaging. *Arch. Gen. Psychiatry* 55, 1097–1103.

120. Callicott, J. H., Mattay, V. S., Bertolino, A., Finn, K., Coppola, R., Frank, J. A., et al. (1999). Physiological characteristics of capacity constraints in working memory as revealed by functional MRI. *Cereb. Cortex* 9, 20–26.

121. Dolan, R. J., Fletcher, P., Frith, C. D., Friston, K. J., Frackowiak, R. S. J., and Grasby, P. M. (1995). Dopaminergic modulation of impaired cognitive activation in the anterior cingulate cortex in schizophrenia. *Nature* 378, 180–182.

122. Karlsson, P., Farde, L., Halldin, C., and Sedvall, G. (2002). PET study of D(1) dopamine receptor binding in neuroleptic-naive patients with schizophrenia. *Am. J. Psychiatry* 159, 761–767.

123. Abi-Dargham, A., Mawlawi, O., Lombardo, I., Gil, R., Martinez, D., Huang, Y., et al. (2002). Prefrontal dopamine D1 receptors and working memory in schizophrenia. *J. Neurosci.* 22, 3708–3719.

124. Goldman-Rakic, P. S., Castner, S. A., Svensson, T. H., Siever, L. J., and Williams, G. V. (2004). Targeting the dopamine D1 receptor in schizophrenia: Insights for cognitive dysfunction. *Psychopharmacology* 174, 3–16.

125. Wong, D. F., Wagner, Jr., H. N., Tune, L. E., Dannals, R. F., Pearlson, G. D., Links, J. M., et al. (1986). Positron emission tomography reveals elevated D2 dopamine receptors in drug-naïve schizophrenics. *Science* 234, 1558–1563.

126. Pearlson, G. D., Wong, D. F., Tune, L. E., Ross, C. A., Chase, G. A., Links, J. M., et al. (1995). In vivo D2 dopamine receptor density in psychotic and nonpsychotic patients with bipolar disorder. *Arch. Gen. Psychiatry* 52, 471–477.

127. Farde, L., Wiesel, F. A., Stone-Elander, S., Halldin, C., Nordstrom, A. L., Hall, H., et al. (1990). D2 dopamine receptors in neuroleptic-naive schizophrenic patients. A

positron emission tomography study with ^{11}C raclopride. *Arch. Gen. Psychiatry* 47, 213–219.

128. Hietala, J., Syvälahti, E., and Vuorio, K. (1991). Striatal dopamine D2 receptor density in neuroleptic-naive schizophrenics studied with positron emission tomography. In *Biological Psychiatry*, Vol. 2, G. Racagni, N. Brunello, and T. Fukuda, Eds. Excerpta Medica, Amsterdam, pp. 386–387.

129. Martinot, J. L., Peron-Magnan, P., and Huret, J. D. (1990). Striatal D2 dopaminergic receptors assessed with positron emission tomography and ^{76}Br-bromospiperone in untreated schizophrenic patients. *Am. J. Psychiatry* 147, 44–50.

130. Martinot, J. L., Paillere-Martinot, M. L., Loc'h, C., Hardy, P., Poirier, M. F., Mazoyer, B., et al. (1991). The estimated density of D2 striatal receptors in schizophrenia. A study with positron emission tomography and ^{76}Br-bromolisuride. *Br. J. Psychiatry* 158, 346–350.

131. Hietala, J., Syvälahti, E., Vuorio, K., Nagren, K., Lehikoinen, P., Ruotsalainen, U., et al. (1994). Striatal D_2 dopamine receptor characteristics in neuroleptic-naive schizophrenic patients studied with positron emission tomography. *Arch. Gen. Psychiatry* 51, 116–123.

132. Laruelle, M., Abi-Dargham, A., van Dyck, C. H., Gil, R., D'Souza, C. D., Erdos, J., et al. (1996). Single photon emission computerized tomography imaging of amphetamine-induced dopamine release in drug-free schizophrenic subjects. *Proc. Natl. Acad. Sci. USA* 93, 235–240.

133. Abi-Dargham, A., Gil, R., Krystal, J., Baldwin, R. M., Seibyl, J. P., Bowers, M., et al. (1998). Increased striatal dopamine transmission in schizophrenia: Confirmation in a second cohort. *Am. J. Psychiatry* 155, 761–767.

134. Laruelle, M., Abi-Dargham, A., Gil, R., Kegeles, L., and Innis, R. (1999). Increased dopamine transmission in schizophrenia: Relationship to illness phases. *Biol. Psychiatry* 46, 56–72.

135. Smith, G. S., Schloesser, R., Brodie, J. D., Dewey, S. L., Logan, J., Vitkun, S. A., Simkowitz, P., Hurley, A., Cooper, T., Volkow, N. D., and Cancro, R. (1998). Glutamate modulation of dopamine measured in vivo with positron emission tomography (PET) and 11C-raclopride in normal human subjects. *Neuropsychopharmacology* 18, 18–25.

136. Kegeles, L. S., Abi-Dargham, A., Zea-Ponce, Y., Rodenhiser-Hill, J., Mann, J. J., Van Heertum, R. L., Cooper, T. B., Carlsson, A., and Laruelle, M. (2000). Modulation of amphetamine-induced striatal dopamine release by ketamine in humans: Implications for schizophrenia. *Biol. Psychiatry* 48, 627–640.

137. Waterhouse, R. N., Slifstein, M., Dumont, F., Zhao, J., Chang, R. C., Sudo, Y., Sultana, A., Balter, A., and Laruelle, M. (2004). In vivo evaluation of [11C]*N*-(2-chloro-5thiomethylphenyl)-*N'*-(3-methoxy-phenyl)-*N'*-methylguanidine ([11C]GMOM) as a potential PET radiotracer for the PCP/NMDA receptor. *Nucl. Med. Biol.* 31, 939–948.

138. Harrison, P. J., and Eastwood, S. L. (2001). Neuropathological studies of synaptic connectivity in the hippocampal formation in schizophrenia. *Hippocampus* 11, 508–519.

139. Bogerts, B. (1993). Recent advances in the neuropathology of schizophrenia. *Schizophr. Bull.* 19, 431–445.

140. Harrison, P. J. (1999). The neuropathology of schizophrenia. A critical review of the data and their interpretation. *Brain* 122, 593–624.

141. Carlsson, A., and Lindquist, M. (1963). Effect of chlorpromazine and haloperidol of formation of 3-methoxytyramine and normetanephrine in mouse brain. *Acta. Pharmacol. Toxicol.* 20, 140–144.
142. Elkashef, A. M., Issa, F., and Wyatt, R. J. (1995). The biochemical basis of schizophrenia. In *Contemporary Issues in the Treatment of Schizophrenia*, C. L. Shriqui, and H. A. Nasrallah, Eds. American Psychiatric Press, Washington, DC, p. 863.
143. Davis, K. L., Kahn, R. S., Ko, G., and Davidson, M. (1991). Dopamine in schizophrenia: A review and reconceptualization. *Am. J. Psychiatry* 148, 1474–1486.
144. Abi-Dargham, A., Rodenhiser, J., Printz, D., Zea-Ponce, Y., Gil, R., Kegeles, L. S., Weiss, R., Cooper, T. B., Mann, J. J., Van Heertum, R. L., Gorman, J. M., and Laruelle, M. (2000). Increased baseline occupancy of D2 receptors by dopamine in schizophrenia. *Proc. Natl. Acad. Sci. USA* 97(14), 8104–8109.
145. Meador-Woodruff, J. H., and Healy, D. J. (2000). Glutamate receptor expression in schizophrenic brain. *Brain Res. Brain Res. Rev.* 31, 288–294.
146. Scarr, E., Beneyto, M., Meador-Woodruff, J. H., and Dean, B. (2005). Cortical glutamatergic markers in schizophrenia. *Neuropsychopharmacology* 30, 1521–1531.
147. Dracheva, S., McGurk, S. R., and Haroutunian, V. (2005). mRNA expression of AMPA receptors and AMPA receptor binding proteins in the cerebral cortex of elderly schizophrenics. *J. Neurosci. Res.* 79(6), 868–878.
148. Ibrahim, H. M., Hogg, A. J., Jr., Healy, D. J., Haroutunian, V., Davis, K. L., and Meador-Woodruff, J. H. (2000). Ionotropic glutamate receptor binding and subunit mRNA expression in thalamic nuclei in schizophrenia. *Am. J. Psychiatry* 157, 1811–1823.
149. Clinton, S. M., Haroutunian, V., Davis, K. L., and Meador-Woodruff, J. H. (2003). Altered transcript expression of NMDA receptor-associated postsynaptic proteins in the thalamus of subjects with schizophrenia. *Am. J. Psychiatry* 160(6), 1100–1109.
150. Moghaddam, B., and Adams, B. W. (1998). Reversal of phencyclidine effects by a group II metabotropic glutamate receptor agonist in rats. *Science* 281, 1349–1352.
151. Krystal, J. H., Abi-Saab, W., Perry, E., D'Souza, D. C., Liu, N., Gueorguieva, R., McDougall, L., Hunsberger, T., Belger, A., Levine, L., and Breier, A. (2005). Preliminary evidence of attenuation of the disruptive effects of the NMDA glutamate receptor antagonist, ketamine, on working memory by pretreatment with the group II metabotropic glutamate receptor agonist, LY354740, in healthy human subjects. *Psychopharmacology (Berl.)* 179, 303–309.
152. Coyle, J. T. (1997). The nagging question of the function of N-acetylaspartylglutamate. *Neurobiol. Dis.* 4, 231–238.
153. Neale, J. H., Bzdega, T., and Wroblewska, B. (2000). N-Acetylaspartylglutamate: The most abundant peptide neurotransmitter in the mammalian central nervous system. *J. Neurochem.* 75, 443–452.
154. Tsai, G., Passani, L. A., Slusher, B. S., Carter, R., Baer, L., Kleinman, J. E., and Coyle, J. T. (1995). Abnormal excitatory neurotransmitter metabolism in schizophrenic brains. *Arch. Gen. Psychiatry* 52, 829–836.
155. Ghose, S., Weickert, C. S., Colvin, S. M., Coyle, J. T., Herman, M. M., Hyde, T. M., and Kleinman, J. E. (2004). Glutamate carboxypeptidase II gene expression in the human frontal and temporal lobe in schizophrenia. *Neuropsychopharmacology* 29, 117–125.
156. Egan, M. F., Straub, R. E., Goldberg, T. E., Yakub, I., Callicott, J. H., Hariri, A. R., Mattay, V. S., Bertolino, A., Hyde, T. M., Shannon-Weickert, C., Akil, M., Crook, J., Vakkalanka, R. K., Balkissoon, R., Gibbs, R. A., Kleinman, J. E., and Weinberger,

D. R. (2004). Variation in GRM3 affects cognition, prefrontal glutamate, and risk for schizophrenia. *Proc. Natl. Acad. Sci. USA* 101, 12604–12609.

157. Lewis, D. A., Volk, D. W., and Hashimoto, T. (2004). Selective alterations in prefrontal cortical GABA neurotransmission in schizophrenia: A novel target for the treatment of working memory dysfunction. *Psychopharmacology (Berl.)* 174, 143–150.

158. Benes, F. M., and Berretta, S. (2001). GABAergic interneurons: Implications for understanding schizophrenia and bipolar disorder. *Neuropsychopharmacology* 25, 1–27.

159. Lewis, D. A., and Lund, J. S. (1990). Heterogeneity of chandelier neurons in monkey neocortex: Corticotropin-releasing factor- and parvalbumin-immunoreactive populations. *J. Comp. Neurol.* 293, 599–615.

160. Lewis, D. A., Hashimoto, T., and Volk, D. W. (2005). Cortical inhibitory neurons and schizophrenia. *Nat. Rev. Neurosci.* 6(4), 312–324.

161. Freedman, D. X. (1975). LSD, psychotogenic procedures, and brain neurohumors. *Psychopharmacol. Bull.* 11, 42–43.

162. Harrison, P. J. (1999). Neurochemical alterations in schizophrenia affecting the putative receptor targets of atypical antipsychotics. Focus on dopamine (D1, D3, D4) and 5-HT2a receptors. *Br. J. Psychiatry Suppl.* 38, 12–22.

163. Marcus, M. M., Nomikos, G. G., and Svensson, T. H. (2000). Effects of atypical antipsychotic drugs on dopamine output in the shell and core of the nucleus accumbens: Role of 5-HT (2A) and alpha(1)-adrenoceptor antagonism. *Eur. Neuropsychopharmacol.* 10, 245–253.

164. Kuroki, T., Meltzer, H. Y., and Ichikawa, J. (2003). 5-HT 2A receptor stimulation by DOI, a 5-HT 2Ã2C receptor agonist, potentiates amphetamine-induced dopamine release in rat medial prefrontal cortex and nucleus accumbens. *Brain Res.* 972, 216–221.

165. de Paulis, T. (2001). M-100907 (Aventis). *Curr. Opin. Investig. Drugs* 2, 123–132.

166. Hughes, J. R., Hatsukami, D. K., Mitchell, J. E., and Dahlgren, L. A. (1986). Prevalence of smoking among psychiatric outpatients. *Am. J. Psychiatry.* 143, 993–997.

167. Benwell, M. E. M., Balfour, D. J. K., and Anderson, J. M. (1988). Evidence that tobacco smoking increases the density of (−)-[^{3}H]nicotine binding sites in human brain. *J. Neurochem.* 50, 1243–1247.

168. Wonnacott, S. (1990). The paradox of nicotinic acetylcholine receptor up-regulation by nicotine. *Trends Pharmacol. Sci.* 11, 216–219.

169. Hyde, T. M., and Crook, J. M. (2001). Cholinergic systems and schizophrenia: Primary pathology or epiphenomena? *J. Chem Neuroanat.* 22(1/2), 53–63.

170. Stefansson, H., Sigurdsson, E., Steinthorsdottir, V., Bjornsdottir, S., Sigmundsson, T., Ghosh, S., et al. (2002). Neuregulin 1 and susceptibility to schizophrenia. *Am. J. Hum. Genet.* 71, 877–892.

171. Schwab, S. G., Knapp, M., Mondabon, S., Hallmayer, J., Borrmann-Hassenbach, M., Albus, M., et al. (2003). Support for association of schizophrenia with genetic variation in the 6p22.3 gene, dysbindin, in sib-pair families with linkage and in an additional sample of triad families. *Am. J. Hum. Genet.* 72, 185–190.

172. Chumakov, I., Blumenfeld, M., Guerassimenko, O., Cavarec, L., Palicio, M., Abderrahim, H., et al. (2002). Genetic and physiological data implicating the new human gene G72 and the gene for D-amino acid oxidase in schizophrenia. *Proc. Natl. Acad. Sci. USA* 99, 13675–13680.

173. Chowdari, K. V., Mirnics, K., Semwal, P., Wood, J., Lawrence, E., Bhatia, T., et al. (2002). Association and linkage analyses of RGS4 polymorphisms in schizophrenia. *Hum. Mol. Genet.* 11, 1373–1380.

174. Liu, H., Heath, S. C., Sobin, C., Roos, J. L., Galke, B. L., Blundell, M. L., et al. (2002). Genetic variation at the 22q11 PRODH2DGCR6 locus presents an unusual pattern and increases susceptibility to schizophrenia. *Proc. Natl. Acad. Sci. USA* 99, 3717–3722.

175. Egan, M. F., Goldberg, T. E., Kolachana, B. S., Callicott, J. H., Mazzanti, C. M., Straub, R. E., et al. (2001). Effect of COMT Val108158 Met genotype on frontal lobe function and risk for schizophrenia. *Proc. Natl. Acad. Sci. USA* 98, 6917–6922.

176. Shifman, S., Bronstein, M., Sternfeld, M., Pisante-Shalom, A., Lev-Lehman, E., Weizman, A., et al. (2002). A highly significant association between a COMT haplotype and schizophrenia. *Am. J. Hum. Genet.* 71, 1296–1302.

177. Harrison, P. J., and Owen, M. (2003). Genes for schizophrenia? Recent findings and their pathophysiological implications. *Lancet* 361, 417–419.

178. Harrison, P. J., and Weinberger, D. (2005). Schizophrenia genes, gene expression, and neuropathology: On the matter of their convergence. *Mol. Psychiatry* 10, 40–68.

179. Avila, M. T., Hong, E., and Thaker, G. K. (2002). Current progress in schizophrenia research. Eye movement abnormalities in schizophrenia: What is the nature of the deficit? *J. Nerv. Men. Dis.* 190, 479–480.

180. Ross, R. G., Olincy, A., Mikulich, S. K., Radant, A. D., Harris, J. G., Waldo, M., et al. (2002). Admixture analysis of smooth pursuit eye movements in probands with schizophrenia and their relatives suggests gain and leading saccades are potential endophenotypes. *Psychophysiology* 39, 809–819.

181. Sweeney, J. A., Luna, B., Srinivasagam, N. M., Keshavan, M. S., Schooler, N. R., Haas, G. L., et al. (1998). Eye tracking abnormalities in schizophrenia: Evidence for dysfunction in the frontal eye fields. *Biol. Psychiatry* 44, 698–708.

182. Braff, D. L., and Geyer, M. A. (1990). Sensorimotor gating and schizophrenia. Human and animal model studies. *Arch. Gen. Psychiatry* 47, 181–188.

183. Swerdlow, N. R., and Geyer, M. A. (1998). Using an animal model of deficient sensorimotor gating to study the pathophysiology and new treatments of schizophrenia. *Schizophr. Bull.* 24, 285–301.

184. Freedman, R. (2003). Electrophysiological phenotypes. *Meth. Mol. Med.* 77, 215–225.

185. Gottesman, I. I., and Gould, T. (2003). The endophenotype concept in psychiatry: Etymology and strategic intentions. *Am. J. Psychiatry* 160, 636–645.

186. Tregellas, J. R., Tanabe, J. L., Miller, D. E., Ross, R. G., Olincy, A., and Freedman, R. (2004). Neurobiology of smooth pursuit eye movement deficits in schizophrenia: An fMRI study. *Am. J. Psychiatry* 161, 315–321.

187. Thaker, G. K., Ross, D. E., Cassady, S. L., Adami, H. M., Medoff, D. R., and Sherr, J. (2000). Saccadic eye movement abnormalities in relatives of patients with schizophrenia. *Schizophr. Res.* 45, 235–244.

188. Thaker, G. K., Nguyen, J. A., and Tamminga, C. A. (1989). Increased saccadic distractibility in tardive dyskinesia: Functional evidence for subcortical GABA dysfunction. *Biol. Psychiatry* 25, 49–59.

189. Swerdlow, N. R., Braff, D. L., Taaid, N., and Geyer, M. A. (1994). Assessing the validity of an animal model of deficient sensorimotor gating in schizophrenic patients. *Arch. Gen. Psychiatry* 51, 139–154.

190. Swerdlow, N. R., Braff, D. L., and Geyer, M. A. (1999). Cross-species studies of sensorimotor gating of the startle reflex. *Ann. NY Acad. Sci.* 877, 202–216.

191. Olton, D. S., and Samuelson, R. J. (1976). Remembrances of places passed: Spatial memory in rats. *J. Exp. Psychol. Anim. Behav. Proc.* 2, 97–116.

192. Castner, S. A., Goldman-Rakic, P. S., and Williams, G. V. (2004). Animal models of working memory: Insights for targeting cognitive dysfunction in schizophrenia. *Psychopharm. (Berl.)* 174, 111–125.

193. Saykin, A. J., Gur, R. C., Gur, R. E., Mozley, P. D., Mozley, L. H., Resnick, S. M., Kester, D. B., and Stafiniak, P. (1991). Neuropsychological function in schizophrenia. Selective impairment in memory and learning. *Arch. Gen. Psychiatry* 48, 618–624.

194. Saykin, A. J., Shtasel, D. L., Gur, R. E., Kester, D. B., Mozley, L. H., Stafiniak, P., and Gur, R. C. (1994). Neuropsychological deficits in neuroleptic naive patients with first-episode schizophrenia. *Arch. Gen. Psychiatry* 51, 124–131.

195. Heinrichs, R. W., and Zakzanis, K. K. (1998). Neurocognitive deficit in schizophrenia: A quantitative review of the evidence. *Neuropsychology* 12, 426–445.

196. Eichenbaum, H. (1998). Using olfaction to study memory. *Ann. NY Acad. Sci.* 855, 657–669.

197. Titone, D., Ditman, T., Holzman, P. S., Eichenbaum, H., and Levy, D. L. (2004). Transitive inference in schizophrenia: Impairments in relational memory organization. *Schizophr. Res.* 68, 235–247.

198. Dusek, J. A., and Eichenbaum, H. (1997). The hippocampus and memory for orderly stimulus relations. *Proc. Natl. Acad. Sci. USA* 94, 7109–7114.

199. Rosvold, H. E., Mirsky, A. F., Sarason, I., Bransome, E. D., and Beck, L. H. (1956). A continuous performance test of brain damage. *J. Consult. Psychol.* 20, 343–350.

200. Cohen, J. D., Barch, D. M., Carter, C., and Servan-Schreiber, D. (1999). Context-processing deficits in schizophrenia: Converging evidence from three theoretically motivated cognitive tasks. *J. Abnorm. Psychol.* 108(1), 120–133.

201. Chudasama, Y., and Robbins, T. W. (2004). Psychopharmacological approaches to modulating attention in the five-choice serial reaction time task: Implications for schizophrenia. *Psychopharmacology (Berl.)* 174, 86–98.

202. Muir, J. L., Everitt, B. J., and Robbins, T. W. (1996). The cerebral cortex of the rat and visual attentional function: Dissociable effects of mediofrontal, cingulate, anterior dorsolateral, and parietal cortex lesions on a five-choice serial reaction time task. *Cereb. Cortex* 6, 470–481.

203. Robbins, T. W. (2000). From arousal to cognition: The integrative position of the prefrontal cortex. *Prog. Brain Res.* 126, 469–483.

204. Bluthe, R. M., and Dantzer, R. (1993). Role of the vomeronasal system in vasopressinergic modulation of social recognition in rats. *Brain Res.* 604, 205–210.

205. Thor, D. H., and Holloway, W. R. (1982). Anosmia and play fighting behavior in prepubescent male and female rats. *Physiol. Behav.* 29, 281–285.

206. Kuperberg, G., and Heckers, S. (2000). Schizophrenia and cognitive function. *Curr. Opin. Neurobiol.* 10(2), 205–210.

207. Gao, X. M., Elmer, G., Cooper, T., and Tamminga, C. A. (submitted). Social memory in mice: Disruption with an NMDA antagonist and reversal with antipsychotics.

208. Young, L. J. (2002). The neurobiology of social recognition, approach, and avoidance. *Biol. Psychiatry* 51, 18–26.

209. Carter, C. S., Williams, J. R., Witt, D. M., and Insel, T. R. (1992). Oxytocin and social bonding. *Ann. NY Acad. Sci.* 652, 204–211.

210. Mohn, A. R., Gainetdinov, R. R., Caron, M. G., and Koller, B. H. (1998). Mice with reduced NMDA receptor expression display behaviors related to schizophrenia. *Cell* 98, 427–436.

211. Brody, S. A., Conquet, F., and Geyer, M. A. (2003). Disruption of prepulse inhibition in mice lacking mGluR1. *Eur. J. Neurosci.* 18, 3361–3366.
212. Brody, S. A., Dulawa, S. C., Conquet, F., and Geyer, M. A. (2004). Assessment of a prepulse inhibition deficit in a mutant mouse lacking mGlu5 receptors. *Mol. Psychiatry* 9(1), 35–41.
213. Holmes, A., Lachowicz, J. E., and Sibley, D. R. (2004). Phenotypic analysis of dopamine receptor knockout mice; recent insights into the functional specificity of dopamine receptor subtypes. *Neuropharmacology* 47, 1117–1134.
214. Lahdesmaki, J., Sallinen, J., MacDonald, E., and Scheinin, M. (2004). Alpha2A-adrenoceptors are important modulators of the effects of D-amphetamine on startle reactivity and brain monoamines. *Neuropsychopharmacology* 29, 1282–1293.
215. Erbel-Sieler, C., Dudley, C., Zhou, Y., Wu, X., Estill, S. J., Han, T., Diaz-Arrastia, R., Brunskill, E. W., Potter, S. S., and McKnight, S. L. (2004). Behavioral and regulatory abnormalities in mice deficient in the NPAS1 and NPAS3 transcription factors. *Proc. Natl. Acad. Sci.* 101, 13648–13653.
216. Javitt, D. C., and Zukin, S. R. (1991). Recent advances in the phencyclidine model of schizophrenia. *Am. J. Psychiatry* 148, 1301–1308.
217. Luby, E. D., Cohen, B. D., Rosenbaum, G., Gottlieb, J. S., and Kelley, R. (1959). Study of a new schizophrenomimetic drug: Sernyl. *Arch. Neurol. Psychiatry* 81, 363–369.
218. Krystal, J. H., Karper, L. P., Seibyl, J. P., Freeman, G. K., Delaney, R., Bremner, J. D., Heninger, G. R., Bowers, M. B., Jr., and Charney, D. S. (1994). Subanesthetic effects of the noncompetitive NMDA antagonist, ketamine, in humans. Psychotomimetic, perceptual, cognitive, and neuroendocrine responses. *Arch. Gen. Psychiatry* 51, 199–214.
219. Malhotra, A. K., Pinals, D. A., Weingartner, H., Sirocco, K., Missar, C. D., Pickar, D., and Breier, A. (1996). NMDA receptor function and human cognition: The effects of ketamine in healthy volunteers. *Neuropsychopharmacology* 14, 301–307.
220. Lahti, A. C., Weiler, M. A., Tamara Michaelidis, B. A., Parwani, A., and Tamminga, C. A. (2001). Effects of ketamine in normal and schizophrenic volunteers. *Neuropsychopharmacology* 25, 455–467.
221. Bakshi, V. P., and Geyer, M. A. (1995). Antagonism of phencyclidine-induced deficits in prepulse inhibition by the putative atypical antipsychotic olanzapine. *Psychopharmacology* 122, 198–201.
222. Bakshi, V. P., Swerdlow, N. R., and Geyer, M. A. (1994). Clozapine antagonizes phencyclidine-induced deficits in sensorimotor gating of the startle response. *J. Pharm. Exp. Ther.* 271, 787–794.
223. Castellani, S., and Adams, P. M. (1981). Acute and chronic phencyclidine effects on locomotor activity, stereotypy and ataxia in rats. *Eur. J. Pharm.* 73, 143–154.
224. Haggerty, G. C., Forney, R. B., and Johnson, J. M. (1984). The effect of a single administration of phencyclidine on behavior in the rat over a 21-day period. *Toxicol. Appl. Pharm.* 75, 444–453.
225. Kesner, R. P., Hardy, J. D., and Calder, L. D. (1981). Phencyclidine and behavior: I. Sensory-motor function, activity level, taste aversion and water intake. *Pharm. Biochem. Behav.* 15, 7–13.
226. Lehmann-Masten, V. D., and Geyer, M. A. (1991). Spatial and temporal patterning distinguishes the locomotor activating effects of dizocilpine and phencyclidine in rats. *Neuropharmacology* 30, 629–636.

227. Murray, T. F., and Horita, A. (1979). Phencyclidine-induced stereotyped behavior in rats: Dose response effects and antagonism by neuroleptics. *Life Sci.* 24, 2217–2226.
228. Sams-Dodd, F. (1995). Distinct effects of D-amphetamine and phencyclidine on the social behaviour of rats. *Behav. Pharm.* 6, 55–65.
229. Sams-Dodd, F. (1996). Phencyclidine-induced stereotyped behavior and social isolation in rats: A possible animal model of schizophrenia. *Behav. Pharm.* 7, 3–23.
230. Kesner, R. P., and Davis, M. (1993). Phencyclidine disrupts acquisition and retention performance within a spatial continuous recognition memory task. *Pharm. Biochem. Behav.* 44, 419–424.
231. Sams-Dodd, F. (1995). Automation of the social interaction test by a video-tracking system: Behavioural effects of repeated phencyclidine treatment. *J. Neurosci. Meth.* 59, 157–167.
232. Cartmell, J., Monn, J. A., and Schoepp, D. D. (2000). Attenuation of specific PCP-evoked behaviors by the potent mGlu2/3 receptor agonist, LY379268 and comparison with the atypical antipsychotic, clozapine. *Psychopharm. (Berl.)* 148, 423–429.
233. Carlsson, A. (1995). The dopamine theory revisited. In *Schizophrenia*, S. R. Hirsch and D. R. Weinberger, Eds. Blackwell Science, Oxford, pp. 379–400.
234. Seiden, L. S., Sabol, K. E., and Ricaurte, G. A. (1993). Amphetamine: Effects on catecholamine systems and behavior. *Annu. Rev. Pharmacol. Toxicol.* 33, 639–677.
235. Snyder, S. H. (1973). Amphetamine psychosis: A "model" schizophrenia mediated by catecholamines. *Am. J. Psychiatry* 130(1), 61–67.
236. Sams-Dodd, F. (1998). Effects of continuous D-amphetamine and phencyclidine administration on social behaviour, stereotyped behaviour, and locomotor activity in rats. *Neuropsychopharmacology* 19, 18–25.
237. D'Souza, D. C., Abi-Saab, W. M., Madonick, S., Forselius-Bielen, K., Doersch, A., Braley, G., Gueorguieva, R., Cooper, T. B., and Krystal, J. H. (2005). Delta-9-tetrahydrocannabinol effects in schizophrenia: Implications for cognition, psychosis, and addiction. *Biol. Psychiatry* 57, 594–608.
238. Fadda, P., Robinson, L., Fratta, W., Pertwee, R. G., and Riedel, G. (2004). Differential effects of THC- or CBD-rich cannabis extracts on working memory in rats. *Neuropharmacology* 47, 1170–1179.
239. Fujiwara, M., and Egashira, N. (2004). New perspectives in the studies on endocannabinoid and cannabis: Abnormal behaviors associate with CB1 cannabinoid receptor and development of therapeutic application. *J. Pharmacol. Sci.* 96, 362–366.
240. Chaperon, F., and Thiebot, M. H. (1999). Behavioral effects of cannabinoid agents in animals. *Crit. Rev. Neurobiol.* 13, 243–281.
241. Varvel, S. A., Hamm, R. J., Martin, B. R., and Lichtman, A. H. (2001). Differential effects of delta 9-THC on spatial reference and working memory in mice. *Psychopharm. (Berl.)* 157, 142–150.
242. Gourevitch, R., Rocher, C., Le Pen, G., Krebs, M. O., and Jay, T. M. (2004). Working memory deficits in adult rats after prenatal disruption of neurogenesis. *Behav. Pharmacol.* 15, 287–292.
243. Flagstad, P., Glenthoj, B. Y., and Didriksen, M. (2005). Cognitive deficits caused by late gestational disruption of neurogenesis in rats: A preclinical model of schizophrenia. *Neuropsychopharmacology* 30, 250–260.
244. Selemon, L. D., Wang, L., Nebel, M. B., Csernansky, J. G., Goldman-Rakic, P. S., and Rakic, P. (2005). Direct and indirect effects of fetal irradiation on cortical gray and white matter volume in the macaque. *Biol. Psychiatry* 57(1), 83–90.

245. Lipska, B. K., Jaskiw, G. E., and Weinberger, D. R. (1993). Postpubertal emergence of hyperresponsiveness to stress and to amphetamine after neonatal excitotoxic hippocampal damage: A potential animal model of schizophrenia. *Neuropsychopharmacology* 9, 67–75.
246. Lipska, B. K., and Weinberger, D. R. (1993). Delayed effects of neonatal hippocampal damage on haloperidol-induced catalepsy and apomorphine-induced stereotypic behaviors in the rat. *Brain Res. Dev. Brain Res.* 75, 213–222.
247. Lipska, B. K., Swerdlow, N. R., Geyer, M. A., Jaskiw, G. E., Braff, D. L., and Weinberger, D. R. (1995). Neonatal excitotoxic hippocampal damage in rats causes post-pubertal changes in prepulse inhibition of startle and its disruption by apomorphine. *Psychopharmacology (Berl.)* 122, 35–43.
248. Sams-Dodd, F., Lipska, B. K., and Weinberger, D. R. (1997). Neonatal lesions of the rat ventral hippocampus result in hyperlocomotion and deficits in social behaviour in adulthood. *Psychopharmacology (Berl.)* 132(3), 303–310.
249. Flores, G., Wood, G. K., Liang, J. J., Quirion, R., and Srivastava, L. K. (1996). Enhanced amphetamine sensitivity and increased expression of dopamine D2 receptors in postpubertal rats after neonatal excitotoxic lesions of the medial prefrontal cortex. *J. Neurosci.* 16(22), 7366–7375.

8

DOPAMINE AND GLUTAMATE HYPOTHESES OF SCHIZOPHRENIA

BITA MOGHADDAM AND HOUMAN HOMAYOUN
University of Pittsburgh, Pittsburgh, Pennsylvania

8.1	Introduction	283
8.2	Dopamine Hypothesis	284
	8.2.1 History	284
	8.2.2 Pathological Evidence	285
	8.2.3 Imaging Evidence	285
	8.2.4 Genetic Evidence	286
	8.2.5 Pharmacological Evidence	287
	8.2.6 Evolution of Dopamine Hypothesis: Cortical Versus Striatal Dopamine	287
8.3	Glutamate Theory of Schizophrenia	289
	8.3.1 History	289
	8.3.2 Pathological Evidence	291
	8.3.3 Imaging Evidence	292
	8.3.4 Genetic Evidence	293
	8.3.5 Pharmacological Evidence	294
8.4	Consolidating Glutamate and Dopamine Hypotheses of Schizophrenia	295
	References	297

8.1 INTRODUCTION

Discovery of the first generation of antipsychotic drugs in the 1950s is often credited with the birth of neuronally based approaches to explain the etiology and the pathophysiology of schizophrenia. While at the time this discovery presented a major conceptual shift from the Freudian psychosocial approach to explaining schizophrenia, it is important to note that the pre-Freudian ideas about schizophrenia (*dementia praecox*) were eerily similar to our current concepts and understandings of the disease, specifically, that the etiology is dependent on genetic predisposition [1] and that the primary pathophysiology may involve cortical dysfunction [2, 3]. This is apparent in many texts and research papers written on mental illness at the turn of

---

Handbook of Contemporary Neuropharmacology, Edited by David R. Sibley, Israel Hanin, Michael Kuhar, and Phil Skolnick. Copyright © 2007 John Wiley & Sons, Inc.

the century where, in describing the "etiology" of the disease, statements like "in the causation of dementia praecox the hereditary factor is the most important: the other factors are, for the most part, contributory or excitatory" [4, p.16] or "the importance of heredity as a factor concerned in the etiology of schizophrenia has long been recognized" [5, p.77] were the norm. Similarly, the leading pathological theories about schizophrenia by Mott, Kraeplin, and Alzeimer included gliosis of the cortex and dissociated activity of the afferent and efferent neurons causing an imbalance of "pyramidal" activity [6, 7]. Given this historical context, our approach in this chapter on dopamine and glutamate hypotheses of schizophrenia has been to focus on the evolution of these theories. Recent advances in postmortem, imaging, and genetic fields clearly indicate that schizophrenia is not caused by abnormalities in a single gene, a single neurotransmitter or receptor, or a single brain region. Dopamine and glutamate hypotheses of schizophrenia, although narrowly defined at conception, have evolved to accommodate these most recent neuroscientific findings and thus remain two of the most influential theories in the field.

8.2 DOPAMINE HYPOTHESIS

8.2.1 History

The dopamine hypothesis of schizophrenia, in its original form, stated that a hyperactive dopamine transmission is responsible for the psychotic features of the disease [8]. This theory was consistent with the then newly emerged concept that neurochemical imbalances in the brain may be responsible for major psychiatric disorders [9–12]. A few years earlier, clinical studies with chlorpromazine [13] and reserpine [14, 15] had demonstrated, for the first time, the effectiveness of pharmacotherapy in treating psychotic symptoms of schizophrenia. Subsequent animal studies showed that reserpine, which was later found to inhibit the vesicular monoamine transporter protein (VMAT), increased tissue levels of serotonin and norepinephrine (these studies did not assess the levels of dopamine as dopamine neurons had not yet been discovered). These findings led to the hypothesis that schizophrenia was associated with a state of monoamine deficiency and that neuroleptics ameliorated this condition by increasing the release of serotonin and norepinephrine [9]. Upon discovering the dopamine neurons, Carlsson and Lindquist found that chlorpromazine and another antipsychotic drug haloperidol increased the metabolite levels of dopamine, suggesting that these drugs increase the turnover rate of this neurotransmitter [8]. The authors then proposed that this increased turnover was a *compensatory* mechanism that was secondary to the blockade of dopamine receptors. The idea that inhibition of dopamine receptors, as opposed to enhancing monoamine release, mediates the actions of neuroleptics gained acceptance after the identification of two different subtypes of dopamine receptors, D_1 and D_2, and became the prominent theory of the field after the seminal finding that all antipsychotic drugs block the dopamine D_2 receptors with affinities that correlate with their clinical efficacy [16, 17]. Concurrent with these studies, it was found that psychostimulants that increase dopamine neurotransmission, either through release of endogenous dopamine [18–20] or through direct activation of dopamine receptors [21–23], had psychotomimetic properties in nonschizophrenics and exacerbated symptoms in patients with schizophrenia. Together, these findings lend a great deal of support for Carlsson and Lindquist's initial idea that antipsychotic drugs help to alleviate a hyperactive dopamine system and led to intense efforts to find direct evidence for a disrupted dopamine transmission in schizophrenia. However, the substantial body of research, spreading over five decades, which has been undertaken to address this fundamental issue has not yet provided direct evidence that overactivation of the dopamine system accounts for the spectrum of symptoms that are associated with schizophrenia. But these studies have found many interesting, albeit subtle, changes in some dopamine systems in schizophrenia which have prompted the formulation of more elaborate ideas about dopaminergic abnormalities in schizophrenia.

8.2.2 Pathological Evidence

Over 50 years of intense research has failed to show postmortem dopamine-related abnormalities that would be consistent with a hyperactive dopamine state in schizophrenia. Although several studies have reported an increase in striatal D_2 receptor density in postmortem schizophrenic tissues [24–27], the interpretation of these results is confounded by the fact that chronic antipsychotic treatment can upregulate D_2 receptors [28]. Other dopamine-related findings in postmortem schizophrenic brains include (1) a lack of change in striatal and prefrontal cortex (PFC) D_1 receptor density and messenger RNA (mRNA) levels [29–34]; (2) a reported increase in striatal D_3 receptor number [35] that was not associated with change in striatal D_3 receptor mRNA levels [30]; (3) an increase in striatal D_4 receptor density [36–38] that was not confirmed by other studies [39–41]; (4) a lack of change [42, 43] (but also see [44]) in the expression of D_4 mRNA levels in the PFC; (5) a lack of change in striatal dopamine transporter (DAT) density [33, 45–47]; and (6) unaltered activity of striatal dopamine-related enzymes such as tyrosine hydroxylase (TH), dopamine β-hyroxylase, and catechol-O-methyl transferase (COMT) [48]. Moreover, limited and inconsistent changes in the concentration of tissue dopamine and its metabolites have been reported in schizophrenic brains [49, 50]. Collectively, these negative findings have engendered speculations that dopaminergic abnormalities in schizophrenics may involve subtle and activity-dependent abnormalities that cannot be detected in postmortem tissues.

8.2.3 Imaging Evidence

New evidence from in vivo imaging studies has been instrumental in advancing our knowledge of the dynamics of the dopamine systems in schizophrenia. In general, imaging studies have the advantage of allowing investigators to control for the effects of treatment, to correlate the abnormalities with clinical symptoms, and to study the in vivo functional dynamics of dopamine release. For example, imaging studies in untreated drug-naive schizophrenic patients have addressed the confounding effect of previous neuroleptic treatment on striatal dopamine receptor density. While two studies reported increased striatal D_2 receptor density in schizophrenia [51, 52], a meta-analysis of 17 studies reported a relatively small (12%) increase in the density of these receptors [53], leading to the consensus that it is unlikely that such an inconsistent and weak effect on D_2 receptor density would be the primary cause of schizophrenic pathology. The imaging findings with other dopamine receptor subtypes have also been inconsistent. For example, a high-profile study reporting an increase in the density of D_1 receptors in the PFC of schizophrenics [54] subsequently was not replicated [55]. On the other hand, interesting and consistent results have emerged from investigations of the functional dynamics of dopamine release in schizophrenia. For example, positron emission tomography (PET) studies following administration of radiolabeled dopamine substrates such as dopa or fluorodopa have shown that patients with schizophrenia have a higher rate of dopamine synthesis than normal controls [56–59]. Others, using PET and single-photon-emission computerized tomography imaging during an amphetamine challenge to assess the release of endogenous dopamine, have found a higher level of dopamine release in response to amphetamine in patients with schizophrenia compared to normal controls [60, 61]. Interestingly, this effect was associated with acute exacerbations of psychotic symptoms but could not be detected when patients were in a phase of symptom stabilization [62]. A recent report of increased baseline occupancy of striatal D_2 receptors in schizophrenics is of special interest [63], though this finding remains to be replicated. Together, these recent findings have strengthened the link between dopaminergic hyperactivity and positive symptoms of schizophrenia [50, 64] but have not established a primary role for dopamine abnormality in this disorder. Another important PET study measured D_1 receptor availability in drug-naive or drug-free patients and reported that D_1 receptor antagonist binding potential was significantly elevated in dorsolateral PFC of patients with schizophrenia [65]. This measure demonstrated an increased availability of D_1 receptors which would result from reduced, as opposed to increased, dopaminergic neurotransmission. Implications of this dichotomy are discussed later.

8.2.4 Genetic Evidence

Schizophrenia is a multifactorial disease with a complex mode of inheritance [66]. There has been limited convergence of evidence on dopamine-associated genetic loci that may be associated with schizophrenia. Positive reports of D_3 receptor gene polymorphism associated with schizophrenia [67, 68] were not confirmed in other association or linkage studies [69, 70]. Nonetheless, a recent meta-analysis of genetic studies has shown a small degree of association for the D_3 receptor gene [71]. Linkage studies involving genes for other dopamine receptors as well as dopamine related proteins have been mostly negative or ambiguous [69, 72]. One exception, however, involves the gene that encodes for the enzyme COMT. This is an extracellular degradative enzyme that converts dopamine to its aldehyde derivative and, therefore, plays a critical role in regulating the extracellular levels of dopamine [73]. The COMT gene is on 22q11, which is considered a chromosomal "hot spot" for genes that are associated with increased vulnerability to develop schizophrenia [74]. A common functional polymorphism on this gene ($Val^{108}/^{158}Met$) accounts for up to a fourfold variation in enzymatic activity and the subsequent dopamine metabolism. In patients with schizophrenia this polymorphism may predict 4% of the variance in performance on cognitive tasks, such as the Wisconsin card sort task (WCST), that are dependent on the proper functioning of cortical dopamine [75]. Subsequent studies have replicated the effects of COMT genotype on PFC cortical function [76, 77]. However, a recent meta-analysis failed to show a significant association of COMT polymorphism with schizophrenia [71]. While this COMT polymorphism may not have a substantial influence on the pathophysiology of schizophrenia, its convincing influence on cognitive function suggests that it may contribute to poor cognitive capacity of some patients with schizophrenia [2].

8.2.5 Pharmacological Evidence

In the absence of direct evidence for dopamine hyperactivity in schizophrenia, the pharmacological profile of antipsychotic drugs continues to provide the strongest support for a hyperdopaminergic state in schizophrenia. Imaging studies have established a link between D_2 receptor occupancy and clinical efficacy of antipsychotic drugs (see [78, 79] for review). While all clinically efficacious antipsychotic drugs lead to significant D_2 receptor occupancy, the imaging studies have failed to establish a direct relationship between the degree of striatal D_2 receptor occupancy and the clinical efficacy of antipsychotic drugs [80–82], primarily because ample D_2 receptor occupancy is observed in patients who do not respond to conventional antipsychotic treatment [81]. This fact has reinforced the idea that D_2 occupancy may be necessary but not sufficient for treatment of schizophrenia and has led to suggestions that co-occupation of D_2 with other receptors such as the dopamine D_3 [83] or D_4 [84, 85], the serotonin 5-HT_2 [86] or 5-HT_{1A} [87], and the α-noradrenergic [88] receptors may lead to more efficacious treatment. On the other hand, Kapur and Seeman [89] have argued that optimal modulation of D_2 receptors involving factors such as rate of dissociation, and not complementary actions on other receptors, is the key to clinical efficacy of atypical antipsychotics. In addition to D_2 receptor antagonism, other manipulations of dopaminergic transmission have been explored as potential therapeutic strategies in schizophrenia. Some researchers have attempted to develop a therapeutic strategy based on pure D_4 receptor antagonism [90] primarily because the atypical antipsychotic drug clozapine has preferential affinity for D_4 over D_2 receptors. However, clinical trials with two selective D_4 blockers, sonepiprazole and L-745,870, have been disappointing [90, 91]. Others have suggested that partial D_2 receptor agonists may be used as dopaminergic stabilizers to antagonize the excessive activation of the dopaminergic system without inducing a hypodopaminergic state that has been associated with serious motor and motivational side effects of current drugs [92, 93]. Preliminary studies with the partial D_2 agonist (−)-3PPP have produced positive results [94, 95]. Another drug in this class, aripiprazole, has been approved recently for clinical use and early results on the clinical efficacy and side-effect profile of this drug appear promising [96–98]. Whether this superior profile is mainly due to dopaminergic modulation remains a matter of debate because aripiprazole also modulates serotonin 5-HT_{1A} and 5-HT_{2A} receptors [99]. Interestingly, the selective dopamine D_2/D_3 receptor antagonist amisulpride was recently introduced as the first atypical antipsychotic that does not have a significant affinity for 5-HT_{2A} or other serotonin receptors. Ongoing clinical trials with this drug will allow for a better assessment of the exclusive contribution of dopaminergic effects to the therapeutic profile of antipsychotic drugs [100, 101].

8.2.6 Evolution of Dopamine Hypothesis: Cortical Versus Striatal Dopamine

An increased understanding of the principles that govern higher cognitive functions has led to formulation of more elaborate versions of the dopamine hypothesis of schizophrenia. This progress has been made in the larger framework of a "systems neuroscience" approach to complex psychiatric disorders, where (1) distinct behavioral components of a clinical syndrome are considered and (2) relevant molecular, cellular, and circuit-based data from "normal" (human or animal) subjects are applied to define mechanisms that subserve these behavioral components. In the context of schizophrenia, applying this approach has been useful in elucidating mechanisms that may underlie the cognitive and negative symptoms of this disorder. The most notable insight has come from studies that have characterized the role of PFC in maintaining cognitive functions that are relevant to schizophrenia. In general, numerous imaging studies have shown that several subregions of the PFC are activated during performance of cognitive tasks that require working memory or set shifting [102–106]. In patients with schizophrenia, which generally exhibit impaired working memory, this task-dependent activation of cortical activity is diminished (see [73] for a review). Seminal work by Goldman-Rakic and coinvestigators has shown that a key neuronal system in the PFC for maintaining working memory is the dopaminergic projection to this region [107–110]. In particular, optimal activation of PFC dopamine D_1 receptors, a subtype that is abundant in the cortical regions [111], appears to be critical for working memory performance (see [112] for a review). These primate studies have been critical in generating the hypothesis that a deficiency in cortical dopamine transmission may underlie the cognitive deficits of schizophrenia [113, 114].

A number of clinical studies also suggest a role for cortical dopamine dysfunction in schizophrenia. For example, a direct relationship between decreased metabolic activity in PFC and reduced cerebrospinal fluid (CSF) concentration of homovanillic acid, the major metabolite of cortical dopamine, has been reported in schizophrenic patients during their performance of cognition tasks [115, 116]. Furthermore, Akil and coinvestigators [117, 118] have reported a significant reduction in the length of cortical axons that are immunoreactive for tyrosine-hydroxylase, a finding that would be consistent with reduced catecholaminergic innervation in the PFC. While the low density of D_2 receptors in the PFC has not allowed for reliable PET measurements with D_2-selective ligands, several studies have reported interesting changes in D_1 receptor occupancy in patients with schizophrenia. The first report was by Okubo et al. [54], who demonstrated a positive correlation between the increased density of D_1 receptors in PFC of patients and performance on the WCST. A more recent PET study using a superior D_1 receptor ligand has reported a contrasting finding of increased, rather than decreased, D_1 receptor binding in drug-free and drug-naive schizophrenia patients, which showed a positive correlation with performance in a working memory task [65]. Notably, the same investigators have provided evidence from rodent experiments that the clinical findings may reflect a compensatory upregulation of D_1 receptors following sustained dopaminergic depletion, an interpretation that would fit with a deficit in PFC dopamine activity [119, 120].

Collectively, these findings have led to a more elaborate bidirectional dopamine hypothesis proposing that schizophrenia may be associated with a concomitant cortical hypodopaminergia, which presumably contributes to negative and cognitive symptoms of schizophrenia through reduced D_1 receptor activity, and a subcortical hyperdopaminergia, which leads to positive symptoms through overactivation of D_2 receptors [50, 114]. This revised theory offers a mechanism that explains not only psychosis but also the cognitive symptoms of schizophrenia and has encouraged development of therapeutics that may specifically target these symptoms. Furthermore, this framework has prompted systems-oriented clinical research in schizophrenia which is helping to increase our knowledge of the pathophysiology of the disease. For example, Bertolino and coinvestigators [121, 122] have shown that N-acetylaspartate (NAA), an imaging marker of neuronal functional integrity, is negatively correlated, in dorsolateral PFC, with striatal dopamine release in schizophrenia. Meyer-Lindberg et al. [123], using double measures of regional cerebral blood flow and fluorodopa uptake in schizophrenic subjects during performance of the WCST, corroborated the relationship between hypoactivation of PFC and increased striatal dopamine utilization during a working memory task.

Pharmacological studies using dopamine receptor agonists in primates have supported the notion that activation of D_1 receptor function may be useful for treating cognitive deficits in some animal models [124–126]. While therapeutic efficacy of D_1 receptor agonists remains to be validated, this pharmacological strategy has been indirectly tested in several studies demonstrating that administration of nonspecific dopamine agonists, such as amphetamine or apomorphine, to patients with schizophrenia improves working memory performance and PFC signal-to-noise ratio [127–129].

8.3 GLUTAMATE THEORY OF SCHIZOPHRENIA

8.3.1 History

Unlike the dopamine hypothesis, which was not based on actual dopaminergic abnormalities and was formed to accommodate the mechanism of action of antipsychotic drugs, the idea of a glutamatergic hypofunction was first generated because postmortem and CSF data from patients with schizophrenia were suggestive of a dysregulated excitatory amino acid system [130, 131]. This theory, however, did not gain acceptance at the time because, first, subsequent studies did not confirm the findings of Kim and coinvestigators [132–134] and, second, our limited knowledge of the function and behavioral pharmacology of the glutamate system at the time dictated that a dysfunctional glutamate system would result in overt toxicity and developmental abnormalities as opposed to the subtle and regionally specific cellular changes that occur in schizophrenia. A major revival of the glutamate theory occurred with the discovery that the well-known psychotomimetic drug phencyclidine ("angel dust") is a selective noncompetitive blocker of N-methyl-D-aspartate (NMDA) glutamate receptors [135–138]. This agent produces an acute psychotic episode with high resemblance to the spectrum of schizophrenic symptoms and profoundly exacerbates preexisting symptoms of schizophrenia in patients [139–142]. Recent clinical trials using ketamine and analogs, Federal Drug Administration (FDA)–approved blockers of NMDA receptors, have carefully characterized the profile of symptoms induced in healthy subjected by this class of compounds [143–146]. The range of symptoms produced by these agents resemble positive (delusion and hallucination), negative (avolition, apathy, and blunted affect), and cognitive (deficits in attention, memory, and abstract reasoning) symptoms of schizophrenia as well as disruptions in smooth-pursuit eye movements and prepulse inhibition of the startle response [143–150]. Moreover, administration of low doses of ketamine to patients with schizophrenia precipitates the expression of acute psychosis incorporating symptoms that are similar in content to patients' preexisting experience [140, 151–153]. Collectively, these studies have made a strong case for an NMDA receptor deficiency in schizophrenia because they demonstrated that an NMDA receptor antagonist produces a behavioral syndrome that resembles symptoms of schizophrenia far better than dopamine agonists do [154].

NMDA receptors play an essential role in the development of neural pathways, including the critical process of the pruning of cortical connections during adolescence [155, 156], making them a likely contributor to the hypothesized developmental malfunctions in schizophrenia [157, 158]. Given the pharmacological and developmental evidence, it was suggested that a hypoglutamatergic state, probably at the level of NMDA receptors, might account for some aspects of schizophrenia, particularly the cognitive and negative symptoms that are closely associated with frontal cortical function [154, 159, 160]. During the past decade, this theory has been further modified to account for the complexity of glutamatergic transmission and its interactions with other neurotransmitter systems, especially dopamine and γ-aminobutyric acid (GABA) [161–166]. Here, we will first briefly review the main elements of the glutamate system and then discuss the evidence for a glutamatergic dysregulation in schizophrenia.

In general, glutamate receptors can be classified into two broad families: ionotropic and metabotropic receptors. Ionotropic glutamate receptors are classified into three broad subtypes according to their preferential agonists: the NMDA, kainate, and α-amino-3-hydroxy-5-methylisoxazole-4-propionic acid (AMPA) receptors. Binding of glutamate to these receptors stimulates Ca^{2+} entry into neurons through channels formed either by the receptor itself (as is the case with the NMDA receptor subtype) or by opening voltage-sensitive Ca^{2+} channels that are on the cell membrane. The AMPA receptors are composed of at least four subunits derived from a family of four genes termed *GluR1* to *GluR4*. Kainate receptors are thought to be composed of five identical subunits (homomers) derived from genes termed *GluR5* to *GluR7* and *KA1* and *KA2*. The NMDA receptor is a heteromeric complex composed of four or five subunits derived from seven genes, *NR1*, *NR2A* to *NR2D*, *NR3A* and *NR3B* [167]. The *NR1* subunit, which has several isoforms, is an obligate subunit. Nearly all neurons express AMPA and NMDA receptors, and it is estimated that glutamate ionotropic receptors mediate nearly 50% of all synaptic transmission in the mammalian central nervous system. The more recently discovered metabotropic glutamate receptors [168] have a distinct mechanism of action and use G-protein-coupled synaptic transduction mechanisms, similar to those used by the monoamine neurotransmitters, to indirectly regulate the electrical signaling. This mechanism is in contrast to rapid excitation and opening of ion channels by ionotropic glutamate receptors, which is a more suitable mechanism for pharmacological targets. At least eight metabotropic glutamate receptors have been cloned (termed mGlu1 to mGlu8). These receptors share no sequence homology with other known receptors in the nervous system, suggesting that they are members of a new receptor gene family. The eight subtypes of mGlu receptors are currently classified into three groups (termed groups I–III) based on amino acid sequence homology and transduction mechanisms. Group I (mGlu1 and mGlu5) metabotropic receptors activate the enzyme phospholipase C, which in turn results in the breakdown of membrane phospholipid to the second messengers inositol triphosphate or diacylglycerol. Groups II (mGlu2 and mGlu3) and III (mGlu4, mGlu6, mGlu7, and mGlu8) metabotropic receptors downregulate the enzyme adenylate cyclase and result in reduced synthesis of the second messenger cyclic adenosine monophosphate (cAMP).

8.3.2 Pathological Evidence

In general, the direct evidence for glutamatergic involvement in schizophrenia is abundant and converges on several principles. First, abnormalities in various components of glutamatergic systems, including the NMDA receptor, have been reported in schizophrenic brain samples. Second, these abnormalities follow a region-specific pattern with the most impressive accumulation of evidence being so far reported from temporal and frontal cortices, limbic regions, and thalamus, with limited evidence found in striatum.

Several groups have reported altered densities of kainate and AMPA glutamate receptors in postmortem schizophrenic brains [169–173]. Harrison and coinvestigators reported decreases in AMPA receptor binding in CA3 and CA4 subfields of hippocampus [170, 172]. These findings are consistent with reports of reduced expression of GluR1 and GluR2 protein or mRNA levels in similar regions [172, 174–176]. In contrast to the temporal lobe regions, the reported changes in frontal cortex and striatal regions have been small [177]. Consistent decreases in AMPA GluR1 and GluR2 expression have also been reported in the thalamus [178]. Collectively, these data suggest that in schizophrenics' brains there are decreases in the expression of several AMPA receptor subunits and in AMPA receptor binding in the medial temporal lobe and the thalamus.

Several other studies have examined kainate receptor binding or mRNA levels [131, 179–183]. In general, these studies follow the same pattern of change as in AMPA receptor expression, suggesting reduced levels of expression in temporal lobe regions. Furthermore, a recent study reported increased transcript levels of GluR5 (a kainate subunit) in substantia nigra in schizophrenia [167].

Studies on NMDA receptor density in cortical, striatal, and temporal lobe structures have led to less consistent results (see [169] for a review). However, more recent data indicate that part of the earlier inconsistencies may be due to alterations in the subunit composition of NMDA receptors. The earliest report in the literature using [^{3}H]MK801 described increased binding in the putamen but not in the frontal cortex or temporal lobe [171]. Similar increases were reported using [^{3}H]D-aspartate [184] but another study failed to replicate the finding in putamen [180]. Studies using [^{3}H]TCP (which, similar to MK801, binds to the phencyclidine site on the NMDA receptor complex) have also resulted in conflicting observations with either no change [185] or an increase in binding in orbitofrontal cortex being reported [186].

More recent studies have examined the expression of NMDA receptor subunits in schizophrenic brain and have reported several region-specific results. There are reports of increased temporal and PFC expression of NR1 [187–189]. However, an older study [190] had found no major changes in any of the NMDA receptor subunits in PFC with the exception of a higher ratio of NR2D to the other NR2 subunits. In the thalamus, a significant reduction in NR1, NR2A, NR2B, and NR2CR subunits have been reported [178, 191, 192]. Other reports demonstrated a downregulation of

NR1 in the superior temporal gyrus, hippocampus [182, 193], and thalamus [178] and upregulation of NR2B subunit in the superior temporal cortex [188]. A recent study also reported a decrease in NR1 subunit expression in substantia nigra [167].

Studies examining the expression of the family of metabotropic glutamate receptors have only recently begun, and although there are only a few published studies in this area [194, 195], this is likely to be an active field of research in the future. So far, an increase in mGluR5 in orbitofrontal cortex has been reported [194].

In addition to glutamate receptors, Coyle and coinvestigators [196] have reported postmortem abnormalities in the expression of the neuropeptide N-acetylaspartyl glutamate (NAAG), which is considered an endogenous ligand for some subtypes of glutamate receptors. This reported increase in the levels of NAAG as well as a decrease in its catabolic enzyme NAALADase in the PFC and hippocampus may reflect alteration in glutamate neurotransmission in schizophrenia [197]. Abnormalities of other indices of glutamate transmission, such as a decrease in vesicular transporter 1, have also been reported in the medial temporal cortex of schizophrenic brains [198]. In the thalamus, an increase in excitatory amino acid transporters EAAT1 and EAAT2 and vesicular glutamate transporter VGLUT2 and in the NMDA receptor-associated proteins NF-L, PSD95, and SAP102 has been reported [199–201].

Another approach has been to investigate mechanisms that indirectly affect the NMDA receptor function, including those that involve the glycine modulatory site on this receptor. Preliminary evidence suggests that the levels of endogenous agonists (glycine and D-serine) and antagonist (kynurenic acid) for this site may have been altered in schizophrenia. This includes reports of decreased serum levels of D-serine [202] and glycine [203] and increased CSF levels of kynurenic acid [204–206] in patients with schizophrenia.

Pathological evidence of abnormalities in structural organization of frontal cortices in schizophrenia may be an indirect indicator of disruption in the main mode of chemical communication (glutamatergic transmission) in this region. Accordingly, abnormalities in a range of structural parameters, including gray matter volume [207–212], cortical thickness [213], cortical gyrification [214, 215], hippocampal shape [216, 217], neocortical and hippocampal pyramidal cell size [218–226], and dendritic spine number and arborization [227–230], have been reported in schizophrenia. Furthermore, several groups have reported the presence of aberrantly located or clustered neurons in enthorhinal cortex [231–233] and neocortical white matter [234–239] of schizophrenic brains, findings that fit the idea of an early neurodevelopmental problem in cortical areas. While these pathological abnormalities should be interpreted with caution because of the relatively small effect of sizes and inconsistencies in reported changes in any single parameter, together they further support the involvement of the cortical and thalamic glutamatergic system in the pathophysiology of schizophrenia.

8.3.3 Imaging Evidence

Unlike the monoamine systems, selective glutamate receptor ligands for clinical imaging studies have not been fully developed for routine use in healthy and patient volunteers [240]. As a result, most of the imaging evidence regarding a link between glutamate and schizophrenia is indirect. This includes evidence of abnormal functional connectivity in frontotemporal cortices during working memory tasks in schizophrenic patients [241–247]. In addition, an impaired recruitment of hippocampus during a memory recollection task [248] and an abnormal frontotemporal interaction during a semantic processing task [249] have been reported in schizophrenic patients. Offering another indirect line of evidence, Kegeles et al. [250] used SPECT and proton magnetic resonance spectroscopy (MRS) to study, in normal subjects, the effect of an experimental state of NMDA receptor hypofunction (induced by ketamine) on amphetamine-induced striatal dopamine release, a measure previously reported to be enhanced in schizophrenia [60] (see Section 8.2). They found an increase in raclopride displacement, interpreted as enhanced dopamine release, by an NMDA receptor antagonist. This finding is similar to observations in schizophrenic patients and suggests that NMDA receptor hypofunction may explain the enhanced dopaminergic response to amphetamine challenge in schizophrenia.

8.3.4 Genetic Evidence

While there is limited evidence for the direct involvement of a glutamate receptor gene in schizophrenia (see [251, 252] for a review), recent genetic studies offer a novel insight for possible pathophysiological processes that converge on glutamate-related targets (see below). A linkage study with a genetically isolated African population suggested that a NR1 subunit polymorphism might be associated with predisposition to develop schizophrenia [253]. Other studies, however, have so far reported lack of association with polymorphisms for genes encoding for NR1, NR2B, GluR5, mGluR7, and mGluR8 [254–257]. So far, the most interesting link to a glutamate receptor gene has been suggested for mGluR3 (*GRM3*) in three independent association studies [258–260]. Egan and coinvestigators [258] have shown that a variation in this gene can affect performance on working memory and attention tasks and on functional magnetic resonance imaging (fMRI) activation of dorsolateral PFC and hippocampus in both schizophrenic patients and normal controls. Interestingly, the agonists of type II mGlu receptors (including mGluR2 and mGluR3) can reverse the adverse behavioral, cognitive, and electrophysiological effects of NMDA receptor antagonists [261, 262]. However, further investigation on the role of this candidate gene is required since there are reports of unaltered GRM3 mRNA level in PFC and thalamus of schizophrenic patients [194, 195, 263].

Regardless of direct involvement of glutamate receptor genes, most of the candidate genes that have emerged from recent association and linkage studies are functionally linked to glutamatergic transmission (see [166, 264] for a review). These genes include, but are not limited to, neurogelin 1 (*NRG1*), regulator of G-protein signaling 4 (*RGS4*), G72, dysbindin (*DTNBP1*), *PPP3CC*, disrupted-in-schizophrenia 1 (*DISC1*), and proline dehydrogenase (*PRODH2*). All of these candidate genes may interact with the glutamatergic transmission and function at various postsynaptic levels. For example, *NRG1* regulates the expression of glutamate receptor subunits and directly activates ErbB4, a tyrosine kinase that regulates the kinetic properties of NMDA receptor [265, 266]. *RGS4* can inhibit the mGlu5 receptor transmission through negative regulation of G-protein signaling [267–269]. G72 interacts with the enzyme D-amino acid oxidase (DAAO) (see above) that reduces the synaptic availability of D-serine through oxidizing it [270, 271]. Dysbindin recruits nitric oxide synthase (NOS), which in turn affects NMDA receptor activity [272].

PPP3CC encodes a subunit of calcineurin that is considered essential for some types of NMDA receptor–mediated plasticity [273]. Implication of these genes has prompted the suggestion that they may functionally converge at the level of microcircuit information processing, particularly involving NMDA receptor pathways [166, 264].

8.3.5 Pharmacological Evidence

It is plausible that the next generation of antipsychotic therapies may eventually emerge from current research on glutamatergic transmission. In contrast to the dopamine field that was originally derived by the effectiveness of serendipitously discovered drugs, glutamate-based therapeutics would conceptualize the efforts to translate current neuroscientific ideas into clinical treatments. However, the progress in this field has been slowed by the widespread distribution of major glutamate receptors such as NMDA or AMPA receptors and their involvement in key functions such as learning and memory, raising the concerns that drugs that directly target these receptors may be associated with serious side effects. To tackle this caveat, some researchers have attempted to use coagonists of NMDA receptor that bind to its glycine site and increase the frequency of NMDA-gated channel opening [274–278]. Basic research has indicated that the glycine modulatory site on NMDA receptor is not saturated in vivo and thus glycine and related molecules such as D-serine and D-cycloserine may be able to ameliorate the NMDA receptor hypofunction (see [279] for a review). Early clinical trials have indicated that this strategy may alleviate the negative and perhaps cognitive symptoms of schizophrenia [276, 280–285]. However, these agents do not appear to have antipsychotic efficacy and their effectiveness as adjuvant therapy remains to be established [286–289]. Notably, a recent meta-analysis of the randomized controlled trials in schizophrenic subjects showed a moderate amelioration of negative symptoms by glycine and D-serine without any significant effect on other symptoms [290]. Meanwhile, some have suggested that a positive modulation of the glycine site may best be achieved through manipulating the molecular pathways that regulate the turnover of its endogenous ligands. For example, it is known that the availability of glycine is dependent on the activity of glycine transporter 1 (GlyT1) [291, 292], while the availability of D-serine is determined by the activity of serine racemase and the degrading enzyme DAAO [293]. Thus, efforts are underway to develop inhibitors of GlyT1 and serine racemase in order to increase the in vivo availability of glycine and D-serine, respectively [278, 279, 294, 295]. Another line of potential therapies that is currently under investigation is based on fine tuning glutamate transmission through metabotropic glutamate receptors [296, 297]. In this regard, one promising strategy may be based on functional potentiation of postsynaptic mGlu5 receptors that show synergistic interactions with NMDA receptors in regulation of behavior and cognition in animal studies [298–301]. Findings from these studies predict that activation of mGlu5 receptors may ameliorate the presumed state of NMDA receptor deficiency in schizophrenia. However, the rapid desensitization rate of mGlu5 receptors makes it unlikely that direct agonists of these receptors may have persistent therapeutic effectiveness. Instead, recently developed positive allosteric modulators of mGlu5 receptor function may offer a more efficacious strategy [302–304], a promise backed by recent reports in experimental models [305, 306, 306a]. Alternatively, preclinical studies have shown that the agonists of group II mGlu receptors may inhibit the adverse effects of NMDA receptor antagonists on behavior, working memory, and PFC function [261, 262, 307], suggesting the therapeutic potential of this strategy for schizophrenia. A key finding was that NMDA receptor antagonists lead to an excessive increase in PFC glutamatergic transmission through non-NMDA receptors [308], leading to the assumption that agents such as activators of presynaptic group II mGlu autoreceptors that can block this aberrant activity may prove beneficial to relieve the presumed states of cortical malfunction. Accordingly, a recent clinical study in healthy human subjects treated with ketamine offered the first proof of concept that activation of group II mGluRs may ameliorate cognitive dysfunction in the context of NMDA hypofunction [309]. The same principle, normalizing an inappropriate pattern of cortical activity, may underlie the reported effectiveness of lamotrigine, an anticonvulsant agent with cation channel blockade properties, in ketamine-treated subjects [310, 311]. Correspondingly, preliminary reports of the advantageous effects of lamotrigine adjunctive therapy in schizophrenia have been published [312–314].

Another approach has been to develop agents that reduce the rate of desensitization and therefore potentiate the function of AMPA glutamate receptors as "cognitive enhancers" since these agents can improve learning and memory in animal models [315–318]. Preliminary results with this class of agents, called "AMPAkines," suggest that boosting glutamatergic transmission may indeed be beneficial for the core cognitive deficits in schizophrenia [319]. However, these drugs may be in particular worthy as adjuvant to current therapies [319, 320], rather than for single-agent therapy [321].

Given that our approach to treating schizophrenia has not fundamentally changed for 50 years and the acute need to develop more efficacious drugs for treatment of nonpsychotic symptoms of schizophrenia, in particular the enduring cognitive deficits of the disease, there has been a surge of interest in developing and testing "novel" glutamatergic drugs in animal models and in human subjects. Hence, the next decade promises to be an exciting time for the field because, for the first time, drugs that are designed based on pathophysiological mechanisms and are not merely prototypes of existing neuroleptics may be developed.

8.4 CONSOLIDATING GLUTAMATE AND DOPAMINE HYPOTHESES OF SCHIZOPHRENIA

Given the dominance of the dopamine hypothesis, the original attempts to consolidate these theories focused on proving that NMDA receptor deficiency is associated with dopamine hyperactivity. Earlier release studies examining dopamine turnover or measuring the uptake of labeled dopamine showed that NMDA receptor antagonists increase the release of striatal dopamine [322–324]. This finding contributed to the first version of an integrated dopamine–glutamate theory, suggesting that NMDA receptor hypofunction may represent a paradigm that simulates the presumed dopamine hyperfunction in schizophrenia [154, 325, 326]. This interpretation, however, could not account for the fact that NMDA receptor antagonists induce a far wider range of schizophrenia-like symptoms than the dopaminergic models. Thus, the theory was modified to distinguish a role for cortical versus subcortical glutamate–dopamine interactions for induction of negative and cognitive versus positive symptoms [50, 114, 160]. However, subsequent work using microdialysis or imaging methodologies showed that behaviorally relevant doses of NMDA antagonists do not increase dopamine release in rodents, primates, or humans [327–330]. Furthermore, behavioral studies demonstrated that the dopamine system is neither necessary [331] nor sufficient [327] for maintenance of the aberrant behavioral effects of the NMDA receptor antagonists. This and the abundance of postmortem and genetic findings supporting a role for the glutamate system in the etiology and pathophysiology of schizophrenia have led to the proposal that the primary abnormalities in schizophrenia may involve the synaptic signaling machinery in cortical regions [2, 92, 332] and that a dopaminergic abnormality may be a consequence of cortical dysregulation of dopamine neurons. Interestingly, contrary to years of assertion that the PFC stimulates dopamine neuronal activity [333, 334], recent anatomical studies have demonstrated that cortical projections do not synapse directly onto mesostriatal dopamine neurons [335]. Furthermore, stimulation of PFC neurons at physiological frequencies actually decreases dopamine release in the ventral striatum [336]. This suggests that the PFC exerts an inhibitory influence over subcortical dopamine presumably through indirect activation of GABA neurons [336, 337]. Thus, reduced glutamatergic function in the PFC may remove this inhibitory influence and lead to an abnormally overactive subcortical dopamine system in schizophrenia. Recent electrophysiological studies recording from PFC neurons in behaving rodents, in fact, show that a state of NMDA deficiency can lead to reduced burst activity of cortical neurons [338].

Given the lack of direct evidence for a dopaminergic abnormality in schizophrenia, an alternative hypothesis has been that antipsychotic drugs, which are D_2 receptor antagonists, work by modifying the function of cortical (glutamatergic) neurons [166]. A substantial body of evidence demonstrates that dopamine modulates cortical and subcortical glutamatergic transmission [339–345]. Notably, electrophysiological studies have revealed a delicate modulatory effect for dopamine on the electrical conductance of cortical excitatory neurons, that is, neither excitatory nor inhibitory, but rather is a gating effect that depends on the activity state of target neurons [341, 344, 345]. Furthermore, D_2 receptors may regulate the temporal organization of electrical activity in PFC [343]. The D_2 receptors also inhibit the release of glutamate [346, 347], suggesting that blockade of D_2 receptors by antipsychotic drugs can overcome a putative state of glutamate deficiency. In support of this mechanism, electrophysiological studies have shown that antipsychotic agents, particularly clozapine, exert positive modulatory effects on the NMDA receptor function in PFC and may attenuate the blockade of these receptors by phencyclidine [348–351]. Interestingly, a recent study in behaving animals suggests that clozapine can reverse the disruptive effects of NMDA receptor blockers on cortical firing in correlation with behavior. This reversal may be a result of fine-tuning of cortical activity as clozapine increased the activity of the neurons with low baseline firing rates and decreased the activity of neurons with higher firing rates [351a].

Another hypothesis has been that dopamine and glutamate interactions may occur at the postsynaptic level and through the intricate postsynaptic intracellular mechanisms known to mediate crosstalks between these transmitter systems [352, 353]. Taken together, these modified scenarios would explain the lack of strong pathological and genetic evidence for the involvement of dopamine in the pathophysiology of schizophrenia despite the clinical effectiveness of dopamine-based drugs. Instead, they emphasize the importance of viewing schizophrenia as a constellation of molecular and cellular processes that may functionally converge at the circuitry level, most probably downstream from corticolimbic NMDA receptors. One implication of these models is that polytransmitter theories, incorporating interactions between dopamine, glutamate, and other major neurotransmitter systems, have replaced the existing monotransmitter theories [342]. An important example in this case is the PFC GABAergic system which has been strongly linked to schizophrenia (see [354, 355] for a review). It has been hypothesized that disruptions in GABA-mediated inhibitory tone of cortical interneurons may contribute to decrease the signal-to-noise ratio in cortical circuitry in schizophrenia [341, 342], paving the way for the sort of functional degradation that occurs in the NMDA antagonist model [338, 356].

Rapid progress in the fields of imaging, psychiatric genetics, and postmortem molecular analysis of brain tissues is likely to help continue the evolution of dopamine and glutamate hypotheses of schizophrenia. While one hopes that for a devastating disease like schizophrenia hypotheses will soon be replaced by concrete data and effective cures, the concerted efforts of researchers in conceptualizing theoretical bases of schizophrenia has been, and will continue to be, instrumental in developing a better understanding of the mechanisms underlying schizophrenic disorders and efforts to develop a new generation of more effective treatments.

REFERENCES

1. Kendler, K. (2003). The genetics of schizophrenia: Chromosomal deletions, attentional disturbances, and spectrum boundaries. *Am. J. Psychiatry* 160, 1549–1553.
2. Winterer, G., and Weinberger, D. (2004). Genes, dopamine and cortical signal-to-noise ratio in schizophrenia. *Trends Neurosci.* 27, 683–690.
3. Lewis, D., Glantz, L., Pierri, J., and Sweet, R. (2003). Altered cortical glutamate neurotransmission in schizophrenia: Evidence from morphological studies of pyramidal neurons. *Ann. NY Acad. Sci.* 1003, 102–112.
4. Norman, H. J. (1928). *Mental Disorders.* E. & S. Livingstone, Edinburgh.
5. Barrett, A. (1927). Heredity relations in schizophrenia. *Am. J. Psychiatry* 83, 77–104.
6. Cole, R. (1924). *Mental Disease: A Text Book of Psychiatry for Medical Students and Practitioners.* University of London Press, London.
7. Stoddart, W. (1926). *Mind and Its Disorders.* Blackston's Son and Co., Philadelphia.
8. Carlsson, A., and Lindqvist, M. (1963). Effect of chlorpromazine or haloperidol on formation of 3-methoxytyramine and normetanephrine in mouse brain. *Acta Pharmacol. Toxicol.* 20, 140–144.
9. Brodie, T. M. (1959). Psychopharmacology: an evaluation. In *Biological Psychiatry*, J. H. Masserman, Ed. Grune and Stratton, New York, pp. 264–268.
10. Hoch, P. H., and Solomon, G. (1952). Experimental induction of psychosis. In *The Biology of Mental Health and Disease*, P. B. Cobb, Ed., Hoeber, New York.
11. Frankenburg, F. (1994). History of the development of antipsychotic medication. *Psychiatr. Clin. North Am.* 17, 531–540.

12. Delay, J., and Deniker, P. (1955). Neuroleptic effects of chlorpromazine in therapeutics of neuropsychiatry. *J. Clin. Exp. Psychopathol.* 16, 104–111.

13. Delay, J., Deniker, P., and Ropert, R. (1956). Study of 300 case histories of psychotic patients treated with chlorpromazine in closed wards since 1952. *Encephale* 45, 528–535.

14. Kline, N., and Stanley, A. (1955). Use of reserpine in a neuropsychiatric hospital. *Ann. NY Acad. Sci.* 61, 85–91.

15. Hollister, L., Krieger, G., Kringel, A., and Roberts, R. (1955). Treatment of chronic schizophrenic reactions with reserpine. *Ann. NY Acad. Sci.* 61, 92–100.

16. Seeman, P., and Lee, T. (1975). Antipsychotic drugs: Direct correlation between clinical potency and presynaptic action on dopamine neurons. *Science* 188, 1217–1219.

17. Creese, I., Burt, D., and Snyder, S. (1976). Dopamine receptor binding predicts clinical and pharmacological potencies of antischizophrenic drugs. *Science* 192, 481–483.

18. Snyder, S. (1973). Amphetamine psychosis: A "model" schizophrenia mediated by catecholamines. *Am. J. Psychiatry* 130, 61–67.

19. Snyder, S., Banerjee, S., and Yamamura, H. (1974). Drugs, neurotransmitters and schizophrenia. *Science* 184, 1243–1253.

20. Angrist, B., Sathananthan, G., Wilk, S., and Gershon, S. (1974). Amphetamine psychosis: Behavioral and biochemical aspects. *J. Psychiatry Res.* 11, 13–23.

21. Lipper, S. (1976). Letter: Psychosis in patient on bromocriptine and levodopa with carbidopa. *Lancet* 2, 571–572.

22. Angrist, B., and van Kammen, D. P. (1984). CNS stimulants as a tool in the study of schizophrenia. *Trends Neurosci.* 7, 388–390.

23. Lieberman, J., Kane, J., and Alvir, J. (1987). Provocative tests with psychostimulant drugs in schizophrenia. *Psychopharmacology* 91, 415–433.

24. Lee, T., Seeman, P., Tourtellotte, W., Farley, I., and Hornykeiwicz, O. (1978). Binding of ^{3}H-neuroleptics and ^{3}H-apomorphine in schizophrenic brains. *Nature* 274, 897–900.

25. Owen, F., Cross, A., Crow, T., Longden, A., Poulter, M., and Riley, G. (1978). Increased dopamine-receptor sensitivity in schizophrenia. *Lancet* 2, 223–226.

26. Seeman, P., Ulpian, C., Bergeron, C., Riederer, P., Jellinger, K., Gabriel, E., Reynolds, G., and Tourtellotte, W. (1984). Bimodal distribution of dopamine receptor densities in brains of schizophrenics. *Science* 225, 728–731.

27. Mita, T., Hanada, S., Nishino, N., Kuno, T., Nakai, H., Yamadori, T., Mizoi, Y., and Tanaka, C. (1986). Decreased serotonin S2 and increased dopamine D2 receptors in chronic schizophrenics. *Biol. Psychiatry* 21, 1407–1414.

28. Burt, D., Creese, I., and Snyder, S. (1977). Antischizophrenic drugs: Chronic treatment elevates dopamine receptor binding in brain. *Science* 196, 326–328.

29. Laruelle, M., Casanova, M. F., Weinberger, D. R., and Kleinman, J. E. (1990). Postmortem study of the dopaminergic D1 receptors in the dorsolateral prefrontal cortex of schizophrenics and controls. *Schizophr. Res.* 3, 30–31.

30. Meador-Woodruff, J., Haroutunian, V., Powchik, P., Davidson, M., Davis, K., and Watson, S. (1997). Dopamine receptor transcript expression in striatum and prefrontal and occipital cortex. Focal abnormalities in orbitofrontal cortex in schizophrenia. *Arch. Gen. Psychiatry* 54, 1089–1095.

31. Seeman, P. (1987). Dopamine receptors and the dopamine hypothesis of schizophrenia. *Synapse* 1, 133–152.

32. Pimoule, C., Schoemaker, H., Reynolds, G., and Langer, S. (1985). [^{3}H] SCH 23390 labeled D1 dopamine receptors are unchanged in schizophrenia and Parkinson's disease. *Eur. J. Pharmacol.* 114, 235–237.

33. Knable, M., Hyde, T., Herman, M., Carter, J., Bigelow, L., and Kleinman, J. (1994). Quantitative autoradiography of dopamine-D1 receptors, D2 receptors, and dopamine uptake sites in postmortem striatal specimens from schizophrenic patients. *Biol. Psychiatry* 36, 827–835.

34. Czudek, C., and Reynolds, G. (1989). [^{3}H] GBR 12935 binding to the dopamine uptake site in post-mortem brain tissue in schizophrenia. *J. Neural Transmiss.* 77, 227–230.

35. Gurevich, E., Bordelon, Y., Shapiro, R., Arnold, S., Gur, R., and Joyce, J. (1997). Mesolimbic dopamine D3 receptors and use of antipsychotics in patients with schizophrenia. A postmortem study. *Arch. Gen. Psychiatry* 54, 225–232.

36. Seeman, P., Guan, H., and Van Tol, H. (1993). Dopamine D4 receptors elevated in schizophrenia. *Nature* 365, 441–445.

37. Murray, A., Hyde, T., Knable, M., Herman, M., Bigelow, L., Carter, J., Weinberger, D., and Kleinman, J. (1995). Distribution of putative D4 dopamine receptors in postmortem striatum from patients with schizophrenia. *J. Neurosci.* 15, 2186–2191.

38. Sumiyoshi, T., Stockmeier, C., Overholser, J., Thompson, P., and Meltzer, H. (1995). Dopamine D4 receptors and effects of guanine nucleotides on [^{3}H] raclopride binding in postmortem caudate nucleus of subjects with schizophrenia or major depression. *Brain Res.* 681, 109–116.

39. Lahti, R., Roberts, R., Cochrane, E., Primus, R., Gallager, D., Conley, R., Tamminga, C., and Cabib, S. (1998). Direct determination of dopamine D4 receptors in normal and schizophrenic postmortem brain tissue: A [^{3}H] NGD-94-1 study. *Mol. Psychiatry* 3, 528–533.

40. Lahti, R., Roberts, R., Conley, R., Cochrane, E., Mutin, A., and Tamminga, C. (1996). D2-type dopamine receptors in postmortem human brain sections from normal and schizophrenic subjects. *Neuroreport* 7, 1945–1948.

41. Reynolds, G., and Mason, S. (1994). Are striatal dopamine D4 receptors increased in schizophrenia? *J. Neurochem.* 63, 1576–1577.

42. Mulcrone, J., and Kerwin, R. (1996). No difference in the expression of the D4 gene in post-mortem frontal cortex from controls and schizophrenics. *Neurosci. Lett.* 29, 163–166.

43. Roberts, D., Balderson, D., Pickering-Brown, S., Deakin, J., and Owen, F. (1996). The relative abundance of dopamine D4 receptor mRNA in post mortem brains of schizophrenics and controls. *Schizophr. Res.* 20, 171–174.

44. Stefanis, N., Bresnick, J., Kerwin, R., Schofield, W., and McAllister, G. (1998). Elevation of D4 dopamine receptor mRNA in postmortem schizophrenic brain. *Brain Res. Mol. Brain Res.* 53, 112–119.

45. Hirai, M., Kitamura, N., Hashimoto, T., Nakai, T., Mita, T., Shirakawa, O., Yamadori, T., Amano, T., Noguchi-Kuno, S., and Tanaka, C. (1988). [^{3}H] GBR-12935 binding sites in human striatal membranes: Binding characteristics and changes in parkinsonians and schizophrenics. *Jpn. J. Pharmacol.* 47, 237–243.

46. Joyce, J., Lexow, N., Bird, E., and Winokur, A. (1988). Organization of dopamine D1 and D2 receptors in human striatum: Receptor autoradiographic studies in Huntington's disease and schizophrenia. *Synapse* 2, 546–557.

47. Pearce, R., Seeman, P., Jellinger, K., and Tourtellotte, W. (1990). Dopamine uptake sites and dopamine receptors in Parkinson's disease and schizophrenia. *Eur. Neurol.* 30(Suppl. 1), 9–14.

48. Crow, T., Baker, H., Cross, A., Joseph, M., Lofthouse, R., Longden, A., Owen, F., Riley, G., Glover, V., and Killpack, W. (1979). Monoamine mechanisms in chronic schizophrenia: Post-mortem neurochemical findings. *Br. J. Psychiatry* 134, 249–256.
49. Reynolds, G. P. (1989). Beyond the dopamine hypothesis. The neurochemical pathology of schizophrenia. *Br. J. Psychiatry* 155, 305–316.
50. Davis, K. L., Kahn, R. S., Ko, G., and Davidson, M. (1991). Dopamine in schizophrenia: A review and reconceptualization. *Am. J. Psychiatry* 148, 1474–1486.
51. Crawley, J., Owens, D., Crow, T., Poulter, M., Johnstone, E., Smith, T., Oldland, S., Veall, N., Owen, F., and Zanelli, G. (1986). Dopamine D2 receptors in schizophrenia studied in vivo. *Lancet* 2, 224–225.
52. Wong, D., Wagner, H. J., Tune, L., Dannals, R., Pearlson, G., Links, J., Tamminga, C., Broussolle, E., Ravert, H., and Wilson, A. (1986). Positron emission tomography reveals elevated D2 dopamine receptors in drug-naive schizophrenics. *Science* 234, 1558–1563.
53. Laruelle, M. (2003). Dopamine transmission in the schizophrenic brain. In *Schizophrenia*, S. R. Hirsch and D. R.Weinberger, Eds. Blackwell Science, Malden.
54. Okubo, Y., Suhara, T., Suzuki, K., Kobayashi, K., Inoue, O., Terasaki, O., Someya, Y., Sassa, T., Sudo, Y., Matsushima, E., Iyo, M., Tateno, Y., and Toru, M. (1997). Decreased prefrontal dopamine D1 receptors in schizophrenia revealed by PET. *Nature* 385, 634–636.
55. Karlsson, P., Farde, L., Halldin, C., and Sedvall, G. (2002). PET study of D(1) dopamine receptor binding in neuroleptic-naive patients with schizophrenia. *Am. J. Psychiatry* 159, 761–767.
56. Hietala, J., Syvalahti, E., Vuorio, K., Nagren, K., Lehikoinen, P., Ruotsalainen, U., Rakkolainen, V., Lehtinen, V., and Wegelius, U. (1994). Striatal D2 dopamine receptor characteristics in neuroleptic-naive schizophrenic patients studied with positron emission tomography. *Arch. Gen. Psychiatry* 51, 116–123.
57. Reith, J., Benkelfat, C., Sherwin, A., Yasuhara, Y., Kuwabara, H., Andermann, F., Bachneff, S., Cumming, P., Diksic, M., Dyve, S., Etienne, P., Evans, A. C., Lal, S., Shevell, M., Savard, G., Wong, D. F., Chouinard, G., and Gjedde, A. (1994). Elevated dopa decarboxylase activity in living brain of patients with psychosis. *Proc. Nat. Acad. Sci. USA* 91, 11651–11654.
58. Dao-Castellana, M., Paillere-Martinot, M., Hantraye, P., Attar-Levy, D., Remy, P., Crouzel, C., Artiges, E., Feline, A., Syrota, A., and Martinot, J. (1997). Presynaptic dopaminergic function in the striatum of schizophrenic patients. *Schizophr. Res.* 23, 167–174.
59. Lindstrom, L., Gefvert, O., Hagberg, G., Lundberg, T., Bergstrom, M., Hartvig, P., and Langstrom, B. (1999). Increased dopamine synthesis rate in medial prefrontal cortex and striatum in schizophrenia indicated by L-(beta-^{11}C) DOPA and PET. *Biol. Psychiatry* 46, 681–688.
60. Laruelle, M., Abi-Dargham, A., van Dyck, C., Gil, R., D'Souza, C., Erdos, J., McCance, E., Rosenblatt, W., Fingado, C., Zoghbi, S., Baldwin, R., Seibyl, J., Krystal, J., Charney, D., and Innis, R. (1996). SPECT imaging of amphetamine-induced dopamine release in drug-free schizophrenic subjects. *Proc. Nat. Acad. Sci. USA* 93, 9235–9340.
61. Breier, A., Su, T. P., Saunders, R., Carson, R. E., Kolachana, B. S., de Bartolomeis, A., Weinberger, D. R., Weisenfeld, N., Malhotra, A. K., Eckelman, W. C., and Pickar, D. (1997). Schizophrenia is associated with elevated amphetamine-induced synaptic

dopamine concentrations: Evidence from a novel positron emission tomography method. *Proc. Nat. Acad. Sci. USA* 94, 2569–2574.

62. Laruelle, M., Abi-Dargham, A., Gil, R., Kegeles, L., and Innis, R. (1999). Increased dopamine transmission in schizophrenia: Relationship to illness phases. *Biol. Psychiatry* 46, 56–72.

63. Abi-Dargham, A., Rodenhiser, J., Printz, D., Zea-Ponce, Y., Gil, R., Kegeles, L., Weiss, R., Cooper, T., Mann, J., Van Heertum, R., Gorman, J., Laruelle, M. (2000). Increased baseline occupancy of D2 receptors by dopamine in schizophrenia. *Proc. Nat. Acad. Sci. USA* 97, 8104–8109.

64. Davidson, M., and Davis, K. (1988). A comparison of plasma homovanillic acid concentrations in schizophrenic patients and normal controls. *Arch. Gen. Psychiatry* 45, 561–563.

65. Abi-Dargham, A., Mawlawi, O., Lombardo, I., Gil, R., Martinez, D., Huang, Y., Hwang, D., Keilp, J., Kochan, L., Van Heertum, R., Gorman, J., L, M (2002). Prefrontal dopamine D1 receptors and working memory in schizophrenia. *J. Neurosci.* 22, 3708–3719.

66. Weinberger, D. R. (1997). The biological basis of schizophrenia: New directions. *J. Clin. Psychiatry* 58(Suppl. 10), 22–27.

67. Crocq, M., Mant, R., Asherson, P., Williams, J., Hode, Y., Mayerova, A., Collier, D., Lannfelt, L., Sokoloff, P., and Schwartz, J. (1992). Association between schizophrenia and homozygosity at the dopamine D3 receptor gene. *J. Med. Genet.* 29, 858–860.

68. Griffon, N., Crocq, M., Pilon, C., Martres, M., Mayerova, A., Uyanik, G., Burgert, E., Duval, F., Macher, J., Javoy-Agid, F., Tamminga, C., Schwartz, J., and Sokoloff, P. (1996). Dopamine D3 receptor gene: Organization, transcript variants, and polymorphism associated with schizophrenia. *Am. J. Med. Genet.* 67, 63–70.

69. Coon, H., Byerley, W., Holik, J., Hoff, M., Myles-Worsley, M., Lannfelt, L., Sokoloff, P., Schwartz, J., Waldo, M., and Freedman, R. et al. (1993). Linkage analysis of schizophrenia with five dopamine receptor genes in nine pedigrees. *Am. J. Hum. Genet.* 52, 327–334.

70. Jonsson, E., Lannfelt, L., Sokoloff, P., Schwartz, J., and Sedvall, G. (1993). Lack of association between schizophrenia and alleles in the dopamine D3 receptor gene. *Acta. Psychiatr. Scand.* 87, 345–349.

71. Lohmueller, K., Pearce, C., Pike, M., Lander, E., and Hirschhorn, J. (2003). Meta-analysis of genetic association studies supports a contribution of common variants to susceptibility to common disease. *Nat. Genet.* 33, 177–182.

72. Barr, C., Kennedy, J., Lichter, J., Van Tol, H., Wetterberg, L., Livak, K., and Kidd, K. (1993). Alleles at the dopamine D4 receptor locus do not contribute to the genetic susceptibility to schizophrenia in a large Swedish kindred. *Am. J. Med. Genet.* 48, 218–222.

73. Heinz, A., Romero, B., Gallinat, J., Juckel, G., and Weinberger, D. (2003). Molecular brain imaging and the neurobiology and genetics of schizophrenia. *Pharmacology* 36(Suppl 3), S152–S157.

74. Karayiorgou, M., and Gogos, J. (1997). A turning point in schizophrenia genetics. *Neuron* 19, 967–979.

75. Egan, M., Goldberg, T., Kolachana, B., Callicott, J., Mazzanti, C., Straub, R., Goldman, D., and Weinberger, D. (2001). Effect of COMT Val108/158 Met genotype on frontal lobe function and risk for schizophrenia. *Proc. Nat. Acad. Sci. USA* 98, 6917–6922.

76. Weinberger, D. R., Egan, M. F., Bertolino, A., Callicott, J. H., Mattay, V. S., Lipska, B. K., Berman, K. F., and Goldberg, T. E. (2001). Prefrontal neurons and the genetics of schizophrenia. *Biol. Psychiatry* 50, 825–844.
77. Harrison, P., and Weinberger, D. (2005). Schizophrenia genes, gene expression, and neuropathology: On the matter of their convergence. *Mol. Psychiatry* 10, 40–68.
78. Kapur, S., Zipursky, R., and Remington, G. (1999). Clinical and theoretical implications of 5-HT2 and D2 receptor occupancy of clozapine, risperidone, and olanzapine in schizophrenia. *Am. J. Psychiatry* 156, 286–293.
79. Nyberg, S., Nilsson, U., Okubo, Y., Halldin, C., and Farde, L. (1998). Implications of brain imaging for the management of schizophrenia. *Int. Clin. Psychopharmacol.* 13(Suppl. 3), S15–S20.
80. Pilowsky, L., Costa, D., Ell, P., Murray, R., Verhoeff, N., and Kerwin, R. (1992). Clozapine, single photon emission tomography, and the D2 dopamine receptor blockade hypothesis of schizophrenia. *Lancet* 340, 199–202.
81. Pilowsky, L., Costa, D., Ell, P., Murray, R., Verhoeff, N., and Kerwin, R. (1993). Antipsychotic medication, D2 dopamine receptor blockade and clinical response: A 123I IBZM SPET (single photon emission tomography) study. *Psychol. Med.* 23, 791–797.
82. Wolkin, A., Barouche, F., Wolf, A., Rotrosen, J., Fowler, J., Shiue, C., Cooper, T., and Brodie, J. (1989). Dopamine blockade and clinical response: Evidence for two biological subgroups of schizophrenia. *Am. J. Psychiatry* 146, 905–908.
83. Schwartz, J., Diaz, J., Pilon, C., and Sokoloff, P. (2000). Possible implications of the dopamine D(3) receptor in schizophrenia and in antipsychotic drug actions. *Brain Res. Brain Res. Rev.* 31, 277–287.
84. van Tol, H., Bunzow, J., Guan, H. -C., Sunahara, R., Seeman, P., Niznik, H., and Civelli, O. (1991). Cloning of the gene for a human dopamine D4 receptor with high affinity for the antipsychotic clozapine. *Nature* 350, 610–614.
85. Seeman, P., Tallerico, T., Corbett, R., Van Tol, H., and Kamboj, R. (1997). Role of dopamine D2, D4 and serotonin(2A) receptors in antipsychotic and anticataleptic action. *J. Psychopharmacol.* 11, 15–17.
86. Meltzer, H. Y., Matsubara, S., and Lee, J. C. (1989). Classification of typical and atypical antipsychotic drugs on the basis of dopamine D-1, D-2 and serotonin2 pKi values. *J. Pharmacol. Exp. Ther.* 251, 238–246.
87. Meltzer, H. Y. (1999). Treatment of schizophrenia and spectrum disorders: Pharmacotherapy, psychosocial treatments, and neurotransmitter interactions. *Biol. Psychiatry* 46, 1321–1327.
88. Svensson, T. (2003). Alpha-adrenoceptor modulation hypothesis of antipsychotic atypicality. *Biol. Psychiatry* 27, 1145–1158.
89. Kapur, S., and Seeman, P. (2001). Does fast dissociation from the dopamine D(2) receptor explain the action of atypical antipsychotics?: A new hypothesis. *Am. J. Psychiatry* 158, 360–369.
90. Corrigan, M., Gallen, C., Bonura, M., and Merchant, K. (2004). Effectiveness of the selective D4 antagonist sonepiprazole in schizophrenia: A placebo-controlled trial. *Biol. Psychiatry* 55, 445–451.
91. Kramer, M., Last, B., Getson, A., and Reines, S. (1997). The effects of a selective D4 dopamine receptor antagonist (L-745,870) in acutely psychotic inpatients with schizophrenia. D4 Dopamine Antagonist Group. *Arch. Gen. Psychiatry* 54, 567–572.
92. Carlsson, A., Waters, N., and Carlsson, M. (1999). Neurotransmitter interactions in schizophrenia: Therapeutic implications. *Biol. Psychiatry* 46, 1388–1395.

93. Tamminga, C., and Carlsson, A. (2002). Partial dopamine agonists and dopaminergic stabilizers, in the treatment of psychosis. *Curr. Drug Targets CNS Neurol. Disord.* 1, 141–147.
94. Tamminga, C. (2002). Partial dopamine agonists in the treatment of psychosis. *J. Neural Transmiss.* 109, 411–420.
95. Naber, D., Gaussares, C., Moeglen, J., Tremmel, L., and Bailey, P. (1992). Efficacy and tolerability of SDZ HDC 912, a partial dopamine D2 agonist, in the treatment of schizophrenia. In *Novel Antipsychotic Drugs*, H. Y.Meltzer, Ed. Raven, New York, pp. 99–107.
96. Naber, D., and Lambert, M. (2004). Aripiprazole: A new atypical antipsychotic with a different pharmacological mechanism. *Prog. Neuropsychopharmacol. Biol. Psychiatry* 28, 1213–1219.
97. Kane, J., Carson, W., Saha, A., McQuade, R., Ingenito, G., Zimbroff, D., and Ali, M. (2002). Efficacy and safety of aripiprazole and haloperidol versus placebo in patients with schizophrenia and schizoaffective disorder. *J. Clin. Psychiatry* 63, 763–771.
98. DeLeon, A., Patel, N., and Crismon, M. (2004). Aripiprazole: A comprehensive review of its pharmacology, clinical efficacy, and tolerability. *Clin. Ther.* 26, 649–666.
99. Davis, J., and Chen, N. (2004). Dose response and dose equivalence of antipsychotics. *J. Clin. Psychopharmacol.* 24, 192–208.
100. Mortimer, A., Martin, S., Loo, H., Peuskens, J., and Group, S. S. (2004). A double-blind, randomized comparative trial of amisulpride versus olanzapine for 6 months in the treatment of schizophrenia. *Int. Clin. Psychopharmacol.* 19, 63–69.
101. Wagner, M., Quednow, B., Westheide, J., Schlaepfer, T., Maier, W., and Kuhn, K. (2005). Cognitive improvement in schizophrenic patients does not require a serotonergic mechanism: Randomized controlled trial of olanzapine vs amisulpride. *Neuropsychopharmacology* 30, 381–390.
102. McCarthy, G., Puce, A., Constable, R., Krystal, J., Gore, J., and Goldman-Rakic, P. (1996). Activation of human prefrontal cortex during spatial and nonspatial working memory tasks measured by functional MRI. *Cereb. Cortex* 6, 600–611.
103. Barch, D., Braver, T., Nystrom, L., Forman, S., Noll, D., and Cohen, J. (1997). Dissociating working memory from task difficulty in human prefrontal cortex. *Neuropsychologia* 35, 1373–1380.
104. D'Esposito, M., Postle, B., and Rypma, B. (2000). Prefrontal cortical contributions to working memory: Evidence from event-related fMRI studies. *Exper. Brain Res.* 133, 3–11.
105. Konishi, S., Nakajima, K., Uchida, I., Kameyama, M., Nakahara, K., Sekihara, K., and Miyashita, Y. (1998). Transient activation of inferior prefrontal cortex during cognitive set shifting. *Nat. Neurosci.* 1, 80–84.
106. Volz, H., Gaser, C., Hager, F., Rzanny, R., Mentzel, H., Kreitschmann-Andermahr, I., Kaiser, W., and Sauer, H. (1997). Brain activation during cognitive stimulation with the Wisconsin Card Sorting Test—A functional MRI study on healthy volunteers and schizophrenics. *Psychiatry Res.* 75, 145–157.
107. Goldman-Rakic, P., Lidow, M., Smiley, J., and Williams, M. (1992). The anatomy of dopamine in monkey and human prefrontal cortex. *J. Neural Transmiss.* 36, 163–177.
108. Goldman-Rakic, P. S. (1996). Memory: Recording experience in cells and circuits: diversity in memory research. *Proc. Nat. Acad. Sci. USA* 93, 13435–13447.
109. Gao, W., and Goldman-Rakic, P. (2003). Selective modulation of excitatory and inhibitory microcircuits by dopamine. *Proc. Nat. Acad. Sci. USA* 100, 2836–2841.

110. Brozoski, T. J., Brown, R. M., Rosvold, H. E., and Goldman, P. S. (1979). Cognitive deficit caused by depletion of dopamine in prefrontal cortex of rhesus monkey. *Science* 205, 929–931.

111. Lidow, M. S., Goldman-Rakic, P. S., Gallager, D. W., and Rakic, P. (1991). Distribution of dopaminergic receptors in the primate cerebral cortex: Quantitative autoradiographic analysis using [^{3}H]raclopride, [^{3}H]spiperone and [^{3}H]SCH23390. *Neuroscience* 40, 657–671.

112. Goldman-Rakic, P., Muly, E. R., and Williams, G. (2000). D(1) receptors in prefrontal cells and circuits. *Brain Res. Brain Res. Rev.* 31, 295–301.

113. Goldman-Rakic, P. (1994). Cerebral cortical mechanisms in schizophrenia. *Neuropsychopharmacology* 10, 22S–27S.

114. Weinberger, D. R. (1987). Implications of normal brain development for the pathogenesis of schizophrenia. *Arch. Gen. Psychiatry* 44, 660–669.

115. Weinberger, D. R., Berman, K. F., and Illowsky, B. P. (1988). Physiological dysfunction of dorsolateral prefrontal cortex in schizophrenia III. A new cohort and evidence for a monoaminergic mechanism. *Arch. Gen. Psychiatry* 45, 609–615.

116. Kahn, R., Harvey, P., Davidson, M., Keefe, R., Apter, S., Neale, J., Mohs, R., and Davis, K. (1994). Neuropsychological correlates of central monoamine function in chronic schizophrenia: Relationship between CSF metabolites and cognitive function. *Schizophr. Res.* 11, 217–224.

117. Akil, M., Edgar, C. L., Pierri, J. N., Casali, S., and Lewis, D. A. (2000). Decreased density of tyrosine hydroxylase-immunoreactive axons in the entorhinal cortex of schizophrenic subjects. *Biol. Psychiatry* 47, 361–370.

118. Akil, M., Pierri, J., Whitehead, R., Edgar, C., Mohila, C., Sampson, A., and Lewis, D. (1999). Lamina-specific alterations in the dopamine innervation of the prefrontal cortex in schizophrenic subjects. *Am. J. Psychiatry* 156, 1580–1589.

119. Abi-Dargham, A., and Laruelle, M. (2005). Mechanisms of action of second generation antipsychotic drugs in schizophrenia: Insights from brain imaging studies. *Eur. Psychiatry* 20, 15–27.

120. Guo, N., Hwang, D., Lo, E., Huang, Y., Laruelle, M., and Abi-Dargham, A. (2003). Dopamine depletion and in vivo binding of PET D1 receptor radioligands: Implications for imaging studies in schizophrenia. *Neuropsychopharmacology* 28, 1703–1711.

121. Bertolino, A., Breier, A., Callicott, J. H., Adler, C., Mattay, V. S., Shapiro, M., Frank, J. A., Pickar, D., and Weinberger, D. R. (2000). The relationship between dorsolateral prefrontal neuronal N-acetylaspartate and evoked release of striatal dopamine in schizophrenia. *Neuropsychopharmacology* 22, 125–132.

122. Bertolino, A., Roffman, J. L., Lipska, B. K., Van Gelderen, P., Olson, A., and Weinberger, D. R. (1999). Postpubertal emergence of prefrontal neuronal deficits and altered dopaminergic behaviors in rats with neonatal hippocampal lesions. *Soc. Neurosci. Abstr.* 520.8.

123. Meyer-Lindenberg, A., Miletich, R., Kohn, P., Esposito, G., Carson, R., Quarantelli, M., Weinberger, D., and Berman, K. (2002). Reduced prefrontal activity predicts exaggerated striatal dopaminergic function in schizophrenia. *Nat. Neurosci.* 5, 267–271.

124. Schneider, J., Sun, Z., and Roeltgen, D. (1994). Effects of dihydrexidine, a full dopamine D-1 receptor agonist, on delayed response performance in chronic low dose MPTP-treated monkeys. *Brain Res.* 663, 140–144.

125. Arnsten, A. F., Cai, J. X., Murphy, B. L., and Goldman-Rakic, P. S. (1994). Dopamine D1 receptor mechanisms in the cognitive performance of young adult and aged monkeys. *Psychopharmacology* 116, 143–151.

126. Floresco, S., and Phillips, A. (2001). Delay-dependent modulation of memory retrieval by infusion of a dopamine D1 agonist into the rat medial prefrontal cortex. *Behav. Neurosci.* 115, 934–939.
127. Daniel, D. G., Weinberger, D. R., Jones, D. W., Zigun, J. R., Cippola, R., Handel, S., Bigelow, L. B., Goldberg, T. E., Berman, K. F., and Kleinman, J. E. (1991). The effect of amphetamine on regional cerebral blood flow during cognitive activation in schizophrenia. *J. Neurosci.* 11, 1907–1917.
128. Mattay, V., Berman, K., Ostrem, J., Esposito, G., Van Horn, J., Bigelow, L., and Weinberger, D. (1996). Dextroamphetamine enhances "Neural-network specfic" physiological signals: A positron-emission tomography rCBF study. *J. Neurosci.* 16, 4816–4822.
129. Dolan, R., Fletcher, P., Frith, C., Friston, K., Frackowiak, R., and Grasby, P. (1995). Dopaminergic modulation of impaired cognitive activation in the anterior cingulate cortex in schizophrenia. *Nature* 378, 180–182.
130. Kim, J., Kornhuber, H., Schmid-Burgk, W., and Holzmuller, B. (1980). Low cerebrospinal fluid glutamate in schizophrenic patients and a new hypothesis on schizophrenia. *Neurosci. Lett.* 20, 379–382.
131. Deakin, J., Slater, P., Simpson, M., Gilchrist, A., and Skan, W. et al. 1989). Frontal cortical and left temporal glutamatergic dysfunction in schizophrenia. *J. Neurosci.* 52, 1781–1786.
132. Gattaz, W. F., Gattaz, D., and Beckmann, H. (1982). Glutamate in schizophrenics and healthy controls. *Arch. Psychiatr. Nervenkrankheiten.* 231, 221–225.
133. Perry, T. L. (1982). Normal cerebrospinal fluid and brain glutamate levels in schizophrenia do not support the hypothesis of glutamatergic neuronal dysfunction. *Neurosci. Lett.* 28, 81–85.
134. Korpi, E. R., Kaufmann, C. A., Marnela, K. M., and Weinberger, D. R. (1987). Cerebrospinal fluid amino acid concentrations in chronic schizophrenia. *Psychiatry Res.* 20, 337–345.
135. Lodge, D., and Anis, N. A. (1982). Effects of phencyclidine on excitatory amino acid activation of spinal interneurones in the cat. *Eur. J. Pharmacol.* 77, 203–204.
136. Javitt, D. C., Jotkowitz, A., Sircar, R., and Zukin, S. R. (1987). Non-competitive regulation of phencyclidine/sigma-receptors by the N-methyl-D-aspartate receptor antagonist D-($-$)-2-amino-5-phosphonovaleric acid. *Neurosci. Lett.* 78, 193–198.
137. Sircar, R., Ludvig, N., Zukin, S. R., and Moshe, S. L. (1987). Down-regulation of hippocampal phencyclidine (PCP) receptors following amygdala kindling. *Eur. J. Pharmacol.* 141, 167–168.
138. Wong, E. H., Knight, A. R., and Woodruff, G. N. (1988). [^{3}H] MK-801 labels a site on the N-methyl-D-aspartate receptor channel complex in rat brain membranes. *J. Neurochem.* 50, 274–281.
139. Luby, E., Cohen, B., Rosenbaum, G., Gottlieb, J., and Kelley, R. (1959). Study of a new schizophrenomimetic drug-sernyl. *Am. Med. Assoc. Arch. Neurol. Psychiatry* 81, 363–369.
140. Itil, T., Keskiner, A., Kiremitci, N., and Holden, J. M. C. (1967). Effect of phencyclidine in chronic schizophrenics. *Can. Psychiatr. Assoc. J.* 12, 209–212.
141. Bakker, C. B., and Amini, F. B. (1961). Observations on the psychotomimetic effects of sernyl. *Comp. Psychiatry* 2, 269–280.
142. Aniline, O., and Pitts, F. N.Jr. (1982). Phencyclidine (PCP): A review and perspectives. *Crit. Rev. Toxicol.* 10, 145–177.

143. Krystal, J. H., Karper, L. P., Seibyl, J. P., Freeman, G. K., Delaney, R., Bremner, J. D., Heninger, G. R., Bowers, M., and Charney, D. S. (1994). Subanesthetic effects of the noncompetitive NMDA antagonist, ketamine, in humans: Psychotomimetic, perceptual, cognitive, and neuroendocrine responses. *Arch. Gen. Psychiatry* 51, 199–214.

144. Malhotra, A. K., Pinals, D. A., Weingartner, H., Sirocco, K., Missar, C. D., Pickar, D., and Breier, A. (1996). NMDA receptor function and human cognition: The effects of ketamine in healthy volunteers. *Neuropsychopharmacology* 14, 301–307.

145. Adler, C. M., Malhotra, A. K., Elman, I., Goldberg, T., Egan, M., Pickar, D., and Breier, A. (1999). Comparison of ketamine-induced thought disorder in healthy volunteers and thought disorder in schizophrenia. *Am. J. Psychiatry* 156, 1646–1649.

146. Newcomer, J. W., Farber, N. B., Jevtovic-Todorovic, V., Selke, G., Melson, A. K., Hershcy, T., Craft, S., and Olney, J. W. (1999). Ketamine-induced NMDA receptor hypofunction as a model of memory impairment and psychosis. *Neuropsychopharmacology* 20, 106–118.

147. Oye, N., Paulson, O., and Maurset, A. (1992). Effects of ketamine on sensory perception: Evidence for a role of N-methyl-D-asparate receptors. *J. Pharmacol. Exp. Ther.* 260, 1209–1213.

148. Abi-Saab, W. M., D'Souza, D. C., Moghaddam, B., and Krystal, J. H. (1998). The NMDA antagonist model for schizophrenia: Promise and pitfalls. *Pharmacopsychiatry* 31, 104–109.

149. Lahti, A., Weiler, M., Tamara Michaelidis, B., Parwani, A., and Tamminga, C. (2001). Effects of ketamine in normal and schizophrenic volunteers. *Neuropsychopharmacology* 25, 455–467.

150. Ghoneim, M., Hinrichs, J., Mewaldt, S., and Petersen, R. (1985). Ketamine: Behavioral effects of subanesthetic doses. *J. Clin. Psychopharmacol.* 5, 70–77.

151. Lahti, A. C., Holocomb, H. H., Medoff, D. R., Tamminga, C. A., (1995). Ketamine activates psychosis and alters limbic blood flow in schizophrenia. *Neuroreport* 6, 869–872.

152. Lahti, A. C., Koffel, B., LaPorte, D., and Tamminga, C. A. (1995). Subanesthetic doses of ketamine stimulate psychosis in schizophrenia. *Neuropsychopharmacology* 13, 9–19.

153. Malhotra, A. K., Pinals, D. A., Adler, C. M., Elman, I., Clifton, A., Pickar, D., and Breier, A. (1997). Ketamine-induced exacerbation of psychotic symptoms and cognitive impairment in neuroleptic-free schizophrenics. *Neuropsychopharmacology* 17, 141–150.

154. Javitt, D. C., and Zukin, S. R. (1991). Recent advances in the phencyclidine model of schizophrenia. *Am. J. Psychiatry* 148, 1301–1308.

155. Marenco, S., and Weinberger, D. (2000). The neurodevelopmental hypothesis of schizophrenia: Following a trail of evidence from cradle to grave. *Dev. Psychopathol.* 12, 501–527.

156. McGlashan, T., and Hoffman, R. (2000). Schizophrenia as a disorder of developmentally reduced synaptic connectivity. *Arch. Gen. Psychiatry* 57, 637–648.

157. Roberts, G. W. (1990). Schizophrenia: The cellular biology of a functional psychosis. *Trends Neurosci.* 13, 207–211.

158. Harrison, P. J. (1997). Schizophrenia: A disorder of neurodevelopment? *Curr. Opin. Neurobiol.* 7, 285–289.

159. Olney, J. W. (1990). Excitotoxic amino acids and neuropsychiatric disorders. *Annu. Rev. Pharmacol. Toxicol.* 30, 47–71.

160. Carlsson, M., and Carlsson, A. (1990). Interactions between glutamatergic and monoaminergic systems within the basal ganglia—Implications for schizophrenia and Parkinson's disease. *Trends Neurosci.* 13, 272–276.

161. Olney, J., and Farber, N. (1995). Glutamate receptor dysfunction and schizophrenia. *Arch. Gen. Psychiatry* 52, 998–1007.

162. Tamminga, C. A. (1998). Schizophrenia and glutamatergic transmission. *Crit. Rev. Neurobiol.* 12, 21–36.

163. Krystal, J. H., D'Souza, D. C., Belge, A., Anand, A., Charney, D. S., Aghajanian, G. K., and Moghaddam, B. (1999). Therapeutic implications of the hyperglutamatergic effects of NMDA antagonists. *Neuropsychopharmacology* 21, S143–S157.

164. Goff, D. C., and Coyle, J. T. (2001). The emerging role of glutamate in the pathophysiology and treatment of schizophrenia. *Am. J. Psychiatry* 158, 1367–1377.

165. Grace, A. (1991). Phasic versus tonic dopamine release and modulation of dopamine system responsivity: A hypothesis for the etiology of schizophrenia. *Neuroscience* 41, 1–24.

166. Moghaddam, B. (2003). Bringing order to the glutamate chaos in schizophrenia. *Neuron* 40, 881–884.

167. Mueller, H., Haroutunian, V., Davis, K., and Meador-Woodruff, J. (2004). Expression of the ionotropic glutamate receptor subunits and NMDA receptor-associated intracellular proteins in the substantia nigra in schizophrenia. *Brain Res. Mol. Brain Res.* 121, 60–69.

168. Conn, J. P., and Pin, J. P. (1997). Pharmacology and functions of metabotropic glutamate receptors. *Annu. Rev. Pharmacol. Toxicol.* 37, 205–237.

169. Meador-Woodruff, J. H., and Healy, D. J. (2000). Glutamate receptor expression in schizophrenic brain. *Brain Res. Brain Res. Rev.* 31, 288–294.

170. Kerwin, R., Patel, S., and Meldrum, B. (1990). Quantitative autoradiographic analysis of glutamate binding sites in the hippocampal formation in normal and schizophrenic brain post mortem. *Neuroscience* 39, 25–32.

171. Kornhuber, J., Mack-Burkhardt, F., Riederer, P., Hebenstreit, G., Reynolds, G., Andrews, H., and Beckmann, H. (1989). [^{3}H]MK-801 binding sites in postmortem brain regions of schizophrenic patients. *J. Neural Transmiss.* 77, 231–236.

172. Harrison, P. J., McLaughlin, D., and Kerwin, R. W. (1991). Decreased hippocampal expression of a glutamate receptor gene in schizophrenia. *Lancet* 337, 450–452.

173. Kerwin, R., Patel, S., Meldrum, B., Czudek, C., and Reynolds, G. (1988). Asymmetrical loss of glutamate receptor subtype in left hippocampus in schizophrenia. *Lancet* 1, 583–584.

174. Eastwood, S. L., and Harrison, P. J. (1995). Decreased synaptophysin in the medial temporal lobe in schizophrenia demonstrated using immunoautoradiography. *Neuroscience* 69, 339–343.

175. Eastwood, S. L., Kerwin, R. W., and Harrison, P. J. (1997). Immunoautoradiographic evidence for a loss of α–amino-3-hydroxy-5-methyl-4-isoxazole propionate-preferring non-*N*-methyl-D-asparate glutamate receptors within the medial temporal lobe in schizophrenia. *Biol. Psychiatry* 41, 636–643.

176. Healy, D. J., Haroutunian, V., Powchik, P., Davidson, M., Davis, K. L., Watson, S. J., and Meador-Woodruff, J. H. (1998). AMPA receptor binding and subunit mRNA expression in prefrontal cortex and striatum of elderly schizophrenics. *Neuropsychopharmacology* 19, 278–286.

177. Noga, J. T., Hyde, T. M., Bachus, S. E., Herman, M. M., and Kleinman, J. E. (2001). AMPA receptor binding in the dorsolateral prefrontal cortex of schizophrenics and controls. *Schizophr. Res.* 48, 361–363.

178. Ibrahim, H. M., Hogg, A. J.Jr., Healy, D. J., Haroutunian, V., Davis, K. L., and Meador-Woodruff, J. H. (2000). Ionotropic glutamate receptor binding and subunit mRNA expression in thalamic nuclei in schizophrenia. *Am. J. Psychiatry* 157, 1811–1823.

179. Nishikawa, T., Takashima, M., and Toru, M. (1983). Increased [^{3}H]kainic acid binding in the prefrontal cortex in schizophrenia. *Neurosci. Lett.* 40, 245–250.

180. Noga, J. T., Hyde, T. M., Herman, M. M., Spurney, C. F., Bigelow, L. B., Weinberger, D. R., and Kleinman, J. E. (1997). Glutamate receptors in the postmortem striatum of schizophrenic, suicide, and control brains. *Synapse* 27, 168–176.

181. Porter, R. H., Eastwood, S. L., and Harrison, P. J. (1997). Distribution of kainate receptor subunit mRNAs in human hippocampus, neocortex and cerebellum, and bilateral reduction of hippocampal GluR6 and KA2 transcripts in schizophrenia. *Brain Res.* 751, 217–231.

182. Sokolov, B. P. (1998). Expression of NMDAR1, GluR1, GluR7, and KA1 glutamate receptor mRNAs is decreased in frontal cortex of "neuroleptic-free" schizophrenics: Evidence on reversible up-regulation by typical neuroleptics. *J. Neurochem.* 71, 2454–2464.

183. Meador-Woodruff, J. H., Davis, K. L., and Haroutunian, V. (2001). Abnormal kainate receptor expression in prefrontal cortex in schizophrenia. *Neuropsychopharmacology* 24, 545–552.

184. Aparicio-Legarza, M. I., Cutts, A. J., Davis, B., and Reynolds, G. P. (1997). Deficits of [^{3}H] D-aspartate binding to glutamate uptake sites in striatal and accumbens tissue in patients with schizophrenia. *Neurosci. Lett.* 232, 13–16.

185. Weissman, A. D., Casanova, M. F., Kleinman, J. E., London, E. D., and De Souza, E. B. (1991). Selective loss of cerebral cortical sigma, but not PCP binding sites in schizophrenia. *Biol. Psychiatry* 29, 41–54.

186. Simpson, M. D., Slater, P., Royston, M. C., and Deakin, J. F. W. (1992). Regionally selective deficits in uptake sites for glutamate and gamma-aminobutyric acid in the basal ganglia in schizophrenia. *Psychiatry Res.* 42, 273–282.

187. Dracheva, S., Marras, S., Elhakem, S., Kramer, F., Davis, K., and Haroutunian, V. (2001). *N*-methyl-D-aspartic acid receptor expression in the dorsolateral prefrontal cortex of elderly patients with schizophrenia. *Am. J. Psychiatry* 158, 1400–1410.

188. Grimwood, S., Slater, P., Deakin, J. F., and Hutson, P. H. (1999). NR2B-containing NMDA receptors are up-regulated in temporal cortex in schizophrenia. *Neuroreport* 10, 461–465.

189. Le Corre, S., Harper, C., Lopez, P., Ward, P., and Catts, S. (2000). Increased levels of expression of an NMDARI splice variant in the superior temporal gyrus in schizophrenia. *Neuroreport* 11, 983–986.

190. Akbarian, S., Sucher, N. J., Bradley, D., Tafazzoli, A., Trinh, D., Hetrick, W. P., Potkin, S. G., Sandman, C. A., Bunney, W. E.Jr., and Jones, E. G. (1996). Selective alterations in gene expression for NMDA receptor subunits in prefrontal cortex of schizophrenics. *J. Neurosci.* 16, 19–30.

191. Ibrahim, H. M., Healy, D. J., Hogg, A. J.Jr., and Meador-Woodruff, J. H. (2000). Nucleus-specific expression of ionotropic glutamate receptor subunit mRNAs and binding sites in primate thalamus. *Brain Res. Mol. Brain Res.* 79, 1–17.

192. Clinton, S., and Meador-Woodruff, J. (2004). Abnormalities of the NMDA receptor and associated intracellular molecules in the thalamus in schizophrenia and bipolar disorder. *Neuropsychopharmacology* 29, 1353–1362.

193. Gao, X. M., Sakai, K., Roberts, R. C., Conley, R. R., Dean, B., and Tamminga, C. A. (2000). Ionotropic glutamate receptors and expression of *N*-methyl-D-aspartate receptor subunits in subregions of human hippocampus: Effects of schizophrenia. *Am. J. Psychiatry* 157, 1141–1149.

194. Ohnuma, T., Augood, S. J., Arai, H., McKenna, P. J., and Emson, P. C. (1998). Expression of the human excitatory amino acid transporter 2 and metabotropic glutamate receptors 3 and 5 in the prefrontal cortex from normal individuals and patients with schizophrenia. *Brain Res. Mol. Brain Res.* 56, 207–217.

195. Richardson-Burns, S. M., Haroutunian, V., Davis, K. L., Watson, S. J., and Meador-Woodruff, J. H. (2000). Metabotropic glutamate receptor mRNA expression in the schizophrenic thalamus. *Biol. Psychiatry* 47, 22–28.

196. Tsai, G., Passani, L. A., Slusher, B. S., Carter, R., Baer, L., Kleinman, J. E., and Coyle, J. T. (1995). Abnormal excitatory neurotransmitter metabolism in schizophrenic brains. *Arch. Gen. Psychiatry* 52, 829–836.

197. Coyle, J. (1996). The glutamatergic dysfunction hypothesis for schizophrenia. *Harvard Rev. Psychiatry* 3, 241–253.

198. Eastwood, S., and Harrison, P. (2005). Decreased expression of vesicular glutamate transporter 1 and complexin II mRNAs in schizophrenia: Further evidence for a synaptic pathology affecting glutamate neurons. *Schizophr. Res.* 73, 159–172.

199. Clinton, S. M., Haroutunian, V., Davis, K. L., and Meador-Woodruff, J. H. (2003). Altered transcript expression of NMDA receptor-associated postsynaptic proteins in the thalamus of subjects with schizophrenia. *Am. J. Psychiatry* 160, 1100–1109.

200. Smith, R., Haroutunian, V., Davis, K., and Meador-Woodruff, J. (2001). Expression of excitatory amino acid transporter transcripts in the thalamus of subjects with schizophrenia. *Am. J. Psychiatry* 158, 1393–1399.

201. Smith, R., Haroutunian, V., Davis, K., and Meador-Woodruff, J. (2001). Vesicular glutamate transporter transcript expression in the thalamus in schizophrenia. *Neuroreport* 12, 2885–2887.

202. Hashimoto, K., Fukushima, T., Shimizu, E., Komatsu, N., Watanabe, H., Shinoda, N., Nakazato, M., Kumakiri, C., Okada, S., Hasegawa, H., Imai, K., and Iyo, M. (2003). Decreased serum levels of D-serine in patients with schizophrenia: Evidence in support of the *N*-methyl-D-aspartate receptor hypofunction hypothesis of schizophrenia. *Arch. Gen. Psychiatry* 60, 572–576.

203. Sumiyoshi, T., Anil, A., Jin, D., Jayathilake, K., Lee, M., and Meltzer, H. (2004). Plasma glycine and serine levels in schizophrenia compared to normal controls and major depression: Relation to negative symptoms. *Int. J. Neuropsychopharmacol.* 7, 1–8.

204. Erhardt, S., Schwieler, L., and Engberg, G. (2003). Kynurenic acid and schizophrenia. *Adv. Exper. Med. Biol.* 527, 155–165.

205. Erhardt, S., Blennow, K., Nordin, C., Skogh, E., Lindstrom, L., and Engberg, G. (2001). Kynurenic acid levels are elevated in the cerebrospinal fluid of patients with schizophrenia. *Neurosci. Lett.* 313, 96–98.

206. Schwarcz, R., Rassoulpour, A., Wu, H., Medoff, D., Tamminga, C., and Roberts, R. (2001). Increased cortical kynurenate content in schizophrenia. *Biol. Psychiatry* 50, 521–530.

207. Gur, R. E., Turetsky, B. I., Cowell, P. E., Finkelman, C., Maany, V., Grossman, R. I., Arnold, S. E., Bilker, W. B., and Gur, R. C. (2000). Temporolimbic volume reductions in schizophrenia. *Arch. Gen. Psychiatry* 57, 769–775.

208. Gur, R. E., Cowell, P. E., Latshaw, A., Turetsky, B. I., Grossman, R. I., Arnold, S. E., Bilker, W. B., and Gur, R. C. (2000). Reduced dorsal and orbital prefrontal gray matter volumes in schizophrenia. *Arch. Gen. Psychiatry* 57, 761–768.

209. Zipursky, R., Lambe, E., Kapur, S., and Mikulis, D. (1998). Cerebral gray matter volume deficits in first episode psychosis. *Arch. Gen. Psychiatry* 55, 540–546.

210. Szeszko, P., Goldberg, E., Gunduz-Bruce, H., Ashtari, M., Robinson, D., Malhotra, A., Lencz, T., Bates, J., Crandall, D., Kane, J., and Bilder, R. (2003). Smaller anterior hippocampal formation volume in antipsychotic-naive patients with first-episode schizophrenia. *Am. J. Psychiatry* 160, 2190–2197.

211. Yamasue, H., Iwanami, A., Hirayasu, Y., Yamada, H., Abe, O., Kuroki, N., Fukuda, R., Tsujii, K., Aoki, S., Ohtomo, K., Kato, N., and Kasai, K. (2004). Localized volume reduction in prefrontal, temporolimbic, and paralimbic regions in schizophrenia: An MRI parcellation study. *Psychiatry Res.* 131, 195–207.

212. Sanfilipo, M., Lafargue, T., Rusinek, H., Arena, L., Loneragan, C., Lautin, A., Feiner, D., Rotrosen, J., and Wolkin, A. (2000). Volumetric measure of the frontal and temporal lobe regions in schizophrenia: Relationship to negative symptoms. *Arch. Gen. Psychiatry* 57, 471–480.

213. Kuperberg, G., Broome, M., McGuire, P., David, A., Eddy, M., Ozawa, F., Goff, D., West, W., Williams, S., van der Kouwe, A., Salat, D., Dale, A., and Fischl, B. (2003). Regionally localized thinning of the cerebral cortex in schizophrenia. *Arch. Gen. Psychiatry* 60, 878–888.

214. Kulynych, J., Luevano, L., Jones, D., and Weinberger, D. (1997). Cortical abnormality in schizophrenia: An in vivo application of the gyrification index. *Biol. Psychiatry* 41, 995–999.

215. Vogeley, K., Schneider-Axmann, T., Pfeiffer, U., Tepest, R., Bayer, T., Bogerts, B., Honer, W., and Falkai, P. (2000). Disturbed gyrification of the prefrontal region in male schizophrenic patients: A morphometric postmortem study. *Am. J. Psychiatry* 157, 34–39.

216. Casanova, M., and Rothberg, B. (2002). Shape distortion of the hippocampus: A possible explanation of the pyramidal cell disarray reported in schizophrenia. *Schizophr. Res.* 55, 19–24.

217. Csernansky, J., Wang, L., Jones, D., Rastogi-Cruz, D., Posener, J., Heydebrand, G., Miller, J., and Miller, M. (2002). Hippocampal deformities in schizophrenia characterized by high dimensional brain mapping. *Am. J. Psychiatry* 159, 2000–2006.

218. Benes, F. M., McSparren, J., Bird, E. D., SanGiovanni, J. P., and Vincent, S. L. (1991). Deficits in small interneurons in prefrontal and cingulate cortices of schizophrenic and schizoaffective patients. *Arch. Gen. Psychiatry* 48, 996–1001.

219. Arnold, S., Franz, B., Gur, R., Gur, R., Shapiro, R., Moberg, P., and Trojanowski, J. (1995). Smaller neuron size in schizophrenia in hippocampal subfields that mediate cortical-hippocampal interactions. *Am. J. Psychiatry* 152, 738–748.

220. Zaidel, D., Esiri, M., and Harrison, P. (1997). Size, shape, and orientation of neurons in the left and right hippocampus: Investigation of normal asymmetries and alterations in schizophrenia. *Am. J. Psychiatry* 154, 812–818.

221. Zaidel, D., Esiri, M., and Harrison, P. (1997). The hippocampus in schizophrenia: Lateralized increase in neuronal density and altered cytoarchitectural asymmetry. *Psychol. Med.* 27, 703–713.

222. Rajakowska, G., Selemon, L., and Goldman-Rakic, P. (1998). Neuronal and glial somal size in the prefrontal cortex. A postmortem study of schizophrenia and Huntington-disease. *Arch. Gen. Psychiatry* 55, 215–224.

223. Pierri, J. N., Volk, C. L., Auh, S., Sampson, A., and Lewis, D. A. (2003). Somal size of prefrontal cortical pyramidal neurons in schizophrenia: Differential effects across neuronal subpopulations. *Biol. Psychiatry* 54, 111–120.

224. Sweet, R., Pierri, J., Auh, S., Sampson, A., and Lewis, D. (2003). Reduced pyramidal cell somal volume in auditory association cortex of subjects with schizophrenia. *Neuropsychopharmacology* 28, 599–609.

225. Sweet, R., Bergen, S., Sun, Z., Sampson, A., Pierri, J., D, L. (2004). Pyramidal cell size reduction in schizophrenia: Evidence for involvement of auditory feedforward circuits. *Biol. Psychiatry* 55, 1128–1137.

226. Pierri, J., Volk, C., Auh, S., Sampson, A., and Lewis, D. (2001). Decreased somal size of deep layer 3 pyramidal neurons in the prefrontal cortex of subjects with schizophrenia. *Arch. Gen. Psychiatry* 55, 466–473.

227. Garey, L., Ong, W., Patel, T., Kanani, M., Davis, A., Mortimer, A., Barnes, T., and Hirsch, S. (1998). Reduced dendritic spine density on cerebral cortical pyramidal neurons in schizophrenia. *J. Neurol. Neurosurg. Psychiatry* 65, 446–453.

228. Glantz, L., and Lewis, D. (2000). Decreased dendritic spine density on prefrontal cortical pyramidal neurons in schizophrenia. *Arch. Gen. Psychiatry* 57, 65–73.

229. Rosoklija, G., Toomayan, G., Ellis, S., Keilp, J., Mann, J., Latov, N., Hays, A., and Dwork, A. (2000). Structural abnormalities of subicular dendrites in subjects with schizophrenia and mood disorders: Preliminary findings. *Arch. Gen. Psychiatry* 57, 349–356.

230. Black, J., Kodish, I., Grossman, A., Klintsova, A., Orlovskaya, D., Vostrikov, V., Uranova, N., and Greenough, W. (2004). Pathology of layer V pyramidal neurons in the prefrontal cortex of patients with schizophrenia. *Am. J. Psychiatry* 161, 742–744.

231. Arnold, S. E., Hyman, B. T., van Hoesen, G. W., and Damasio, A. R. (1991). Some cytoarchitectural abnormalities of the entorhinal cortex in schizophrenia. *Arch. Gen. Psychiatry* 48, 625–632.

232. Falkai, P., Schneider-Axmann, T., and Honer, W. (2000). Entorhinal cortex pre-alpha cell clusters in schizophrenia: Quantitative evidence of a developmental abnormality. *Biol. Psychiatry* 47, 937–943.

233. Kovalenko, S., Bergmann, A., Schneider-Axmann, T., Ovary, I., Majtenyi, K., Havas, L., Honer, W., Bogerts, B., and Falkai, P. (2003). Regio entorhinalis in schizophrenia: More evidence for migrational disturbances and suggestions for a new biological hypothesis. *Pharmacology* 36(Suppl 3), S158–S161.

234. Akbarian, S., Bunney, W. E.Jr., Potkin, S. G., Wigal, S. B., Hagman, J. O., Sandman, C. A., and Jones, E. G. (1993). Altered distribution of nicotinamide-adenine dinucleotide phosphate-diaphorase cells in frontal lobe of schizophrenics implies disturbances of cortical development. *Arch. Gen. Psychiatry* 50, 169–177.

235. Akbarian, S., Vinuela, A., Kim, J. J., Potkin, S. G., Bunney, W. E.Jr., and Jones, E. G. (1993). Distorted distribution of nicotinamide-adenine dinucleotide phosphate-diaphorase neurons in temporal lobe of schizophrenics implies anomalous cortical development. *Arch. Gen. Psychiatry* 50, 178–187.

236. Akbarian, S., Kim, J., Potkin, S., Hetrick, W., Bunney, W. J., and Jones, E. (1996). Maldistribution of interstitial neurons in prefrontal white matter of the brains of schizophrenic patients. *Arch. Gen. Psychiatry* 53, 425–436.

237. Anderson, S., Volk, D., and Lewis, D. (1996). Increased density of microtubule associated protein 2-immunoreactive neurons in the prefrontal white matter of schizophrenic subjects. *Schizophr. Res.* 19, 111–119.

238. Eastwood, S. (2004). The synaptic pathology of schizophrenia: Is aberrant neurodevelopment and plasticity to blame. *Int. Rev. Neurobiol.* 59, 47–72.

239. Eastwood, S., and Harrison, P. (2003). Interstitial white matter neurons express less reelin and are abnormally distributed in schizophrenia: Towards an integration of molecular and morphologic aspects of the neurodevelopmental hypothesis. *Mol. Psychiatry* 8, 821–831.

240. Bressan, R. A., and Pilowsky, L. S. (2000). Imaging the glutamatergic system in vivo—Relevance to schizophrenia. *Eur. J. Nucl. Med.* 27, 1723–1731.

241. Berman, K. F., Zec, R. F., and Weinberger, D. R. (1986). Physiological dysfunction of dorsolateral prefrontal cortex in schizophrenia, II: Role of neuroleptic treatment, attention, and mental effort. *Arch. Gen. Psychiatry* 43, 126–135.

242. Berman, K. F., Illowsky, B. P., and Weinberger, D. R. (1988). Physiological dysfunction of dorsolateral prefrontal cortex in schizophrenia IV. Further evidence for regional and behavioral specificity. *Arch. Gen. Psychiatry* 45, 616–622.

243. Carter, C. S., Perlstein, W., Ganguli, R., Brar, J., Mintun, M., and Cohen, J. D. (1998). Functional hypofrontality and working memory dysfunction in schizophrenia. *Am. J. Psychiatry* 155, 1285–1287.

244. Meyer-Lindenberg, A., Poline, J. B., Kohn, P. D., Holt, J. L., Egan, M. F., Weinberger, D. R., and Berman, K. F. (2001). Evidence for abnormal cortical functional connectivity during working memory in schizophrenia. *Am. J. Psychiatry* 158, 1809–1817.

245. Barch, D., Carter, C., Braver, T., Sabb, F., MacDonald, A. R., Noll, D., and Cohen, J. (2001). Selective deficits in prefrontal cortex function in medication-naive patients with schizophrenia. *Arch. Gen. Psychiatry* 58, 280–288.

246. Manoach, D., Gollub, R., Benson, E., Searl, M., Goff, D., Halpern, E., Saper, C., and Rauch, S. (2000). Schizophrenic subjects show aberrant fMRI activation of dorsolateral prefrontal cortex and basal ganglia during working memory performance. *Biol. Psychiatry* 48, 99–109.

247. Dolan, R., Fletcher, P., McKenna, P., Friston, K., and Frith, C. (1999). Abnormal neural integration related to cognition in schizophrenia. *Acta Psychiatr. Scand. Suppl.* 395, 58–67.

248. Heckers, S., Rauch, S., Goff, D., Savage, C., Schacter, D., Fischman, A., and Alpert, N. (1998). Impaired recruitment of the hippocampus during conscious recollection in schizophrenia. *Nat. Neurosci.* 1, 318–323.

249. Jennings, J., McIntosh, A., Kapur, S., Zipursky, R., and Houle, S. (1998). Functional network differences in schizophrenia: A rCBF study of semantic processing. *Neuroreport* 9, 1697–1700.

250. Kegeles, L. S., Abi-Dargham, A., Zea-Ponce, Y., Rodenhiser-Hill, J., Mann, J. J., Van Heertum, R. L., Cooper, T. B., Carlsson, A., and Laruelle, M. (2000). Modulation of amphetamine-induced striatal dopamine release by ketamine in humans: Implications for schizophrenia. *Biol. Psychiatry* 48, 627–640.

251. Schiffer, H. (2002). Glutamate receptor genes: Susceptibility factors in schizophrenia and depressive disorders. *Mol. Neurobiol.* 25, 191–212.

252. Collier, D. A., and Li, T. (2003). The genetics of schizophrenia: Glutamate not dopamine? *Eur. J. Pharmacol.* 480, 177–184.

253. Riley, B. P., Tahir, E., Rajagopalan, S., Mogudi-Carter, M., Faure, S., Weissenbach, J., Jenkins, T., and Williamson, R. (1997). A linkage study of the N-methyl-D-aspartate receptor subunit gene loci and schizophrenia in southern African Bantu-speaking families. *Psychiatr. Genet.* 7, 57–74.
254. Pariseau, C., Gregor, P., Myles-Worsley, M., Holik, J., Hoff, M., Waldo, M., Freedman, R., Coon, H., and Byerley, W. (1994). Schizophrenia and glutamate receptor genes. *Psychiatr. Genet.* 4, 161–165.
255. Bray, N. J., Williams, N. M., Bowen, T., Cardno, A. G., Gray, M., Jones, L. A., Murphy, K. C., Sanders, R. D., Spurlock, G., Odonovan, M. C., and Owen, M. J. (2000). No evidence for association between a non-synonymous polymorphism in the gene encoding human metabotropic glutamate receptor 7 and schizophrenia. *Psychiatr. Genet.* 10, 83–86.
256. Nishiguchi, N., Shirakawa, O., Ono, H., Hashimoto, T., and Maeda, K. (2000). Novel polymorphism in the gene region encoding the carboxyl-terminal intracellular domain of the NMDA receptor 2B subunit: Analysis of association with schizophrenia. *Am. J. Psychiatry* 157, 1329–1331.
257. Bolonna, A. A., Kerwin, R. W., Munro, J., Arranz, M. J., and Makoff, A. J. (2001). Polymorphisms in the genes for mGluR types 7 and 8: Association studies with schizophrenia. *Schizophr. Res.* 47, 99–103.
258. Egan, M., Straub, R., Goldberg, T., Yakub, I., Callicott, J., Hariri, A., Mattay, V., Bertolino, A., Hyde, T., Shannon-Weickert, C., Akil, M., Crook, J., Vakkalanka, R., Balkissoon, R., Gibbs, R., Kleinman, J., and Weinberger, D. (2004). Variation in GRM3 affects cognition, prefrontal glutamate, and risk for schizophrenia. *Proc. Nat. Acad. Sci. USA* 101, 12604–12609.
259. Marti, S., Cichon, S., Propping, P., and Nothen, M. (2002). Metabotropic glutamate receptor 3 (GRM3) gene variation is not associated with schizophrenia or bipolar affective disorder in the German population. *Am. J. Med. Genet.* 114, 46–50.
260. Fujii, Y., Shibata, H., Kikuta, R., Makino, C., Tani, A., Hirata, N., Shibata, A., Ninomiya, H., Tashiro, N., and Fukumaki, Y. (2003). Positive associations of polymorphisms in the metabotropic glutamate receptor type 3 gene (GRM3) with schizophrenia. *Psychiatr. Genet.* 13, 71–76.
261. Moghaddam, B., and Adams, B. (1998). Reversal of phencyclidine effects by a group II metabotropic glutamate receptor agonist in rats. *Science* 281, 1349–1352.
262. Homayoun, H., Jackson, M. E., Moghaddam, B., (2005). Activation of metabotropic glutamate 2/3 (mGlu2/3) receptors reverses the effects of NMDA receptor hypofunction on prefrontal cortex unit activity in awake rats. *J. Neurophysiol.* 93, 1989–2001.
263. Crook, J., Akil, M., Law, B., Hyde, T., and Kleinman, J. (2002). Comparative analysis of group II metabotropic glutamate receptor immunoreactivity in Brodmann's area 46 of the dorsolateral prefrontal cortex from patients with schizophrenia and normal subjects. *Mol. Psychiatry* 7, 157–164.
264. Harrison, P. J., and Owen, M. J. (2003). Genes for schizophrenia? Recent findings and their pathophysiological implications[comment]. *Lancet* 361, 417–419.
265. Stefansson, H., Sigurdsson, E., Steinthorsdottir, V., Bjornsdottir, S., Sigmundsson, T., Ghosh, S., Brynjolfsson, J., Gunnarsdottir, S., Ivarsson, O., Chou, T. T., Hjaltason, O., Birgisdottir, B., Jonsson, H., Gudnadottir, V. G., Gudmundsdottir, E., Bjornsson, A., Ingvarsson, B., Ingason, A., Sigfusson, S., Hardardottir, H., Harvey, R. P., Lai, D., Zhou, M., Brunner, D., Mutel, V., Gonzalo, A., Lemke, G., Sainz, J., Johannesson, G., Andresson, T., Gudbjartsson, D., Manolescu, A., Frigge, M. L., Gurney, M. E., Kong, A., Gulcher, J. R., Petursson, H., and Stefansson, K. (2002). Neuregulin 1 and susceptibility to schizophrenia. *Am. J. Hum. Genet.* 71, 877–892.

266. Stefansson, H., Thorgeirsson, T., Gulcher, J., and Stefansson, K. (2003). Neuregulin 1 in schizophrenia: Out of Iceland. *Mol. Psychiatry* 8, 639–640.

267. Saugstad, J. A., Marino, M. J., Folk, J. A., Hepler, J. R., and Conn, P. J. (1998). RGS4 inhibits signaling by group I metabotropic glutamate receptors. *J. Neurosci.* 18, 905–913.

268. Chowdari, K. V., Mirnics, K., Semwal, P., Wood, J., Lawrence, E., Bhatia, T., Deshpande, S. N., Ferrell, K. T. B., R. E., Middleton, F. A., Devlin, B., Levitt, P., Lewis, D. A., Nimgaonkar, V.L., (2002). Association and linkage analyses of RGS4 polymorphisms in schizophrenia. *Hum. Mol. Genet.* 11, 1373–1380.

269. Owen, M., Williams, N., and O'Donovan, M. (2004). The molecular genetics of schizophrenia: New findings promise new insights. *Mol. Psychiatry* 9, 14–27.

270. Chumakov, I., Blumenfeld, M., Guerassimenko, O., Cavarec, L., Palicio, M., Abderrahim, H., Bougueleret, L., Barry, C., Tanaka, H., La Rosa, P., Puech, A., Tahri, N., Cohen-Akenine, A., Delabrosse, S., Lissarrague, S., Picard, F. P., Maurice, K., Essioux, L., Millasseau, P., Grel, P., Debailleul, V., Simon, A. M., Caterina, D., Dufaure, I., Malekzadeh, K., Belova, M., Luan, J. J., Bouillot, M., Sambucy, J. L., Primas, G., Saumier, M., Boubkiri, N., Martin-Saumier, S., Nasroune, M., Peixoto, H., Delaye, A., Pinchot, V., Bastucci, M., Guillou, S., Chevillon, M., Sainz-Fuertes, R., Meguenni, S., Aurich-Costa, J., Cherif, D., Gimalac, A., Van Duijn, C., Gauvreau, D., Ouelette, G., Fortier, I., Realson, J., Sherbatich, T., Riazanskaia, N., Rogaev, E., Raeymaekers, P., Aerssens, J., Konings, F., Luyten, W., Macciardi, F., Sham, P. C., Straub, R. E., Weinberger, D. R., Cohen, N., and Cohen, D. (2002). Genetic and physiological data implicating the new human gene G72 and the gene for D-amino acid oxidase in schizophrenia [comment]. *Proc. Nat. Acad. Sci. USA.* 99, 13675–13680.

271. Schumacher, J., Jamra, R., Freudenberg, J., Becker, T., Ohlraun, S., Otte, A., Tullius, M., Kovalenko, S., Bogaert, A., Maier, W., Rietschel, M., Propping, P., Nothen, M., and Cichon, S. (2004). Examination of G72 and D-amino-acid oxidase as genetic risk factors for schizophrenia and bipolar affective disorder. *Mol. Psychiatry* 9, 203–207.

272. Bredt, D. (1999). Knocking signalling out of the dystrophin complex. *Nat. Cell. Biol.* 1, E89–E91.

273. Gerber, D., Hall, D., Miyakawa, T., Demars, S., Gogos, J., Karayiorgou, M., and Tonegawa, S. (2003). Evidence for association of schizophrenia with genetic variation in the 8p21.3 gene, PPP3CC, encoding the calcineurin gamma subunit. *Proc. Nat. Acad. Sci. USA* 100, 8993–8998.

274. Deutsch, S., Mastropaolo, J., Schwartz, B., Rosse, R., and Morihisa, J. (1989). A "glutamatergic hypothesis" of schizophrenia. Rationale for pharmacotherapy with glycine. *Clin. Neuropharmacol.* 12, 1–13.

275. Goff, D. C., Tsai, G., Manoach, D. S., Flood, J., Darby, D. G., and Coyle, J. T. (1996). D-Cycloserine added to clozapine for patients with schizophrenia. *Am. J. Psychiatry* 153, 1628–1630.

276. Goff, D. C., Tsai, G., Levitt, J., Amico, E., Manoach, D., Schoenfeld, D. A., Hayden, D. L., McCarley, R., and Coyle, J. T. (1999). A placebo-controlled trial of D-cycloserine added to conventional neuroleptics in patients with schizophrenia. [see comments]. *Arch. Gen. Psychiatry* 56, 21–27.

277. Farber, N. B., Newcomer, J. W., and Olney, J. W. (1999). Glycine agonists: What can they teach us about schizophrenia? [letter; comment]. *Arch. Gen. Psychiatry* 56, 13–17.

278. Javitt, D. C. (2002). Glycine modulators in schizophrenia. *Curr. Opin. Investig. Drugs* 3, 1067–1072.

279. Coyle, J., and Tsai, G. (2004). The NMDA receptor glycine modulatory site: A therapeutic target for improving cognition and reducing negative symptoms in schizophrenia. *Psychopharmacology* 174, 32–38.

280. Javitt, D. C., Zylberman, I., Zukin, S. R., Heresco-Levy, U., and Lindenmayer, J. -P. (1994). Amelioration of negative symptoms in schizophrenia by glycine. *Am. J. Psychiatry* 151, 1234–1236.

281. Tsai, G., Yang, P., Chung, L., Lange, N., and Coyle, J. (1998). D-serine added to antipsychotics for the treatment of schizophrenia. *Biol. Psychiatry* 44, 1081–1089.

282. Heresco-Levy, U., Javitt, D., Ermilov, M., Mordel, C., Horowitz, A., and Kelly, D. (1996). Double-blind, placebo-controlled, crossover trial of glycine adjuvant therapy for treatment-resistant schizophrenia. *Br. J. Psychiatry* 169, 610–617.

283. Heresco-Levy, U., Javitt, D., Ermilov, M., Mordel, C., Silipo, G., and Lichtenstein, M. (1999). Efficacy of high-dose glycine in the treatment of enduring negative symptoms of schizophrenia. *Arch. Gen. Psychiatry* 56, 29–36.

284. Heresco-Levy, U., Ermilov, M., Lichtenberg, P., Bar, G., and Javitt, D. (2004). High-dose glycine added to olanzapine and risperidone for the treatment of schizophrenia. *Biol. Psychiatry* 55, 165–171.

285. Evins, A., Fitzgerald, S., Wine, L., Rosselli, R., and Goff, D. (2000). Placebo-controlled trial of glycine added to clozapine in schizophrenia. *Am. J. Psychiatry* 157, 826–828.

286. Goff, D., Henderson, D., Evins, A., and Amico, E. (1999). A placebo-controlled crossover trial of D-cycloserine added to clozapine in patients with schizophrenia. *Biol. Psychiatry* 45, 512–514.

287. Tsai, G., Yang, P., Chung, L., Tsai, I., Tsai, C., and Coyle, J. (1999). D-Serine added to clozapine for the treatment of schizophrenia. *Am. J. Psychiatry* 156, 1822–1825.

288. Duncan, E., Szilagyi, S., Schwartz, M., Bugarski-Kirola, D., Kunzova, A., Negi, S., Stephanides, M., Efferen, T., Angrist, B., Peselow, E., Corwin, J., Gonzenbach, S., and Rotrosen, J. (2004). Effects of D-cycloserine on negative symptoms in schizophrenia. *Schizophr. Res.* 71, 239–248.

289. van Berckel, B., Evenblij, C., van Loon, B., Maas, M., van der Geld, M., Wynne, H., van Ree, J., and Kahn, R. (1999). D-Cycloserine increases positive symptoms in chronic schizophrenic patients when administered in addition to antipsychotics: A double-blind, parallel, placebo-controlled study. *Neuropsychopharmacology* 21, 203–210.

290. Tuominen, H., Tiihonen, J., and Wahlbeck, K. (2005). Glutamatergic drugs for schizophrenia: A systematic review and meta-analysis. *Schizophr. Res.* 72, 225–234.

291. Kim, K., Kingsmore, S., Han, H., Yang-Feng, T., Godinot, N., Seldin, M., Caron, M., and Giros, B. (1994). Cloning of the human glycine transporter type 1: Molecular and pharmacological characterization of novel isoform variants and chromosomal localization of the gene in the human and mouse genomes. *Mol. Pharmacol.* 45, 608–617.

292. Bergeron, R., Meyer, T., Coyle, J., and Greene, R. (1998). Modulation of N-methyl-D-aspartate receptor function by glycine transport. *Proc. Nat. Acad. Sci. USA* 95, 15730–15734.

293. Mothet, J., Parent, A., Wolosker, H., Brady, R. J., Linden, D., Ferris, C., Rogawski, M., and Snyder, S. (2000). D-serine is an endogenous ligand for the glycine site of the N-methyl-D-aspartate receptor. *Proc. Nat. Acad. Sci. USA* 97, 4926–4931.

294. Panizzutti, R., De Miranda, J., Ribeiro, C., Engelender, S., and Wolosker, H. (2001). A new strategy to decrease N-methyl-D-aspartate (NMDA) receptor co-activation: Inhibition of D-serine synthesis by converting serine racemase into an eliminase. *Proc. Nat. Acad. Sci. USA* 98, 5294–5299.

295. Sur, C., and Kinney, G. (2004). The therapeutic potential of glycine transporter-1 inhibitors. *Exp. Opin. Investig. Drugs* 13, 515–521.

296. Marino, M. J., and Conn, P. J. (2002). Direct and indirect modulation of the *N*-methyl-D-aspartate receptor. *Curr. Drug Target CNS Neurol. Disord.* 1, 1–16.

297. Moghaddam, B. (2004). Targeting metabotropic glutamate receptors for treatment of the cognitive symptoms of schizophrenia. *Psychopharmacology (Berl.)* 174, 39–44.

298. Henry, S. A., Lehmann-Masten, V., Gasparini, F., Geyer, M. A., and Markou, A. (2002). The mGluR5 antagonist MPEP, but not the mGluR2/3 agonist LY314582, augments PCP effects on prepulse inhibition and locomotor activity. *Neuropharmacology* 43, 1199–1209.

299. Kinney, G., Burno, M., Campbell, U., Hernandez, L., Rodriguez, D., Bristow, L., and Conn, P. (2003). Metabotropic glutamate subtype 5 receptors modulate locomotor activity and sensorimotor gating in rodents. *J. Pharmacol. Exper. Ther.* 306, 116–123.

300. Campbell, U., Lalwani, K., Hernandez, L., Kinney, G., Conn, P., and Bristow, L. (2004). The mGluR5 antagonist 2-methyl-6-(phenylethynyl)-pyridine (MPEP) potentiates PCP-induced cognitive deficits in rats. *Psychopharmacology (Berl.)* 175, 310–318.

301. Homayoun, H., Stefani, M. R., Adams, B. W., Tamagan, G. D., and Moghaddam, B. (2004). Functional interaction between NMDA and mGlu5 receptors: Effects on working memory, instrumental learning, motor behaviors, and dopamine release. *Neuropsychopharmacology* 29, 1259–1269.

302. Knoflach, F., Mutel, V., Jolidon, S., Kew, J. N., Malherbe, P., Vieira, E., Wichmann, J., and Kemp, J. A. (2001). Positive allosteric modulators of metabotropic glutamate 1 receptor: Characterization, mechanism of action, and binding site. *Proc. Nat. Acad. Sci. USA* 98, 13402–13407;erratum 98(26), 15393.

303. O'Brien, J. A., Lemaire, W., Chen, T. B., Chang, R. S., Jacobson, M. A., Ha, S. N., Lindsley, C. W., Schaffhauser, H. J., Sur, C., Pettibone, D. J., Conn, P. J., and Williams, D. L., Jr. (2003). A family of highly selective allosteric modulators of the metabotropic glutamate receptor subtype 5. *Mol. Pharmacol.* 64, 731–740.

304. Marino, M. J., Williams, D. L., O'Brien, J. A., Valenti, O., McDonald, T. P., Clements, M. K., Wang, R., DiLella, A. G., Hess, J. F., Kinney, G. G., and Conn, P. J. (2003). Allosteric modulation of group III metabotropic glutamate receptor 4: A potential approach to Parkinson's disease treatment. *Proc. Nat. Acad. Sci. USA* 100, 13668–13673.

305. Kinney, G., O'Brien, J., Lemaire, W., Burno, M., Bickel, D., Clements, M., Chen, T., Wisnoski, D., Lindsley, C., Tiller, P., Smith, S., Jacobson, M., Sur, C., Duggan, M., Pettibone, D., Conn, P., and Williams, D. (2004). A novel selective positive allosteric modulator of metabotropic glutamate receptor subtype 5 (mGluR5) has in vivo activity and antipsychotic-like effects in rat behavioral models. *J. Pharmacol. Exper. Ther.* 312, 199–206.

306. Lindsley, C., Wisnoski, D., Leister, W., O'brien, J., Lemaire, W., Williams, D. J., Burno, M., Sur, C., Kinney, G., Pettibone, D., Tiller, P., Smith, S., Duggan, M., Hartman, G., Conn, P., and Huff, J. (2004). Discovery of positive allosteric modulators for the metabotropic glutamate receptor subtype 5 from a series of *N*-(1,3-diphenyl-1*H*-pyrazol-5-yl)benzamides that potentiate receptor function in vivo. *J. Med. Chem.* 47, 5825–5828.

306a. Homayoun, H., and Moghaddam, B. (in press). Fine-tuning of awake prefrontal cortex neurons by clozapine: comparison to haloperidol and N-desmethylclozapine. *Biol. Psychiatry*.

307. Cartmell, J., Monn, J. A., and Schoepp, D. D. (1999). The metabotropic glutamate 2/3 receptor agonists LY354740 and LY379268 selectively attenuate phencyclidine versus d-amphetamine motor behaviors in rats. *J. Pharmacol. Exper. Ther.* 291, 161–170.

308. Moghaddam, B., Adams, B., Verma, A., and Daly, D. (1997). Activation of glutamatergic neurotransmission by ketamine: A novel step in the pathway from NMDA receptor blockade to dopaminergic and cognitive disruptions associated with the prefrontal cortex. *J. Neurosci.* 17, 2921–2927.

309. Krystal, J. H., Abi-Saab, W., Perry, E., D'Souza, D. C., Liu, N., Gueorguieva, R., McDougall, L., Hunsberger, T., Belger, A., Levine, L., and Breier, A. (2005). Preliminary evidence of attenuation of the disruptive effects of the NMDA glutamate receptor antagonist, ketamine, on working memory by pretreatment with the group II metabotropic glutamate receptor agonist, LY354740, in healthy human subjects. *Psychopharmacology (Berl.)* 179, 303–309.

310. Anand, A., Charney, D. S., Oren, D. A., Berman, R. M., Hu, X. S., Cappiello, A., and Krystal, J. H. (2000). Attenuation of the neuropsychiatric effects of ketamine with lamotrigine: Support for hyperglutamatergic effects of *N*-methyl-D-aspartate receptor antagonists. *Arch. Gen. Psychiatry* 57, 270–276.

311. Krystal, J. H., Anand, A., and Moghaddam, B. (2002). Effects of NMDA receptor antagonists: Implications for the pathophysiology of schizophrenia. *Arch. Gen. Psychiatry* 59, 663–664.

312. Tiihonen, J. H. T., Ryynanen, O. P., Repo-Tiihonen, E., Kotilainen, I., Eronen, M., Toivonen, P., Wahlbeck, K., and Putkonen, A. (2003). Lamotrigine in treatment-resistant schizophrenia: A randomized placebo-controlled crossover trial. *Biol. Psychiatry* 54, 1241–1248.

313. Kremer, I., Vass, A., Gorelik, I., Bar, G., Blanaru, M., Javitt, D., and Heresco-Levy, U. (2003). Placebo-controlled trial of lamotrigine added to conventional and atypical antipsychotics in schizophrenia. *Biol. Psychiatry* 56, 441–446.

314. Kolivakis, T., Beauclair, L., Margolese, H., and Chouinard, G. (2004). Long-term lamotrigine adjunctive to antipsychotic monotherapy in schizophrenia: Further evidence. *Can. J. Psychiatry* 49, 280–281.

315. Staubli, U., Rogers, G., and Lynch, G. (1994). Facilitation of glutamate receptors enhances memory. *Proc. Nat. Acad. Sci. USA* 91, 777–781.

316. Larson, J., Lieu, T., Petchpradub, V., LeDuc, B., Ngo, H., Rogers, G., and Lynch, G. (1995). Facilitation of olfactory learning by a modulator of AMPA receptors. *J. Neurosci.* 15, 8023–8030.

317. Hampson, R., Rogers, G., Lynch, G., and Deadwyler, S. (1998). Facilitative effects of the ampakine CX516 on short-term memory in rats: Correlations with hippocampal neuronal activity. *J. Neurosci.* 18, 2748–2763.

318. Hampson, R., Rogers, G., Lynch, G., and Deadwyler, S. (1998). Facilitative effects of the ampakine CX516 on short-term memory in rats: Enhancement of delayed-nonmatch-to-sample performance. *J. Neurosci.* 18, 2740–2747.

319. Goff, D., Leahy, L., Berman, I., Posever, T., Herz, L., Leon, A., Johnson, S., and Lynch, G. (2001). A placebo-controlled pilot study of the ampakine CX516 added to clozapine in schizophrenia. *J. Clin. Psychopharmacol.* 21, 484–487.

320. Johnson, S., Luu, N., Herbst, T., Knapp, R., Lutz, D., Arai, A., Rogers, G., and Lynch, G. (1999). Synergistic interactions between ampakines and antipsychotic drugs. *J. Pharmacol. Exper. Ther.* 289, 392–397.

321. Marenco, S., Egan, M., Goldberg, T., Knable, M., McClure, R., Winterer, G., and Weinberger, D. (2002). Preliminary experience with an ampakine (CX516) as a single agent for the treatment of schizophrenia: A case series. *Schizophr. Res.* 57, 221–226.

322. Doherty, J., Simonovic, M., So, R., and Meltzer, H. (1980). The effect of phencyclidine on dopamine synthesis and metabolism in rat striatum. *Eur. J. Pharmacol.* 65, 139–149.

323. Deutch, A. Y., Tam, S. -Y., Freeman, A. S., Bowers, M. B.Jr., and Roth, R. H. (1987). Mesolimbic and mesocortical dopamine activation induced by phencyclidine: Contrasting pattern to striatal response. *Eur. J. Pharmacol.* 134, 257–264.

324. Carboni, E., Imperato, A., Perezzani, L., and Di Chiara, G. (1989). Amphetamine, cocaine, phencyclidine and nomifensine increase extracellular dopamine concentrations preferentially in the nucleus accumbens of freely moving rats. *Neuroscience* 28, 653–661.

325. Kornhuber, J. (1990). Glutamate and schizophrenia. *Trends Pharmacol. Sci.* 11, 357–359.

326. Carlsson, A. (1988). The current status of the dopamine hypothesis of schizophrenia. *Neuropsychopharmacology* 1, 179–186.

327. Adams, B., and Moghaddam, B. (1998). Corticolimbic dopamine neurotransmission is temporally dissociated from the cognitive and locomotor effects of phencyclidine. *J. Neurosci.* 18, 5545–5554.

328. Adams, B. W., Bradberry, C. W., and Moghaddam, B. (2002). NMDA antagonist effects on striatal dopamine release: Microdialysis studies in awake monkeys. *Synapse* 43, 12–18.

329. Kegeles, L., Martinez, D., Kochan, L., Hwang, D., Huang, Y., Mawlawi, O., Suckow, R., Van Heertum, R., and Laruelle, M. (2002). NMDA antagonist effects on striatal dopamine release: Positron emission tomography studies in humans. *Synapse* 43, 19–29.

330. Aalto, S., Hirvonen, J., Kajander, J., Scheinin, H., Nagren, K., Vilkman, H., Gustafsson, L., Syvalahti, E., and Hietala, J. (2002). Ketamine does not decrease striatal dopamine D2 receptor binding in man. *Psychopharmacology* 164, 401–406.

331. Carlsson, M., and Carlsson, A. (1989). The NMDA antagonist MK-801 causes marked locomotor stimulation in monamine-depleted mice. *J. Neural Transmiss.* 75, 221–226.

332. Lewis, D., and Levitt, P. (2002). Schizophrenia as a disorder of neurodevelopment. *Annu. Rev. Neurosci.* 25, 409–432.

333. Murase, S., Grenhoff, J., Chouvet, G., Gonon, F., and Svensson, T. (1993). Prefrontal cortex regulates burst firing and transmitter release in rat mesolimbic dopamine neurons studied in vivo. *Neurosci. Lett.* 157, 53–56.

334. Taber, M., and Fibiger, H. (1995). Electrical stimulation of the prefrontal cortex increases dopamine release in the nucleus accumbens of the rat: Modulation by metabotropic glutamate receptors. *J. Neurosci.* 15, 3896–3904.

335. Carr, D., and Sesack, S. (2000). Projections from the rat prefrontal cortex to the ventral tegmental area: Target specificity in the synaptic associations with mesoaccumbens and mesocortical neurons. *J. Neurosci.* 20, 3864–3873.

336. Jackson, M. E., Frost, A., and Moghaddam, B. (2001). Stimulation of prefrontal cortex at physiologically relevant frequencies inhibits dopamine release in the nucleus accumbens. *J. Neurochem.* 78, 920–923.

337. Sesack, S., and Carr, D. (2002). Selective prefrontal cortex inputs to dopamine cells: Implications for schizophrenia. *Physiol. Behav.* 77, 513–517.

338. Jackson, M., Homayoun, H., and Moghaddam, B. (2004). NMDA receptor hypofunction produces concomitant firing rate potentiation and burst activity reduction in the prefrontal cortex. *Proc. Nat. Acad. Sci. USA* 101, 6391–6396.

339. Kornhuber, J., and Kornhuber, M. (1986). Presynaptic dopaminergic modulation of cortical input to the striatum. *Life Sci.* 39, 699–674.

340. Maura, G., Giardi, A., and Raiteri, M. (1988). Release-regulating D-2 dopamine receptors are located on striatal glutamatergic nerve terminals. *J. Pharmacol. Exper. Ther.* 247, 680–684.

341. Yang, C., Seamand, J., and Gorelova, N. (1999). Developing a neuronal model for the pathophysiology of schizophrenia based on the nature of electrophysiological actions of dopamine in the prefrontal cortex. *Neuropsychopharmacology* 21, 161–194.

342. Carlsson, A., Waters, N., Holm-Waters, S., Tedroff, J., Nilsson, M., and Carlsson, M. (2001). Interactions between monoamines, glutamate, and GABA in schizophrenia: New evidence. *Annu. Rev. Pharmacol. Toxicol.* 41, 237–260.

343. Wang, Y., and Goldman-Rakic, P. (2004). D2 receptor regulation of synaptic burst firing in prefrontal cortical pyramidal neurons. *Proc. Nat. Acad. Sci. USA* 101, 5093–5098.

344. Tseng, K., and O'Donnell, P. (2004). Dopamine-glutamate interactions controlling prefrontal cortical pyramidal cell excitability involve multiple signaling mechanisms. *J. Neurosci.* 24, 5131–5139.

345. Lavin, A., and Grace, A. (2001). Stimulation of D1-type dopamine receptors enhances excitability in prefrontal cortical pyramidal neurons in a state-dependent manner. *Neuroscience* 104, 335–346.

346. Harte, M., and O'Connor, W. (2004). Evidence for a differential medial prefrontal dopamine D1 and D2 receptor regulation of local and ventral tegmental glutamate and GABA release: A dual probe microdialysis study in the awake rat. *Brain Res.* 1017, 120–129.

347. Kalivas, P., and Duffy, P. (1997). Dopamine regulation of extracellular glutamate in the nucleus accumbens. *Brain Res.* 761, 173–177.

348. Arvanov, V., Liang, X., Schwartz, J., Grossman, S., and Wang, R. (1997). Clozapine and haloperidol modulate N-methyl-D-aspartate- and non-N-methyl-D-aspartate receptor-mediated neurotransmission in rat prefrontal cortical neurons in vitro. *J. Pharmacol. Exper. Ther.* 283, 226–234.

349. Wang, R. Y., and Liang, X. (1998). M100907 and clozapine, but not haloperidol or raclopride, prevent phencyclidine-induced blockade of NMDA responses in pyramidal neurons of the rat medial prefrontal cortical slice. *Neurosychopharmacology* 19, 74–85.

350. Ninan, I., Jardemark, K., and Wang, R. (2003). Differential effects of atypical and typical antipsychotic drugs on N-methyl-D-aspartate- and electrically evoked responses in the pyramidal cells of the rat medial prefrontal cortex. *Synapse* 48, 66–79.

351. Chen, L., and Yang, C. (2002). Interaction of dopamine D1 and NMDA receptors mediates acute clozapine potentiation of glutamate EPSPs in rat prefrontal cortex. *J. Neurophysiol.* 87, 2324–2336.

351a. Lecourtier, L., Homayoun, H., Tamagan, G., and Moghaddam, B. (in press). Positive allosteric modulation of metabotropic glutamate 5 (mGlu5) receptors reverses MK801-induced alteration of neuronal firing in prefrontal cortex. Implications for the treatment of schizophrenia. *Biol. Psychiatry*.

352. Girault, J., and Greengard, P. (2004). The neurobiology of dopamine signaling. *Arch. Neurol.* 61, 641–644.

353. Kelley, A. (2004). Memory and addiction: Shared neural circuitry and molecular mechanisms. *Neuron* 44, 161–179.
354. Lewis, D. A. (2000). GABAergic local circuit neurons and prefrontal cortical dysfunction in schizophrenia. *Brain Res. Brain Res. Rev.* 31, 270–276.
355. Benes, F., and Berretta, S. (2001). GABAergic interneurons: Implications for understanding schizophrenia and bipolar disorder. *Neuropsychopharmacology* 25, 1–27.
356. Greene, R. (2001). Circuit analysis of NMDAR hypofunction in the hippocampus, in vitro, and psychosis of schizophrenia. *Hippocampus* 11, 569–577.

9

MOLECULAR GENETICS OF SCHIZOPHRENIA

LIAM CARROLL, MICHAEL C. O'DONOVAN, AND MICHAEL J. OWEN
Wales College of Medicine, Cardiff University, Cardiff, Wales, United Kingdom

9.1	Genetic Epidemiology	321
	9.1.1 Defining Phenotype for Genetic Research	322
	9.1.2 Are There Clues for Genetics from Epidemiology, Pathophysiology, and Neurobiology?	323
9.2	Molecular Genetic Studies	323
	9.2.1 Linkage Studies	323
	9.2.2 Positional Candidate Genetics	325
9.3	Candidate Genes	325
	9.3.1 Dystrobrevin Binding Protein 1 (DTNBP1)	325
	9.3.2 Neuregulin 1	326
	9.3.3 D-Amino Acid Oxidase (*DAO*) and D-Amino Acid Oxidase Activator (*DAOA*)	327
	9.3.4 Regulator of G-Protein Signaling 4	328
	9.3.5 Others	328
9.4	Chromosomal Abnormalities	328
	9.4.1 Catechol-*O*-Methyltransferase (*COMT*)	328
	9.4.2 PRODH	329
	9.4.3 ZDHHC8	330
	9.4.4 DISC1	330
9.5	Functional Candidate Genes	331
9.6	Functional Implications of Susceptibility Genes	332
9.7	Conclusions	333
	References	333

9.1 GENETIC EPIDEMIOLOGY

The results of numerous family, twin, and adoption studies show conclusively that risk of schizophrenia is increased among the relatives of affected individuals and that

---

Handbook of Contemporary Neuropharmacology, Edited by David R. Sibley, Israel Hanin, Michael Kuhar, and Phil Skolnick. Copyright © 2007 John Wiley & Sons, Inc.

is the result largely of genes rather than shared environment [1–3]. In the children and siblings of individuals with schizophrenia, the increase in risk is around 10-fold and somewhat less than this in parents. The latter finding is probably explained by a reduction in the reproductive opportunities, drive, and possibly fertility of affected individuals. Five recent systematically ascertained studies report monozygotic (MZ) concordance estimated at 41–65% compared with dizygotic (DZ) concordance of 0–28% and an estimate of broad heritability of 85% [4]. The heritability of schizophrenia is one of the highest for any complex genetic disorder. To place it in perspective, it is similar to that of type 1 diabetes (72–88% [5, 6]) but greater than breast cancer (30% [7]), coronary heart disease in males (57% [8]), and type II diabetes (26% [9]).

While the twin and adoption literature leaves little doubt that genes are important, they also point to the importance of environmental factors since the concordance for schizophrenia in MZ twins is typically around 50% and heritability estimates are less than 100%. Moreover, we should also note that risks resulting from gene–environment interactions tend to be attributed to genes in most genetic epidemiological studies.

Genetic epidemiology also tells us that, like other common disorders, schizophrenia has a mode of transmission that is complex and includes the multiple-susceptibility-loci model [10, 11]. However, the number of loci, the risk conferred by each, and the degree of interaction between them remain unknown. Risch [12] has calculated that the data are incompatible with the existence of a single locus conferring a sibling relative risk (λ_s) of more than 3 and, unless extreme epistasis (gene–gene interaction) exists, models with two or three loci of $\lambda_s \leqslant 2$ are more plausible. It should be emphasized that these calculations are based upon the assumption of homogeneity and refer to populationwide λ_s. It is quite possible that alleles of larger effect are operating in some groups of patients, for example families with a high density of illness. However, high-density families are expected to occur by chance even under polygenic inheritance, and their existence does not prove the existence of disease alleles of large effect [11].

9.1.1 Defining Phenotype for Genetic Research

Schizophrenia displays considerable heterogeneity of symptoms, course, and outcome (see Chapter 7). It is possible that this reflects etiological heterogeneity, although if etiologically distinct subgroups do exist, we cannot yet identify them. In spite of this, structured and semistructured interviews together with explicit operational diagnostic criteria permit reliable diagnosis of a syndrome with high heritability. It should then in principle be possible to subject schizophrenia to molecular genetic analysis.

One way of refining the phenotype for genetic studies of complex traits is to define intermediate phenotypes or endophenotypes, that is, traits that are intermediate between susceptibility genes and the clinical phenotype. A number of endophenotypes for schizophrenia have been proposed based upon electrophysiology, pharmacology, psychology, or neuroimaging. Such traits are likely to be essential for understanding how variation in a proven susceptibility gene leads to the clinical phenotype. However, the use of endophenotypes for the identification of disease genes requires that the measures in question are trait, rather than state, variables and compelling evidence from genetic epidemiology that they reflect genetic vulnerability to that disease rather than environmental factors. Promising data are accumulating for some potential endophenotypes for schizophrenia [13], but, in most cases, uncertainties remain.

The situation is further complicated by the fact that we are unable to define the limits of the clinical phenotype to which genetic liability can lead. It clearly extends beyond the core diagnosis of schizophrenia to include a spectrum of disorders, including schizoaffective disorder and schizotypal personality disorder [14, 15]. However, the limits of this spectrum and its relationship to other psychotic disorders, especially bipolar disorder, remain uncertain [16, 17]. Based upon the way the field is progressing, it seems likely that one of the earliest benefits of the identification of susceptibility genes is that the validity of current nosological categories can be further explored. Knowing the genes involved should allow us to dissect the current concept of schizophrenia and help us to understand its relationship to other diagnostic groups.

9.1.2 Are There Clues for Genetics from Epidemiology, Pathophysiology, and Neurobiology?

Epidemiological, pharmacological, and neurobiological studies have made some progress in our general understanding of schizophrenia (see other chapters in this section). The more specific hypotheses based upon abnormalities in neurotransmission, especially dopaminergic and glutaminergic, are very possibly relevant to some of the overt clinical manifestations of the disorder, but with few exceptions, molecular genetic studies predicated on these hypotheses have met with disappointing results. Moreover, many of the leading hypotheses involve rather vague concepts such as neurodevelopment, synaptic dysfunction, and aberrant neuronal connectivity. These concepts are so broad that it is difficult to use them to confidently implicate specific pathophysiological processes or to specify compelling candidate genes. These problems with hypothesis-based approaches have encouraged a number of groups to apply so-called positional genetic approaches for the simple reason that these do not depend upon knowledge of disease pathophysiology.

9.2 MOLECULAR GENETIC STUDIES

9.2.1 Linkage Studies

In contrast with several other common disorders like breast cancer, Alzheimer's disease, Parkinson's disease, and epilepsy, no genetically simple subtypes of schizophrenia have yet been discovered. The results of linkage studies in schizophrenia have often seemed to be disappointing, with positive studies usually falling short of stringent "genomewide" levels of significance and abundant failures to replicate. This is probably attributable to a combination of small genetic effects, inadequate sample sizes, and heterogeneity of causative loci between and within populations [18]. However, as more than 20 genomewide studies have been reported, and sample sizes increased, some consistent patterns have emerged. Linkages that reached genomewide significance on their own according to the criteria set forth by Lander and Kruglyak [19] or those that have received strong support from more than one sample are shown in Figure 9.1.

Recently, two meta-analyses of schizophrenia linkage have been reported. Each used different methods and obtained overlapping but somewhat different results. The study of Badner and Gershon [20] supported the existence of susceptibility genes on chromosomes 8p, 13q, and 22q, while that of Lewis et al. [21] most strongly favored 2q. The latter study also found that the number of loci meeting the aggregate criteria for significance was much greater than expected by chance ($p < 0.001$), with evidence for susceptibility genes on chromosomes 5q, 3p, 11q, 6p, 1q, 22q, 8p, 20q, and 14p.

The linkage data therefore support the predictions made by Risch [12] on the basis of genetic epidemiological findings; that is, the evidence is consistent with the existence of multiple susceptibility alleles of moderate effect. Nevertheless, it is also possible that loci of larger effect exist in specific samples of large multiply affected families. Of course, the proof that a positive linkage is correct comes when the disease gene has been identified. Happily, recent years have finally seen a number of breakthroughs in post-linkage positional cloning.

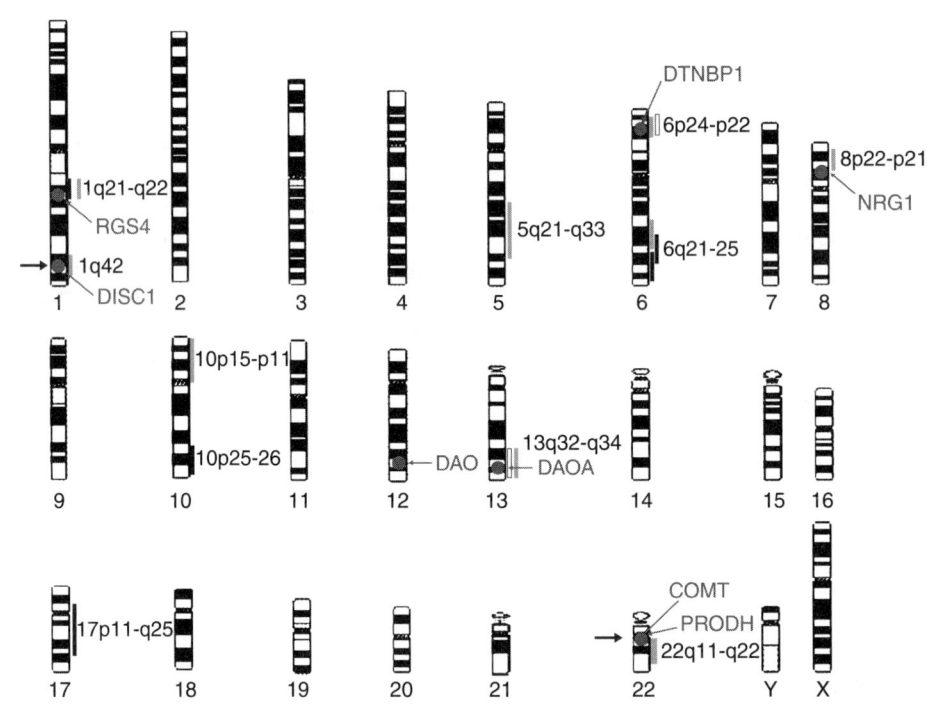

Figure 9.1 Ideogram showing chromosomal regions of linkage to schizophrenia and candidate genes that may be associated. Vertical bars denote regions where evidence for linkage has been found in more than one study (green) and where linkage has reached genomewide significance (red) according to the criteria of Lander and Kruglyak [19]. Arrows (red) identify regions where chromosomal abnormalities are involved with schizophrenia. The chromosomal positions of the major candidate genes discussed in this chapter are also displayed. (See color insert.)

9.2.2 Positional Candidate Genetics

Previously, the economics and practicalities of hunting a susceptibility gene within a linked chromosomal region dictated that one should have virtually definitive evidence that the linkage was a true positive. With recent improvements in our knowledge of genome anatomy and in genome analysis technology, the task of positional cloning has been transformed and favors bolder endeavors. These considerations, together with the convergence of some positive linkage findings, have led to a number of detailed mapping studies of linked regions which have in turn implicated specific genes. However, the quality of the data has been variable and a number of putative susceptibility genes have yet to be clearly replicated. Here, we focus on the genes where, at the time of writing, there are published follow-up studies or where we are aware of data that allow judgment about whether the gene is likely to be a true positive. In making these judgments, we have primarily been influenced by the strength of the genetic evidence for association to the clinical phenotype. We have given no weight to claims that a SNP (single-nucleotide polymorphism) is functional or that the gene has plausibility by virtue of patterns of expression or participation in relevant pathophysiological pathways. These are key properties of true susceptibility variants, but the number of SNPs in genes that meet the above criteria is so vast that such evidence cannot be used to prop up weak genetic findings. We have also given little weight to associations with putative endophenotypes, be they based on electrophysiology, pharmacology, psychology, or neuroimaging or performed in humans or modeled in animals. Such studies are likely to be essential for understanding how variation in a proven susceptibility gene leads to the clinical phenotype. However, for the de novo identification of disease genes, unless it is known with a very high degree of confidence that an endophenotype in question does actually index genetic risk for disorder, a considerable amount of uncertainty inevitably must accompany its use.

9.3 CANDIDATE GENES

9.3.1 Dystrobrevin Binding Protein 1 (DTNBP1)

Chromosome 6p22.3 is one of the most consistently reported linkage regions for schizophrenia (Fig. 9.1). After detailed studies designed to follow up their original findings of linkage in Irish pedigrees, Straub and colleagues [22] reported evidence for genetic association between schizophrenia and markers in the *DTNBP1* or dysbindin gene which maps to this region. Significant associations to markers and haplotypes have subsequently been found by several other research groups in independent populations of schizophrenics (e.g., [23–29]) which have included samples that do not show significant linkage to the 6p region. Although not unexpectedly there have also been some samples in association has not been found [9, 26, 30], the evidence now strongly favors *DTNBP1* as a susceptibility gene for schizophrenia and possibly a more general psychotic phenotype [32]. However, the associated haplotypes have differed between studies, suggesting possible allelic heterogeneity or, alternatively, population differences in the linkage disequilibrium structure across the gene [23].

As yet, no causative variant has been identified, and the absence of associated nonsynonymous alleles after systematic mutation detection of the exons [25] suggests that disease susceptibility depends upon variation affecting messenger RNA (mRNA) expression or processing. The latter possibility is *directly* supported by evidence for as-yet-unknown cis-acting alleles affecting *DTNBP1* expression in the human brain [33] that may reside upon haplotypes reported to be overrepresented in schizophrenics [37] and also by two recent studies showing reduced levels of expression of the mRNA [34] and protein [35] in post-mortem brain samples from patients with schizophrenia. This hypothesis needs to be tested by studying the relationship between the various associated haplotypes and RNA abundance, but identification of the risk variant, or variants, will require high-resolution work, including the identification and analysis of all polymorphisms across *DTNBP1*, possibly in multiple populations.

Dysbindin binds both α- and β-dystrobrevin, which are components of the dystrophin glycoprotein complex. The dystrophin complex is found in the sarcolemma of muscle but is also located in postsynaptic densities in a number of brain areas, particularly mossy fiber synaptic terminals in the cerebellum and hippocampus. Its location initially suggested that variation in *DTNBP1* might confer risk of schizophrenia by mediating effects on *postsynaptic* structure and function [22]. However, dysbindin has been shown to be part of a complex that influences the activity of presynaptic intracellular vesicles [36]. Talbot and colleagues [35] have recently shown that the presynaptic dystrobrevin-independent fraction of dysbindin is reduced in schizophrenic brain within certain intrinsic glutamatergic neurons of the hippocampus. Talbot and colleagues also observed that in schizophrenic brain reduced dysbindin expression was associated with increased expression of the vesicular glutamate transporter type 1. Taken together with the further observation that reduction in *DTNBP1* expression [27] is associated with reduced glutamate release in vitro, the findings so far are compatible with the hypothesis that *DTNBP1* might confer risk by altering presynaptic glutamate function.

9.3.2 Neuregulin 1

Neuregulin (*NRG1*) was first implicated in schizophrenia in an Icelandic sample [38]. Association analysis across a schizophrenia linkage region on 8p21–22 revealed highly significant evidence for association between schizophrenia and a multimarker haplotype at the 5′ end of *NRG1*. Strong evidence for association with the same at-risk haplotype was subsequently found in a large sample from Scotland [39] and weakly replicated in a U.K. sample [40]. Further positive findings have emerged from Irish [41], Bulgarian (Kirov et al., unpublished), Chinese [30, 42–44], and South African [30] samples that largely implicate the 5′ region of the gene. However, some negative findings have also been reported [30, 45–47], notably in Irish, Japanese, U.S. and South African populations. Only the two deCODE studies and our own U.K. study have implicated the specific Icelandic haplotype, perhaps reflecting differences in the LD (linkage disequilibrium) structure across *NRG1* in European and Asian samples (e.g., [44]) and emphasizing the fact that the associated variants, even if true positives, are not the causative ones.

Despite detailed resequencing [38], it has not yet proven possible to identify specific susceptibility variants, but the Icelandic haplotype points to the 5′ end of the gene, once again suggesting that altered expression or perhaps mRNA splicing might be involved. It is even formally possible at this stage that *NRG1* is not itself the susceptibility gene, as intron 1 contains another expressed sequence [41] whose function is unknown. However, insofar as it is possible to model schizophrenia in animals, behavioral analyses of *NRG1* hypomorphic mice support the view that the association is related to altered *NRG1* function or expression [48]. More direct evidence suggesting that altered expression, and in particular altered expression of the ratios of different *NRG1* transcripts, might be involved in the pathogenesis of schizophrenia is also beginning to accumulate [49].

Just as for *DTNBP1*, the pathological pathways by which altered *NRG1* function might lead to schizophrenia are unclear. *NRG1* encodes many mRNA species, which in turn translate into numerous proteins with multifarious functions. At the time it was implicated as a susceptibility gene for schizophrenia, it was thought to encode around 15 proteins with a diverse range of functions in the brain, including cell–cell signaling, ErbB receptor interactions, axon guidance, synaptogenesis, glial differentiation, myelination, and glutamatergic neurotransmission [50]. Any, or perhaps a combination of several of these, could be involved. Moreover, to further complicate matters, a number of novel exons that encode novel *NRG1* isoforms whose functions are currently unknown have recently been identified [51].

9.3.3 D-Amino Acid Oxidase (*DAO*) and D-Amino Acid Oxidase Activator (*DAOA*)

Chumakov and colleagues [52] undertook association mapping in the schizophrenia linkage region on chromosome 13q22–34. They found evidence for association to markers around two novel genes they termed *G72* and *G30* in French Canadian and Russian populations. *G72* and *G30* are overlapping but transcribed in opposite directions. Little is known of *G30* other than that it is transcribed in the brain. *G72* is a primate-specific gene expressed in the caudate and amygdala. Using yeast two-hybrid analysis, Chumakov and colleagues reported evidence for physical interaction between *G72* and *DAO*. *DAO* is expressed in human brain where it oxidizes D-serine, a potent activator of NMDA glutamate receptors. Coincubation of *G72* and *DAO* in vitro revealed a functional interaction between the two, with *G72* enhancing the activity of *DAO*, and consequently, *G72* has now been named *DAOA*. In the same study, *DAO* polymorphisms were shown to be associated with schizophrenia in the Canadian sample only, and analysis of *DAOA* and *DAO* variants revealed modest evidence for a statistical interaction between the loci and disease risk. Given the three levels of interaction, the authors concluded that both genes influence risk of schizophrenia through a similar pathway and that this effect is likely to be mediated through altered NMDA (*N*-methyl-D-aspartate) receptor function.

Associations between *DAOA* and schizophrenia have subsequently been reported in samples from Germany [53], China [54, 55], and both the United States and South Africa [30] and in Askenazi Jews [56] and a small sample of very early onset psychosis subjects from the United States [57]. As before, and conceivably for similar reasons, there is no consensus concerning the specific risk alleles or haplotypes across studies. At present, the published genetic evidence in support of both of these genes is weaker than for *DTNBP1* and *NRG1* and stronger for *DAOA* than *DAO*; indeed, so far, only a German group [53] has reported (weak) evidence in favor of *DAO*. Nevertheless further research is clearly required given reports of association of *DAOA* with bipolar disorder and psychosis [57, 58] suggesting that the gene might be a susceptibility locus for some aspect of psychopathology that is present in both schizophrenia and bipolar disorder.

9.3.4 Regulator of G-Protein Signaling 4

RGS4 maps to a putative linkage region on chromosome 1q22, but it was targeted for genetic analysis [59] following a microarray-based gene expression study in which decreased *RGS4* expression was found in schizophrenic postmortem brain [60]. Evidence for association between schizophrenia and haplotypes at the 5' end of the gene was found in two samples from the United States, and while not providing significant evidence alone, inclusion of a sample from India added to the overall level of support [59]. Analysis of a Brazilian sample has not provided support [61], but positive findings with both single markers and haplotypes have been reported in samples from the United Kingdom and Ireland [62–64]. The level of support for each has been modest and the pattern of association different between samples. Currently, our view is that the evidence for RGS4 is interesting but far from convincing, and the results of a meta-analysis being coordinated by the original group to which the present authors have contributed are now keenly awaited.

In terms of possible mechanisms of action, RGS4 is a negative regulator of G-protein-coupled receptors. The relationship between RGS molecules and receptor function is a promiscuous one, but of possible interest to schizophrenia is the evidence that RGS4 modulates activity at certain serotonergic [65] and metabotropic glutamatergic receptors [66], while its own expression is modulated by dopaminergic transmission [67]. Moreover, RGS4 interacts with ErbB3 [68], which may be of relevance as ErbB3 is a *neuregulin 1* receptor whose expression is downregulated in schizophrenic brains [50]. Interestingly, variation between *RGS4* has also recently been associated with reduction in dorsolateral prefrontal cortex gray matter volume [69], a finding of possible relevance given that reduction in prefrontal gray matter is well documented in schizophrenics (e.g., [70]).

9.3.5 Others

Association has been claimed between schizophrenia and *CAPON* (C-terminal PDZ domain ligand of neuronal nitric oxide synthase) [71], *PPP3CC* (protein phosphatase 3, catalytic subunit) [72], *TRAR4* (trace amine receptor 4) [73], and enthoprotin [74], which map respectively to putative linkage regions on 1q22, 8p21.3, 6q23.2, and 5q33. As discussed in the original articles, each of these genes can be plausibly related to candidate pathophysiologies of schizophrenia, but at the time of writing, we are not aware of any robust replication data to support these hypotheses, although *CAPON* has received some support in a Chinese sample [75].

9.4 CHROMOSOMAL ABNORMALITIES

9.4.1 Catechol-*O*-Methyltransferase (*COMT*)

There have been numerous reports of associations between schizophrenia and chromosomal abnormalities [76], but with two exceptions none provides convincing evidence for the location of a susceptibility gene. Several studies have shown that adults with 22q11 deletions have a high risk for schizophrenia [77–79], with the largest study of adult patients to date ($n = 50$) estimating this at 24% [79]. The deletion cannot account for a high proportion of schizophrenic cases [80], but reports of linkage to 22q11 [20, 21] suggest that variants in genes mapping to this region might contribute to more typical cases. Current candidates include *COMT*, proline dehydrogenase (*PRODH*), and zinc finger– and DHHC domain–containing protein 8 (*ZDHHC8*).

COMT has been intensively studied because of its key role in dopamine catabolism. Most studies have focused upon a valine-to-methionine change at codon 158 of the brain predominant membrane-bound form of COMT (MB-COMT) and codon 108 of the soluble form (S-COMT). The valine allele confers higher activity and thermal stability to COMT [81] and has been fairly consistently associated with reduced performance in tests of frontal lobe function [82, 83]. The results in schizophrenia have been mixed, with recent meta-analyses [84] reporting no overall evidence for association.

Since the preparation of the meta-analysis, an Israeli study of over 700 cases reported strong evidence for association between haplotypes, including the *val158* allele and two flanking, non coding SNPs [85]. As in an earlier study [86] the evidence from haplotypes was stronger than for the valine allele alone, suggesting that *COMT* may well be a susceptibility gene for schizophrenia but that the effect is not attributable to the *val/met* variant. We have been unable to replicate association with any of the SNPs or haplotypes, including the *val/met* polymorphism in a study of more than 2800 individuals, including almost 1200 schizophrenics [87], but two other groups [81, 88] have recently reported rather different haplotype associations at *COMT* in Irish and U.S. samples, respectively. As for the Israeli study, haplotypes carrying the *val158* allele exhibited stronger evidence for association than did that allele alone, while in the second study, the strongest findings included markers spanning the 3' end of the armadillo repeat deleted in the velocardiofacial syndrome gene (*ARVCF*). The latter has also been implicated in an earlier study [86] and its transcribed genomic sequence overlaps with *COMT* [89]. While the picture is confused, we consider that the evidence does not support a role for *val/met 158* in susceptibility to schizophrenia, although a small effect cannot be excluded, nor can a role in phenotype modification. However, it remains a strong possibility that variation elsewhere in *COMT*, or *ARVCF*, confers susceptibility.

9.4.2 PRODH

PRODH is another functional candidate gene given that a loss-of-function mutant mouse exhibits behavioral abnormalities in sensorimotor gating that are analogous to those observed in schizophrenics [90] and because proline dehydrogenase influences the availability of glutamate. Evidence in favor of association between SNPs in *PRODH* has been reported [91, 92], but arguing against this, we were unable to replicate either of these findings in large case-control and family-based association samples ([93] and G. Kirov et al., unpublished). Moreover, discrepancies in allele labeling between the two positive studies reduces, though does not abolish, the support provided to the former by the latter. One of the studies [91] also suggested association between a number of *PRODH* missense variants and schizophrenia while a separate study reported both heterozygous deletion of the entire *PRODH* gene in a family that included two schizophrenic subjects and missense variants in 3 of 63 schizophrenic patients studied [94]. However, we [93] and (in a follow-up of their own study [94]) Jacquet and colleagues [95] observed a range of missense mutations to be equally common in schizophrenic cases and controls, while *PRODH* deletions were reported not to be associated with schizophrenia in a very large sample of Japanese subjects [96]. Interestingly, while the study of Jacquet and colleagues [95] failed to provide evidence for their hypothesis of association between schizophrenia and hyperprolinemia (a consequence of loss-of-function *PRODH* mutations), they did find evidence for association between schizoaffective disorder and *PRODH*. Whether this is a chance finding or a finding of relevance to the discrepancies between existing data is at present unknown.

9.4.3 ZDHHC8

Finally, there is evidence that a SNP (rs175174) in *ZDHHC8*, a gene which encodes a putative transmembrane palmitoyl transferase, might directly confer susceptibility to schizophrenia by affecting the splicing of *ZDHHC8* mRNA [97]. Interestingly, association was only observed in females [97]. The genetic evidence was not strong but gained support from the observation of a similar sexual dimorphism in mice homozygous for a knockout of this gene, with females but not males, displaying the phenotypes modeling aspects of schizophrenia. Unfortunately, of the two published attempts at replication so far, one found the opposite allele to be associated in a Han Chinese sample and no evidence for a gender effect [98] and the other, in a relatively large Japanese case–control study, failed to find any association [99]. Recently in collaboration with colleagues in Bonn [100] we investigated rs175174 in four schizophrenia samples including a Bulgarian proband/parent sample (474 trios) and three case–control panels of European origin (1028 patients, 1253 controls). The results did not support the hypothesis that genetic variation at rs175174 is associated with increased risk for schizophrenia nor did they suggest the presence of gender-specific differences. Overall, the current evidence fails to support the hypothesis that SNP rs175174 in intron 4 of *ZDHHC8* directly influences susceptibility to schizophrenia. However, although unlikely in our opinion, it remains possible that susceptibility to schizophrenia is conferred by another genetic variant or variants in *ZDHHC8* that are in LD with rs175174 in the U.S. and South African samples studied by Mukai and colleagues [97] and the Han Chinese sample studied by Chen and colleagues [98] but not in the samples from Bulgaria, Germany, Poland, Sweden, and Japan [99, 100].

9.4.4 DISC1

The other major finding based upon a chromosomal abnormality comes from an extended pedigree in which a balanced chromosomal translocation (1;11)(q42;q14.3) showed strong evidence for linkage to a fairly broad phenotype consisting of schizophrenia, bipolar disorder, and recurrent depression [101]. The translocation was found to disrupt two genes on chromosome 1 which were on this basis called disrupted in schizophrenia 1 and 2 (*DISC1* and *DISC2* [101, 102]). No known genes mapped within the chromosome 11 disruption. *DISC2* contains no open reading frame and may regulate *DISC1* expression via antisense RNA [102]. Interestingly *DISC1* and *2* are located close to the chromosome 1 markers implicated in two Finnish linkage studies [103, 104] (Fig. 9.1). It has been suggested that truncation of *DISC1* in the translocation family might contribute to schizophrenia by affecting neuronal functions dependent upon intact cytoskeletal regulation such as neuronal migration, neurite architecture, and intracellular transport [105, 106]. While these are interesting hypotheses, it is important to remember that translocations can exert effects on genes other than those directly disrupted. For example, there are several mechanisms by which a translocation can influence the expression of neighboring genes. Thus, in order to unequivocally implicate *DISC1* and/or *2* in the pathogenesis of schizophrenia, it is necessary to identify in another population mutations or polymorphisms that are not in strong LD with neighboring genes but which are associated with schizophrenia. Four published studies have attempted to do this. Negative studies were reported by the Edinburgh group that originally identified *DISC1 and 2* [107] and by a group who focused on the 5' end of the gene in a large Japanese sample [108]. In contrast, positive findings have been reported in a large Finnish study [109] while haplotypic associations were found in U.S. samples with schizophrenia, schizoaffective disorder, and bipolar disorder [110]. At present, the genetic evidence in favor of *DISC1* as a susceptibility gene is gaining momentum but, in our view, is not yet compelling. Interestingly, if *DISC1* is a true susceptibility gene, it appears to confer risk for phenotypes including schizoaffective disorder, bipolar disorder, and major depression as well as schizophrenia [110]. Given the range of phenotypes associated with the translocation in the original study, despite its name, this should not be that surprising.

9.5 FUNCTIONAL CANDIDATE GENES

There is a huge schizophrenia candidate gene literature consisting of negative findings or positive findings that have either not been replicated or have seemed so unconvincing that there have been no attempts to do so. While most of the reported positives are unlikely to stand the test of time, neither can we conclude that any gene has been effectively excluded, given that most have not been studied exhaustively in large samples through a combination of detailed sequencing of exons, introns, and large regions of 5' and 3' flanking sequences combined with exhaustive genotyping. However, meta-analyses do at least suggest that the dopamine receptors *DRD3* [111] and *DRD2* [112] and the serotonergic receptor *HTR2A* [113] might confer risk. The effect sizes, if any, are extremely small [odds ratio (OR) < 1.2] and difficult to confirm, but if the associations are true, the findings provide some support for the view that altered dopaminergic and serotonergic function might be a primary event in schizophrenia susceptibility. If the putative associations are the result of LD between the assayed markers and the true susceptibility variant, it is possible that the latter might contribute somewhat more, depending upon the degree of LD between the two.

Despite the accumulating evidence for abnormalities of glutamatergic neurotransmission in schizophrenia, by and large, analysis of glutamatergic genes as functional candidates for schizophrenia has failed to produce consistent positive findings. However, recently claims have been made that variation in *GRM3* (the gene encoding metabotropic glutamate receptor type 3) might confer risk to schizophrenia. *GRM3* was first implicated in a case–control study of German patients. However, as only one SNP was significantly associated in one out of the three groups of patients studied [114], the authors concluded against a role for this gene in schizophrenia. Fujii and colleagues [115] genotyped six SNPs in a small case–control sample from

Japan. They found significant association with one SNP and a three-marker haplotype containing this SNP. Egan et al. [116] genotyped seven SNPs, including the two implicated in the previous reports, in a family based association study. Weak evidence for overtransmission to cases was observed for one SNP; however, this was not one of the SNPs implicated previously and the result failed to replicate in a second sample. A haplotype including this SNP was also overtransmitted to cases, but this finding has yet to be replicated. The authors presented further data relating the single putatively associated GRM3 SNP to cognitive, fMRI, MRS, and neurochemical variables. They argued that these data converge on the conclusion that *GRM3* affects prefrontal and hippocampal physiology, cognition, and risk for schizophrenia by altering glutamate neurotransmission. However, the genetic data implicating *GRM3* as a susceptibility gene for schizophrenia remain weak, although the findings of Egan and colleagues [116] clearly suggest that further study is warranted.

9.6 FUNCTIONAL IMPLICATIONS OF SUSCEPTIBILITY GENES

In our view the evidence now strongly implicates *DTNBP1* and *NRG1* as susceptibility genes for schizophrenia, while the data for *DAO, DAOA, DISC1,* and *RGS4* are promising but not yet compelling. Even in the most convincing cases, the risk haplotypes appear to be associated with small effect sizes [odds ratio (OR) < 2.5] and, although this is difficult to determine, do not appear to fully explain the linkage findings that prompted each study. This could suggest that the associated polymorphisms/haplotypes are only in weak LD with the true pathogenic variants, that the linkages reflect variation at more than one susceptibility site in the same gene (or in multiple genes in the area of linkage), or that in some cases, despite the statistical evidence, the associations are spurious. Work in this area highlights how difficult it can be to determine what comprises a clear replication of associations that are based on LD, especially those based upon associations with haplotypes rather than single markers [117]. It is by no means certain that support requires the same pattern of association to be obtained or, conversely, that a negative finding can be regarded as a failure to replicate only if the associated allele or haplotype from the original study is examined. Detailed follow-up studies, including de novo mutation detection and detailed genotyping in large samples drawn from different populations, with the aim of answering these questions are now required.

For most geneticists, the purpose of disease gene identification is to enhance our understanding of pathogenesis. Thus it is now important that we identify the specific mechanisms by which the recently implicated genes alter the risk of schizophrenia and the molecular and cognitive processes that link these primary events to psychopathology. Already, it has been noted that several of the genes encode proteins that potentially impact on the function of glutamatergic synapses which might therefore be the location of the primary abnormality [118–120]. The possible importance of synaptic abnormalities in schizophrenia had already been recognized [121] and the recent genetic data suggest that there might at last be convergence between the genetics of schizophrenia and its neurobiology. However, there are several reasons for remaining cautious. First, the genetic evidence is not yet definitive and we have not identified the specific pathogenic variants, much less the pathogenic mechanisms. Second, if we consider the two best-supported genes, *NRG1* encodes proteins with multiple functions of potential relevance to alternative hypotheses of schizophrenia, for example, aberrant myelination [50] while the function(s) of dysbindin are still obscure. Third, the widely held assumption that schizophrenia is a heterogeneous disorder with more that one core pathophysiology may well be correct. If this is so, then attempts to fit the data into a unified theory, while attractive and parsimonious, will ultimately prove futile. It is therefore vital that there is no letup in the hunt for novel schizophrenia genes, the finding of which will allow us to test existing and to generate novel hypotheses of pathogenesis.

9.7 CONCLUSIONS

Molecular genetic studies of schizophrenia are built upon the firm foundations of reliable diagnostic methodology and a wealth of genetic epidemiological data. The fact that most, if not all, disease genes apparently have only moderate or small effect sizes has proved challenging, as it has in the study of other common diseases. However, the sample and technological resources combined with the reagents generated by the Human Genome Project have begun to permit what appears finally to be genuine progress. A number of potential regions of linkage and two associated chromosomal abnormalities have been identified, and accumulating evidence favors several positional candidate genes, although in no case has the causative variant(s) been identified. These findings suggest that the positional genetic approach to schizophrenia is at last bearing fruit. As in most respects the task of positional cloning is becoming simpler, there are grounds for considerable optimism that genetics will continue to provide crucial insights into the aetiology of schizophrenia.

REFERENCES

1. Gottesman, I. I. (1991). *Schizophrenia Genesis*. W. H. Freeman, New York.
2. Kendler, K. S. (2000). Schizophrenia: Genetics. In *Kaplan and Sadock's Comprehensive Textbook of Psychiatry*, Vol. 1, 7th ed. B. J. Sadock and V. A. Sadock, Eds. Lippincott, Williams & Wilkins, Philadelphia, pp. 1147–1159.
3. McGuffin, P. O. M., O'Donovan, M. C., Thapar, A., and Gottesman, I. I. (1994). Schizophrenia. In *Seminars in Psychiatric Genetics*. Royal College of Psychiatrists, London, pp. 87–109.
4. Cardno, A. G., and Gottesman, I. I. (2000). Twin studies of schizophrenia: From bow-and-arrow concordances to star wars Mx and functional genomics. *Am. J. Med. Genet.* 97, 12–17.
5. Hyttinen, V., Kaprio, J., Kinnunen, L., Koskenvuo, M., and Tuomilehto, J. (2003). Genetic liability of type 1 diabetes and the onset age among 22,650 young Finnish twin pairs: A nationwide follow-up study. *Diabetes* 52, 1052–1055.
6. Kyvik, K. O., Green, A., and Beck-Nielsen, H. (1995). Concordance rates of insulin dependent diabetes mellitus: A population based study of young Danish twins. *BMJ* 91, 913–917.
7. Locatelli, I., Lichtenstein, P., and Yashin, A. I. (2004). The heritability of breast cancer: A Bayesian correlated frailty model applied to Swedish twins data. *Twin Res.* 7, 182–191.

8. Zdravkovic, S., Wienke, A., Pedersen, N. L., Marenberg, M. E., Yashin, A. I., and De Faire, U. (2002). Heritability of death from coronary heart disease: A 36-year follow-up of 20 966 Swedish twins. *J. Intern. Med.* 252, 247–254.
9. Poulsen, P., Kyvik, K. O., Vaag, A., and Beck-Nielsen, H. (1999). Heritability of type II (non-insulin-dependent) diabetes mellitus and abnormal glucose tolerance—a population-based twin study. *Diabetologia* 42, 139–145.
10. Gottesman, I. I., and Shields, J. (1967). A polygenic theory of schizophrenia. *Proc. Natl. Acad. Sci. USA* 58, 199–205.
11. McGue, M., and Gottesman, I. I., et al. (1989). A single dominant gene still cannot account for the transmission of schizophrenia. *Arch. Gen. Psychiatry* 46, 478–480.
12. Risch, N. (1990). Genetic linkage and complex diseases, with special reference to psychiatric disorders. *Genet. Epidemiol.* 7, 3–16; discussion 17–45.
13. Gottesman, I. I., and Gould, T. D. (2003). The endophenotype concept in psychiatry: Etymology and strategic intentions. *Am. J. Psychiatry* 160, 636–645.
14. Farmer, A. E., McGuffin, P., and Gottesman, I. I. (1987). Twin concordance for DSM-III schizophrenia. Scrutinizing the validity of the definition. *Arch. Gen. Psychiatry* 44, 634–641.
15. Kendler, K. S., Neale, M. C., and Walsh, D. (1995). Evaluating the spectrum concept of schizophrenia in the Roscommon Family Study. *Am. J. Psychiatry* 152, 749–754.
16. Kendler, K. S., Karkowski, L. M., and Walsh, D. (1998). The structure of psychosis: Latent class analysis of probands from the Roscommon Family Study. *Arch. Gen. Psychiatry* 55, 492–499.
17. Tienari, P., Wynne, L. C., Moring, J., Laksy, K., Nieminen, P., Sorri, A., Lahti, I., Wahlberg, K. E., Naarala, M., Kurki-Suonio, K., Saarento, O., Koistinen, P., Tarvainen, T., Hakko, H., and Miettunen, J. (2000). Finnish adoptive family study: Sample selection and adoptee DSM-III-R diagnoses. *Acta Psychiatr. Scand.* 101, 433–443.
18. Suarez, B. K., Hampe, C. L., and Van Erdewegh, P. (1994). Problems in replicating linkage claims in psychiatry. In *Genetic Approaches to Mental Disorders*. E. S. Gershon and C. R. Cloninger, Eds. American Psychiatric Press, Washington, DC, pp. 23–46.
19. Lander, E., and Kruglyak, L. (1995). Genetic dissection of complex traits: Guidelines for interpreting and reporting linkage results. *Nat. Genet.* 11, 241–247.
20. Badner, J. A., and Gershon, E. S. (2002). Meta-analysis of whole-genome linkage scans of bipolar disorder and schizophrenia. *Mol. Psychiatry* 7, 405–411.
21. Lewis, C. M., Levinson, D. F., Wise, L. H., DeLisi, L. E., Straub, R. E., Hovatta, I., Williams, N. M., Schwab, S. G., Pulver, A. E., Faraone, S. V., Brzustowicz, L. M., Kaufmann, C. A., Garver, D. L., Gurling, H. M., Lindholm, E., Coon, H., Moises, H. W., Byerley, W., Shaw, S. H., Mesen, A., Sherrington, R., O'Neill, F. A., Walsh, D., Kendler, K. S., Ekelund, J., Paunio, T., Lonnqvist, J., Peltonen, L., O'Donovan, M. C., Owen, M. J., Wildenauer, D. B., Maier, W., Nestadt, G., Blouin, J. L., Antonarakis, S. E., Mowry, B. J., Silverman, J. M., Crowe, R. R., Cloninger, C. R., Tsuang, M. T., Malaspina, D., Harkavy-Friedman, J. M., Svrakic, D. M., Bassett, A. S., Holcomb, J., Kalsi, G., McQuillin, A., Brynjolfson, J., Sigmundsson, T., Petursson, H., Jazin, E., Zoega, T., and Helgason, T. (2003). Genome scan meta-analysis of schizophrenia and bipolar disorder, part II: Schizophrenia. *Am. J. Hum. Genet.* 73, 34–48.
22. Straub, R. E., Jiang, Y., MacLean, C. J., Ma, Y., Webb, B. T., Myakishev, M. V., Harris-Kerr, C., Wormley, B., Sadek, H., Kadambi, B., Cesare, A. J., Gibberman, A., Wang, X., O'Neill, F. A., Walsh, D., and Kendler, K. S. (2002). Genetic variation in the 6p22.3 gene DTNBP1, the human ortholog of the mouse dysbindin gene, is associated with schizophrenia. *Am. J. Hum. Genet.* 71, 337–348.

23. Schwab, S. G., Knapp, M., Mondabon, S., Hallmayer, J., Borrmann-Hassenbach, M., Albus, M., Lerer, B., Rietschel, M., Trixler, M., Maier, W., and Wildenauer, D. B. (2003). Support for association of schizophrenia with genetic variation in the 6p22.3 gene, dysbindin, in sib-pair families with linkage and in an additional sample of triad families. *Am. J. Hum. Genet.* 72, 185–190.
24. Tang, J. X., Zhou, J., Fan, J. B., Li, X. W., Shi, Y. Y., Gu, N. F., Feng, G. Y., Xing, Y. L., Shi, J. G., and He, L. (2003). Family-based association study of DTNBP1 in 6p22.3 and schizophrenia. *Mol. Psychiatry* 8, 717–718.
25. Williams, N. M., Preece, A., Morris, D. W., Spurlock, G., Bray, N. J., Stephens, M., Norton, N., Williams, H., Clement, M., Dwyer, S., Curran, C., Wilkinson, J., Moskvina, V., Waddington, J. L., Gill, M., Corvin, A. P., Zammit, S., Kirov, G., Owen, M. J., and O'Donovan, M. C. (2004). Identification in 2 independent samples of a novel schizophrenia risk haplotype of the dystrobrevin binding protein gene (DTNBP1). *Arch. Gen. Psychiatry* 61, 336–344.
26. Van Den Bogaert, A., Schumacher, J., Schulze, T. G., Otte, A. C., Ohlraun, S., Kovalenko, S., Becker, T., Freudenberg, J., Jonsson, E. G., Mattila-Evenden, M., Sedvall, G. C., Czerski, P. M., Kapelski, P., Hauser, J., Maier, W., Rietschel, M., Propping, P., Nothen, M. M., and Cichon, S. (2003). The DTNBP1 (dysbindin) gene contributes to schizophrenia, depending on family history of the disease. *Am. J. Hum. Genet.* 73, 1438–1443.
27. Numakawa, T., Yagasaki, Y., Ishimoto, T., Okada, T., Suzuki, T., Iwata, N., Ozaki, N., Taguchi, T., Tatsumi, M., Kamijima, K., Straub, R. E., Weinberger, D. R., Kunugi, H., and Hashimoto, R. (2004). Evidence of novel neuronal functions of dysbindin, a susceptibility gene for schizophrenia. *Hum. Mol. Genet.* 13, 2699–2708.
28. Funke, B., Finn, C. T., Plocik, A. M., Lake, S., DeRosse, P., Kane, J. M., Kucherlapati, R., and Malhotra, A. K. (2004). Association of the DTNBP1 locus with schizophrenia in a U.S. population. *Am. J. Hum. Genet.* 75, 891–898.
29. Kirov, G., Ivanov, D., Williams, N. M., Preece, A., Nikolov, I., Milev, R., Koleva, S., Dimitrova, A., Toncheva, D., O'Donovan, M. C., and Owen, M. J. (2004). Strong evidence for association between the dystrobrevin binding protein 1 gene (DTNBP1) and schizophrenia in 488 parent-offspring trios from Bulgaria. *Biol. Psychiatry* 55, 971–975.
30. Hall, D., Gogos, J. A., and Karayiorgou, M. (2004). The contribution of three strong candidate schizophrenia susceptibility genes in demographically distinct populations. *Genes Brain Behav.* 3, 240–248.
31. Morris, D. W., McGhee, K. A., Schwaiger, S., Scully, P., Quinn, J., Meagher, D., Waddington, J. L., Gill, M., and Corvin, A. P. (2003). No evidence for association of the dysbindin gene [DTNBP1] with schizophrenia in an Irish population-based study. *Schizophr. Res.* 60, 167–172.
32. Raybould, R., Green, E. K., MacGregor, S., Gordon-Smith, K., Heron, J., Hyde, S., Caesar, S., Nikolov, I., Williams, N., Jones, L., O'Donovan, M. C., Owen, M. J., Jones, I., Kirov, G., and Craddock, N. (2005). Bipolar disorder and polymorphisms in the dysbindin gene (DTNBP1). *Biol. Psychiatry* 57, 696–701.
33. Bray, N. J., Buckland, P. R., Owen, M. J., and O'Donovan, M. C. (2003). Cis-acting variation in the expression of a high proportion of genes in human brain. *Hum. Genet.* 113, 149–153.
34. Weickert, C. S., Straub, R. E., McClintock, B. W., Matsumoto, M., Hashimoto, R., Hyde, T. M., Herman, M. M., Weinberger, D. R., and Kleinman, J. E. (2004). Human dysbindin (DTNBP1) gene expression in normal brain and in schizophrenic prefrontal cortex and midbrain. *Arch. Gen. Psychiatry* 61, 544–555.

35. Talbot, K., Eidem, W. L., Tinsley, C. L., Benson, M. A., Thompson, E. W., Smith, R. J., Hahn, C. G., Siegel, S. J., Trojanowski, J. Q., Gur, R. E., Blake, D. J., and Arnold, S. E. (2004). Dysbindin-1 is reduced in intrinsic, glutamatergic terminals of the hippocampal formation in schizophrenia. *J. Clin. Invest.* 113, 1353–1363.

36. Li, W., Zhang, Q., Oiso, N., Novak, E. K., Gautam, R., O'Brien, E. P., Tinsley, C. L., Blake, D. J., Spritz, R. A., Copeland, N. G., Jenkins, N. A., Amato, D., Roe, B. A., Starcevic, M., Dell'Angelica, E. C., Elliott, R. W., Mishra, V., Kingsmore, S. F., Paylor, R. E., and Swank, R. T. (2003). Hermansky-Pudlak syndrome type 7 (HPS-7) results from mutant dysbindin, a member of the biogenesis of lysosome-related organelles complex 1 (BLOC-1). *Nat. Genet.* 35, 84–89.

37. Bray, N. J., Preece, A., Williams, N. M., Moskvina, V., Buckland, P. R., Owen, M. J., and O'Donovan, M. C. (2005). Haplotypes at the dystrobrevin binding protein 1 (DTNBP1) gene locus mediate risk for schizophrenia through reduced DTNBP1 expression. *Hum. Mol. Genet.* 14, 1947–1954.

38. Stefansson, H., Sigurdsson, E., Steinthorsdottir, V., Bjornsdottir, S., Sigmundsson, T., Ghosh, S., Brynjolfsson, J., Gunnarsdottir, S., Ivarsson, O., Chou, T. T., Hjaltason, O., Birgisdottir, B., Jonsson, H., Gudnadottir, V. G., Gudmundsdottir, E., Bjornsson, A., Ingvarsson, B., Ingason, A., Sigfusson, S., Hardardottir, H., Harvey, R. P., Lai, D., Zhou, M., Brunner, D., Mutel, V., Gonzalo, A., Lemke, G., Sainz, J., Johannesson, G., Andresson, T., Gudbjartsson, D., Manolescu, A., Frigge, M. L., Gurney, M. E., Kong, A., Gulcher, J. R., Petursson, H., and Stefansson, K. (2002). Neuregulin 1 and susceptibility to schizophrenia. *Am. J. Hum. Genet.* 71, 877–892.

39. Stefansson, H., Sarginson, J., Kong, A., Yates, P., Steinthorsdottir, V., Gudfinnsson, E., Gunnarsdottir, S., Walker, N., Petursson, H., Crombie, C., Ingason, A., Gulcher, J. R., Stefansson, K., and St Clair, D. (2003). Association of neuregulin 1 with schizophrenia confirmed in a Scottish population. *Am. J. Hum. Genet.* 72, 83–87.

40. Williams, N. M., Preece, A., Spurlock, G., Norton, N., Williams, H. J., Zammit, S., O'Donovan, M. C., and Owen, M. J. (2003). Support for genetic variation in neuregulin 1 and susceptibility to schizophrenia. *Mol. Psychiatry* 8, 485–487.

41. Corvin, A. P., Morris, D. W., McGhee, K., Schwaiger, S., Scully, P., Quinn, J., Meagher, D., Clair, D. S., Waddington, J. L., and Gill, M. (2004). Confirmation and refinement of an "at-risk" haplotype for schizophrenia suggests the EST cluster, Hs.97362, as a potential susceptibility gene at the neuregulin-1 locus. *Mol. Psychiatry* 9, 208–213.

42. Yang, J. Z., Si, T. M., Ruan, Y., Ling, Y. S., Han, Y. H., Wang, X. L., Zhou, M., Zhang, H. Y., Kong, Q. M., Liu, C., Zhang, D. R., Yu, Y. Q., Liu, S. Z., Ju, G. Z., Shu, L., Ma, D. L., and Zhang, D. (2003). Association study of neuregulin 1 gene with schizophrenia. *Mol. Psychiatry* 8, 706–709.

43. Tang, J. X., Chen, W. Y., He, G., Zhou, J., Gu, N. F., Feng, G. Y., and He, L. (2004). Polymorphisms within 5' end of the neuregulin 1 gene are genetically associated with schizophrenia in the Chinese population. *Mol. Psychiatry* 9, 11–12.

44. Zhao, X., Shi, Y., Tang, J., Tang, R., Yu, L., Gu, N., Feng, G., Zhu, S., Liu, H., Xing, Y., Zhao, S., Sang, H., Guan, Y., St Clair, D., and He, L. (2004). A case control and family based association study of the neuregulin1 gene and schizophrenia. *J. Med. Genet.* 41, 9–34.

45. Iwata, N., Suzuki, T., Ikeda, M., Kitajima, T., Yamanouchi, Y., Inada, T., and Ozaki, N. (2004). No association with the neuregulin 1 haplotype to Japanese schizophrenia. *Mol. Psychiatry* 9, 126–127.

46. Thiselton, D. L., Webb, B. T., Neale, B. M., Ribble, R. C., O'Neill, F. A., Walsh, D., Riley, B. P., and Kendler, K. S. (2004). No evidence for linkage or association of

neuregulin-1 (NRG1) with disease in the Irish study of high-density schizophrenia families (ISHDSF). *Mol. Psychiatry* 9, 777–783; image 729.

47. Hong, C. J., Huo, S. J., Liao, D. L., Lee, K., Wu, J. Y., and Tsai, S. J. (2004). Case-control and family-based association studies between the neuregulin 1 (Arg38Gln) polymorphism and schizophrenia. *Neurosci. Lett.* 366, 158–161.

48. Stefansson, H., Steinthorsdottir, V., Thorgeirsson, T. E., Gulcher, J. R., and Stefansson, K. (2004). Neuregulin 1 and schizophrenia. *Ann. Med.* 36, 62–71.

49. Hashimoto, R., Straub, R. E., Weickert, C. S., Hyde, T. M., Kleinman, J. E., and Weinberger, D. R. (2004). Expression analysis of neuregulin-1 in the dorsolateral prefrontal cortex in schizophrenia. *Mol. Psychiatry* 9, 299–307.

50. Corfas, G., Roy, K., and Buxbaum, J. D. (2004). Neuregulin 1-erbB signaling and the molecular/cellular basis of schizophrenia. *Nat. Neurosci.* 7, 575–580.

51. Steinthorsdottir, V., Stefansson, H., Ghosh, S., Birgisdottir, B., Bjornsdottir, S., Fasquel, A. C., Olafsson, O., Stefansson, K., and Gulcher, J. R. (2004). Multiple novel transcription initiation sites for NRG1. *Gene* 342, 97–105.

52. Chumakov, I., Blumenfeld, M., Guerassimenko, O., Cavarec, L., Palicio, M., Abderrahim, H., Bougueleret, L., Barry, C., Tanaka, H., La Rosa, P., Puech, A., Tahri, N., Cohen-Akenine, A., Delabrosse, S., Lissarrague, S., Picard, F. P., Maurice, K., Essioux, L., Millasseau, P., Grel, P., Debailleul, V., Simon, A. M., Caterina, D., Dufaure, I., Malekzadeh, K., Belova, M., Luan, J. J., Bouillot, M., Sambucy, J. L., Primas, G., Saumier, M., Boubkiri, N., Martin-Saumier, S., Nasroune, M., Peixoto, H., Delaye, A., Pinchot, V., Bastucci, M., Guillou, S., Chevillon, M., Sainz-Fuertes, R., Meguenni, S., Aurich-Costa, J., Cherif, D., Gimalac, A., Van Duijn, C., Gauvreau, D., Ouellette, G., Fortier, I., Raelson, J., Sherbatich, T., Riazanskaia, N., Rogaev, E., Raeymaekers, P., Aerssens, J., Konings, F., Luyten, W., Macciardi, F., Sham, P. C., Straub, R. E., Weinberger, D. R., Cohen, N., and Cohen, D. (2002). Genetic and physiological data implicating the new human gene G72 and the gene for D-amino acid oxidase in schizophrenia. *Proc. Natl. Acad. Sci. USA* 99, 13675–13680.

53. Schumacher, J., Jamra, R. A., Freudenberg, J., Becker, T., Ohlraun, S., Otte, A. C., Tullius, M., Kovalenko, S., Bogaert, A. V., Maier, W., Rietschel, M., Propping, P., Nothen, M. M., and Cichon, S. (2004). Examination of G72 and D-amino-acid oxidase as genetic risk factors for schizophrenia and bipolar affective disorder. *Mol. Psychiatry* 9, 203–207.

54. Zou, F., Li, C., Duan, S., Zheng, Y., Gu, N., Feng, G., Xing, Y., Shi, J., and He, L. (2005). A family-based study of the association between the G72/G30 genes and schizophrenia in the Chinese population. *Schizophr. Res.* 73, 257–261.

55. Wang, X., He, G., Gu, N., Yang, J., Tang, J., Chen, Q., Liu, X., Shen, Y., Qian, X., Lin, W., Duan, Y., Feng, G., and He, L. (2004). Association of G72/G30 with schizophrenia in the Chinese population. *Biochem. Biophys. Res. Commun.* 99, 1281–1286.

56. Korostishevsky, M., Kaganovich, M., Cholostoy, A., Ashkenazi, M., Ratner, Y., Dahary, D., Bernstein, J., Bening-Abu-Shach, U., Ben-Asher, E., Lancet, D., Ritsner, M., and Navon, R. (2004). Is the G72/G30 locus associated with schizophrenia? Single nucleotide polymorphisms, haplotypes, and gene expression analysis. *Biol. Psychiatry* 56, 169–176.

57. Addington, A. M., Gornick, M., Sporn, A. L., Gogtay, N., Greenstein, D., Lenane, M., Gochman, P., Baker, N., Balkissoon, R., Vakkalanka, R. K., Weinberger, D. R., Straub, R. E., and Rapoport, J. L. (2004). Polymorphisms in the 13q33.2 gene G72/G30 are associated with childhood-onset schizophrenia and psychosis not otherwise specified. *Biol. Psychiatry* 55, 976–980.

58. Hattori, E., Liu, C., Badner, J. A., Bonner, T. I., Christian, S. L., Maheshwari, M., Detera-Wadleigh, S. D., Gibbs, R. A., and Gershon, E. S. (2003). Polymorphisms at the G72/G30 gene locus, on 13q33, are associated with bipolar disorder in two independent pedigree series. *Am. J. Hum. Genet.* 72, 119–1140.

59. Chowdari, K. V., Mirnics, K., Semwal, P., Wood, J., Lawrence, E., Bhatia, T., Deshpande, S. N., Thelma, B. K., Ferrell, R. E., Middleton, F. A., Devlin, B., Levitt, P., Lewis, D. A., and Nimgaonkar, V. L. (2002). Association and linkage analyses of RGS4 polymorphisms in schizophrenia. *Hum. Mol. Genet.* 11, 1372–1380. Erratum in *Hum. Mol. Genet.* 12, 1781.

60. Mirnics, K., Middleton, F. A., Lewis, D. A., and Levitt, P. (2001). Analysis of complex brain disorders with gene expression microarrays: Schizophrenia as a disease of the synapse. *Trends Neurosci.* 24, 479–486.

61. Cordeiro, Q., Talkowski, M. E., Chowdari, K. V., Wood, J., Nimgaonkar, V., and Vallada, H. (2005). Association and linkage analysis of RGS4 polymorphisms with schizophrenia and bipolar disorder in Brazil. *Genes Brain Behav.* 4, 45–50.

62. Chen, X., Dunham, C., Kendler, S., Wang, X., O'Neill, F. A., Walsh, D., and Kendler, K. S. (2004). Regulator of G-protein signaling 4 (RGS4) gene is associated with schizophrenia in Irish high density families. *Am. J. Med. Genet. B. Neuropsychiatr. Genet.* 129, 23–26.

63. Morris, D. W., Rodgers, A., McGhee, K. A., Schwaiger, S., Scully, P., Quinn, J., Meagher, D., Waddington, J. L., Gill, M., and Corvin, A. P. (2004). Confirming RGS4 as a susceptibility gene for schizophrenia. *Am. J. Med. Genet. B. Neuropsychiatr. Genet.* 125, 50–53.

64. Williams, N. M., Preece, A., Spurlock, G., Norton, N., Williams, H. J., McCreadie, R. G., Buckland, P., Sharkey, V., Chowdari, K. V., Zammit, S., Nimgaonkar, V., Kirov, G., Owen, M. J., and O'Donovan, M. C. (2004). Support for RGS4 as a susceptibility gene for schizophrenia. *Biol. Psychiatry* 55, 192–195.

65. Beyer, C. E., Ghavami, A., Lin, Q., Sung, A., Rhodes, K. J., Dawson, L. A., Schechter, L. E., and Young, K. H. (2004). Regulators of G-protein signaling 4: Modulation of 5-HT(1A)-mediated neurotransmitter release in vivo. *Brain Res.* 1022, 214–220.

66. De Blasi, A., Conn, P. J., Pin, J., and Nicoletti, F. (2001). Molecular determinants of metabotropic glutamate receptor signaling. *Trends Pharmacol. Sci.* 22, 114–120.

67. Taymans, J. M., Kia, H. K., Claes, R., Cruz, C., Leysen, J., and Langlois, X. (2004). Dopamine receptor-mediated regulation of RGS2 and RGS4 mRNA differentially depends on ascending dopamine projections and time. *Eur. J. Neurosci.* 19, 2249–2260.

68. Thaminy, S., Auerbach, D., Arnoldo, A., and Stagljar, I. (2003). Identification of novel ErbB3-interacting factors using the split-ubiquitin membrane yeast two-hybrid system. *Genome. Res.* 13, 1744–1753.

69. Prasad, K. M., Chowdari, K. V., Nimgaonkar, V. L., Talkowski, M. E., Lewis, D. A., and Keshavan, M. S. (2005). Genetic polymorphisms of the RGS4 and dorsolateral prefrontal cortex morphometry among first episode schizophrenia patients. *Mol. Psychiatry* 10, 213–219.

70. Shenton, M. E., Dickey, C. C., Frumin, M., and McCarley, R. W. (2001). A review of MRI findings in schizophrenia. *Schizophr. Res.* 49, 1–52.

71. Brzustowicz, L. M., Simone, J., Mohseni, P., Hayter, J. E., Hodgkinson, K. A., Chow, E. W., and Bassett, A. S. (2004). Linkage disequilibrium mapping of schizophrenia susceptibility to the CAPON region of chromosome 1q22. *Am. J. Hum. Genet.* 74, 1057–1063.

72. Gerber, D. J., Hall, D., Miyakawa, T., Demars, S., Gogos, J. A., Karayiorgou, M., and Tonegawa, S. (2003). Evidence for association of schizophrenia with genetic variation in the 8p21.3 gene, PPP3CC, encoding the calcineurin gamma subunit. *Proc. Natl. Acad. Sci. USA* 100, 8993–8998.

73. Duan, J., Martinez, M., Sanders, A. R., Hou, C., Saitou, N., Kitano, T., Mowry, B. J., Crowe, R. R., Silverman, J. M., Levinson, D. F., and Gejman, P. V. (2004). Polymorphisms in the trace amine receptor 4 (TRAR4) gene on chromosome 6q23.2 are associated with susceptibility to schizophrenia. *Am. J. Hum. Genet.* 75, 624–638.

74. Pimm, J., McQuillin, A., Thirumalai, S., Lawrence, J., Quested, D., Bass, N., Lamb, G., Moorey, H., Datta, S. R., Kalsi, G., Badacsonyi, A., Kelly, K., Morgan, J., Punukollu, B., Curtis, D., and Gurling, H. (2005). The epsin 4 gene on chromosome 5q, which encodes the clathrin-associated protein enthoprotin, is involved in the genetic susceptibility to schizophrenia. *Am. J. Hum. Genet.* 76, 902–907.

75. Zheng, Y., Li, H., Qin, W., Chen, W., Duan, Y., Xiao, Y., Li, C., Zhang, J., Li, X., Feng, G., and He, L. (2005). Association of the carboxyl-terminal PDZ ligand of neuronal nitric oxide synthase gene with schizophrenia in the Chinese Han population. *Biochem. Biophys. Res. Commun.* 328, 809–815.

76. MacIntyre, D. J., Blackwood, D. H., Porteous, D. J., Pickard, B. S., and Muir, W. J. (2003). Chromosomal abnormalities and mental illness. *Mol. Psychiatry* 8, 275–287.

77. Pulver, A. E., Nestadt, G., Goldberg, R., Shprintzen, R. J., Lamacz, M., Wolyniec, P. S., Morrow, B., Karayiorgou, M., Antonarakis, S. E., Housman, D., et al. (1994). Psychotic illness in patients diagnosed with velo-cardio-facial syndrome and their relatives. *J. Nerv. Ment. Dis.* 182, 476–478.

78. Bassett, A. S., Hodgkinson, K., Chow, E. W., Correia, S., Scutt, L. E., and Weksberg, R. (1998). 22q11 deletion syndrome in adults with schizophrenia. *Am. J. Med. Genet.* 81, 328–337.

79. Murphy, K. C., Jones, L. A., and Owen, M. J. (1999). High rates of schizophrenia in adults with velo-cardio-facial syndrome. *Arch. Gen. Psychiatry* 56, 940–945.

80. Ivanov, D., Kirov, G., Norton, N., Williams, H. J., Williams, N. M., Nikolov, I., Tzwetkova, R., Stambolova, S. M., Murphy, K. C., Toncheva, D., Thapar, A., O'Donovan, M. C., and Owen, M. J. (2003). Chromosome 22q11 deletions, velo-cardio-facial syndrome and early-onset psychosis. Molecular genetic study. *Br. J. Psychiatry* 183, 409–413.

81. Chen, X., Wang, X., O'Neill, A. F., Walsh, D., and Kendler, K. S. (2004). Variants in the catechol-O-methyltransferase (COMT) gene are associated with schizophrenia in Irish high-density families. *Mol. Psychiatry* 9, 962–967.

82. Egan, M. F., Goldberg, T. E., Kolachana, B. S., Callicott, J. H., Mazzanti, C. M., Straub, R. E., Goldman, D., and Weinberger, D. R. (2001). Effect of COMT Val108/158 Met genotype on frontal lobe function and risk for schizophrenia. *Proc. Natl. Acad. Sci. USA* 98, 6917–6922.

83. Malhotra, A. K., Kestler, L. J., Mazzanti, C., Bates, J. A., Goldberg, T., and Goldman, D. (2002). A functional polymorphism in the COMT gene and performance on a test of prefrontal cognition. *Am. J. Psychiatry* 159, 652–654.

84. Glatt, S. J., Faraone, S. V., and Tsuang, M. T. (2003). Association between a functional catechol *O*-methyltransferase gene polymorphism and schizophrenia: Meta-analysis of case-control and family-based studies. *Am. J. Psychiatry* 160, 469–476.

85. Shifman, S., Bronstein, M., Sternfeld, M., Pisante-Shalom, A., Lev-Lehman, E., Weizman, A., Reznik, I., Spivak, B., Grisaru, N., Karp, L., Schiffer, R., Kotler, M., Strous, R. D., Swartz-Vanetik, M., Knobler, H. Y., Shinar, E., Beckmann, J. S., Yakir, B.,

Risch, N., Zak, N. B., and Darvasi, A. (2002). A highly significant association between a COMT haplotype and schizophrenia. *Am. J. Hum. Genet.* 71, 1296–1302.

86. Li, T., Ball, D., Zhao, J., Murray, R. M., Liu, X., Sham, P. C., and Collier, D. A. (2000). Family-based linkage disequilibrium mapping using SNP marker haplotypes: Application to a potential locus for schizophrenia at chromosome 22q11. *Mol. Psychiatry* 5, 452.

87. Williams, H. J., Glaser, B., Williams, N. M., Norton, N., Zammit, S., MacGregor, S., Kirov, G. K., Owen, M. J., and O'Donovan, M. C. (2005). No association between schizophrenia and polymorphisms in COMT in two large samples. *Am. J. Psychiatry* 162, 1736–1738.

88. Sanders, A. R., Rusu, I., Duan, J., Vander Molen, J. E., Hou, C., Schwab, S. G., Wildenauer, D. B., Martinez, M., and Gejman, P. V. (2005). Haplotypic association spanning the 22q11.21 genes COMT and ARVCF with schizophrenia. *Mol. Psychiatry* 10, 353–365.

89. Bray, N. J., Buckland, P. R., Williams, N. M., Williams, H. J., Norton, N., Owen, M. J., and O'Donovan, M. C. (2003). A haplotype implicated in schizophrenia susceptibility is associated with reduced COMT expression in human brain. *Am. J. Hum. Genet.* 73, 152–161.

90. Gogos, J. A., Santha, M., Takacs, Z., Beck, K. D., Luine, V., Lucas, L. R., Nadler, J. V., and Karayiorgou, M. (1999). The gene encoding proline dehydrogenase modulates sensorimotor gating in mice. *Nat. Genet.* 21, 434–439.

91. Liu, H., Heath, S. C., Sobin, C., Roos, J. L., Galke, B. L., Blundell, M. L., Lenane, M., Robertson, B., Wijsman, E. M., Rapoport, J. L., Gogos, J. A., and Karayiorgou, M. (2002). Genetic variation at the 22q11 PRODH2/DGCR6 locus presents an unusual pattern and increases susceptibility to schizophrenia. *Proc. Natl. Acad. Sci. USA* 99, 3717–3722.

92. Li, T., Ma, X., Sham, P. C., Sun, X., Hu, X., Wang, Q., Meng, H., Deng, W., Liu, X., Murray, R. M., and Collier, D. A. (2004). Evidence for association between novel polymorphisms in the PRODH gene and schizophrenia in a Chinese population. *Am. J. Med. Genet. B. Neuropsychiatr. Genet.* 129, 13–15.

93. Williams, H. J., Williams, N., Spurlock, G., Norton, N., Ivanov, D., McCreadie, R. G., Preece, A., Sharkey, V., Jones, S., Zammit, S., Nikolov, I., Kehaiov, I., Thapar, A., Murphy, K. C., Kirov, G., Owen, M. J., and O'Donovan, M. C. (2003). Association between PRODH and schizophrenia is not confirmed. *Mol. Psychiatry* 8, 644–645.

94. Jacquet, H., Raux, G., Thibaut, F., Hecketsweiler, B., Houy, E., Demilly, C., Haouzir, S., Allio, G., Fouldrin, G., Drouin, V., Bou, J., Petit, M., Campion, D., and Frebourg, T. (2002). PRODH mutations and hyperprolinemia in a subset of schizophrenic patients. *Hum. Mol. Genet.* 11, 2243–2249.

95. Jacquet, H., Demily, C., Houy, E., Hecketsweiler, B., Bou, J., Raux, G., Lerond, J., Allio, G., Haouzir, S., Tillaux, A., Bellegou, C., Fouldrin, G., Delamillieure, P., Menard, J. F., Dollfus, S., D'Amato, T., Petit, M., Thibaut, F., Frebourg, T., and Campion, D. (2005). Hyperprolinemia is a risk factor for schizaffective disorder. *Mol. Psychiatry* 10, 479–485.

96. Ohtsuki, T., Tanaka, S., Ishiguro, H., Noguchi, E., Arinami, T., Tanabe, E., Yara, K., Okubo, T., Takahashi, S., Matsuura, M., Sakai, T., Muto, M., Kojima, T., Matsushima, E., Toru, M., and Inada, T. (2004). Failure to find association between PRODH deletion and schizophrenia. *Schizophr. Res.* 67, 111–113.

97. Mukai, J., Liu, H., Burt, R. A., Swor, D. E., Lai, W. S., Karayiorgou, M., and Gogos, J. A. (2004). Evidence that the gene encoding ZDHHC8 contributes to the risk of schizophrenia. *Nat. Genet.* 36, 725–79.

98. Chen, W. Y., Shi, Y. Y., Zheng, Y. L., Zhao, X. Z., Zhang, G. J., Chen, S. Q., Yang, P. D., and He, L. (2004). Case-control study and transmission disequilibrium test provide consistent evidence for association between schizophrenia and genetic variation in the 22q11 gene ZDHHC8. *Hum. Mol. Genet.* 13, 2991–2995.

99. Saito, S., Ikeda, M., Iwata, N., Suzuki, T., Kitajima, T., Yamanouchi, Y., Kinoshita, Y., Takahashi, N., Inada, T., and Ozaki, N. (2005). No association was found between a functional SNP in ZDHHC8 and schizophrenia in a Japanese case-control population. *Neurosci. Lett.* 374, 21–24.

100. Glaser, B., Schumacher, J., Williams, H. J., Jamra, R. A., Ianakiev, N., Milev, R., Ohlraun, S., Schulze, T. G., Czerski, P. M., Hauser, J., Jonsson, E. G., Sedvall, G. C., Klopp, N., Illig, T., Becker, T., Propiing, P., Williams, N. M., Cichon, S., Kirov, G., Rietschel, M., Murphy, K. C., O'Donovan, M. C., Nothen, M. M., and Owen, M. J. (2005). No association between the putative functional ZDHHC8 single nucleotide polymorphism rs175174 and schizophrenia in large European samples. *Biol. Psychiatry* 58, 78–80.

101. Blackwood, D. H., Fordyce, A., Walker, M. T., St Clair, D. M., Porteous, D. J., and Muir, W. J. (2001). Schizophrenia and affective disorders—Cosegregation with a translocation at chromosome 1q42 that directly disrupts brain-expressed genes: Clinical and P300 findings in a family. *Am. J. Hum. Genet.* 69, 428–433.

102. Millar, J. K., Wilson-Annan, J. C., Anderson, S., Christie, S., Taylor, M. S., Semple, C. A., Devon, R. S., Clair, D. M., Muir, W. J., Blackwood, D. H., and Porteous, D. J. (2000). Disruption of two novel genes by a translocation co-segregating with schizophrenia. *Hum. Mol. Genet.* 9, 1415–1423.

103. Ekelund, J., Hennah, W., Hiekkalinna, T., Parker, A., Meyer, J., Lonnqvist, J., and Peltonen, L. (2004). Replication of 1q42 linkage in Finnish schizophrenia pedigrees. *Mol. Psychiatry* 9, 1037–1041.

104. Ekelund, J., Hovatta, I., Parker, A., Paunio, T., Varilo, T., Martin, R., Suhonen, J., Ellonen, P., Chan, G., Sinsheimer, J. S., Sobel, E., Juvonen, H., Arajarvi, R., Partonen, T., Suvisaari, J., Lonnqvist, J., Meyer, J., and Peltonen, L. (2001). Chromosome 1 loci in Finnish schizophrenia families. *Hum. Mol. Genet.* 10, 1611–1617.

105. Miyoshi, K., Honda, A., Baba, K., Taniguchi, M., Oono, K., Fujita, T., Kuroda, S., Katayama, T., and Tohyama, M. (2003). Disrupted-in-schizophrenia 1, a candidate gene for schizophrenia, participates in neurite outgrowth. *Mol. Psychiatry* 8, 685–694.

106. Ozeki, Y., Tomoda, T., Kleiderlein, J., Kamiya, A., Bord, L., Fujii, K., Okawa, M., Yamada, N., Hatten, M. E., Snyder, S. H., Ross, C. A., and Sawa, A. (2003). disrupted-in-schizophrenia-1 (DISC-1): Mutant truncation prevents binding to NudE-like (NUDEL) and inhibits neurite outgrowth. *Proc. Natl. Acad. Sci. USA* 100, 289–294.

107. Devon, R. S., Anderson, S., Teague, P. W., Burgess, P., Kipari, T. M., Semple, C. A., Millar, J. K., Muir, W. J., Murray, V., Pelosi, A. J., Blackwood, D. H., and Porteous, D. J. (2001). Identification of polymorphisms within disrupted in schizophrenia 1 and disrupted in schizophrenia 2, and an investigation of their association with schizophrenia and bipolar affective disorder. *Psychiatr. Genet.* 11, 71–78.

108. Kockelkorn, T. T., Arai, M., Matsumoto, H., Fukuda, N., Yamada, K., Minabe, Y., Toyota, T., Ujike, H., Sora, I., Mori, N., Yoshikawa, T., and Itokawa, M. (2004). Association study of polymorphisms in the 5′ upstream region of human DISC1 gene with schizophrenia. *Neurosci. Lett.* 368, 41–45.

109. Hennah, W., Varilo, T., Kestila, M., Paunio, T., Arajarvi, R., Haukka, J., Parker, A., Martin, R., Levitzky, S., Partonen, T., Meyer, J., Lonnqvist, J., Peltonen, L., and Ekelund, J. (2003). Haplotype transmission analysis provides evidence of association

for DISC1 to schizophrenia and suggests sex-dependent effects. *Hum. Mol. Genet.* 12, 951–959.

110. Hodgkinson, C. A., Goldman, D., Jaeger, J., Persaud, S., Kane, J. M., Lipsky, R. H., and Malhotra, A. K. (2004). Disrupted in schizophrenia 1 (DISC1): Association with schizophrenia, schizoaffective disorder, and bipolar disorder. *Am. J. Hum. Genet.* 75, 862–872.

111. Jonsson, E. G., Flyckt, L., Burgert, E., Crocq, M. A., Forslund, K., Mattila-Evenden, M., Rylander, G., Asberg, M., Nimgaonkar, V. L., Edman, G., Bjerkenstedt, L., Wiesel, F. A., and Sedvall, G. C. (2003). Dopamine D3 receptor gene Ser9Gly variant and schizophrenia: Association study and meta-analysis. *Psychiatr. Genet.* 13, 1–12.

112. Glatt, S. J., Faraone, S. V., and Tsuang, M. T. (2003). Meta-analysis identifies an association between the dopamine D2 receptor gene and schizophrenia. *Mol. Psychiatry* 8, 911–915.

113. Abdolmaleky, H. M., Faraone, S. V., Glatt, S. J., and Tsuang, M. T. (2004). Meta-analysis of association between the T102C polymorphism of the 5HT2a receptor gene and schizophrenia. *Schizophr. Res.* 67, 53–62.

114. Marti, S. B., Cichon, S., Propping, P., and Nothen, M. (2002). Metabotropic glutamate receptor 3 (GRM3) gene variation is not associated with schizophrenia or bipolar affective disorder in the German population. *Am. J. Med. Genet.* 114, 46–50.

115. Fujii, Y., Shibata, H., Kikuta, R., Makino, C., Tani, A., Hirata, N., Shibata, A., Ninomiya, H., Tashiro, N., and Fukumaki, Y. (2003). Positive associations of polymorphisms in the metabotropic glutamate receptor type 3 gene (GRM3) with schizophrenia. *Psychiatr. Genet.* 13, 71–76.

116. Egan, M. F., Straub, R. E., Goldberg, T. E., Yakub, I., Callicott, J. H., Hariri, A. R., Mattay, V. S., Bertolino, A., Hyde, T. M., Shannon-Weickert, C., Akil, M., Crook, J., Vakkalanka, R. K., Balkissoon, R., Gibbs, R. A., Kleinman, J. E., and Weinberger, D. R. (2004). Variation in GRM3 affects cognition, prefrontal glutamate, and risk for schizophrenia. *Proc. Natl. Acad. Sci. USA* 101, 12604–12609.

117. Neale, B. M., and Sham, P. C. (2004). The future of association studies: Gene-based analysis and replication. *Am. J. Hum. Genet.* 75, 353–362.

118. Harrison, P. J., and Owen, M. J. (2003). Genes for schizophrenia? Recent findings and their pathophysiological implications. *Lancet* 361, 417–419.

119. Moghaddam, B. (2003). Bringing order to the glutamate chaos in schizophrenia. *Neuron* 40, 881–884.

120. Harrison, P. J., and Weinberger, D. R. (2005). Schizophrenia genes, gene expression, and neuropathology: On the matter of their convergence. *Mol. Psychiatry* 10, 40–68; image 45.

121. Moises, H. W., Zoega, T., and Gottesman, I. I. (2002). The glial growth factors deficiency and synaptic destabilization hypothesis of schizophrenia. *BMC Psychiatry* 2, 8.

10

POSTMORTEM BRAIN STUDIES: FOCUS ON SUSCEPTIBILITY GENES IN SCHIZOPHRENIA

Shiny V. Mathew, Shruti N. Mitkus, Barbara K. Lipska, Thomas M. Hyde, and Joel E. Kleinman

National Institute of Mental Health, National Institutes of Health, Bethesda, Maryland

10.1	Introduction	343
10.2	Approaches to Identify Susceptibility genes in Schizophrenia	344
	10.2.1 *COMT*	347
	10.2.2 *DTNBP1*	348
	10.2.3 *GRM3*	349
	10.2.4 *DISC1*	349
	10.2.5 *NRG1*	350
	10.2.6 *GAD1*	350
	10.2.7 *RGS4*	351
10.3	Molecular Interactions of Schizophrenia Susceptibility Genes	351
	10.3.1 *DISC1*	351
	10.3.2 *DTNBP1*	352
	10.3.3 *NRG1*	353
10.4	Conclusions	355
References		356

10.1 INTRODUCTION

Schizophrenia is a syndrome characterized by psychotic symptoms (hallucinations, delusions, thought disorder) and cognitive impairment, with a prevalence rate approaching 1% worldwide. Over 100 years of neuropathology research has failed to identify a pathomnemonic lesion in the brains of schizophrenic patients. Nevertheless, important facts dictating the direction of a number of neuropathological studies have arisen from research efforts in related areas.

First and foremost is the evidence that schizophrenia has a clear genetic component. Results from twin and adoption studies show a heritability estimate

---

Handbook of Contemporary Neuropharmacology, Edited by David R. Sibley, Israel Hanin, Michael Kuhar, and Phil Skolnick. Copyright © 2007 John Wiley & Sons, Inc.

for schizophrenia of 70–90% [1–3]. However, analysis of recurrence risk estimates in families with one or more affected individuals clearly argues against schizophrenia being a single-gene disorder even with the possibility of incomplete penetrance [4]. Alternatively, the mode of transmission for schizophrenia is complex and multifactorial with the possibility of a number of genes conferring varying degrees of susceptibility. With this in mind, efforts have been directed at identifying allelic variants in genes that may confer increased risk for schizophrenia.

The identification of allelic variation in susceptibility genes that increase the risk for schizophrenia is only a first step in elucidating the pathophysiology. Exactly how susceptibility genes lead to schizophrenia remains largely unknown. A neurodevelopmental hypothesis argues that schizophrenia is the result of in utero events that lead to changes in neurogenesis, neuronal migration, and synaptic plasticity [5]. An alternative hypothesis of neurodegeneration proposes that schizophrenia is the result of neuronal loss or gliosis that occurs during aging [6]. For the most part, the latter theory has languished in part due to studies showing that such pathological hallmarks are only found in schizophrenia associated with dementia [6]. Still a third line of inquiry suggests that schizophrenia is a progressive developmental disorder with aberrant neuronal pruning during development that continues into early adulthood [7]. A better understanding of the pathophysiology associated with schizophrenia susceptibility genes may elucidate which, if any, of these hypotheses is correct.

Studies on the neurochemical basis of schizophrenia implicate many neurotransmitter systems, including dopamine, glutamate, γ-aminobutyric acid (GABA), and acetylcholine. During the last five decades, the dopamine system has been the central focus of schizophrenia research. The focus on dopamine relies largely on the fact that antipsychotics used to treat schizophrenia correlate with their ability to block D_2 receptors [8, 9]. A revised "dopamine hypothesis" posits that a hypofunction of the D_1 receptors in the prefrontal cortex (PFC) coexist with increased subcortical dopamine associated with D_2 receptors [10–12]. An alternative hypothesis based on the psychomimetic properties of phencyclidine (PCP), an N-methyl-D-aspartate (NMDA) receptor antagonist, has implicated the glutamate neurons and is supported by neuroimaging and postmortem studies [13, 14]. A number of other postmortem studies implicate GABA inhibitory neurons in the neuropathology of schizophrenia [15–18]. Last but not least, both muscarinic (M) and nicotinic acetylcholine receptors [19] have also been postulated in the pathophysiology of schizophrenia [20, 21]. Again the identification of schizophrenia susceptibility genes may be the best evidence that multiple neurotransmitter systems are implicated in schizophrenia.

Identification of allelic variation in genes that increase risk for schizophrenia may implicate specific neurotransmitter systems and pathological processes. Moreover, this knowledge may elucidate molecular pathways involved in the pathophysiology of the syndrome that may alter both our diagnostic systems and lead to new therapeutic targets.

10.2 APPROACHES TO IDENTIFY SUSCEPTIBILITY GENES IN SCHIZOPHRENIA

With the high heritability estimates for schizophrenia, genetic researchers have postulated that there are a number of susceptibility genes, each conferring increased risk for the disorder. The search for the genetic component of schizophrenia has primarily employed linkage analysis and association studies.

The aim of linkage studies is to identify regions of the genome that are cotransmitted with the disease in the affected individual but not in unaffected family members. Using polymorphic DNA markers distributed along each chromosome it is determined which DNA marker is cotransmitted with the disease due to its close physical proximity to the disease-causing gene. Once a candidate chromosomal locus harboring the disease gene is identified, fine mapping of this putative disease-linked region is then performed in order to pinpoint the disease-causing gene. Although this technique has been used with great success in identifying distinct chromosomal regions in the genome that may play a role in schizophrenia (Table 10.1), there are a number of limitations to linkage analysis. Due to the lack of a large number of

TABLE 10.1 Schizophrenia Susceptibility Genes Identified by Linkage Analysis and Association Studies

Gene	Location	Linkage Studies	Association Studies
COMT	22q11	[194]	[44]
			[41]
			[39]
			[195]
			[42]
GRM3	7q21–22	[99]	[106, 196]
			[197]
DTNBP1	6p22.3	[198]	[202]
		[199]	[203]
		[200]	[204]
		[201]	[205]
			[93]
DRD2	11q23.2	[200]	[82]
		[206]	[77, 79, 80]
		[207]	
DISC1	4q42.2	[99, 208]	[212]
		[209]	[213]
		[149]	[214]
		[210]	
		[211]	
NRG1	8p21–22	[179, 215]	[216–219]
AKT1	14q32.33	[220]	[96]
		[221]	[222]
GAD1	2q31	[202]	[223]
RGS4	1q23.1	[157]	[138]
			[224]
			[225–227]
			[228]

families with multiple affected individuals, ascertainment differences, broad phenotypic definitions, ethnic and environmental variations, and sparse polymorphic DNA markers, it is not surprising that linkage studies have not been an unmitigated success in the identification of schizophrenia susceptibility genes [22].

Chromosomal location by linkage analysis and fine mapping of the region followed by association studies of the genes present in this chromosomal region are designed to identify alleles of certain genes that are more common among individuals with the disorder than in the general population. Association studies are typically carried out by selecting specific polymorphisms in candidate genes that are thought to be correlated with the disease based on location and/or function and then determining the allelic frequency in affected versus unaffected individuals. Although useful, association studies are limited by the fact that the actual disease-causing polymorphisms have to be identified and then tested in affected versus unaffected individuals [23]. Since little is known about the neurobiology of complex mental disorders, picking truly relevant causative genes for association studies is inherently challenging. This difficulty is further increased when interpreting polymorphisms in noncoding regions that are not ultimately translated to a protein product. Moreover, inadequate patient–control matching, small sample size, and differences in allelic frequencies between different populations further contribute to the observed discrepancies in findings on the same gene by different groups.

Another method used to identify disease genes is analysis of cytogenetic abnormalities found more often in patients than in unaffected individuals. These chromosomal abnormalities such as translocations and large-scale deletions/duplications may be helpful if the affected chromosomal region harbors genes that contribute to the disease when their function is disrupted. Although there have been numerous reports on chromosomal anomalies associated with schizophrenia [24, 25], only two have provided convincing evidence that is supported by linkage data. The first is the identification of *DISC1* by a balanced reciprocal translocation [(1;11)(q42;q14.3)] in a large Scottish family with multiple individuals affected with schizophrenia and other psychiatric disorders [26, 27]. The second finding of interest is the association of schizophrenia with velocardiofacial syndrome (VCFS), which is caused by interstitial deletions of chromosome 22q11. In addition to a large number of physical anomalies associated with VCFS, patients with this disorder have a dramatic increase in the risk of psychosis, particularly schizophrenia [27–31]. It has been hypothesized that the deleted chromosomal region in VCFS may harbor schizophrenia susceptibility genes.

As is evident, over the last decade a large number of association studies have implicated numerous genes in the pathophysiology of schizophrenia. As an alternative to discussing all of these implicated genes in-depth, for the purpose of this postmortem brain studies review, we will concentrate on genes that fulfill the following criteria: First, the gene should be located on a chromosomal region implicated by linkage analysis. Second, there should be at least three positive association studies with the gene and schizophrenia in ethnically homogeneous populations [32]. Third, there should be data from postmortem molecular studies on expression of messenger RNA (mRNA) or protein available for the gene, particularly from regions of the brain implicated in schizophrenia. Finally, the gene product should have some functional significance for schizophrenia either at the time of neuronal development or in adult brain; that is, it would be expected to relate to prevalent schizophrenia hypotheses such as the neurodevelopmental hypothesis and dopamine hypothesis. Based on these criteria we will review the following genes in detail: *COMT*, *DTNBP1*, *GRM3*, *DISC1*, *NRG1*, *GAD1*, and *RGS4*. Some of the linkage and association studies implicating these genes are listed in Table 10.1.

10.2.1 *COMT*

Catechol-O-methyl transferase (*COMT*) is a 27-kb gene located on chromosome 22q11 and encodes for a protein crucial for the enzymatic degradation of dopamine. This gene is composed of six exons: exons 1 and 2 are noncoding while exon 3 contains codons for two distinct promoters giving rise to two functionally different transcription products [33]. The short, 1.3-kb human mRNA produces the soluble isoform (S-COMT) while the longer 1.5-kb human mRNA produces the membrane-bound isoform (MB-COMT) [34]. Of these, the MB-COMT predominates in the human brain while S-COMT is found peripherally [33, 35, 36]. In the human brain, COMT mRNA is highly expressed in the prefrontal cortex, striatum, and midbrain [35] while electron microscopy studies have revealed the protein to be present on dendrites in these regions [37, 38].

A number of single-nucleotide polymorphisms (SNPs) in the *COMT* gene have been found to be associated with schizophrenia [39–43]. Only two of these polymorphisms affect COMT enzymatic activity [36]. A P_2 promoter SNP may have an effect on COMT expression as reflected in enzymatic activity in lymphocytes [36].

By far, the SNP with the most effect on the COMT expression and enzymatic activity is a missense mutation in exon 4 of the *COMT* gene yielding a nonsynonymous amino acid change from Val-Met at either position 108 in S-COMT or 158 in MB-COMT [44]. Although the *val* allele is associated with lower mRNA [40] and protein expression [36], it has higher enzymatic activity than the *met* allele [36]. Earlier studies of COMT enzymatic activity in brain found no differences between schizophrenics and controls [45, 46]. More recent postmortem findings also indicate that mRNA and protein expression levels of COMT are unaltered in the dorsolateral prefrontal cortex of schizophrenics [35, 36, 47]. However, an altered mRNA distribution pattern is observed in this region in schizophrenics when compared to controls [35]. Since the difference in frequency of the Val/Met allelic variation between schizophrenic cases and controls is small (approximately 6%), a large number of postmortem brains ($n = 272$) would be necessary to observe a significant difference in the schizophrenics [36]. As a consequence it is possible that the postmortem studies mentioned above were underpowered to observe a significant difference in COMT between schizophrenics and controls.

As dopamine transporters are expressed in low levels in the PFC [48] and thus are thought to play only a small role in synaptic dopamine reuptake in the PFC [49, 50], COMT may be crucial in terminating dopamine neurotransmitter function in PFC. Moreover, those individuals with the homozygous *val* allele in COMT may have lower cortical dopamine levels. Low levels of dopamine in the PFC alters downstream signaling pathways and initiates the synthesis of dopamine subcortically by an observed increase in nigral tyrosine hydroxylase (TH) mRNA in postmortem tissue [51–59].

In addition to COMT and TH, the level of dopamine receptors (DRD2) have also been examined in postmortem schizophrenia in an effort to better understand the role dopamine plays in disease pathology. The psychomimetic effect of dopamine agonists and antipsychotic antagonism at DRD2 [9, 60–62] led to numerous studies of the D_2 receptor in postmortem human brain of schizophrenics and controls. While many studies have reported alterations in the level of D_2 receptors in postmortem tissue [63–68], much of the earlier findings have been challenged by the lack of isoform-specific antibodies and receptor-specific ligands as well as being confounded by antemortem neuroleptic treatment. Even in vivo neuroimaging receptor studies in drug-naive patients, which report an increase of D_2 receptors in the striatum [69], have not been confirmed by others [70–73]. Currently, there is a general consensus from postmortem and neuroimaging studies that D_2-like receptors, particularly the D_2, are increased in the striatum [74, 75], although the etiology of this increase is probably secondary to neuroleptic treatment. A number of association studies have linked DRD2 with schizophrenia [76–82]; however, due to methodological problems in population stratification, the validity of these studies remains doubtful.

10.2.2 DTNBP1

DTNBP1 is a 140-kb gene located on 6p22.3, one of the best-established regions to have emerged from linkage studies of schizophrenia (Table 10.1). *DTNBP1*, is composed of 10 exons and encodes dysbindin 1 protein. Dysbindin mRNA is expressed widely in the brain and has been detected in the frontal and temporal neocortices, hippocampus, caudate, putamen, nucleus accumbens, amygdala, thalamus, and midbrain of the adult human brain [83]. These anatomical expression data are salient because regions such as frontal cortex and hippocampus are strongly implicated in schizophrenia.

Although the precise molecular function of dysbindin protein in the brain has not been determined, dysbindin binds to dystobrevins, which are components of the dystrophin-associated glycoprotein complex (DCG) [84]. DCG is a multiprotein complex that is required for normal functioning of muscle cells, and several DCG-like complexes have been identified in postsynaptic densities in the brain [85]. Alterations of these complexes have been implicated in the cognitive impairment that commonly occurs in patients with Duchenne muscular dystrophy (DMD) [86, 87]. Interestingly, the absence of dystrophin in the *mdx* mouse model of DMD results in altered distribution of dysbindin in the cerebellum [88]. Dysbindin has also been found to be a component of the biogenesis of lysosome-related organelles complex (BLOC)-1 [89], which may play a role in schizophrenia and will be subsequently discussed in greater detail.

Postmortem brain studies have found expression levels of dysbindin mRNA levels to be reduced in the dorsolateral prefrontal cortex of schizophrenics compared to controls [83], and SNPs in three prime untranslated region (3'UTR), intron 3, 5'UTR, and 5' flanking region significantly impact dysbindin mRNA levels in PFC [83]. Dysbindin protein levels are also significantly reduced in the postmortem hippocampus of schizophrenic patients [90]. Dysbindin mRNA levels in human brains are reduced by cis-acting polymorphisms, and a schizophrenia risk haplotype was also found to be associated with reduced DTNBP1 expression in the frontal, parietal, or temporal cortices [91, 92].

Downregulation of dysbindin expression has been found to cause reduced phosphorylation of AKT1 [93]. The serine–threonine protein kinase gene encoded by AKT1 is 32.8 kb in size, located on chromosome 14q32 spanning 14 exons.

AKT1-GSK-3β (glycogen synthase kinase 3β) is a target of lithium and has been implicated in bipolar disorder [94]. In the developing nervous system AKT1 is a critical mediator of growth factor–induced neuronal survival. In situ histochemistry of mouse brain during normal development determined that embryonic AKT1 mRNA levels were high throughout the entire neuroaxis. The level of expression gradually decreased during postnatal development and into adulthood [95]. AKT1 protein levels are reduced in lymphocytes, hippocampus, and PFC of schizophrenics [96]. Reduced phosphorylation of GSK-3β, which is a target of AKT1, was also detected in lymphocytes and frontal cortex lysates [96]. GSK-3β mRNA levels are also reduced in dorsolateral prefrontal cortex (DLPFC) of schizophrenic patients versus controls [97]. Based on these findings, AKT1 may play a role in neurodevelopment and altered postnatal levels of AKT1 and its downstream molecular targets may contribute to increased risk for schizophrenia.

10.2.3 GRM3

GRM3 (human metabotropic glutamate receptor subtype 3) is mapped to chromosome 7q21–22 [98] and is considered a positional and functional candidate gene for schizophrenia based on a genomewide scan [99]. *GRM3* is approximately 220 kb in size and contains six exons [100]. The protein product of the gene is assembled into a membrane-bound receptor coupled to second-messenger pathways and allows for a decrease in glutamate release [101, 102]. GRM3 is widely distributed in the DLPFC, thalamus, and hippocampus. However, neither the mRNA nor protein expression was altered in schizophrenics relative to controls in any of these regions [103–105]. In our laboratory, in vivo functional magnetic resonance imaging (MRI) testing has revealed that an intronic SNP in the *GRM3* gene is associated with poor hippocampal and prefrontal functions [106]. This study also reports that the same intronic SNP is associated with a lower mRNA expression in the postmortem brain tissue of the excitatory amino acid transporter 2 (EAAT2), a modulator of synaptic glutamate levels. Additionally, a number of splice variants of *GRM3* have been detected in the human brain [107].

10.2.4 DISC1

DISC1 is a 414.3-kb gene located on chromosome 1q42.2 and consists of 13 exons. As mentioned above, *DISC1* was originally identified as a candidate gene for schizophrenia in a large Scottish family, in which a balanced translocation involving chromosomes 1 and 11 was strongly linked to schizophrenia, schizoaffective disorder, bipolar affective disorder, and recurrent major depression [26]. In this family, carriers of the translocation were found to have reduced P300 amplitude, which is observed in some patients with schizophrenia [27]. Subsequent association studies identified a number of polymorphisms in the *DISC1* gene associated with schizophrenia and affective disorder (Table 10.1).

In the adult mouse brain, DISC1 is expressed widely including the olfactory bulb, cortex, hippocampus, hypothalamus, cerebellum, and brain stem. During development, DISC1 protein is detected at all stages, from embryonic day 10 (E10) to 6 months old, with two significant peaks of protein expression of one of the *DISC1* isoforms at E13.5 and postnatal day 35 [108]. Interestingly, these time points correspond to periods of active neurogenesis and puberty in the mouse. These results suggest that DISC1 may play a critical role in brain development, lending support to the neurodevelopmental hypothesis of schizophrenia [108]. Although the precise function of DISC1 in the brain is unknown, a number of DISC1-interacting partners have been identified, including FEZ1, NUDEL, and LIS1, which are known to play a role in neuronal development and functioning. Postmortem studies have detected altered subcellular distribution of DISC1 in patients with psychosis and alcohol/substance abuse, with increased ratios of nuclear to cytoplasmic DISC1 protein levels in patients [109]. Although DISC1 mRNA expression is unchanged in postmortem human brains of patients with schizophrenia, the expression of DISC1-interacting proteins NUDEL, FEZ1, and LIS1 mRNA is significantly reduced in schizophrenic tissue in both the DLPFC and hippocampus [110]. Altered interactions between DISC1 and its binding partners have also been investigated in order to understand more accurately the biology of *DISC1* as a schizophrenia susceptibility gene.

10.2.5 *NRG1*

Neuregulins are a family of widely expressed growth and differentiation factors. The neuregulin gene family consists of four genes (*NRG1* to *NRG4*). *NRG1* is approximately 1.125 Mb in size and contains at least 21 exons and 9 potential promoters [111]. Thus far six distinct isoforms and at least 16 splice variants have been reported [111, 112]. While *NRG2*, *NRG3*, and *NRG4* are found only in adult tissue, *NRG1* type I isoform is expressed early in development, type II is expressed late in development, and type III is expressed in peripheral sensory and motor neurons as well as in the brain [113]. The newly discovered isoform types IV–VI [111] have an unknown anatomical distribution and functions. In the developing and adult human brain, NRG1 mRNA and protein are present in the hippocampus, cerebellum, neocortex, and some subcortical nuclei [114]. NRG1 type I expression is increased in the DLPFC of schizophrenic patients, while the type II and III levels remain unchanged [115]. Recently, our laboratory has found 5' SNPs in the *NRG1* gene that are associated with a change in the mRNA expression of type I and IV isoforms [116]. Postmortem microarray studies also report a significant reduction in the level of ErbB3 receptors, through which neuregulins indirectly exert their biological effect, in the prefrontal cortex of schizophrenics [117, 118]. However, preliminary in situ hybridization studies done in our laboratories using an ErbB3 probe could not confirm the previous findings [119].

10.2.6 *GAD1*

Glutamic acid decarboxylase (GAD) is the rate-limiting enzyme that converts glutamic acid to GABA, an inhibitory neurotransmitter in the brain. *GAD1* gene is 45 kb in size, contains 16 exons [120], and is mapped to chromosome 2q31 [121]. Alternative splicing of this gene results in two products, the predominant 67-kD form and a less abundant 25-kD form. GAD67 is concentrated in interneurons and neurons that fire tonically [122] and is involved in the nonvesicular release of GABA [123].

A number of postmortem studies have reported reduced GAD67 mRNA and protein in PFC of schizophrenic patients [15, 17, 18]. On the contrary, GAD67 mRNA was found to be unaltered in the hippocampus of schizophrenic patients [124]. However, one study has found an increase in GAD67 mRNA in the DLPFC [125]. Besides alterations in GAD67, ligand binding and autoradiography studies demonstrate that $GABA_A$ receptors are upregulated in the cingulate cortex, PFCs and hippocampus of schizophrenics [126], while the short isoform of $GABA_A$ γ subunit is downregulated in the DLPFC [127]. This, in addition to other studies on $GABA_A$ receptor binding and immunoreactivity [16, 18, 128–135], provides strong evidence for an overall hypofunction of the GABAergic system.

10.2.7 *RGS4*

Regulator of G-protein signaling 4 (*RGS4*) is a 110-kb gene located on chromosome 1q23.1 spanning 16 exons. RGS4 is involved in neuronal differentiation and is under dopaminergic regulation [136, 137]. Using microarray analysis RGS4 mRNA expression was found to be reduced in the PFC in schizophrenics and controls [138]. These studies were confirmed by in situ hybridization in PFC [138]. Postmortem studies on expression of brain RGS4 mRNA levels detected highest levels in the cortical layers, with moderate levels observed in the parahippocampal gyrus. Inner layers of the frontal cortex, which is implicated in schizophrenia, also showed dense labeling [139]. Given these findings, *RGS4* continues to be an interesting candidate gene for schizophrenia.

10.3 MOLECULAR INTERACTIONS OF SCHIZOPHRENIA SUSCEPTIBILITY GENES

As discussed in the previous sections, the neuropathology of schizophrenia involves a number of susceptibility genes. Many of these susceptibility genes, alone, may exert only a small effect on the disease pathology but working via molecular partners may converge to share a common pathway leading to disease. In the past, much of the attention had been focused on convergent anatomical pathway involving neurotransmitters such as dopamine, glutamate, and GABA. In this section, our attention is focused on those susceptibility genes that have been shown to interact through molecular partners in animal models or artificial in vitro systems. This will then be followed by our hypotheses of how these interactions may play a role in schizophrenia with evidence from postmortem studies whenever available.

10.3.1 *DISC1*

As mentioned earlier, *DISC1* was identified by a chromosomal translocation in a large Scottish family and is considered a susceptibility gene for schizophrenia by a number of association studies. In an effort to understand the cellular function of DISC1, yeast-two hybrid studies have been used to identify molecular interactors of DISC1. It was found that DISC1 has numerous binding partners, including NUDEL, FEZ1, ATF4/5, MAP1A [140–142]. NUDEL is a component of a pathway involved in cytoplasmic dynein movement and is involved in neurofilament assembly, neuronal migration, and development of neurite morphology [143–148]. Overexpression of truncated DISC1 protein inhibits neurite outgrowth in PC12 cells, suggesting that the DISC1–NUDEL complex may be involved in neuronal outgrowth [141, 148, 149]. The predicted peptide product resulting from the Scottish translocation removes the interaction domain for NUDEL. The defective DISC1–NUDEL complex may be a cause of neurodevelopmental abnormalities in schizophrenia [150]. Recently, it has been shown that NUDEL oligopeptidase activity is under tight regulation through binding to DISC1 since a mutation very close to the DISC1 binding site of NUDEL abolishes this activity [151]. Interestingly, NUDEL cleaves a number of neuropeptides in vitro, some of which have previously been implicated in the pathophysiology of schizophrenia, including neurotensin (NT) (reviewed in [152, 153]). Postmortem studies have revealed increased NT levels in the frontal cortex [154] and decreased NT binding in the entorhinal cortex in schizophrenic patients compared to controls [155]. NT receptor agonists may be potential antipsychotics; thus inhibition of NUDEL could lead to increase in local concentration of NT, which may have an antipsychotic effect [151]. Cell culture studies in cortical neurons have found evidence that DISC1 may colocalize with mitochondrial markers and that its subcellular targeting is independent of the NUDEL binding site [149]. Hayashi et al. have also demonstrated that DISC1 and NUDEL bind in a neurodevelopmentally regulated manner and form a trimolecular complex with another protein, lissencephaly 1 (LIS1). LIS1 is involved in neuronal migration and corticogenesis. Although the function of this complex is currently unknown, it is thought to play a role in dynein-mediated motor transport [151].

Another interacting partner of DISC1 is the fasciculation and elongation protein zeta-1 (FEZ1), which is a mammalian homolog of the *Caenorhabditis elegans* UNC-76 protein, involved in axonal outgrowth and fasciculation. Miyoshi et al. demonstrated that DISC1 participates in neurite extension through its C-terminal interaction with FEZ1 [156]. The chromosomal location for FEZ1 was previously implicated in a schizophrenia linkage analysis, although results from different populations vary in significance [157]. A modest association between schizophrenia and FEZ1 polymorphisms has been detected in a subset of Japanese patients [158].

An interesting hypothesis is that altered expression of DISC1 and/or its molecular partners NUDEL, FEZ1, and LIS1 may underlie its pathogenic role in schizophrenia and explain its genetic association [110]. Although DISC1 mRNA expression is unchanged in postmortem human brains of patients with schizophrenia and there is no association with previously identified risk SNPs, the expression of NUDEL, FEZ1, and LIS1 mRNA is significantly reduced in schizophrenic tissue in both the DLPFC and hippocampus and the expression of each gene showed association with a high-risk DISC1 polymorphism [110]. These data implicate genetically linked abnormalities in the DISC1 molecular pathway in the pathophysiology of schizophrenia. Given its role in brain development and plasticity via its interaction with a number of different proteins, *DISC1* remains a candidate gene for schizophrenia and an understanding of its exact mechanistic role in neuronal pathways may shed more light on the disease.

10.3.2 *DTNBP1*

Over the last decade the involvement of *DTNBP1* gene, which encodes dysbindin protein, with schizophrenia has been demonstrated by a large number of association studies and several postmortem findings. However, only recently have we begun to understand the role of dysbindin in the brain and the biological pathways that may be affected by disruption of DTNBP1 function.

Dysbindin overexpression and knockdown experiments using rat cortical cells suggest that dysbindin regulates the expression of synaptosomal-associated protein 25 (SNAP25) and synapsin I proteins in the presynaptic machinery [93, 158]. SNAP25 is a molecular component of the SNARE (soluble N-ethyl-maleimide-sensitive factor attachment protein receptors) protein complex, which is involved in intracellular vesicle trafficking and neurotransmitter release [159]. Synapsin I is localized to synaptic vesicles that are both docked and located away from the plasma membrane [159]. Reduction in protein levels of SNAP25 in the frontal cortex [160] and synapsin I in the hippocampus [161] has been reported in patients with schizophrenia, although other studies have found no change in SNAP25 [162]. Dysbindin also influences extracellular glutamate levels and glutamate release [93]. As discussed earlier, hypofunction of the glutamatergic neurotransmitter system has been implicated in schizophrenia [163].

Numakawa et al. reported that overexpression of dysbindin protected cortical neurons from cell death upon serum deprivation [93, 163]. This effect was mediated through the phosphoinositol 3 (PI3)–kinase–AKT signaling pathway. Downregulation of dysbindin expression caused reduced phosphorylation of AKT [93]. Independently, impaired PI3–kinase–AKT signaling in schizophrenia has also been observed in the PFC [96]. Reduced dysbindin expression in the schizophrenic brain [83, 90] may contribute to the impairment in AKT signaling. Disrupted dysbindin–AKT signaling might cause increased cell vulnerability and neuronal loss in vulnerable brain regions leading to the onset of schizophrenia symptoms [93]. These data establish a role for dysbindin in regulating neuronal cell viability.

Biogenesis of lysosome-related organelles complex-1 (BLOC1) is a ubiquitously expressed aggregation of interacting proteins required for the biogenesis of specialized lysosome-related organelles. This complex is linked to the secretory and endocytic pathways for cellular protein and lipid trafficking [164]. BLOC1 is comprised of several interacting proteins, including pallidin, muted, cappuccino, and dysbindin. Several of the genes that make up the BLOC1 complex are defective in the genetic disorder called Hermansky–Pudlak syndrome (HPS) [165–167]. Mutations in dysbindin cause a form of HPS called HPS7 [89]. A mouse model for HPS, the Sandy mouse, has a deleted *DTNBP1* gene and expresses no dysbindin [89]. This mouse model could be a powerful tool for investigating the function of dysbindin in the brain in vivo. Although the precise biological role of dysbindin in the BLOC1 complex is still unknown, it might be involved with endocytic vesicle docking and fusion. Presynaptic protein expression, glutamate release, AKT phosphorylation, and neuronal viability may also be assessed in vivo using this mouse model.

10.3.3 *NRG1*

Rodent studies have shown NRG1 to function in a converging neurochemical pathway with glutamatergic, cholinergic, and GABAergic receptor systems [168–172]. As molecules located intracellularly, membrane bound, and released into the synapse, neuregulins exert their effects by acting as ligands for three receptors, ErbB2, ErbB3, and ErbB4, which are tyrosine kinases belonging to the epidermal growth factor (EGF) receptor–related family [173]. The ErbB4, in particular, has been shown to be associated with postsynaptic density-95 (PSD-95) and NMDA receptors [174]. PSD-95, like the NMDA receptor subunits, is altered in schizophrenia [175–177] and is reported to enhance NRG1 signaling by ErbB4 dimerization [178]. Additional evidence for a molecular interaction between NRG1 and NMDA receptors has been shown in cerebellar granule cell culture, where the more biologically active β_1 isoform of NRG1 increases the levels of the NR2C subunit of the NMDA receptors [169]. More recently, the same isoform has been shown to cause ErbB dimerization resulting in increased intracellular Ca^{2+} and activation of extracellular regulated kinase (ERK) in the pyramidal neurons of the rat PFC. This downstream cascade is then thought to enhance the actin depolymerization, leading to internalization of NR1 subunits, downregulation of NMDA receptors, and a decrease in NMDA receptor–mediated current [168]. Mice lacking one copy of the *NRG1* gene showed decreased NMDA receptor binding and behavioral features related to schizophrenia [179]. These results are suggestive of the hypothesis that polymorphisms in the *NRG1* gene may lead to deficits in glutamate signaling, offering an explanation of the concept of glutamate hypofunction in schizophrenia.

Neuregulins were initially discovered as acetylcholine receptor inducing activity at the neuromuscular junction, but less is known about their effect on brain nicotinic acetylcholine receptors (nAChRs). Both high- and low-affinity nAChRs are reported to be decreased in the hippocampus, thalamus, and PFC of schizophrenics [19, 180–184]. In cultured hippocampal neurons, the NRG1 isoform β_1 was shown to increase presynaptic neurotransmitter release and to increase the number of surface membrane α_7 nAChRs [171]. Although the exact mechanism is unknown, the upregulation of nAChRs by NRG1 is presumed to occur via intracellular cascade involving ErbB4 receptors due to the colocalization of both of these receptors onto GABA interneurons in the hippocampus [174, 178, 185]. Another isoform of NRG1, the type III, is a membrane-bound bidirectional molecule which is thought to also alter nAChRs. When the extracellular portion of this isoform binds ErbB4 receptors, an intracellular cascade occurs in both the NRG1- and ErbB4-expressing neurons. Back signaling, which occurs in the NRG1-expressing neuron, is accompanied by proteolytic release and translocation of NRG1 intracellular domain into the nucleus, leading to changes in gene expression and resistance to apoptosis [186]. This back signaling in sensory neurons stimulates a redistribution of the nAChR α_7 from a diffuse somatodendritic location to a punctate axonal distribution [187]. In support of this, heterozygous mice of type III isoform have deficits in prepulse inhibition with a decrease in α_7-subunit binding [188]. Concurrently, our own postmortem studies lend support for the interaction of NRG1 and nAChRs by the finding that 5′ NRG1 SNPs identified in the original disease haplotype [179] are associated with altered α_7-subunit receptor binding in the human DLPFC [189].

The immunoglobulin (Ig) NRG isoform has been shown to increase levels of the β_2-subunit protein of the GABA receptors in cerebellar granule cell culture [172]. Furthermore, binding of NRG1 with ErbB4 receptor kinase is necessary for upregulation of GABA receptors [172, 190]. Because the β_2 subunits are responsible for targeting the whole receptor to the cell surface [191, 192], Rieff and colleagues [172] suggest that NRG1 may be responsible for the total number of functional receptors at the postsynaptic terminal. In contrast, infusion of the Ig isoform of NRG1 decreases the mRNA expression of the $GABA_A$ α subunits in hippocampal slices [193]. This report suggests that NRG1 may cause a downregulation of the GABAergic synaptic activity. The variability in the regulation of receptor subunits reviewed above indicates the diversity of the functions served by NRG1 in various brain regions. Most importantly in schizophrenia, the search should be focused on methods to elucidate the function of NRG1 in those brain regions known to be involved, such as the hippocampus, DLPFC, and midbrain.

10.4 CONCLUSIONS

Schizophrenia is a devastating neuropsychiatric disorder the genetics of which has been under extensive investigation for several decades. Despite being an exceedingly complex disease in terms of both etiology and pathogenesis, recent research is finally shedding light on schizophrenia susceptibility genes. Linkage analysis using families with multiple affected individuals has identified regions of the genome that are cotransmitted with the disease and may harbor genes involved in the pathogenesis of schizophrenia. To narrow the chromosomal regions implicated by linkage analysis, association studies using candidate gene analysis have identified a number of genes that may increase susceptibility to schizophrenia. Postmortem brain studies of these genes (such as *COMT, DTNBP1, GRM3, DISC1, NRG1, GAD1,* and *RGS4*) suggest that there are at least four neuronal systems implicated in the pathophysiology of schizophrenia. (1) Genes such as *COMT, GRM3,* and *GAD1* involve dopamine, glutamate, and GABA neurons, and it is conceivable that convergent interactions between these genes may be abnormal in schizophrenia. (2) *DTNBP1*, which encodes dysbindin protein, is involved in the presynaptic machinery and influences extracellular glutamate levels. Dysbindin influences cellular secretory and endocytic pathways responsible for protein and lipid trafficking through its involvement with the BLOC1 protein complex. (3) *DISC1* and its binding partners *FEZ1, NUDEL,* and *LIS1* are involved in cytoplasmic dynein movement, neurofilament assembly, neuronal migration, and neurite morphology and may play a role in the neurodevelopmental deficits observed in schizophrenia. (4) Neuregulins, encoded by *NRG1*, are involved in the maintenance of synaptic plasticity by regulating excitatory (glutamate, ACH) and inhibitory (GABA) neurotransmitters, and a disruption in their function, particularly during development, may contribute to schizophrenia.

Although the precise neurobiological cause of schizophrenia continues to be unknown, the abundance of evidence regarding susceptibility genes for schizophrenia cannot be dismissed. Susceptibility genes may provide important insights into the pathogenesis of schizophrenia. Identification of the molecular and cellular mechanisms that link susceptibility genes to the neurobiological functioning of the brain continues to be a major focus of research. It is conceivable that of the multitude of genes expressed in the brain, some of the susceptibility genes identified would have an effect on one another by either direct molecular binding or indirect upstream functioning. As evidence for the functioning of the various susceptibility genes increases, it may be determined that these genes operate in a convergent molecular pathway affecting neural development and synaptic plasticity. The disruption of multiple genes within this pathway may lead to the development of schizophrenia. Such a convergent biochemical pathway may also be an attractive target for therapeutic intervention.

Despite tremendous advances in schizophrenia research, numerous questions remain unanswered. Future studies are needed to analyze the abundance, distribution, developmental expression patterns, and perhaps most importantly molecular function and abnormalities in schizophrenia susceptibility genes. Data from these studies will not only offer insights into the functions of numerous neurobiological pathways in healthy individuals but also provide a mechanistic link between the genetics and the neurobiology of schizophrenia and other mental illnesses. Further identification of new schizophrenia susceptibility genes, dissection of the molecular pathways involved, discovery of the underlying causative defect in the schizophrenic brain, and ultimately development of better therapeutic strategies are important future goals of schizophrenia research that can be advanced by the study of postmortem brains.

REFERENCES

1. Kendler, K. S. (1983). Overview: a current perspective on twin studies of schizophrenia. *Am. J. Psychiatry* 140(11), 1413–1425.
2. Kendler, K. S., et al. (1994). An epidemiologic, clinical, and family study of simple schizophrenia in County Roscommon, Ireland. *Am. J. Psychiatry* 151(1), 27–34.
3. Tsuang, M. T., Gilbertson, M. W., and Faraone, S. V. (1991). The genetics of schizophrenia. Current knowledge and future directions. *Schizophr. Res.* 4(2), 157–171.
4. Risch, N. (1990). Linkage strategies for genetically complex traits. II. The power of affected relative pairs. *Am. J. Hum. Genet.* 46(2), 229–241.
5. Harrison, P. J., and Weinberger, D. R. (2005). Schizophrenia genes, gene expression, and neuropathology: On the matter of their convergence. *Mol. Psychiatry* 10(4), 420.
6. Murray, R. M. (1994). Neurodevelopmental schizophrenia: The rediscovery of dementia praecox. *Br. J. Psychiatry Suppl.* 165(25), 6–12.
7. de Haan, L., and Bakker, J. M. (2004). Overview of neuropathological theories of schizophrenia: From degeneration to progressive developmental disorder. *Psychopathology* 37(1), 1–7.
8. Seeman, P., and Lee, T. (1975). Antipsychotic drugs: Direct correlation between clinical potency and presynaptic action on dopamine neurons. *Science* 188(4194), 1217–1219.
9. Creese, I., Burt, D. R., and Snyder, S. H. (1976). Dopamine receptor binding predicts clinical and pharmacological potencies of antischizophrenic drugs. *Science* 192(4238), 481–483.
10. Pycock, C. J., Kerwin, R. W., and Carter, C. J. (1980). Effect of lesion of cortical dopamine terminals on subcortical dopamine receptors in rats. *Nature* 286(5768), 74–76.
11. Weinberger, D. R., Berman, K. F., and Chase, T. N. (1988). Mesocortical dopaminergic function and human cognition. *Ann. N.Y. Acad. Sci.* 537, 330–338.
12. Weinberger, D. R., et al. (2001). Prefrontal neurons and the genetics of schizophrenia. *Biol. Psychiatry* 50(11), 825–844.
13. Laruelle, M., Kegeles, L. S., and Abi-Dargham, A. (2003). Glutamate, dopamine, and schizophrenia: From pathophysiology to treatment. *Ann. N. Y. Acad. Sci.* 1003, 138–158.
14. Kegeles, L. S., et al. (2000). Modulation of amphetamine-induced striatal dopamine release by ketamine in humans: Implications for schizophrenia. *Biol. Psychiatry* 48(7), 627–640.

15. Akbarian, S., et al. (1995). GABAA receptor subunit gene expression in human prefrontal cortex: comparison of schizophrenics and controls. *Cereb. Cortex* 5(6), 550–560.
16. Benes, F. M., et al. (1996). Up-regulation of GABAA receptor binding on neurons of the prefrontal cortex in schizophrenic subjects. *Neuroscience* 75(4), 1021–1031.
17. Guidotti, A., et al. (2000). Decrease in reelin and glutamic acid decarboxylase67 (GAD67) expression in schizophrenia and bipolar disorder: A postmortem brain study. *Arch. Gen. Psychiatry* 57(11), 1061–1069.
18. Volk, D. W., et al. (2000). Decreased glutamic acid decarboxylase67 messenger RNA expression in a subset of prefrontal cortical gamma-aminobutyric acid neurons in subjects with schizophrenia. *Arch. Gen. Psychiatry* 57(3), 237–245.
19. Freedman, R., Adams, C. E., and Leonard, S. (2000). The alpha7-nicotinic acetylcholine receptor and the pathology of hippocampal interneurons in schizophrenia. *J. Chem. Neuroanat* 20(3–4), 299–306.
20. Tandon, R. (1999). Cholinergic aspects of schizophrenia. *Br. J. Psychiatry Suppl.* 37, 7–11.
21. Friedman, J. I. (2004). Cholinergic targets for cognitive enhancement in schizophrenia: Focus on cholinesterase inhibitors and muscarinic agonists. *Psychopharmacology (Berl.)* 174(1), 45–53.
22. Owen, M. J., Williams, N. M., and O'Donovan, M. C. (2004). The molecular genetics of schizophrenia: New findings promise new insights. *Mol. Psychiatry* 9(1), 14–27.
23. Owen, M. J., Holmans, P., and McGuffin, P. (1997). Association studies in psychiatric genetics. *Mol. Psychiatry* 2(4), 270–273.
24. Bassett A. S., Chow, E. W., and Weksberg, R. (2000). Chromosomal abnormalities and schizophrenia. *Am. J. Med. Genet.* 97(1), 45–51.
25. MacIntyre, D. J., et al. (2003). Chromosomal abnormalities and mental illness. *Mol. Psychiatry* 8(3), 275–287.
26. St Clair, D., et al. (1990). Association within a family of a balanced autosomal translocation with major mental illness. *Lancet* 336(8706), 13–16.
27. Blackwood, D. H., et al. (2001). Schizophrenia and affective disorders—cosegregation with a translocation at chromosome 1q42 that directly disrupts brain-expressed genes: clinical and P300 findings in a family. *Am. J. Hum. Genet.* 69(2), 428–433.
28. Pulver, A. E., et al. (1994). Psychotic illness in patients diagnosed with velo-cardio-facial syndrome and their relatives. *J. Nerv. Ment. Dis.* 182(8), 476–478.
29. Shprintzen, R. J., et al. (1992). Late-onset psychosis in the velo-cardio-facial syndrome. *Am. J. Med. Genet.* 42(1), 141–142.
30. Papolos, D. F., et al. (1996). Bipolar spectrum disorders in patients diagnosed with velo-cardio-facial syndrome: Does a hemizygous deletion of chromosome 22q11 result in bipolar affective disorder? *Am. J. Psychiatry* 153(12), 1541–1547.
31. Murphy, K. C., Jones, L. A., and Owen, M. J. (1999). High rates of schizophrenia in adults with velo-cardio-facial syndrome. *Arch. Gen. Psychiatry* 56(10), 940–945.
32. Lander, E. S. (1988). Splitting schizophrenia. *Nature* 336(6195), 105–106.
33. Tenhunen, J., et al. (1994). Genomic organization of the human catechol O-methyltransferase gene and its expression from two distinct promoters. *Eur. J. Biochem.* 223(3), 1049–1059.
34. Mannisto, P. T., and Kaakkola, S. (1999). Catechol-O-methyltransferase (COMT): biochemistry, molecular biology, pharmacology, and clinical efficacy of the new selective COMT inhibitors. *Pharmacol. Rev.* 51(4), 593–628.

35. Matsumoto, M., et al. (2003). Catechol O-methyltransferase (COMT) mRNA expression in the dorsolateral prefrontal cortex of patients with schizophrenia. *Neuropsychopharmacology* 28(8), 1521–1530.
36. Chen, J., et al. (2004). Functional analysis of genetic variation in catechol-O-methyltransferase (COMT): Effects on mRNA, protein, and enzyme activity in postmortem human brain. *Am. J. Hum. Genet.* 75(5), 807–821.
37. Kastner, A., et al. (1994). Immunohistochemical study of catechol-O-methyltransferase in the human mesostriatal system. *Neuroscience* 62(2), 449–457.
38. Karhunen, T., et al. (1995). Catechol-O-methyltransferase (COMT) in rat brain: Immunoelectron microscopic study with an antiserum against rat recombinant COMT protein. *Neurosci. Lett.* 187(1), 57–60.
39. Shifman, S., et al. (2002). A highly significant association between a COMT haplotype and schizophrenia. *Am. J. Hum. Genet.* 71(6), 1296–1302.
40. Palmatier, M. A., et al. (2004). COMT haplotypes suggest P2 promoter region relevance for schizophrenia. *Mol. Psychiatry* 9(9), 859–870.
41. Li, T., et al. (1996). Preferential transmission of the high activity allele of COMT in schizophrenia. *Psychiatr. Genet.* 6(3), 131–133.
42. Lee, S. G., et al. (2005). Association of Ala72Ser polymorphism with COMT enzyme activity and the risk of schizophrenia in Koreans. *Hum. Genet.* 116(4), 319–328.
43. Bray, N. J., et al. (2003). A haplotype implicated in schizophrenia susceptibility is associated with reduced COMT expression in human brain. *Am. J. Hum. Genet.* 73(1), 152–161.
44. Lotta, T., et al. (1995). Kinetics of human soluble and membrane-bound catechol O-methyltransferase: A revised mechanism and description of the thermolabile variant of the enzyme. *Biochemistry* 34(13), 4202–4210.
45. Murphy, D. L., and Wyatt, R. J. (1975). Neurotransmitter-related enzymes in the major psychiatric disorders: I. Catechol-O-methyl transferase, monoamine oxidase in the affective disorders, and factors affecting some behaviorally correlated enzyme activities. *Res. Publ. Assoc. Res. Nerv. Ment. Dis.* 54, 277–288.
46. Cross, A. J., et al. (1978). The activities of brain dopamine-beta-hydroxylase and catechol-O-methyl transferase in schizophrenics and controls. *Psychopharmacology (Berl.)* 59(2), 117–121.
47. Tunbridge, E., et al. (2004). Catechol-O-methyltransferase (COMT) and proline dehydrogenase (PRODH) mRNAs in the dorsolateral prefrontal cortex in schizophrenia, bipolar disorder, and major depression. *Synapse* 51(2), 112–118.
48. Lewis, D. A., et al. (2001). Dopamine transporter immunoreactivity in monkey cerebral cortex: Regional, laminar, and ultrastructural localization. *J. Comp. Neurol.* 432(1), 119–136.
49. Moron, J. A., et al. (2002). Dopamine uptake through the norepinephrine transporter in brain regions with low levels of the dopamine transporter: Evidence from knock-out mouse lines. *J. Neurosci.* 22(2), 389–395.
50. Mazei, M. S., et al. (2002). Effects of catecholamine uptake blockers in the caudate-putamen and subregions of the medial prefrontal cortex of the rat. *Brain Res.* 936(1–2), 58–67.
51. Tank, A. W., et al. (1998). Regulation of tyrosine hydroxylase gene expression by transsynaptic mechanisms and cell-cell contact. *Adv. Pharmacol.* 42, 25–29.
52. Roberts, A. C., et al. (1994). 6-Hydroxydopamine lesions of the prefrontal cortex in monkeys enhance performance on an analog of the Wisconsin Card Sort Test: Possible interactions with subcortical dopamine. *J. Neurosci.* 14(5 Pt 1), 2531–2544.

53. Nagatsu, T. (1995). Tyrosine hydroxylase: Human isoforms, structure and regulation in physiology and pathology. *Essays Biochem.* 30, 15–35.
54. Kumer, S. C., and Vrana, K. E. (1996). Intricate regulation of tyrosine hydroxylase activity and gene expression. *J. Neurochem.* 67(2), 443–462.
55. Kolachana, B. S., Saunders, R. C., and Weinberger, D. R. (1995). Augmentation of prefrontal cortical monoaminergic activity inhibits dopamine release in the caudate nucleus: An in vivo neurochemical assessment in the rhesus monkey. *Neuroscience* 69(3), 859–868.
56. Huotari, M., et al. (2002). Brain catecholamine metabolism in catechol-O-methyltransferase (COMT)-deficient mice. *Eur. J. Neurosci.* 15(2), 246–256.
57. Gogos, J. A., et al. (1998). Catechol-O-methyltransferase-deficient mice exhibit sexually dimorphic changes in catecholamine levels and behavior. *Proc. Natl. Acad. Sci. U.S.A.* 95(17), 9991–9996.
58. Bertolino, A., et al. (2000). The relationship between dorsolateral prefrontal neuronal N-acetylaspartate and evoked release of striatal dopamine in schizophrenia. *Neuropsychopharmacology* 22(2), 125–132.
59. Akil, M., et al. (2003). Catechol-O-methyltransferase genotype and dopamine regulation in the human brain. *J. Neurosci.* 23(6), 2008–2013.
60. Seeman, P., et al. (1976). Antipsychotic drug doses and neuroleptic/dopamine receptors. *Nature* 261(5562), 717–719.
61. Creese, I., Burt, D. R., and Snyder, S. H. (1996). Dopamine receptor binding predicts clinical and pharmacological potencies of antischizophrenic drugs. *J. Neuropsychiatry Clin. Neurosci.* 8(2), 223–226.
62. Seeman, P., et al. (1975). Brain receptors for antipsychotic drugs and dopamine: Direct binding assays. *Proc. Natl. Acad. Sci. U.S.A.* 72(11), 4376–4380.
63. Owen, F., et al. (1978). Increased dopamine-receptor sensitivity in schizophrenia. *Lancet* 2(8083), 223–226.
64. Mita, T., et al. (1986). Decreased serotonin S2 and increased dopamine D2 receptors in chronic schizophrenics. *Biol. Psychiatry* 21(14), 1407–1414.
65. Lee, T., and Seeman, P. (1980). Abnormal neuroleptic/dopamine receptors in schizophrenia. *Adv. Biochem. Psychopharmacol.* 21, 435–442.
66. Reynolds, G. P. (1981). Dopamine receptors in post-mortem schizophrenic brains. *Lancet* 1(8232), 1261.
67. Cross, A. J., Crow, T. J., and Owen, F. (1981). 3H-Flupenthixol binding in post-mortem brains of schizophrenics: Evidence for a selective increase in dopamine D2 receptors. *Psychopharmacology (Berl.)* 74(2), 122–124.
68. Mackay, A. V., et al. (1980). Dopaminergic abnormalities in postmortem schizophrenic brain. *Adv. Biochem. Psychopharmacol.* 24, 325–333.
69. Wong, D. F., et al. (1986). Positron emission tomography reveals elevated D2 dopamine receptors in drug-naive schizophrenics. *Science* 234(4783), 1558–1563.
70. Kampman, O., et al. (2003). Dopamine receptor D2 -141C insertion/deletion polymorphism in a Finnish population with schizophrenia. *Psychiatry Res.* 121(1), 89–92.
71. Hovatta, I., et al. (1994). Linkage analysis in two schizophrenic families originating from a restricted subpopulation of Finland. *Psychiatr. Genet.* 4(3), 143–152.
72. Farde, L., et al. (1990). D2 dopamine receptors in neuroleptic-naive schizophrenic patients. A positron emission tomography study with [11C]raclopride. *Arch. Gen. Psychiatry* 47(3), 213–219.

73. Farde, L., et al. (1987). No D2 receptor increase in PET study of schizophrenia. *Arch. Gen. Psychiatry* 44(7), 671–672.
74. Seeman, P., et al. (1997). Dopamine D2-like sites in schizophrenia, but not in Alzheimer's, Huntington's, or control brains, for [3H]benzquinoline. *Synapse* 25(2), 137–146.
75. Knable, M. B., et al. (1997). Altered dopaminergic function and negative symptoms in drug-free patients with schizophrenia. [123I]-iodobenzamide SPECT study. *Br. J. Psychiatry* 171, 574–577.
76. Jonsson, E. G., et al. (1999). Association between a promoter polymorphism in the dopamine D2 receptor gene and schizophrenia. *Schizophr. Res.* 40(1), 31–36.
77. Arinami, T., et al. (1994). Association of dopamine D2 receptor molecular variant with schizophrenia. *Lancet* 343(8899), 703–704.
78. Virgos, C., et al. (2001). Association study of schizophrenia with polymorphisms at six candidate genes. *Schizophr. Res.* 49(1/2), 65–71.
79. Breen, G., et al. (1999). -141 C del/ins polymorphism of the dopamine receptor 2 gene is associated with schizophrenia in a British population. *Am. J. Med. Genet.* 88(4), 407–410.
80. Jonsson, E. G., et al. (2003). Dopamine D2 receptor gene Ser311Cys variant and schizophrenia: Association study and meta-analysis. *Am. J. Med. Genet. B. Neuropsychiatr. Genet.* 119(1), 28–34.
81. Glatt, S. J., Faraone, S. V., and Tsuang, M. T. (2003). Meta-analysis identifies an association between the dopamine D2 receptor gene and schizophrenia. *Mol. Psychiatry* 8(11), 911–915.
82. Dubertret, C., et al. (2004). The 3′ region of the DRD2 gene is involved in genetic susceptibility to schizophrenia. *Schizophr. Res.* 67(1), 75–85.
83. Weickert, C. S., et al. (2004). Human dysbindin (DTNBP1) gene expression in normal brain and in schizophrenic prefrontal cortex and midbrain. *Arch. Gen. Psychiatry* 61(6), 544–555.
84. Blake, D. J., et al. (2002). Function and genetics of dystrophin and dystrophin-related proteins in muscle. *Physiol. Rev.* 82(2), 291–329.
85. Blake, D. J., et al. (1999). Different dystrophin-like complexes are expressed in neurons and glia. *J. Cell. Biol.* 147(3), 645–658.
86. Blake, D. J., and Kroger, S. (2000). The neurobiology of duchenne muscular dystrophy: Learning lessons from muscle? *Trends Neurosci.* 23(3), 92–99.
87. Benson, M. A., et al. (2001). Dysbindin, a novel coiled-coil-containing protein that interacts with the dystrobrevins in muscle and brain. *J. Biol. Chem.* 276(26), 24232–24241.
88. Sillitoe, R. V., et al. (2003). Abnormal dysbindin expression in cerebellar mossy fiber synapses in the mdx mouse model of Duchenne muscular dystrophy. *J. Neurosci.* 23(16), 6576–6585.
89. Li, W., et al. (2003). Hermansky-Pudlak syndrome type 7 (HPS-7) results from mutant dysbindin, a member of the biogenesis of lysosome-related organelles complex 1 (BLOC-1). *Nat. Genet.* 35(1), 84–89.
90. Talbot, K., et al. (2004). Dysbindin-1 is reduced in intrinsic, glutamatergic terminals of the hippocampal formation in schizophrenia. *J. Clin. Invest.* 113(9), 1353–1363.
91. Bray, N. J., et al. (2005). Haplotypes at the dystrobrevin binding protein 1 (DTNBP1) gene locus mediate risk for schizophrenia through reduced DTNBP1 expression. *Hum. Mol. Genet.* 14(14), 1947–1954.

92. Bray, N. J., et al. (2003). Cis-acting variation in the expression of a high proportion of genes in human brain. *Hum. Genet.* 113(2), 149–153.
93. Numakawa, T., et al. (2004). Evidence of novel neuronal functions of dysbindin, a susceptibility gene for schizophrenia. *Hum. Mol. Genet.* 13(21), 2699–2708.
94. Coyle, J. T., and Duman, R. S. (2003). Finding the intracellular signaling pathways affected by mood disorder treatments. *Neuron* 38(2), 157–160.
95. Owada, Y., et al. (1997). Expression of mRNA for Akt, serine-threonine protein kinase, in the brain during development and its transient enhancement following axotomy of hypoglossal nerve. *J. Mol. Neurosci.* 9(1), 27–33.
96. Emamian, E. S., et al. (2004). Convergent evidence for impaired AKT1-GSK3beta signaling in schizophrenia. *Nat. Genet.* 36(2), 131–137.
97. Kozlovsky, N., et al. (2004). Reduced GSK-3beta mRNA levels in postmortem dorsolateral prefrontal cortex of schizophrenic patients. *J. Neural. Transm.* 111(12), 1583–1592.
98. Scherer, S. W., et al. (1996). Localization of two metabotropic glutamate receptor genes, GRM3 and GRM8, to human chromosome 7q. *Genomics* 31(2), 230–233.
99. Ekelund, J., et al. (2000). Genome-wide scan for schizophrenia in the Finnish population: Evidence for a locus on chromosome 7q22. *Hum. Mol. Genet.* 9(7), 1049–1057.
100. Corti, C., et al. (2001). Identification and characterization of the promoter region of the GRM3 gene. *Biochem. Biophys. Res. Commun.* 286(2), 381–387.
101. Lovinger, D. M., and McCool, B. A. (1995). Metabotropic glutamate receptor-mediated presynaptic depression at corticostriatal synapses involves mGLuR2 or 3. *J. Neurophysiol.* 73(3), 1076–1083.
102. Battaglia, G., Monn, J. A., and Schoepp, D. D (1997). In vivo inhibition of veratridine-evoked release of striatal excitatory amino acids by the group II metabotropic glutamate receptor agonist LY354740 in rats. *Neurosci. Lett.* 229(3), 161–164.
103. Ohnuma, T., et al. (1998). Expression of the human excitatory amino acid transporter 2 and metabotropic glutamate receptors 3 and 5 in the prefrontal cortex from normal individuals and patients with schizophrenia. *Brain Res. Mol. Brain Res.* 56(1/2), 207–217.
104. Crook, J. M., et al. (2002). Comparative analysis of group II metabotropic glutamate receptor immunoreactivity in Brodmann's area 46 of the dorsolateral prefrontal cortex from patients with schizophrenia and normal subjects. *Mol. Psychiatry* 7(2), 157–164.
105. Richardson-Burns, S. M., et al. (2000). Metabotropic glutamate receptor mRNA expression in the schizophrenic thalamus. *Biol. Psychiatry* 47(1), 22–28.
106. Egan, M. F., et al. (2004). Variation in GRM3 affects cognition, prefrontal glutamate, and risk for schizophrenia. *Proc. Natl. Acad. Sci. U.S.A.* 101(34), 12604–12609.
107. Sartorius, L., et al. (2006). Alternative splicing of human metabotropic glutamate receptor 3. *J. Neurochem.* 96(4), 1139–1148.
108. Schurov, I. L., et al. (2004). Expression of disrupted in schizophrenia 1 (DISC1) protein in the adult and developing mouse brain indicates its role in neurodevelopment. *Mol. Psychiatry* 9(12), 1100–1110.
109. Sawamura, N., et al. (2005). A form of DISC1 enriched in nucleus: Altered subcellular distribution in orbitofrontal cortex in psychosis and substance/alcohol abuse. *Proc. Natl. Acad. Sci. U.S.A.* 102(4), 1187–1192.
110. Lipska, B. K., et al. (2006). Expression of DISC1 binding partners is reduced in schizophrenia and associated with DISC1 SNPs. *Hum. Mol. Genet.* 15(8), 1245–1258.

111. Steinthorsdottir, V., et al. (2004). Multiple novel transcription initiation sites for NRG1. *Gene* 342(1), 97–105.
112. Falls, D. L. (2003). Neuregulins and the neuromuscular system: 10 years of answers and questions. *J. Neurocytol.* 32(5–8), 619–647.
113. Garratt, A. N., Britsch, S., and Birchmeier, C. (2000). Neuregulin, a factor with many functions in the life of a schwann cell. *Bioessays* 22(11), 987–996.
114. Law, A. J., et al. (2003). Expression of NMDA receptor NR1, NR2A and NR2B subunit mRNAs during development of the human hippocampal formation. *Eur. J. Neurosci.* 18(5), 1197–1205.
115. Hashimoto, R., et al. (2004). Expression analysis of neuregulin-1 in the dorsolateral prefrontal cortex in schizophrenia. *Mol. Psychiatry* 9(3), 299–307.
116. Law, A. J., et al. (2006). Neuregulin 1 transcripts are differentially expressed in schizophrenia and regulated by 5' SNPs associated with the disease. *Proc. Natl. Acad. Sci. U.S.A.* 103(17), 6747–6752.
117. Tkachev, D., et al. (2003). Oligodendrocyte dysfunction in schizophrenia and bipolar disorder. *Lancet* 362(9386), 798–805.
118. Hakak, Y., et al. (2001). Genome-wide expression analysis reveals dysregulation of myelination-related genes in chronic schizophrenia. *Proc. Natl. Acad. Sci. U.S.A.* 98(8), 4746–4751.
119. Beltaifa, S., et al. (2005). Expression levels and cellular localization of ErbB receptor mRNA in the dorsolateral prefrontal cortex in schizophrenia. *J. Neuropath. Exp. Neurol.* 64(5): 437.
120. Bu, D. F., and Tobin, A. J. (1994). The exon-intron organization of the genes (GAD1 and GAD2) encoding two human glutamate decarboxylases (GAD67 and GAD65) suggests that they derive from a common ancestral GAD. *Genomics* 21(1), 222–228.
121. Bu, D. F., et al. (1992). Two human glutamate decarboxylases, 65-kDa GAD and 67-kDa GAD, are each encoded by a single gene. *Proc. Natl. Acad. Sci. U.S.A.* 89(6), 2115–2119.
122. Esclapez, M., et al. (1994). Comparative localization of two forms of glutamic acid decarboxylase and their mRNAs in rat brain supports the concept of functional differences between the forms. *J. Neurosci.* 14(3 Pt 2), 1834–1855.
123. Reetz, A., et al. (1991). GABA and pancreatic beta-cells: Colocalization of glutamic acid decarboxylase (GAD) and GABA with synaptic-like microvesicles suggests their role in GABA storage and secretion. *Embo. J.* 10(5), 1275–1284.
124. Heckers, S., et al. (2002). Differential hippocampal expression of glutamic acid decarboxylase 65 and 67 messenger RNA in bipolar disorder and schizophrenia. *Arch. Gen. Psychiatry* 59(6), 521–529.
125. Dracheva, S., et al. (2004). GAD67 and GAD65 mRNA and protein expression in cerebrocortical regions of elderly patients with schizophrenia. *J. Neurosci. Res.* 76(4), 581–592.
126. Benes, F. M., and Berretta, S. (2001). GABAergic interneurons: Implications for understanding schizophrenia and bipolar disorder. *Neuropsychopharmacology* 25(1), 1–27.
127. Huntsman, M. M., et al. (1998). Altered ratios of alternatively spliced long and short gamma2 subunit mRNAs of the gamma-amino butyrate type A receptor in prefrontal cortex of schizophrenics. *Proc. Natl. Acad. Sci. U.S.A.* 95(25), 15066–15071.
128. Hanada, S., et al. (1987). [3H]muscimol binding sites increased in autopsied brains of chronic schizophrenics. *Life Sci.* 40(3), 259–266.

129. Benes, F. M., et al. (1996). Differences in the subregional and cellular distribution of GABAA receptor binding in the hippocampal formation of schizophrenic brain. *Synapse* 22(4), 338–349.

130. Impagnatiello, F., et al. (1998). A decrease of reelin expression as a putative vulnerability factor in schizophrenia. *Proc. Natl. Acad. Sci. U.S.A.* 95(26), 15718–15723.

131. Ishikawa, M., et al. (2004). GABAA receptor gamma subunits in the prefrontal cortex of patients with schizophrenia and bipolar disorder. *Neuroreport* 15(11), 1809–1812.

132. Ishikawa, M., et al. (2004). Immunohistochemical and immunoblot study of GABA(A) alpha1 and beta2/3 subunits in the prefrontal cortex of subjects with schizophrenia and bipolar disorder. *Neurosci. Res.* 50(1), 77–84.

133. Dean, B., et al. (1999). Changes in serotonin2A and GABA(A) receptors in schizophrenia: Studies on the human dorsolateral prefrontal cortex. *J. Neurochem.* 72(4), 1593–1599.

134. Dean, B. (2004). The neurobiology of bipolar disorder: Findings using human postmortem central nervous system tissue. *Aust. N. Z. J. Psychiatry* 38(3), 135–140.

135. Volk, D. W., et al. (2002). Reciprocal alterations in pre- and postsynaptic inhibitory markers at chandelier cell inputs to pyramidal neurons in schizophrenia. *Cereb. Cortex* 12(10), 1063–1070.

136. Taymans, J. M., et al. (2004). Dopamine receptor-mediated regulation of RGS2 and RGS4 mRNA differentially depends on ascending dopamine projections and time. *Eur. J. Neurosci.* 19(8), 2249–2260.

137. Grillet, N., et al. (2003). Dynamic expression of RGS4 in the developing nervous system and regulation by the neural type-specific transcription factor Phox2b. *J. Neurosci.* 23(33), 10613–10621.

138. Mirnics, K., et al. (2001). Disease-specific changes in regulator of G-protein signaling 4 (RGS4) expression in schizophrenia. *Mol. Psychiatry* 6(3), 293–301.

139. Erdely, H. A., et al. (2004). Regional expression of RGS4 mRNA in human brain. *Eur. J. Neurosci.* 19(11), 3125–3128.

140. Morris, J. A., et al. (2003). DISC1 (Disrupted-In-Schizophrenia 1) is a centrosome-associated protein that interacts with MAP1A, MIPT3, ATF4/5 and NUDEL: Regulation and loss of interaction with mutation. *Hum. Mol. Genet.* 12(13), 1591–1608.

141. Ozeki, Y., et al. (2003). Disrupted-in-Schizophrenia-1 (DISC-1): Mutant truncation prevents binding to NudE-like (NUDEL) and inhibits neurite outgrowth. *Proc. Natl. Aca. Sci. U.S.A.* 100(1), 289–294.

142. Millar, J. K., Christie, S., and Porteous, D. J. (2003). Yeast two-hybrid screens implicate DISC1 in brain development and function. *Biochem. Biophys. Res. Commun.* 311(4), 1019–1025.

143. Niethammer, M., et al. (2000). NUDEL is a novel Cdk5 substrate that associates with LIS1 and cytoplasmic dynein. *Neuron* 28(3), 697–711.

144. Sasaki, S., et al. (2000). A LIS1/NUDEL/cytoplasmic dynein heavy chain complex in the developing and adult nervous system. *Neuron* 28(3), 681–696.

145. Sweeney, K. J., Prokscha, A., and Eichele, G. (2001). NudE-L, a novel Lis1-interacting protein, belongs to a family of vertebrate coiled-coil proteins. *Mech. Dev.* 101(1–2), 21–33.

146. Nguyen, M. D., et al. (2004). A NUDEL-dependent mechanism of neurofilament assembly regulates the integrity of CNS neurons. *Nat. Cell. Biol.* 6(7), 595–608.

147. Feng, Y., and Walsh, C. A. (2004). Mitotic spindle regulation by Nde1 controls cerebral cortical size. *Neuron* 44(2), 279–293.
148. Shu, T., et al. (2004). Ndel1 operates in a common pathway with LIS1 and cytoplasmic dynein to regulate cortical neuronal positioning. *Neuron* 44(2), 263–277.
149. Brandon, N. J., et al. (2005). Subcellular targeting of DISC1 is dependent on a domain independent from the Nudel binding site. *Mol. Cell Neurosci.* 28(4), 613–624.
150. Brandon, N. J., et al. (2004). Disrupted in Schizophrenia 1 and Nudel form a neurodevelopmentally regulated protein complex: Implications for schizophrenia and other major neurological disorders. *Mol. Cell Neurosci.* 25(1), 42–55.
151. Hayashi, M. A., et al. (2005). Inhibition of NUDEL (nuclear distribution element-like)-oligopeptidase activity by disrupted-in-schizophrenia 1. *Proc. Natl. Acad. Sci. U.S.A.* 102(10), 3828–3833.
152. Caceda, R., Kinkead, B., and Nemeroff, C. B. (2003). Do neurotensin receptor agonists represent a novel class of antipsychotic drugs? *Semin. Clin. Neuropsychiatry* 8(2), 94–108.
153. Kinkead, B., and Nemeroff, C. B. (1994). The effects of typical and atypical antipsychotic drugs on neurotensin-containing neurons in the central nervous system. *J. Clin. Psychiatry* 55(Suppl. B), 30–32.
154. Nemeroff, C. B., et al. (1983). Regional brain concentrations of neuropeptides in Huntington's chorea and schizophrenia. *Science* 221(4614), 972–975.
155. Wolf, S. S., et al. (1995). Autoradiographic characterization of neurotensin receptors in the entorhinal cortex of schizophrenic patients and control subjects. *J. Neural. Transm. Gen. Sect.* 102(1), 55–65.
156. Miyoshi, K., et al. (2003). Disrupted-In-Schizophrenia 1, a candidate gene for schizophrenia, participates in neurite outgrowth. *Mol. Psychiatry* 8(7), 685–694.
157. Lewis, C. M., et al. (2003). Genome scan meta-analysis of schizophrenia and bipolar disorder, part II: Schizophrenia. *Am. J. Hum. Genet.* 73(1), 34–48.
158. Yamada, K., et al. (2004). Association analysis of FEZ1 variants with schizophrenia in Japanese cohorts. *Biol. Psychiatry* 56(9), 683–690.
159. Turner, K. M., Burgoyne, R. D., and Morgan, A. (1999). Protein phosphorylation and the regulation of synaptic membrane traffic. *Trends Neurosci.* 22(10), 459–464.
160. Honer, W. G., et al. (2002). Abnormalities of SNARE mechanism proteins in anterior frontal cortex in severe mental illness. *Cereb Cortex* 12(4), 349–356.
161. Vawter, M. P., et al. (2002). Reduction of synapsin in the hippocampus of patients with bipolar disorder and schizophrenia. *Mol. Psychiatry* 7(6), 571–578.
162. Halim, N. D., et al. (2003). Presynaptic proteins in the prefrontal cortex of patients with schizophrenia and rats with abnormal prefrontal development. *Mol. Psychiatry* 8(9), 797–810.
163. Tsai, G., and Coyle, J. T. (2002). Glutamatergic mechanisms in schizophrenia. *Annu. Rev. Pharmacol. Toxicol.* 42, 165–179.
164. Dell'Angelica E. C. (2004). The building BLOC(k)s of lysosomes and related organelles. *Curr. Opin. Cell Biol.* 16(4), 458–464.
165. Falcon-Perez, J. M., and Dell'Angelica, E. C. (2002). The pallidin (Pldn) gene and the role of SNARE proteins in melanosome biogenesis. *Pigment Cell Res.* 15(2), 82–86.
166. Moriyama, K., and Bonifacino, J. S. (2002). Pallidin is a component of a multi-protein complex involved in the biogenesis of lysosome-related organelles. *Traffic* 3(9), 666–677.

167. Ciciotte, S. L., et al. (2003). Cappuccino, a mouse model of Hermansky-Pudlak syndrome, encodes a novel protein that is part of the pallidin-muted complex (BLOC-1). *Blood* 101(11), 4402–4407.
168. Gu, Z., et al. (2005). Regulation of NMDA receptors by neuregulin signaling in prefrontal cortex. *J. Neurosci.* 25(20), 4974–4984.
169. Ozaki, M., et al. (1997). Neuregulin-beta induces expression of an NMDA-receptor subunit. *Nature* 390(6661), 691–694.
170. Yang, X., et al. (1998). A cysteine-rich isoform of neuregulin controls the level of expression of neuronal nicotinic receptor channels during synaptogenesis. *Neuron* 20(2), 255–270.
171. Liu, Y., et al. (2001). Neuregulins increase alpha7 nicotinic acetylcholine receptors and enhance excitatory synaptic transmission in GABAergic interneurons of the hippocampus. *J. Neurosci.* 21(15), 5660–5669.
172. Rieff, H. I., et al. (1999). Neuregulin induces GABA(A) receptor subunit expression and neurite outgrowth in cerebellar granule cells. *J. Neurosci.* 19(24), 10757–10766.
173. Corfas, G., Roy, K., and Buxbaum, J. D. (2004). Neuregulin 1-erbB signaling and the molecular/cellular basis of schizophrenia. *Nat. Neurosci.* 7(6), 575–580.
174. Garcia, R. A., Vasudevan, K., and Buonanno, A. (2000). The neuregulin receptor ErbB-4 interacts with PDZ-containing proteins at neuronal synapses. *Proc. Natl. Acad. Sci. U.S.A.* 97(7), 3596–3601.
175. Dracheva, S., et al. (2001). N-methyl-D-aspartic acid receptor expression in the dorsolateral prefrontal cortex of elderly patients with schizophrenia. *Am. J. Psychiatry* 158(9), 1400–1410.
176. Ohnuma, T., et al. (2000). Gene expression of PSD95 in prefrontal cortex and hippocampus in schizophrenia. *Neuroreport* 11(14), 3133–3137.
177. Gao, X. M., et al. (2000). Ionotropic glutamate receptors and expression of N-methyl-D-aspartate receptor subunits in subregions of human hippocampus: Effects of schizophrenia. *Am. J. Psychiatry* 157(7), 1141–1149.
178. Huang, Y. Z., et al. (2000). Regulation of neuregulin signaling by PSD-95 interacting with ErbB4 at CNS synapses. *Neuron* 26(2), 443–455.
179. Stefansson, H., et al. (2002). Neuregulin 1 and susceptibility to schizophrenia. *Am. J. Hum. Genet.* 71(4), 877–892.
180. Breese, C. R., et al. (2000). Abnormal regulation of high affinity nicotinic receptors in subjects with schizophrenia. *Neuropsychopharmacology* 23(4), 351–364.
181. Guan, Z. Z., et al. (2000). Decreased protein levels of nicotinic receptor subunits in the hippocampus and temporal cortex of patients with Alzheimer's disease. *J. Neurochem.* 74(1), 237–243.
182. Court, J., et al. (1999). Neuronal nicotinic receptors in dementia with Lewy bodies and schizophrenia: Alpha-bungarotoxin and nicotine binding in the thalamus. *J. Neurochem.* 73(4), 1590–1597.
183. Spurden, D. P., et al. (1997). Nicotinic receptor distribution in the human thalamus: Autoradiographical localization of [3H]nicotine and [125I] alpha-bungarotoxin binding. *J. Chem. Neuroanat.* 13(2), 105–113.
184. Guan, Z. Z., et al. (1999). Decreased protein level of nicotinic receptor alpha7 subunit in the frontal cortex from schizophrenic brain. *Neuroreport* 10(8), 1779–1782.
185. Fox, I. J., and Kornblum, H. I. (2005). Developmental profile of ErbB receptors in murine central nervous system: Implications for functional interactions. *J. Neurosci. Res.* 79(5), 584–597.

186. Bao, J., et al. (2003). Back signaling by the Nrg-1 intracellular domain. *J. Cell. Biol.* 161(6), 1133–1141.
187. Hancock, M. L., et al. (2004). Type III neuregulin 1 bi-directional signaling regulates alpha7 nicotinic acetylcholine receptors expression and axonal targeting. *Soc. Neurosci. Abstr.*
188. Chen, Y. J., et al. (2004). Mice haplo-insufficient for cysteine-rich domain containing neuroregulin I have impaired prepulse inhibition, an endophenotypes related to schizophrenia. *Soc. Neurosci. Abstr.*
189. Mathew, S. V., et al. (2006). Association of NRG1 SNPs with ^{125}I α-bungerotoxin binding sites in the dorsolateral prefrontal cortex in schizophenia. *Soc. Neurosci. Abstr.*
190. Xie, F., Raetzman, L. T., and Siegel, R. E. (2004). Neuregulin induces GABAA receptor beta2 subunit expression in cultured rat cerebellar granule neurons by activating multiple signaling pathways. *J. Neurochem.* 90(6), 1521–1529.
191. Connolly, C. N., et al. (1996). Assembly and cell surface expression of heteromeric and homomeric gamma-aminobutyric acid type A receptors. *J. Biol. Chem.* 271(1), 89–96.
192. Connor, J. X., Boileau, A. J., and Czajkowski, C. (1998). A GABAA receptor alpha1 subunit tagged with green fluorescent protein requires a beta subunit for functional surface expression. *J. Biol. Chem.* 273(44), 28906–28911.
193. Okada, M., and Corfas, G. (2004). Neuregulin1 downregulates postsynaptic GABAA receptors at the hippocampal inhibitory synapse. *Hippocampus* 14(3), 337–344.
194. Kunugi, H., et al. (1997). Catechol-O-methyltransferase polymorphisms and schizophrenia: a transmission disequilibrium study in multiply affected families. *Psychiatr. Genet.* 7(3), 97–101.
195. Egan, M. F., and Goldberg, T. E. (2003). Intermediate cognitive phenotypes associated with schizophrenia. *Methods Mol. Med.* 77, 163–197.
196. Fujii, Y., et al. (2003). Positive associations of polymorphisms in the metabotropic glutamate receptor type 3 gene (GRM3) with schizophrenia. *Psychiatr. Genet.* 13(2), 71–76.
197. Chen, Q., et al. (2005). A case-control study of the relationship between the metabotropic glutamate receptor 3 gene and schizophrenia in the Chinese population. *Schizophr. Res.* 73(1), 21–26.
198. Straub, R. E., et al. (1995). A potential vulnerability locus for schizophrenia on chromosome 6p24-22: evidence for genetic heterogeneity. *Nat. Genet.* 11(3), 287–293.
199. Moises, H. W., et al. (1995). Potential linkage disequilibrium between schizophrenia and locus D22S278 on the long arm of chromosome 22. *Am. J. Med. Genet.* 60(5), 465–467.
200. Maziade, M., et al. (1995). Linkage results on 11Q21-22 in Eastern Quebec pedigrees densely affected by schizophrenia. *Am. J. Med. Genet.* 60(6), 522–528.
201. Schwab, S. G., et al. (2000). A genome-wide autosomal screen for schizophrenia susceptibility loci in 71 families with affected siblings: Support for loci on chromosome 10p and 6. *Mol. Psychiatry* 5(6), 638–649.
202. Straub, R. E., et al. (2002). Genome-wide scans of three independent sets of 90 Irish multiplex schizophrenia families and follow-up of selected regions in all families provides evidence for multiple susceptibility genes. *Mol. Psychiatry* 7(6), 542–559.
203. Schwab, S. G., et al. (2003). Support for association of schizophrenia with genetic variation in the 6p22.3 gene, dysbindin, in sib-pair families with linkage and in an additional sample of triad families. *Am. J. Hum. Genet.* 72(1), 185–190.

204. Kirov, G., et al. (2004). Strong evidence for association between the dystrobrevin binding protein 1 gene (DTNBP1) and schizophrenia in 488 parent-offspring trios from Bulgaria. *Biol. Psychiatry* 55(10), 971–975.
205. Williams, N. M., et al. (2004). Identification in 2 independent samples of a novel schizophrenia risk haplotype of the dystrobrevin binding protein gene (DTNBP1). *Arch. Gen. Psychiatry* 61(4), 336–344.
206. Levinson, D. F., et al. (1998). Genome scan of schizophrenia. *Am. J. Psychiatry* 155(6), 741–750.
207. Gurling, H. M., et al. (2001). Genomewide genetic linkage analysis confirms the presence of susceptibility loci for schizophrenia, on chromosomes 1q32.2, 5q33.2, and 8p21-22 and provides support for linkage to schizophrenia, on chromosomes 11q23.3-24 and 20q12.1-11.23. *Am. J. Hum. Genet.* 68(3), 661–673.
208. Ekelund, J., et al. (2001). Chromosome 1 loci in Finnish schizophrenia families. *Hum. Mol. Genet.* 10(15), 1611–1617.
209. Hennah, W., et al. (2003). Haplotype transmission analysis provides evidence of association for DISC1 to schizophrenia and suggests sex-dependent effects. *Hum. Mol. Genet.* 12(23), 3151–3159.
210. Curtis, D., et al. (2003). Genome scan of pedigrees multiply affected with bipolar disorder provides further support for the presence of a susceptibility locus on chromosome 12q23-q24, and suggests the presence of additional loci on 1p and 1q. *Psychiatr. Genet.* 13(2), 77–84.
211. Hwu, H. G., et al. (2003). Linkage of schizophrenia with chromosome 1q loci in Taiwanese families. *Mol. Psychiatry* 8(4), 445–452.
212. Thomson, P. A., et al. (2005). Association between the TRAX/DISC locus and both bipolar disorder and schizophrenia in the Scottish population. *Mol. Psychiatry* 10(7), 657–668.
213. Hodgkinson, C. A., et al. (2004). Disrupted in schizophrenia 1 (DISC1): Association with schizophrenia, schizoaffective disorder, and bipolar disorder. *Am. J. Hum. Genet.* 75(5), 862–872.
214. Gasperoni, T. L., et al. (2003). Genetic linkage and association between chromosome 1q and working memory function in schizophrenia. *Am. J. Med. Genet. B. Neuropsychiatr. Genet.* 116(1), 8–16.
215. Stefansson, H., et al. (2003). Neuregulin 1 in schizophrenia: out of Iceland. *Mol. Psychiatry* 8(7), 639–640.
216. Stefansson, H., et al. (2003). Association of neuregulin 1 with schizophrenia confirmed in a Scottish population. *Am. J. Hum. Genet.* 72(1), 83–87.
217. Williams, N. M., et al. (2003). Support for genetic variation in neuregulin 1 and susceptibility to schizophrenia. *Mol. Psychiatry* 8(5), 485–487.
218. Tang, J. X., et al. (2004). Polymorphisms within 5′ end of the Neuregulin 1 gene are genetically associated with schizophrenia in the Chinese population. *Mol. Psychiatry* 9(1), 11–12.
219. Liu, C. M., et al. (2005). Linkage evidence of schizophrenia to loci near neuregulin 1 gene on chromosome 8p21 in Taiwanese families. *Am. J. Med. Genet. B. Neuropsychiatr. Genet.* 134(1), 79–83.
220. Chiu, Y. F., et al. (2002). Genetic heterogeneity in schizophrenia II: Conditional analyses of affected schizophrenia sibling pairs provide evidence for an interaction between markers on chromosome 8p and 14q. *Mol. Psychiatry* 7(6), 658–664.

221. Liu, J., et al. (2003). Evidence for a putative bipolar disorder locus on 2p13-16 and other potential loci on 4q31, 7q34, 8q13, 9q31, 10q21-24, 13q32, 14q21 and 17q11-12. *Mol. Psychiatry* 8(3), 333–342.
222. Ikeda, M., et al. (2004). Association of AKT1 with schizophrenia confirmed in a Japanese population. *Biol. Psychiatry* 56(9), 698–700.
223. Addington, A. M., et al. (2005). GAD1 (2q31.1), which encodes glutamic acid decarboxylase (GAD67), is associated with childhood-onset schizophrenia and cortical gray matter volume loss. *Mol. Psychiatry* 10(6), 581–588.
224. Chowdari, K. V., et al. (2002). Association and linkage analyses of RGS4 polymorphisms in schizophrenia. *Hum. Mol. Genet.* 11(12), 1373–1380.
225. Williams, N. M., et al. (2004). Support for RGS4 as a susceptibility gene for schizophrenia. *Biol. Psychiatry* 55(2), 192–195.
226. Morris, D. W., et al. (2004). Confirming RGS4 as a susceptibility gene for schizophrenia. *Am. J. Med. Genet. B. Neuropsychiatr. Genet.* 125(1), 50–53.
227. Chen, X., et al. (2004). Regulator of G-protein signaling 4 (RGS4) gene is associated with schizophrenia in Irish high density families. *Am. J. Med. Genet. B. Neuropsychiatr. Genet.* 129(1), 23–26.
228. Prasad, K. M., et al. (2005). Genetic polymorphisms of the RGS4 and dorsolateral prefrontal cortex morphometry among first episode schizophrenia patients. *Mol. Psychiatry* 10(2), 213–219.

11

PHARMACOTHERAPY OF SCHIZOPHRENIA

ZAFAR SHARIF[1], SEIYA MIYAMOTO[2], AND JEFFREY A. LIEBERMAN[3]

[1]*College of Physicians and Surgeons, Columbia University; Lieber Schizophrenia Research Clinic, New York State Psychiatric Institute, New York, New York;* [2]*St. Marianna School of Medicine, Kawasaki City, Kanagawa Prefecture, Japan; and* [3]*College of Physicians and Surgeons, Columbia University; Lieber Center for Schizophrenia Research, New York State Psychiatric Institute, New York, New York*

11.1	Introduction	370
11.2	Neurochemical Hypotheses of Schizophrenia	371
	11.2.1 Dopamine Hypothesis	371
	11.2.2 Glutamate (NMDA Receptor Hypofunction) Hypothesis	373
	11.2.3 Integration of Dopamine and Glutamate Hypotheses	374
11.3	Hypothesized Mechanisms of Action of Antipsychotics	376
	11.3.1 D_2 Receptor Occupancy and Antipsychotic Effect	376
	11.3.2 High 5-HT_{2A} versus D_2 affinity	378
	11.3.3 D_2 Occupancy Thresholds and Rapid Dissociation	378
	11.3.4 Highly Selective D_2/D_3 Antagonism, D_4 Antagonism, and Regional Specificity	380
	11.3.5 Role of D_1 Receptors and Other Mechanisms	380
	11.3.6 Synthesis	381
11.4	Clinical Profiles of Antipsychotic Drugs	383
	11.4.1 First-Generation or Conventional Antipsychotics	383
	11.4.2 Second-Generation or Atypical Antipsychotics	383
	11.4.3 Safety and Tolerability	387
11.5	Drugs in Development and Future Directions	388
	11.5.1 Drugs Acting Directly or Indirectly on Dopamine System	389
	11.5.2 D_4 Antagonists	390
	11.5.3 D_3 Antagonist	390
	11.5.4 D_1 Agonists and Antagonists	390
	11.5.5 Neurotensin Agonist/Antagonist	390
	11.5.6 Neurokinin Antagonists	391
	11.5.7 Drugs Acting on Glutamate System	391
	11.5.8 Noradrenergic Agents	393
	11.5.9 Cholinergic Agents	393
	11.5.10 Other Agents	394
11.6	Conclusion	394
References		395

Handbook of Contemporary Neuropharmacology, Edited by David R. Sibley, Israel Hanin, Michael Kuhar, and Phil Skolnick. Copyright © 2007 John Wiley & Sons, Inc.

11.1 INTRODUCTION

It has been over half a century since effective treatment for psychosis was introduced into clinical practice. Chlorpromazine was the first of several antipsychotics, now called conventional or first-generation antipsychotics (FGAs), which revolutionized the treatment of psychotic disorders and enabled large numbers of individuals afflicted with these illnesses to be discharged from chronic care institutions and be cared for in the community. However, the high rate of extrapyramidal symptoms (EPSs) at therapeutic doses of these drugs was a major impediment to patient acceptability [1], and efficacy limitations such as minimal or no improvement of cognitive deficits, negative symptoms, and mood symptoms resulted in a substantial number of patients not tolerating these medications, not responding to them, or refusing to take them.

The second major step in the treatment of psychosis was the discovery of clozapine in 1958. Because of the risk of agranulocytosis, clozapine remained relatively obscure until the seminal study by Kane et al. [2] convincingly demonstrated its superior efficacy to chlorpromazine in treatment-resistant patients. Clozapine was reintroduced in the United States in 1990 under strict blood-monitoring requirements to mitigate the risk of agranulocytosis. Numerous studies have since confirmed its superior efficacy in patients with treatment-resistant schizophrenia [3, 4] and its broader spectrum of efficacy, including improvement in cognition [5], aggressivity [6], mood stabilization [7–9], and suicide risk reduction [10]. But perhaps the most important aspect of the clinical profile of clozapine is that it almost never causes parkinsonian-type side effects. For decades it was felt that the antipsychotic effect of antipsychotics and their propensity to induce parkinsonian-type side effects were inextricably linked; that is, to get an antipsychotic effect, it was necessary to increase the dose of the drug to the point of impairment of fine motor control. This, so-called neuroleptic threshold concept was essentially invalidated by the observed clinical profile of clozapine.

The "atypical" clinical profile of clozapine spurred the development of safer alternatives that would preserve the "atypicality" of clozapine and eliminate the agranulocytosis risk. The second-generation antipsychotics (SGAs), all introduced within the last decade or so, are also commonly referred to as atypical antipsychotics (risperidone, olanzapine, quetiapine, ziprasidone, and aripiprazole). Other agents not approved in the United States that have atypical properties include amisulpiride, zotepine, and sertindole (withdrawn from clinical use because of QT prolongation). Although there is debate as to what constitutes atypicality, the defining feature of this class of medications is the separation of the dose that results in a therapeutic effect from that which is associated with an increasing risk of EPSs. All SGAs meet this definition, but there are substantial differences in clinical profiles within the group. Unfortunately, the progress made in reducing motor side-effect burden with SGAs is tempered by their increased liability for causing weight gain (especially clozapine and olanzapine) and metabolic side effects, including increased risk of diabetes and dyslipidemia. The efficacy of these newer agents on psychotic symptoms has not been proven to be substantially different from conventional antipsychotics [11, 12], although one meta-analysis demonstrated a modest efficacy advantage for some of the SGAs [13]. The literature suggests incremental gains in cognitive function [14], relapse prevention [15–17], and negative symptoms [18, 19].

Despite the proven utility of antipsychotics in the management of schizophrenia, much remains to be deciphered about their differential clinical profiles, their mechanisms of action, and the pathophysiological substrates of the disease states in which they are used. In this chapter we will begin by briefly reviewing the two predominant theories of the proposed neurochemical dysregulation in schizophrenia; this will provide the conceptual framework for the rest of the chapter. We will then discuss and critique the various theories that attempt to explain the mechanism of action of antipsychotics, summarize the literature on their efficacy and side-effect profiles, and review strategies and targets for future drug development.

11.2 NEUROCHEMICAL HYPOTHESES OF SCHIZOPHRENIA

This review will cover the current status and the salient research relevant to the dopamine and glutamate dysfunction hypotheses of schizophrenia but is not meant to be an exhaustive review of the data. Readers are referred elsewhere for more detailed information [20–23; see also other chapters in this part].

11.2.1 Dopamine Hypothesis

The dopamine hypothesis of schizophrenia was proposed more than 40 years ago by Carlsson and Lindquist [24], who showed that haloperidol and chlorpromazine increased the turnover of brain monoamines as reflected by an increase in their metabolites. They proposed that these drugs acted on monoamine receptor targets in brain causing a secondary compensatory increase in monoamine turnover. Numerous studies have documented that dopamine-releasing drugs such as amphetamine are capable of inducing a paranoid psychotic state in normal control subjects that closely resembles paranoid schizophrenia [25, 26]. Additionally, psychotic symptoms are exacerbated in approximately 40% of schizophrenic patients after receiving smaller doses of such stimulants that are not psychotogenic in normals [27, 28]. Moreover, data suggest that patients who show such symptom exacerbation upon stimulant challenge are at increased risk for acute relapse if not taking antipsychotics [29–31]. In 1967 Van Rossum [32] was the first to hypothesize that the therapeutic effects of antipsychotics were related to their action on dopamine (DA) receptors. However, it was not until the mid 1970s that these receptors were actually identified and the actions of these drugs linked to D_2 receptors [33, 34]. Advances in functional brain-imaging [single-photon emission computerized tomography (SPECT) and positron emission tomography (PET)] technology in the past 20 years have provided in vivo evidence in support of the dopamine hypothesis, at least in the pathogenesis of psychotic symptoms.

Wong et al. [35] using [^{11}C]-N-methyl-spiperone were the first to study in vivo D_2 receptor density in the striatum of patients with schizophrenia and found a substantial elevation compared to normal control subjects. Most subsequent studies, however, failed to replicate this finding [23]. One factor frequently quoted as impacting the results in D_2 receptor quantification studies is the upregulation of these receptors following antipsychotic treatment, a fact well established in the animal literature. The usual drug-free period prior to imaging is two to three weeks, but it is not precisely known if this is enough time for complete reversal of upregulation secondary to antipsychotic therapy. Other factors, such as small sample size, differences in receptor ligands used in different studies, and their susceptibility to competition from endogenous dopamine for the D_2 receptors, may also have contributed to these inconsistent results [23, 36, 37]. However, when all the PET and SPECT studies that have addressed this question are pooled, the effect size of increased D_2 receptor densities in schizophrenia was 0.51 ± 0.76 [standard deviation (SD)] [23]. The probability of yielding this effect size under the null hypothesis of "no difference" is <0.05 [23]. This translates to a 12% increase in D_2 receptor density parameters in patients with schizophrenia, an increase that is significant compared to controls, although not of the magnitude reported in postmortem studies [23].

The state of presynaptic DA synthesis in the striatum of patients with schizophrenia has also been investigated. Seven studies [38–44] have examined dopa-decarboxylase (a non-rate-limiting enzyme in the synthesis of DA) in patients with schizophrenia, and most demonstrated a higher accumulation of radioligand labeled 3,4-dihydroxy-L-phenylalanine (DOPA), suggestive of increased dopamine synthesis. Increased DA synthesis, however, does not necessarily imply increased DA release into the synapse. In a series of elegant experiments using SPECT and PET, Laruelle et al. [45] and Breier et al. [46] found that an intravenous amphetamine challenge in drug-naïve/drug-withdrawn patients with schizophrenia resulted in a greater *decrease* in radioligand binding relative to baseline as compared to normals, suggesting a relatively greater release of DA upon amphetamine stimulation in schizophrenia. As expected, the increase in DA release following amphetamine was associated with transient worsening of psychotic symptoms. Furthermore, the severity of baseline psychotic symptoms was correlated with baseline DA level as well as the magnitude of DA release upon amphetamine challenge and subsequent treatment response. However, the magnitude of DA release accounted for only 30% of the variability in the psychotic response [23]. Finally, higher challenge-induced DA release was found in most but not all patients in acute relapse and was not demonstrable in stable outpatients.

Although these seminal studies confirmed a dysregulation in the synaptic control of DA in at least some patients with schizophrenia in response to an exogenous pharmacological challenge, they did not provide information on the natural state of the DA synapse. Another productive strategy to indirectly assess intrasynaptic DA has utilized two PET studies to quantify D_2 receptor occupancy before and after two days of treatment with α-methylparatyrosine (AMPT), which acutely depletes DA; the extent of the *increase* in D_2 radioligand binding from baseline to post-AMPT treatment is an indirect quantitative measure of intrasynaptic DA concentration at baseline; that is, the greater the increase in D_2 binding following DA depletion, the greater the baseline occupancy of D_2 receptors by DA. Using this strategy in acutely relapsed medication-naïve or medication-free patients, Abi-Dargham et al. [47] found a statistically greater increase in D_2 binding following DA depletion in patients with schizophrenia compared to healthy age- and sex-matched controls. These observations suggest that in acute exacerbation schizophrenia is associated with higher intrasynaptic DA levels compared to normal controls. Psychotic symptoms improved upon DA depletion (cf. experience with reserpine in the 1950s), and the increase in radioligand binding in the striatum was correlated with the degree of improvement of psychotic symptoms. If these observations are confirmed, it would provide direct proof of the DA hypothesis that increased DA transmission is, at least in part, responsible for psychotic symptoms [23]. It is important to reiterate that these conclusions of increased subcortical DA transmission in schizophrenia are based on group data and individual patients may fall within the normal range of DA transmission parameters.

Thus far we have focused on DA transmission indices in subcortical regions and their relation to psychosis. Another brain region implicated in the pathophysiology of schizophrenia, especially with regards to cognitive dysfunction and negative symptoms, is the dorsolateral prefrontal cortex (DLPFC) [48]. A few PET studies have examined the density of D_1 receptors in the prefrontal cortex (PFC), where this is the predominant DA receptor subtype. The results have been conflicting. Okubo et al. [49] demonstrated a *decrease* of D_1 receptors in the PFC, Abi-Dargham et al. [50] found an *increase* in D_1 receptors in the DLPFC, while Karlsson et al. [51] were unable to demonstrate a difference from normals in D_1 receptor density in any subcortical or neocortical region that was examined. Receptor ligand differences have been proposed as accounting for these discrepancies [52]. Interestingly, despite variable outcomes in D_1 receptor densities in the DLPFC in the above studies, all found an association between D_1 binding and various cognitive measures and/or negative symptoms. Potential D_1 receptor dysfunction is especially relevant for the pathophysiology of schizophrenia given the postulated role for this receptor in mediating critical aspects of cognitive function [53] and the ability of a full D_1-like agonist (ABT431) to reverse working memory deficits that emerge after long-term treatment with antipsychotics in nonhuman primates [54]. Functional brain-imaging studies in patients with schizophrenia have consistently demonstrated a hypometabolic state in the DLPFC which is correlated with poor performance on cognitive tasks and negative symptomatology [55].

Further support for DA dysfunction in the PFC comes from studies that have evaluated cognitive function in carriers of the valine allele of catechol-*O*-methyltranferase (COMT), an enzyme involved in DA degradation. This type of gene polymorphism increases the activity (methylation of dopamine) of COMT fourfold compared to the methionine allele, presumably resulting in lower functional DA levels in the PFC of people who carry the *Val* allele. Subjects with valine gene polymorphism demonstrate worse performance on cognitive tests of PFC function compared to the methionine allele carriers [56–59].

Thus, all these observations point in the direction that there is reduced DA function in the DLPFC of schizophrenia patients, although the exact nature of the pathophysiology underlying this perturbation (D_1 receptor dysregulation, decreased presynaptic DA release, excessive degradation of DA, or secondary to some other factor) is yet to be identified.

In summary, the literature reviewed above suggests, in its simplest form, that schizophrenia is associated with a functional *increase* in subcortical dopamine transmission which correlates with psychotic symptoms and is evident at illness onset and in acute exacerbation but not in stable outpatients, as well as a functional *decrease* in dopamine transmission in the PFC that appears to underlie deficits in cognition and negative symptomatology.

11.2.2 Glutamate (NMDA Receptor Hypofunction) Hypothesis

The second dominant pathophysiological hypothesis of schizophrenia is the glutamatergic dysfunction hypothesis. Glutamate acts on two families of receptors: ionotropic receptors, which are rapid excitatory on–off cation channels, and metabotropic receptors, which are G-protein coupled. The ionotropic receptors are further subdivided into the kainate receptor, the α-amino-3-hydroxy-5-methylisoxazole-4-proprionic acid (AMPA) receptor, and the N-methyl-D-aspartate (NMDA) receptor. The NMDA receptor is equipped with an ion channel regulating the penetration of calcium and other cations into the neuron. PCP binds to a specific site in this channel, thereby blocking the function of the receptor. Glycine, a coagonist, binds to the strychnine-insensitive binding site and enables glutamate to open the ion channel.

The glutamatergic dysfunction hypothesis evolved from observations that phencyclidine (PCP), a noncompetitive antagonist at the NMDA receptor, could induce a psychotic state in normals that was accompanied by negative symptoms and cognitive deficits that were similar to those seen in patients with schizophrenia [60, 61]. Subanesthetic doses of another noncompetitive NMDA receptor antagonist, ketamine, have also been shown to faithfully induce the spectrum of psychopathology of schizophrenia when administered to normal control subjects [62, 63]. Jentsch and Roth [64] contend that long-term repeated exposure to PCP (as opposed to acute exposure) faithfully mimics the various abnormalities observed in patients with schizophrenia, including positive symptoms, negative symptoms, and cognitive dysfunction, as well as hypofrontality in cerebral blood flow in functional brain-imaging studies. Patients with schizophrenia were found to be more sensitive to the deleterious effects of ketamine and demonstrated a worsening of positive and negative symptoms and cognitive deficits [65–67]. These observations led to the hypothesis that NMDA receptor hypofunction might be involved in the pathophysiology of schizophrenia [62, 68–70]. Farber and colleagues have hypothesized that decreased functioning of NMDA receptors leads to reduced inhibitory output from γ-aminobutric acid (GABA)–ergic interneurons and consequent increased cortical glutamatergic excitatory output to limbic regions leading to symptoms of schizophrenia. Consistent with the NMDA receptor hypofunction hypothesis is the observation that glutamatergic agonist drugs such as glycine and D-serine have shown promising results in treatment of patients with schizophrenia; these will be reviewed later. Lastly, postmortem studies have identified abnormalities of glutamate receptor density in the PFC, thalamus, and temporal lobe of patients with schizophrenia [71–73].

11.2.3 Integration of Dopamine and Glutamate Hypotheses

There is substantial evidence of reciprocal interactions between the glutamatergic and DA systems. Acute administration of ketamine to normal volunteers resulted in substantial increase in striatal DA release as measured by reduction in [^{11}C] raclopride binding using PET imaging [74–76]. Chronic NMDA receptor antagonist administration *increases* subcortical DA release, particularly in the nucleus accumbens, and *decreases* mesocortical DA transmission in animals [64]. Chronic administration of NMDA receptor antagonists also results in decreased expression of the DA D_1 receptor messenger RNA (mRNA) in the PFC of rats and monkeys [64, 77, 78]; as mentioned above, the D_1 receptor has been shown to be critical for working memory function [53].

Various possible disturbances in the corticostriatal–thalamic–cortical loops that connect the PFC to subcortical structures have been postulated to account for increased subcortical DA transmission in the context of reduced PFC activity and to attempt to integrate the DA and glutamate dysfunction hypotheses (see [23] for a review and synthesis). Weinberger postulated in 1986 [79], based on the seminal work of Pycock et al. [80], that dysregulation of subcortical DA function in schizophrenia may be secondary to a failure of the PFC to adequately inhibit subcortical transmission. Mesocortical DA input has the net effect of inhibiting subcortical DA release through feedback loops. This is mediated in part by DA stimulation of GABAergic interneurons in the cortex which inhibit excitatory glutamate corticostriatal input to ventral tegmental area (VTA) DA neurons. Reduced DA input to the PFC (or dysfunctional DA transmission in the PFC because of impaired D_1 receptor function) would result in increased excitatory glutamatergic output to VTA DA neurons and increased subcortical DA transmission.

A second mechanism proposed to account for increased subcortical DA transmission in the context of PFC dysfunction was proposed by Carlsson [81]. He described a model in which the PFC modulates subcortical DA transmission via an excitatory pathway (direct corticostriatal glutamatergic pathway) and an inhibitory pathway (indirect via intermediate midbrain GABAergic neurons), with the inhibitory pathway normally in slight dominance. Subtle NMDA receptor hypofunction would be predicted to result in reduced stimulation of the midbrain GABAergic interneurons (indirect pathway) which would normally inhibit the midbrain DA neurons. The release of VTA DA neurons from the normal inhibitory GABAergic input would result in increased subcortical DA transmission.

The third hypothesized mechanism of dysfunction in the corticostraital–thalamic–cortical circuitry involves the GABAergic neurons in the PFC that exert tonic inhibitory control over excitatory glutamatergic projections to the VTA DA neurons. A primary deficiency in PFC GABAergic neurotransmission would release the glutamatergic corticostriatal neurons from inhibition and thereby directly stimulate VTA DA neurons into overactivity. Consistent with this proposed GABAergic functional deficiency are the results of several postmortem studies that demonstrate an alteration of GABAergic function in the PFC of patients with schizophrenia (reviewed in [23]).

The preceding brief conceptual overview of the neurochemical pathophysiology of schizophrenia highlights several possible strategies for targeting therapeutic interventions for this disorder. Psychotic symptoms, presumably secondary to increased subcortical DA transmission, could be addressed from several directions: by selective D_2 antagonism in limbic regions; by increasing DA transmission in the PFC (e.g., reducing the rate of DA degradation, increasing DA release, or blocking reuptake); by augmenting GABAergic action in the PFC; or by modulating NMDA receptor/glutamatergic function in the PFC. Negative symptoms and cognitive deficits may respond to interventions that increase PFC DA activity (by direct D_1 stimulation, reducing the rate of DA degradation, increasing DA release, or blocking reuptake). These strategies, of course, need not be mutually exclusive, and a combination of various interventions that target disturbed neural circuits at various points may provide *maximal* benefit to most patients and relief to those with treatment-resistant illness.

Finally, a disease as complex and clinically varied as schizophrenia is not likely to result from a simple dysregulation in one neurotransmitter system [82]. The variability in the exact nature and magnitude of the neural-based dysfunction in schizophrenia and its interaction with normal maturational/developmental brain processes [48], coupled with the variability inherent in the dynamic interaction of an individual with his or her environment, are likely to collectively contribute to the clinical heterogeneity of the disorder across individuals and within the same individual in different stages (first episode vs. chronic) and phases (relapse vs. remission) of the illness. Whether schizophrenia is the result of a single insult that simultaneously disrupts the development and/or function of multiple neurotransmitter systems or neural circuits or the consequence of an insult that primarily disrupts one system with all other observed perturbations occurring secondarily as a compensatory response is not yet known. The precise answer to this question, however, may not be as pertinent to clinical progress as is a thorough understanding of normal brain circuitry and the homeostatic mechanisms that maintain stability among the various neural circuits which are the underpinnings of normal human emotion and cognition and how these homeostatic mechanisms are disrupted in schizophrenia. This knowledge will surely provide us with numerous opportunities to correct an imbalanced neural network(s) at multiple prospective loci irrespective of the exact nature and neuropathological location of the primary insult responsible for the disorder.

11.3 HYPOTHESIZED MECHANISMS OF ACTION OF ANTIPSYCHOTICS

We will begin with a review of the evidence in support of D_2 receptor antagonism of antipsychotics as the fundamental action that underlies their therapeutic effect on psychosis. We will then review the various theories that have been postulated to account for the atypical profile of SGAs and review the evidence for other receptor actions of antipsychotic drugs and how that may relate to their efficacy profiles.

11.3.1 D_2 Receptor Occupancy and Antipsychotic Effect

A consistent observation that has stood the test of time about antipsychotic drug treatment is that every clinically effective antipsychotic reduces DA transmission to some extent; drugs that do not have never been shown to have antipsychotic effect. More specifically, the primary receptor target implicated in antipsychotic effect, as well as the induction of EPS and prolactin elevation, is the D_2 receptor. Recent examples of non-D_2 antagonists that failed in clinical trials in schizophrenia are MDL-100907 [serotonin type 2A (5-HT$_{2A}$) antagonist] [83], L-745,870 (D_4 antagonist) [84], fananserin (5-HT$_{2A}$ and D_4 antagonist) [85], and SCH-39166 and NNC-01-0687 (D_1 receptor antagonists) [86–88].

Dopamine receptors exist in two broad families, D_1-like (D_1 and D_5) and D_2-like ($D_{2,long/short}$, D_3, D_4). The D_1 receptor has widespread distribution and is the predominant DA receptor in the PFC, while the D_5 receptor is localized in specific corticolimbic regions. The D_2 receptor has both presynaptic (autoreceptor) and postsynaptic location, and its distribution is in mesostriatal–limbic regions; it also mediates prolactin release in the pituitary. The D_3 and D_4 receptors have low-density corticolimbic distribution, with the D3 receptor additionally exhibiting presynaptic autoreceptor location (see [89] for review). Seeman [90] was the first to directly associate the therapeutic actions of antipsychotic drugs to the D_2 receptor. He demonstrated a strong correlation between in vitro affinities of antipsychotic drugs for the D_2 receptor and their clinical potencies [34], although at that time the various subtypes of the D_2 family had not been identified. Recent studies, however, using cloned cell lines have confirmed that clinical antipsychotic potencies correlate generally with their affinities for the D_2 receptor expressed independently of D_3 and D_4 subtypes [90, 91].

The advent of functional brain-imaging techniques (SPECT and PET) in the late 1980s gave the opportunity to address in vivo the nature of the exact relationship between D_2 receptor occupancy and the three cardinal properties of FGAs: antipsychotic effect, EPS, and prolactin elevation. Farde et al. [92] using PET and [^{11}C] raclopride as the radiotracer, evaluated in vivo D_2 receptor occupancy by various FGAs and clozapine and found D_2 receptor occupancies in the range of 70–89% and 38–63% in FGA- and clozapine-treated patients, respectively. Patients who had acute EPSs had significantly higher D_2 receptor occupancies. Nordstrom et al. [93] confirmed that lower D_2 receptor occupancy was required for antipsychotic effect than for induction of EPS. Subsequently, Kapur et al. [94] confirmed in a low-dose haloperidol study in patients in first-episode schizophrenia that occupancy thresholds of 65, 72, and 78% were related to antipsychotic affect, prolactin elevation, and EPSs, respectively. These and other studies have found that there was a wide variation in D_2 receptor occupancy among patients on the same dose of drug and that the thresholds, although generally accurate, were not invariably reliable in predicting clinical events. For example, a few patients responded to FGAs at low D_2 occupancy, while other subjects with $>65\%$ D_2 occupancy did not exhibit a response [94–96]. Similarly, on occasion, occupancy $>72\%$ was not associated with prolactin elevation or occupancy $>78\%$ was not associated with EPS [94]. The D_2 receptor occupancy also did not correlate with improvement (or lack thereof) of negative symptoms or cognitive deficits. Despite these limitations of not accounting for *all* clinical scenarios observed in patients with schizophrenia, the importance of this work cannot be underestimated as these data directly link in vivo D_2 receptor occupancy to antipsychotic effect, prolactin elevation, and EPSs.

Another question that has recently been addressed in the literature is the time to onset of antipsychotic effect. It has been a long-held belief that onset of antipsychotic effect is delayed by one to two weeks after initiation of treatment, and "depolarization inactivation" of dopamine neurons which occurs over about a two-week time frame (see [97] for a review) has been proposed as the underlying mechanism responsible for this delay. Kuhar and Joyce [98] proposed that drug-induced changes in protein synthesis or degradation following changes in gene expression could also explain the delay. However, a recent article by Agid et al. [99] questions the very existence of the delay in onset of antipsychotic effect. They reported a meta-analysis of 42 double-blind comparator-controlled studies and found that antipsychotic effect was evident within the first week of treatment and improvement in the first two weeks was greater than during any subsequent two-week period. Kapur et al. [100] reported that onset of specific antipsychotic effect was evident within the first 24 h in a double-blind placebo-controlled study comparing intramuscular olanzapine to intramuscular haloperidol and that improvement in psychosis was independent of change in agitation and excitement. Abi-Dargham also observed rapid improvement in psychotic symptoms upon DA depletion with α-methyl-*para*-tyrosine [47]. These observations are intriguing and clearly warrant further investigation. If true, they again support a direct role for DA in the mediation of psychosis and antidopaminergic activity in antipsychotic effect.

With the introduction of the second-generation antipsychotics, functional brain-imaging techniques were used to address the question of the underlying mechanism of atypicality. That the level of D_2 receptor occupancy was important in atypicality had been suggested by the work of Farde in 1992 [92], in which clozapine demonstrated lower D_2 receptor occupancy as compared to FGAs.

Two major theories have been postulated to account for an atypical profile; relatively higher 5-HT_{2A} versus D_2 antagonism and relative ease of staying below the $\sim 80\%$ D_2 occupancy threshold for EPSs with SGAs because of their loose binding (lower affinity) to the D_2 receptor.

11.3.2 High 5-HT_{2A} versus D_2 affinity

Meltzer [101] (also see Chapter 12 by Meltzer) proposed that higher 5-HT_{2A} versus D_2 receptor affinity conferred an atypical profile. This was based on observations that a higher in vitro 5-HT_{2A} relative to D_2 affinity distinguished the atypical antipsychotic class. 5-HT_{2A} antagonism can increase DA transmission in the nigrostriatal pathway and thereby mitigate the risk of EPSs and may also contribute to improvement of negative symptoms and cognitive dysfunction by increasing DA release in the PFC [101]. However, there are critical limitations to the "serotonin/dopamine" theory of atypicality of SGAs (reviewed in [102]): many FGAs (chlorpromazine, loxapine) have high 5-HT_{2A} affinity [103] and do not have an atypical profile; amisulpiride has no appreciable affinity for the 5-HT_{2A} receptor, and aripiprazole has higher D_2 compared to 5-HT_{2A} affinity, and yet both have atypical profiles; risperidone and olanzapine demonstrate high 5-HT_{2A} receptor occupancy at doses that are not antipsychotic (therefore 5-HT_{2A} antagonism per se cannot account for antipsychotic effect), and as the dose of these drugs is increased beyond the usual therapeutic range, the risk of EPSs increases despite saturation of the 5-HT_{2A} receptor system; the relative ratios of 5-HT_{2A}/D_2 receptor affinities of the SGAs do not predict their clinical EPS liability, for example, risperidone has the highest and quetiapine the lowest 5-HT_{2A}/D_2 ratio, but most clinicians would concur (and the data show [11, 104, 105]) that the EPS liability of risperidone is greater than that of quetiapine. Additionally, at equivalent D2 receptor occupancies, risperidone and haloperidol are associated with comparable EPS liability [106]. Thus, high 5-HT_{2A} affinity may contribute to modulating DA in the striatum and PFC, but high 5-HT_{2A} occupancy does not protect from EPSs if D_2 occupancy is greater than the EPS threshold. The 5-HT_{2A}/D_2 hypothesis therefore does not satisfactorily explain atypicality [107].

11.3.3 D_2 Occupancy Thresholds and Rapid Dissociation

The second major hypothesis put forth to account for atypicality is the loose binding, or low affinity, of SGAs for the D_2 receptor as compared to FGAs [108–110]. This builds on the observation by Farde and Nordstrom (see above) that higher D_2 receptor occupancy was observed with FGAs compared to clozapine and was correlated with increased risk of EPSs. PET imaging studies with SGAs have demonstrated that at clinically therapeutic doses these drugs occupy between 50 and 75% of D_2 receptors [92, 111–117]. On the other hand, FGAs occupy in excess of 75% of available D_2 receptors at therapeutic doses [92, 94]. Lower D_2 receptor occupancy in and of itself would account for the lower EPS liability of SGAs if the proposed EPS threshold of $> \sim 80\%$ D_2 receptor occupancy is true. Kapur and Seeman [110], in a further elaboration of this concept, suggested that rapid dissociation of SGAs from the D_2 receptor is the fundamental underlying molecular property that accounts for atypicality. They propose that the most important aspect of the affinity of a drug for the D_2 receptor is not how rapidly it binds to a receptor but how rapidly it dissociates from that receptor. The rate at which a drug dissociates from the receptor, or its k_{off}, is the most important determinant of how the drug and DA compete for the receptor. In a unit of time, a drug with fast k_{off} goes on and off a receptor much more frequently than a drug with a slow k_{off}. The faster the k_{off}, the more quickly the drug responds to DA surges, allowing for a more physiological DA transmission [110]. They conclude that this relationship between fast k_{off} and low affinity is the critical underlying molecular feature that explains how low affinity at the D_2 receptor leads to the atypical antipsychotic profile.

Another feature of atypicality that is exhibited by all SGAs except risperidone and amisulpiride is minimal elevation of serum prolactin. However, prolactin elevation has been shown to occur with all SGAs, but for most, it is transient and rapidly returns to baseline several hours after the last dose [118]. This has also been attributed to rapid dissociation of SGAs (fast k_{off}) from D_2 receptors in the anterior pituitary. Risperidone-induced elevation of serum prolactin has been attributed, at least in part, to higher peripheral compared to central distribution of its active metabolite 9-OH risperidone, leading to excessive D_2 blockade in the anterior pituitary which lies outside the blood–brain barrier [102].

In terms of D_2 receptor occupancy profiles, clozapine and quetiapine differ from ziprasidone, risperidone, olanzapine, amisulpiride, and aripiprazole, as they never exceed approximately 60–70% D_2 receptor occupancy even at the highest therapeutic doses. Because these drugs rapidly dissociate from the D_2 receptor, the level of occupancy rapidly drops off after the last dose (300–600 mg/day quetiapine or 350 mg/day clozapine used in these studies) such that 12 h later it is only 20% for quetiapine and 55% for clozapine [113, 115, 119]. A possible downside of rapid dissociation of clozapine and quetiapine from D_2 receptors could be the rapid emergence of psychotic symptoms upon drug discontinuation [120]. Although initially ziprasidone was found to have substantial D_2 receptor occupancy at low doses (20- and 40-mg single doses) in healthy volunteers [121], a recent study [122] found that 60% D_2 occupancy was not achieved until plasma levels corresponding to a 120-mg/day dose were reached, suggesting the optimal dose of this drug is 120 mg/day or higher. The predicted dose based on PET imaging of ≥ 120 mg/day is consistent with the clinical trial data for this drug [123–125]. Risperidone and olanzapine demonstrate increasing D_2 occupancy with increasing dose and also are associated with dose-related risk of EPSs [126]. The only SGA that does not appear to fit into the D_2 threshold schema is aripiprazole, a mixed DA partial agonist/antagonist [127]. In a study of 15 healthy men [128] who were treated with aripiprazole for a duration of two weeks, it was found that a dose of 2 mg/day of aripiprazole occupied between 70 and 80% of the striatal D_2-like DA receptors. When the dose was increased to 30 mg/day, the receptor occupancy increased to almost 95% in the putamen, yet no associated EPS was evident as would be predicted for all other antipsychotics based on the $> 80\%$ D_2 occupancy threshold. The lack of EPS with aripiprazole has been attributed to its agonist activity at D_2

receptors. Similarly, the lack of efficacy in the presence of adequate D2 receptor occupancy at the 2 mg/day dose is also not consistent with the 65% threshold hypothesis of efficacy [127] and could be accounted for by the partial agonist activity of aripiprazole at the D-2 receptor.

Thus both the 5-HT$_{2A}$/D$_2$ and D$_2$ receptor occupancy threshold/rapid dissociation theories have limitations as to their ability to account for *all* aspects of the disease or clinical profiles of *all* antipsychotics. These limitations, however, do not diminish the tremendous contribution made by these hypotheses to our understanding of antipsychotic drug action and drug development.

11.3.4 Highly Selective D$_2$/D$_3$ Antagonism, D$_4$ Antagonism, and Regional Specificity

Amisulpiride is a unique antipsychotic in that it is a highly selective, low-affinity antagonist at D$_2$/D$_3$ receptors. It has no activity at the D$_1$ or any other receptor. Low doses of amisulpiride (50–100 mg/day) occupy only 4–26% of striatal D$_2$ receptors [129] and seem to improve negative symptoms [130], while higher doses of 200–800 mg/day occupy 38–76% of D$_2$ receptors [129] and are effective against both positive and negative symptoms [131, 132]. It has been hypothesized that at low doses amisulpiride preferentially antagonizes presynaptic D$_2$/D$_3$ receptors, causing an increase in DA transmission in the PFC accounting for its efficacy in negative symptoms [133].

Another property of some antipsychotics that has been proposed to account for an atypical profile is D$_4$ receptor antagonism. The D$_4$ hypothesis grew out of observations of the receptor binding profile of clozapine (D$_4$ affinity > D$_2$) and the localization of this receptor in corticolimbic regions. However, this hypothesis has not withstood the test of time, and a study of a D$_4$ receptor antagonists L-745,870 not only did not demonstrate antipsychotic efficacy or EPS but was associated with worsening compared to placebo [84]. Sonepiprazole, a selective D$_4$ antagonist, yielded a negative outcome in a large double-blind, placebo-controlled randomized trial in 467 inpatients with schizophrenia in acute relapse [134]. Fananserin, a mixed 5-HT$_{2A}$ and D$_4$ antagonist, was also found to be without antipsychotic effect [85]. Also, quetiapine and amisulpiride do not have D$_4$ affinity but have an atypical profile [135, 136].

Regionally specific preferential binding of SGAs to DA tracts projecting to the limbic region (as opposed to motor striatal projections) has also been proposed as a mechanism contributing to an atypical profile. Numerous studies in animals have found a selective effect of SGAs on A10 versus A9 DA neurons and inducing early gene expression in the nucleus accumbens and medial striatum as opposed to the dorsolateral striatum [137–140]. In humans, several SPECT and PET studies have demonstrated this regional specificity for clozapine, risperidone, olanzapine, amisulpiride, quetiapine, and sertindole [112, 141–146], although other studies using more rigorous analytical methods [52] have found no regional specificity for clozapine or risperidone [147, 148]. Further evaluation of this attribute is required to confirm its existence in humans and identify its underpinnings; its significance is evident as it raises the possibility of spatial targeting of drugs in the future.

11.3.5 Role of D$_1$ Receptors and Other Mechanisms

Activity at other receptors has also been postulated to mediate antipsychotic or other effects of antipsychotics, such as improvement in mood, cognition, and negative symptoms. As described in Section 11.2.1, the D_1 receptor in the PFC is critically important in working memory function. Long-term FGA treatment induced working memory deficits in nonhuman primates that were reversed by brief treatment with a full D_1 agonist, and the beneficial effects were maintained over an extended period of time [54]. As working memory deficits have been consistently documented in patients with schizophrenia [149], drugs that have D_1 agonist activity might be particularly useful to target such a deficiency. No currently available antipsychotic has D_1 agonist activity.

Preclinical studies suggest that 5-HT_{2A} antagonism in the presence of D_2 antagonism results in increased DA release in the PFC, an effect that might be mediated by 5-HT_{1A} agonism [150]. Aripiprazole, clozapine, ziprasidone, and quetiapine are all partial agonists at the 5-HT_{1A} receptor. Clozapine, olanzapine, risperidone, and ziprasidone, but not haloperidol, increased prefrontal DA release [151–153]. Irrespective of the exact mechanism, increased prefrontal DA release in the PFC with the SGAs might contribute to improvement in negative symptoms, depressive symptoms, and cognitive dysfunction. Most SGAs, but not the FGAs, also increase release of acetylcholine in the PFC, which might lead to improved cognitive function [154]. Ziprasidone is also a norepinephrine and 5-HT reuptake inhibitor, and since the norepinephrine transporter is also functional in DA reuptake in the PFC, it is possible that this is another mechanism by which ziprasidone may increase DA transmission in the PFC. Zotepine also inhibits norepinephrine reuptake.

Lastly, some of the SGAs, but not the FGAs, have been shown to modulate NMDA receptor function at the cellular and behavioral levels in preclinical animal models [155–159]. Clozapine and olanzapine, but not haloperidol or raclopride, inhibit the electrophysiological effects of PCP in brain slices [158, 160, 161] and attenuate NMDA receptor antagonist–induced deficits in prepulse inhibition [155, 162]. As these drugs do not directly interact with the glutamatergic system, it is not clearly understood how they might be exerting their influence. One possibility for clozapine was recently highlighted in the report by Sur et al. [163] which showed that the active metabolite of clozapine, N-desmethylclozapine, can potentiate hippocampal NMDA currents by its M_1 agonist activity.

11.3.6 Synthesis

From the above review several preliminary conclusions can be drawn about the mechanisms of action of antipsychotic drugs and the basis of atypicality: (1) D_2 receptor antagonism is the fundamental property of antipsychotic drugs that underlies their antipsychotic effect; (2) continuous D_2 receptor antagonism is not required for antipsychotic effect, but how intermittent this antagonism can be without losing antipsychotic efficacy is not known; (3) different thresholds of D_2 receptor occupancy are predictive of antipsychotic effect, prolactin elevation, and EPS liability; (4) D_2 antagonism alone does not explain antipsychotic effect across all patients, that is, patients may fail to respond despite adequate D_2 blockade; (5) 5-HT_{2A} receptor antagonism and activity at other 5-HT receptors (e.g., 5-HT_{1A}) contributes to clinical profiles of most but not all SGAs (amisulpiride is an exception); (6) activity at receptors other than or in addition to DA receptors will probably be required for amelioration of negative symptoms, depressive symptoms, and cognitive dysfunction as well as for patients with treatment-resistant illness; and (7) there is substantial variability among the SGAs in receptor binding and clinical profiles—they are not members of one class.

Lastly, on a cautionary note, although remarkable advances have been made in the neurosciences over the past two decades, it is important to guard against overinterpretation of findings about the mechanisms that underlie the antipsychotic effect. There are limitations to our current conceptualizations of the receptor or intracellular basis of efficacy and side effects of antipsychotics. Studies done at a cellular level clearly do not reflect what happens in intact neural circuits of living animals. As an illustration, the output of a neuron in an intact neural circuit in response to an input may be influenced by its basal activity state and what other stimulatory or inhibitory inputs it receives at that time—the same input may result in opposite outputs depending on these and other factors. Not surprisingly, conflicting or unexpected results are not uncommon when ideas generated from basic science are taken to behavioral animal models and then to human disease states. We also know that the same receptor type may mediate completely different actions at different locations in the brain, for example, the D_2 receptor mediating antipsychotic effect, EPSs, and influence over prolactin secretion. What makes these receptors behave differently in different brain regions is not exactly known, and will this knowledge, once it accumulates, be able to guide us in developing strategies for spatial targeting of drugs? Additionally, although the relationships between degree of receptor occupancy in vivo and clinical effect has received recent attention, the temporal component of this interaction has not been rigorously evaluated. Is it better (or worse) to occupy 50–60% of D_2 receptors for 20% of the time (quetiapine) or 60% of the receptors for 100% of the time (or any combination thereof)? As noted earlier, an occasional patient may improve at low D_2 receptor occupancies. A study by Nyberg et al. [164] found that D_2 receptor occupancy for patients taking monthly injections of haloperidol decanoate dropped from 73% (60–82%) at week 1 postinjection to 52% (20–74%) at week 4. Also, the 25-mg biweekly dose of the long-acting injectable formulation of risperidone demonstrated robust efficacy [165] but was associated with only 25–48% D_2 receptor occupancy at trough plasma levels at steady state [166]. Similarly, in the long-term outpatient trial of Fleischakker et al. [167], 25 mg biweekly was found to be an effective dose. These observations are compatible with several mutually nonexclusive scenarios: (a) that a substantially lower level of D_2 occupancy than the proposed ~65% threshold may be compatible with antipsychotic effect (at least in a some patients); (b) that, similar to the profile of clozapine and quetiapine, D_2 receptor occupancy with long-acting injectables exceeds the antipsychotic threshold only transiently, although with these formulations the time frame during which the antipsychotic threshold is exceeded is in days (not hours) followed by several days of "subtherapeutic" D_2 receptor occupancy; and, lastly, (c) that a lower level of D_2 receptor occupancy may be sufficient for maintenance of antipsychotic effect as compared to the 60–70% postulated for treatment of acute exacerbation. The last scenario is consistent with the finding by Laruelle et al. [168] that stable patients (as opposed to those in acute relapse) did not exhibit abnormal DA release upon an amphetamine challenge; yet we know that patients remain vulnerable to relapse secondary to perturbation of the DA system in response to stress. These and other relevant clinical questions will need to be addressed over the coming years.

11.4 CLINICAL PROFILES OF ANTIPSYCHOTIC DRUGS

11.4.1 First-Generation or Conventional Antipsychotics

The FGAs (phenothiazines, butyrophenones, thioxanthines) had been the mainstay of treatment for psychotic disorders from the early 1950s until the introduction of the first-line SGAs in the early 1990s. Their primary efficacy domain is in psychotic symptoms and they demonstrate minimal efficacy against negative symptoms and cognitive dysfunction and may actually worsen depressive symptomatology [169, 170]. About a third of patients in acute exacerbation have minimal response to these medications, and another 50% have a partial response [171, 172]. There are no significant efficacy differences among FGAs (reviewed in [173]). Until recently, the only long-acting injectable formulations available were of the FGAs; risperidone is now available in a long-acting injectable form (Risperdal Consta). The FGAs were routinely used in doses that were excessive leading to high rates of movement disorders, secondary negative symptoms, and further cognitive impairment because of anticholinergic effect of the drug itself or the anticholinergics prescribed to mitigate EPSs. Their side-effect profile included acute EPSs, tardive dyskinesia (TD), neuroleptic malignant syndrome, sedation, anticholinergic side effects, weight gain, and prolactin-induced side effects. The rates of acute EPSs in first-episode patients at therapeutic doses were as high as 70% [174], while TD risk was approximately 5% per year of exposure in the not elderly [175] and 25–30% per year in the elderly [176]. The high risk of TD, a potentially irreversible movement disorder, and the high rates of acute EPSs were the major motivating factors for psychiatrists to switch patients to SGAs when they became available beginning in the early 1990s.

11.4.2 Second-Generation or Atypical Antipsychotics

There is a wealth of double-blind placebo- and active comparator-controlled studies of the SGAs, most of them conducted to obtain regulatory approval. Such studies, among others, have been included in several recently published meta-analyses [11–13, 177] of the efficacy and safety/tolerability of SGAs compared to FGAs and SGAs compared to each other. In general, these studies did not include treatment-resistant patients, were conducted mostly in patients in acute exacerbation, were of relatively short duration, and assessed limited efficacy and safety outcome measures. Also, since most of the studies in these meta-analyses were sponsored by manufacturers of the new agents, it can be safely stated that the designs were at best neutral and at worst stacked to favor the new agent. Usually these design flaws were reflected in a higher than necessary dose of the comparator FGA, which would be expected to negatively influence dropout rates (because of increased risk of side effects), negative and depressive symptom ratings (because of EPSs that may mimic negative/depressive symptoms), and cognitive function (because of higher use of adjunctive anticholinergic medication to ameliorate EPSs).

The first meta-analysis by Leucht [11] included studies on risperidone, olanzapine, quetiapine, and sertindole. They found a very modest efficacy advantage on total symptomatology for risperidone and olanzapine compared to haloperidol (effect size r values of 0.06 and 0.07, respectively), with no difference for quetiapine and sertindole. On negative symptoms both olanzapine and risperidone were superior to haloperidol, but again the effect size was very small. Sertindole was no different from haloperidol in the treatment of negative symptoms, and quetiapine in one study [178] was equivalent to chlorpromazine while in another [105] it was actually statistically *inferior* to haloperidol. Compared to haloperidol, all SGAs were associated with lower anticholinergic use, although the effect was weakest for risperidone. Interestingly, in a double-blind sertindole study that used a low 4-mg/day dose of haloperidol there was still a statistically higher use of anticholinergic medication in this group of patients compared to pooled sertindole dose groups, suggesting that even at relatively low doses high-potency FGAs are associated with significant EPS liability [11]. In two studies that used either a midpotency or low-potency FGA comparator (perphenazine, chlorpromazine), no difference in concomitant anticholinergic use was found compared to the SGA group. Because of lack of efficacy, dropout rates were statistically lower only for olanzapine compared to haloperidol; olanzapine also demonstrated lower dropout rates because of adverse events. Quetiapine had lower dropout rates compared to haloperidol related to adverse events and did not differ in dropouts for lack of efficacy; risperidone did not show an advantage over haloperidol in dropout rates related to either lack of efficacy or adverse events. This meta-analysis therefore suggested minor efficacy advantages for olanzapine and risperidone, moderate overall tolerability advantage for quetiapine and olanzapine, and a lower EPS liability as reflected in lower anticholinergic use for all the SGAs compared to haloperidol. However, in a second meta-analysis by Leucht [177] comparing SGAs to only low-potency FGAs, no advantage on EPS liability was seen for the SGAs (other than clozapine), although a moderate superiority in efficacy was documented for the SGAs.

The meta-analysis by Geddes et al. [12] was even less optimistic. They included 52 randomized trials with a total of 12,649 patients treated with risperidone, clozapine, olanzapine, quetiapine, amisulpiride, and sertindole. Overall, they found that SGAs had slightly superior efficacy and better tolerability and a lower risk of causing EPSs. However, when they controlled for comparator dose of the FGAs and separately analyzed data for patients who received 12 mg/day of haloperidol equivalents or less, all advantages of SGAs except for a modest EPS advantage disappeared. Essentially the conclusion from this meta-analysis was that other than a slight superiority on EPS profile, all other differences in outcomes between SGAs and FGAs could be accounted for by a higher than necessary dose of the comparator FGA.

The last meta-analysis conducted by Davis et al. [13] included 124 randomized trials of 10 SGAs versus FGAs and 18 trials comparing different SGAs. They found significantly greater effect size for efficacy for clozapine (0.49), risperidone (0.25), olanzapine (0.21), and amisulpiride (0.29). The mean effect sizes for the above drugs (other than clozapine) corresponded to about a four- to six-point advantage on the PANSS compared to FGAs. For perspective, the difference between these SGAs and the FGA comparator group was about half as much further improvement over that seen with FGAs compared to placebo. The effect size of efficacy of clozapine versus FGAs was double that of other SGAs versus FGAs. Quetiapine, sertindole, ziprasidone, aripiprazole, and remoxipride demonstrated similar efficacy as FGAs. Significance for superior efficacy for zotepine depended on the statistical method used and was significant with one method and just missed significance with another. Distinct from the results of the Geddes meta-analysis, Davis et al. did not find that the dose of the comparator FGAs had any effect on the outcome of their analysis. A sub-meta-analysis of studies comparing SGAs to each other did not reveal statistical differences among them on efficacy profiles. However, clozapine was superior to risperidone if studies that used a low dose of clozapine were excluded from the analysis. The Davis meta-analysis did not address safety and tolerability issues.

Thus, collectively these meta-analyses suggest an EPS advantage for the SGAs (although the dose of FGAs was higher than necessary in many studies and there were minor differences among the SGAs) and probable superior overall symptom efficacy for clozapine, risperidone, olanzapine, and amisulpiride over FGAs, with clozapine demonstrating the most robust difference.

The claimed superiority of SGAs over FGAs on negative symptoms is even more problematic to address, because some features of EPSs caused by FGAs (flat affect, bradykinesia—so-called *secondary* negative symptoms) may be impossible to distinguish from the *primary* negative symptoms of the disease [179–182]. Additionally, negative symptoms could also be secondary to positive symptoms, depressive symptoms, and environmental deprivation [183, 184]. Modest differences have been demonstrated for risperidone and olanzapine compared to FGAs [18, 19] on negative-symptom improvement using path-analytic methods that attempt to remove the influence of psychotic, depressive, and extrapyramidal symptoms on negative symptomatology. These results should not engender significant enthusiasm as the analyses were performed post hoc and the most effective dose of the SGA was chosen—the gain in negative-symptom improvement, most of it in secondary negative symptoms, is modest at best.

Similarly, the superiority of SGAs on cognitive function improvement relative to FGAs is not well established. Impairments in cognitive test performance in patients on FGAs may result from EPSs, anticholinergic effects, and sedative effects, on top of what is due to the underlying disease process [185–187]. The improvement seen in cognitive function with SGAs may at least in part be attributable to elimination or relative reduction of some of these deleterious effects of FGAs. Additionally, optimal dosing of FGAs is of critical importance in these studies as excessive dose may result in sedation and impairment of motor function secondary to EPSs that negatively impacts performance on timed tests. In general, the SGAs have demonstrated improvement in verbal fluency, digit symbol substitution, executive function, and fine motor control [5, 188], and a meta-analysis by Keefe et al. [189] found a significant overall advantage for SGAs on cognitive test performance. However, in a prospective two-year study Green et al. [190] found no advantage on cognitive functioning for risperidone (mean dose 6 mg/day) compared to haloperidol (mean dose 5 mg/day) in stable outpatients with schizophrenia. Similarly, a recent double-blind randomized 12-week trial [191] comparing olanzapine (mean dose 9.6 mg/day) with low-dose haloperidol (4.6 mg/day) found that both drugs improved verbal fluency, motor function, working memory, verbal memory, and vigilance to a similar degree in primary analysis. On secondary analysis, a minor advantage was noted for olanzapine, but statistical significance levels were not corrected for in multiple analyses that were conducted to yield this conclusion. Thus the differences in cognitive improvement with SGAs versus FGAs, if both are dosed appropriately, appear to be minor. Further research is needed to definitively address this issue.

The potential of some of the SGAs to delay relapse as compared to FGAs has also been evaluated. In a double-blind randomized trial comparing risperidone to haloperidol and utilizing appropriate doses of both drugs, Csernansky et al. [192] found that risperidone was associated with a significantly lower risk for relapse by study endpoint (Kaplan-Meier estimates of relapse risk were 34 vs. 60%, respectively). Data are also available for olanzapine in maintaining long-term therapeutic effect [17]. The data from the extension phases of three double-blind studies comparing olanzapine to haloperidol were pooled to form one group for each drug. Olanzapine-treated subjects experienced less relapse ($p = 0.034$), and the Kaplan-Meier estimated one-year risk of relapse was 19.7% with olanzapine and 28% with haloperidol. Finally, in a meta-analysis of relapse prevention studies comparing SGAs to FGAs conducted by Leucht [193], the rate of relapse and overall treatment failure were modestly but significantly lower with the newer drugs. Methodological limitations identified by the authors that need to be addressed in future relapse prevention studies included the choice of comparator FGA, use of appropriate doses, application of clinically relevant relapse criteria, and monitoring of adherence. Collectively, these data suggest that the SGAs are associated with a modest reduction in relapse risk, although methodological limitations of the studies conducted thus far dampen this conclusion.

The use of SGAs is now routine in the treatment of first-episode patients because of their lower EPS burden, slightly superior symptom domain efficacy, and probable superiority in relapse prevention. At a neurochemical level, SGAs, based on the evidence from animal literature, may have effects on the NMDA system that are different from those of FGAs (see Section 11.3), thus providing another avenue for assertion of therapeutic effect distinct from direct D_2 antagonism. If the pathophysiology of schizophrenia is progressive, modulation of the glutamatergic system by SGAs may lead to better long-term outcomes [194]. Two recent studies [16, 195] of olanzapine and risperidone in first-episode patients have demonstrated that in treatment of acute phase of the illness both drugs were comparable to haloperidol in efficacy. However, at the last observation point (12 weeks) in the olanzapine study, significantly more patients were still in treatment in the olanzapine arm versus the haloperidol arm (67 vs. 54%). Similarly, in the risperidone-versus-haloperidol trial, which used appropriate doses for both drugs (~ 3 mg/day), relapse rates were 42 and 55% for risperidone- and haloperidol-treated patients, respectively, over a median follow-up period of 206 days. Additionally, risperidone was associated with a significantly longer median time to relapse (466 days for risperidone- vs. 205 days for haloperidol-treated patients). The advantage for risperidone in reducing relapse risk was evident even though both groups had comparable symptom improvement. Both SGAs were superior to haloperidol in EPS liability; olanzapine caused more weight gain and risperidone more prolactin elevation compared to haloperidol. Weight gain was initially greater with risperidone compared to haloperidol, but at study endpoint there was no difference. These studies therefore support the use of SGAs in the first episode of the illness, not because of superior acute treatment efficacy but due to modestly better long-term relapse outcomes.

Another area of significant importance in schizophrenia treatment research is the study of the prodromal period preceding the onset of psychosis. The usual time from onset of frank psychotic symptoms to treatment initiation is one year, but when the prodromal period is taken into account, the average delay is three years [196]. There is widespread interest in evaluating the utility of various interventions in the prodromal stage of schizophrenia before the onset of overt psychosis. The broad goals of these efforts are to develop systems for early recognition of psychosis in high-risk individuals and develop strategies for secondary prevention—specifically, does intervention during the prodromal period reduce the risk of developing overt psychotic symptomatology, and in those who do develop the illness, do these interventions alter the course or severity of the illness? Research in this area is in its early stages. McGorry et al. [197] reported on a randomized, controlled, nonblinded trial in 59 "ultra-high-risk" individuals at late prodromal stages close to psychosis onset. They compared low-dose risperidone treatment (mean dose 1.3 mg/day) combined with cognitive behavior therapy to routine clinical care over a six-month period followed by six months of needs-based care. Significantly fewer subjects in the risperidone group had transitioned into psychosis at the six-month time point, and in those subjects who had been compliant with risperidone, the benefits extended through the ensuing six-month extension period even though risperidone had been stopped. It is however not possible from this study to determine the relative contribution of risperidone or the cognitive behavior therapy to the reduced risk of transition into psychosis [197]. Early psychosis recognition and intervention programs are being developed in several countries and we await the results of this important work.

Lastly, in treatment-resistant schizophrenia the evidence in support of clozapine is most robust and it is the only antipsychotic specifically approved by the U.S. Food and Drug Administration (FDA) for this indication as well as for reduction of suicide risk. In a review of seven studies Chakos et al. [4] found clozapine to be superior in efficacy to FGAs, produced less EPSs, and was associated with better compliance. The double-blind, randomized, active comparator-controlled (olanzapine) study that led to the suicide risk reduction indication for clozapine [10] included 980 patients who were at relatively higher risk of suicide that were followed for up to two years,. Approximately 25% of patients had treatment-resistant schizophrenia. Suicidal behavior was significantly less in patients treated with clozapine versus olanzapine as reflected by fewer clozapine-treated patients attempting suicide (34 vs. 55; $p = 0.03$), requiring hospitalizations (82 vs. 107; $p = 0.05$) or rescue interventions to prevent suicide (118 vs. 155; $p = 0.01$), or requiring concomitant treatment with antidepressants (221 vs. 258; $p = 0.01$) or anxiolytics or soporifics (301 vs. 331; $p = 0.03$). Clozapine remains a uniquely effective drug, especially for treatment-resistant schizophrenia, and its importance to contemporary antipsychotic research is evident in the fact that all theories of the neurochemical underpinnings of atypicality evolved from observations and research on its biochemical and clinical profiles.

11.4.3 Safety and Tolerability

The biggest advance in side-effect profiles of SGAs is the lower risk of acute EPSs. Among the types of EPSs, acute dystonias are very rare with SGAs, while akathisia still occurs with all the newer agents. Within the group, clozapine and quetiapine have the lowest (almost absent risk) of parkinsonism, while amisulpiride, risperidone, and olanzapine are associated with dose-related parkinsonism. Ziprasidone and aripiprazole can also occasionally induce EPSs, although it is not clear if there is a dose relationship with these drugs. Lower rates of TD have also been reported with risperidone compared to haloperidol (0.6 vs. 4.1%, respectively) in a one-year double-blind study [192] and for olanzapine compared to haloperidol (0.5 vs. 7.4%, respectively) [198]. Weight gain has emerged as a major problem with some of the SGAs [199]. Olanzapine and clozapine are most notorious in this respect, and in some patients, rapid and massive weight gain can occur. Quetiapine and risperidone are intermediate in weight gain liability, while ziprasidone and aripiprazole rarely cause significant weight gain [200]. Weight gain in patients with schizophrenia is especially problematic as these patients are usually overweight at baseline, have high rates of smoking, and are usually physically inactive. This combination of risk factors topped off by an increased risk of glucose dysregulation and hyperlipidemia reported to varying degrees with these agents [200] can create a potentially fatal constellation of risk factors for cardiovascular disease and stroke. These adverse effects in their entirety may well be worse than tardive dyskinesia, which was the major concern for FGAs [201]. The diabetes risk appears to be greatest for clozapine and olanzapine, less for risperidone and quetiapine, and lowest for ziprasidone and aripiprazole [200]. Risperidone causes sustained prolactin elevation, and therefore patients who previously developed prolactin-induced side effects (galactorrhea, gynecomastia, menstrual irregularities, and sexual dysfunction) on older agents should be tried on other SGAs. Ziprasidone is associated with QT prolongation, although the significance of this in patients with no other risk factors is not clear. Clozapine, in addition to agranulocytosis risk and other side effects mentioned previously, is associated with significant orthostasis, seizures (dose related), myocarditis, constipation (at times severe), and various other side effects, making it a challenging drug to use in clinical practice. Recently, the FDA issued a black-boxed warning of increased death rate in elderly patients with dementia who were prescribed SGAs. This was based on a review of data from 17 placebo-controlled trials of SGAs (risperidone, olanzapine, aripiprazole, quetiapine) involving 5106 elderly patients with dementia-related psychosis. The results showed an approximate 1.6-fold increase in death rate with SGAs compared to placebo. The warning is applicable to all SGAs marketed in the United States. No controlled data are available for FGAs as regards to this risk. Additionally, from the same studies, an increased risk of stroke and other cerebrovascular adverse events were noted for risperidone, olanzapine, and aripiprazole (approximately 2–3 times greater rate of these events in drug vs. placebo). Data were not available for the other SGAs.

In summary, incremental gains have been made with the SGAs in terms of efficacy, but clozapine still remains unchallenged in its robust efficacy profile, especially in treatment-resistant patients. Significant reduction in the EPS burden with SGAs, however, is offset by problematic side effects of weight gain, diabetes, and hyperlipidemia.

11.5 DRUGS IN DEVELOPMENT AND FUTURE DIRECTIONS

This section will review drugs that are currently in clinical development or in preclinical evaluation as well as potential future interventional targets, some of which are relatively speculative at this time.

11.5.1 Drugs Acting Directly or Indirectly on Dopamine System

Asenapine is a 5-HT_{2A}/D_2 antagonist that is being jointly developed by Pfizer and Organon and is in phase III clinical trials. Early data from previous trials show good tolerability and superior efficacy when tested against a placebo. No information is available in the public domain about the nature or the methods of the study.

Bifeprunox is in phase III clinical trials. It is a partial DA agonist/antagonist as well as a 5-HT_{1A} receptor agonist. Early results report little to no weight gain and no cardiac or EPS effects. No further information is available.

Iloperidone is being developed by Titan Pharmaceuticals (currently in phase III FDA clinical trials) after being dropped by Novartis due to concerns that the drug may increase the QT interval. Iloperidone displays high affinity for norepinephrine α_1 adrenoceptors and DA D_3 and 5-HT_{2A} receptors and intermediate affinity for norepinephrine α_{2C} adrenoceptors and DA D_2 and D_4 and 5-HT_{1A}, 5-HT_{1B}, 5-HT_{2C}, and 5-HT_6 receptors [202]. This broad receptor profile makes it an interesting drug, although it has been in development for more than 10 years. In patients with schizophrenia treated with iloperidone, a low incidence of EPSs and weight gain has been shown. Data from phase II trials demonstrated efficacy in patients at doses of 8 mg/day and tolerability was good up to 32 mg/day [203].

Paliperidone extended release is the active metabolite (9-OH risperidone) of risperidone. It is a 5-HT_{2A}/D_2 antagonist and is being developed by Johnson and Johnson. No specific research information was found on this compound.

Ocaperidone has approximately equivalent antagonism of 5-HT_{2A} and D_2 DA receptors. It is nearing the end of phase II clinical trials.

Modafinil, a drug currently used to treat narcolepsy, is now being examined for its potential to improve cognitive symptoms and working memory in schizophrenia patients. The mechanism of action is still not entirely clear, although it appears that modafinil induces wakefulness through activation of sleep/wake centers in the hypothalamus and increases DA levels in the PFC. Turner [204] studied 20 chronic schizophrenic patients in a double-blind, randomized, placebo-controlled crossover study using a 200-mg dose of modafinil. Improvement was seen on short-term verbal memory span, with trends toward improved visual memory and spatial planning. This was accompanied by reduced response latency on the spatial planning task. Significant improvement in attentional set shifting was seen in schizophrenic patients, despite no effect of modafinil being seen in healthy volunteers or attention-deficit hyperactivity disorder (ADHD) patients on this task. Modafinil is currently in phase II clinical trials to test whether it improves working memory in schizophrenia patients with COMT gene variations.

Tolcapone is a COMT reversible inhibitor that acts in the PFC of the brain. By inhibiting the catabolism of DA it may be beneficial for the cognitive deficits associated with schizophrenia, especially working memory. Its measurable effects in rat brains include an increase in DA neurotransmitter levels in the PFC but not in the striatum [205], and it has been shown to improve cognitive dysfunction in advanced Parkinson's disease [206]. It can cause severe liver dysfunction and has been removed from the market in several countries. It is currently being evaluated in a National Institute of Mental Health (NIMH) placebo-controlled trial in patients with schizophrenia and normal controls with and without the high-risk COMT alleles.

11.5.2 D$_4$ Antagonists

The negative studies for the highly selective D$_4$ antagonist L-745,870 [84], the 5-HT$_{2A}$/D$_4$ antagonist finanserin [85], and sonepiprazole [134] were described earlier. The D$_4$ story does not look optimistic, at least in monotherapy.

11.5.3 D$_3$ Antagonist

The D$_3$ receptor has corticolimbic distribution and is of interest because most antipsychotics have high affinity for this receptor [207]. In a postmortem study of schizophrenia, D$_3$ receptors were increased in the limbic striatum of drug-free patients, while it was normal in those treated with antipsychotics [208]. D$_3$ antagonists have been developed (S33084, SB-277011-A, AVE5997), but there are only limited animal behavioral data at this time. Controlled trials of D$_3$ antagonists will help clarify the differential contributions of the D$_2$ and D$_3$ receptor in the mediation of antipsychotic effect.

11.5.4 D$_1$ Agonists and Antagonists

The relevance of this receptor to cognitive function was covered earlier in the chapter. In the early 1990s there was interest in D$_1$ receptor antagonists as possible antipsychotic agents because they were active in preclinical models predictive of antipsychotic effect [91]. However, clinical trials of SCH-39166 [86, 87] and NNC-01-0687 [88] demonstrated no antipsychotic activity. On the other hand, there is substantial interest in D$_1$ agonists for their potential role in cognitive enhancement, and positive results have been obtained in nonhuman primates [54]. DAR 0100 (dihydrexidine) is a high-affinity short-acting D$_1$ agonist that has been studied in Parkinson's disease [209] and is currently being tested as a treatment for cognitive deficits in schizophrenia.

11.5.5 Neurotensin Agonist/Antagonist

Neurotensin, an endogenous neuropeptide, is colocalized with DA neurons that project specifically to the PFC and nucleus accumbens and it acts as a modulator of DA function [210]. Neurotensin was proposed to have potential antipsychotic activity more than two decades ago [211] (see [212] for a review). The problem with developing neurotensin agonist/antagonists is their rapid degradation by peptidases and difficulty crossing the blood–brain barrier. Centrally administered neurotensin demonstrates behavioral and biochemical effects very similar to antipsychotics [213]. A recent placebo- and haloperidol-controlled randomized trial to evaluate the utility of four potential novel agents in the treatment of schizophrenia included the neurotensin (NTS1) antagonist SR 48692 as one of the agents [214]. It did not demonstrate any therapeutic effect. However, it has been proposed that neurotensin *agonists* may be more relevant to the treatment of schizophrenia [215]. Richelson et al. [215] have developed a neurotensin agonist, (2s)-2-amino-3-(1H-4-indoyl) propanoic acid, that is resistant to peptidases and enters the brain if injected outside the brain. It is currently in preclinical toxicology testing.

11.5.6 Neurokinin Antagonists

Neurokinin 3 (NK3) receptors appear to regulate midbrain DA activity [216, 217]. A NK3 antagonist in development as potential treatment for schizophrenia is osanetant [218]. In the study of four novel compounds referred to above, Meltzer et al. [214] found that patients treated with SR 142801 demonstrated significant global and psychotic symptom improvement, though not of the same magnitude seen in the haloperidol group.

11.5.7 Drugs Acting on Glutamate System

If NMDA receptor hypofunction contributes to the pathophysiology of schizophrenia, then drugs that enhance NMDA receptor function could potentially be useful in the treatment of this disorder. Various strategies are being employed to modulate the glutamatergic system. Glycine is an obligatory coagonist at the NMDA receptor, and this site represents an interesting target for NMDA receptor augmentation. Studies with glycine have yielded mixed results with very high dose studies showing some benefit (see [20] for a review). This probably results from poor brain penetration of glycine. More optimistic results have been obtained with the glycine site agonists D-cycloserine and D-serine when they are added to ongoing antipsychotic treatment (except when added to clozapine). Patients demonstrated improvement in negative and cognitive symptoms, but less so on positive and depressive symptomatology. D-Serine appears to be the most promising as it has better permeability at the blood–brain barrier than glycine and does not have the partial agonist properties of D-cycloserine. In an eight-week addon trial of D-serine in treatment-resistant patients with schizophrenia, D-serine treatment was associated with improvement in negative, cognitive, and positive symptomatology [219]. In the first systematic review and meta-analysis of glutamatergic drugs for schizophrenia, Tuominen [220] found a beneficial treatment effect on negative symptoms of schizophrenia only for add-on treatment with glycine and D-serine. The average improvement on the PANSS-negative subscale was a modest four points. There was also a trend toward positive effect on cognitive symptoms for glycine and D-serine, although further trials are needed to confirm this finding [220]. In this review D-cycloserine was not found to be helpful in schizophrenia and may even have been detrimental.

Another approach to augmentation of glycine at the NMDA receptor is to inhibit its reuptake, thereby increasing intrasynaptic concentration of glycine. A couple of glycine transporter inhibitors (sarcosine, glycyldodecylamide) show some potential in animal models for antipsychotic effect [221–224]. In a recent six-week double-blind, placebo-controlled addon trial of sarcosine for the treatment of schizophrenia, significant improvement in positive, negative, and cognitive symptoms was evident in the sarcosine group [225].

Glutamate reuptake inhibitors can control glutamatergic transmission by removal of glutamate from the synapse. Postmortem studies in schizophrenia have revealed alterations in gene expression of glutamate transporters [226, 227]. Theoretically glutamate reuptake inhibitors could have potential utility in schizophrenia, although no such agent is currently in testing.

There is also interest in group II metabotropic glutamate receptors (mGluR2/3) which are presynaptically located and may function as autoreceptors regulating glutamate release [228, 229]. Inconsistent results in behavioral animal models have been obtained thus far with mGluR2/3 agonists ([229]). However, in a preliminary human trial in normal subjects, the mGluR2/3 agonist LY354740 attenuated ketamine-induced working memory impairment [230].

The non-NMDA ionotropic glutamate receptors, AMPA, and kainate receptors could potentially mediate some of the behavioral effects of increased glutamate release seen following NMDA antagonism with drugs such as ketamine. Antagonists at these receptors have been shown to reverse some of the deficits induced by NMDA antagonism in pharmacological and behavioral animal models [231–234]. These data suggest that AMPA/kainate receptor antagonists could potentially have utility for the treatment of cognitive deficits [231]. In contrast to the agents discussed above, ampakines *augment* AMPA receptor function and enhance long-term potentiation, learning, and memory in rodents [235, 236]. It is suggested [20] that ampakines, by potentiating AMPA receptor–induced depolarization, indirectly enhance NMDA receptor function. CX516, the first member of this class, synergistically blocked methamphetamine-induced rearing behavior in rats when it was added to clozapine and to conventional antipsychotic agents, an effect believed to predict antipsychotic efficacy [237]. In preliminary human trials in patients with schizophrenia, CX516 improved cognitive and negative symptoms in patients who were also taking clozapine [238]. However, in a recent double-blind, placebo-controlled small study of patients with schizophrenia who were partially refractory to treatment with FGAs, CX516 in monotherapy did not produce impressive effects on positive and cognitive symptoms [239].

Memantine is a noncompetitive NMDA receptor antagonist. Although speculative, it is possible that memantine, by antagonizing NMDA receptors on GABAergic interneurons in the PFC, could potentially reduce the GABAergic (inhibitory) input to the glutamatergic neurons resulting in an increased glutamatergic output. Forrest Pharmaceuticals is currently sponsoring a phase II double-blind, placebo-controlled efficacy and safety trial of memantine added on to atypical antipsychotics in patients with schizophrenia.

Lamotrigine added to ongoing antipsychotic treatment has yielded some positive outcomes. Kremer et al. [240] conducted a 10-week, double-blind, placebo-controlled study in 38 treatment-resistant schizophrenia inpatients receiving conventional and atypical antipsychotics. Patients were randomized in a 2 : 1 ratio to receive adjuvant treatment with lamotrigine, gradually titrated to a 400-mg/day dose, or placebo. Of these, 31 completed the trial. In primary last observation carried forward analysis, no statistically significant between-group differences were observed; however, completer analyses revealed that lamotrigine treatment resulted in significant reductions in positive and general psychopathology symptoms; no significant differences in lamotrigine effects were noted between conventional versus atypical antipsychotics. In a double-blind, placebo-controlled add-on crossover trial involving 34 hospitalized treatment-resistant patients on clozapine Tiihonen [241] found that 200 mg/day lamotrigine was effective in reducing positive and general psychopathological symptoms, whereas no improvement was observed in negative symptoms. The positive impact of lamotrigine on psychotic symptoms may be mediated by DA modulation. Lamotrigine has been demonstrated to reduce DA levels in the striatum of mice presumably by inhibition of tyrosine hydroxylase, thereby reducing DA synthesis [242]. Lamotrigine also reduces glutamate release and in a controlled study of normal volunteers was shown to reduce the extent of neuropsychiatric disruptions in response to ketamine [243]. Lamotrigine is now in phase III clinical trials as an adjunctive treatment for schizophrenia.

11.5.8 Noradrenergic Agents

Norepinephrine plays an important role in cognition in the PFC mediated by α_2 receptors [244–248]. The α_2 agonist clonidine has been shown to improve PFC-mediated cognitive function in patients with schizophrenia [249]. Guanfacine, a selective α_2 agonist, when added to risperidone or FGAs in a four-week placebo-controlled trial, resulted in significant improvement in tasks of working memory and attention, but only in the risperidone-treated subjects [250]. Thus, α_2 agonism may mediate improvement in some aspects of the cognitive function in schizophrenia. On the other hand, clozapine and risperidone are potent α_2 *antagonists*. Litman et al. [251, 252] reported that the addition of idazoxan, an α_2 antagonist to FGAs produced a "clozapine-like" profile. Antagonism at the α_2 receptors therefore, may contribute to the "antipsychotic" efficacy profile of antipsychotics.

11.5.9 Cholinergic Agents

The α_7 nicotinic acetylcholine receptor (nAChR) modulates auditory gating and has been shown to be reduced in certain brain regions of patients with schizophrenia in postmortem studies, and genetic studies link the α_7 nAChR gene to sensory processing deficits in schizophrenia (reviewed in [253]). Agonists at the α_7 nAChR are in development for clinical trials in schizophrenia.

The α_4-β_2 nAChR represents more than 90% of the high-affinity nicotinic binding sites in the rat brain and is believed to play an important role in the actions of nicotine. SIB-1553A is an agonist at this receptor that appears to enhance performance in spatial and nonspatial working memory and reference memory in aged rodents and monkeys [254, 255]. These observations make α_4-β_2 nAChR agonists interesting candidates for evaluation in the treatment of cognitive dysfunction in schizophrenia.

Galantamine is a positive allosteric modulator of nAChRs and also an acetylcholinesterase inhibitor. The allosteric interaction essentially amplifies the action of acetylcholine at pre- and postsynaptic nicotinic receptors. Presynaptic nAChRs are capable of modulating the release of acetylcholine, glutamate, GABA, and 5-HT. Case reports suggest that adjuvant galantamine improves negative symptoms in schizophrenia [256, 257]. An exploratory phase II study of galantamine in patients with schizophrenia who were smokers was recently completed in Canada. The results are not yet known.

A recent double-blind trial of donepezil, a reversible acetylcholinesterase inhibitor, did not show any positive effect when added to risperidone on cognitive function associated with schizophrenia [258].

Lastly, it is well known that cholinergic muscarinic receptors modulate dopaminergic and glutamatergic neurons (reviewed in [259]). Recently the *N*-desmethyl metabolite of clozapine was found to have potent partial agonist activity at this receptor, and it was demonstrated that it could potentiate NMDA currents in the hippocampus [163]. Examples of M_1 agonists include xanomeline and the M_2/M_4

agonists PTAC and BuTAC (reviewed in [259]). Xanomeline has been shown to have positive effects on cognitive and psychotic symptoms in Alzheimer's disease patients. Accumulating data suggest that muscarinic partial agonists might be efficacious in treating not only positive but also negative and cognitive symptoms of schizophrenia.

11.5.10 Other Agents

Acute cannabis intoxication can produce schizophrenia-like symptoms [260] and long-term use may induce "negative" symptoms [261]. These and other observations have led to a cannabinoid hypothesis of schizophrenia [262]. A cannabinoid CB1 antagonist (SR141716) recently failed to reveal any therapeutic effects in the four-novel-compound double-blind, placebo- and haloperidol-controlled six-week study of Meltzer et al. [214].

Other attempts at increasing dopamine in the PFC have included double-blind augmentation trials of the monoamine oxidase type B (MAO_B) inhibitor selegiline [263] and DA reuptake blocker mazindol [264], both of which did not yield a positive outcome on the primary outcome measure of improvement of negative symptoms.

Neurosteroids such as dehydroepiandrosterone (DHEA) and its sulfate derivative (DHEA-S) have demonstrated positive outcomes in case reports [265–267] and one double-blind study [268] as an adjunct to antipsychotic treatment, with improvement in negative, depressive, and anxiety symptoms, especially in women. Further studies with these and other neurosteroids are ongoing.

11.6 CONCLUSION

The last 15 years have been a period of rapid advance in our knowledge about the pathophysiology of schizophrenia, the mechanisms of actions of our drugs, and the number of potential therapies that are in development. An important area that was not covered here is pharmacogenomics (see [269, 270]) in which the relationships between specific genetic polymorphisms and the pharmacokinetic, pharmacodynamic, and clinical profiles of a drug are identified in populations of patients. This line of research will allow a more precise matching of patients with the drugs that they are more likely to respond to and/or better tolerate. At this time, we do not have reliable objective predictors of drug response or side-effect vulnerability.

Schizophrenia is a disease of multiple symptom domains and tremendous inter individual variability in clinical presentation and course. Currently we treat patients with one type of medication which is effective primarily against psychotic symptoms. As we get effective treatments for negative symptoms and cognitive dysfunction, it will likely be routine for a patient to be treated with a combination of drugs individually targeting the specific domains of psychopathology in that individual. The treatments for acute-phase illness will likely be different from maintenance strategies, either qualitatively or quantitatively.

Lastly, we are already moving beyond receptor pharmacology to the exploration of intracellular mechanisms of signal transduction, signaling pathways, and the factors that influence gene expression. Eventually, a thorough understanding of the factors that underlie cell development, plasticity, and resilience may enable us to develop entirely new classes of pharmacotherapeutic agents that exert their effects intracellularly, and we may ultimately be able to stop deterioration and even reverse cumulative morbidity in schizophrenia, the most disabling of mental illnesses.

REFERENCES

1. Van Putten, T. (1974). Why do schizophrenic patients refuse to take their drugs? *Arch. Gen. Psychiatry* 31(1), 67–72.
2. Kane, J., et al. (1988). Clozapine for the treatment-resistant schizophrenic. A double-blind comparison with chlorpromazine. *Arch. Gen. Psychiatry* 45(9), 789–796.
3. Lieberman, J. A., et al. (1994). Clinical effects of clozapine in chronic schizophrenia: Response to treatment and predictors of outcome. *Am. J. Psychiatry* 151(12), 1744–1752.
4. Chakos, M., et al. (2001). Effectiveness of second-generation antipsychotics in patients with treatment-resistant schizophrenia: A review and meta-analysis of randomized trials. *Am. J. Psychiatry* 158(4), 518–526.
5. Meltzer, H. Y., and McGurk, S. R. (1999). The effects of clozapine, risperidone, and olanzapine on cognitive function in schizophrenia. *Schizophr. Bull.* 25(2), 233–255.
6. Volavka, J. (1999). The effects of clozapine on aggression and substance abuse in schizophrenic patients. *J. Clin. Psychiatry* 60(Suppl.12), 43–46.
7. Suppes, T., Phillips, K. A., and Judd, C. R. (1994). Clozapine treatment of non-psychotic rapid cycling bipolar disorder: A report of three cases. *Biol. Psychiatry* 36(5), 338–340.
8. Zarate, C. A., Jr., Tohen, M., and Baldessarini, R. J. (1995). Clozapine in severe mood disorders. *J. Clin. Psychiatry* 56(9), 411–417.
9. Zarate, C. A., Jr., et al. (1995). Is clozapine a mood stabilizer?. *J. Clin. Psychiatry* 56(3), 108–112.
10. Meltzer, H. Y., et al. (2003). Clozapine treatment for suicidality in schizophrenia: International Suicide Prevention Trial (InterSePT). [see comment]. *Arch. Gen. Psychiatry* 60(1), 82–91; erratum 60(7), 735.
11. Leucht, S., et al. (1999). Efficacy and extrapyramidal side-effects of the new antipsychotics olanzapine, quetiapine, risperidone, and sertindole compared to conventional antipsychotics and placebo. A meta-analysis of randomized controlled trials. *Schizophr. Res.* 35(1), 51–68.
12. Geddes, J., et al. (2000). Atypical antipsychotics in the treatment of schizophrenia: Systematic overview and meta-regression analysis. *BMJ* 321(7273), 1371–1376.
13. Davis, J. M., Chen, N., and Glick, I. D. (2003). A meta-analysis of the efficacy of second-generation antipsychotics. *Arch. Gen. Psychiatry* 60(6), 553–564.
14. Meltzer, H. Y., and Sumiyoshi, T. (2003). Atypical antipsychotic drugs improve cognition in schizophrenia. *Biol. Psychiatry* 53(3), 265–267.
15. Csernansky, J., Okamoto, A. (2000). Risperidone vs haloperidol for prevention of relapse in schizophrenia and schizoaffective disorders: A long-term double-blind comparison. Paper presented at the Tenth Biennial Winter Workshop on Schizophrenia, Davos, Switzerland.
16. Schooler, N., et al. (2005). Risperidone and haloperidol in first-episode psychosis: A long-term randomized trial. *Am. J. Psychiatry* 162(5), 947–953.
17. Tran, P. V., et al. (1998). Oral olanzapine versus oral haloperidol in the maintenance treatment of schizophrenia and related psychoses. *Br. J. Psychiatry* 172, 499–505.

18. Tollefson, G. D., and Sanger, T. M. (1997). Negative symptoms: A path analytic approach to a double-blind, placebo- and haloperidol-controlled clinical trial with olanzapine. *Am. J. Psychiatry* 154(4), 466–474.

19. Moller, H. J., et al. (1995). A path-analytical approach to differentiate between direct and indirect drug effects on negative symptoms in schizophrenic patients. A reevaluation of the North American risperidone study. *Eur. Arch. Psychiatry Clin. Neurosci.* 245(1), 45–49.

20. Goff, D. C., and Coyle, J. T. (2001). The emerging role of glutamate in the pathophysiology and treatment of schizophrenia. *Am. J. Psychiatry* 158(9), 1367–1377.

21. Harrison, P. J., and Weinberger, D. R. (2005). Schizophrenia genes, gene expression, and neuropathology: On the matter of their convergence. *Mol. Psychiatry* 10(1), 40–68, image 5; erratum 10(4), 420.

22. Frankle, W. G., Lerma, J., and Laruelle, M. (2003). The synaptic hypothesis of schizophrenia. *Neuron* 39(2), 205–216.

23. Laruelle, M., Hirsch, S. R., Weinberger, D. R. (2003). Dopamine transmission in the schizophrenic brain. In *Schizophrenia*, 2nd ed. S. R. Hirsch and D. R. Weinberger, Eds. Blackwell Science, Oxford, pp. 365–387.

24. Carlsson, A., and Lindqvist, M. (1963). Effect of chlorpromazine or haloperidol on formation of 3methoxytyramine and normetanephrine in mouse brain. *Acta Pharmacol. Toxicol.* 20, 140–144.

25. Griffith, J. D., et al. (1972). Dextroamphetamine: Evaluation of psychomimetic properties in man. *Arch. Gen. Psychiatry* 26, 97–100.

26. Angrist, B. M., and Gershon, S. (1970). The phenomenology of experimentally induced amphetamine psychosis—Preliminary observations. *Biol. Psychiatry* 2(2), 95–107.

27. Lieberman, J. A., Kane, J. M., and Alvir, J. A. J. (1987). Provocative tests with psychostimulant drugs in schizophrenia. *Psychopharmacology (Berl.)* 91, 415–433.

28. Janowsky, D. S., et al. (1973). Provocation of schizophrenic symptoms by intravenous administration of methylphenidate. *Arch. Gen. Psychiatry* 28(2), 185–191.

29. Van Kammen, D. P., Docherty, J. P., and Bunney, W. E., Jr., (1982). Prediction of early relapse after pimozide discontinuation by response to d-amphetamine during pimozide treatment. *Biol. Psychiatry* 17(2), 233–242.

30. Angrist, B., et al. (1985). Amphetamine response and relapse risk after depot neuroleptic discontinuation. *Psychopharmacology* 85(3), 277–283.

31. Lieberman, J.A., et al. (1987). Prediction of relapse in schizophrenia. *Arch. Gen. Psychiatry* 44(7), 597–603.

32. van Rossum, J. (1967). The significance of dopamine-receptor blockade for the action of neuroleptic drugs. In *Neuropsychopharmacology, Proceedings of the Fifth Collegium Internationale Neuropsychopharmacologicum*, H. Brille, et al. Eds. Excerpta Medica, Amsterdam pp. 321–329.

33. Creese, I., Burt, D. R., and Snyder, S. H. (1976). Dopamine receptor binding predicts clinical and pharmacological potencies of antischizophrenic drugs. *Science* 192, 480–483.

34. Seeman, P., et al. (1976). Antipsychotic drug doses and neuroleptic/dopamine receptors. *Nature* 261, 717–719.

35. Wong, D. F., et al. (1986). Positron emission tomography reveals elevated D2 dopamine receptors in drug-naive schizophrenics. *Science* 234(4783), 1558–1563.

36. Seeman, P., Guan, H. C., and Niznik, H. B. (1989). Endogenous dopamine lowers the dopamine D2 receptor density as measured by [3H]raclopride: Implications for positron emission tomography of the human brain. *Synapse* 3(1), 96–97.

37. Seeman, P. (1988). Brain dopamine receptors in schizophrenia: PET problems. *Arch. Gen. Psychiatry* 45(6), 598–600; erratum (1989), 46(1), 99.
38. Reith, J., et al. (1994). Elevated dopa decarboxylase activity in living brain of patients with psychosis. *Proc. Nat. Acad. Sci. USA* 91(24), 11651–11654.
39. Hietala, J., et al. (1995). Presynaptic dopamine function in striatum of neuroleptic-naive schizophrenic patients. *Lancet* 346(8983), 1130–1131.
40. Dao-Castellana, M. H., et al. (1997). Presynaptic dopaminergic function in the striatum of schizophrenic patients. *Schizophr. Res.* 23(2), 167–174.
41. Lindstrom, L. H., et al. (1999). Increased dopamine synthesis rate in medial prefrontal cortex and striatum in schizophrenia indicated by L-(beta-11C) DOPA and PET. *Biol. Psychiatry* 46(5), 681–688.
42. Hietala, J., et al. (1999). Depressive symptoms and presynaptic dopamine function in neuroleptic-naive schizophrenia. *Schizophr. Res.* 35(1), 41–50.
43. McGowan, S., et al. (2004). Presynaptic dopaminergic dysfunction in schizophrenia: A positron emission tomographic [18F]fluorodopa study. *Arch. Gen. Psychiatry* 61(2), 134–142.
44. Meyer-Lindenberg, A., et al. (2002). Reduced prefrontal activity predicts exaggerated striatal dopaminergic function in schizophrenia. *Nat. Neurosci.* 5(3), 267–271.
45. Laruelle, M., et al. (1996). Single photon emission computerized tomography imaging of amphetamine-induced dopamine release in drug-free schizophrenic subjects. *Proc. Natl. Acad. Sci. USA* 93, 9235–9240.
46. Breier, A., et al. (1997). Schizophrenia is associated with elevated amphetamine-induced synaptic dopamine concentrations evidence from a novel positron emission tomography method. *Proc. Natl. Acad. Sci. USA* 94, 2569–2574.
47. Abi-Dargham, A., et al. (2000). Increased baseline occupancy of D2 receptors by dopamine in schizophrenia. *Proc. Natl. Acad. Sci. USA* 97(14), 8104–8109.
48. Weinberger, D.R. (1987). Implications of normal brain development for the pathogenesis of schizophrenia. *Arch. Gen. Psychiatry* 44(7), 660–669.
49. Okubo, Y., et al. (1997). Decreased prefrontal dopamine D1 receptors in schizophrenia revealed by PET. *Nature* 385(6617), 634–636.
50. Abi-Dargham, A., et al. (2002). Prefrontal dopamine D1 receptors and working memory in schizophrenia. *J. Neurosci.* 22(9), 3708–3719.
51. Karlsson, P., et al. (2002). PET study of D(1) dopamine receptor binding in neuroleptic-naive patients with schizophrenia. *Am. J. Psychiatry* 159(5), 761–767.
52. Abi-Dargham, A., and Laruelle, M. (2005). Mechanisms of action of second generation antipsychotic drugs in schizophrenia: Insights from brain imaging studies. *Eur. Psychiatry* 20(1), 15–27.
53. Goldman-Rakic, P. S., et al. (2004). Targeting the dopamine D1 receptor in schizophrenia: Insights for cognitive dysfunction. *Psychopharmacology* 174(1), 3–16.
54. Castner, S. A., Williams, G. V., and Goldman-Rakic, P. S. (2000). Reversal of antipsychotic-induced working memory deficits by short-term dopamine D1 receptor stimulation [see comment]. *Science* 287(5460), 2020–2022.
55. Knable, M. B., and Weinberger, D. R. (1997). Dopamine, the prefrontal cortex and schizophrenia. *J. Psychopharmacol.* 11(2), 123–131.
56. Egan, M. F., et al. (2001). Effect of COMT Val108/158 Met genotype on frontal lobe function and risk for schizophrenia. *Proc.Nat. Acad. Sci. USA* 98(12), 6917–6922.
57. Weinberger, D. R., et al. (2001). Prefrontal neurons and the genetics of schizophrenia. *Biol. Psychiatry* 50(11), 825–844.

58. Bilder, R. M., et al. (2002). Neurocognitive correlates of the COMT Val(158)Met polymorphism in chronic schizophrenia. *Biol. Psychiatry* 52(7), 701–707.
59. Malhotra, A. K., et al. (2002). A functional polymorphism in the COMT gene and performance on a test of prefrontal cognition. *Am. J. Psychiatry* 159(4), 652–654.
60. Luby, E. D., et al. (1959). Study of a new schizophrenomimetic drug; Sernyl. *AMA Arch. Neurol. Psychiatry* 81(3), 363–369.
61. Snyder, S. H. (1980). Phencyclidine. *Nature* 285(5764), 355–356.
62. Krystal, J. H., et al. (1994). Subanesthetic effects of the noncompetitive NMDA antagonist, ketamine, in humans. Psychotomimetic, perceptual, cognitive, and neuroendocrine responses. *Arch. Gen. Psychiatry* 51(3), 199–214.
63. Malhotra, A. K., et al. (1996). NMDA receptor function and human cognition - The effects of ketamine in healthy volunteers. *Neuropsychopharmacology* 14, 301–307.
64. Jentsch, J. D., and Roth, R. H. (1999). The neuropsychopharmacology of phencyclidine: From NMDA receptor hypofunction to the dopamine hypothesis of schizophrenia. *Neuropsychopharmacology* 20(3), 201–225.
65. Itil, T., et al. (1967). Effect of phencyclidine in chronic schizophrenics. *Can. Psychiatr. Assoc. J.* 12(2), 209–212.
66. Malhotra, A. K., et al. (1997). Ketamine-induced exacerbation of psychotic symptoms and cognitive impairment in neuroleptic-free schizophrenics. *Neuropsychopharmacology* 17, 141–150.
67. Lahti, A. C., et al. (2001). Effects of ketamine in normal and schizophrenic volunteers. *Neuropsychopharmacology* 25(4), 455–467.
68. Deutsch, S. I., et al. (1989). A "glutamatergic hypothesis" of schizophrenia. *Rationale for pharmacotherapy with glycine. Clin. Neuropharmacol.* 12(1), 1–13.
69. Javitt, D. C., and Zukin, S. R. (1991). Recent advances in the phencyclidine model of schizophrenia. *Am. J. Psychiatry* 148(10), 1301–1308.
70. Olney, J. W., and Farber, N. B. (1995). Glutamate receptor dysfunction and schizophrenia. *Arch. Gen. Psychiatry* 52, 998–1007.
71. Ibrahim, H. M., et al. (2000). Ionotropic glutamate receptor binding and subunit mRNA expression in thalamic nuclei in schizophrenia [see comment]. *Am. J. Psychiatry* 157(11), 1811–1823.
72. Meador-Woodruff, J. H., and Healy, D. J. (2000). Glutamate receptor expression in schizophrenic brain. *Brain Res. Brain Res. Rev.* 31(2/3), 288–294.
73. Gao, X. M., et al. (2000). Ionotropic glutamate receptors and expression of N-methyl-D-aspartate receptor subunits in subregions of human hippocampus: Effects of schizophrenia. *Am. J. Psychiatry* 157(7), 1141–1149.
74. Breier, A., et al. (1998). Effects of NMDA antagonism on striatal dopamine release in healthy subjects—Application of a novel PET approach. *Synapse* 29(2), 142–147.
75. Smith, G. S., et al. (1998). Glutamate modulation of dopamine measured in vivo with positron emission tomography (PET) and C-11-raclopride in normal human subjects. *Neuropsychopharmacology* 18, 18–25.
76. Vollenweider, F. X., et al. (2000). Effects of (S)-ketamine on striatal dopamine: A [11C]raclopride PET study of a model psychosis in humans. *J. Psychiatr. Res.* 34(1), 35–43.
77. Healy, D. J., and Meador-Woodruff, J. H. (1996). Dopamine receptor gene expression in hippocampus is differentially regulated by the NMDA receptor antagonist MK-801. *Eur. J. Pharmacology* 306(1/3), 257–264.

78. Healy, D. J., and Meador-Woodruff, J. H. (1996). Differential regulation, by MK-801, of dopamine receptor gene expression in rat nigrostriatal and mesocorticolimbic systems. *Brain Res.* 708(1/2), 38–44.
79. Weinberger, D. R., Berman, K. F., and Zec, R. F. (1986). Physiologic dysfunction of dorsolateral prefrontal cortex in schizophrenia. I. Regional cerebral blood flow evidence. *Arch. Gen. Psychiatry* 43(2), 114–124.
80. Pycock, C. J., Kerwin, R. W., and Carter, C. J. (1980). Effect of lesion of cortical dopamine terminals on subcortical dopamine receptors in rats. *Nature* 286(5768), 74–76.
81. Carlsson, A., et al. (1999). A glutamatergic deficiency model of schizophrenia. *Br. J. Psychiatry Suppl.* (37), 2–6.
82. Duncan, G. E., Sheitman, B. B., and Lieberman, J. A. (1999). An integrated view of pathophysiological models of schizophrenia. *Brain Res. Rev.* 29(2/3), 250–264.
83. Carlsson, A. (2000). Focusing on dopaminergic stabilizers and 5-HT2A receptor antagonists. *Curr. Opin. CPNS Investing Drugs* 2(1), 22–24.
84. Kramer, M. S., et al. (1997). The effects of a selective D4 dopamine receptor antagonist (L-745,870) in acutely psychotic inpatients with schizophrenia. D4 Dopamine Antagonist Group. *Arch. Gen. Psychiatry* 54(6), 567–572.
85. Truffinet, P., et al. (1999). Placebo-controlled study of the D4/5-HT2A antagonist fananserin in the treatment of schizophrenia. *Am. J. Psychiatry* 156(3), 419–425.
86. Karlsson, P., et al. (1995). Lack of apparent antipsychotic effect of the D1-dopamine receptor antagonist SCH39166 in acutely ill schizophrenic patients. *Psychopharmacology (Berl.)* 121(3), 309–316.
87. Den Boer, J. A., et al. (1995). Differential effects of the D1-DA receptor antagonist SCH39166 on positive and negative symptoms of schizophrenia. *Psychopharmacology (Berl.)* 121(3), 317–322.
88. Karle, J., et al. (1995). NNC 01-0687, a selective dopamine D1 receptor antagonist, in the treatment of schizophrenia. *Psychopharmacology (Berl.)* 121(3), 328–329.
89. Waddington, J. L., Kapur, S., and Remington, G. J. (2003). The neuroscience and clinical psychopharmacology of first- and second-generation antipsychotic drugs. In *Schizophrenia*, 2nd ed., S. R. Hirsch and D. R. Weinberger Eds., Blackwell Science, Oxford, pp. 421–441.
90. Seeman, P. (1992). Dopamine receptor sequences. Therapeutic levels of neuroleptics occupy D2 receptors, clozapine occupies D4. *Neuropsychopharmacology* 7(4), 261–284.
91. Waddington, J. L., Barnes, T. R. E. (1993). Pre- and postsynaptic D1 to D5 dopamine receptor mechanisms in relation to antipsychotic activity. In *Antipsychotic Drugs and Their Side Effects*. T. R. E. Barnes, Ed. Academic, London, pp. 65–85.
92. Farde, L., et al. (1992). Positron emission tomographic analysis of central D1 and D2 dopamine receptor occupancy in patients treated with classical neuroleptics and clozapine. Relation to extrapyramidal side effects. *Arch. Gen. Psychiatry* 49(7), 538–544.
93. Nordstrom, A. L., et al. (1993). Central D2-dopamine receptor occupancy in relation to antipsychotic drug effects: A double-blind PET study of schizophrenic patients. *Biol. Psychiatry* 33(4), 227–235.
94. Kapur, S., et al. (2000). Relationship between dopamine D2 occupancy, clinical response, and side effects: A double-blind PET study of first-episode schizophrenia. *Am. J. Psychiatry* 157(4), 514–520.
95. Wolkin, A., et al. (1989). Dopamine blockade and clinical response: Evidence for two biological subgroups of schizophrenia. *Am. J. Psychiatry* 146(7), 905–908.

96. Coppens, H. J., et al. (1991). High central D2-dopamine receptor occupancy as assessed with positron emission tomography in medicated but therapy-resistant schizophrenic patients. *Biol. Psychiatry* 29(7), 629–634.

97. Grace, A. A., et al. (1997). Dopamine-cell depolarization block as a model for the therapeutic actions of antipsychotic drugs. *Trends Neurosci.* 20(1), 31–37.

98. Kuhar, M. J., and Joyce, A. R. (2001). Slow onset of CNS drugs: Can changes in protein concentration account for the delay?. *Trends Pharmacol. Sci.* 22(9), 450–456.

99. Agid, O., et al. (2003). Delayed-onset hypothesis of antipsychotic action: A hypothesis tested and rejected. *Arch. Gen. Psychiatry* 60(12), 1228–1235.

100. Kapur, S., et al. (2005). Evidence for onset of antipsychotic effects within the first 24 hours of treatment. *Am. J. Psychiatry* 162(5), 939–946.

101. Meltzer, H. Y., Matsubara, S., and Lee, J. C. (1989). Classification of typical and atypical antipsychotic drugs on the basis of dopamine D1, D2 and Serotonin2 pKi values. *J. Pharmacol. Exp. Ther.* 251, 238–246.

102. Kapur, S., and Mamo, D. (2003). Half a century of antipsychotics and still a central role for dopamine D2 receptors. *Prog. Neuro-Psychopharmacol. Biol. Psychiatry* 27(7), 1081–1090.

103. Seeman, P. (2002). Atypical antipsychotics: Mechanism of action. *Can. J. Psychiatry* 47(1), 27–38.

104. Marder, S. R., and Meibach, R. C. (1994). Risperidone in the treatment of schizophrenia. *Am. J. Psychiatry* 151(6), 825–835.

105. Arvanitis, L. A., Miller, B. G. The Seroquel Trial 13 Study (1997). Multiple fixed doses of "Seroquel" (quetiapine) in patients with acute exacerbation of schizophrenia: A comparison with haloperidol and placebo. *Biol. Psychiatry* **42**(4), 233-246.

106. Knable, M. B., et al. (1997). Extrapyramidal side effects with risperidone and haloperidol at comparable D2 receptor occupancy levels. *Psychiatry Res.* 75(2), 91–101.

107. Kapur, S., and Remington, G. (2001). Dopamine D(2) receptors and their role in atypical antipsychotic action: Still necessary and may even be sufficient. *Biol Psychiatry* 50(11), 873–883.

108. Hartvig, P., et al. (1986). Receptor binding of N-(methyl-11C) clozapine in the brain of rhesus monkey studied by positron emission tomography (PET). *Psychopharmacology* 89(2), 248–252.

109. Seeman, P., and Tallerico, T. (1998). Antipsychotic drugs which elicit little or no parkinsonism bind more loosely than dopamine to brain D2 receptors, yet occupy high levels of these receptors. *Mol. Psychiatry* 3(2), 123–134.

110. Kapur, S., and Seeman, P. (2001). Does fast dissociation from the dopamine d(2) receptor explain the action of atypical antipsychotics?: A new hypothesis. *Am. J. Psychiatry* 158(3), 360–369.

111. Pickar, D., et al. (1996). Individual variation in D2 dopamine receptor occupancy in clozapine-treated patients. *Am. J. Psychiatry* 153(12), 1571–1578.

112. Xiberas, X., et al. (2001). In vivo extrastriatal and striatal D2 dopamine receptor blockade by amisulpride in schizophrenia. *J. Clin. Psychopharmacol.* 21(2), 207–214.

113. Gefvert, O., et al. (1998). Time course of central nervous dopamine-D2 and 5-HT2 receptor blockade and plasma drug concentrations after discontinuation of quetiapine (Seroquel) in patients with schizophrenia. *Psychopharmacology* 135(2), 119–126.

114. Tauscher-Wisniewski, S., et al. (2002). Quetiapine: An effective antipsychotic in first-episode schizophrenia despite only transiently high dopamine-2 receptor blockade. *J. Clin. Psychiatry* 63(11), 992–997.
115. Kapur, S., et al. (2000). A positron emission tomography study of quetiapine in schizophrenia: A preliminary finding of an antipsychotic effect with only transiently high dopamine D2 receptor occupancy. *Arch. Gen. Psychiatry* 57(6), 553–559.
116. Kapur, S., Zipursky, R. B., and Remington, G. (1999). Clinical and theoretical implications of 5-HT2 and D2 receptor occupancy of clozapine, risperidone, and olanzapine in schizophrenia. *Am. J. Psychiatry* 156(2), 286–293.
117. Frankle, W. G., et al. (2004). Occupancy of dopamine D2 receptors by the atypical antipsychotic drugs risperidone and olanzapine: Theoretical implications. *Psychopharmacology* 175(4), 473–480.
118. Turrone, P., et al. (2002). Elevation of prolactin levels by atypical antipsychotics. *Am. J. Psychiatry* 159(1), 133–135.
119. Jones, H. M., and Pilowsky, L. S. (2002). Dopamine and antipsychotic drug action revisited. *Br. J. Psychiatry* 181, 271–275.
120. Seeman, P., and Tallerico, T. (1999). Rapid release of antipsychotic drugs from dopamine D2 receptors: An explanation for low receptor occupancy and early clinical relapse upon withdrawal of clozapine or quetiapine. *Am. J. Psychiatry* 156(6), 876–884.
121. Bench, C. J., et al. (1993). Dose dependent occupancy of central dopamine D2 receptors by the novel neuroleptic CP-88,059-01: A study using positron emission tomography and 11C-raclopride. *Psychopharmacology (Berl.)* 112(2/3), 308–314.
122. Mamo, D., et al. (2004). A PET study of dopamine D2 and serotonin 5-HT2 receptor occupancy in patients with schizophrenia treated with therapeutic doses of ziprasidone. *Am. J. Psychiatry* 161(5), 818–825.
123. Daniel, D. G., et al. (1999). Ziprasidone 80 mg/day and 160 mg/day in the acute exacerbation of schizophrenia and schizoaffective disorder: A 6-week placebo-controlled trial. *Neuropsychopharmacology* 20(5), 491–505.
124. Keck, P., Jr., et al. (1998). Ziprasidone 40 and 120 mg/day in the acute exacerbation of schizophrenia and schizoaffective disorder: A 4-week placebo-controlled trial. *Psychopharmacology (Berl.)* 140(2), 173–184.
125. Keck, P. E., Jr., et al. (2001). Ziprasidone in the short-term treatment of patients with schizoaffective disorder: Results from two double-blind, placebo-controlled, multicenter studies. *J. Clin. Psychopharmacol.* 21(1), 27–35.
126. Kasper, S. (1998). Risperidone and olanzapine: Optimal dosing for efficacy and tolerability in patients with schizophrenia. *Int. Clin. Psychopharmacol.* 13(6), 253–262.
127. Grunder, G., Carlsson, A., and Wong, D. F. (2003). Mechanism of new antipsychotic medications: Occupancy is not just antagonism. *Arch. Gen. Psychiatry* 60(10), 974–977.
128. Yokoi, F., et al. (2002). Dopamine D2 and D3 receptor occupancy in normal humans treated with the antipsychotic drug aripiprazole (OPC 14597): A study using positron emission tomography and [11C]raclopride. *Neuropsychopharmacology* 27(2), 248–259.
129. Martinot, J. L., et al. (1996). In vivo characteristics of dopamine D2 receptor occupancy by amisulpride in schizophrenia. *Psychopharmacology (Berl.)* 124(1/2), 154–158.
130. Danion, J. M., Rein, W., and Fleurot, O. (1999). Improvement of schizophrenic patients with primary negative symptoms treated with amisulpride. Amisulpride Study Group. *Am. J. Psychiatry* 156(4), 610–616.
131. Coulouvrat, C., and Dondey-Nouvel, L. (1999). Safety of amisulpride (Solian): A review of 11 clinical studies. *Int. Clin. Psychopharmacol.* 14(4), 209–218.

132. Colonna, L., et al. (2000). Long-term safety and efficacy of amisulpride in subchronic or chronic schizophrenia. Amisulpride Study Group. *Int. Clin. Psychopharmacol.* 15(1), 13–22.

133. Scatton, B., and Sanger, D. J. (2000). Pharmacological and molecular targets in the search for novel antipsychotics. *Behav. Pharmacol.* 11(3/4), 243–256.

134. Corrigan, M. H., et al. (2004). Effectiveness of the selective D4 antagonist sonepiprazole in schizophrenia: A placebo-controlled trial. *Biol. Psychiatry* 55(5), 445–451.

135. Seeman, P., Corbett, R., and Van Tol, H. H. (1997). Atypical neuroleptics have low affinity for dopamine D2 receptors or are selective for D4 receptors. *Neuropsychopharmacology* 16(2), 93–110; discussion 111–135.

136. Scatton, B., et al. (1997). Amisulpride: From animal pharmacology to therapeutic action. *Int. Clin. Psychopharmacol.* 12(Suppl.2), S29–S36.

137. Deutch, A. Y., lee, M. C., and Iadarola, M. J. (1992). Regionally specific effects of atypical antipsychotic drugs on striatal Fos expression: The nucleus accumbens shell as a locus of antipsychotic action. *Mol. Cell. Neurosci.* 3, 332–341.

138. Robertson, G. S., Matsumura, H., and Fibiger, H. C. (1994). Induction patterns of neuroleptic-induced Fos-like immunoreactivity as predictors of atypical antipsychotic activity. *J. Pharmacol. Exp. Ther.* 271, 1058–1066.

139. White, F. J., and Wang, R. Y. (1983). Differential effects of classical and atypical antipsychotic drugs on A9 and A10 dopamine neurons. *Science* 221(4615), 1054–1057.

140. Di Giovanni, G., et al. (1998). Effects of acute and repeated administration of amisulpride, a dopamine D2/D3 receptor antagonist, on the electrical activity of midbrain dopaminergic neurons. *J. Pharmacol. & Exp. Ther.* 287(1), 51–57.

141. Bigliani, V., et al. (2000). Striatal and temporal cortical D2/D3 receptor occupancy by olanzapine and sertindole in vivo: A [123I]epidepride single photon emission tomography (SPET) study. *Psychopharmacology (Berl.)* 150(2), 132–140.

142. Bressan, R. A., et al. (2003). Is regionally selective D2/D3 dopamine occupancy sufficient for atypical antipsychotic effect? An in vivo quantitative [123I]epidepride SPET study of amisulpride-treated patients. *Am. J. Psychiatry* 160(8), 1413–1420.

143. Bressan, R. A., et al. (2003). Optimizing limbic selective D2/D3 receptor occupancy by risperidone: a [123I]-epidepride SPET study. *J. Clin. Psychopharmacol.* 23(1), 5–14.

144. Pilowsky, L. S., et al. (1997). Limbic selectivity of clozapine [letter]. *Lancet* 350(9076), 490–491.

145. Stephenson, C. M., et al. (2000). Striatal and extra-striatal D(2)/D(3) dopamine receptor occupancy by quetiapine in vivo. [(123)I]-epidepride single photon emission tomography (SPET) study. *Br. J. Psychiatry J. Ment. Sci.* 177, 408–415.

146. Xiberas, X., et al. (2001). Extrastriatal and striatal D(2) dopamine receptor blockade with haloperidol or new antipsychotic drugs in patients with schizophrenia. *Br. J. Psychiatry* 179, 503–508.

147. Talvik, M., et al. (2001). No support for regional selectivity in clozapine-treated patients: A PET study with [(11)C]raclopride and [(11)C]FLB 457. *Am. J. Psychiatry* 158(6), 926–930.

148. Yasuno, F., et al. (2001). Dose relationship of limbic-cortical D2-dopamine receptor occupancy with risperidone. *Psychopharmacologia* 154(1), 112–114.

149. Sharma, T., and Antonova, L. (2003). Cognitive function in schizophrenia. Deficits, functional consequences, and future treatment. *Psychiatr. Clin. North Am.* 26(1), 25–40.

150. Ichikawa, J., et al. (2001). 5-HT(2A) and D(2) receptor blockade increases cortical DA release via 5-HT(1A) receptor activation: A possible mechanism of atypical antipsychotic-induced cortical dopamine release. *J. Neurochem.* 76(5), 1521–1531.

151. Li, X. M., et al. (1998). Olanzapine increases in vivo dopamine and norepinephrine release in rat prefrontal cortex, nucleus accumbens and striatum. *Psychopharmacology (Berl.)* 136(2), 153–161.

152. Moghaddam, B., and Bunney, B. S. (1990). Utilization of microdialysis for assessing the release of mesotelencephalic dopamine following clozapine and other antipsychotic drugs. *Prog. Neuro.-Psychopharmacol. Biol. Psychiatry* 14(Suppl.), S51–S57.

153. Kuroki, T., Meltzer, H. Y., and Ichikawa, J. (1999). Effects of antipsychotic drugs on extracellular dopamine levels in rat medial prefrontal cortex and nucleus accumbens. *J. Pharmacol. Exp. Ther.* 288(2), 774–781.

154. Ichikawa, J., et al. (2002). Atypical, but not typical, antipsychotic drugs increase cortical acetylcholine release without an effect in the nucleus accumbens or striatum. *Neuropsychopharmacology* 26(3), 325–339.

155. Bakshi, V. P., and Geyer, M. A. (1995). Antagonism of phencyclidine-induced deficits in prepulse inhibition by the putative atypical antipsychotic olanzapine. *Psychopharmacology (Berl.)* 122(2), 198–201.

156. Corbett, R., et al. (1995). Antipsychotic agents antagonize non-competitive N-methyl-D-aspartate antagonist-induced behaviors. *Psychopharmacology (Berl.)* 120, 67–74.

157. Duncan, G. E., et al. (1998). Differential effects of clozapine and haloperidol on ketamine-induced brain metabolic activation. *Brain Res.* 812, 65–75.

158. Wang, R. Y., and Liang, X. (1998). M100907 and clozapine, but not haloperidol or raclopride, prevent phencyclidine-induced blockade of NMDA responses in pyramidal neurons of the rat medial prefrontal cortical slice. *Neuropsychopharmacology* 19(1), 74–85.

159. Duncan, G. E., et al. (2000). Comparison of the effects of clozapine, risperidone, and olanzapine on ketamine-induced alterations in regional brain metabolism. *J. Pharmacol. Exp. Ther.* 293(1), 8–14.

160. Arvanov, V. L., et al. (1997). Clozapine and haloperidol modulate N-methyl-D-aspartate- and non-N-methyl-D-aspartate receptor-mediated neurotransmission in rat prefrontal cortical neurons in vitro. *J. Pharmacol. Exp. Ther.* 283(1), 226–234.

161. Arvanov, V. L., and Wang, R. Y. (1999). Clozapine, but not haloperidol, prevents the functional hyperactivity of N-methyl-D-aspartate receptors in rat cortical neurons induced by subchronic administration of phencyclidine. *J. Pharmacol. Exp. Ther.* 289(2), 1000–1006.

162. Bakshi, V. P., Swerdlow, N. R., and Geyer, M. A. (1994). Clozapine antagonizes phencyclidine-induced deficits in sensorimotor gating of the startle response. *J. Pharmacol. Exp. Ther.* 271, 787–794.

163. Sur, C., et al. (2003). N-Desmethylclozapine, an allosteric agonist at muscarinic 1 receptor, potentiates N-methyl-D-aspartate receptor activity. *Proc. Natl. Acad. Sci. USA* 100(23), 13674–13679.

164. Nyberg, S., et al. (1995). D2 dopamine receptor occupancy during low-dose treatment with haloperidol decanoate. *Am. J. Psychiatry* 152(2), 173–178.

165. Kane, J. M., et al. (2003). Long-acting injectable risperidone: Efficacy and safety of the first long-acting atypical antipsychotic. *Am. J. Psychiatry* 160(6), 1125–1132.

166. Gefvert, O., et al. (2005). Pharmacokinetics and D2 receptor occupancy of long-acting injectable risperidone (Risperdal Consta) in patients with schizophrenia. *Int. J. Neuropsychopharmacol.* 8(1), 27–36.

167. Fleischhacker, W. W., et al. (2003). Treatment of schizophrenia with long-acting injectable risperidone: A 12-month open-label trial of the first long-acting second-generation antipsychotic. *J. Clin. Psychiatry* 64(10), 1250–1257.
168. Laruelle, M., et al. (1999). Increased dopamine transmission in schizophrenia: Relationship to illness phases. *Biol. Psychiatry* 46(1), 56–72.
169. Harrow, M., et al. (1994). Depression in schizophrenia: Are neuroleptics, akinesia, or anhedonia involved? *Schizophr. Bull.* 20(2), 327–338.
170. Voruganti, L., and Awad, A. G. (2004). Neuroleptic dysphoria: Towards a new synthesis. *Psychopharmacology* 171(2), 121–132.
171. Kane, J. M. (1989). The current status of neuroleptic therapy. *J. Clin. Psychiatry* 50, 322–328.
172. Fleischhacker, W. W. (1995). New drugs for the treatment of schizophrenic patients. *Acta. Psychiatr. Scand. (Suppl.)* 388, 24–30.
173. Miyamoto, S., et al., (2002). Therapeutics of schizophrenia. In *Neuropsychopharmacology: The Fifth Generation of Progress*, K. L. Davis, D. Charney, J. T. Coyle, and C. Nemeroff, Eds. Lippincott Williams & Wilkins, Philadelphia, pp. 775–807.
174. Chakos, M. H., et al. (1992). Incidence and correlates of acute extrapyramidal symptoms in first episode of schizophrenia. *Psychopharmacol. Bull.* 28(1), 81–86.
175. Kane, J. M., Woerner, M., and Lieberman, J. (1985). Tardive dyskinesia: Prevalence, incidence, and risk factors. *Psychopharmacol. Suppl.* 2, 72–78.
176. Woerner, M. G., et al. (1998). Prospective study of tardive dyskinesia in the elderly: Rates and risk factors. *Am. J. Psychiatry* 155(11), 1521–1528.
177. Leucht, S., et al. (2003). New generation antipsychotics versus low-potency conventional antipsychotics: A systematic review and meta-analysis. *Lancet* 361(9369), 1581–1589.
178. Peuskens, J., and Link, C. G. (1997). A comparison of quetiapine and chlorpromazine in the treatment of schizophrenia. *Acta Psychiatr. Scand.* 96(4), 265–273.
179. Remington, G., and Kapur, S. (2000). Atypical antipsychotics: Are some more atypical than others? *Psychopharmacology (Berl.)* 148, 3–15.
180. Kane, J. M., et al., (2001). Second generation antipsychotics in the treatment of schizophrenia: Clozapine. In *Current Issues in the Psychopharmacology of Schizophrenia*, A. Breir, F. Bymaster, and P. Tran, Eds. Lippincott Williams & Wilkins Healthcare, Philadelphia, pp. 209–223.
181. Carpenter, W. T., Jr., et al. (1995). Patient response and resource management: Another view of clozapine treatment of schizophrenia. *Am. J. Psychiatry* 152(6), 827–832.
182. Conley, R., Gounaris, C., and Tamminga, C. (1994). Clozapine response varies in deficit versus non-deficit schizophrenic subjects. *Biol. Psychiatry* 35, 746–747.
183. Buchanan, R. W., and Gold, J. M. (1996). Negative symptoms: Diagnosis, treatment and prognosis. *Int. Clin. Psychopharmacol.* 11(Suppl.2), 3–11.
184. Collaborative Working Group on Clinical Trial (1998). Assessing the effects of atypical antipsychotics on negative symptoms. Collaborative Working Group on Clinical Trial Evaluations. *J. Clin. Psychiatry* 59(Suppl.12), 28–34.
185. Mortimer, A. M. (1997). Cognitive function in schizophrenia—Do neuroleptics make a difference? *Pharmacol. Biochem. Behav.* 56(4), 789–795.
186. Velligan, D. I., and Miller, A. L. (1999). Cognitive dysfunction in schizophrenia and its importance to outcome: The place of atypical antipsychotics in treatment. *J. Clin. Psychiatry* 60(Suppl.23), 25–28.

187. Green, M. F., and Braff, D. L. (2001). Translating the basic and clinical cognitive neuroscience of schizophrenia to drug development and clinical trials of antipsychotic medications. *Biol. Psychiatry* 49(4), 374–384.

188. Green, M. F., et al. (1997). Does risperidone improve verbal working memory in treatment-resistant schizophrenia? *Am. J. Psychiatry* 154(6), 799–804.

189. Keefe, R. S. E., et al. (1999). The effects of atypical antipsychotic drugs on neurocognitive impairment in schizophrenia: A review and meta-analysis. *Schizophr. Bull.* 25(2), 201–222.

190. Green, M. F., et al. (2002). The neurocognitive effects of low-dose haloperidol: A two-year comparison with risperidone. *Biol. Psychiatry* 51(12), 972–978.

191. Keefe, R. S. E., et al. (2004). Comparative effect of atypical and conventional antipsychotic drugs on neurocognition in first-episode psychosis: A randomized, double-blind trial of olanzapine versus low doses of haloperidol. *Am. J. Psychiatry* 161(6), 985–995.

192. Csernansky, J. G., Mahmoud, R., and Brenner, R. (2002). A comparison of risperidone and haloperidol for the prevention of relapse in patients with schizophrenia. *N. Engl. J. Med.* 346(1), 16–22.

193. Leucht, S., et al. (2003). Relapse prevention in schizophrenia with new-generation antipsychotics: A systematic review and exploratory meta-analysis of randomized, controlled trials. *Am. J. Psychiatry* 160(7), 1209–1222.

194. Lieberman, J. A., et al. (2001). The early stages of schizophrenia: Speculations on pathogenesis, pathophysiology, and therapeutic approaches. *Biol. Psychiatry* 50(11), 884–897.

195. Lieberman, J. A., et al. (2003). Comparative efficacy and safety of atypical and conventional antipsychotic drugs in first-episode psychosis: A randomized, double-blind trial of olanzapine versus haloperidol. *Am. J. Psychiatry* 160(8), 1396–1404.

196. McGlashan, T. H. (1996). Early detection and intervention in schizophrenia: Research. *Schizophr. Bull.* 22(2), 327–345.

197. McGorry, P. D., et al. (2002). Randomized controlled trial of interventions designed to reduce the risk of progression to first-episode psychosis in a clinical sample with subthreshold symptoms. *Arch. Gen. Psychiatry* 59(10), 921–928.

198. Beasley, C. M., et al. (1999). Randomised double-blind comparison of the incidence of tardive dyskinesia in patients with schizophrenia during long-term treatment with olanzapine or haloperidol [see comment]. *Br. J. Psychiatry* 174, 23–30.

199. Allison, D. B., et al. (1999). Antipsychotic-induced weight gain: A comprehensive research synthesis. *Am. J. Psychiatry* 156(11), 1686–1696.

200. Newcomer, J. W. (2005). Second-generation (atypical) antipsychotics and metabolic effects: A comprehensive literature review. *CNS Drugs* 19(Suppl.1), 1–93.

201. Casey, D. E., et al. (2004). Antipsychotic-induced weight gain and metabolic abnormalities: Implications for increased mortality in patients with schizophrenia. *J. Clin. Psychiatry* 65(Suppl.7), 4–18; quiz 19–20.

202. Kalkman, H. O., Subramanian, N., and Hoyer, D. (2001). Extended radioligand binding profile of iloperidone: A broad spectrum dopamine/serotonin/norepinephrine receptor antagonist for the management of psychotic disorders. *Neuropsychopharmacology* 25(6), 904–914.

203. Jain, K. K. (2000). An assessment of iloperidone for the treatment of schizophrenia. *Exp. Opin. Investig. Drugs* 9(12), 2935–2943.

204. Turner, D. C., et al. (2004). Modafinil improves cognition and attentional set shifting in patients with chronic schizophrenia. *Neuropsychopharmacology* 29(7), 1363–1373.

205. Liljequist, R., et al. (1997). Catechol O-methyltransferase inhibitor tolcapone has minor influence on performance in experimental memory models in rats. *Behav. Brain Res.* 82(2), 195–202.

206. Gasparini, M., et al. (1997). Cognitive improvement during Tolcapone treatment in Parkinson's disease. *J. Neural Transm.* 104(8/9), 887–894.

207. Schwartz, J. C., et al. (2000). Possible implications of the dopamine D(3) receptor in schizophrenia and in antipsychotic drug actions. *Brain Res. Brain Res. Rev.* 31(2/3), 277–287.

208. Gurevich, E. V., et al. (1997). Mesolimbic dopamine D3 receptors and use of antipsychotics in patients with schizophrenia. A postmortem study. *Arch. Gen. Psychiatry* 54(3), 225–232.

209. Blanchet, P. J., et al. (1998). Effects of the full dopamine D1 receptor agonist dihydrexidine in Parkinson's disease. *Clin. Neuropharmacol.* 21(6), 339–343.

210. Kasckow, J., and Nemeroff, C. B. (1991). The neurobiology of neurotensin: Focus on neurotensin-dopamine interactions. *Regul. Peptides* 36(2), 153–164.

211. Nemeroff, C. B. (1980). Neurotensin: Perchance an endogenous neuroleptic? *Biol. Psychiatry* 15(2), 283–302.

212. Binder, E. B., et al. (2001). The role of neurotensin in the pathophysiology of schizophrenia and the mechanism of action of antipsychotic drugs. *Biol. Psychiatry* 50(11), 856–872.

213. Kinkead, B., and Nemeroff, C. B. (2002). Neurotensin: An endogenous antipsychotic?. *Curr. Opin. Pharmacol.* 2(1), 99–103.

214. Meltzer, H. Y., et al. (2004). Placebo-controlled evaluation of four novel compounds for the treatment of schizophrenia and schizoaffective disorder [see comment]. *Am. J. Psychiatry* 161(6), 975–984.

215. Richelson, E., Fredrickson, P. A., and Boules, M. M. (2005). Neurotensin receptor agonists and antagonists for schizophrenia [comment]. *Am. J. Psychiatry* 162(3), 633–634; author reply 635.

216. Gueudet, C., et al. (1999). Blockade of neurokinin3 receptors antagonizes drug-induced population response and depolarization block of midbrain dopamine neurons in guinea pigs. *Synapse* 33(1), 71–79.

217. Marco, N., et al. (1998). Activation of dopaminergic and cholinergic neurotransmission by tachykinin NK3 receptor stimulation: An in vivo microdialysis approach in guinea pig. *Neuropeptides* 32(5), 481–488.

218. Kamali, F. (2001). Osanetant Sanofi-Synthelabo. *Curr. Opin. Investig. Drugs* 2(7), 950–956.

219. Tsai, G., et al. (1998). D-Serine added to antipsychotics for the treatment of schizophrenia. *Biol. Psychiatry* 44, 1081–1089.

220. Tuominen, H. J., Tiihonen, J., and Wahlbeck, K. (2005). Glutamatergic drugs for schizophrenia: A systematic review and meta-analysis. *Schizophr. Res.* 72(2/3), 225–234.

221. Bergeron, R., et al. (1998). Modulation of N-methyl-D-aspartate receptor function by glycine transport. *Proc. Natl. Acad. Sci. USA* 95(26), 15730–15734.

222. Berger, A. J., Dieudonne, S., and Ascher, P. (1998). Glycine uptake governs glycine site occupancy at NMDA receptors of excitatory synapses. *J. Neurophysiol.* 80(6), 3336–3340.

223. Javitt, D. C., et al. (1997). Reversal of phencyclidine-induced hyperactivity by glycine and the glycine uptake inhibitor glycyldodecylamide. *Neuropsychopharmacology* 17(3), 202–204.

224. Javitt, D. C., and Frusciante, M. (1997). Glycyldodecylamide, a phencyclidine behavioral antagonist, blocks cortical glycine uptake: Implications for schizophrenia and substance abuse. *Psychopharmacology (Berl.)* 129(1), 96–98.

225. Tsai, G., et al. (2004). Glycine transporter I inhibitor, *N*-methylglycine (sarcosine), added to antipsychotics for the treatment of schizophrenia. *Biol. Psychiatry* 55(5), 452–456.

226. Smith, R. E., et al. (2001). Expression of excitatory amino acid transporter transcripts in the thalamus of subjects with schizophrenia. *Am. J. Psychiatry* 158(9), 1393–1399.

227. McCullumsmith, R. E., and Meador-Woodruff, J. H. (2002). Striatal excitatory amino acid transporter transcript expression in schizophrenia, bipolar disorder, and major depressive disorder. *Neuropsychopharmacology* 26(3), 368–375.

228. Rowley, M., Bristow, L. J., and Hutson, P. H. (2001). Current and novel approaches to the drug treatment of schizophrenia. *J. Med. Chem.* 44(4), 477–501.

229. Chavez-Noriega, L. E., Schaffhauser, H., and Campbell, U. C. (2002). Metabotropic glutamate receptors: Potential drug targets for the treatment of schizophrenia. *Curr. Drug Target CNS. Neurol. Disord.* 1(3), 261–281.

230. Krystal, J. H., et al. (2005). Preliminary evidence of attenuation of the disruptive effects of the NMDA glutamate receptor antagonist, ketamine, on working memory by pretreatment with the group II metabotropic glutamate receptor agonist, LY354740, in healthy human subjects. *Psychopharmacology* 179(1), 303–309.

231. Moghaddam, B., et al. (1997). Activation of glutamatergic neurotransmission by ketamine—A novel step in the pathway from NMDA receptor blockade to dopaminergic and cognitive disruptions associated with the prefrontal cortex. *J. Neurosci.* 17, 2921–2927.

232. Bubser, M., et al. (1992). Differential behavioral and neurochemical effects of competitive and non-competitive NMDA receptor antagonists in rats. *Eur. J. Pharmacol.* 229, 75–82.

233. Hauber, W., and Andersen, R. (1993). The non-NMDA glutamate receptor antagonist GYKI 52466 counteracts locomotor stimulation and anticataleptic activity induced by the NMDA antagonist dizocilpine. *Naunyn Schmiedebergs Arch. Pharmacol.* 348, 486–490.

234. Willins, D. L., et al. (1993). The role of dopamine and AMPA/kainate receptors in the nucleus accumbens in the hypermotility response to MK801. *Pharmacol. Biochem. Behav.* 46, 881–887.

235. Hampson, R. E., et al. (1998). Facilitative effects of the ampakine CX516 on short-term memory in rats: Correlations with hippocampal neuronal activity. *J. Neurosci.* 18(7), 2748–2763.

236. Hampson, R. E., et al. (1998). Facilitative effects of the ampakine CX516 on short-term memory in rats: Enhancement of delayed-nonmatch-to-sample performance. *J. Neurosci.* 18(7), 2740–2747.

237. Johnson, S. A., et al. (1999). Synergistic interactions between ampakines and antipsychotic drugs. *J. Pharmacol. Exp. Ther.* 289(1), 392–397.

238. Goff, D., et al. (1999). A preliminary dose-escalation trial of CX 516 (ampakine) added to clozapine in schizophrenia. *Schizophr. Res.* 36(1/3), 280.

239. Marenco, S., et al. (2002). Preliminary experience with an ampakine (CX516) as a single agent for the treatment of schizophrenia: A case series. *Schizophr. Res.* 57(2/3), 221–226.
240. Kremer, I., et al. (2004). Placebo-controlled trial of lamotrigine added to conventional and atypical antipsychotics in schizophrenia. *Biol. Psychiatry* 56(6), 441–446.
241. Tiihonen, J., et al. (2003). Lamotrigine in treatment-resistant schizophrenia: A randomized placebo-controlled crossover trial. *Biol. Psychiatry* 54(11), 1241–1248.
242. Vriend, J., and Alexiuk, N. A. (1997). Lamotrigine inhibits the in situ activity of tyrosine hydroxylase in striatum of audiogenic seizure-prone and audiogenic seizure-resistant Balb/c mice. *Life Sci.* 61(25), 2467–2474.
243. Anand, A., et al. (2000). Attenuation of the neuropsychiatric effects of ketamine with lamotrigine: Support for hyperglutamatergic effects of N-methyl-D-aspartate receptor antagonists. *Arch. Gen. Psychiatry* 57(3), 270–276.
244. Goldman-Rakic, P. S., Lidow, M. S., and Gallager, D. W. (1990). Overlap of dopaminergic, adrenergic, and serotoninergic receptors and complementarity of their subtypes in primate prefrontal cortex. *J. Neurosci.* 10(7), 2125–2138.
245. Arnsten, A. F., Steere, J. C., and Hunt, R. D. (1996). The contribution of alpha 2-noradrenergic mechanisms of prefrontal cortical cognitive function. Potential significance for attention-deficit hyperactivity disorder. *Arch. Gen. Psychiatry* 53(5), 448–455.
246. Friedman, J. I., Temporini, H., and Davis, K. L. (1999). Pharmacologic strategies for augmenting cognitive performance in schizophrenia. *Biol. Psychiatry* 45(1), 1–16.
247. Friedman, J. I., Adler, D. N., and Davis, K. L. (1999). The role of norepinephrine in the pathophysiology of cognitive disorders: Potential applications to the treatment of cognitive dysfunction in schizophrenia and Alzheimer's disease. *Biol. Psychiatry* 46(9), 1243–1252.
248. Coull, J. T. (1994). Pharmacological manipulations of the alpha 2-noradrenergic system. Effects on cognition. *Drugs & Aging* 5(2), 116–126.
249. Fields, R. B., et al. (1988). Clonidine improves memory function in schizophrenia independently from change in psychosis. Preliminary findings. *Schizoph. Res.* 1(6), 417–423.
250. Friedman, J. I., et al. (2001). Guanfacine treatment of cognitive impairment in schizophrenia. *Neuropsychopharmacology* 25(3), 402–409.
251. Litman, R. E., et al. (1993). Idazoxan, an alpha 2 antagonist, augments fluphenazine in schizophrenic patients: A pilot study. *J. Clin. Psychopharmacol.* 13(4), 264–267.
252. Litman, R. E., et al. (1996). Idazoxan and response to typical neuroleptics in treatment-resistant schizophrenia. Comparison with the atypical neuroleptic, clozapine. *Br. J. Psychiatry* 168(5), 571–579.
253. Adler, L. E., et al. (1998). Schizophrenia, sensory gating, and nicotinic receptors. *Schizophr. Bull.* 24(2), 189–202.
254. Bontempi, B., et al. (2001). SIB-1553A, (+/−)-4-[[2-(1-methyl-2-pyrrolidinyl)ethyl]thio]phenol hydrochloride, a subtype-selective ligand for nicotinic acetylcholine receptors with putative cognitive-enhancing properties: Effects on working and reference memory performances in aged rodents and nonhuman primates. *J. Pharmacol. Exp. Ther.* 299(1), 297–306.
255. Lloyd, G. K., et al. (1998). The potential of subtype-selective neuronal nicotinic acetylcholine receptor agonists as therapeutic agents. *Life Sci.* 62(17/18), 1601–1606.
256. Allen, T. B., and McEvoy, J. P. (2002). Galantamine for treatment-resistant schizophrenia. *Am. J. Psychiatry* 159(7), 1244–1245.

257. Rosse, R. B., and Deutsch, S. I. (2002). Adjuvant galantamine administration improves negative symptoms in a patient with treatment-refractory schizophrenia. *Clin. Neuropharmacol.* 25(5), 272–275.
258. Friedman, J. I., et al. (2002). A double blind placebo controlled trial of donepezil adjunctive treatment to risperidone for the cognitive impairment of schizophrenia. *Biol. Psychiatry* 51(5), 349–357.
259. Bymaster, F. P., et al., (2001). Possible role of muscarinic receptor agonists as therapeutic agents for psychosis. In *Current Issues in the Psychopharmacology of Schizophrenia*, A. Breir, F. Bymaster, and P. Tran, Eds. Lippincott Williams & Wilkins Healthcare, Philadelphia, pp. 333–348.
260. Chopra, G. S., and Smith, J. W. (1974). Psychotic reactions following cannabis use in East Indians. *Arch. Gen. Psychiatry* 30(1), 24–27.
261. Andreasson, S., et al. (1987). Cannabis and schizophrenia. A longitudinal study of Swedish conscripts. *Lancet* 2(8574), 1483–1486.
262. Emrich, H. M., Leweke, F. M., and Schneider, U. (1997). Towards a cannabinoid hypothesis of schizophrenia: Cognitive impairments due to dysregulation of the endogenous cannabinoid system. *Pharmacol. Biochem. Behav.* 56(4), 803–807.
263. Jungerman, T., Rabinowitz, D., and Klein, E. (1999). Deprenyl augmentation for treating negative symptoms of schizophrenia: A double-blind, controlled study. *J. Clin. Psychopharmacol.* 19(6), 522–525.
264. Carpenter, W.T., Jr., et al. (2000). Mazindol treatment of negative symptoms. *Neuropsychopharmacology* 23(4), 365–374.
265. Strauss, E. B., et al. (1952). Use of dehydroisoandrosterone in psychiatric treatment: A preliminary survey. *Br. Med. J.* 2(4775), 64–66.
266. Sands, D. E. (1954). Further studies on endocrine treatment in adolescence and early adult life. *J. Ment. Sci.* 100, 211–219.
267. Strauss, E. B., and Stevenson, W. A. H. (1955). Use of dehydroisoandrosterone in psychiatric practice. *J. Neurol. Neurosurg. Psychiatry* 18, 137–144.
268. Strous, R. D., et al. (2003). Dehydroepiandrosterone augmentation in the management of negative, depressive, and anxiety symptoms in schizophrenia. *Arch. Gen. Psychiatry* 60(2), 133–141.
269. Basile, V. S., et al., (2001). Application of pharmacogenetics to schizophrenia: Emerging insights from studies of clozapine response and tardive dyskinesia. In *Current Issues in the Psychopharmacology of Schizophrenia*. Lippincott Williams & Wilkins Healthcare, Philadelphia, pp. 85–110.
270. Arranz, M. J., and Kerwin, R. W. (2003). Advances in the pharmacogenetic prediction of antipsychotic response. *Toxicology* 192(1), 33–35.

12

ATYPICAL ANTIPSYCHOTIC DRUGS: MECHANISM OF ACTION

HERBERT Y. MELTZER
Vanderbilt University School of Medicine, Nashville, Tennessee

12.1	Introduction: Distinction Between Typical and Atypical Antipsychotic Drugs	411
12.2	Clozapine and Related Drugs: Dopamine D_2 Receptor Blockade	412
12.3	D_1, D_3, and D_4 Receptors: Substituted Benzamides	415
12.4	Partial Dopamine Agonists	416
12.5	Role of 5-HT_{2A}, 5-HT_{2C}, 5-HT_{1A}, and Other 5-HT Receptors	417
12.6	Atypical Antipsychotics and 5-HT_{2A} Receptor	418
12.7	5-HT_{2A} Receptor Blockade, Enhancement of Cortical DA Efflux, and Cognitive Function in Schizophrenia	421
12.8	5-HT_{2A} Receptor Blockade and Extrapyramidal Function	422
12.9	Role of 5-HT_{2C} Receptor in Antipsychotic Drug Action: 5-HT_{2A} and 5-HT_{2C} Interactions	422
12.10	Role of 5-HT_{1A} Receptor in Antipsychotic Drug Action: 5-HT_{1A} and 5-HT_{2A} Interactions	424
12.11	Role of 5-HT_6 Receptor	425
12.12	Role of Serotonin Release in Antipsychotic Drug Action	426
12.13	α_2- and α_1-Adrenergic Mechanisms and Atypical APDs	426
12.14	Glutamatergic Mechanisms	427
12.15	Cholinergic Mechanisms	429
12.16	Neurokinin 3 Receptors	430
12.17	Neurogenesis	430
12.18	Conclusions	431
Acknowledgments		431
References		431

12.1 INTRODUCTION: DISTINCTION BETWEEN TYPICAL AND ATYPICAL ANTIPSYCHOTIC DRUGS

Antipsychotic drugs (APDs), by definition, suppress hallucinations and delusions, which are core features of schizophrenia as well as other neuropsychiatric disorders with psychotic features. Those APDs which produce catalepsy in rodents and extrapyramidal side effects (EPS) in humans within the same dose range (e.g.,

---

Handbook of Contemporary Neuropharmacology, Edited by David R. Sibley, Israel Hanin, Michael Kuhar, and Phil Skolnick. Copyright © 2007 John Wiley & Sons, Inc.

chlorpromazine and haloperidol) are called typical APDs or neuroleptics. Acute EPSs (parkinsonism, dystonias, neuroleptic malignant syndrome) and delayed EPSs (tardive dyskinesia, tardive dystonia) represent disturbing and sometimes life-threatening side effects which interfere greatly with the patient's quality of life and compliance with treatment. Clozapine, discovered five years after chlorpromazine, was the first APD which did not produce catalepsy and virtually no EPSs. Because of this dissociation between antipsychotic efficacy and EPSs, clozapine was called an *atypical* APD. This name has persisted, although some clinical investigators incorrectly refer to typical APDs as first-generation antipsychotics and to clozapine and all subsequent atypical APDs as second-generation antipsychotics, even though many typical APDs which are still in use were discovered and introduced 5–10 years *after* clozapine (e.g., molindone and thiothixene) [1].

As will be discussed, there are important clinical differences between typical and atypical APDs beyond EPS liability. Clozapine (but not all other atypical APDs) was found to be effective to treat delusions and hallucinations in 60–70% of the 30% of patients with schizophrenia who have persistent psychotic symptoms despite treatment with typical APDs [2, 3] or with other atypical APDs [4]. Clozapine produces agranulocytosis in about 1% of patients [5]. For this reason, it has generally been used only in patients who do not respond to or cannot tolerate other APDs [3]. Atypical APDs are also able to modestly improve negative symptoms compared with typical APDs [6]. The advantage for efficacy for some atypical APDs over typical APDs has recently been challenged in a large, pragmatic clinical trial that had fewer constraints on patient population than most previous studies [7]. Most importantly, they have been reported to improve some domains of cognition in patients with schizophrenia [8, 9]. However, the advantages for cognition are modest, not apparent in all domains, and further research is needed to establish definitively that they do have an advantage over typical neuroleptic drugs to improve cognition. The advantage of greater efficacy for these components of schizophrenia coupled with advantages for EPS, both acute and chronic (e.g., tardive dyskinesia), has led to this group of compounds becoming the most widely prescribed APDs in all countries where they are freely available.

There are now numerous types of atypical APDs. As indicated in Table 12.1, there are at least seven subtypes of atypical APDs which have been identified, although not all are clinically available and, indeed, the efficacy of some of these agents is still not adequately established. In addition, there are many other proposed atypical APD mechanisms which cannot be reviewed here for space limitations.

As can be seen in Table 12.1, there is a diversity of mechanisms which are now believed to be able to achieve some degree of control of psychosis with significant sparing of EPSs. This review will consider current information on the mechanism of action of these drugs, concentrating on clozapine and related drugs because most is known about its actions.

12.2 CLOZAPINE AND RELATED DRUGS: DOPAMINE D_2 RECEPTOR BLOCKADE

There are numerous theories of why clozapine is atypical, that is, produces low EPSs at clinically effective doses. Historically, the low EPSs due to clozapine were

TABLE 12.1 Atypical Antipsychotic Drugs

Clozapine-like serotonin (5-HT$_{2A}$)/D$_2$
Receptor antagonists/inverse agonists
  Asenapine
  Clozapine
  Lurasidone
  Melperone
  N-Desmethylclozapine
  Olanzapine
  Paliperidone
  Perospirone
  Quetiapine
  Risperidone
  Sertindole
  Ziprasdione
  Zotepine

Partial dopamine agonists
  Ariprazole
  Bifeprunox

5-HT$_{2A/2C}$ antagonists
  SR43469B
  ACP 103
  M100907

D$_2$ antagonists/5-HT$_{1A}$ agonists
  SLV313
  SSR181507
  S16924

Substituted benzamides
  Amisulpride
  Remoxipride

Muscarinic agonists
  Xanomeline
  N-Desmethylclozapine

Neurokinin 3 antagonists
  Osanetant
  Talnetant

attributed to its relatively weak affinity for the D$_2$ receptor, its antimuscarinic properties, its lack of effect on the firing of nigro striatal dopamine (DA) neurons compared to ventral tegmental (VTA) DA neurons, or to D$_1$ receptor antagonism (see [10, 11] for a review). The typical APDs have been suggested to diminish psychotic symptoms by blockade of D$_2$ receptors in mesolimbic nuclei, especially the nucleus accumbens (NAC), stria terminalis, and extended amygdala, while blockade of D$_2$ receptors in the caudate/putamen (dorsal striatum) has been shown to be the major basis for parkinsonism and other EPSs (see [10] for review). For the typical APDs, there is a very high correlation between the estimated therapeutic dose of these drugs and their affinity for the D_2 receptor [12, 13]. Actions of these agents at other receptors (e.g., M_1 muscarinic receptors, histamine H_1 receptors, and α_1 and α_2 adrenoceptors) have been thought to contribute to side effects such as drowsiness, weight gain, and constipation rather than efficacy.

Positron emission tomography (PET) studies utilizing ^{11}C-raclopride as the ligand have shown that occupancy of 65–80% of striatal D_2 receptors is required for an antipsychotic action by typical APDs and risperidone or olanzapine and that $\geq 80\%$ occupancy is associated with EPSs (see [14, 15] for a review). However, clozapine and quetiapine are effective at lower occupancies of D_2 receptors than typical and other atypical APDs listed with it in Table 12.1 (e.g., risperidone, olanzapine, and ziprasidone), implying some mechanism other than D_2 receptor blockade is contributing to their low-side-effect profile and perhaps their efficacy as well [14, 16–19]. However, caution is needed in interpreting these studies because they do not assess the occupancy of VTA, ventral striatal, or cortical D_2 receptors, all of which are more likely to be related to antipsychotic action than is the dorsal striatum, which is the region of interest in studies using ^{11}C-raclopride in the first generation of PET studies. This ligand is much less useful than high-affinity substituted benzamides which have been developed more recently. Kessler et al. [20] performed [^{18}F]fallypride PET studies in six schizophrenic subjects treated with olanzapine and six treated with haloperidol to examine the occupancy of striatal and extrastriatal D_2/D_3 receptors. [^{18}F]setoperone PET studies were performed in seven olanzapine-treated subjects to determine 5-HT$_{2A}$ receptor occupancy. Occupancy of DA D_2 receptors by olanzapine was not significantly different from that seen with haloperidol in the putamen, ventral striatum, medial thalamus, amygdala, or temporal cortex, that is, 67.5–78.2% occupancy; no preferential occupancy of DA D_2 receptors was seen in the ventral striatum, medial thalamus, amygdala, or temporal cortex. There was significantly lower occupancy of substantia nigra (SN)/VTA D_2 receptors in olanzapine- than haloperidol-treated subjects, that is, 40.2 versus 59.3% ($p = 0.01$); in olanzapine-treated subjects, the SN/VTA DA D_2 receptor occupancy was significantly lower than that seen in the putamen, that is, 40.2 versus 69.2% ($p = 0.01$). Sparing of SN/VTA DA D_2 receptor occupancy was suggested to contribute to the low incidence of EPSs in the olanzapine-treated patients. Similar results have now been obtained with clozapine- and quetiapine-treated patients [21]. Clozapine, the most effective of these agents, was found to produce the lowest occupancy of SN/VTA D_2 receptors. It is not possible to resolve the SN and VTA binding. Thus, it could be that binding by the atypical APDs to either or both regions is reduced. In any case, it does not seem likely that this alone could account for all the differences between typical and atypical APDs. Grunder et al. [22] studied the occupancy of extrastriatal D_2/D_3 DA receptors by clozapine using [^{18}F]fallypride in 15 patients with schizophrenia. Mean D_2/D_3 receptor occupancy was statistically significantly higher in cortical (inferior temporal cortex 55%) than in striatal regions (putamen 36%, caudate 43%, $p < 0.005$). Occupancy of cortical receptors approached 60% with plasma clozapine levels in the range of 350–400 ng/mL, which corresponds to the threshold for antipsychotic efficacy of clozapine. These authors concluded that extrastriatal D_2/D_3 receptor binding of clozapine may be more relevant to its antipsychotic actions than striatal binding.

It has been suggested that atypicality may be due to rapid dissociation from the DA D_2 receptor due to its relatively easy displacement by surges of endogenous DA [23, 24]. It has also been proposed that rapid and extensive displacement of clozapine and quetiapine from binding sites by endogenous DA accounts for the low occupancy of striatal D_2 receptors by these drugs [23]. However, it is not clear on what basis these agents achieve their antipsychotic action if they are equally easily displaced from limbic D_2 receptors. Moreover, numerous atypical APDs (e.g., sertindole, risperidone, asenapine, and ziprasidone) are comparable to haloperidol in their rate of dissociation from the D_2 receptor, based upon their equally high affinity for that receptor. Thus, this theory fails to account for the atypical profile of these high-D_2-affinity atypical APDs. However, relatively easy displacement from D_2 receptors of low-D_2-affinity atypical APDs such as clozapine and quetiapine could contribute to their very low risk of EPSs and greater tolerability in patients with Parkinson's disease. Seeman [25] has proposed the fast-off theory as the basis for the atypical features of amisulpride, but it is difficult to understand what distinguishes it from other D_2/D_3 antagonists which are not atypical. The fast-off theory has had no apparent impact on the process of antipsychotic drug discovery development and, thus, has not met that important clinical test. This is in marked contrast to the hypothesis, to be discussed, that atypicality is related to the combination of a partial decrease in dopaminergic function coupled to blockade of 5-HT_{2A} receptors or stimulation of 5-HT_{1A} receptors [26, 27].

12.3 D_1, D_3, AND D_4 RECEPTORS: SUBSTITUTED BENZAMIDES

The central nervous system (CNS) contains four subtypes of DA receptor other than the D_2 receptor, the D_1, D_3, D_4, and D_5 receptors. Whether these DA receptors play a role in the action of current antipsychotic drugs or are potential targets for future ones is poorly understood. Phenothiazine and thiothanthines, but not butyrophenones such as haloperidol or substituted benzamides such as amisulpride, are effective D_1 antagonists. Clozapine is a D_1 partial agonist [28] and has a greater extent of occupancy of D_1 receptors than any other antipsychotic drug [16]. There is some indirect evidence that the ability of the atypical APDs to improve cognition in schizophrenia may be mediated through effects on D_1 receptors via their role in long-term potentiation [29]. Specific D_1 receptor antagonists have been evaluated in the treatment of schizophrenia, but no clear evidence of beneficial therapeutic activity was obtained in pilot studies [30, 31].

The cloning of the D_4 receptor provoked much interest in the possibility that this was a key mechanism in the action of atypical APDs. This idea first originated from the observation that clozapine differed from other antipsychotics in having significantly higher affinity for the D_4 than for the D_2 receptor [32], a finding not supported by a number of other studies. Interest in the D_4 receptor as a target for antipsychotic drugs has waned after the completion of three negative randomized clinical trials with D_4 receptor antagonists fananserin [33], L-745,870 [34], and sonepiprazole [35].

Schwartz et al. [36] have suggested that the D_3 receptor, which is relatively highly expressed in limbic and cortical areas, may represent an important target for antipsychotic drugs which generally have similar affinities for D_2 and D_3 receptors. Clozapine has modest affinity for D_3 receptors although most of the other atypical

APDs related to clozapine do not. The discriminative stimulus for clozapine sometimes but not always generalizes to D_3 antagonists [37]. SB-277011-A has high affinity and selectivity for the D_3 receptor and good brain bioavailability [38]. This compound was active in preventing isolation-induced deficits in prepulse inhibition (PPI), a putative animal model for antipsychotic activity, but was not effective to block either amphetamine- or phencyclidine (PCP)–induced locomotor activity, which has much more validity in that regard [38]. However, subchronic administration of SB-277011-A selectively decreased the firing rate of VTA but not nigrostriatal DA neurons in the rat, indicating a clozapine-like profile [39]. In a microdialysis study in rats, the acute administration of SB-277011-A significantly increased extracellular levels of DA, norepinephrine (NE), and acetylcholine (ACh) without affecting levels of 5-HT in the anterior cingulate region of the medial PFC (mPFC). As will be discussed, this is similar to the profile we and others have reported with clozapine and other atypical APDs [40, 41]. Clinical trials of selective D_3 antagonists have not yet been reported.

The substituted benzamides are an interesting group of APDs and like the butyrophenones may include both typical and atypical APDs. The prototype is sulpiride, which is generally thought of as a typical APD, while the drug in widespread use in Europe but not the United States is amisulpride [42]. It has been suggested that the low EPS profile of sulpiride and amisulpride is due to selective antagonism of D_2/D_3 receptors in the mesocortico/limbic system [43]. Using single-proton emission computerized tomography (SPECT) with [123 I] epidepride as the ligand, eight amisulpride-treated patients (mean dose 406 mg/day) showed moderate levels of D_2/D_3 receptor occupancy in the striatum (56%) and significantly higher levels in the thalamus (78%) and temporal cortex (82% [44]). This finding suggests that modest striatal D_2 receptor occupancy and preferential occupancy of limbic cortical dopamine D_2/D_3 receptors may be major factors which explain the therapeutic efficacy and low-EPS profile of amisulpride. However, the risk of tardive dyskinesia with sulpiride is higher than that with other typical APDs [45]. On the other hand, the risk with amisulpride has been reported to be in the same range as other atypical APDs [46]. However, no differences in the mechanism of action of these two drugs have been reported as yet, suggesting there is some additional feature of the pharmacology of amisulpride that has yet to be identified. Another contrast is that sulpiride has been reported to impair cognitive functioning in normal volunteers [47] while amisulpride has been reported to improve some aspects of cognition in schizophrenia, but the data are very limited and did not involve a control group [48]. The clinical profile of amisulpride and its mechanism of action are worthy of more extensive investigation.

12.4 PARTIAL DOPAMINE AGONISTS

Most antipsychotic drugs which have affinity for D_2 and D_3 receptors are inverse agonists at both receptors [49]. However, some are partial D_2/D_3 agonists, for example, aripiprazole, bifeprunox [50], and N-desmethylclozapine (NDMC), the major metabolite of clozapine [49, 51, 52]. Partial agonists, by definition, produce lesser activation of the D_2/D_3 receptors than the full agonist and as such will produce smaller functional responses than the endogenous neurotransmitter [53]. Partial agonists are particularly more potent as agonists when there is high receptor reserve. Thus, DA partial agonists are more likely to stimulate DA autoreceptors than postsynaptic DA receptors. Because of this, they diminish dopaminergic stimulation through a dual mechanism: suppression of the release of DA by stimulating autoreceptors and blocking the response to the full agonist at postsynaptic receptors. There have been many attempts to develop DA autoreceptor agonists for the treatment of schizophrenia but all failed until recently, when DA partial agonists, which also had 5-HT$_{2A}$ inverse agonist or 5-HT$_{1A}$ partial agonist properties or both, were tested and were found to be effective and tolerable. Thus aripiprazole, an approved atypical antipsychotic drug [51], is a D$_2$ partial agonist and both a 5-HT$_{2A}$ inverse agonist and 5-HT$_{1A}$ partial agonist. Bifeprunox is a partial agonist at both the D$_2$ and 5-HT$_{1A}$ receptors only, with no 5-HT$_{2A}$ antagonist properties [50]. It is in phase III testing as an antipsychotic drug. Both drugs produce minimal EPSs at clinically effective doses. As agonists, both suppress serum prolactin levels. Aripiprazole, but not bifeprunox, has been reported to reverse deficits in social interaction in rats produced by the NMDA receptor antagonist PCP [52]. The contribution of 5-HT$_{2A}$ inverse agonism or 5-HT$_{1A}$ partial agonism to their efficacy will be discussed subsequently. Functional selectivity of some DA agonists, including partial agonists, for specific types of DA receptors (e.g., autoreceptors vs. postsynaptic D$_2$ receptors) [54, 55] has been demonstrated, that is, differential activation of different isoforms of a D$_2$ receptor, thus implying variable "intrinsic activity" of an agonist [56]. Whether aripiprazole or bifeprunox also demonstrate functional selectivity for D$_2$ or D$_3$ receptors and whether this contributes to their atypical antipsychotic properties remain to be seen. Li et al. [57] have reported that aripiprazole, at a dose of 0.3 mg/kg, which corresponds to clinically effective doses, can increase the release of DA in the rat mPFC and hippocampus. These results have been replicated [58]. It will be of interest to determine if there are any partial DA agonists, with no significant affinity for 5-HT$_{2A}$ or 5-HT$_{1A}$ receptor which are effective and tolerable APDs or whether some other potentiating mechanism (e.g., M$_1$ agonism, to be discussed) is needed.

12.5 ROLE OF 5-HT$_{2A}$, 5-HT$_{2C}$, 5-HT$_{1A}$, AND OTHER 5-HT RECEPTORS

Clozapine and a group of other atypical antipsychotic drugs have a greater affinity for 5-HT$_{2A}$ than D$_2$ receptors [26, 59, 60]. The hypothesis that a relatively high affinity for the 5-HT$_{2A}$ receptor compared to their affinities for the D$_2$ receptor was the basis for the difference between atypical and typical APDs contributed to the development of the newer antipsychotic agents listed above, all of which support the previously mentioned hypothesis of high affinity for 5-HT$_{2A}$ and low affinity for D$_2$ receptors [59, 60]. However, other 5-HT receptors may be important in the action of clozapine and other recently introduced antipsychotic agents or of potential value for developing more effective or better tolerated antipsychotic agents. These include 5-HT$_{1A}$, 5-HT$_{2A}$, 5-HT$_{2C}$, 5-HT$_3$, 5-HT$_6$, and 5-HT$_7$ receptors [61]. While some of the atypical APDs developed on the basis of the 5-HT$_{2A}$/D$_2$ hypothesis also have affinities for 5-HT$_{2C}$, 5-HT$_3$, 5-HT$_6$ or 5-HT$_7$ receptors in the same range as that for the 5-HT$_{2A}$ receptor, this is not characteristic of all of these agents and, thus, it is not likely that affinities for these receptors are primary factors contributing to the low-EPS profile of the entire class of agents [60, 62, 63]. However, this does not rule out that actions at various 5-HT receptor contribute to low-EPS effects of specific drugs or other actions, for example, cognitive improvement or improvement in negative symptoms.

12.6 ATYPICAL ANTIPSYCHOTICS AND 5-HT$_{2A}$ RECEPTOR

5-HT$_{2A}$ receptors have been implicated in the genesis of as well as the treatment of psychosis, negative symptoms, mood disturbance, and EPSs. The hallucinogenic effect of indole hallucinogens has been related to stimulation of 5-HT$_{2A}$ rather than 5-HT$_{2C}$ receptors [64]. Numerous studies have examined the density of 5-HT$_{2A}$ receptors in various cortical regions of patients with schizophrenia with decreased [65, 66], increased [67], or normal levels reported. It is well established that some typical and atypical APDs can decrease the density of 5-HT$_{2A}$ receptors [68] so the postmortem results noted above may be related to drug treatment. A PET study in never-medicated patients with schizophrenia confirmed this decrease in cortical 5-HT$_{2A}$ receptor density [69], but other studies which were not exclusively with never-medicated patients found no decrease in 5-HT$_{2A}$ receptors in the cortex of patients with schizophrenia [70, 71]. Further study of this important issue is warranted. The antipsychotic effect of clozapine and other atypical ADPs has been attributed, in part, to its ability to block excessive 5-HT$_{2A}$ receptor stimulation without excessive blockade of D$_2$ receptors [26]. This conclusion is consistent with the high occupancy of 5-HT$_{2A}$ receptors produced by clozapine at clinically effective doses and its low occupancy of D$_2$ receptors (in the 30–50% range as measured with the [^{3}H]raclopride), the latter being significantly below the 80–100% occupancy usually produced by typical neuroleptic drugs [16, 21, 72]. The occupancy of 5-HT$_{2A}$ and D$_2$ receptors has been studied with other atypical APDs such as risperidone, olanzapine, sertindole, and quetiapine with results similar to those of clozapine; all are more potent 5-HT$_{2A}$ inverse agonists and D$_2$ antagonists at appropriate doses, but less so than clozapine. Some of these agents (e.g., risperidone) produce high D$_2$ occupancy at moderately high doses [18, 72] but do not cause the level of EPSs associated with such high levels of occupancy when produced by typical APDs. The most likely reason for this difference is the blockade of 5-HT$_{2A}$ receptors by the atypical APDs.

The bell-shaped dose–response curve of risperidone, with higher doses being less effective than lower doses [73], suggests that excessive D$_2$ receptor antagonism may diminish some of the beneficial effects of 5-HT$_{2A}$ receptor blockade [63]. This is supported by two recent studies in which risperidone was added to clozapine treatment of partial responders in placebo-controlled randomized clinical trials. Placebo was generally superior to or equal to risperidone in a number of outcome measures [74, 75]. The highly selective 5-HT$_{2A}$ inverse agonist M100907, formerly MDL 100907, has been found in a controlled study to have some efficacy for treating positive and negative symptoms in hospitalized schizophrenic patients [76]. However, because it was less effective than haloperidol, no further testing in schizophrenia followed. Nevertheless, the concept that 5-HT$_{2A}$ receptor blockade may be useful to treat some forms of psychosis, especially when combined with weak D$_2$ receptor blockade, is deserving of further testing. The 5-HT$_{2A/2C}$ selective antagonist SR46349B [77] was recently reported to be nearly as effective as haloperidol in treating patients with schizophrenia in a double-blind clinical trial [78]. NRA0045, which has potent 5-HT$_{2A}$, D$_4$, and α$_1$ but negligible D$_2$ or D$_3$ receptor blockade, has been found to have atypical antipsychotic properties in rodents [79, 80]. The selective 5-HT$_{2A/2C}$ inverse agonist ACP 103 [81, 82] is being tested as monotherapy in the treatment of 3,4-dihydroxy-L-phenylalanine (L-DOPA) psychosis and schizophrenia. Low doses of three atypical APDs, clozapine, quetiapine, and melperone [83], are effective and tolerable in the treatment of L-DOPA psychosis. We have proposed that this is due to their 5-HT$_{2A}$ receptor blockade, sparing D$_2$ receptors [84]. The role of 5-HT$_{2A}$ receptor blockade in the action of clozapine and possibly other drugs with potent 5-HT$_{2A}$ affinities is supported by the evidence that the *His452Tyr* allele of the 5-HT$_{2A}$ receptor, which is present in 10–12% of the population, is associated with a higher frequency of poor response to clozapine [85]. In addition, the T102C single-nucleotide polymorphism has been reported to be related to response to clozapine [86]. Taken together, the evidence from clinical trial data suggests that 5-HT$_{2A}$ receptor blockade may contribute to antipsychotic drug action.

There is additional evidence consistent with the relevance of 5-HT$_{2A}$ receptor blockade for APD action. Thus, M100907, or other selective 5-HT$_{2A}$ receptor inverse agonist, either alone or in combination with selective antagonists of other receptors, has been found to be effective in various animal models of psychosis. These include (a) blockade of amphetamine-induced locomotor activity and inhibition of the firing of VTA dopaminergic neurons [87]; (b) blockade of PCP- and dizocilpin (MK-801-)-induced locomotor activity [88, 89]; (c) blockade of MK-801-induced prepulse inhibition [90]; and (d) antipsychotic-like activity in the paw test [91], among others. Of particular interest is the report of Wadenberg et al. [92] that the combination of an ED 50 dose of raclopride, a D$_2$ receptor antagonist, and M100907, but not M100907 alone, was effective in blocking the conditioned avoidance response. They concluded that 5-HT$_{2A}$ antagonism alone could not achieve an antipsychotic action but that minimal blockade of D$_2$ receptors was required to achieve such an effect. This corresponds much more closely to the apparent clinical situation than does the models above where M100907 alone was effective, for example, blockade of PCP- or MK-801-induced locomotor activity. ACP 103 is another selective 5-HT$_{2A/2C}$ inverse agonist [93] which has been shown to potentiate the effect of haloperidol and risperidone to enhance cortical DA efflux in rats [94]. Gardell et al. [95] have recently reported that ACP 103 reduced the dose of haloperidol and risperidone required for activity in the amphetamine- or MK-801-induced hyperactivity models and suppressed haloperidol-induced hyperprolactinemia in mice.

Additional evidence for the greater importance of 5-HT$_{2A}$ and D$_2$ receptor interactions in the regulation of mesocorticolimbic versus nigrostriatal DAergic activity comes from two studies of Olijslagers et al. [96, 97] using midbrain rat slices and electrophysiological recording of the activity of A9 and A10 DA neurons. They first reported that 5-HT (20 µM) in combination with quinpirole (30 nM), a D$_2$ agonist, enhanced the reduction of the firing rate in both A9 and A10 DA neurons. compared to quinpirole (30 nM) alone. However, the 5-HT$_{2A/2C}$ agonist 1-(2,5-dimethoxy-4-iodophenyl)-2-aminopropane (DOI, 500 nM) enhanced quinpirole-induced reduction of firing rate in the A10 but not A9 DA neurons. The selective 5-HT$_{2A}$ receptor antagonist MDL100907 and the selective 5-HT$_{2C}$ receptor antagonist SB242084 (50 and 500 nM) both abolished the enhancement of quinpirole-induced reduction by either 5-HT or DOI, suggesting the involvement of direct and indirect (possibly via interneurons) modulation pathways in A10. $5-HT_{2A}$ receptors have been localized on the cell bodies of the A10 DA and other nondopaminergic VTA neurons [98].

Olanzapine and clozapine, two atypical APDs, more potently reversed the amphetamine-induced inhibition in A10 neurons compared to A9 neurons [96]. Olijslagers et al. [96] also reported that risperidone (0.03 and 0.1 μM) reversed amphetamine-induced inhibition of firing activity similarly in A9 and A10. Risperidone has a higher affinity for D_2 relative to $5-HT_{2A}$ receptors than either clozapine or olanzapine. The dopamine D_2 receptor antagonist $(-)$sulpiride (0.05 and 1 μM) reversed the amphetamine (10 μM)–induced inhibition of firing activity in A9 and A10 neurons. However, the selective $5-HT_{2A}$ receptor antagonist M100907 (0.05 μM), strongly enhanced the reversal of amphetamine-induced inhibition by $(-)$sulpiride in A10, but its effectiveness to enhance the effect of sulpiride was much less in A9 DA neurons. They suggested that $5-HT_{2A}$ in combination with DA D_2 receptor antagonism may play a role in atypical APD differential effects on nigrostriatal and mesocorticolimbic DAergic activity, leading to some of the clinical differences between typical and atypical APDs.

The $5-HT_{2A}$ and $5-HT_{1A}$ agonist psilocybin has been reported to impair cognitive function in normal volunteers [99]. Increased dopaminergic activity in the NAC and other mesolimbic and possibly cortical regions may contribute to positive symptoms, including formal thought disorder. The $5-HT_{2A/2C}$ agonist DOI, which is hallucinogenic in humans, itself had no effect on basal DA release, potentiated amphetamine-induced DA release, and attenuated the ability of apomorphine, a direct-acting $D_{1/2/3}$ agonist, to decrease DA release in the striatum [100]. There is now considerable evidence from both behavioral and neurochemical studies involving N-methyl-D-aspartate (NMDA) antagonists such as PCP and MK-801 that $5-HT_{2A}$ receptors modulate activate but not basal mesolimbic DAergic function [88, 101, 102]. Thus, stimulated DA release (e.g., with stress) may be increased in the forebrain terminal regions secondary to enhanced stimulation of $5-HT_{2A}$ receptors. Agents which block the effect of excessive but not basal $5-HT_{2A}$ receptor stimulation may be the most useful clinically. M100907 has been found to diminish the increase in DA efflux in the NAC produced by haloperidol [103] or S-sulpiride [27]. M100907 infused directly into the mPFCs resulted in a concentration-dependent blockade of $K(+)$-stimulated DA release and also blocked increases in DA release produced by the systemic administration of DOI. Thus, local $5-HT_{2A}$ antagonism has an inhibitory effect on stimulated DA release and suggest that cortical $5-HT_{2A}$ receptors potentiate the phasic release of mesocortical DA [104]. The local (in the mPFC) and systemic administration of DOI increased the firing rate and burst firing of DA neurons and DA release in the VTA and mPFC [105]. The increase in VTA DA release was mimicked by the electrical stimulation of the mPFC. The effects of DOI were reversed by M100907. These results indicate that the activity of VTA DA neurons is under the excitatory control of mPFC $5-HT_{2A}$ receptors. Taken together, these data suggest that blockade of cortical $5-HT_{2A}$ receptors, by itself, may have antipsychotic action when dopaminergic activity is slightly to moderately increased. More studies are needed to define the ability of $5-HT_{2A}$ receptor antagonists to potentiate the action of low doses of D_2 receptor blockers in animal models as well as the clinic. Jakab and Goldman-Rakic [106] have demonstrated that $5-HT_{2A}$ receptors are located on most cortical pyramidal neurons, especially those above and below layer

IV, as well as on many (γ-aminobutric acid) (GABA)–ergic interneurons known to specialize in the perisomatic inhibition of pyramidal cells: large- and medium-size parvalbumin- and calbindin-containing interneurons. Together they may play a crucial role in psychosis by virtue of their ability to modulate intracortical and cortical–subcortical glutamatergic neurotransmission. This could contribute to the ability of 5-HT$_{2A}$ inverse agonists, including those atypical APDs which are potent in this regard, to attenuate some of the behavioral effects of PCP and ketamine.

12.7 5-HT$_{2A}$ RECEPTOR BLOCKADE, ENHANCEMENT OF CORTICAL DA EFFLUX, AND COGNITIVE FUNCTION IN SCHIZOPHRENIA

As previously mentioned, clozapine and related atypical APDs (e.g., risperidone and olanzapine) have been shown to modestly improve selected areas of cognitive function in most patients with schizophrenia [9]. The effect of these agents on cognition may be dependent, in part, upon their ability to increase the release of DA in PFC and hippocampus, which depends, in part, on their serotonergic actions [107, 107a]. We have found that the combination of a saturating dose of a 5-HT$_{2A}$ inverse agonist/antagonist and a dose of D$_2$ antagonist which only partially blocks D$_2$ receptors leads to increased DA release in the frontal cortex [94, 108, 109]. The 5-HT$_{2A}$ receptor blockers do not potentiate D$_2$ receptor blockade when the dose of the latter is saturating [108]. This is consistent with the hypothesis that at clinical doses atypical APDs achieve partial blockade of D$_2$ receptors relative to 5-HT$_{2A}$ receptor blockade. In addition, the atypical APDs enhance efflux of ACh in the PFC and hippocampus of rodents [110–113]. It is possible that this effect may also contribute to their ability to improve cognition.

5-HT$_{2C}$, 5-HT$_3$, 5-HT$_{1A}$, and 5-HT$_4$ receptors have also been reported to have significant effects on ACh release in the rat PFC [114–118]. Impairment of working memory in humans following administration of the 5-HT$_{1A}$ agonist flesinoxan has been reported [119]. Sumiyoshi et al. [120], on the other hand, have found that tandospirone, a 5-HT$_{1A}$ partial agonist, can improve other domains of cognition in patients with schizophrenia treated with typical neuroleptic drugs.

Brain-derived neurotrophic factor (BDNF) regulates survival, differentiation, synaptic strength, and neuronal morphology in the cerebral cortex and hippocampus in frontal and other cortical areas while decreasing its expression in the dentate gyrus granule cell layer. The BDNF gene *Val66Met* polymorphism has been reported to be associated with schizophrenia and response to clozapine [121]. It has recently been demonstrated that stimulation of 5-HT$_{2A}$ receptors by the 5-HT$_{2A/2C}$ agonist DOI and stress increases the expression of BDNF in cortex and hippocampus [122]. These effects were blocked by the 5-HT$_{2A}$ antagonist M100907 and ritanserin, respectively, which by themselves did not have any effect in these regions. Electrophysiological studies with slices from rats following chronic treatment with clozapine or haloperidol showed that chronic clozapine but not haloperidol treatment resulted in an attenuation of the effect of the activation of 5-HT$_{2A}$ receptors without changing response to 5-HT$_{1A}$ and 5-HT$_4$ receptor activation. These data are consistent with the hypothesis that chronic clozapine selectively attenuates 5-HT-mediated excitation in neuronal circuitry of the frontal cortex while leaving 5-HT-mediated inhibition intact [123]. Clozapine and olanzapine upregulated BDNF messenger RNA (mRNA) expression in CA1, CA3, and dentate gyrus regions of the rat hippocampus whereas haloperidol (1 mg/kg) downregulated BDNF mRNA expression in both CA1 ($p<0.05$) and dentate gyrus ($p<0.01$) regions [124]. Neither acute nor chronic clozapine treatment significantly affected the expression of BDNF mRNA in various brain areas. However, the NMDA antagonist MK-801 (5 mg/kg; 4 h) significantly increased BDNF mRNA in the entorhinal cortex, an effect which was attenuated by pre-treatment with clozapine and haloperidol [125]. These data suggest that clozapine-like atypical APDs, via their 5-HT_{2A} antagonism, might modulate the activity of BDNF and possibly other growth factors.

Transcription factors of the Nur family (Nurr1, Nur77, and Nor-1) are orphan nuclear receptors that have been associated with DA neurotransmission. Nurr1 is involved in midbrain DA neuron development. Nur77 and Nor-1 are expressed in dopaminoceptive areas such as the striatum, NAC, and PFC. Modulation of Nur77 and Nor-1 mRNA expression by antipsychotics can be used to calculate an index that is predictive of the typical or atypical profile of antipsychotic drugs [126]. Inductions of Nur by antipsychotic drugs was correlated with DA D_2 receptor in the striatum and NAC. The 5-HT_{2A}/D_2 affinity ratio of antipsychotics also predicted these patterns of inductions. These data suggest that typical and atypical APDs might induce distinct Nur-dependent transcriptional activities, which may contribute to their pharmacological effects.

12.8 5-HT_{2A} RECEPTOR BLOCKADE AND EXTRAPYRAMIDAL FUNCTION

Several lines of evidence suggest that potent 5-HT_{2A} receptor blockade is relevant to the low-EPS profile of clozapine but that 5-HT_{2A} receptor blockade by itself cannot explain the low-EPS liability of these agents. In order to test the role of 5-HT_{2A} receptor blockade, Meltzer et al. [26] studied a group of compounds which had antipsychotic activity in human or animal models that are thought to be predictive of antipsychotic activity and which produced less EPSs in humans or weak catalepsy in animals. The ratio of affinity for 5-HT_{2A} to D_2 receptors was the best predictor of atypicality [26]. This continues to be supported by further research [11]. Ishikane et al. [127] reported that M100907 is able to block haloperidol-induced catalepsy only at low doses of haloperidol. Weiner et al. [128] profiled antipsychotic drugs for functional activity at 33 of the 36 known human monoaminergic G-protein-coupled receptors using the mammalian cell-based functional assay Receptor Selection and Amplification Technology (R-SAT). Competitive antagonism of D_2 receptors and inverse agonism of 5-HT_{2A} receptors were nearly uniform throughout this class, with typical agents demonstrating low 5-HT_{2A}/D_2 ratios and atypical agents demonstrating high ratios.

12.9 ROLE OF 5-HT_{2C} RECEPTOR IN ANTIPSYCHOTIC DRUG ACTION: 5-HT_{2A} AND 5-HT_{2C} INTERACTIONS

There has been extensive consideration given to the role of 5-HT_{2C} receptors in the action of atypical APDs. The 5-HT_{2C} receptor is found throughout the CNS, including the VTA and the NAC [129]. The 5-HT$_{2C}$ receptor is constituitively active, meaing it is activated even in the absence of agonist [130, 131]. The *Ser23Cys* single-nucleotide polymorphism of the *HTR2C* receptor gene has been reported to be predictive of response to clozapine [132]. The *HTR2C* receptor gene undergoes extensive RNA editing in the brain, which leaves open the possibility that there are multiple forms of the receptor in brain [133]. This in turn suggests the *HTR2C* gene may be very important to epigenetic events which may influence the course of schizophrenia and response to treatment [134, 135]. Because of the development of specific 5-HT$_{2C}$ agonists, inverse agonists, and antagonists, it has been possible to obtain evidence for a tonic inhibitory action of 5-HT$_{2C}$ receptors on the burst firing of mesolimbic and mesocortical dopaminergic neurons. Thus, the firing rate of VTA DA neurons is inhibited or increased by 5-HT$_{2C}$ agonists or antagonists, respectively. This is consistent with microdialysis studies which show that 5-HT$_{2C}$ antagonists increase extracellular concentrations of DA in the NAC and mPFC [101, 136, 137]. These studies establish that the 5-HT$_{2C}$ receptor is most important for regulation of tonic DA release. We have recently reported that the combination of the 5-HT$_{2C}$ neutral antagonist SB242984 1.0 mg/kg and low- or high-dose haloperidol enhanced the release of cortical and NAC DA in rats using microdialysis [82]. SB242084 0.2 mg/kg produced significant increase in DA efflux in the NAC, not the mPFC. The extent of both 5-HT$_{2C}$ and 5-HT$_{2A}$ receptor blockade, in relation to D2 receptor blockade, may be a key factor in the relative ability of atypical APDs to preferentially increase cortical DA efflux compared to NAC DA efflux [82].

Early studies found no significant differences between groups of atypical APDs, and typical neuroleptics with regard to the affinity for 5-HT$_{2C}$ receptor or the difference between 5-HT$_{2C}$ and D$_2$ affinities have been reported [60, 62, 138]. A large group of atypical antipsychotic drugs (sertindole, clozapine, olanzapine, ziprasidone, risperidone, zotepine, tiospirone, fluperlapine, tenilapine) displayed potent inverse agonist activity at rat and human 5-HT$_{2C}$ receptors [139]. Typical antipsychotic drugs of various chemical classes did not. Several typical antipsychotic drugs (chlorpromazine, thioridazine, spiperone, thiothixene) displayed neutral antagonist activity by reversing clozapine inverse agonism. These data are consistent with the concept that 5-HT$_{2C}$ receptor blockade of constitutive and stimulated 5-HT$_{2C}$ receptor stimulation may play a role in the action of atypical APDs and be involved in the etiology of schizophrenia and other forms of psychosis. Chronic sertindole but not clozapine downregulated cortical 5-HT$_{2C}$ receptors [140]. 5-HT$_{2C}$ receptor antagonism appears to have useful effects on certain types of memory impairment. Thus, SB-200646 antagonized memory impairment due to some 5-HT$_{2A/AC}$ agonists and dizocilpine but not scopolamine [141]. Of the approved atypical APDs, some have equivalent affinities for the 5-HT$_{2A}$ and 5-HT$_{2C}$ receptors (clozapine, olanzapine, sertindole) while others are more selective for the 5-HT$_{2A}$ receptor (risperidone, quetiapine, ziprasidone). This difference roughly corresponds with potential to produce weight gain in that clozapine and olanzapine cause the greatest weight gain, quetiapine intermediate, and aripiprazole, bifeprunox, risperidone, and ziprasidone the least. The 759T polymorphism in the promoter region of the 5-HT$_{2C}$ receptor gene has been found to be associated with clozapine-induced weight gain, response to clozapine, and tardive dyskinesia [134].

An interesting aspect of the 5-HT$_{2C}$ receptor with regard to antipsychotic action is that 5-HT$_{2C}$ antagonism may be functionally opposed to 5-HT$_{2A}$ antagonism.

Meltzer et al. [142] reported that atypical APDs were more likely to be weak 5-HT$_{2C}$ and potent 5-HT$_{2A}$ antagonists compared to typical neuroleptic drugs. There is some evidence for a functional antagonism of these two receptors which may be expressed on the same neurons. Thus, Martin et al. [89] found that ritanserin, a mixed 5-HT$_{2A/2C}$ antagonist, blocked the ability of M100907 to antagonize the effect of MK-801 to increase locomotor activity in mice.

12.10 ROLE OF 5-HT$_{1A}$ RECEPTOR IN ANTIPSYCHOTIC DRUG ACTION: 5-HT$_{1A}$ AND 5-HT$_{2A}$ INTERACTIONS

5-HT$_{1A}$ receptors are located pre- and postsynaptically. The presynaptic 5-HT$_{1A}$ receptor is an autoreceptor located on cell bodies of raphe neurons; stimulation leads to inhibition of firing of 5-HT neurons. Stimulation of postsynaptic 5-HT$_{1A}$ receptors leads to hyperpolarization of pyramidal neurons, opposite to the effect of stimulation of 5-HT$_{2A}$ receptors. Approximately 60% of rat PFC glutamatergic cells were found to have 5-HT$_{1A}$ mRNA, as did approximately 25% of generalized anxiety disorder (GAD)–expressing cells [143]. 5-HT$_{1A}$ receptor agonists have effects similar to 5-HT$_{2A}$ receptor inverse agonists in a variety of functions [144, 145]. A few examples will be given. For example, DOI injected bilaterally into the rat mPFC elicited a dose-dependent head-twitch response. This effect is inhibited by the 5-HT$_{1A}$ agonist 8-OH-DPAT as well as the 5-HT$_{2A}$ inverse agonists M100907 and ketanserin. Ahlenius [146] first suggested that stimulation of 5-HT$_{1A}$ receptors might produce an antipsychotic-like action on the basis of behavioral studies in animals using the direct 5-HT$_{1A}$ agonist 8-OH-DPAT. Subsequent studies demonstrated that 8-OH-DPAT enhanced the antipsychotic-like effect of the D$_2$/D$_3$ antagonist raclopride [147] and of haloperidol [148] and antagonized the catalepsy induced by the D$_1$ agonist SCH23390 in rats [149]. The beneficial effect of 5-HT$_{1A}$ agonists appears to be mediated by inhibition of median raphe serotonergic neurons [150]. Ichikawa and Meltzer [151] demonstrated that 8-OH-DPAT inhibited the ability of clozapine and low-dose risperidone, but not haloperidol, to increase extracellular DA levels in the NAC and the striatum of conscious rats. The effect in the NAC would be expected to enhance the antipsychotic effect of these agents by reducing dopaminergic activity in this region which is believed to participate in the generation of psychotic symptoms. Several atypical APDs are partial agonist at the 5-HT$_{1A}$ receptor, including aripiprazole, bifeprunox, clozapine, ziprasidone, quetiapine, and tiospirone. Their affinities for the 5-HT$_{1A}$ receptor were similar to their affinities at the human D$_2$ receptor [152]. The ability of atypical APDs to increase DA efflux in the rat PFC and hippocampus is blocked, in part, by WAY-100635, a 5-HT$_{1A}$ antagonist [27, 113, 153, 154]. This effect of 5-HT$_{1A}$ receptors appears to be mediated by 5-HT$_{1A}$ receptors in the PFC as it is blocked by local injection of a 5-HT$_{1A}$ antagonist in the mPFC or by transection of cortical connections to the VTA [155]. These findings suggest that the combination of D$_2$ antagonism and 5-HT$_{1A}$ agonism should produce an atypical antipsychotic agent [155a]. S16924 is an example of such a compound, and it has atypical properties very similar to those of clozapine in a variety of animal models [137]. The 5-HT$_{1A}$ partial agonist S15535 enhanced the release of ACh in rat mPFC [156]. However, there is little evidence so far that the increase in ACh efflux in mPFC or hippocampus produced by atypical antipsychotic drugs is related to their direct or indirect 5-HT$_{1A}$ agonism [111, 113]. Bruins et al. [52] have suggested that the balance of activity at D$_2$ and 5-HT$_{1A}$ receptors is important for the ability of antipsychotic drugs to reverse the deficit in social interaction, a putative model of negative symptoms, in rats.

12.11 ROLE OF 5-HT$_6$ RECEPTOR

Recent interest in the 5-HT$_6$ receptor in relation to the action of APDs has been based, in part, on the finding that some APDs, including the atypical APDs clozapine, olanzapine, and sertindole, as well as some antidepressant agents (e.g., clomipramine and amitriptyline), are relatively potent 5-HT$_6$ receptor antagonists [62, 157–160]. Regional analysis of receptor binding and the expression of 5-HT$_6$ receptor mRNA revealed the highest levels are found in the striatum, olfactory tubercle, NAC, cerebral cortex, and subfields of the hippocampus [157, 161–164]. Together, these data on expression and localization suggest possible involvement of 5-HT$_6$ receptors in cognitive, affective, and motor function.

It has been reported that clozapine, the prototypical antipsychotic drug, but not haloperidol, significantly decreased 5-HT$_6$ receptor expression in all subfields of the hippocampus [165]. As clozapine has a greater effect than haloperidol to improve some aspects of cognition in schizophrenia, it was suggested that downregulation of this receptor in the hippocampus might contribute to the ability of clozapine to enhance cognition [165]. This hypothesis is supported by a series of behavioral studies which demonstrate that the 5-HT$_6$ receptors may be involved in learning and memory [166–173]. These data suggest that 5-HT$_6$ receptor stimulation may interfere with learning and long-term memory function and the potential role for 5-HT$_6$ receptor antagonists for the enhancement of cognition in patients with schizophrenia. The high affinity of some atypical antipsychotic drugs for 5-HT$_6$ receptors and the localization of 5-HT$_6$ receptor in limbic and cortical regions of the brain suggest that 5-HT$_6$ receptors also play a role in the mechanism of action and pathophysiology of some aspects of schizophrenia. Minabe et al. [174] reported that high but not low doses of the selective 5-HT$_6$ receptor antagonist SB-271046 given acutely suppressed the firing rate of VTA DA neurons. Chronic administration altered the pattern of firing of these neurons, which are highly relevant to schizophrenia in a manner which differed from that of either typical or atypical APDs. It was suggested that clinical study of this type of agent would be of interest to determine its role, if any, in the treatment of schizophrenia. There has been only limited study of the role of the 5-HT$_6$ receptors in the modulation of DA or ACh release, which might be relevant to their ability to improve cognition, and the results have been inconsistent. 5-HT$_6$ receptor antagonists have been reported to increase extracellular ACh efflux in the cortex or hippocampus in two studies [175, 176], However, another 5-HT$_6$ receptor antagonist RO 04-6790 failed to do so [112].

The 5-HT$_6$ receptor antagonist SB-271046, which has been shown to be effective in enhancing cognitive function in models of learning and memory [167, 169], had no effect on DA efflux in either the frontal cortex or dorsal hippocampus [177]. However, a recent study reported that SB-271046 produced a significant increase in DA release in the rat mPFC [178]. Pouzet et al. [179] found that SB-271046 dose dependently inhibited *d*-amphetamine-induced suppression of prepulse inhibition

(PPI), consistent with an antipsychotic action. However, Leng et al. [180] found no effect of two other 5-HT_6 antagonists in latent inhibition (LI) or PPI models in which clozapine was active. The 5-HT_6 receptor antagonist N-[4-methoxy-3-(4-methyl-1-piperazinyl)-phenyl]-5-chloro-3-methylbenzo-thiophene-2-yl sulfonamide monohydrochloride (SB-258510A) has been reported to produce greater potentiation of amphetamine-induced increase in extracellular DA release in the mPFC than the NAC [181]. Another 5-HT_6 receptor antagonist, SB-271046, potentiated amphetamine-induced DA release in the striatum [182]. Li et al. (in preparation) found that SB-399885, 3 and 10 mg/kg, a selective 5-HT_6 receptor antagonist, had no effect on cortical DA efflux but slightly increased hippocampal DA efflux in freely moving rats. However, SB-399885, 3 mg/kg, significantly potentiated the ability of haloperidol, a D_2 receptor antagonist, at a dose of 0.1 mg/kg, to increase DA release in the hippocampus but not the mPFC. SB-399885 also potentiated risperidone-, 1.0 mg/kg, induced DA efflux in both hippocampus and mPFC. These results suggest that the combined blockade of 5-HT_6 and D_2 receptor may contribute to the potentiation of haloperidol- or risperidone-induced DA efflux in the mPFC and hippocampus. In addition, other microdialysis studies suggest that the 5-HT_6 receptor may interact with DA mechanisms in the rat mPFC as antisense oligonucleotides partially antagonized the fluoxetine-induced cortical DA release [183]. Taken together these data suggest that 5-HT_6 receptors may have modulatory influence on DA efflux in the mPFC and hippocampus and, hence, may contribute to some of the clinical benefits of atypical APDs. 5-HT_6 receptor antagonists may also be useful as augmenting agents to improve cognitive dysfunction in schizophrenia. There is, however, insufficient evidence to conclude that they will be first-line treatments for the psychosis of schizophrenia.

12.12 ROLE OF SEROTONIN RELEASE IN ANTIPSYCHOTIC DRUG ACTION

The antagonism of multiple 5-HT receptors by clozapine would be expected to enhance the release of 5-HT by feedback mechanisms. Ichikawa et al. [184] reported that clozapine (20 mg/kg) and risperidone (1 mg/kg) but not olanzapine significantly increased extracellular 5-HT levels in the NAC and mPFC, respectively, whereas amperozide (1 and 10 mg/kg) increased extracellular 5-HT levels in both regions. Hertel et al. [185] reported similar results with risperidone and suggested that this might be relevant to its ability to improve negative symptoms. The enhancement of 5-HT efflux in the PFC may contribute to the ability of these agents to improve mood disorders and cognition [184]. Bortolozzi et al. [186] reported that clozapine blocked the efflux of cortical 5-HT produced by the hallucinogen DOI in rat brain by both 5-HT_{2A}- and α_1-adrenoceptor-dependent mechanisms.

12.13 α_2- AND α_1-ADRENERGIC MECHANISMS AND ATYPICAL APDS

Many, but not all, of the atypical APDs which are multireceptor antagonists are also potent antagonists of α_1 or α_2 adrenoceptors or both. Thus, risperidone 9-hydroxyrisperidone, clozapine, olanzapine, zotepine, quetiapine, ORG-5222 (asenapine), sertindole, and ziprasidone are potent α_1 antagonists [60]. Svensson [187] has suggested that blockade of α_1 adrenoceptors by APDs may contribute to suppression of positive symptoms whereas α_2 adrenoceptor blockade may be involved in relief of negative and cognitive symptoms. He postulates that α_1 adrenoceptor blockade may act by suppressing, at the presynaptic level, striatal hyperdopaminergia, and α_2 adrenoceptor blockade may act by augmenting and improving prefrontal dopaminergic functioning. Prazosin, an α_1 adrenoceptor antagonist, can, in the presence of weak D_2 receptor blockade, block the conditioned avoidance response [188] and has, similar to clozapine and other atypical APDs, been shown to increase DA efflux in the shell but not the core of the NAC, signifying a limbic rather than a striatal effect of α_1 antagonism [189]. These authors also suggested that α_1 antagonism may explain the atypical properties of sertindole which has as high an occupancy of D_2 receptors as typical APDs [190]. All of the atypical agents mentioned above are also potent α_2 antagonists with the exception of zotepine and sertindole. Kalkman et al. [191] have raised the possibility that the α_{2C} subtype may be particularly relevant to the anticataleptic actions of clozapine and iloperidone. However, McAllister and Rey [192] were unable to reverse the effects of loxapine or haloperidol on catalepsy with α_2 antagonists and showed that the effect of clozapine to reverse loxapine-induced increase in catalepsy was due to its anticholinergic rather than its adrencoeptor blocking properties.

The addition of idazoxan, an α_2 antagonist, to fluphenazine, a typical neuroleptic, was reported by Litman et al. [193] to have efficacy comparable to clozapine in a small group of neuroleptic-resistant patients with SCH. These results need to be replicated. Polymorphisms of the α_1 and α_2 receptors have been reported not to predict response to clozapine [194]. In this regard, it is of interest that idazoxan has been shown to preferentially increase DA efflux in the rat mPFC by an action at the terminal area [195]. This effect appears to be independent of dopaminergic activity. Subsequently, it was reported that the combination of raclopride, a D_2 antagonist, and idazoxan [196] produced a dose-dependent increase in NE in the mPFC of rats, as does systemic administration of clozapine, risperidone, ziprasidone, and olanzapine but also haloperidol [197]. This effect was closely coupled to the increase in DA efflux. Stimulation of α_2 receptors in cortex has been postulated to improve some types of cognitive function, for example, executive functions [198, 199]. Atypical antipsychotic drugs block α_2 receptors as noted above and would be expected to compromise cognitive function on this basis. However, these drugs also enhance the release of NE along with DA, which could overcome the effects of α_2 blockade. In fact, the atypical antipsychotic drugs have their least beneficial effect on executive function [9].

12.14 GLUTAMATERGIC MECHANISMS

Glutamate is the predominant excitatory neurotransmitter in the mammalian CNS. There are two types of glutamate receptors (GluRs): ionotroic GluRs, which are postsynaptic, mutimeric ligand-gated ion channels classified into three groups related to group-selective agonists—NMDA, amino-3-hydroxy-5-methyl-isoxazole-4-proprionic acid (AMPA) and kainite receptors— and metabotropic GluRs (mGluRs), which are members of family C of the G-protein-coupled receptors. None of the currently available APDs have a high affinity for any of the ionotropic or metabotropic GluRs. Because of some similarities between the behavioral effects of NMDA receptor antagonists PCP and ketamine to the cognitive, negative, and positive symptoms of schizophrenia, it has been suggested that hypoglutamatergic function might contribute to schizophrenia [15, 200]. Laruelle et al. [201] summarized data for dopaminergic–glutamatergic interactions and proposed that hypoglutamatergic cortical function might lead to increased mesolimbic dopaminergic stimulation while diminution of mesolimbic dopamine function might reverse hypoglutamatergia. There have been numerous in vivo microdialysis studies of the effect of haloperidol and clozapine, as well as other antipsychotic drugs, to modulate the efflux of glutamate in cortex or striatum. The results are very mixed, reflecting differences in dosages, duration of treatment, use of anesthesia, and difficulty in separating glutamate efflux that is neuronally based from that due to the amino acid compartment [202]. Chronic treatment with haloperidol for six weeks followed by its withdrawal for four days elevated the basal, but not the veratridine-stimulated, extracellular levels of glutamate and aspartate [203] and enhanced the activity of cortical neurons. In contrast, six-week treatment with clozapine lowered both the basal and the stimulated levels of glutamate and aspartate but had no effect on the activity of cortical neurons. In a study of the effect of these two antipsychotic drugs on glutamate release from nerve terminals isolated from rat PFC, Yang and Wang [204] found that both haloperidol and clozapine inhibited glutamate release by ion-channel activities which influence nerve terminal excitability. At the present time, this effect of antipsychotic drugs on glutamate release cannot be related to their actions with any degree of confidence.

However, behavioral studies involving two models of cognitive impairment in schizophrenia, PPI and LI, provide more robust evidence that glutamatergic mechanisms may be important to the action of antipsychotic drugs. PPI of the startle response provides a measure of the ability of the organism to attenuate its response to repeated sensory input. The diminished response to sound- or air pulse-induced startle is usually used to test this reflex. Latent inhibition is a measure of the capacity to ignore irrelevant (nonreinforced) stimuli. Both PPI and LI are disrupted in schizophrenia. Treatment with NMDA receptor antagonists such as MK-801 or PCP can disrupt PPI and LI. Atypical antipsychotic drugs such as clozapine are more effective than typical antipsychotic drugs to reverse PPI [205, 206] or LI [207]. A recent study found no difference between typical and atypical APDs in reducing startle magnitude and increasing PPI in a mouse line which expresses low levels of the NMDA R1 subunit of the NMDA receptor [208]. The ability of drugs to reverse PCP-induced PPI disruption is correlated to their affinity for $5\text{-}HT_{2A}$, not D_2 receptors [209]. Interestingly, the $5\text{-}HT_{2A}$ antagonist M100907 and the α_1-adrenergic antagonist prazosin are also effective to reverse PPI deficits induced by NMDA receptor antagonists [205] but the α_2 antagonist RX821002, the M_1/M_4 muscarinic antagonist pirenzepine, or the $GABA\text{-}_A$ antagonist pitrazepin had no effect on basal or PCP-impaired PPI in mice [210]. As previously mentioned, $5\text{-}HT_{2A}$ receptors on cortical glutamatergic pyramidal neurons and GABAergic interneurons may have a key role in modulating glutamatergic function [143]. It has been suggested that the hallucinogenic action of $5\text{-}HT_{2A}$ agonists such as DOI is mediated by mGluR2/3-induced glutamate release as the head shakes induced by DOI are blocked by the mGluR2/3 agonist LY354740 and potentiated by the mGluR2/3 antagonist

LY341495 [211]. The combination of raclopride, a D_2 antagonist, and idazoxan, an α_2 antagonist, also was ineffective to block PCP-induced disruption of PPI [212]. Neonatal ventral hippocampal (NVH) lesions in rats induce behavioral abnormalities in adult rats that have some correspondence to cognitive deficits and negative symptoms in patients with schizophrenia, including deficits in PPI. Clozapine, olanzapine, and risperidone, but not haloperidol, reversed the deficit in PPI produced by an NVH lesion, possibly by enhancing glutamatergic function [213].

There is some evidence for a possible role of mGluR5 in schizophrenia [214]. mGluR2 agonists [215, 216] and positive allosteric modulators of the mGlurR5 [217] have been shown to have activity in various animal models of antipsychotic activity, but there is no direct evidence that the current generation of atypical antipsychotic drugs act through either mechanism. Thus, neither clozapine nor raclopride were able to attenuate the PPI deficit in mGluR5 knockout mice [214].

12.15 CHOLINERGIC MECHANISMS

The concept of muscarinic agonism as a first-line treatment for schizophrenia was initiated by studies with xanomeline, which is a M_1/M_4 agonist or partial agonist. It was found to have some antipsychotic effects in patients with Alzheimer's disease or schizophrenia [218]. Preclinical studies with xanomeline and a closely related compound sabcomeline indicated it had the profile of an atypical APD, blocking conditioned avoidance response and producing minimal EPSs [219, 220]. Sabcomeline and possibly xanomeline also have indirect effects on D_2 receptor binding in the mouse striatum, as revealed by changes in the availability of D_2 receptors [221]. NDMC, the major metabolite of clozapine, has been reported to be an effective M_1 agonist in vitro [median effective concentration (EC_{50}) of 100 nM with 80% efficacy (relative to carbachol)] as well as in vivo [222, 223]. The M_1 agonist activity of NDMC is blocked by anticholinergic drugs and clozapine [222, 223]. These results confirm that NDMC is a potent, efficacious, M_1 receptor agonist, distinguishing it from the M_1 receptor antagonist properties of clozapine. No other antipsychotic has potent M_1 agonist properties [223, 224]. Clozapine is, in fact, a very weak partial agonist at M_1 receptors, a more efficacious agonist at M_2 and M_4 receptors, and to lack agonist activity at M_3 and M_5 receptors. NDMC also displayed high-potency interactions with all five human muscarinic receptors, but with increased agonist efficacy at M_1, M_4, and M_5 receptors when compared to clozapine. In contrast, olanzapine and N-desmethylolanzapine, both structurally related to clozapine and NDMC, lack agonist activity at human muscarinic receptors [223].

Li et al. [236] have reported that NDMC enhances DA and ACh efflux in the mPFC and hippocampus. Clozapine blocks the effects of NDMC on cortical and hippocampal ACh efflux and on hippocampal DA efflux [82]. The M_1 antagonist telenzepine also blocked the effect of NDMC on DA and ACh efflux. These results suggest that clozapine, acting through its predominant metabolite NDMC, may function as a direct-acting muscarinic receptor agonist in vivo. During pharmacotherapy with clozapine, the agonist actions of NDMC would be attenuated by the antagonistic actions of the parent compound. Thus, high NDMC levels, and particularly high NDMC/clozapine ratios, would increase agonist efficacy at muscarinic receptors, as predicted by mass action and by agonist/antagonist mixing studies [225]. Clinical data support this notion. Not only does clozapine therapy usually lack the traditional anti cholinergic side effects of dry mouth, blurred vision, and urinary retention common to classical muscarinic antagonists, but also it is unique in its ability to frequently produce sialorrhea, an effect that can be blocked by the muscarinic antagonist pirenzepine [226]. Thus, the muscarinic receptor agonist activity of NDMC likely mediates this peripheral effect. The muscarinic agonist properties of NDMC may underlie some of the unique central effects of treatment with clozapine. If this hypothesis is correct, NDMC/clozapine ratios should be a better predictor of therapeutic response to clozapine, particularly for cognition, than absolute clozapine levels. As predicted, higher NDMC/clozapine ratios predicted improvement in multiple measures of cognition as well as negative symptoms [223]. Some other recent reports [227, 228] all suggest that the NDMC/clozapine ratio is a better predictor of clinical response to clozapine than clozapine levels alone and support the hypothesis that NDMC is a critical mediator of clozapine action.

12.16 NEUROKININ 3 RECEPTORS

The possible involvement of neurokinin 3 (NK_3) receptors in antipsychotic drug action has been recently reviewed [229]. The NK_3 antagonists osanetant and talnetant have been tested in schizophrenia. Osanetant showed some efficacy to treat positive symptoms with no evidence of EPSs in randomized, placebo- and haloperidol-controlled trials, indicating it met the criteria for an atypical APD [78]. Talnetant is in phase 2 testing but no results have been reported as of yet. Should either or both of these two agents prove clinically effective as monotherapy or as addon therapy, it would be a major advance in the treatment of schizophrenia. Preclincal data suggest that NK_3 receptor antagonism achieves its antipsychotic efficacy by inhibition of dopaminergic activity via an indirect mechanism [230].

12.17 NEUROGENESIS

The evidence for the loss of neurons and decreased neuropil in schizophrenia [231] provided the initial impetus for the investigation of a possible role of antipsychotic drugs in schizophrenia [232]. In a review of the effects of antipsychotic drugs on neuroplasticity, these authors concluded that the ability of long-term treatment with antipsychotic drugs to induce anatomical and molecular changes in the brain may be relevant to their antipsychotic properties. Imaging studies which indicate that atypical but not typical antipsychotic drugs slow the loss of cortical volume in schizophrenia is compatible with the view that neurogenesis may be, at least, a component of the action of atypical antipsychotic drugs [233]. Preclinical studies have added some evidence for this hypothesis. Atypical but not typical APDs risperidone and olanzapine increase the number of newly generated call in the subventricular zone [234]. Wang et al. [235] reported that three-week treatment with olanzapine but not haloperidol produced slight evidence for cortical and dorsal striatal neurogenesis but none in the NAC. They concluded that neurogenesis did not play a significant role in the effects of olanzapine on cortical function. Further study in this regard is still of interest, however.

12.18 CONCLUSIONS

Atypical APDs are those APDs which produce an antipsychotic effect at doses which cause minimal EPSs compared to typical APDs. Any other clinical feature of the atypical APDs is not part of the core definition, even if the bases for the additional clinical effect are related to the same pharmacological principles. Thus, lack of prolactin elevation is not a core feature of an atypical APD, even though it, like low EPSs, may be related to potent 5-HT_{2A} antagonism relative to weaker D_2 antagonism. The advantage to patients of having antipsychotic drugs with reduced risk parkinsonism and tardive dyskinesia are adequate reasons for making these drugs the first-line treatment for schizophrenia and bipolar disorder. There are now two established classes of atypical APDs: multireceptor antagonists which have a common serotonergic profile (e.g., clozapine) and partial DA agonists (e.g., aripiprazole). All clinically viable examples of these two classes of agents involve both a dopaminergic and serotonergic profile. 5-HT_{1A} partial agonism may be a functional substitute for 5-HT_{2A} antagonism. There is strong evidence for the role of 5-HT_{2A} receptor antagonism and 5-HT_{1A} partial agonism as a sufficient if not necessary feature of an atypical APD, in conjunction with no more than moderate D_2 receptor blockade whether it be the result of direct blockade or partial agonism. Studies are underway to determine if selective $5\text{-HT}_{2A/2C}$ antagonists are sufficient to treat some forms of psychosis without supplemental D_2 receptor blockade. 5-HT_6 antagonism may also facilitate some of the clinical advantages of those atypical APDs, which are potent 5-HT_6 antagonists. 5-HT_{2C} receptor blockade is a feature of some atypical APDs, but its contribution to their mechanism of action is unclear at the present time. Rapid dissociation from the D_2 receptor is not a core feature of most examples of these two classes of APDs but may contribute to the low EPS profile of clozapine and quetiapine. There are five other groups of drugs which may be atypical APDs. These include substituted benzamides, of which there are two main examples, amisulpride and remoxipride; selective $5\text{-HT}_{2A/2C}$ inverse agonists; $D_2/5\text{-HT}_{1A}$ partial agonists; NK_3 antagonists; and M_1 agonists or partial agonists, of which there is only one available and that is not specific for M_1. These mechanisms of atypicality are promising and need to be further studied. There are no atypical APDs, as of yet, which have come from intensive study of D_1, D_3, or D_4 mechanisms. There are also no atypical APDs which primarily act through glutamatergic mechanisms, despite intensive effort to date to develop them and the fact that the multireceptor antagonists have been shown to act, in part, by modulating glutamatergic pathways.

ACKNOWLEDGMENTS

This work was supported by grants from grants from the Ritter Foundation, the Prentiss Foundation, and the William K. Warren Foundation. Herbert Meltzer is the Bixler, May, Johnson Professor of Psychiatry.

REFERENCES

1. Meltzer, H. Y. (2000). An atypical compound by any other name is still an atypical. *Psychopharmacology* 148(1), 16–19.

2. Kane, J., Honigfeld, G., Singer, J., and Meltzer, H. (1988). Clozapine for the treatment-resistant schizophrenic. A double-blind comparison with chlorpromazine. *Arch. Gen. Psychiatry* 45, 789–796.
3. Meltzer, H. Y. (1997). Treatment-resistant schizophrenia — The role of clozapine. *Curr. Med. Res. Opin.* 14(2), 1–20.
4. McEvoy, J. P., Lieberman, J. A., Stroup, T. S., Davis, S. M., Meltzer, H. Y., Rosenheck, R. A., Swartz, M. S., Perkins, D. O., Keefe, R. S. E., Davis, C. E., Severe, J., and Hsiao, J. K., for the CATIE Investigators (2006). Effectiveness of clozapine versus olanzapine, quetiapine or risperidone in patients with chronic schizophrenia who failed prior atypical antipsychotic treatment. *Am. J. Psychiatry* 163(4), 600–610.
5. Gerson, S. L., and Meltzer, H. (1992). Mechanisms of clozapine-induced agranulocytosis. *Drug Safety* 7(Suppl. 1), 17–25.
6. Serretti, A., De Ronchi, D., Lorenzi, C., and Berardi, D. (2004). New antipsychotics and schizophrenia: A review on efficacy and side effects. *Curr. Med. Chem.* 11(3), 343–358.
7. Lieberman, J. A., Stroup, T. S., McEvoy, J. P., Swartz, M. S., Rosenheck, R. A., Perkins, D. O., Keefe, R. S. E., Davis, S. M., Davis, C. E., Lebowitz, B. D., Severe, J., and Hsiao, J. K. (2005). For the Clinical Antipsychotic Trials of Intervention Effectiveness (CATIE) investigators (2005): Effectiveness of antipsychotic drugs in patients with chronic schizophrenia. *N. Eng. J. Med.* 353, 1209–1223.
8. Meltzer, H. Y., and McGurk, S. R. (1999). The effects of clozapine, risperidone, and olanzapine on cognitive function in schizophrenia. *Schizophr. Bull.* 25, 233–255.
9. Woodward, N. D., Purdon, S. E., Meltzer, H. Y., and Zald, D. H. (2005). A meta-analysis of neuropsychological change to clozapine, olanzapine, quetiapine, and risperidone in schizophrenia. *Int. J. Neuropsychopharmacology* 8(3), 457–472.
10. Meltzer, H. Y., and Stahl, S. M. (1976). The dopamine hypothesis of schizophrenia: A review. *Schizophr. Bull.* 2, 19–76.
11. Meltzer, H. Y. (2002). Mechanism of action of atypical antipsychotic drugs. In *Neuropsychopharmacology: The fifth generation of progress*, K. L. Davis, D. Charney, J. T. Coyle and C. Nemeroff, Eds. Lippincott Williams & Wilkins, Philadelphia pp. 819–832.
12. Creese, I., Burt, D. R., and Snyder, S. H. (1976). Dopamine receptor binding predicts clinical and pharmacological potencies of antischizophrenic drugs. *Science* 192, 481–483.
13. Seeman, P., Lee, T., Chau-Wong, M., and Wong, K. (1976). Antipsychotic drug doses and neuroleptic/dopamine receptors. *Nature* 261, 717–719.
14. Kapur, S., Remington, G., Zipursky, R. B., Wilson, A. A., and Houle, S. (1995). The D2 dopamine receptor occupancy of risperidone and its relationship to extrapyramidal symptoms: A PET study. *Life Sci.* 57, PL103–PL107.
15. Miyamoto, S., Duncan, G. E., Marx, C. E., and Lieberman, J. A. (2005). Treatments for schizophrenia: A critical review of pharmacology and mechanisms of action of antipsychotic drugs. *Mol. Psychiatry* 10, 79–104.
16. Farde, L., Nordstrom, A. L., Wiesel, F. A., Pauli, S., Halldin, C., and Sedvall, G. (1992). Positron emission tomographic analysis of central D1 and D2 dopamine receptor occupancy in patients treated with classical neuroleptics and clozapine. Relation to extrapyramidal side effects. *Arch. Gen. Psychiatry* 49, 538–544.
17. Talvik, M., Nordstrom, A. L., Nyberg, S., Olsson, H., Halldin, C., and Farde, L. (2001). No support for regional selectivity in clozapine-treated patients: A PET study with [(11)C]raclopride and (11)C]FLB 457. *Am. J. Psychiatry* 158(6), 926–930.

18. Kapur, S., Zipursky, R., Jones, C., Shammi, C. S., Remington, G., and Seeman, P. (2000). A positron emission tomography study of quetiapine in schizophrenia: A preliminary finding of an antipsychotic effect with only transiently high dopamine D2 receptor occupancy. *Arch. Gen. Psychiatry* 57, 553–559.

19. Mamo, D., Kapur, S., Shammi, C. M., Papatheodorou, G., Mann, S., Therrien, F., and Remington, G. (2004). A PET study of dopamine D2 and serotonin 5-HT2 receptor occupancy in patients with schizophrenia treated with therapeutic doses of ziprasidone. *Am. J. Psychiatry* 161, 818–825.

20. Kessler, R. M., Ansari, M. S., Riccardi, P., Li, R., Jayathilake, K., Dawant, B., and Meltzer, H. Y. (2005). Occupancy of striatal and extrastriatal dopamine D(2)/D(3) receptors by olanzapine and haloperidol. *Neuropsychopharmacology* 30(12), 2283–2289.

21. Kessler, R. M., Sib Ansari, M., Riccardi, P., Li, R., Jayathilake, K., Dawant, B., and Meltzer, H. Y., (in press). Occupancy of extrastriatal dopamine D2 receptors by clozapine and quetiapine. *Neuropsychopharmacology*.

22. Grunder, G., Landvogt, C., Vernaleken, Buchholz, H.-G., Ondracek, J., Siessmeier, Hartter, S., Schreckenberger, M., Stoeter, P., Hiemke, C., Rosch, F., Wong, D. F., Bartenstein, P. (2006). The striatal and extrastriatal D2/3 receptor-binding profile of clozapine in patients with schizophrenia. *Neuropsychopharmacology* 31(5), 1027–1035.

23. Seeman, P., and Tallerico, T. (1999). Rapid release of antipsychotic drugs from dopamine D2 receptors: An explanation for low receptor occupancy and early clinical relapse upon withdrawal of clozapine or quetiapine. *Am. J. Psychiatry* 156, 876–884.

24. Kapur, S., and Seeman, P. (2000). Antipsychotic agents differ in how fast they come off the dopamine D2 receptors. Implications for atypical antipsychotic action. *J. Psychiatry Neurosci.* 25, 161–166.

25. Seeman, P. (2002). Atypical antipsychotics: Mechanism of action. *Can. J. Psychiatry* 47(1), 27–38.

26. Meltzer, H. Y., Matsubara, S., and Lee, J. C. (1989). Classification of typical and atypical antipsychotic drugs on the basis of dopamine D-1, D-2 and serotonin2 pKi values. *J. Pharmacol. Exp. Ther.* 251, 238–246.

27. Ichikawa, J., Ishii, H., Bonaccorso, S., Fowler, W. L., O'Laughlin, I. A., and Meltzer, H. Y. (2001). 5-HT(2A) and D(2) receptor blockade increases cortical DA release via 5-HT(1A) receptor activation: A possible mechanism of atypical antipsychotic-induced cortical dopamine release. *J. Neurochem.* 76(5), 1521–1531.

28. Salmi, P., Karlsson, T., and Ahlenius, S. (1994). Antagonism by SCH 23390 of clozapine-induced hypothermia in the rat. *Eur. J. Pharmacol.* 253(1/2), 67–73.

29. Jay, T. M., Rocher, C., Hotte, M., Naudon, L., Gurden, H., and Spedding, M. (2004). Plasticity at hippocampal to prefrontal cortex synapses is impaired by loss of dopamine and stress: Importance for psychiatric diseases. *Neurotox. Res.* 6, 233–244.

30. Gessa, G. L., Canu, A., Del Zompo, M., Burrai, C., and Serra, G. (1991). Lack of acute antipsychotic effect of Sch 23390, a selective dopamine D1 receptor antagonist. *Lancet* 337(8745), 854–855.

31. Karlsson, P., Smith, L., Farde, L., Harnryd, C., Sedvall, G., and Wiesel, F. A. (1995). Lack of apparent antipsychotic effect of the D1-dopamine receptor antagonist SCH39166 in acutely ill schizophrenic patients. *Psychopharmacology* 121(3), 309–916.

32. Van Tol, H. H., Bunzow, J. R., Guan, H. C., Sunahara, R. K., Seeman, P., Niznik, H. B., and Civelli, O. (1991). Cloning of the gene for a human dopamine D4 receptor with high affinity for the antipsychotic clozapine. *Nature* 350, 610–614.

33. Truffinet, P., Tamminga, C. A., Fabre, L. F., Meltzer, H. Y., Riviere, M. E., and Papillon-Downey, C. (1999). A placebo controlled study of the $D_4/5\text{-}HT_{2A}$ antagonist fananserin in the treatment of schizophrenia. *Am. J. Psychiatry* 156(3), 419–425.
34. Kramer, M. S., Last, B., Getson, A., and Reines, S. A. (1997). The effects of a selective D4 dopamine receptor antagonist (L-745,870) in acutely psychotic inpatients with schizophrenia. D4 Dopamine Antagonist Group. *Arch. Gen. Psychiatry* 54, 567–572.
35. Corrigan, M. H., Gallen, C. C., Bonura, M. L., and Merchant, K. M. (2004). Sonepiprazole Study Group. Effectiveness of the selective D4 antagonist sonepiprazole in schizophrenia: A placebo-controlled trial. *Biol. Psychiatry* 55(5), 445–451.
36. Schwartz, J. C., Diaz, J., Pilon, C., and Sokoloff, P. (2000). Possible implications of the dopamine D(3) receptor in schizophrenia and in antipsychotic drug actions. *Brain Res. Brain Res. Rev.* 31, 277–287.
37. Goudie, A. J., Baker, L. E., Smith, J. A., Prus, A. J., Svensson, K. A., Cortes-Burgos, L. A., Wong, E. H., and Haadsma-Svensson, S. (2001). Common discriminative stimulus properties in rats of muscarinic antagonists, clozapine and the D3 preferring antagonist PNU-99194a: An analysis of possible mechanisms. *Behav. Pharmacology* 12, 303–315.
38. Reavill, C., Taylor, S. G., Wood, M. D., Ashmeade, T., Austin, N. E., Avenell, K. Y., Boyfield, I., Branch, C. L., Cilia, J., Coldwell, M. C., Hadley, M. S., Hunter, A. J., Jeffrey, P., Jewitt, F., Johnson, C. N., Jones, D. N., Medhurst, A. D., Middlemiss, D. N., Nash, D. J., Riley, G. J., Routledge, C., Stemp, G., Thewlis, K. M., Trail, B., Vong, A. K., and Hagan, J. J. (2000). Pharmacological actions of a novel, high-affinity, and selective human dopamine D(3) receptor antagonist, SB-277011-A. *J. Pharmacol. Exp. Ther.* 294, 1154–1165.
39. Ashby, C. R., Jr., Minabe, Y., Stemp, G., Hagan, J. J., and Middlemiss, D. N. (2000). Acute and chronic administration of the selective D(3) receptor antagonist SB-277011-A alters activity of midbrain dopamine neurons in rats: An in vivo electrophysiological study. *J. Pharmacol. Exp. Ther.* 294, 1166–1174.
40. Moghaddam, B., and Bunney, B. S. (1990). Acute effects of typical and atypical antipsychotic drugs on the release of dopamine from prefrontal cortex, nucleus accumbens, and striatum of the rat: An in vivo microdialysis study. *J. Neurochem.* 54, 1755–1760.
41. Kuroki, T., Meltzer, H. Y., Ichikawa, J. (1999). Effects of antipsychotic drugs on extracellular dopamine levels in rat medial prefrontal cortex and nucleus accumbens. *J. Pharmacol. Expl. Thera.* 288(2), 774–781.
42. Sechter, D., Peuskens, J., Fleurot, O., Rein, W., Lecrubier, Y., and Amisullpride Study Group (2002). Amisulpride vs. risperidone in chronic schizophrenia: Results of a 6-month double-blind study. *Neuropsychopharmacology* 27(6), 1071–1081.
43. Pani L., and Gessa, G. L. (2002). The substituted benzamides and their clinical potential on dysthymia and on the negative symptoms of schizophrenia. *Mol. Psychiatry* 7(3), 247–253.
44. Bressan, R. A., Erlandsson, K., Jones, H. M., Mulligan, R., Flanagan, R. J., Ell, P. J., and Pilowsky, L. S., (2003). Is regionally selective D2/D3 dopamine occupancy sufficient for atypical antipsychotic effect? An in vivo quantitative [123I]epidepride SPET study of amisulpride-treated patients. *Am. J. Psychiatry* 160(8), 1413–1420.
45. Jimenez-Jimenez, F. J., Garcia-Ruiz, P. J., and Molina, J. A. (1997). Drug-induced movement disorders. *Drug Safety* 16(3), 180–204.
46. Correll, C. U., Leucht, S., and Kane, J. M. (2004). Lower risk for tardive dyskinesia associated with second-generation antipsychotics: A systematic review of 1-year studies. *Am. J. Psychiatry* 161(3), 414–425.

47. Mehta, M. A., Manes, F. F., Magnolfi, G., Sahakian, B. J., and Robbins, T. W. (2004). Impaired set-shifting and dissociable effects on tests of spatial working memory following the dopamine D2 receptor antagonist sulpiride in human volunteers. *Psychopharmacology* 176(3/4), 331–342.
48. Wagner, M., Quednow, B. B., Westheide, J., Schlaepfer, T. E., Maier, W., and Kuhn, K. U. (2005). Cognitive improvement in schizophrenic patients does not require a serotonergic mechanism: Randomized controlled trial of olanzapine vs amisulpride. *Neuropsychopharmacology* 30(2), 381–390.
49. Burstein, E. S., Ma, J., Wong, S., Gao, Y., Pham, E., Knapp, A. E., Nash, N. R., Olsson, R., Davis, R. E., Hacksell, U., Weiner, D. M., and Brann, M. R. (2005). Intrinsic efficacy of antipsychotics at human D2, D3, and D4 dopamine receptors: Identification of the clozapine metabolite N-desmethylclozapine as a D2/D3 partial agonist. *J. Pharmacol. Exp. Ther.* 315, 1278–1287.
50. Hertel, P., Husum, H., Marquis, K., Herremans, A. H. J., and Hesselink, M. B. (2006). Bifeprunox: A new atypical antipsychotic with in vivo, agonistic activity at the 5-HT1A receptor. *Sch. Res.* 81(Suppl.), 83.
51. Swainston Harrison, T., and Perry, C. M. (2004). Aripiprazole: A review of its use in schizophrenia and schizoaffective disorder. *Drugs* 64(15), 1715–1736.
52. Bruins Slot, L. A., Kleven, M. S., and Newman-Tancredi, A. (2005). Effects of novel antipsychotics with mixed D(2) antagonist/5-HT(1A) agonist properties on PCP-induced social interaction deficits in the rat. *Neuropharmacology* 49(7), 996–1006.
53. Tamminga, C. A. (2002). Partial dopamine agonists in the treatment of psychosis. *J. Neural Transm.* 109(3), 411–420.
54. Mottola, D. M., Kilts, J. D., Lewis, M. M., Connery, H. S., Walker, Q. D., Jones, S. R., Booth, R. G., Hyslop, D. K., Piercey, M., Wightman, R. M., Lawler, C. P., Nichols, D. E., and Mailman, R. B. (2002). Functional selectivity of dopamine receptor agonists. I. Selective activation of postsynaptic dopamine D2 receptors linked to adenylate cyclase. *J. Pharmacol. Exp. Ther.* 301(3), 1166–1178.
55. Ryman-Rasmussen, J. P., Nichols, D. E., and Mailman, R. B. (2005). Differential activation of adenylate cyclase and receptor internalization by novel dopamine D1 receptor agonists. *Mol. Pharmacol.* 68(4), 1039–1048.
56. Kilts, J. D., Connery, H. S., Arrington, E. G., Lewis, M. M., Lawler, C. P., Oxford, G. S., O'Malley, K. L., Todd, R. D., Blake, B. L., Nichols, D. E., and Mailman, R. B. (2002). Functional selectivity of dopamine receptor agonists. II. Actions of dihydrexidine in D2L receptor-transfected MN9D cells and pituitary lactotrophs. *J. Pharmacol. Exp. Ther.* 301(3), 1179–1189.
57. Li, Z., Ichikawa, J., Dai, J., and Meltzer, H. Y., (2004). Aripiprazole, a novel antipsychotic drug, preferentially increases dopamine release in the prefrontal cortex and hippocampus in rat brain. *Eur. J. Pharmacol.* 493(1–3), 75–83.
58. Zocchi, A., Fabbri, D., and Heidbreder, C. A. (2005). Aripiprazole increases dopamine but not noradrenaline and serotonin levels in the mouse prefrontal cortex. *Neurosci. Lett.* 387(3), 157–161.
59. Altar, C. A., Wasley, A. M., Neale, R. F., and Stone, G. A. (1986). Typical and atypical antipsychotic occupancy of D2 and S2 receptors: An autoradiographic analysis in rat brain. *Brain Res. Bull.* 16, 517–525.
60. Schotte, A., Janssen, P. F., Gommeren, W., Luyten, W. H., Van Gompel, P., Lesage, A. S., De Loore, K., and Leysen, J. E. (1996). Risperidone compared with new and reference antipsychotic drugs: In vitro and in vivo receptor binding. *Psychopharmacology* 124, 57–73.

61. Meltzer, H. Y., and Nash, J. F. (1991). Effects of antipsychotic drugs on serotonin receptors. *Pharmacol. Rev.* 43, 587–604.
62. Roth, B. L., Craigo, S. C., Choudhary, M. S., Uluer, A., Monsma, F. J., Jr., Shen, Y., Meltzer, H. Y., and Sibley, D. R. (1994). Binding of typical and atypical antipsychotic agents to 5-hydroxytryptamine-6 and 5-hydroxytryptamine-7 receptors. *J. Pharmacol. Exp. Ther.* 268, 1403–1410.
63. Meltzer, H. Y., and Fatemi, S. H. (1996). The role of serotonin in schizophrenia and the mechanism of action on anti-psychotic drugs. In *Serotonergic Mechanisms in Antipsychotic Treatment*, J. M. Kane, H. J. Moller and F. Awouters, Eds. Marcel Decker, New York, pp. 77–107.
64. Fiorella, D., Rabin, R. A., and Winter, J. C., (1995). Role of 5-HT2A and 5-HT2C receptors in the stimulus effects of hallucinogenic drugs. II: Reassessment of LSD false positives. *Psychopharmacol.* 121(3), 357–363.
65. Arora, R. C., and Meltzer, H. Y. (1991). Serotonin2 (5-HT2) receptor binding in the frontal cortex of schizophrenic patients. *J. Neural Transm. Genet. Sect.* 85, 19–29.
66. Burnet, P. W., Eastwood, S. L., and Harrison, P. J. (1996). 5-HT1A and 5-HT2A receptor mRNAs and binding site densities are differentially altered in schizophrenia. *Neuropsychopharmacology* 15, 442–455.
67. Joyce, J. N., Shane, A., Lexow, N., Winokur, A., Casanova, M. F., and Kleinman, J. E. (1993). Serotonin uptake sites and serotonin receptors are altered in the limbic system of schizophrenics. *Neuropsychopharmacology* 8, 315–336.
68. Matsubara, S., and Meltzer, H. Y. (1989). Effect of typical and atypical antipsychotic drugs on 5-HT2 receptor density in rat cerebral cortex. *Life Sci.* 45(15), 1397–1406.
69. Ngan, E. T., Yatham, L. N., Ruth, T. J., and Liddle, P. F. (2000). Decreased serotonin 2A receptor densities in neuroleptic-naive patients with schizophrenia: A PET study using [(18)F]setoperone. *Am. J. Psychiatry* 157, 1016–1018.
70. Trichard, C., Paillere-Martinot, M. L., Attar-Levy, D., Blin, J., Feline, A., and Martinot, J. L. (1998). No serotonin 5-HT2A receptor density abnormality in the cortex of schizophrenic patients studied with PET. *Schizophr. Res.* 31, 13–17.
71. Verhoeff, N. P., Meyer, J. H., Kecojevic, A., Hussey, D., Lewis, R., Tauscher, J., Zipursky, R. B., and Kapur, S. (2000). A voxel-by-voxel analysis of [18F]setoperone PET data shows no substantial serotonin 5-HT(2A) receptor changes in schizophrenia. *Psychiatry Res.* 99, 123–135.
72. Kapur, S., and Remington, G. (1996). Serotonin-dopamine interaction and its relevance to schizophrenia. *Am. J. Psychiarty* 153, 466–476.
73. Marder, S. R. and Meibach, R. C. (1994). Risperidone in the treatment of schizophrenia. *Am. J. Psychiatry* 151(16), 825–835.
74. Anil Yagcioglu, A. E., Kivircik Akdede, B. B., Turgut, T. I., Tumuklu, M., Yazici, M. K., Alptekin, K., Ertugrul, A., Jayathilake, K., Gogus, A., Tunca, Z., and Meltzer, H. Y. (2005). A double-blind controlled study of adjunctive treatment with risperidone in schizophrenic patients partially responsive to clozapine: Efficacy and safety. *J. Clin. Psychiatry* 66, 63–72.
75. Honer, W. G., Thornton, A. E., Chen, E. Y., Chan, R. C., Wong, J. O., Bergmann, A., Falkai, P., Pomarol-Clotet, E., McKenna, P. J., Stip, E., Williams, R., MacEwan, G. W., Wasan, K., and Procyshyn, R. (2006). Clozapine and Risperidone Enhancement (CARE) Study Group. Clozapine alone versus clozapine and risperidone with refractory schizophrenia. *N. Engl. J. Med.* 354, 472–482.
76. Shipley, J. (1998). M100907 phase IIB trial. Paper presented at the Hoechst Marion Roussel Conference on M100907. West Palm Beach, FL.

77. Rinaldi-Carmona, M., Congy, C., Santucci, V., Simiand, J., Gautret, B., Neliat, G., Labeeuw, B., Le Fur, G., Soubrié, P. G., and Breliere, J. C. (1992). Biochemical and pharmacological properties of SR 46349B, a new potent and selective 5-hydroxytryptamine$_2$ receptor antagonists. *J. Pharmacol. Exp. Ther.* 262, 759–768.
78. Meltzer, H. Y., Arvanitis, L., Bauer, D., Rein, W., and Meta-Trial Study Group. (2004). Placebo-controlled evaluation of four novel compounds for the treatment of schizophrenia and schizoaffective disorder. *Am. J. Psychiatry* 161(6), 975–984.
79. Okuyama, S., Chaki, S., Kawashima, N., Suzuki, Y., Ogawa, S., Kumagai, T., Nakazato, A., Nagamine, M., Yamaguchi, K., and Tomisawa, K. (1997). The atypical antipsychotic profile of NRA0045, a novel dopamine D4 and 5-hydroxytryptamine2A receptor antagonist, in rats. *Br. J. Pharmacol.* 121(3), 515–525.
80. Okuyama, S., Chaki, S., Yoshikawa, R., Suzuki, Y., Ogawa, S., Imagawa, Y., Kawashima, N., Ikeda, Y., Kumagai, T., Nakazato, A., Nagamine, M., and Tomisawa, K. (1997). In vitro and in vivo characterization of the dopamine D4 receptor, serotonin 5-HT2A receptor and alpha-1 adrenoceptor antagonist (R)-(+)-2-amino-4-(4-fluorophenyl)-5-[1-[4-(4-fluorophenyl)-4-oxobutyl] pyrrolidin-3-yl]thiazole (NRA0045). *J. Pharmacol. Expl. Ther.* 282(1), 56–63.
81. Vanover, K. E., Weiner, D. M., Makhay, M., Veinbergs, I., Gardell, L. R., Lameh, J., Del Tredici, A. L., Piu, F., Schiffer, H. H., Ott, T. R., Burstein, E. S., Uldam, A. K., Thygesen, M. B., Schlienger, N., Anderson, C. M., Son, T. Y., Harvey, S. C., Powell, S. B., Geyer, M. A., Tolf, B. R., Brann, M. R., and Davis, R. E. (2006). Pharmacological and behavioral profile of N-(4-fluorophenylmethyl)-N-(1-methylpiperidin-4-yl)-N'-(4-(2-methylpropyloxy)phenylmethyl) carbamide (2R,3R)-dihydroxybutanedioate (2:1) (ACP-103), a novel 5-hydroxytryptamine(2A) receptor inverse agonist. *J. Pharmacol. Exp. Thera.* 317(2), 910–918.
82. Li, Z., Huang, M., Prus, A., Ichikawa, J., Dai, J., and Meltzer, H. Y. (2005). Effect of the 5-HT$_{2c}$ receptor antagonist SB242084 in combination with haloperidol and the 5-HT$_{2a/2c}$ inverse agonist ACP103 on dopamine (DA) efflux in rat brain. *Neurosci. Abstr.* 914.8.
83. Barbato, L., Monge, A., Stocchi, F., and Nordera, G. (1996). Melperone in the treatment of iatrogenic psychosis in Parkinson's disease. *Funct. Neurol.* 11(4), 201–207.
84. Meltzer, H. Y. (1995). Role of serotonin in the action of atypical antipsychotic drugs. *Clin. Neurosci.* 3(2), 64–75.
85. Masellis, M., Basile, V., Meltzer, H. Y., Lieberman, J. A., Sevy, S., Macciardi, F. M., Cola, P., Howard, A., Badri, F., Nothen, M. M., Kalow, W., and Kennedy, J. L. (1998). Serotonin subtype 2 receptor genes and clinical response to clozapine in schizophrenia patients. *Neuropsychopharmacology* 19, 123–132.
86. Arranz, M., Collier, D., Sodhi, M., Ball, D., Roberts, G., Price, J., Sham, P., and Kerwin, R. (1995). Association between clozapine response and allelic variation in 5-HT2A receptor gene. *Lancet* 346(8970), 281–282.
87. Schmidt, C. J., Sorensen, S. M., Kehne, J. H., Carr, A. A., and Palfreyman, M. G. (1995). The role of 5-HT$_{2A}$ receptors in antipsychotic activity. *Life Sci.* 56, 2209–2222.
88. Gleason, S. D., and Shannon, H. E. (1997). Blockade of phencyclidine-induced hyperlocomotion by olanzapine, clozapine and serotonin receptor subtype selective antagonists in mice. *Psychopharmacology (Berl.)* 129, 79–84.
89. Martin, P., Waters, N., Carlsson, A., and Carlsson, M. L. (1997). The apparent antipsychotic action of the 5-HT2a receptor antagonist M100907 in a mouse model of schizophrenia is counteracted by ritanserin. *J. Neural Transm.* 104, 561–564.

90. Varty, G. B., and Higgins, G. A. (1995). Reversal of dizocilpine-induced disruption of prepulse inhibition of an acoustic startle response by the 5-HT2 receptor antagonist ketanserin. *Eur. J. Pharmacol.* 287, 201–205.

91. Prinssen, E. P., Ellenbroek, B. A., and Cools, A. R. (1994). Combined antagonism of adrenoceptors and dopamine and 5-HT receptors underlies the atypical profile of clozapine. *Eur. J. Pharmacol.* 262, 167–170.

92. Wadenberg, M. L., Hicks, P. B., Richter, J. T., and Young, K. A. (1998). Enhancement of antipsychoticlike properties of raclopride in rats using the selective serotonin2A receptor antagonist MDL 100,907. *Biol. Psychiatry* 44, 508–515.

93. Vanover, K. E., Weiner, D. M., Makhay, M., Veinbergs, I., Gardell, L. R., Lameh, J., Del Tredici, A. L., Piu, F., Schiffer, H. H., Ott, T. R., Burstein, E. S., Uldam, A. K., Thygesen, M. B., Schlienger, N., Andersson, C. M., Son, T. Y., Harvey, S. C., Powell, S. B., Gcyer, M. A., Tolf, B. R., Brann, M. R., and Davis, R. E. (2006). Pharmacological and behavioral profile of N-(4-fluorophenylmethyl)-N-(1-methylpiperidin-4-yl)-N'-(4-(2-methylpropyloxy)phenylmethyl)carbamide (2R,3R)-dihydroxybutanedioate (2:1) (ACP-103), a novel 5-hydroxytryptamine(2A) receptor inverse agonist. *J. Pharmacol. Exp. Thera.* 317(2), 910–918.

94. Huang, M., Li, Z., Prus, A. J., Ichikawa, J., Dai, J., and Meltzer, H. Y. (2005). 5-HT$_{2a}$ and 5-HT$_{2c}$ receptor antagonism enhances risperidone-induced dopamine (da) efflux in rat medial prefrontal cortex (mpfc) and diminishes it in the nucleus accumbens (NAC). *Neurosci. Abstr.* 914, 10.

95. Gardell, L. R., Barido, R. E., Pounds, L., Johnson, R. E., Anderson, G. T., Veinbergs, I., Bonhaus, D. W., Hacksell, U., Brann, M. R., Davis, R. E., and Vanover, K. E. (2006). ACP = 103, a novel 5-HT@A receptor inverse agonist, improves the efficacy and side effect profile of haloperidol in experimental models. *Sch. Res.* 81(Suppl.), 49.

96. Olijslagers, J. E., Perlstein, B., Werkman, T. R., McCreary, A. C., Siarey, R., Kruse, C. G., and Wadman, W. J. (2005). The role of 5-HT(2A) receptor antagonism in amphetamine-induced inhibition of A10 dopamine neurons in vitro. *Eur. J. Pharmacol.* 520(1/3), 77–85.

97. Olijslagers, J. E., Werkman, T. R., McCreary, A. C., Siarey, R., Kruse, C. G., and Wadman, W. J. (2004). 5-HT2 receptors differentially modulate dopamine-mediated auto-inhibition in A9 and A10 midbrain areas of the rat. *Neuropharmacology* 46(4), 504–510.

98. Doherty, M. D., and Pickel, V. M. (2000). Ultrastructural localization of the serotonin 2A receptor in dopaminergic neurons in the ventral tegmental area. *Brain Res.* 864(2), 176–185.

99. Hasler, F., Grimberg, U., Benz, M. A., Huber, T., and Vollenweider, F. X. (2004). Acute psychological and physiological effects of psilocybin in healthy humans: A double-blind, placebo-controlled dose-effect study. *Psychopharmacology* 172(2), 145–156.

100. Ichikawa, J., and Meltzer, H. Y. (1995). DOI, a 5-HT2A/2C receptor agonist, potentiates amphetamine-induced dopamine release in rat striatum. *Brain Res.* 698, 204–208.

101. De Deurwaerdere, P., and Spampinato, U. (1999). Role of serotonin(2A) and serotonin(2B/2C) receptor subtypes in the control of accumbal and striatal dopamine release elicited in vivo by dorsal raphe nucleus electrical stimulation. *J. Neurochem.* 73(3), 1033–1042.

102. Carlsson, M. L., Martin, P., Nilsson, M., Sorensen, S. M., Carlsson, A., Waters, S., and Waters, N. (1999). The 5-HT2A receptor antagonist M100907 is more effective in counteracting NMDA antagonist than dopamine agonist-induced hyperactivity in mice. *J. Neural. Transm. (Budapest)* 106, 123–129.

103. Liegeois, J. F., Ichikawa, J., and Meltzer, H. Y. (2002). 5-HT(2A) receptor antagonism potentiates haloperidol-induced dopamine release in rat medial prefrontal cortex and inhibits that in the nucleus accumbens in a dose-dependent manner. *Brain Res.* 947(2), 157–165.

104. Pehek, E. A., McFarlane, H. G., Maguschak, K., Price, B., and Pluto, C. P. (2001). M100,907, a selective 5-HT(2A) antagonist, attenuates dopamine release in the rat medial prefrontal cortex. *Brain Res.* 888(1), 51–59.

105. Bortolozzi, A., Diaz-Mataix, L., Scorza, M. C., Celada, P., and Artigas, F. (2005). The activation of 5-HT receptors in prefrontal cortex enhances dopaminergic activity. *J. Neurochem.* 95, 1597–1607.

106. Jakab, R. L., and Goldman-Rakic, P. S. (1998). 5-Hydroxytryptamine2A serotonin receptors in the primate cerebral cortex: Possible site of action of hallucinogenic and antipsychotic drugs in pyramidal cell apical dendrites. *Proc. Natl. Acad. Sci. USA* 95, 735–740.

107. Kuroki, T., Meltzer, H. Y., and Ichikawa, J. (1999). Effects of antipsychotic drugs on extracellular dopamine levels in rat medial prefrontal cortex and nucleus accumbens. *J. Pharmacol. Exp. Thera.* 288(2), 774–781.

107a. Li, X. M., Perry, K. W., Wong, D. T., and Bymaster, F. P. (1998). Olanzapine increases in vivo dopamine and norepinephrine release in rat prefrontal cortex, nucleus accumbens and striatum. *Psychopharmacology (Berl.)* 136, 153–161.

108. Liegeois, J.-F., Ichikawa, J., and Meltzer, H. Y. (2002). 5HT$_{2A}$ receptor antagonism potentiates haloperidol-induced dopamine release in rat medial prefrontal cortex and inhibits that in the nucleus accumbens in a dose-dependent manner. *Brain Res.* 947, 157–165.

109. Bonaccorso, S., Meltzer, H. Y., Li, Z., Dai, J., Alboszta, A. R., and Ichikawa, J. (2002). SR46349-B, a 5-HT (2A/2C) receptor antagonist, potentiates haloperidol-induced dopamine release in rat medial prefrontal cortex and nucleus accumbens. *Neuropsychopharmacology* 27, 430–441.

110. Parada, M. A., Hernandez, L., Puig de Parada, M., Rada, P., and Murzi, E. (1997). Selective action of acute systemic clozapine on acetylcholine release in the rat prefrontal cortex by reference to the nucleus accumbens and striatum. *J. Pharmacol. Exp. Ther.* 281, 582–588.

111. Ichikawa, J., Li, Z., Dai, J., and Meltzer, H. Y. (2002). Atypical antipsychotic drugs, quetiapine, iloperidone, and melperone, preferentially increase dopamine and acetylcholine release in rat medial prefrontal cortex: Role of 5-HT1A receptor agonism. *Brain Res.* 956(2), 349–357.

112. Shirazi-Southall, S., Rodriguez, D. E., and Nomikos, G. G. (2002). Effects of typical and atypical antipsychotics and receptor selective compounds on acetylcholine efflux in the hippocampus of the rat. *Neuropsychopharmacology* 26(5), 583–594.

113. Chung, Y. C., Li, Z., Dai, J., Meltzer, H. Y., and Ichikawa, J. (2004). Clozapine increases both acetylcholine and dopamine release in rat ventral hippocampus: role of 5-HT1A receptor agonism. *Brain Res.* 1023, 54–63.

114. Consolo, S., Arnaboldi, S., Giorgi, S., Russi, G., and Ladinsky, H. (1994). 5-HT4 receptor stimulation facilitates acetylcholine release in rat frontal cortex. *Neuroreport* 5, 1230–1232.

115. Consolo, S., Bertorelli, R., Russi, G., Zambelli, M., and Ladinsky, H. (1994). Serotonergic facilitation of acetylcholine release in vivo from rat dorsal hippocampus via serotonin 5-HT3 receptors. *J. Neurochem.* 62(6), 2254–2261.

116. Consolo, S., Ramponi, S., Ladinsky, H., and Baldi, G. (1996). A critical role for D1 receptors in the 5-HT1A-mediated facilitation of in vivo acetylcholine release in rat frontal cortex. *Brain Res.* 707, 320–323.

117. Zhelyazkova-Savova, M., Giovannini, M. G., and Pepeu, G. (1997). Increase of cortical acetylcholine release after systemic administration of chlorophenylpiperazine in the rat: An in vivo microdialysis study. *Neurosci. Lett.* 236(3), 151–154.

118. Zhelyazkova-Savova, M., Giovannini, M. G., and Pepeu, G. (1999). Systemic chlorophenylpiperazine increases acetylcholine release from rat hippocampus—implication of 5-HT2C receptors. *Pharmacol. Res.* 40, 165–170.

119. Herremans, A. H., Hijzen, T. H., Olivier, B., and Slangen, J. L. (1995). Cholinergic drug effects on a delayed conditional discrimination task in the rat. *Behav. Neurosci.* 109, 426–435.

120. Sumiyoshi, T., Matsui, M., Nohara, S., Yamashita, I., Kurachi, M., Sumiyoshi, C., Jayathilake, K. and Meltzer, H. Y. (2001). Enhancement of cognitive performance in schizophrenia by addition of tandospirone to neuroleptic treatment. *Am. J. Psychiatry* 158(10), 1722–1725.

121. Hong, C. J., Yu, Y. W., Lin, C. H., and Tsai, S. J. (2003). An association study of a brain-derived neurotrophic factor Val66Met polymorphism and clozapine response of schizophrenic patients. *Neurosci. Lett.* 349, 206–208.

122. Vaidya, V. A., Marek, G. J., Aghajanian, G. K., and Duman, R. S. (1997). 5-HT2A receptor-mediated regulation of brain-derived neurotrophic factor mRNA in the hippocampus and the neocortex. *J. Neurosci.* 17, 2785–2795.

123. Zahorodna, A., Bobula, B., Grzegorzewska, M., Tokarski, K., and Hess, G. (2004). The influence of repeated administration of clozapine and haloperidol on the effects of the activation of 5-HT(1A), 5-HT(2) and 5-HT(4) receptors in rat frontal cortex. *J. Physiol. Pharmacol.* 55(2), 371–379.

124. Bai, O., Chlan-Fourney, J., Bowen, R., Keegan, D., and Li, X. M. (2003). Expression of brain-derived neurotrophic factor mRNA in rat hippocampus after treatment with antipsychotic drugs. *J. Neurosci. Res.* 71, 127–131.

125. Linden, A. M., Vaisanen, J., Lakso, M., Nawa, H., Wong, G., and Castren, E. (2000). Expression of neurotrophins BDNF and NT-3, and their receptors in rat brain after administration of antipsychotic and psychotropic agents. *J. Mol. Neurosci.* 14, 27–37.

126. Maheux, J., Ethier, I., Rouillard, C., and Levesque, D. (2005). Induction patterns of transcription factors of the nur family (nurr1, nur77, and nor-1) by typical and atypical antipsychotics in the mouse brain: Implication for their mechanism of action. *J. Pharmacol. Exp. Ther.* 313, 460–473.

127. Ishikane, T., Kusumi, I., Matsubara, R., Matsubara, S., and Koyama, T. (1997). Effects of serotonergic agents on the up-regulation of dopamine D2 receptors induced by haloperidol in rat striatum. *Eur. J. Pharmacol.* 321, 163–169.

128. Weiner, D. M., Burstein, E. S., Nash, N., Croston, G. E., Currier, E. A., Vanover, K. E., Harvey, S. C., Donohue, E., Hansen, H. C., Andersson, C. M., Spalding, T. A., Gibson, D. F. C., Krebs-Thomson, K., Powell, S. B., Geyer, M. A., Hacksell, U., and Brann, M. R. (2001). 5-Hydroxytryptamine2A receptor inverse agonists as antipsychotics. *J. Pharmacol. Exp. Ther.* 299, 268–276.

129. Pazos, A., Probst, A., and Palacios, J. M. (1987). Serotonin receptors in the human brain--IV. Autoradiographic mapping of serotonin-2 receptors. *J. Neurosci.* 21, 123–139.

130. Barker, E. L., Westphal, R. S., Schmidt, D., and Sanders-Bush, E. (1994). Constitutively active 5-hydroxytryptamine2C receptors reveal novel inverse agonist activity of receptor ligands. *J. Biol. Chem.* 269, 11687–11690.

131. De Deurwaerdere, P., Navailles, S., Berg, K. A., Clarke, W. P., and Spampinato, U. (2004). Constitutive activity of the serotonin2C receptor inhibits in vivo dopamine release in the rat striatum and nucleus accumbens. *Neuroscience* 24(13), 3235–3241.

132. Sodhi, M. S., Arranz, M. J., Curtis, D., Ball, D. M., Sham, P., Roberts, G. W., Price, J., Collier, D. A., and Kerwin, R. W. (1995). Association between clozapine response and allelic variation in the 5-HT2C receptor gene. *Neuroreport* 7(1), 169–172.

133. Niswender, C. M., Copeland, S. C., Herrick-Davis, K., Emeson, R. B., and Sanders-Bush, E. (1999). RNA editing of the human serotonin 5-hydroxytryptamine 2C receptor silences constitutive activity. *J. Biol. Chem.* 274(14), 9472–9478.

134. Reynolds, G. P., Templeman, L. A., and Zhang, Z. J. (2005). The role of 5-HT2C receptor polymorphisms in the pharmacogenetics of antipsychotic drug treatment. *Prog. Neuro-Psychopharmacol. Biol. Psychiatry* 29(6), 1021–1028.

135. Sodhi, M. S., Airey, D. C., Lambert, W., Burnet, P. W., Harrison, P. J., and Sanders-Bush, E. (2005). A rapid new assay to detect RNA editing reveals antipsychotic-induced changes in serotonin-2C transcripts. *Mol. Pharmacol.* 68(3), 711–719.

136. Di Matteo, V., Di Giovanni, G., Di Mascio, M., and Esposito, E. (1999). SB 242084, a selective serotonin2C receptor antagonist, increases dopaminergic transmission in the mesolimbic system. *Neuropharmacology* 38(8), 1195–1205.

137. Millan, M. J., Gobert, A., Newman-Tancredi, A., Audinot, V., Lejeune, F., Rivet, J. M., Cussac, D., Nicolas, J. P., Muller, O., and Lavielle, G. (1998). S 16924 ((R)-2-[1-[2-(2,3-dihydro-benzo[1,4] dioxin-5-yloxy)-ethyl]-pyrrolidin-3yl]-1-(4-fluoro-phenyl)-ethanone), a novel, potential antipsychotic with marked serotonin (5-HT)1A agonist properties: I. Receptorial and neurochemical profile in comparison with clozapine and haloperidol. *J. Pharmacol. Exp. Ther.* 286, 1341–1355.

138. Roth, B. L., Ciaranello, R. D., and Meltzer, H. Y. (1992). Binding of typical and atypical antipsychotic agents to transiently expressed 5-HT1C receptors. *J. Pharmacol. Exp. Ther.* 260, 1361–1365.

139. Herrick-Davis, K., Grinde, E., and Teitler, M. (2000). Inverse agonist activity of atypical antipsychotic drugs at human 5-hydroxytryptamine2C receptors. *J. Pharmacol. Exp. Ther.* 295(1), 226–232.

140. Hietala, J., Kuonnamaki, M., Palvimaki, E. P., Laakso, A., Majasuo, H., and Syvalahti, E. (2001). Sertindole is a serotonin 5-HT2c inverse agonist and decreases agonist but not antagonist binding to 5-HT2c receptors after chronic treatment. *Psychopharmacology* 157(2), 180–187.

141. Meneses, A. (2002). Involvement of 5-HT(2A/2B/2C) receptors on memory formation: Simple agonism, antagonism, or inverse agonism? *Cell. Mol. Neurobiol.* 22(5/6), 675–688.

142. Meltzer, H. Y., Kennedy, J., Dai, J., Parsa, M., and Riley, D. (1995). Plasma clozapine levels and the treatment of L-DOPA-induced psychosis in Parkinson's disease. A high potency effect of clozapine. *Neuropsychopharmacology* 12, 39–45.

143. Santana, N., Bortolozzi, A., Serrats, J., Mengod, G., and Artigas, F. (2004). Expression of serotonin1A and serotonin2A receptors in pyramidal and GABAergic neurons of the rat prefrontal cortex. *Cerebr. Cortex* 14(10), 1100–1109.

144. Darmani, N. A., Martin, B. R., Pandey, U., and Glennon, R. A. (1990). Do functional relationships exist between 5-HT1A and 5-HT2 receptors? *Pharmacol. Biochem. Behav.* 36, 901–906.

145. Meltzer, H. Y., and Maes, M. (1995). Pindolol pretreatment blocks stimulation by meta-chlorophenylpiperazine of prolactin but not cortisol secretion in normal men. *Psychiatry Res.* 58, 89–98.
146. Ahlenius, S. (1989). Antipsychotic-like properties of the 5-HT1A agonist 8-OH-DPAT in the rat. *Pharmacol. Toxicol.* 64(1), 3–5.
147. Wadenberg, M. L., and Ahlenius, S. (1991). Antipsychotic-like profile of combined treatment with raclopride and 8-OH-DPAT in the rat: Enhancement of antipsychotic-like effects without catalepsy. *J. Neural Transm. Genet. Sect.* 83, 43–53.
148. Prinssen, E. P., Kleven, M. S., and Koek, W. (1996). Effects of dopamine antagonists in a two-way active avoidance procedure in rats: Interactions with 8-OH-DPAT, ritanserin, and prazosin. *Psychopharmacology (Berl.)* 128, 191–197.
149. Wadenberg, M. L. (1992). Antagonism by 8-OH-DPAT, but not ritanserin, of catalepsy induced by SCH 23390 in the rat. *J. Neural Transm. Genet. Sect.* 89, 49–59.
150. Wadenberg, M. L., and Hillegaart, V. (1995). Stimulation of median, but nor dorsal, raphe 5-HT$_{1A}$ autoreceptors by the local application of 8-OH-DPAT reverses raclopride-induced catalepsy in the rat. *Neuropharmacology* 34, 495–499.
151. Ichikawa, J., and Meltzer, H. Y. (2000). The effect of serotonin(1A) receptor agonism on antipsychotic drug-induced dopamine release in rat striatum and nucleus accumbens. *Brain Res.* 858(2), 252–263.
152. Newman-Tancredi, A., Gavaudan, S., Conte, C., Chaput, C., Touzard, M., Verriele, L., Audinot, V., and Millan, M. J. (1998). Agonist and antagonist actions of antipsychotic agents at 5-HT1A receptors: A [35S]GTPgammaS binding study. *Eur. J. Pharmacol.* 355, 245–256.
153. Rollema, H., Lu, Y., Schmidt, A. W., and Zorn, S. H. (1997). Clozapine increases dopamine release in prefrontal cortex by 5-HT1A receptor activation. *Eur. J. Pharmacol,* 338, R3–R5.
154. Ichikawa, J., Dai, J., O'Laughlin, I. A., Dai, J., Fowler, W., and Meltzer, H. Y. (2002). Atypical, but not typical, antipsychotic drugs selectively increase acetylcholine release in rat medial prefrontal cortex, nucleus accumbens and striatum. *Neuropsychopharmacology* 26(3), 325–339.
155. Diaz-Mataix, L., Scorza, M. C., Bortolozzi, A., Toth, M., Celada, P., and Artigas, F., (2005). Involvement of 5-HT1A receptors in prefrontal cortex in the modulation of dopaminergic activity: Role in atypical antipsychotic action. *J. Neurosci.* 25(47), 10831–10843.
155a. Boulay, D., Depoortere, R., Louis, C., Perrault, G., Griebel, G., and Soubrie, P. (2004). SSR181507, a putative atypical antipsychotic with dopamine D2 antagonist and 5-HT1A agonist activities: Improvement of social interaction deficits induced by phencyclidine in rats. *Neuropharmacology* 46, 1121–1129.
156. Millan, M. J., Gobert, A., Roux, S., Porsolt, R., Meneses, A., Carli, M., Di Cara, B., Jaffard, R., Rivet, J. M., Lestage, P., Mocaer, E., Peglion, J. L., and Dekeyne, A. (2004). The serotonin1A receptor partial agonist S15535 [4-(benzodioxan-5-yl)1-(indan-2-yl)piperazine] enhances cholinergic transmission and cognitive function in rodents: A combined neurochemical and behavioral analysis. *J. Pharmacol. Exp. Ther.* 311, 190–203.
157. Monsma, F. J., Jr., Shen, Y., Ward, R. P., Hamblin, M. W., and Sibley, D. R. (1993). Cloning and expression of a novel serotonin receptor with high affinity for tricyclic psychotropic drugs. *Mol. Pharmacol.* 43, 320–327.
158. Kohen, R., Metcalf, M. A., Khan, N., Druck, T., Huebner, K., Lachowicz, J. E., Meltzer, H. Y., Sibley, D. R., Roth, B. L., and Hamblin, M. W. (1996). Cloning,

characterization, and chromosomal localization of a human 5-HT6 serotonin receptor. *J. Neurochem.* 66, 47–56.

159. Boess, F. G., Monsma, F. G., Jr., Carolo, C., Meyer, V., Rudler, A., Zwingelstein, C., and Sleight, A. J. (1997). Functional and radioligand binding characterization of rat 5-HT6 receptors stably expressed in HEK293 cells. *Neuropharmacol* 36(4–5), 713–720.

160. Arnt, J., and Skarsfeldt, T. (1998). Do novel antipsychotics have similar pharmacological characteristics? A review of the evidence. *Neuropsychopharmacology* 18, 63–101.

161. Ruat, M., Traiffort, E., Arrang, J. M., Tardivel-Lacombe, J., Diaz, J., Leurs, R., and Schwartz, J. C. (1993). A novel rat serotonin (5-HT6) receptor: Molecular cloning, localization and stimulation of cAMP accumulation. *Biochem. Biophys. Res. Commun.* 193, 268–276.

162. Gerard, C., el Mestikawy, S., Lebrand, C., Adrien, J., Ruat, M., Traiffort, E., Hamon, M., and Martres, M. P. (1996). Quantitative RT-PCR distribution of serotonin 5-HT6 receptor mRNA in the central nervous system of control or 5,7-dihydroxytryptamine-treated rats. *Synapse* 23, 164–173.

163. Gerard, C., Martres, M. P., Lefevre, K., Miquel, M. C., Verge, D., Lanfumey, L., Doucet, E., Hamon, M., and el Mestikawy, S. (1997). Immuno-localization of serotonin 5-HT6 receptor-like material in the rat central nervous system. *Brain Res.* 746, 207–219.

164. Hamon, M., Doucet, E., Lefevre, K., Miquel, M. C., Lanfumey, L., Insausti, R., Frechilla, D., Del Rio, J., and Verge, D. (1999). Antibodies and antisense oligonucleotide for probing the distribution and putative functions of central 5-HT6 receptors. *Neuropsychopharmacology* 21(2, Suppl.), 68S–76S.

165. Frederick, J. A., and Meador-Woodruff, J. H. (1999). Effects of clozapine and haloperidol on 5-HT6 receptor mRNA levels in rat brain. *Schizophr. Res.* 38, 7–12.

166. Bentley, J. C., Sleight, A. J., Marsden, C. A., and Fone, K. C. F. (1997). 5-HT6 antisense oligonucleotide i.c.v. affects rat performance in the water maze and feeding. *J. Psychopharmacol.* 11, 864.

168. Huber, G., Maerz, W., Martin, J. R., Malherbe, P., Richards, J. G., Sueoka, N., Ohm, T., and Hoffmann, M. M. (2000). Characterization of transgenic mice expressing apolipoprotein E4 (C112R) and apolipoprotein E4 (L28P; C112R). *Neuroscience* 101, 211–218.

167. Rogers, D. C., Robinson, T. L., Quilter, A. J., Routledge, C., and Hagan, J. J. (1999). Cognitive enhancement effects of the selective 5-HT6 antagonist SB-271046. *Br. J. Pharmacol.* 127, 22P.

169. Rogers, D. C., and Hagan, J. J. (2001). 5-HT6 receptor antagonists enhance retention of a water maze task in the rat. *Psychopharmacology (Berl.)* 158, 114–119.

170. Meneses, A. (2001). Effects of the 5-HT(6) receptor antagonist Ro 04-6790 on learning consolidation. *Behav. Brain Res.* 118, 107–110.

170a. Woolley, M. L., Bentley, J. C., Sleight, A. J., Marsden, C. A., and Fone, K. C. (2001). A role for 5-HT6 receptors in retention of spatial learning in the Morris water maze. *Neuropharmacology* 41, 210–219.

171. Stean, T. O., Hirst, W. D., Thomas, D. R., Price, G. W., Rogers, D., Riley, G., Bromidge, S. M., Serafinowska, H. T., Smith, D. R., Bartlett, S., Deeks, N., Duxon, M., and Upton, N. (2002). Pharmacological profile of SB-357134: A potent, selective, brain penetrant, and orally active 5-HT(6) receptor antagonist. *Pharmacol. Biochem. Behav.* 71, 645–367.

172. Woolley, M. L., Marsden, C. A., Sleight, A. J., and Fone, K. C. (2003). Reversal of a cholinergic-induced deficit in a rodent model of recognition memory by the selective 5-HT6 receptor antagonist, Ro 04-6790. *Psychopharmacology (Berl.)* 170, 358–367.

173. Lieben, C. K., Blokland, A., Sik, A., Sung, E., van Nieuwenhuizen, P., and Schreiber, R. (2005). The selective 5-HT6 receptor antagonist Ro4368554 restores memory performance in cholinergic and serotonergic models of memory deficiency in the rat. *Neuropsychopharmacology* 30(12), 2169–2179.

174. Minabe, Y., Shirayama, Y., Hashimoto, K., Routledge, C., Hagan, J. J., and Ashby, C. R., Jr. (2004). Effect of the acute and chronic administration of the selective 5-HT6 receptor antagonist SB-271046 on the activity of midbrain dopamine neurons in rats: An in vivo electrophysiological study. *Synapse* 52(1), 20–28.

175. Sleight, A. J., Consolo, S., Martin, J. R., Boess, J. C., Bentley, J. C., and Bourson, A. (1999). 5-HT6 receptors: Functional correlates and potential therapeutic indications. *Behav. Pharmacol.* 10, S86–S87.

176. Riemer, C., Borroni, E., Levet-Trafit, B., Martin, J. R., Poli, S., Porter, R. H., and Bos, M. (2003). Influence of the 5-HT6 receptor on acetylcholine release in the cortex: Pharmacological characterization of 4-(2-bromo-6-pyrrolidin-1-ylpyridine-4-sulfonyl)-phenylamine, a potent and selective 5-HT6 receptor antagonist. *J. Med. Chem.* 46(7), 1273–1276.

177. Dawson, L. A., Nguyen, H. Q., and Li, P. (2001). The 5-HT(6) receptor antagonist SB-271046 selectively enhances excitatory neurotransmission in the rat frontal cortex and hippocampus. *Neuropsychopharmacology* 25, 662–668.

178. Lacroix, L. P., Dawson, L. A., Hagan, J. J., and Heidbreder, C. A. (2004). 5-HT6 receptor antagonist SB-271046 enhances extracellular levels of monoamines in the rat medial prefrontal cortex. *Synapse* 51, 158–164.

179. Pouzet, B., Didriksen, M., and Arnt, J. (2002). Effects of the 5-HT(6) receptor antagonist, SB-271046, in animal models for schizophrenia. *Pharmacol. Biochem. Behav.* 71(4), 635–643.

180. Leng, A., Ouagazzal, A., Feldon, J., and Higgins, G. A. (2003). Effect of the 5-HT6 receptor antagonists Ro04-6790 and Ro65-7199 on latent inhibition and prepulse inhibition in the rat: Comparison to clozapine. *Pharmacol. Biochem. Behav.* 75(2), 281–288.

181. Frantz, K. J., Hansson, K. J., Stouffer, D. G., and Parsons, L. H. (2002). 5-HT(6) receptor antagonism potentiates the behavioral and neurochemical effects of amphetamine but not cocaine. *Neuropharmacology* 42, 170–180.

182. Dawson, L. A., Nguyen, H. Q., and Li, P. (2003). Potentiation of amphetamine-induced changes in dopamine and 5-HT by a 5-HT(6) receptor antagonist. *Brain Res. Bull.* 59, 513–521.

183. Matsumoto, M., Togashi, H., Mori, K., Ueno, K., Miyamoto, A., and Yoshioka, M. (1999). Characterization of endogenous serotonin-mediated regulation of dopamine release in the rat prefrontal cortex. *Eur. J. Pharmacol.* 383, 39–48.

184. Ichikawa, J., Kuroki, T., Dai, J., and Meltzer, H. Y. (1998). Effect of antipsychotic drugs on extracellular serotonin levels in rat medial prefrontal cortex and nucleus accumbens. *Eur. J. Pharmacol.* 351, 163–171.

185. Hertel, P., Nomikos, G. G., Schilstrom, B., Arborelius, L., and Svensson, T. H. (1997). Risperidone dose-dependently increases extracellular concentrations of serotonin in the rat frontal cortex: Role of alpha 2-adrenoceptor antagonism. *Neuropsychopharmacology* 17, 44–55.

186. Bortolozzi, A., Amargos-Bosch, M., Adell, A., Diaz-Mataix, L., Serrats, J., Pons, S., and Artigas, F. (2003). In vivo modulation of 5-hydroxytryptamine release in mouse prefrontal cortex by local 5-HT (2A) receptors: Effect of antipsychotic drugs. *Eur. J. Neurosci.* 18, 1235–1246.

187. Svensson, T. H. (2003). Alpha-adrenoceptor modulation hypothesis of antipsychotic atypicality. *Prog. Neuro-Psychopharmacol. Biol. Psychiatry* 27, 1145–1158.

188. Wadenberg, M. L., Hertel, P., Fernholm, R., Hygge Blakeman, K., Ahlenius, S., and Svensson, T. H. (2000). Enhancement of antipsychotic-like effects by combined treatment with the alpha1-adrenoceptor antagonist prazosin and the dopamine D2 receptor antagonist raclopride in rats. *J. Neural Transm.* 107(10), 1229–1238.

189. Marcus, M. M., Nomikos, G. G., and Svensson, T. H. (2000). Effects of atypical antipsychotic drugs on dopamine output in the shell and core of the nucleus accumbens: Role of 5-HT(2A) and alpha(1)-adrenoceptor antagonism. *Eur. Neuropsychopharmacol.* 10(4), 245–253.

190. Pilowsky, L. S., O'Connell, P., Davies, N., Busatto, G. F., Costa, D. C., Murray, R. M., Ell, P. J., and Kerwin, R. W. (1997). In vivo effects on striatal dopamine D2 receptor binding by the novel atypical antipsychotic drug sertindole—A 123I IBZM single photon emission tomography (SPET) study. *Psychopharmacology* 130(2), 152–158.

191. Kalkman, H. O., Neumann, V., Hoyer, D., and Tricklebank, M. D. (1998). The role of alpha2-adrenoceptor antagonism in the anti-cataleptic properties of the atypical neuroleptic agent, clozapine, in the rat. *Br. J. Pharmacol.* 124, 1550–1556.

192. McAllister, K. H., and Rey, B. (1999). Clozapne reversal of the deficits in coordinated movement induced by D2 receptor blockade does not depend upon antagonism of alpha2 adrenoceptors. *Naunyn Schmiedebergs Arch. Pharmacol.* 360, 603–608.

193. Litman, R. E., Su, T. P., Potter, W. Z., Hong, W. W., and Pickar, D. (1996). Idazoxan and response to typical neuroleptics in treatment-resistant schizophrenia. Comparison with the atypical neuroleptic, clozapine. *Br. J. Psychiatry* 168(5), 571–579.

194. Bolonna, A. A., Arranz, M. J., Munro, J., Osborne, S., Petouni, M., Martinez, M., and Kerwin, R. W. (2000). No influence of adrenergic receptor polymorphisms on schizophrenia and antipsychotic response. *Neurosci. Lett.* 280, 65–68.

195. Hertel, P., Nomikos, G. G., and Svensson, T. H. (1999). Idazoxan preferentially increases dopamine output in the rat medial prefrontal cortex at the nerve terminal level. *Eur. J. Pharmacol.* 371, 153–158.

196. Hertel, P., Fagerquist, M. V., and Svensson, T. H. (1999). Enhanced cortical dopamine output and antipsychotic-like effects of raclopride by alpha2 adrenoceptor blockade. *Science* 286, 105–107.

197. Westerink, B. H., de Boer, P., de Vries, J. B., Kruse, C. G., and Long, S. K. (1998). Antipsychotic drugs induce similar effects on the release of dopamine and noradrenaline in the medial prefrontal cortex of the rat brain. *Eur. J. Pharmacol.* 361, 27–33.

198. Arnsten, A. F., Steere, J. C., Jentsch, D. J., and Li, B. M. (1998). Noradrenergic influences on prefrontal cortical cognitive function: Opposing actions at postjunctional alpha 1 versus alpha 2-adrenergic receptors. *Adv. Pharmacol.* 42, 764–767.

199. Arnsten, A. F., and Li, B. M. (2005). Neurobiology of executive functions: Catecholamine influences on prefrontal cortical functions. *Biol. Psychiatry* 57(11), 1377–1384.

200. Carlsson, M., and Carlsson, A. (1990). Interactions between glutamatergic and monoaminergic systems within the basal ganglia–Implications for schizophrenia and Parkinson's disease. *Trends Neurosci.* 13, 272–276.

201. Laruelle, M., Frankle, W. G., Narendran, R., Kegeles, L. S., and Abi-Dargham, A. (2005). Mechanism of action of antipsychotic drugs: From dopamine D(2) receptor antagonism to glutamate NMDA facilitation. *Clin. Ther.* 27(Suppl. A), S16–S24.

202. Yamamoto, B. K., Pehek, E. A., and Meltzer, H. Y. (1994). Brain region effects of clozapine on amino acid and monoamine transmission. *J. Clin. Psychiatry* 55(Suppl. B), 8–14.

203. Pietraszek, M., Golembiowska, K., Bijak, M., Ossowska, K., and Wolfarth, S. (2002). Differential effects of chronic haloperidol and clozapine administration on glutamatergic transmission in the fronto-parietal cortex in rats: Microdialysis and electrophysiological studies. *Naunyn Schmiedebergs Arch. Pharmacol.* 366(5), 417–424.

204. Yang, T. T., and Wang, S. J. (2005). Effects of haloperidol and clozapine on glutamate release from nerve terminals isolated from rat prefrontal cortex. *Synapse* 56, 12–20.

205. Geyer, M. A., Krebs-Thomson, K., Braff, D. L., and Swerdlow, N. R. (2001). Pharmacological studies of prepulse inhibition models of sensorimotor gating deficits in schizophrenia: A decade in review. *Psychopharmacology (Berl.)* 156, 117–154.

206. Linn, G. S., Negi, S. S., Gerum, S. V., and Javitt, D. C. (2003). Reversal of phencyclidine-induced prepulse inhibition deficits by clozapine in monkeys. *Psychopharmacol.* 169(3–4), 234–239.

207. Lipina, T., Labrie, V., Weiner, I., and Roder, J. (2005). Modulators of the glycine site on NMDA receptors, D-serine and ALX 5407, display similar beneficial effects to clozapine in mouse models of schizophrenia. *Psychopharmacology (Berl.)* 179(1), 54–67.

208. Duncan, G. E., Moy, S. S., Lieberman, J. A., and Koller, B. H. (2006). Effects of haloperidol, clozapine, and quetiapine on sersorimotor gating in a genetifc module of reduced NMDA receptor Function. *Psychopharmacology* 184, 190–200.

209. Yamada, S., Harano, M., Annoh, N., Nakamura, K., and Tanaka, M. (1999). Involvement of serotonin 2A receptors in phencyclidine-induced disruption of prepulse inhibition of the acoustic startle in rats. *Biol. Psychiatry* 46, 832–838.

210. Bakshi, V. P., and Geyer, M. A. (1997). Phencyclidine-induced deficits in prepulse inhibition of startle are blocked by prazosin, an alpha-1 noradrenergic antagonist. *J. Pharmacol. Exp. Ther.* 283, 666–674.

211. Gewirtz, J. C., and Marek, G. J. (2000). Behavioral evidence for interactions between a hallucinogenic drug and group II metabotropic glutamate receptors. *Neuropsychopharmacology* 23(5), 569–576.

212. Ballmaier, M., Zoli, M., Mazzoncini, R., Gennarelli, M., and Spano, F. (2001). Combined alpha 2-adrenergic/D2 dopamine receptor blockade fails to reproduce the ability of clozapine to reverse phencyclidine-induced deficits in prepulse inhibition of startle. *Psychopharmacology (Berl.)* 159, 105–110.

213. Le Pen, G., and Moreau, J. L. (2002). Disruption of prepulse inhibition of startle reflex in a neurodevelopmental model of schizophrenia: Reversal by clozapine, olanzapine and risperidone but not by haloperidol. *Neuropsychopharmacology* 27, 1–11.

214. Brody, S. A., Dulawa, S. C., Conquet, F., and Geyer, M. A. (2004). Assessment of a prepulse inhibition deficit in a mutant mouse lacking mGlu5 receptors. *Mol. Psychiatry* 9, 35–41.

215. Moghaddam, B., and Adams, B. W. (1998). Reversal of phencyclidine effects by a group II metabotropic glutamate receptor agonist in rats. *Science* 281, 1349–1352.

216. Swanson, C. J., and Schoepp, D. D. (2002). The group II metabotropic glutamate receptor agonist (−)-2-oxa-4-aminobicyclo[3.1.0.]hexane-4,6-dicarboxylate (LY379268)

and clozapine reverse phencyclidine-induced behaviors in monoamine-depleted rats. *J. Pharmacol. Exp. Ther.* 303, 919–927.

217. Kinney, G. G., O'Brien, J. A., Lemaire, W., Burno, M., Bickel, D. J., Clements, M. K., Chen, T. B., Wisnoski, D. D., Lindsley, C. W., Tiller, P. R., Smith, S., Jacobson, M. A., Sur, C., Duggan, M. E., Pettibone, D. J., Conn, P. J., and Williams, D. L., Jr. (2005). A novel selective positive allosteric modulator of metabotropic glutamate receptor subtype 5 has in vivo activity and antipsychotic-like effects in rat behavioral models. *J. Pharmacol. Exp. Ther.* 313, 199–206.

218. Bymaster, F. P., Felder, C., Ahmed, S., and McKinzie, D. (2002). Muscarinic receptors as a target for drugs treating schizophrenia. *Curr. Drug Targets CNS Neurol. Disord.* 1(2), 163–181.

219. Shannon, H. E., Rasmussen, K., Bymaster, F. P., Hart, J. C., Peters, S. C., Swedberg, M. D., Jeppesen, L., Sheardown, M. J., Sauerberg, P., and Fink-Jensen, A. (2000). Xanomeline, an M(1)/M(4) preferring muscarinic cholinergic receptor agonist, produces antipsychotic-like activity in rats and mice. *Schizophr. Res.* 42(3), 249–259.

220. Jones, C. K., Eberle, E. L., Shaw, D. B., McKinzie, D. L., and Shannon, H. E. (2005). Pharmacologic interactions between the muscarinic cholinergic and dopaminergic systems in the modulation of prepulse inhibition in rats. *J. Pharmacol. Exp. Ther.* 312(3), 1055–1063.

221. Hosoi, R., Kobayashi, K., Ishida, J., Yamaguchi, M., and Inoue, O. (2003). Effect of sabcomeline on muscarinic and dopamine receptor binding in intact mouse brain. *Annl. Nucl. Med.* 17(2), 123–130.

222. Sur, C., Mallorga, P. J., Wittmann, M., Jacobson, M. A., Pascarella, D., Williams, J. B., Brandish, P. E., Pettibone, D. J., Scolnick, E. M., and Conn, P. J. (2003). N-Desmethylclozapine, an allosteric agonist at muscarinic 1 receptor, potentiates N-methyl-D-aspartate receptor activity. *Proc. Nat. Acad. Sci. USA* 100(23), 13674–13679.

223. Weiner, D. M., Meltzer, H. Y., Veinbergs, I., Donohue, E. M., Spalding, T. A., Smith, T. T., Mohell, N., Harvey, S. C., Lameh, J., Nash, N., Vanover, K. E., Olsson, R., Jayathilake, K., Lee, M., Levey, A. I., Hacksell, U., Burstein, E. S., Davis, R. E., and Brann, M. R. (2004). The role of M1 muscarinic receptor agonism of N-desmethylclozapine in the unique clinical effects of clozapine. *Psychopharmacology* 177(1/2), 207–216.

224. Davies, M. A., Compton-Toth, B. A., Hufeisen, S. J., Meltzer, H. Y., and Roth, B. L. (2005). The highly efficacious actions of N-desmethylclozapine at muscarinic receptors are unique and not a common property of either typical or atypical antipsychotic drugs: Is M1 agonism a pre-requisite for mimicking clozapine's actions?. *Psychopharmacology* 178(4), 451–460.

225. Brauner-Osborne, H., Ebert, B., Brann, M. R., Falch, E. and Krogsgaard-Larsen, P. (1996). Functional partial agonism at cloned human muscarinic acetylcholine receptors. *Eur. J. Pharmacol.* 313(1–2), 145–150.

226. Schneider, B., Weigmann, H., Hiemke, C., Weber, B., and Fritze, J. (2004). Reduction of clozapine-induced hypersalivation by pirenzepine is safe. *Pharmacopsychiatry* 37(2), 43–45.

227. Frazier, J. A., Cohen, L. G., Jacobsen, L., Grothe, D., Flood, J., Baldessarini, R. J., Piscitelli, S., Kim, G. S., and Rapoport, J. L. (2003). Clozapine pharmacokinetics in children and adolescents with childhood-onset schizophrenia. *J. Clin. Psychopharmacology* 23(1), 87–91.

228. Mauri, M. C., Volonteri, L. S., Dell'Osso, B., Regispani, F., Papa, P., Baldi, M., and Bareggi, S. R. (2003). Predictors of clinical outcome in schizophrenic patients responding to clozapine. *J. Clin. Psychopharmacol.* 23(6), 660–664.

229. Spooren, W., Riemer, C., and Meltzer, H. (2005). Opinion: NK3 receptor antagonists: The next generation of antipsychotics? *Nat. Rev. Drug Discov.* 4(12), 967–975.
230. Spooren, W., Riemer, C., and Meltzer, H., (2005). Opinion: NK3 receptor antagonists: The next generation of antipsychotics? *Nat. Rev. Drug Discov.* 4(12), 967–975.
231. Selemon, L. D., Kleinman, J. E., Herman, M. M., and Goldman-Rakic, P. S. (2002). Smaller frontal gray matter volume in postmortem schizophrenic brains. *Am. J. Psychiatry* 159, 1983–1991.
232. Konradi, C., and Heckers, S. (2001). Antipsychotic drugs and neuroplasticity: insights into the treatment and neurobiology of schizophrenia. *Biol. Psychiatry* 50, 729–742.
233. Lieberman, J. A., Tollefson, G. D., Charles, C., Zipursky, R., Sharma, T., Kahn, R. S., Keefe, R. S., Green, A. I., Gur, R. E., McEvoy, J., Perkins, D., Hamer, R. M., Gu, H., Tohen, M., and HGDH Study Group. (2005). Antipsychotic drug effects on brain morphology in first-episode psychosis. *Arch. Gen. Psychiatry* 62, 361–370.
234. Wakade, C. G., Mahadik, S. P., Waller, J. L., and Chiu, F. C. (2002). Atypical neuroleptics stimulate neurogenesis in adult rat brain. *J. Neurosci. Res.* 69, 72–79.
235. Wang, H. D., Dunnavant, F. D., Jarman, T., and Deutch, A. Y. (2004). Effects of antipsychotic drugs on neurogenesis in the forebrain of the adult rat. *Neuropsychopharmacology* 29(7), 1230–1238.
236. Li, Z., Huang, M., Ichikawa, J., Dai, J., and Meltzer, H. Y. (2005). *N*-Desmethylclozapine, a major metabolite of clozapine, increases cortical acetylcholine and dopamine release in vivo via stimulation of M1 muscarinic receptors. *Neuropsychopharmacology* 30(11), 1986–1995.

PART III

Substance Abuse and Addictive Disorders

13

INTRODUCTION TO ADDICTIVE DISORDERS: IMPLICATIONS FOR PHARMACOTHERAPIES

MARY JEANNE KREEK
Rockefeller University, New York, New York

13.1	History of Pharmacotherapies	451
13.2	Vulnerability to Develop a Specific Addiction	457
13.3	Reward, Modulation, and CounterModulation of Reward and their Role in Specific Addictions	458
Acknowledgment		459
References		459

13.1 HISTORY OF PHARMACOTHERAPIES

Although a few clinical and also laboratory-based research groups had addressed specific problems related to addictions from 1890 to 1964 and over that same time period a variety of different approaches, including some use of diverse chemicals as "medications," by the early 1960s there was still no clear understanding of the bases of addictions and no consistent approach to their management, other than incarceration. Our original research team first coalesced at The Rockefeller University in very early 1964, led by Vincent P. Dole, a clinical and laboratory investigator of metabolism who up to that time had focused on hypertension and lipid disorders. Included in the group was the late Marie Nyswander, a psychiatrist who had written the very sensitive book *The Addict as a Patient*, and also this author (then a second-year postgraduate trainee having completed medical school and aimed toward a life in academic research medicine). The first task on which we focused was a definition and hypothesis related to addiction. After studying all available written materials of a variety of types and, probably more importantly, getting directly involved in interviewing scores of primarily heroin addicts, a paradigm shift in thinking very rapidly evolved. Thus, by the time we became immersed in our basic clinical research studies in the early spring of 1964 at the Rockefeller Hospital [primarily a National

Handbook of Contemporary Neuropharmacology, Edited by David R. Sibley, Israel Hanin, Michael Kuhar, and Phil Skolnick. Copyright © 2007 John Wiley & Sons, Inc.

Institutes of Health (NIH)–supported General Clinical Research Center], we formulated the following hypothesis: "Heroin (opiate) addiction is a disease–a 'metabolic disease' of the brain, with resultant behaviors of 'drug hunger' and drug self-administration, despite negative consequences to self and others. Heroin addiction is not simply a criminal behavior or due alone to any social personality or some other personality disorders" (paraphrased from the original research paper of 1966 covering clinical laboratory-based research performed in 1964 and presented before the Association of American Physicians (AAP) in 1966 [1, 2]. At that time, Dole decided to change his focus to the enormous social problem of heroin addiction, which he clearly saw as a medical problem with definable "metabolic" bases.

In the first few months of our research together, we had two simple goals. The first was to develop a pharmacotherapy to treat heroin addiction combined with the best behavioral therapeutic approaches, including rigorous but humane counseling as well as psychological and psychiatric and medical care as needed. The second goal was to attempt to define the physiological bases of such treatment if in fact we found one which was successful. At the time of our earliest work, there were no analytical laboratory techniques to measure plasma or even urine levels of methadone, heroin or its major metabolite morphine, or any other opiate like compound, and there were no precise molecular definitions for sites of action of these opiates. Nevertheless, it was known by qualitative work that heroin was metabolized primarily to morphine, at that time (and still) the most commonly used opioid for analgesia purposes which was administered only by parenteral (intravenous or subcutaneous) routes because of poor bioavailability after oral administration. The majority of heroin addicts used heroin by the intravenous route, although a few began use by a nasal route ("snorting") and later by a subcutaneous route ("skin popping") and ultimately by the intravenous route ("main lining"). These three routes of administration are still the most commonly used for many drugs of abuse, with an additional route of smoking or snorting ("freebase"). Extensive laboratory and also clinical work had been conducted on opioid analgesics. The concept of specific opiate receptor binding sites had been introduced by three groups in particular: Martin at the U.S. Public Health Service (PHS) Hospital, then in Lexington, Kentucky; Collier, in England; and our group, headed by Dole, at The Rockefeller University. All three research teams postulated that there were specific opiate receptors. The original work done to pursue that concept, from the 1960s to 1973, has been extensively reviewed, including, in part, in some of our own reviews [3–10].

In our first search for a pharmacotherapeutic agent, we wanted a medication which would be orally effective, to simplify pharmacotherapeutics; a compound with a slow onset of action, since even at that time rapid onset of action was directly related to the euphoria-producing effects of a drug of abuse (and now appreciated to be directly related to the "reinforcing" or "rewarding" effects of a drug of abuse); and a compound with a slow offset of action, to prevent the rapid precipitation of the physiological signs and symptoms of withdrawal in a tolerant and physically dependent individual, since opiates and some other addictive agents, such as barbiturates and alcohol, do produce physical as well as psychic dependence. Early on in our work, we also developed the concepts that a pharmacological agent should achieve two important therapeutic goals: first, a medication should reduce or eliminate all signs and symptoms of opiate withdrawal and, second, it should significantly reduce or eliminate all significant illicit drug "craving" and seeking and also self-administration.

There were then a very limited number of opiate analgesics approved for administration by the oral route. One of these was an infrequently used analgesic, methadone, a very simple synthetic organic diphenyl-heptanone, which had been synthesized by German chemists during World War II but which never had been studied in the clinic. When it was brought to the United States, two pain groups studied this medication and found that when delivered to opiate-naïve individuals, its duration of action with respect to analgesia was approximately the same as morphine, but further, when multiple doses of methadone were given per day, as was the practice with the short-acting available morphine, objective signs of respiratory depression began to appear, suggesting an impending opiate overdose. However, all of these studies were conducted in opioid-naïve subjects; many years later, it became fully appreciated that methadone is the opioid analgesic of choice when delivered orally in most cases of chronic pain, such as cancer-related pain, due to its long duration of action and minimal peak effects and also since it is possible to add additional short-acting opiates to sustained methadone treatment to manage recrudescence of acute pain. However, such use is done in persons receiving opiates on a chronic basis; methadone is not usually the appropriate first opiate to use in analgesia management in opiate-naïve individuals.

In a series of studies which have been published and reviewed extensively elsewhere, we found that methadone is orally effective, that beginning at low doses not to exceed 20–40 mg/day in long-term opioid-dependent heroin addicts, and then gradually increasing the doses over a period of four to eight weeks to a full treatment dose of 80–120 mg/day, no euphoric effects were noted and signs and symptoms were completely prevented [1, 2]. Further, in rigorous four-week studies, each conducted in a double-blind random-order Latin square design, we determined that a dose of 80–100 mg/day of methadone delivered orally, as just described, completely prevents all perception as well as objectively measured signs and symptoms of a superimposed short-acting opiate such as heroin or hydromorphone. In further single-blind studies, we found that to overcome this "narcotic blockade," it is essential to superimpose 200 mg of pure heroin intravenously on the daily oral dose (80–120 mg) of methadone treatment [1–10]. During the next eight years, two different groups developed sensitive analytical techniques using gas liquid chromatography to measure plasma as well as urine levels of methadone and its metabolites. Both our laboratory and that of Charles Inturrisi published independent studies showing that the half-life in humans of racemic methadone is 24 h. (of note and importance for laboratory-based investigators, we learned in other studies that the half-life of methadone in rats is around 90 min and in mice around 60 min) [11–14].

In 1964, after the initial clinical laboratory studies, prospective studies were initiated and later special studies were carried out to determine the physiological effects, medical safety, and effectiveness of methadone; other studies were published in the early 1970s and led to the Food and Drug Administration (FDA) approval of methadone for use in the maintenance treatment of heroin and other short-acting opiate addiction by 1973 [15–19]. Later, long-term follow-up studies were conducted of a randomly selected group of methadone-maintained patients from the early treatment cohorts previously studied who had been in continuous treatment for 11–18 years [20]. Thus, the medical safety as well as physiological effects of methadone were rigorously studied from its first use, with the first subject included in data on both safety and effectiveness (reviewed in [1–10; 13–28]).

Natural History of Drug Abuse and Addictions

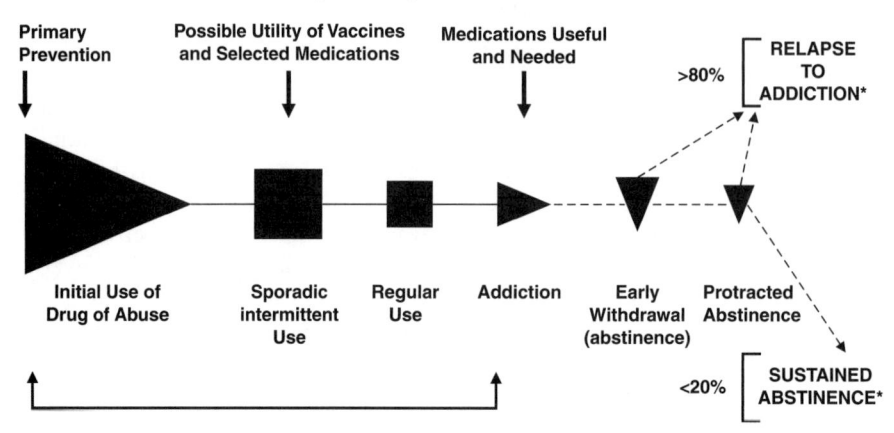

```
Primary          Possible Utility of Vaccines    Medications Useful
Prevention       and Selected Medications        and Needed                      RELAPSE
    ↓                    ↓                           ↓              >80%         TO
                                                                                 ADDICTION*

 Initial Use of      Sporadic      Regular    Addiction    Early       Protracted
 Drug of Abuse      intermittent    Use                   Withdrawal    Abstinence
                       Use                               (abstinence)
                                                                           <20%   SUSTAINED
                                                                                  ABSTINENCE*
```

SHORT ACTING OPIOIDS: 1 in 3 to 1 in 5 who ever self-administer progress to addiction
COCAINE: 1 in 8 to 1 in 15 who ever self-administer progress to addiction
ALCOHOL: 1 in 8 to 1 in 15 who ever self-administer progress to addiction
* with no medications

Figure 13.1 Natural history of drug abuse and addictions.(Adapted from Kreek et al., *Nature Reviews Drug Discovery*, 2002.)

The regulations covering methadone maintenance treatment which were promulgated in 1973 have been modified only once, in 1983 [26]. For entry into methadone maintenance treatment, these regulations define far more severe heroin addiction than the criteria in the fourth edition of the *Diagnostic and Statistical Manual of Mental Disorders* (DSM-IV) of "opiate dependence" or addiction. The federal regulation guidelines still demand that a person be regularly using heroin or another short-acting opiate daily for one year or more prior to entry in methadone maintenance treatment. In numerous laboratory models and in some careful clinical studies, it has been shown that each major drug of abuse administered on a chronic basis causes specific objective changes in the brain and brain function. Also, the relapse rate after medication-free treatment remains extraordinarily high (over 80%) in persons who have been addicted for that length of time. Therefore the Institute of Medicine of the National Academy of Sciences, after a series of extensive meetings, recommended in 1995 that the guidelines be altered to demand only six months or even less of daily self-administration prior to entry into methadone, or λ-α-acetyl methadol (LAAM), maintenance treatment [26]. This regulation, however, has still not changed, but most early federal regulations have been dropped. The previous regulation of the initial maximum daily oral dose of methadone was 120 mg/day for many years, subsequently increased to 150 mg/day and currently with no defined upper limit because of the dramatic increase in the purity of heroin. Also, office-based maintenance treatment using methadone is allowed at the federal level now; the only provision is that initially addicts have to be admitted by a standard opioid treatment clinic, that is, a methadone maintenance or other clinic configured by the original methadone guidelines prior to transferral to a doctor's office for continuing care. However, the duration that subjects have to be in such an organized clinic and the achievements made in their steps to recovery have not been defined. We have reviewed these recent guidelines elsewhere [15]. These regulations are still far more restrictive than those which currently pertain for another opioid partial agonist treatment, that is, treatment with the partial agonist buprenorphine, with or without the combination of naloxone.

Overall, at this time, there are approximately 212,000 persons in methadone maintenance treatment in the United States and over half a million worldwide. The voluntary retention in good clinics which use adequate doses of methadone (usually 80–150 mg/day), along with adequate counseling and psychological and psychiatric care remains over 50%, with excellent clinics still achieving over 80% voluntary retention at one year [3, 4, 9, 10, 29]. The actions of methadone treatment were early established to include prevention of withdrawal symptoms and reduction or elimination of "drug hunger" or drug craving. It was established in early clinical laboratory studies and reproduced by many groups over the last 40 years that methadone blocks the euphoric effect of superimposed short-acting narcotics. Also, further studies, including our prospective and special medical studies and medical safety and many subsequent studies, have shown that steady-dose methadone treatment allows normalization of physiology disrupted by long-term heroin use. The mechanism of action was hypothesized and then established by the time the specific opiate receptors were clearly defined to exist in 1973. It was established by then newly developed analytical techniques that methadone provides steady levels of this opioid at the specific opiate receptor sites. Subsequent work in the 1970s established that there are μ-opioid receptors where heroin, morphine, and methadone primarily act. More recent work by several groups have shown that methadone is a full μ-opioid agonist, not a partial agonist, and further that after binding to μ-opioid receptors methadone undergoes immediate internalization bound to the receptor, similar to the physiological handling of β-endorphin, enkephalin, and other μ-opioid receptor-directed

Factors Contributing to Vulnerability to Develop a Specific Addiction
use of the drug of abuse essential (100%)

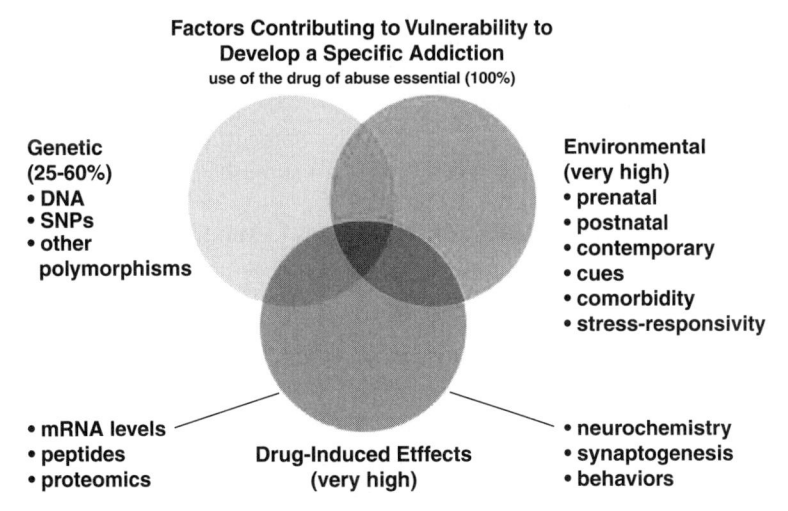

Genetic (25-60%)
- DNA
- SNPs
- other polymorphisms

Environmental (very high)
- prenatal
- postnatal
- contemporary
- cues
- comorbidity
- stress-responsivity

- mRNA levels
- peptides
- proteomics

Drug-Induced Etffects (very high)

- neurochemistry
- synaptogenesis
- behaviors

Figure 13.2 Factors contributing to vulnerability to develop a specific addiction. (Adapted from Kreek et al., *Nature Reviews Drug Discovery*, 2002.) (See color insert.)

endogenous opioids. This is in sharp contrast with most exogenous synthetic or natural plant opioids, which bind to the receptors but then prevent the receptor from rapidly internalizing. In addition, it has been shown both in laboratory studies and more recently in human studies that the two enantiomers of methadone have modest N-methyl-D-aspartate (NMDA) receptor antagonism which would be expected to slow or attenuate the development for opioid tolerance. Our early stable isotope mass spectrometry research showed that the two enantiomers of methadone are metabolized at very different rates, with the active enantiomer l(R) having a half-life of over 36 h in humans and the inactive d(S) enantiomer having a half-life of around 16 h, findings confirmed more recently by several groups. In contrast, it has been shown that heroin has a half-life of only 3 min in humans. Its first and active metabolite, 6-acetyl-morphine, has a half-life of 30 min in humans, and its major metabolite, morphine, and its major active metabolite, morphine-6-glucoronide, have half-lives of 4 and 6 h, respectively (reviewed in [4, 9, 10, 13, 15, 16]).

Several other pharmacological treatments for opiate addiction have been developed, including LAAM, a full agonist which is biotransformed to two active metabolites conferring an even longer half-life in humans than methadone, and buprenorphine, a μ-opioid receptor partial agonist which must be administered sublingually because of its essentially complete "first-pass" effect, that is, biotransformation by the liver after oral administration, and also an opioid which gives a rapid onset of action if used or abused by a parenteral route. This led to the development of a better sublingual formulation, combining buprenorphine with naloxone, which has no adverse effect when administered by this route but would blunt the peak effects of buprenorphine if this formulation were abused in a parenteral route. Each of these compounds has been studied extensively and is effective in the long-term, maintained management of heroin and other slow-acting opiate addiction. However, the maximum dose of buprenorphine which gives any increased opiate effect in humans, because it is a partial agonist, is around 24–32 mg sublingually, equivalent to a maximal 60–70 mg of methadone, a lower dose than shown in many studies over 40 years to be essential for most unselected heroin addicts. The use of each of these compounds in treatment of heroin and other opiate addiction has been reviewed in many articles and will be addressed in Chapter 19 (reviewed in [8, 10, 13, 15, 16, 30]).

Figure. 13.1 presents a history of the development of drug abuse and drug addiction after first self-exposure. It has been well established that primary prevention can be extremely effective, but it is most effective prior to any initial use of a drug of abuse. In the future, vaccines of a variety of types (several now under development specifically for nicotine, cocaine, and heroin) and also some selected medications may have possible utility after the initial sporadic, intermittent use of a drug of abuse occurs. However, regular use, although continuing in only a limited proportion of those who initiate use of a drug of abuse, leads in most cases to addiction. At that point, medications are useful and, in fact, needed. If no targeted specific medications are available, repeated studies over the past 70 years (such as the first outcome studies performed at the PHS facility for opiate addicts in Lexington, Kentucky, after its opening in the mid-1930s) have shown that over 80% of persons meeting any established national (e.g., DSM-IV) or international criteria for addiction will ultimately relapse to an addiction and, in most cases, to the specific initial predominant addiction. Again, according to repeated studies in which the proper denominator is used, that is, all persons entering into any form of management or treatment, less than 20% will respond with sustained abstinence to drug-free, medication-free treatment for one year or more. Therefore, targeted specific medications are needed, and, further, many studies have shown such medications are most effective, by far, when administered in conjunction with behavioral treatments, including counseling and psychological or psychiatric care, as needed (e.g., [4, 5, 8–10, 15, 16, 26, 28–35]). Reviews of many different epidemiological studies over the years as well as our own meta-analyses have shown that approximately 1 in 3 to 1 in 5 who ever self-administer a short-acting opiate, such as heroin, will progress to addiction; approximately 1 in 8 to 1 in 15 who ever self-administer cocaine will progress to cocaine addiction, and roughly 1 in 8 to 1 in 15 who ever self-administer alcohol will progress to alcoholism (see Fig. 13.1 [in 16]).

The chapters in this section will address specific drugs or classes of drugs. In each case, what is known about the nature of each addiction at a molecular, neurobiological, behavioral, and/or global level will be discussed followed by proven or projected interventions with a focus on pharmacotherapeutic interventions either available now or under various stages of development. The chapters will focus on a specific type of addiction, including alcohol abuse and addiction, nicotine abuse and addiction, psychostimulant abuse and addiction, 3, 4 methylenedioxymethamphetamine (MDMA ["Ecstasy"]) and other "club" drug abuse and addiction, and marijuana abuse and addiction.

13.2 VULNERABILITY TO DEVELOP A SPECIFIC ADDICTION

We have defined three domains of factors which may contribute to developing a specific addiction (see Fig. 13.2). These include personal factors such as comorbidity with psychiatric or medical illnesses and also responsivity of an individual along with prenatal and postnatal events, contemporary events, cues or set and setting, and environmental factors. The second domain comprises drug-induced factors; we hypothesized in the mid-1980s that each drug of abuse would profoundly alter molecular events in the brain. Our laboratory and many others worldwide now have joined in an effort which has clearly defined that each major drug of abuse, when administered on a chronic (though usually not acute) basis and in an addiction-like pattern or mode, will cause significant and persistent changes in the brain, including messenger RNA (mRNA) levels, resulting peptides, proteomics, integrated neurochemistry, synaptogenesis, possibly even neurogenesis, and resultant behaviors. Further, our group and others have shown that although many acute effects occur, many of these rapidly disappear and new alterations occur after subacute or chronic administration, some of which may be long-term persistent (or possibly permanent) after cessation of exposure to a drug of abuse. Third and finally, it has been clearly shown that genetic factors play a role and make a 25–60% contribution to the risk for development of specific addictions, as well as any addiction. These genetic factors undoubtedly will include a variety of single nucleotide polymorphisms (SNPs) and other types of polymorphisms of many genes acting in concert to increase vulnerability to develop addiction [36–46]. Essentially all investigators in the area hypothesize that addictions will be complex, not just simple, genetic disorders, that is, involving multiple variants of multiple genes. Moreover, it should be clearly understood that different individuals will have different combinations of these gene variants, in part due to the profound allelic frequency differences of many variants in different ethnic groups, in part due to genetic factors contributing to comorbidity, including differences in drug metabolism as well as psychiatric and some types of medical comorbidity, and in part, because many of the variants will ultimately be shown to be functional, may have very different kinds of impacts on the resultant peptides. Gene variants could include actually changing peptide structure if the gene variant is in the coding region of a gene, or altering amounts of message, and therefore peptide amounts produced, especially if the variants are in critical locations of the 5′ promoter region as well as certain intronic and 3′ regions. Thus, environmental, drug-induced, and genetic factors all may contribute to the vulnerability to develop a specific addiction in an individual (see Fig. 13.2). These changes have been discussed in detail in many recent and earlier review articles ([3, 4, 6–10, 14, 16, 24, 25, 27, 28, 31–34, 36–59]).

13.3 REWARD, MODULATION, AND COUNTERMODULATION OF REWARD AND THEIR ROLE IN SPECIFIC ADDICTIONS

It has been well established by innumerable groups that drugs of abuse have rewarding or reinforcing effects in the context of use which strengthen the perception and, more importantly, the memory of euphoria or pleasure. In addition, each of these effects uses some natural molecular–neurobiological neurotransmitter or transporter systems, including established neural pathways. However, distortions develop in both the absolute and relative amounts of each neurotransmitter, receptor, and downstream single-transduction event component as well as the neuropathways, and possibly synaptogenesis and neurogenesis get altered in the development of "reward," with the associated processes of learning and memory. The natural modulators of each of these systems begin to play a role and they too may become exaggerated, leading to countermodulation of the so-called "rewarding" effects of each drug of abuse, which also contributes to the abnormal status which often persists in the drug-free and medication-free state.

Using a variety of models, much work has been done worldwide on what may be the specific components of both reward, and modulation and countermodulation of reward. Clearly, the majority of studies have pointed to the intermediate-acting monoamine neurotransmitter dopamine as being central to reward. However, two other monaminergic systems, the serotonin and norepinephrine systems, have been shown to be also involved. Our laboratory and many others have also shown unequivocally that the μ-opioid receptor system is involved in reward. There are increasing numbers of studies showing that whereas for some drugs of abuse the dopaminergic system may dominate, for other drugs of abuse the μ-opioidergic system may predominate. Further, it has been shown that the dopaminergic system is involved in some of the effects of all drugs of abuse, but, unexpectedly, our group and others have shown that the endogenous μ-opioidergic system is also involved to a certain extent in most, if not all, of the rewarding properties of drugs of abuse (reviewed in [6–9, 14, 16, 24, 27, 28, 32–34, 36, 38–41, 44]).

Immediate modulators include the usual rapid-acting and stimulatory neurotransmitter systems, including, but not exclusively, the γ-aminobutyric acid (GABA)–ergic and glutamatergic systems, as well as the much slower neuropeptide cannabinoid systems and others. However, distortion of these systems also occurs. Our group and others have shown that the natural dynorphin opioid peptides acting at the κ-opioid receptors play a major role in countermodulation through their ability to reduce dopaminergic tone. Similarly, orphanin-nociceptin FQ, acting at its specific opioid-like but non-opioid receptors, plays a role similar to that of dynorphin acting at the κ-opioid receptors, with modulation of dopaminergic tone. Further, this latter system has also been shown to alter stress responsivity (see below).

One of the initial hypotheses of our laboratory was that an atypical response to stress and stressors may contribute to the persistence of and relapse to a specific addiction, and further, in some individuals, atypical stress responsivity existing a priori on a genetic or environmental basis may contribute to the initial acquisition of an addiction [6, 9, 10, 14, 18, 19, 21, 24, 25, 28, 47–51]. Many studies from our laboratory in humans, including genetics studies as well as basic molecular neuroendocrine studies, have given strong support to this hypothesis. Similarly, in work from our laboratory and innumerable other laboratories, using a variety of animal models, it has been shown that stress responsivity plays a central role both in the acquisition of drug abuse and in the relapse to self-administration or "reinstatement" of drug abuse. Again, these studies have been reported in both early and very recent papers from our laboratory and in some of our review articles [47–59].

Therefore the rewarding or reinforcing effects of drugs of abuse coupled with modulation and countermodulation in the context of specific environments and the specific genetic fabric of each individual and especially with the predictable chronic drug effects which may persist after drug use has ceased all contribute to the acquisition, persistence and perpetuation of an addiction, and some contribute to learning and memory and thus behaviors in the medication-free, drug-free state, despite aggressive counseling and behavioral treatments. These persistent changes in the brain and resultant behaviors may lead to relapse and thus perpetuation of addiction; these topics will be considered in the chapters that follow. Each site of action and alteration provides potential targets for pharmacological intervention as well as increasingly selective behavioral interventions. However, it is now clear that specific pharmacotherapies will be needed for most persons suffering from specific addictive diseases.

ACKNOWLEDGMENT

Funding support was received from the National Institutes of Health—National Institute on Drug Abuse Research Scientific Award Grant K05-DA00049, the National Institutes of Health—National Institute on Drug Abuse Research Center Grant P60-DA05130, the National Institutes of Health—National Center for Research Resources (NCRR) General Clinical Research Center Grant M01-RR00102, and the New York State Office of Alcoholism and Substance Abuse Services. I would also like to thank Susan Russo for help with preparation of the manuscript.

REFERENCES

1. Dole, V. P., Nyswander, M. E., and Kreek, M. J. (1966). Narcotic blockade: A medical technique for stopping heroin use by addicts. *Trans. Assoc. Am. Phys.* 79, 122–136.

2. Dole, V. P., Nyswander, M. E., and Kreek, M. J. (1966). Narcotic blockade. *Arch. Intern. Med.* 118, 304–309.
3. Kreek, M. J. (1990). Historical and medical aspects of methadone maintenance treatment: Effectiveness in treatment of heroin addiction and implications of such treatment in the setting of the AIDS epidemic. In *Evaluation of Different Programmes for Treatment of Drug Addicts*, C. Adamsson, B. Jansson, U. Rydberg, and C. Westrin, Eds. Medicinska Forskningsradet, Stockholm, pp. 61–76.
4. Kreek, M. J. (1991). Using methadone effectively: Achieving goals by application of laboratory, clinical, and evaluation research and by development of innovative programs In *Improving Drug Abuse Treatment: National Institute of Drug Abuse Research Monograph Series 106*, DHHS Pub. No. (ADM)91-1704, R. Pickens, C. Leukefeld, and C. R. Schuster, Eds. U.S. Government Printing Office, Washington, DC, pp. 245–266.
5. Kreek, M. J. (1992) Epilogue: A personal retrospective and prospective viewpoint. In *State Methadone Maintenance Treatment Guidelines*. Center for Substance Abuse Treatment, U.S. Department of Health and Human Services, Public Health Service, Substance Abuse and Mental Health Services Administration, pp. 255–272.
6. Kreek, M. J. (1996). Opioid receptors: Some perspectives from early studies of their role in normal physiology, stress responsivity and in specific addictive diseases. *J. Neurochem. Res.* 21, 1469–1488.
7. Kreek, M. J. (1997). Opiate and cocaine addictions: Challenge for pharmacotherapies. *Pharm. Biochem. Behav.* 57, 551–569.
8. Kreek, M. J. (1997). Clinical update of opioid agonist and partial agonist medications for the maintenance treatment of opioid addiction. *Semin. Neurosci.* 9, 140–157.
9. Kreek, M. J. (2000). Opiates, opioids, SNP's and the addictions: Nathan B. Eddy Memorial Award for lifetime excellence in drug abuse research lecture. In *Problems of Drug Dependence, 1999; Proceedings of the 61st Annual Scientific Meeting of the College on Problems of Drug Dependence: National Institute of Drug Abuse Research Monograph Series 180*. DHHS Pub. No. (ADM)00-4737, L. S. Harris, Ed. U.S. Government Printing Office, Washington, DC, pp. 3–22.
10. Kreek, M. J. (2000). Methadone-related opioid agonist pharmacotherapy for heroin addiction: History, recent molecular and neurochemical research and the future in main stream medicine. *Ann. NY Acad. Sci.* 909, 186–216.
11. Kreek, M. J. (1973). Plasma and urine levels of methadone. *NY State J. Med.* 73, 2773–2777.
12. Kreek, M. J., Gutjahr, C. L., Garfield, J. W., Bowen, D. V., and Field, F. H. (1976). Drug interactions with methadone. *Ann. NY Acad. Sci.* 281, 350–371.
13. Kreek, M. J. (1996). Long-term pharmacotherapy for opiate (primarily heroin) addiction: Opiate agonists. In *Pharmacological Aspects of Drug Dependence: Toward an Integrated Neurobehavioral Approach*, C. R. Schuster and M. J. Kuhar, Eds. Springer-Verlag, Berlin pp. 487–562.
14. Kreek, M. J. (1996). Opiates, opioids and addiction. *Mol. Psychiatry* 1, 232–254.
15. Kreek, M. J., and Vocci, F. J. (2002). History and current status of opioid maintenance treatments: Blending conference session. *J. Subst. Abuse Treat.* 23, 93–105.
16. Kreek, M. J., LaForge, K. S., and Butelman, E. (2002). Pharmacotherapy of addictions. *Nat. Rev. Drug Discov.* 1, 710–726.
17. Kreek, M. J., Dodes, L., Kane, S., Knobler, J., and Martin, R. (1972). Long-term methadone maintenance therapy: Effects on liver function. *Ann. Intern. Med.* 77, 598–602.

18. Kreek, M. J. (1972). Medical safety, side effects and toxicity of methadone. In *Proceedings of the Fourth National Conference on Methadone Treatment*. National Association for the Prevention of Addiction to Narcotics (NAPAN)-NIMH, New York, pp. 171–174.
19. Kreek, M. J. (1973). Medical safety and side effects of methadone in tolerant individuals. *JAMA* 223, 665–668.
20. Novick, D. M., Richman, B. L., Friedman, J. M., Friedman, J. E., Fried, C., Wilson, J. P., Townley, A., and Kreek, M. J. (1993). The medical status of methadone maintained patients in treatment for 11-18 years. *Drug Alcohol Depend.* 33, 235–245.
21. Kreek, M. J. (1973). Physiological implications of methadone treatment. In *Methadone Treatment Manual*, U.S. Government Printing Office, Washington, DC, pp. 85–91.
22. Kreek, M. J. (1975). Methadone maintenance treatment for chronic opiate addiction. In *Medical Aspects of Drug Abuse*, R. Richter, Ed. Harper & Row, New York pp. 167–185.
23. Kreek, M. J. (1986). Exogenous opioids: Drug-disease interactions. In *Advances in Pain Research and Therapy*, K. M. Foley and C. R. Inturrisi, Eds. Raven Press, New York pp. 201–210.
24. Kreek, M. J. (1987). Multiple drug abuse patterns and medical consequences. In *Psychopharmacology: The Third Generation of Progress*, H. Y. Meltzer, Ed. Raven Press, New York pp. 1597–1604.
25. Kreek, M. J. (1992). Rationale for maintenance pharmacotherapy of opiate dependence. In *Addictive States. Association for Research in Nervous and Mental Disease*, C. P. O'Brien and J. H. Jaffe, Eds. Raven Press, Ltd, New York pp. 205–230.
26. Rettig, R. A., and Yarmolinsky, A., Eds. 1995). *Federal Regulation of Methadone Treatment*. National Academy of Sciences, National Academy Press, Washington, DC.
27. Kreek, M. J. (2001). Drug addictions: Molecular and cellular endpoints. *Ann. NY Acad. Sci.* 937, 27–49.
28. Kreek, M. J. (2002). Molecular and cellular neurobiology and pathophysiology of opiate addiction. In *Neuropsychopharmacology: The Fifth Generation of Progress*, K. L. Davis, Ed. Lippincott Williams & Wilkins, Philadelphia pp. 1491–1506.
29. Adelson, M. O., Hayward, R., Bodner, G., Bleich, A., Gelkopf, M., and Kreek, M. J. (2000). Replication of an effective opiate addiction pharmacotherapeutic treatment model: Minimal need for modification in a different country. *J. Maint. Addict.* 1, 5–13.
30. Kreek, M. J. (1996). Long-term pharmacotherapy for opiate (primarily heroin) addiction: Opioid antagonists and partial agonists. In *Pharmacological Aspects of Drug Dependence: Toward an Integrated Neurobehavioral Approach*. C. R. Schuster and M. J. Kuhar, Eds. Springer-Verlag, Berlin pp. 563–598.
31. Novick, D. M., Khan, I., and Kreek, M. J. (1986). Acquired immunodeficiency syndrome and infection with hepatitis viruses in individuals abusing drugs by injection. *U. N. Bull. Narcotics* 38, 15–25.
32. Kreek, M. J. (1999). Gender differences in the effects of opiates and cocaine: Treatment implications. In *Gender and Its Effects on Psychopathology*, E. Frank, Ed. American Psychiatric Press, Washington, DC, pp. 281–299.
33. Mathieu-Kia, A.-M., Kellogg, S. H., Butelman, E. R., and Kreek, M. J. (2002). Nicotine addiction: Insights from recent animal studies. *Psychopharmacology (Berl.)* 162, 102–118.
34. Kreek, M. J. (1996). Cocaine, dopamine and the endogenous opioid system. *J. Addict. Dis.* 15, 73–96.

35. Borg, L., and Kreek, M. J. (2003). The pharmacology of opioids. In *Principles of Addiction Medicine*, 3rd ed, A. W. Graham, T. K. Schultz, M. F. Mayo-Smith, R. K. Ries, and B. B. Wilford, Eds. Chevy Chase, MD: American Society of Addiction Medicine, , pp. 141–153.

36. Kreek, M. J. (2006). Endorphins, gene polymorphisms, stress responsivity, and special addictions: Selected topics. In *Cell biology of Addiction*, B. Madras, C. M. Colvis, and J. D. Pollock, et al., Eds. Cold Spring Harbor Laboratory Press, Cold Spring Harbor, NY, pp. 63–92.

37. Kreek, M. J. (2003). Neurobiological basis for use of opioid agonist maintenance in the treatment of heroin addiction. In *Maintenance Treatment of Heroin Addiction— Evidence at the Crossroads*, H. Waal and E. Haga, Eds. Cappelen Akademisk Forlag, Oslo, pp. 10–39.

38. Kreek, M. J., Schlussman, S. D., Bart, G., LaForge, K. S., and Butelman, E. R. (2004). Evolving perspectives on neurobiological research on the addictions: Celebration of the 30th anniversary of NIDA. *Neuropharmacology* 47, 324–344.

39. Yuferov, V., Nielsen, D. A., Butelman, E. R., and Kreek, M. J. (2005). Microarray studies of psychostimulant-induced changes in gene expression. *Addict. Biol.* 10, 101–118.

40. Bond, C., LaForge, K. S., Tian, M., Melia, D., Zhang, S., Borg, L., Gong, J., Schluger, J., Strong, J. A., Leal, S. M., Tischfield, J. A., Kreek, M. J., and Yu, L. (1998). Single nucleotide polymorphism in the human mu opioid receptor gene alters beta-endorphin binding and activity: Possible implications for opiate addiction. *Proc. Natl. Acad. Sci. USA* 95, 9608–9613.

41. LaForge, K. S., Yuferov, V., and Kreek, M. J. (2000). Opioid receptor and peptide gene polymorphisms: Potential implications for addictions. *Eur. J. Pharmacol.* 410, 249–268.

42. LaForge, K. S., Kreek, M. J., Uhl, G. R., Sora, I., Yu, L., Befort, K., Filliol, D., Favier, V., Hoehe, M., Kieffer, B. L., and Höllt, V. (2000). Symposium XIII: Allelic polymorphism of human opioid receptors: Functional studies: Genetic contributions to protection from, or vulnerability to, addictive diseases. In *Problems of Drug Dependence, 1999; Proceedings of the 61st Annual Scientific Meeting of the College on Problems of Drug Dependence. National Institute of Drug Abuse Research Monograph Series 180*, NIH Pub. No. (ADM)00-4737, Harris, L. S., Ed. U.S. Department of Health and Human Services, National Institutes of Health, Bethesda, MD, pp. 47–50.

43. Kreek, M. J. (2002). Gene diversity in the endorphin system: SNPs, chips and possible implications In *The Genomic Revolution: Unveiling the Unity of Life*, M. Yudell and R. DeSalle, Eds. National Academy Press/Joseph Henry Press, Washington, DC, pp. 97–108.

44. Kreek, M. J., Nielsen, D. A., and LaForge, K. S. (2004). Genes associated with addiction: Alcoholism, opiate and cocaine addiction. *Neuromol. Med.* 5, 85–108.

45. Kreek, M. J., Bart, G., Lilly, C., LaForge, K. S., and Nielsen, D. (2005). Pharmacogenetics and human molecular genetics of opiate and cocaine addictions and their treatments. *Pharmacol. Rev.* 57, 1–26.

46. Kreek, M. J., Nielsen, D. A., Butelman, E. R., and LaForge, K. S. (2005). Genetics influences on impulsivity, risk-taking, stress responsivity, and vulnerability to drug abuse and addiction. *Nat. Neurosci.* 8, 1450–1457.

47. Kreek, M. J., and Hartman, N. (1982). Chronic use of opioids and antipsychotic drugs: Side effects, effects on endogenous opioids and toxicity. *Ann. NY Acad. Sci.* 398, 151–172.

48. Kreek, M. J., Wardlaw, S. L., Hartman, N., Raghunath, J., Friedman, J., Schneider, B., and Frantz, A. G. (1983). Circadian rhythms and levels of beta-endorphin, ACTH, and cortisol during chronic methadone maintenance treatment in humans. *Life Sci.* 33, 409–411.
49. Kreek, M. J., Ragunath, J., Plevy, S., Hamer, D., Schneider, B., and Hartman, N. (1984). ACTH, cortisol and beta-endorphin response to metyrapone testing during chronic methadone maintenance treatment in humans. *Neuropeptides* 5, 277–278.
50. Novick, D. M., Ochshorn, M., Ghali, V., Croxson, T. S., Mercer, W. D., Chiorazzi, N., and Kreek, M. J. (1989). Natural killer cell activity and lymphocyte subsets in parenteral heroin abusers and long-term methadone maintenance patients. *J. Pharmacol. Exp. Ther.* 250, 606–610.
51. Culpepper-Morgan, J. A., and Kreek, M. J. (1997). Hypothalamic-pituitary-adrenal axis hypersensitivity to naloxone in opioid dependence: A case of naloxone induced withdrawal. *Metabolism* 46, 130–134.
52. Kreek, M. J., and Koob, G. F. (1998). Drug dependence: Stress and dysregulation of brain reward pathways. *Drug Alcohol Depend.* 51, 23–47.
53. Kreek, M. J., Borg, L., Zhou, Y., and Schluger, J. (2002). Relationships between endocrine functions and substance abuse syndromes: Heroin and related short-acting opiates in addiction contrasted with methadone and other long-acting opioid agonists used in pharmacotherapy of addiction. In *Hormones, Brain and Behavior*, D. Pfaff, Ed. Academic Press, San Diego, CA, pp. 781–830.
54. O'Malley, S. S., Krishnan-Sarin, S., Farren, C., Sinha, R., and Kreek, M. J. (2002). Naltrexone decreases craving and alcohol self-administration in alcohol dependent subjects and activates the hypothalamo-pituitary-adrenocortical axis. *Psychopharmacology (Berl.)* 160, 19–29.
55. King, A. C., Schluger, J., Gunduz, M., Borg, L., Perret, G., Ho, A., and Kreek, M. J. (2002). Hypothalamic-pituitary-adrenocortical (HPA) axis response and biotransformation of oral naltrexone: Preliminary examination of relationship to family history of alcoholism. *Neuropsychopharmacology* 26, 778–788.
56. Zhou, Y., Bendor, J. T., Yuferov, V., Schlussman, S. D., Ho, A., and Kreek, M. J. (2005). Amygdalar vasopressin mRNA increases in acute cocaine withdrawal: Evidence for opioid receptor modulation. *Neuroscience* 134, 1391–1397.
57. Sinha, R., Garcia, M., Paliwal, P., Kreek, M. J., and Rounsaville, B. J. (2006). Stress-induced cocaine craving and HPA responses predict cocaine relapse outcomes. *Arch. Gen. Psychiatry* 63, 324–331.
58. Aouizerate, B., Ho, A., Schluger, J. H., Perret, G., Borg, L., Le Moal, M., Piazza, P. V., and Kreek, M. J. (2006). Glucocorticoid negative feedback in methadone maintained former heroin addicts with ongoing cocaine dependence: Dose-response to dexamethasone suppression. *Addict Biol.* 11, 84–96.
59. Koob, G., and Kreek, M. J. (in press). Stress, dysregulation of drug reward pathways and the transition to drug dependence. *Am. J. Psychiatry*.

14

DOPAMINERGIC AND GABAERGIC REGULATION OF ALCOHOL-MOTIVATED BEHAVIORS: NOVEL NEUROANATOMICAL SUBSTRATES

HARRY L. JUNE[1] AND WILLIAM J. A. EILER II[2]

[1]*University of Maryland School of Medicine, Baltimore, Maryland and* [2]*Indiana University-Purdue University, Indianapolis, Indiana*

14.1	Introduction	466
14.2	Optimal Animal Model to Study Neuroanatomical Substrates of Alcohol Self-Administration Behaviors	466
14.3	Integrating P Rat Line with Appropriate Behavioral Paradigms and Neuroanatomical Studies to Make Inferences About Novel Neuroanatomical Substrates of Alcohol Self-Administration Behaviors	467
	14.3.1 Appropriate Behavioral Paradigms	467
	14.3.1.1 Reinforcer-Specific Controls	469
	14.3.1.2 Neuroanatomical Controls	469
	14.3.2 Role of CNS Circuitry in Mediating EtOH Self-Administration	470
	14.3.3 Novel Neuroanatomical Substrates Regulating Alcohol Reward	471
14.4	Dopamine Neuronal Systems and Substrates Regulating Alcohol Reward	471
	14.4.1 Dopaminergic Regulation in Alcohol Self-Administration: Review of Previous Research	472
14.5	Novel Dopamine Substrates Regulating Alcohol Reward	473
	14.5.1 Bed Nucleus of Stria Terminalis	473
	14.5.2 Ventral Pallidum	476
	14.5.2.1 Hypothesized Mechanisms of Dopaminergic Regulation in Ventral Pallidum Regulating Alcohol-Motivated Behaviors	478
	14.5.3 Lateral Hypothalamus	481
	14.5.3.1 D_2 Dopaminergic Regulation of Alcohol-Motivated Behaviors in LH: Hypothesized Mechanisms	481
	14.5.4 Summary	485
14.6	Molecular Biology of the $GABA_A$ BDZ Receptor	487
	14.6.1 Commonalities of Alcohol and Modulators of the $GABA_A$ BDZ Systems	487
	14.6.2 $GABA_A$ BDZ Modulation of EtOH Self-Administration: Studies Using Systematic Application of Probes	488
	14.6.2.1 Significance of Systemic Studies	492

Handbook of Contemporary Neuropharmacology, Edited by David R. Sibley, Israel Hanin, Michael Kuhar, and Phil Skolnick. Copyright © 2007 John Wiley & Sons, Inc.

	14.6.3 Site-Specific Microinjection Studies: Manipulation of $GABA_A$ BDZ Receptor Complex in Modifying EtOH Self-Administration	493
	14.6.4 Studies Supporting Hypothesis That GABA–DA Interactions Regulate Alcohol-Motivated Behaviors: GABAergic Modulation of DA Function	496
	14.6.5 Conceptual Framework for Hypothesis Generation and Interpretation of GABA–DA Interaction in Alcohol Drinking Behavior	497
	14.6.6 Novel CNS GABAergic Substrates Regulating Alcohol-Motivated Behaviors	498
	14.6.7 Ligands with Preferential Selectivities for $GABA_A$ Receptors Containing α_1 Subunit ($GABA_{A1}$ Receptors)	498
	14.6.8 Efficacies of βCCt and 3PBC in Modulating GABA Responses in Recombinant $GABA_{A1,2,3,5}$ Receptors	499
14.7	Employing Ligands with Preferential Selectivities for α_1 Subunit Containing $GABA_A$ Receptor as Pharmacological Probes to Investigate Novel Alcohol Reward Substrates	501
	14.7.1 Ventral Pallidum	501
	14.7.2 Systemic Studies	503
	14.7.3 Microinjection Studies	505
14.8	Oral Administration of βCCt or 3PBC Produces Prolonged Reduction on Alcohol Self-Administration: Direct Comparison with Opioid Receptor Antagonist Naltrexone	507
	14.8.1 Oral Efficacy of βCCt and 3PBC in Reducing Anxiety in Alcohol-Preferring Rats	510
14.9	Employing Ligands with Preferential Selectivities for α_5-Subunit-Containing $GABA_A$ Receptors as Pharmacological Probes to Investigate Novel Alcohol Reward Substrates: CA1 and CA3 Hippocampus	511
14.10	Subunit Selectivity versus Intrinsic Efficacy	516
14.11	Conclusions	517
References		518

14.1 INTRODUCTION

Over the past two decades it has become increasingly clear that the disease of alcoholism, like other substance abuse addictions, is a brain disorder. Thus, one of the key objectives of alcoholism research is to understand the neuroanatomical substrates and neurocircuitry within the brain regulating alcohol addiction and dependence in humans. Unfortunately, alcoholism in humans is a complex disorder comprising not only central nervous system (CNS) mechanisms [1] but also social, cultural, and emotional influences [2]. Through basic neuroscience research, scientists in the alcohol field, particularly researchers focused on alcohol self-administration [3–9], are gaining a better understanding of the neuromechanism(s) regulating alcohol drinking behavior. This success has largely been attributable to the development and use of animal models [1].

14.2 OPTIMAL ANIMAL MODEL TO STUDY NEUROANATOMICAL SUBSTRATES OF ALCOHOL SELF-ADMINISTRATION BEHAVIORS

Animal models of alcoholism have provided useful analogs of the human condition, and a number of researchers have employed these models to study the neurobiological factors mediating alcohol self-administration. As noted by Li (see [1], p. 36), such models are useful only "when they reveal some aspects of the complex process to yield understanding about the human condition." Thus, to model the human condition, with specific considerations of criteria of alcoholism of the fourth edition of the *Diagnostic and Statistical Manual of Mental Disorders* (DSM-IV), genetically selective breeding of rats that initiate excessive alcohol drinking has produced an unequivocal impact in the field of alcoholism research. Exemplary of the genetically selected rodent is the alcohol-preferring (P) and high alcohol drinking (HAD) rat lines developed by Indiana University's Alcohol Research Center. One of the primary criteria for an animal model of alcoholism [10], similar to the DSM-IV criterion in humans, is that individuals/rodents will work at high levels to obtain alcohol and that a great deal of time is spent in activities necessary to obtain alcohol. This criterion for alcoholism attests to the reinforcing strength/efficacy of alcohol as an abused substance. In comparison to most genetically selected rodent models of alcohol drinking, the efficacy profile of the Indiana selected rat models, particularly the P line in the operant paradigm, far exceeds that of the other rodent models (see [4, 11–13]). Thus, to model the human condition of alcohol abuse, in the present review, we have primarily selected as subjects the P rats, and the HAD rats to a lesser degree. Further, the P rat line has been shown to satisfy most of the criteria for an animal model of human alcohol abuse [10] to the satisfaction of the alcohol research community [8]. While the criteria have been discussed at length in the excellent review by McBride and Li [1], a brief summary of these findings is warranted to provide the reader with the rationale for using the P rat as subjects in the study of neurobiological mechanisms underlying alcohol self-administration behaviors. Other summaries in relation to the P rat line as an optimal model of the human condition of alcoholism/abuse can also be found in the literature [3, 8, 11]. Nevertheless, the P rat will: (1) voluntarily consume 5–8 g/kg of alcohol to attain blood alcohol concentrations of 50–200 mg%; (2) lever press for alcohol orally in concentrations of 10–40%, despite the fact that water and food are concurrently available; (3) drink alcohol for its pharmacological effect and not solely because of its taste, smell, or caloric properties as evidenced by self-administration of alcohol intragastrically and intracranially by P rats; (4) develop both metabolic and functional tolerance with free-choice alcohol drinking; and (5) develop physical dependence and signs of withdrawal following removal of alcohol after periods of chronic consumption. Taken together, the P rat line is among the best, albeit not perfect, models of human alcoholism [1].

14.3 INTEGRATING P RAT LINE WITH APPROPRIATE BEHAVIORAL PARADIGMS AND NEUROANATOMICAL STUDIES TO MAKE INFERENCES ABOUT NOVEL NEUROANATOMICAL SUBSTRATES OF ALCOHOL SELF-ADMINISTRATION BEHAVIORS

14.3.1 Appropriate Behavioral Paradigms

A variety of procedures have been successfully used to motivate rodents to orally self-administer alcohol [4]. The most widely used and accepted method in the alcohol field, particularly with outbred rats, is the sucrose-fading technique developed by Samson [14, 15]. Over the years, researchers have validated as well as modified this procedure for both limited (e.g., 10–60 min) and more prolonged exposure periods (e.g., 2–4 h) [15, 16]. Modifications to the procedure wherein non-food- and water-deprived rats trained to initiate ethanal (EtOH) responding are allowed to obtain water or EtOH by responding at one of two levers have produced an operant choice paradigm that can be used to investigate the neuropharmacological bases of alcoholism [4, 17]. Other modifications of the procedure include a two-lever design wherein nondeprived rats lever press for alcohol on one lever and a highly palatable/isocaloric solution on the other (see [18, 19]). Some of the important features incorporated in this model include: (a) maintenance of responding for EtOH as a measure of EtOH reinforcement; (b) an index of preference for EtOH over water, independent of the absolute amounts of EtOH consumed; (c) a control for nonspecific drug effects on ingestive behaviors; (d) dissociation of the pharmacological motivation from consummatory processes; and (e) measurement of significant blood alcohol concentration (BAC) levels (see [4], also [17]).

In addition to the sucrose-fading technique, a number of laboratories have developed other procedures wherein pharmacologically relevant EtOH concentrations are obtained after training rats to orally ingest alcohol. Such techniques have been used in the home cage with both outbred rats [20–22] and rats selectively bred for alcohol consumption [1, 8]. For example, the ascending two-bottle water choice [20, 21] and the sweetened cocktail solution procedures [22] have been reported to produce EtOH intake levels in outbred rats that result in pharmacologically relevant EtOH concentrations. In addition, variations in the 24-h home cage model using limited-access procedures (e.g., 30–240 min) have been quite effective in producing significant alcohol levels and have been employed extensively in studying the neurobiological mechanisms of alcohol drinking, even in alcohol selectively bred rodents (Ps, HADs) [23–26]. Unfortunately, the investigator has little control over the contingent relations between responses and ingestion in this home cage model. Roberts and colleagues [27] suggested employing the home cage as the only reinforcing model "is potentially confounded by palatability." As in studies of other abused drugs, the most appropriate instrument is the operant conditioning chamber where the contingency between responding and drinking can be specified and the volume of liquid ingested per completed schedule unit can be controlled. The operant methodology is especially important in analyzing complex dose–response relationships of a test agent [28, 29] and when examining the effects of a test agent on EtOH and another concurrently available reinforcer [5, 28, 30–33]. Finally, when the 24-h access model is employed, it is difficult to determine pharmacologically relevant BACs, since the scheduled drinking bout(s) is often difficult to ascertain. BACs are important when trying to determine the neuromechanism of action of EtOH [34–36]. Hence, the operant paradigm has a number of advantages over simple home cage drinking procedures in rats and mice [4, 27].

As noted above, the most widely used and accepted method of initiating operant responding for alcohol drinking in outbred and alcohol selected rats is the sucrose-fading technique [14]. The merits of this initiation procedure have been discussed in several previous reviews [1, 4]. However, while a number of laboratories are currently evaluating the efficacy of pharmacological treatments on scheduled controlled responding using the Samson procedure, studies in which specific controls are used for rate dependency and the postingestional properties of the test solutions are generally lacking in the alcohol literature. As a result, many published reports are very difficult to interpret in relation to the selectivity of a test agent reducing alcohol drinking on the one hand, and the degree to which inferences can be made from these studies to neural mechanisms of action on the other. It is important to note that selectivity for alcohol drinking is a very important concern in self-administration studies given that most studies in the literature report that test compounds "all" reduce motivated responding for alcohol. Elevations in alcohol-motivated behaviors, particularly within the operant chamber in non-food- or water-deprived rodents, have generally not been reported in the alcohol literature. Thus, to eliminate confounding of results/interpretation, it is important to use *rigorous reinforcer control procedures* in alcohol self-administration research. While a thorough review of these procedures is beyond the scope of this chapter, below we provide a brief review of protocols that can be used to optimize data interpretation in rodent alcohol-self-administration research. For more details on these procedures, the interested reader should consult the protocols outlined in June [4].

14.3.1.1 Reinforcer-Specific Controls. First, to investigate the capacity of a pharmacological agent to produce dose and time course effects when rats are presented with EtOH as the sole reinforcer, rodents should be given the EtOH solution on a fixed-ratio (FR) schedule, preferably an FR4 or FR6. Second, the capacity of a pharmacological agent to produce dose and time course effects when rats are presented with a palatable reinforcer (e.g., saccharin, sucrose) as the sole reinforcer on an FR schedule should also be determined. When the data are interpreted, one is able to make inferences as to whether antagonism is specific to EtOH-motivated behaviors. Third, the researcher should evaluate the capacity of a pharmacological agent to produce dose and time course effects when a concurrent schedule procedure is employed under an FR schedule [37]. Because basal response rates should be equal or near equal between groups in this protocol, the concurrent schedule will address the issue of whether the capacity of an agent to decrease EtOH and not saccharin reinforcement is due to differences in reinforcing efficacy (i.e., strength). Finally, the capacity of a pharmacological agent to produce dose and time course effects under a concurrent FR schedule procedure when two isocaloric alternative solutions are presented should be evaluated. The caloric consideration is important insofar as the calories contained in alcohol could contribute substantially to its motivating properties [32], independent of the CNS pharmacological effects. It should also be noted that Bodnar and his colleagues [38, 39] have reported a differential regulation of caloric compared with noncaloric reinforcers within the opioid systems. Thus, the CNS substrates which regulate a particular type of palatable ingesta may be different. It is well established that an isocaloric concurrent procedure for alcohol and the alternative solution may produce different response rates and profiles (see [40]).

14.3.1.2 Neuroanatomical Controls. Although reinforcer-specific controls add immensely in making inferences about pharmacological probes in investigating neuroanatomical substrates of alcohol-motivated behaviors, equally important is the use of neuroanatomical controls. Such studies are rarely performed in published reports in the alcohol field. CNS substrates are primarily studied in alcohol research using microinjection procedures (i.e., intracerebral drug delivery) [1, 9]. Generally, there are two types of neuroanatomical control groups that will assist in data interpretation (see [4]). First, a researcher may use a "region-specific" control wherein a second infusion is performed 1–2 mm away from the designated brain site. The second infusion may be given rostral, caudal, ventral, or dorsal to the designated brain site. Studies that attempt to compare the anterior and posterior ventral tegmental area (VTA) or the nucleus accumbens (NAcc) shell and core or the NAcc and ventral striatum are also examples of "region-specific" comparisons. For illustrative examples of such control procedures, studies by Nowak et al. [41] and June et al. [19, 29] should be reviewed. Alternatively, a researcher may also use an entirely different locus as the control site. This type of control is referred to as an "alternate region" control. The alternate region control is particularly important when different receptor populations or subunit configurations are of interest. Such controls are illustrated in the work by Eiler et al. [42] wherein the caudate putamen was used as an alternative locus in investigating the dorsal bed nucleus of the stria terminalis. Harvey et al. [37] also used the alternate region design wherein the NAcc and caudate putamen were used as control loci in investigating the ventral pallidum, a putative drug reward substrate ventral to the NAcc [43].

In summary, this section has provided information pertaining to the P rat as a model of alcoholism. The model has a number of advantages over other currently available models, and with the exception of variables relating to psychosocial and cultural factors which influence drinking, the P rat satisfies the DSM-IV criteria reasonably well for the condition of alcoholism in humans [1]. Besides having an "optimal animal model," both reinforcer (i.e., pertaining to ingesta) and neuroanatomical control procedures were discussed and suggested to be critical in making direct inferences about putative neuromechanisms of alcohol-motivated behaviors. We propose that integration of the ideal animal model combined with systematic utilization of reinforcer and neuroanatomical specific control designs is a multi-disciplinary approach which provides a researcher with a wealth of data for systematic evaluation and interpretation of pharmacological probes to understand the neuromechanisms regulating alcohol-motivated behaviors.

14.3.2 Role of CNS Circuitry in Mediating EtOH Self-Administration

An understanding of the neuroanatomical substrates, neurocircuitry, and interaction of the neuronal systems which regulate alcohol drinking is key in the identification of novel targets for drugs to treat alcohol addiction and dependence in humans [19, 37, 44]. While alcohol affects an array of neuronal systems, including opioids, glutamate, γ-aminobutyric acid (GABA), adenosine, serotonin, and the catecholamines [1, 45–47], alcohol also shares common neural substrates, circuitry, and characteristics with other addictive substances. Specifically, alcohol shares the property of increasing dopaminergic activity in the mesocorticolimbic system [48]. Within the mesocorticolimbic system, previous research focused on the VTA of the midbrain and its projection to the limbic forebrain, the NAcc (for a review see [46]). Indeed, prior work in animal models and humans provides evidence that all drugs of abuse converge on this pathway to produce their reinforcing effects ([49]; for a recent review see [50]). However, as discussed in a recent review by Lovinger and Crabbe [44], alcohol abuse and alcoholism have a number of distinct neuronal processes from other substance abuse disorders. For example, recent work has demonstrated that a number of additional brain areas independently or in collaboration with the VTA and NAcc play an important role in regulating alcohol drinking behaviors [46, 51, 52]. Specifically, regions of the extended amygdala circuit [central nucleus of the amygdala, bed nucleus of the stria terminalis, shell of the NAcc, sublenticular substantia innominata (SI)/ventral pallidum] [53, 54], hippocampus, and lateral hypothalamus have all been shown to regulate alcohol drinking ([30, 42, 55, 56]; also for a review see [19]). As noted by Nestler [50], because some of these areas are associated with the traditional memory system, the study of these new substrates could provide information about the cognitive factors and emotional memories which might regulate alcohol drinking and relapse behavior. In addition, because brain areas such as the hypothalamus may play a role in alcohol addiction as well as the so-called natural addictions (e.g., obesity, sex) [57, 58], these areas could provide strategies to understand the common/shared neuronal pathways which regulate the behavioral pathology of alcohol and other consummatory behaviors.

14.3.3 Novel Neuroanatomical Substrates Regulating Alcohol Reward

Research on the substrates and circuitry regulating alcohol self-administration has experienced an enormous growth over the past decade. Several reviews have described this area of inquiry [1, 8, 9, 59]. In many cases, these reviews have provided an exhaustive coverage of the neuronal substrates and systems which have been shown to regulate alcohol-motivated behaviors. In the present review, we will focus exclusively on relatively new findings in the alcohol self-administration literature (many of which were not available or omitted in prior reviews), implicating novel substrates and circuitry within the dopaminergic and GABAergic systems. The *majority* of the recent studies described here have employed rigorus reinforcer and neuroanatomical specific control designs, allowing for more precise inferences about putative alcohol reward mechanisms. The focus on the dopamine (DA) and GABA systems relates to both neuroanatomical topography and established neurochemistry, demonstrating that within several loci in the CNS a neuromodulatory role may exist between the two systems. New findings will be presented demonstrating that exploitation of the GABAergic system indeed represents a vital strategic route for the development of novel prototype ligands to reduce alcohol drinking behavior in human alcoholics. Moreover, we propose that GABA mediates its actions on alcohol self-administration via interaction with the DA system [19, 37]. Hence, in this regard, a review of the literature pertaining to DAergic regulatory control on alcohol self-administration is warranted. Finally, it is clear that a number of other important neuronal systems have been shown to be important in regulating alcohol reward mechanisms, particularly imbalances in corticotropin-releasing factor (CRF) and neuropeptide Y (NPY) [60–63]. A discussion of this literature is beyond the scope of the present review.

14.4 DOPAMINE NEURONAL SYSTEMS AND SUBSTRATES REGULATING ALCOHOL REWARD

According to the DA hypothesis of reward, DA systems directly mediate the rewarding or primary motivational characteristics of natural stimuli such as food, water, and sex as well as various drugs of abuse, including EtOH [57]. The most current research examining the role of DA in the reinforcing properties of EtOH has focused on the interactions of the NAcc and the A10 DA cell body grouping known as the VTA (for a review see [51]). The NAcc receives its extensive DA innervation from the VTA. This DAergic fiber tract is referred to as the mesolimbic pathway (for a review see [64]). Below, we provide a selective review of the early systemic, site-specific microinjection and lesion studies that have been critical in providing support for a dopaminergic regulation in alcohol self-administration research.

14.4.1 Dopaminergic Regulation in Alcohol Self-Administration: Review of Previous Research

A body of research employing systemic injections has implicated DA neurotransmission in alcohol reinforcement. Generally, this research has demonstrated that neurochemical manipulations which increase DA transmission increase EtOH intake and responding, while manipulations that reduce DA transmission reduce responding and intake; however, conflicting reports have emerged (for a review see [1, 9, 17, 51]). Initial studies employing site-specific microinjection methodology evaluated the effects of bilateral infusions of the D_1 antagonist SCH 23390 (0.1–2.0 µg/side) and the D_2 antagonist sulpiride (0.1–2.0 µg/side) into the NAcc of P rats during a 30-min home cage EtOH access period [65]. The D_2 antagonist sulpiride produced a significant dose-dependent increase in alcohol drinking, while no significant effects were seen with SCH 23390. Subsequent studies by Samson and his colleagues [9, 66, 67] have shown that bilateral intra-accumbens infusions of the nonspecific agonist *d*-amphetamine (4–20 µg) or the more selective DA D_2-like (i.e., selectivity toward D_2 compared to D_3 and D_4) agonist quinpirole (1 µg) increased EtOH responding in outbred rats. In this same study, however, higher quinpirole doses (4 and 10 µg) significantly decreased EtOH responding. Samson and his colleagues have also shown that reducing DA neurotransmission in the NAcc directly by local administration of the D_2-like antagonist raclopride [9] or indirectly by infusion of the D_2 agonist quinpirole [66] into the VTA decreased EtOH responding. It should be noted that quinpirole in the VTA inhibits DA cell activity via a proposed feedback of the cell upon itself [68]; hence, it would be predicted that quinpirole would produce effects similar to blockade of DA neurotransmission in the terminal field by raclopride. Indeed, Murphy and his colleagues (see [41]) demonstrated that direct infusion of quinpirole as well as another D_2 agonist quinelorane in the VTA of P rats reduces home cage alcohol but not saccharin drinking. It should be noted that a selective reduction on alcohol was observed in the anterior, but not the posterior, VTA, suggesting that only those D_2 receptors on cell bodies within the anterior VTA selectively regulate alcohol intake [8]. One hypothesis that has been used to explain the effectiveness of DA agonists in decreasing EtOH self-administration is that agonists blunt the reinforcing actions of EtOH by substituting for the DA-enhancing action of the agent. The heightened "hedonic state" produced by DA receptor activation may eliminate the rats' motivation to respond for EtOH [69, 70].

In addition to the pharmacological microinjection studies discussed above, substantial neurochemical evidence supports a role of the mesoaccumbens DA system in mediating EtOH-motivated behaviors [71–73]. These relatively recent neurochemical studies are discussed below. However, not all studies support a direct role for the DA system in alcohol self-administration. Specifically, early neurobehavioral studies with neurotoxic lesions [74–76] suggested that norepinephrine (NE) may play a more important role than DA in EtOH self-administration. Pharmacological manipulations using highly selective DA receptor agents have also failed to alter EtOH self-administration [77]. Nonetheless, it should be noted that these studies used systemic administration, not examining discrete brain loci. Previous work by Rassnick et al. [78] have shown that 6-Hydroxy-Dopamine (6-OHDA) lesions of the NAcc do not block established oral EtOH-reinforced responding on a continuous reinforcement schedule. Rassnick and her colleagues have interpreted these data to mean that the mesoaccumbens pathway is not the only system involved in mediating EtOH reinforcement. Research involving the infusion of DA agonists and antagonists into the NAcc is also equivocal. For example, while Samson and his colleagues demonstrated that DA antagonists infused in the NAcc decrease EtOH-reinforced responding [67], dose-dependent increases were observed by Levy et al. [65] with DA antagonists. While this discrepancy has not been resolved in the current literature, one possible explanation to account for these findings is that altered responses to DA blockade in P rats might result from neurobiological changes in DA systems and cause P rats to initiate rather than suppress responding/intake [1].

14.5 NOVEL DOPAMINE SUBSTRATES REGULATING ALCOHOL REWARD

More recent research has begun to focus on brain substrates other than the NAcc that are innervated by the VTA. Many of these loci have been shown to play a role in mediating the rewarding properties of multiple drugs of abuse [79]. This section examines recent evidence that implicates these new loci in the regulation of EtOH reward. For each locus reviewed, the effects of EtOH on the DA system within the substrate will be discussed, as will any effect DA manipulation has on the mediation of EtOH reinforcement. The first substrate to be discussed is the bed nucleus of the stria terminalis (BST) a forebrain structure innervated by DA within the VTA [80]. The second structure examined is the ventral pallidum (VP), a ventral forebrain structure that receives dopaminergic input from the VTA via the mesopallidal pathway [81, 82]. The final substrate, the lateral hypothalamus (LH), is best known for its control of feeding and drinking behavior [83–85]. It receives innervation from DA neurons originating within the VTA via the mesothalamic pathway [64, 86].

14.5.1 Bed Nucleus of Stria Terminalis

Recent evidence has emerged suggesting that the BST exerts dopaminergic control over the reinforcing properties of EtOH [42, 48]. The BST is perhaps best known as a component of the extended amygdala (EA), a group of forebrain nuclei that exhibit similar morphology, immunoreactivity, and connectivity (including the NAcc shell, central nucleus of the amygdala, and substantia innominata) [53]. As with other members of the EA, the BST receives extensive dopaminergic innervation from the DA cell bodies located within the VTA via the mesolimbic path [87, 88]. DA input from the VTA is received within the BST by a 3:2 ratio of D_1-like to D_2-like DA receptors [80, 89, 90]. Within the BST, several other neurotransmitters (e.g., GABA, glutamate, and various opioid peptides) also facilitate neuronal communication to the other putative alcohol reward substrates of the extended amygdala, such as the NAcc and central nucleus of the amygdala (CeA), as well as other reward areas outside the

EA, such as the VP and the hippocampus [80, 87, 88, 91–93]. The BST has also been found to send GABAergic connections back to the VTA, perhaps to regulate the VTA dopaminergic output [94, 95].

The first study examining the role of the dopaminergic system within the BST on acute EtOH administration was conducted by Carboni and colleagues in 2000 [48]. In this study, Carboni et al. examined DA release in the BST following peripheral administration of various drugs of abuse. To accomplish this, a microdialysis probe was implanted in the anterior BST of male Sprague–Dawley rats. After the recovery phase, the rats were given systemic cocaine, the selective DA reuptake inhibitor GBR12909, morphine, nicotine, and alcohol (0.25 and 0.5 g/kg) (see Fig. 14.1). Their data demonstrated that all drugs led to significant increases in extracellular DA in the BST, lending increased support for a role of the BST in the mediation of drug reward. It should be noted that the 0.25- and 0.5-g/kg alcohol doses represent levels that are obtained during alcohol responding and intake [4]. In addition, these doses typically induce locomotor activation in rodents [96, 97], particularly during the ascending limb of the BAC [96]. Hence, to the extent that the locomotor activational effects in rodents may be a putative model of alcohol-induced euphoria in humans [97, 98], the findings by Carboni and colleagues could have relevance to alcohol's rewarding properties. Nevertheless, Carboni and colleagues [48] suggested that the EtOH-induced increase of DA in the BST might be analogous to the DA release in the NAcc.

While the Carboni et al. study was the first to suggest the DA system within the BST may be involved in EtOH reward, this study obviously does not directly test the

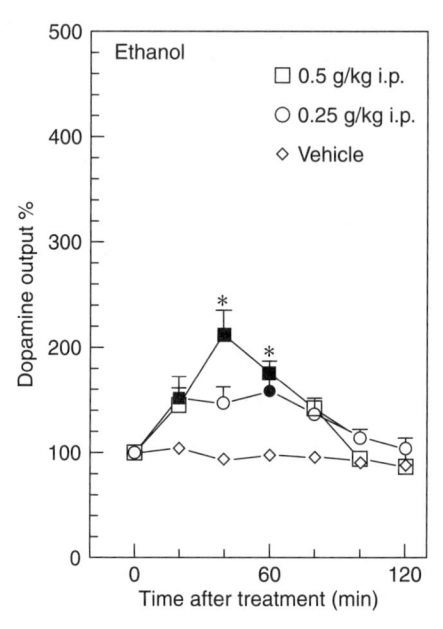

Figure 14.1 Effect of ethanol following intraperitoneal injection of 0.25 and 0.5 g/kg (injected as 10% v/v solution) on dopamine concentration in dialysate obtained by in vivo microdialysis from BST. Each point is the mean [standard error of the mean (SEM)] of at least four determinations. Filled symbols: p, 0.05 from basal values concentration; (*) p, 0.05 from corresponding time point of vehicle group. Adapted from [48].

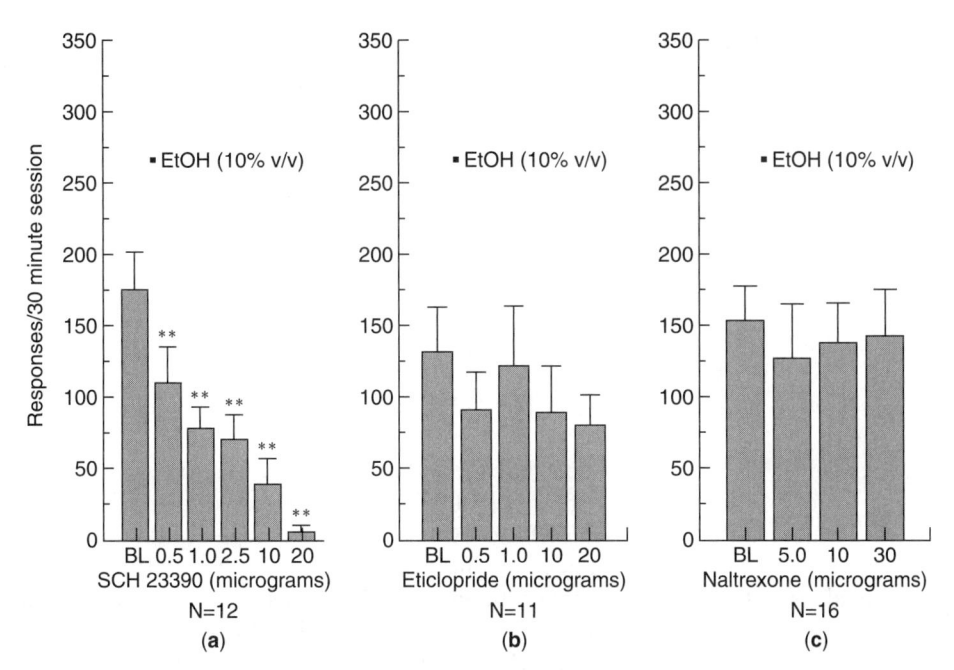

Figure 14.2 (a) Effects of SCH 23390 (0.5–20 μg) following bilateral injection in bed nucleus of stria terminalis (BST) on responding maintained by EtOH (10% v/v). Data are shown as mean ± SEM. (**) $p \leq 0.01$ SCH 23390 vs. baseline (noninfusion and saline infusion controls). (b) Effects of eticlopride (0.5–20 μg) following bilateral injection in BST on responding maintained by EtOH (10% v/v). Data are mean ± SEM. Adapted from Eiler et al., 2003.

hypothesis. Eiler et al. [42] directly investigated the potential role of DA (in the BST) on EtOH reinforcement using the microinfusion technique. To accomplish this, P rats were bilaterally infused with the D_1 receptor antagonist SCH 23390 or D_2-like receptor antagonist eticlopride in the dorsolateral BST following training to lever press for EtOH in an operant paradigm. The results were clear-cut. SCH 23390 produced significant dose reductions on responding maintained by alcohol; however, eticlopride and naltrexone were not effective (Fig. 14.2). These data strongly suggest that EtOH reward is mediated by D_1-like receptors located within the BST. As EtOH consumption at its core is a consumptive, drinking behavior, it is important to determine if the effects of any drug on EtOH are selective or a result of a suppression of drinking behavior in general. To evaluate reinforcer specificity, animals were trained to operantly self-administer sucrose. In contrast to the findings seen with EtOH, the two highest SCH 23390 and eticlopride doses (2.5 and 20.0 μg) significantly reduced sucrose responding; however, naltrexone was not effective. The results of this study were the first to demonstrate that a D_1 DA receptor subtype within the BST plays a significant role in EtOH reinforcement. While the D_1 receptors also appear to have a regulatory role in sucrose reinforcement, the BST appears most sensitive to EtOH reinforcement. In contrast, neither D_2 receptors nor the opioid system plays a role in the regulation of alcohol-rewarding properties in the BST. Similarly, the opioid systems of the BST do not appear significant in mediating the rewarding properties of sweet palatable solutions.

14.5.2 Ventral Pallidum

Increasing evidence implicates the VP as a dompaminoceptive brain region regulating drug reinforcement [99–101]. More recent studies, however, have evaluated the ventral pallidal DA system in regulating alcohol-motivated behaviors. One of the first studies to investigate the role of the VP in EtOH reward was conducted by Melendez and colleagues [102]. This study evaluated the levels of extracellular DA within the VP following intraperitoneal administrations of EtOH. Two groups of Wistar rats were surgically implanted with bilateral microdialysis probes aimed at either the VP and the globus pallidus (GP) or the NAcc and the dorsal striatum (dSTR). EtOH (0.0–2.25 g/kg) produced a dose-dependent increase in extracellular DA in the VP but not the GP, with increases similar to those seen in the VP observed in both the NAcc and the dSTR following a 2.25-g/kg dose of EtOH (Fig. 14.3).

Melendez et al. [102] concluded that these data indicated that the mesopallidal system is more sensitive to the effects of EtOH than the nigropallidal. These data, together with results of the NAcc/dSTR portion of the study, suggest that the ventral regions of the striatopallidal complex are more sensitive to the effects of EtOH than the dorsal aspect. The sensitivity of these ventral circuits is in agreement with research that indicates this circuitry is important in mediating the rewarding effects of various drugs of abuse, including EtOH. Unfortunately, however, unlike the Carboni et al. study [48], the alcohol doses used in this study are exceptionally high, and it is not clear what their relevance to alcohol reward might be. As a result, these data should be interpreted with caution when making inferences to alcohol-rewarding effects.

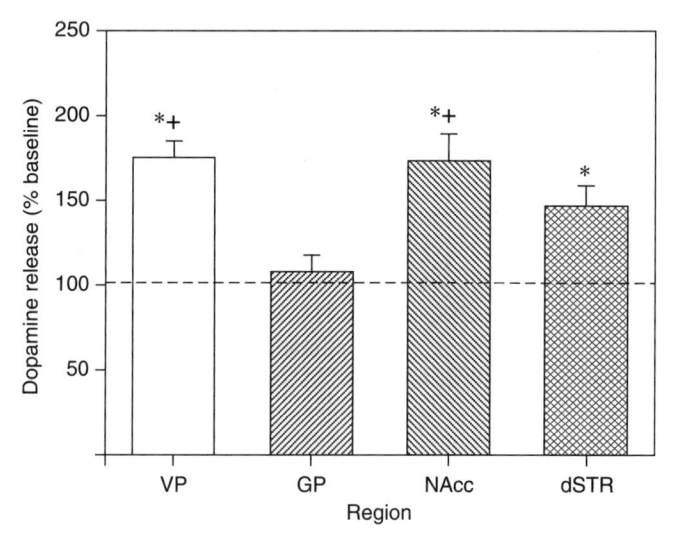

Figure 14.3 Time course effect of sterile saline or 15% (v/v) ethanol at doses of 0.75, 1.5, or 2.25 g/kg on extracellular levels of dopamine in VP and GP of Wistar rats. Values are expressed as percentage of baseline values and represent mean ± SEM. The i.p. administration of saline or 0.75 g/kg failed to significantly alter the extracellular levels of dopamine in either the VP or the GP ($p > 0.05$). (*) $p < 0.05$ as compared to saline (Dunnett's t); (+) $p < 0.05$ as compared to the GP [one-way analys of variance (ANOVA)]. Adapted from Melendez et al., 2003.

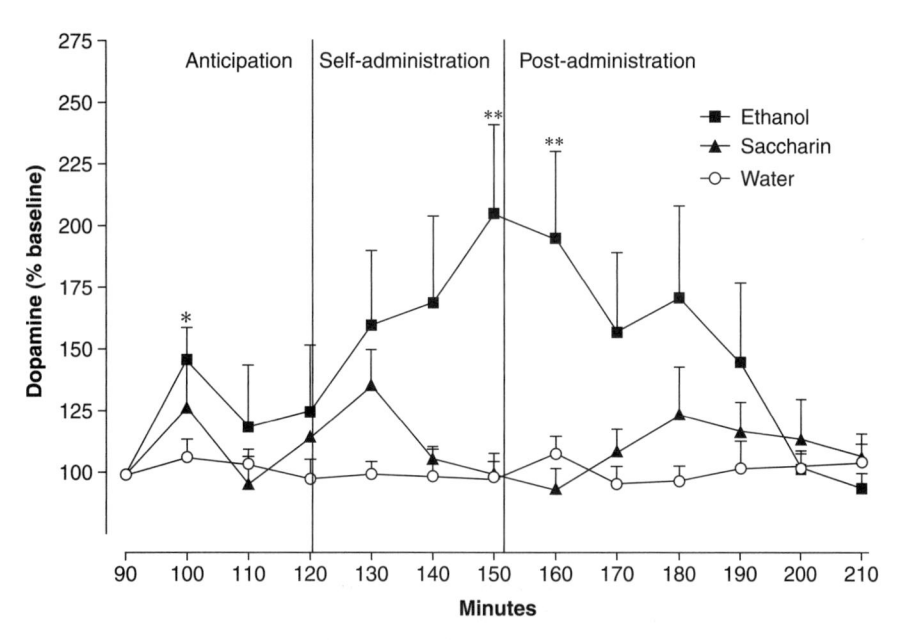

Figure 14.4 Extracellular levels of dopamine in VP of ethanol, saccharin, and water (control) groups expressed as percentage of baseline during anticipation, self-administration, and postadministration periods. Data are means ± SEM. Baseline dialysate levels of dopamine of ethanol, saccharin, and water groups were not significantly different (1.1 ± 0.1, 0.93 ± 0.2, and 0.85 ± 0.1 nM, respectively). (*) $p < 0.05$ compared with values for water; (**) $p < 0.05$ compared with values for water and saccharin with posthoc Tukey *b* test. Adapted from Melendez et al., 2004.

In 2004, Melendez and colleagues continued examining the role of the DA system within the VP on EtOH reward [56]. Female P rats, implanted with guide cannula into the VP, operantly self-administered EtOH, water, or saccharin during a microdialysis session divided into four discrete periods: habituation, anticipation, self-administration, and postadministration. While self-administration of saccharin or water had no effect on DA levels within the VP, the presentation of EtOH led to a marked increase in DA output in the anticipatory phase as well as increases throughout the self-administration phase, which decreased postadministration (see Fig. 14.4). Together, the data revealed that, as with intraperitoneal (i.p.) administration, self-administration of EtOH also led to significant increases in extracellular DA levels within the VP. These data further suggest a role of the VP in the anticipation of EtOH reward as well.

In their most recent study, Melendez and colleagues [26] assessed the effect of D_1 and D_2 DA receptor blockade within the VP on the intake of EtOH in a limited-access home cage paradigm employing similar extracellular DA measurement methods. P rats were separated into two groups and implanted with either bilateral guide cannula in the VP or a unilateral microdialysis probe aimed at the VP. Rats of the microinfusion group initiated EtOH intake during a 60-min limited-access paradigm following the microinjection of either the D_1 antagonist SCH 23390 or the D_2 antagonist sulpiride. Animals in the microdialysis group were evaluated for increases in extracellular DA levels following the reverse dialysis of either SCH 23390 or sulpiride.

In the limited-access/microinfusion portion of the experiment, only the highest tested dose of sulpiride (2.0 μg) was effective, producing an increase in intake. Interestingly, while only the highest dose of sulpiride (200 μM) led to an increase in extracellular DA with the VP, all tested doses (10–200 μM) of SCH 23390 were effective.

The data from the limited-access portion of this study suggest that D_2 receptors within the VP (that may be located on GABAergic neurons) play an important role in the regulation of EtOH reward. Evidence exists that such neurons exit from the VP and innervate the NAcc [103]. It is possible that the blockade of these receptors disinhibit the NAcc or perhaps other reward loci innervated by GABA neurons originating from within the VP. Data from the microdialysis portion of this study seem to support the hypothesis insofar as the minimal increase in extracellular DA suggests that the D_2 receptors within the VP are not acting as autoreceptors. This further strengthens the theory that the increase in intake following D_2 blockade is accomplished by non-dopaminergic neurons. Unlike the D_2 system, the D_1 receptor system within the VP appears to play only a minimal role in the regulation of EtOH reward. Reverse microdialysis of SCH 23390, however, led to significant increases in DA levels within the VP. This finding seems to imply the DA release within the VP is regulated in large part by a yet-undetermined D_1 receptor–mediated inhibitory feedback loop. These data also suggest that while EtOH is capable of increasing extracellular DA within the VP, such an increase fails to alter EtOH intake.

Recently, our laboratory also evaluated the effects of DA receptor blockade within the VP on the self-administration of EtOH [104]. For this study, P rats were implanted with bilateral guide cannula aimed at the VP and trained to operantly self-administer EtOH. SCH 23390 (1.0–40.0 μg) and the D_2-like selective receptor antagonist eticlopride (1.0–40.0 μg) were used for DA receptor blockade. The two highest doses of SCH 23390 (10.0, 40.0 μg) resulted in a marked reduction in lever pressing (Fig. 14.5a). These data implicate the D_1 receptor subtype in the mediation of EtOH, a finding that is somewhat contradictive to that seen in the 2005 Melendez study [26]. Similar to D_1 blockade, eticlopride also led to a reduction in EtOH responding when administered in high doses (20.0–40.0 μg) (Fig. 14.5b). However, when the 10.0-μg dose of eticlopride was microinfused into the VP, it produced a 41% increase in EtOH responding similar to the increases observed by Melendez and colleagues [26]. The overall findings from the research detailed above strongly implicate the VP as an important substrate in the regulation of EtOH self-administration. Microdialysis studies clearly demonstrate that EtOH, whether given via either i.p. injection or self-administration, readily increases DA release within the VP in a manner similar to that seen within the NAcc following exposure to EtOH (see [73]).

14.5.2.1 Hypothesized Mechanisms of Dopaminergic Regulation in Ventral Pallidum Regulating Alcohol-Motivated Behaviors. The precise mechanism(s) responsible for the increase in extracellular DA following EtOH are not clear. Several, hypotheses to explain this phenomenon have been proposed. Melendez et al. [102] suggested that the increased levels of DA within the VP may be higher than those of the GP due to differential sensitivity of the origins of the DA neurons that innervate them. In fact, the DA neurons within the VTA (which contains the cell bodies of the VP DA neurons) have been shown to be five times more sensitive to the effects of EtOH than

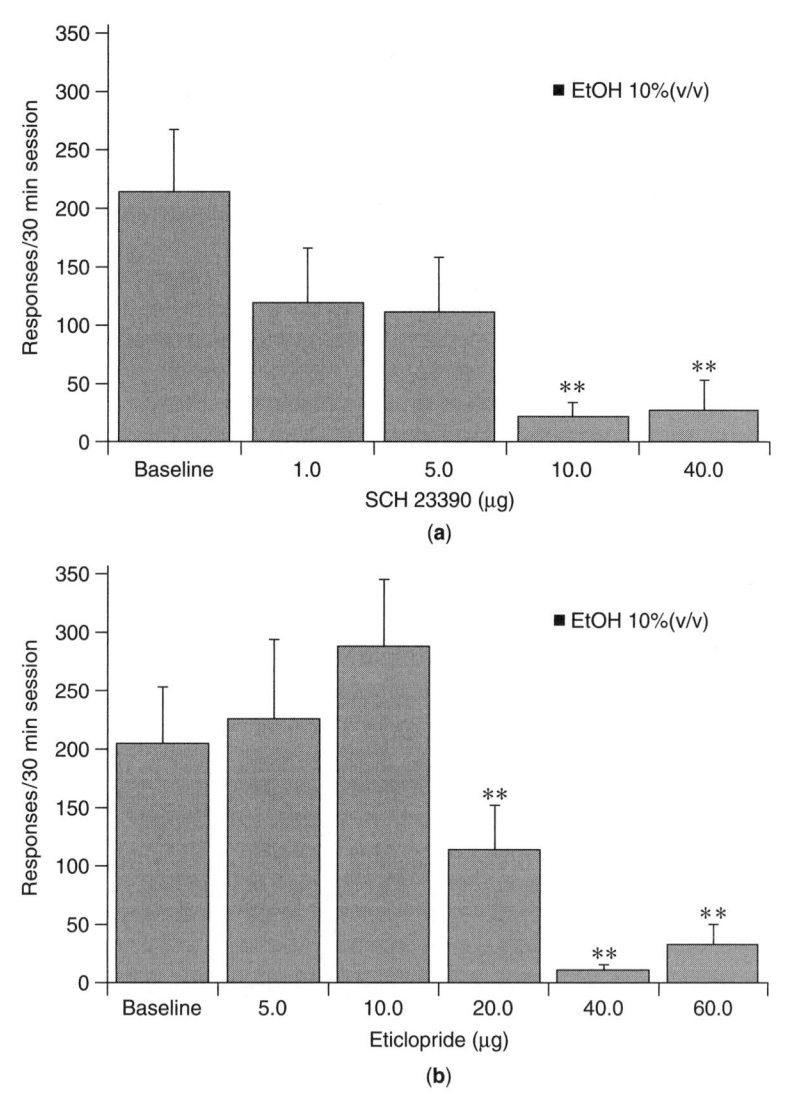

Figure 14.5 (a) Effects of SCH 23390 (1.0–40.0 μg) following bilateral injection in VP on responding maintained by EtOH (10% v/v). Data shown as mean ± SEM. (**) $p \leq 0.01$ SCH 23390 vs. baseline (noninfusion and saline infusion controls). (b) Effects of eticlopride (5.0–60.0 μg) following bilateral injection in VP on responding maintained by EtOH (10% v/v). Data shown as mean ± SEM. Adapted from Foster et al., 2002.

those found in the substantia nigra (SN), which innervates the GP [105]. The sensitivity of these neurons may ultimately be the result of GABAergic inhibition which is higher in the SN. It is also proposed that the differential sensitivity may be due to effects EtOH may have in the terminal fields, that is, that innervation from the striatum may affect the release of DA within the VP and GP. The majority of the striatopallidal neurons are GABAergic, and EtOH may act upon these neurons to regulate DA release. Blockade of both $GABA_A$ and $GABA_B$ receptors within the VP results in increases in extracellular DA within the VP [106]. Further, June and colleagues [19, 37] have previously established a role of $GABA_A$ receptors within the VP in the mediation of EtOH reward. It is also possible that a combination of these two factors could regulate EtOH-related VP DA increases.

The increases in EtOH intake observed by Melendez et al. [26] following D_2 blockade within the VP are compatible with the results seen in other studies involving the self-administration of EtOH [65], amphetamine [107], and cocaine [108]. It is hypothesized that the increase in responding observed is compensatory. Since blockade of the D_2 system may lower the reward efficacy of EtOH, in response the animals self-administer at higher rates in order to compensate for the reduced reinforcement. This hypothesis may be true for a partial blockade produced by lower doses of a D_2 antagonist; however, higher doses lead not to an increase in self-administration but to a decrease. It is possible that as more D_2 receptors are occupied, the reward value of self-administered EtOH reduces even further. While a partial blockade may result in compensatory increases in responding, a more complete blockade may produce such a robust reduction in reward value that the animals no longer possess the necessary motivation to self-administer the drug. As a potential mechanism, Melendez et al. [26] suggest that the D_2 receptors of the VP may reside presynaptically on efferent $GABA_A$ neurons. However, the neuromechanisms regulating these effects are not clearly understood.

Effects on EtOH self-administration produced by the D_1 antagonist SCH 23390 have led to contradictory findings. For example, Melendez [26] reported that while SCH 23390 produced a robust increase in extracellular DA levels within the VP, it had no effect on EtOH intake. However, the study conducted by Foster et al. [104] found that SCH 23390 produced profound reductions in EtOH responding. Melendez suggests that while D_1 blockade does produce profound elevations in DA release within the VP, these increases are not sufficient to influence EtOH drinking behavior. Similar increases within the NAcc also produce no change in EtOH intake [109]. While the DA increase seen following the doses administered in the Melendez study may be insufficient to influence EtOH self-administration, it may be possible that the higher doses used in the Foster study could produce DA levels within the VP that are elevated so that they begin to substitute for the EtOH, thus reducing responding. It is also important to note that the cellular localization of the D_1 receptors within the VP has yet to be determined. It is therefore possible that at higher doses a D_1 antagonist could activate or inhibit pathways that result in the reduction of EtOH reward through a variety of means while still producing increases in extracellular DA within the VP.

Research indicates that the mediation of EtOH reward clearly involves the DA system within the VP. Not only is EtOH capable of producing increases in extracellular DA release within the VP, it also produces anticipatory effects within the VP. Furthermore, both D_1 and D_2 DA receptor subtypes within the VP appear to regulate the reinforcing properties of EtOH, with the D_1 receptors producing a decrease in EtOH self-administration while the D_2 receptors produce biphasic effects with low doses leading to increases and higher doses nearly abolishing EtOH self-administration. Together, the studies presented above suggest that both the D_1 and D_2 receptor subtypes are implicated in the regulation of EtOH self-administration; however, it is clear that while their regulatory control within the VP may be overlapping, there are distinct regulators within the VP which differentiate the two receptors.

14.5.3 Lateral Hypothalamus

The LH, like other reward substrates, receives dopaminergic innervation directly from DA cell bodies located within the VTA as part of the mesencephalic pathway [86, 110, 111]. The LH also contains a number of DA receptors with a higher ratio of D_2 to D_1 receptors [112]. Historically, the DA system within the LH has been implicated in the inhibitory control of both food and water intake [84, 85, 113, 114] as well as inhibiting the locomotor processes associated with the procurement of food and water [115]. This tonic inhibition can be easily removed by local administration of the selective D_2-like antagonist sulpiride, leading to increases in feeding and drinking as well as psychomotor activation [114–116]. The increase in these behaviors, particularly the psychomotor activation, suggests that the LH is in some way involved in mediating the rewarding aspects of eating and drinking along with the initiation of consumptive behaviors that precede intake, as there is often a link sited between the increase in locomotor activity and drug reinforcement [117].

Reward is often associated with the increased release of DA, particularly in brain regions associated with the regulation of the reinforcing properties of various drugs of abuse. Thus, any area that may mediate release of DA into reward areas such as the NAcc may also play a role in the regulation of drug reinforcement. The LH may be one such area. Early studies revealed that electrical stimulation of the LH leads to increased levels of DA and its metabolites within the NAcc [83]. To further investigate the LH's control of DA release within the NAcc, Parada and colleagues [118] examined the effects the D_2 anatagonist sulpiride on the DA release within the NAcc. This study found that sulpiride injected directly into the LH led to a dose-dependent increase in DA release within the NAcc at the highest tested dose (Fig. 14.6). Moreover, this study demonstrated that the Sprague–Dawley rats used would lever press in an operant paradigm for direct infusion of sulpiride into the LH, demonstrating a strong link between increased DA release with the NAcc and the reward value of the D_2 antagonist sulpiride (Fig. 14.7). While the data above suggest that the LH is a prime candidate for a DA-mediated reward locus, research into its role in drug reward has been very limited.

June and his colleagues have examined the role of DA within the LH on the regulation of EtOH reward [119]. In this study, the effects of DA blockade using the D_1 antagonist SCH 23390 and the D_2-like receptor antagonist eticlopride were evaluated following bilateral infusion into the LH of P rats. Reinforcer specificity was determined by evaluation of the antagonist on sucrose-motivated responding. Neuroanatomical specificity in modulating alcohol- and sucrose-motivated behaviors was examined following bilateral injections of both SCH 23990 and eticlopride into the ventral thalamus. Figure 14.8b shows that eticlopride (1–40.0 µg) produced both a dose-related and profound reduction on responding maintained by alcohol. In contrast, Figure 14.8a shows that SCH 23990, the highly selective D_1 antagonist, did not alter alcohol responding (not shown are doses as high as 60 µg). Neither antagonist altered sucrose-maintained responding. Hence, eticlopride produces both reinforcer and neuroanatomical specificity in reducing alcohol drinking behaviors.

14.5.3.1 D_2 Dopaminergic Regulation of Alcohol-Motivated Behaviors in LH: Hypothesized Mechanisms.
The above findings provide compelling data suggesting that blockade of D_2 receptors within the LH leads to a profound reduction in the

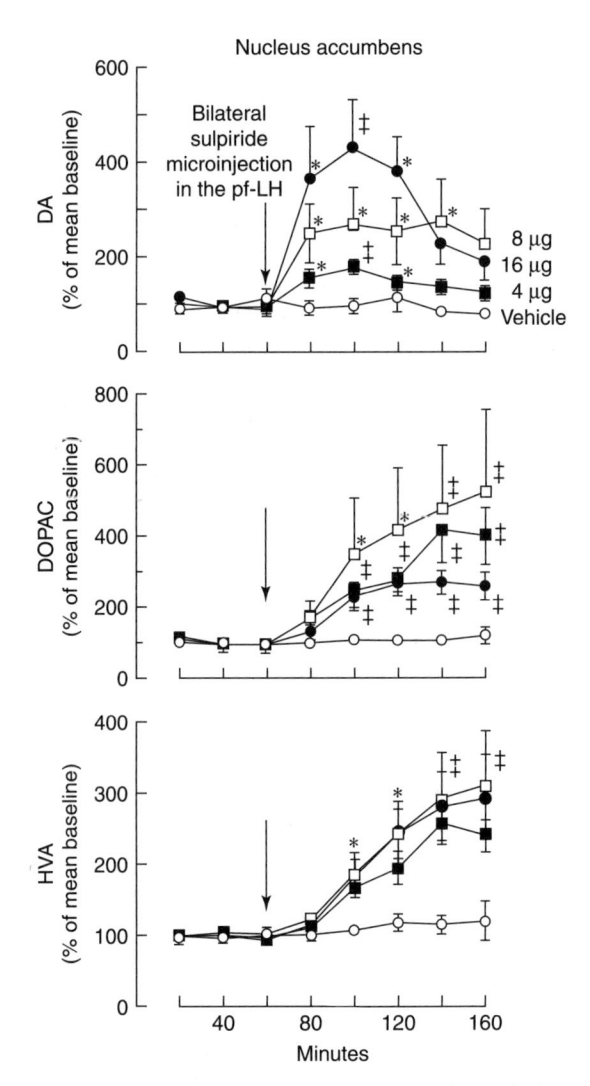

Figure 14.6 Sulpiride injected bilaterally in the prefrontal lateral hypothalamus (pf-LH) increases extracellular DA in NAcc. Curves show extracellular levels of DA (top graph), dihydroxyphenylacetic acid (DOPAC, middle graph), and HVA (bottom graph) in the right NAcc of rats receiving bilateral pf-LH microinjections of sulpiride (filled squares, 4 μg/0.3 μL; open squares, 8 μg/0.3 μL; filled circles, 16 μg/0.3 μL; open circles, 0.3 μL of vehicle). Arrows mark the time of the injection. Symbols indicate statistically significant differences between a data point and its corresponding preinjection level (*) $p<0.01$; ‡, $p<0.001$). Data represent the mean ± SE for four different animals at each dose. Adapted from Parada et al., 1995.

reward efficacy of EtOH. However, this decrease in reward value was not seen for sucrose following either D_1 or D_2 blockade, suggesting that its reward value may be mediated either by a different neurotransmitter system within the LH or in another substrate altogether. As seen with sucrose, D_1 blockade within the LH also failed to reduce responding for the EtOH solution.

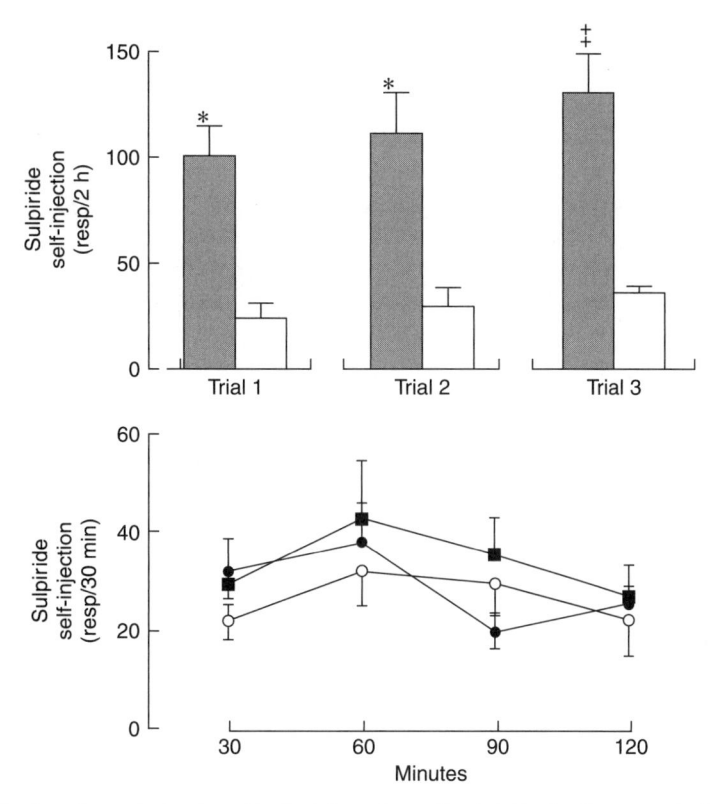

Figure 14.7 Intrahypothalamic self-administration of sulpiride in five rats during sessions (trials) on three different days. Each press of the active lever delivered a 2-s injection of 21.5 ± 1.28 nL of 10 ng/nL sulpiride. Presses on the blank lever were recorded but they did not have any contingent value. Top graph: response frequency on the active lever (filled columns) and the blank lever (open columns) during each session. Symbols indicate significant differences between responses on the active and blank levers (*) $p < 0.01$; ‡, $p < 0.001$). Bottom graph: response frequency on the active lever was consistent in all four 30-min periods during the first (open circles), second (filled circles), and third (filled squares) trials on three different days. Adapted from Parada et al., 1995.

As demonstrated above, the D_1 system produced no change in either EtOH or sucrose responding; however, the absence of effects seen with SCH 23390 may be readily explained. Thus, the LH possesses only a limited number of D_1 receptors [112]. These low numbers may render the D_1 system within the LH ineffective in mediating reinforcement resulting in minimal change in EtOH and sucrose response rates.

While the effects of the D_2 blockade on EtOH self-administration are quite clear, determining the mechanism responsible for this reduction is far more difficult. Nonetheless, plausible explanations are possible. One possible explanation may center around the increased release of accumbal DA previously observed following LH D_2 blockade. As discussed above, D_2 blockade within the LH has been shown to result in increased DA release within the NAcc. This would suggest that such a blockade might in fact increase the reward value of EtOH insofar as increases in

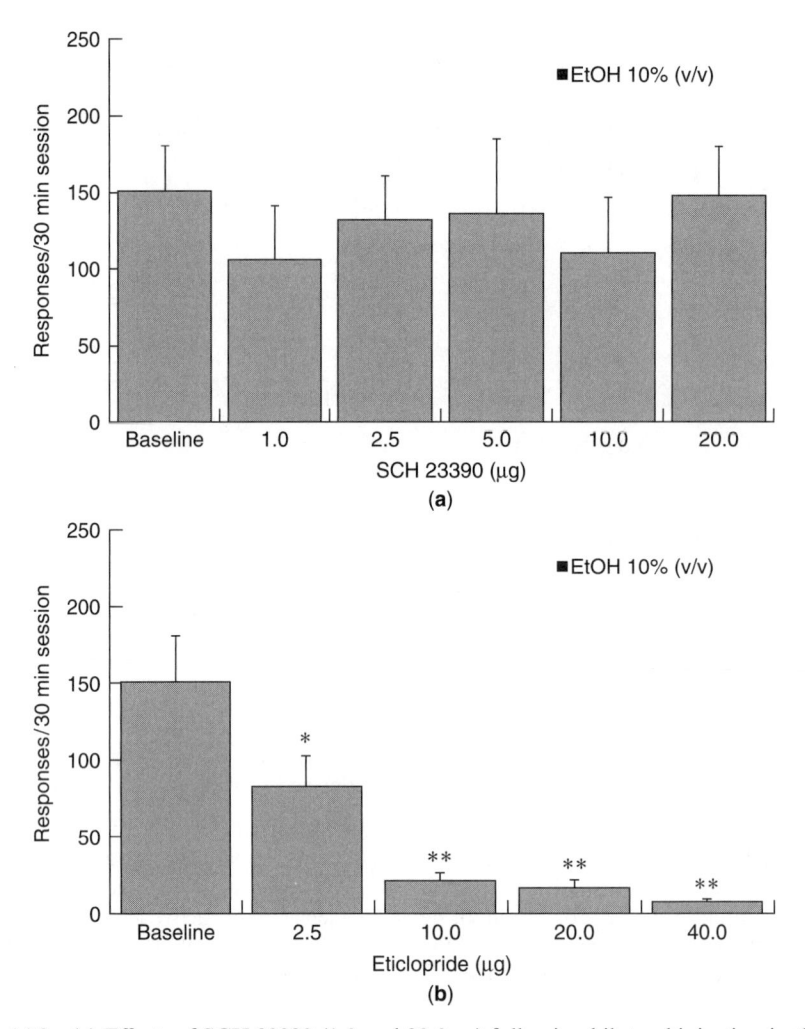

Figure 14.8 (a) Effects of SCH 23390 (1.0 and 20.0 μg) following bilateral injection in the LH on responding maintained by EtOH (10% v/v). Data are shown as mean ± SEM (**) $p < 0.01$ SCH 23390 vs. baseline (noninfusion and saline infusion controls). (b) Effects of eticlopride (2.5–20.0 μg) following bilateral injection in the LH on responding maintained by EtOH (10% v/v). Data shown as mean ± SEM. Adapted from Goergen et al., 2003.

accumbal DA often denote reward efficacy. However, this assumes that the increase in accumbal DA release seen following EtOH self-administration (see [73]) produces an additive effect with the increase in DA release seen with D_2 blockade within the LH [118]. Alternatively, the increased DA release in the NAcc following D_2 blockade within the LH may serve to substitute for the DA release typically seen following EtOH administration. Such a substitution would, in theory, lower the reward value of EtOH resulting in a lowered desire to "work" for the EtOH. This hypothesis, however, fails to explain the effect seen on sucrose consumption. An increase in sucrose responding is expected, because D_2 blockade increases drinking behavior

[114–116]. However, no appreciable change in responding is seen following LH D_2 blockade. It is possible that while the D_2 blockade leads to increased consumptive behaviors, it may not be sufficient to increase the motivation necessary to respond for the sucrose in a self-administration paradigm.

While further research is necessary to identify the mechanisms by which the D_2 antagonist eticlopride reduces EtOH self-administration, it is clear that the D_2 system within the LH strongly regulates the reinforcing properties of EtOH. Indeed, the LH's strong ties to the regulation of the consumptive behaviors of feeding and drinking make it an important site for further EtOH research as alcohol intake can be classified as a drinking behavior. In addition, its clear ability to modulate DA levels within the NAcc may further establish the LH as an important dompaminoceptive substrate regulating not only EtOH reward but also the rewarding properties of various drugs of abuse.

14.5.4 Summary

The neurocircuitry and mechanisms that mediate the propensity to consume EtOH are complex. The focus in EtOH research thus far has clearly been on the DA system of the mesolimbic pathway, particularly the interaction of the NAcc and the VTA. However, evidence has begun to emerge that may shift the focus from the DA system within the NAcc to other substrates that are innervated by DA neurons arising from the VTA DA cell bodies. The purpose of this section has been to describe novel DA substrates that may be involved in the regulation of EtOH reward. To this end, studies involving three DA-innervated substrates—the BST, VP, and LH—were described in the hopes that future research may involve not only the investigation of the NAcc in EtOH reward but also other dopaminoceptive brain loci.

Increases in extracellular DA within the NAcc have been observed in a number of studies following the delivery of EtOH through various routes of administration (see [51]). In fact, it has been generally accepted that an increase in extracellular DA following administration is one way to classify a drug as reinforcing. As demonstrated in the studies reviewed above, EtOH administration is capable of inducing elevated extracellular DA levels in the BST and VP. Intraperitoneally administered EtOH at doses that induce euphoric effects has been shown to increase DA release within the BST [48]. A number of studies of DA release in the VP have been conducted by Melendez and colleagues demonstrating that extracellular DA levels increase within the VP following not only i.p. administration but also self-administration in both operant and limited-access paradigms [26, 56, 102]. This group also observed an increase in DA levels following the reverse microdialysis of the D_1 antagonist SCH [26]. While there are no reports of an increase in extracellular DA within the LH, D_2 blockade within the LH is sufficient to produce increases in NAcc DA levels [118]. Although this is not direct evidence that EtOH can influence DA within the LH, it does show that the LH can effectively modulate DA within a substrate shown to regulate EtOH reward.

While the evaluation of extracellular DA is important in establishing a role of a DA system within a substrate in EtOH reinforcement, it does not provide evidence that the substrate can regulate EtOH reinforcement. One method of determining a more direct regulatory role of DA within a brain structure is via use of DA agonists or antagonists. Using these selective DA agents, it was found that the blockade of the D_1 system within the BST led to robust reductions in EtOH responding with no effect seen with D_2 blockade; therefore, EtOH reinforcement is regulated by D_1 receptor subtypes within the BST [42]. Melendez administered D_1 and D_2 antagonists within the VP via reverse microdialysis and found that the D_1 system had no effect on EtOH reward while blockade of the D_2 system produced increases in intake, suggesting that EtOH reward is mediated by the D_2 receptors within the VP [26]. Different results were seen following microinjection of D_1 and D_2 antagonists into the VP. Using an operant self-administration paradigm, Foster et al. [104] found increases in intake similar to those observed by Melendez, but only at low doses. In contrast, high doses of the D_2 antagonist eticlopride produced robust reductions in EtOH responding. Similar reductions were also observed following the administration of high doses of the D_1 antagonist SCH 23390. These data suggest that EtOH reinforcement may be regulated in a biphasic fashion by D_2 receptors within the VP along with D_1 mediation of reward [104]. The D_2 system also seems to be the regulator of DA reward within the LH. Blockade of the D_2 receptors within the LH led to robust reductions in EtOH responding in a self-administration paradigm [119]. These data demonstrate that while the DA systems in various substrates may mediate EtOH reward efficacy, they do so by the use of differential activation of the D_1 and/or D_2 receptor subtypes.

While the studies discussed in this section detail research on DA's control of EtOH reinforcement in novel substrates, it is important not to discount possible interactions between the DA systems of these brain regions and other neurotransmitter systems. In fact, other studies demonstrate that GABAergic systems can lead to modulation of the effects produced by DA antagonism in both the BST and VP (Eiler et al., unpublished; see also [104]). It is thought that the mechanism of action driving DA regulation of EtOH reinforcement is not simply altering/modulating DA release within key dompaminoceptive loci but is the result of complex interactions between DA and GABA pathways. Clearly, DA interacts with other neuronal systems such as neuropeptides and glutamate [52]. In short, the elucidation of novel DA substrates regulating EtOH reward provides investigators with new challenges in determining the neurocircuitry that mediates EtOH reinforcement.

In summary, evaluating only DA neuroanatomical substrates and systems within the mesolimbic and extended amygdala pathways may limit our understanding of how the complex interactions within these pathways function to control EtOH-reinforced behaviors. Moreover, it is now clear from the work of both Rassnick et al. [78] and Myers and Quarfordt [120] that removal of the mesolimbic DA system does not alter established EtOH self-administration [121]. As such, other neurotransmitters may be differentially involved in various aspects of the reinforcement process. Since it is likely that EtOH-motivated behaviors are mediated by multiple neurochemical systems, the fundamental neuropharmacological information provided by the study of overlapping neuronal systems is essential to understanding the neural processes that regulate EtOH self-administration. In this review, we describe recent studies evaluating the significance of $GABA_A$ receptors in EtOH-seeking behaviors. These studies have advanced our understanding of the neural mechanisms regulating alcohol drinking. Exploitation of compounds selective for specific $GABA_A$ receptor-containing subunits has now led to novel prototype ligands that may have clinical utility in the treatment of alcohol dependence.

14.6 MOLECULAR BIOLOGY OF THE GABA$_A$ BDZ RECEPTOR

GABA is the most abundant inhibitory neurotransmitter present in the mammalian brain. Although there are, to date, at least three unique classes of GABA receptors, the majority of neurobehavioral research on alcoholism has centered on GABA$_A$ receptors, referred to as the GABA$_A$ benzodiazepine (BDZ) receptor complex. This complex has been characterized as a pentameric structure comprised of at least 16 identifiable subunits (α_{1-6}, β_{1-4}, γ_{1-3}, δ, ρ, and ε) in the mammalian CNS [122]. Identifying the various receptor subunits and their function has become increasingly important to gain an understanding of the neurobiological base of alcoholism and treatment target identification. The GABA "system" has been suggested to be the best candidate for a "single" neurotransmitter in regulating the neurobehavioral effects of alcohol [123–125]. Specifically, these effects include alcohol-motivated behaviors [1, 18, 19] as well as the motor-impairing, sedative [28, 124] and anxiolytic [28, 126, 127] properties of alcohol. Here, the neuropharmacological, neuroanatomical, and molecular biological underpinnings of alcohol-motivated behaviors/self-administration are reviewed. The role of the GABA system in other neurobehavioral actions of alcohol has been reviewed elsewhere [124, 128].

14.6.1 Commonalities of Alcohol and Modulators of the GABA$_A$ BDZ Systems

EtOH shares many common behavioral properties with BDZs and barbiturates (e.g., sedation, ataxia, anxiolysis). Similar to BDZs and barbiturates, EtOH potentiates GABA-stimulated Cl$^-$ flux (for a review see [129]). Hence, it has been postulated that EtOH's action at the level of the GABA-coupled Cl$^-$ ion channel may underlie many of its behavioral properties [130–132]. The effects of EtOH are thought to be selective for GABA$_A$ receptors since they are antagonized by negative modulators of GABAergic activity such as BDZ inverse agonists, the GABA$_A$ receptor antagonist bicuculline, and the Cl$^-$ channel blocker picrotoxin [133]. Further, manipulations of central GABAergic activity alters many of the behavioral and physiological effects of EtOH [126, 132, 134, 135], including reinforcement ([78, 136]; also, for a recent review see [19]). Hence, the allosteric modulatory properties of the GABA$_A$ BDZ receptor complex, which allows for neuropharmacological enhancement and reduction of GABAergic function, provides a vehicle to exploit the GABA system to evaluate its significance in regulating alcohol drinking behaviors. Indeed, this neurobehavioral strategy was first demonstrated in the highly cited paper by Suzdak et al. [132] using the partial BDZ inverse agonist RO15-4513. In addition, this neuropharmacological exploitation of the GABA system has been catalyzed by the rapid advances in molecular biology that have resulted in the cloning of key GABA$_A$ receptor subunits [137–140], resulting in knowledge of the heterogeneity and distribution of these receptors [141–143]. For example, substantial research has shown that both the affinities and efficacies of drugs acting at this family of ligand-gated ion channels appear to be defined by subunit composition [137, 144, 145].

The impact of subunit composition on drug action at both recombinant and wild-type GABA$_A$ receptors is best characterized by the chemically diverse class of compounds referred to as the BDZ receptor site ligands [137, 140]. Studies in recombinant GABA$_A$ receptors have shown that the α subunit is the primary determinant of ligand affinity, while the γ subunit affects affinity of a more circumscribed class of compounds, but can dramatically alter ligand efficacy [139, 144–146]. Hence, knowledge of both the affinity and efficacy of BDZ site ligands has permitted the design/development of pharmacological probes to manipulate the GABA BDZ receptor complex to determine the neuromechanism(s) of action of alcohol drinking behaviors. In addition, the development of these ligands has also provided the opportunity to explore and make inferences about the role GABA systems may play in regulating alcohol drinking behaviors (see below).

14.6.2 GABA$_A$ BDZ Modulation of EtOH Self-Administration: Studies Using Systematic Application of Probes

Substantial evidence now suggests that GABA$_A$ receptor–mediated neurotransmission within the mesocorticolimbic system plays a prominent role in regulating EtOH-motivated behaviors (for a recent review see [19]). Early work demonstrated that GABAmimetics decreased voluntary EtOH intake [147–149], while agents like pentobarbital [150] and diazepam [151] were observed to increase EtOH consumption. In addition, subsequent studies by Amit and his colleagues [152, 153] demonstrated that systemically administered tetrahydroisoxazolopyridino (THIP), a GABA agonist, enhances EtOH intake during a 24-h interval. Bretazenil, a partial agonist, has also been observed to increase EtOH intake in AA alcohol-preferring rats [154]. Studies evaluating the role of increased GABA transmission on EtOH-motivated behaviors in the operant chamber, however, have generally resulted in equivocal results on the one hand or no effects on the other. Specifically, Samson and Grant [33], using a concurrent schedule procedure, demonstrated that chlordiazepoxide (CDZ) generally reduced EtOH responding and intake. Rassnick and her colleagues [78] were not able to demonstrate any reliable increases or decreases in EtOH with P and alcohol-non preferring (NP) rats following CDZ (2.5–10 mg/kg) administration. However, using a modified sucrose-fading procedure, Petry [155] demonstrated that low CDZ doses (1–4 mg/kg) significantly and selectively increased EtOH responding, while higher doses (10–20 mg) decreased EtOH responding. In contrast to the equivocal findings evaluating the role of increasing GABA transmission on EtOH self-administration, systemic administration of BDZ inverse agonists [e.g., RO15-4513, FG 7142, methyl-6,7-dimethoxy-4-ethyl-beta-carboline-3-carboxylate (DMCM)] have been consistently reported to reduce EtOH consumption under a variety of self-administration paradigms (for reviews see [156, 157]). For example, RO15-4513 has generally been reported to dose dependently and selectively suppress EtOH intake [7, 156, 158] and responding [78, 159, 160].

Because of the demonstrated selectivity of RO15-4513 in reducing alcohol intake, subsequent work focused on RO19-4603, a related BDZ inverse agonist with a unique pharmacological profile [20, 161]. Unlike RO15-4513, RO19-4603 is an imidazothienodiazepine derivative of RO15-3505 (samazenil), with exceptionally high binding affinity ($K_i = 0.2$ nM) [162]. Figures 14.9a and b show data for P rats ($N = 10$) which initiated EtOH-reinforced responding using a modification of the sucrose-fading procedure under a concurrent FR4 operant schedule for days 1 and 2. RO19-4603 (0.0045–0.3 mg/kg, i.p.) was given 5 min prior to day 1 only. RO19-4603 reduced response-contingent EtOH intake by as much as 97% of controls on day 1, and responding continued to be reduced 24 h post–drug administration by as much as 85% of controls on day 2. CGS 8216, a specific BDZ antagonist, significantly attenuated the RO19-4603 reduction on day 1 and completely reversed the effects on

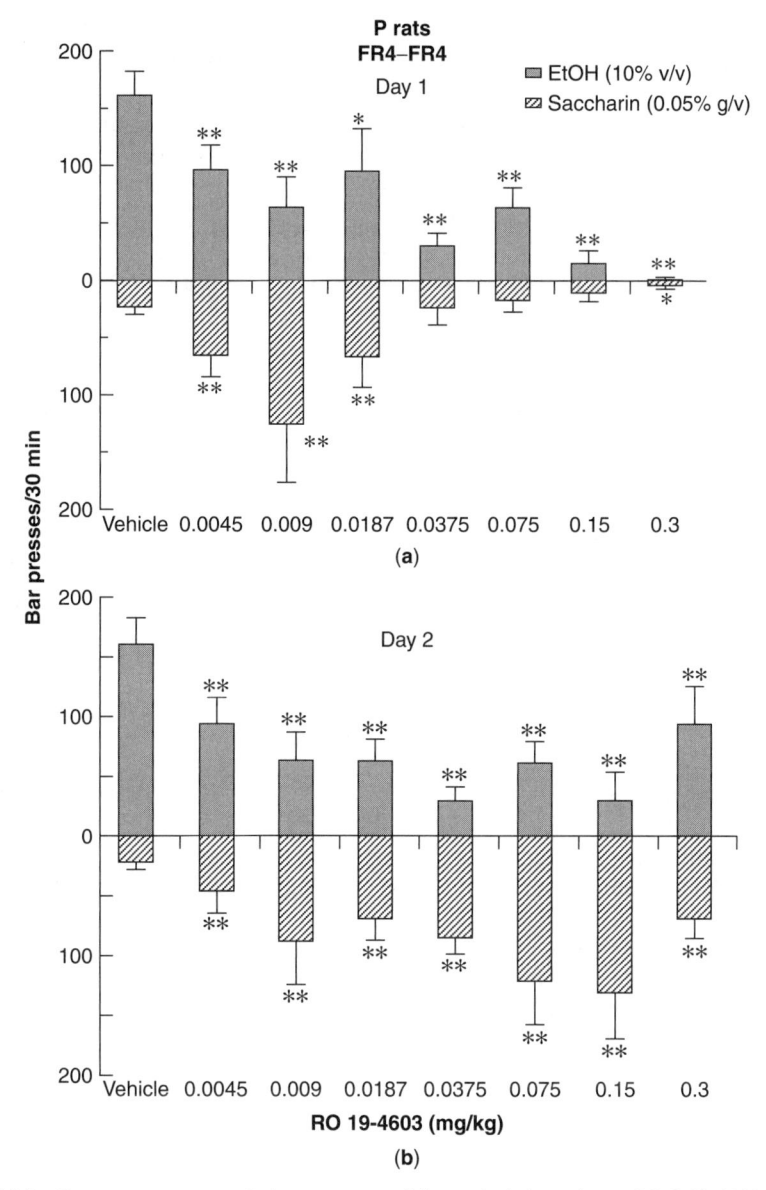

Figure 14.9 Dose–response and time course of i.p. administration of RO19-4603 (0.0045, 0.009, 0.0187, 0.0375, 0.075, 0.15, 0.3 mg/kg) and vehicle given acutely on day 1 (a) and 24 h post–drug administration day 2 (b) on EtOH-reinforced (10% v/v) responding and saccharin-reinforced (0.05% g/v) responding. The RO19-4603 injections were given 5 min prior to test session on day 1 only. RO19-4603 suppressed EtOH–reinforced responding, while the 0.0045-, 0.009-, and 0.0187-mg/kg doses elevated saccharin-reinforced responding on day 1. Day 2 showed suppression of EtOH-reinforced responding and parallel increases of saccharin-reinforced responding for each of the seven doses of RO19-4603. (*) $p < 0.05$ and (**) $p < 0.01$ vs. control vehicle values by ANOVA and post hoc Newman–Keuls test at a corresponding day. Adapted from June et al., 1998.

day 2. Thus, the effects of RO19-4603 may be mediated at the BDZ binding site of the $GABA_A$ BDZ receptor complex. The degree of selectivity of RO19-4603 on EtOH responding, however, could not adequately be determined from this study, primarily because EtOH and saccharin responding were not equated at basal levels; however, analyses of the cumulative records revealed that RO19-4603 produced a dose-dependent decrease in the slope of the cumulative record for EtOH responding while concomitantly producing a dose-dependent increase in the slope for saccharin responding (see Fig. 14.10). Thus, the actions of RO19-4603 "appear" to be mediated via recognition sites at $GABA_A$ BDZ receptors which regulate EtOH reinforcement, and not mechanisms regulating general ingestive behaviors.

In the evaluation of BDZ ligands for their effectiveness to attenuate EtOH responding, June and colleagues have determined if qualitative (i.e., imidazobenzo-diazepinc-selective) and quantitative (affinity for diazepam insensitive (DI) sites; see [144, 162a]) differences exist in a compound's ability to decrease EtOH responding (see [28]). RU 34000 is a novel imidazopyrimidine inverse agonist with relatively low affinity at BDZ receptors ($K_i \sim 0.98\,\mu M$) [163] and little affinity at DI sites [164]. Pharmacokinetic analyses, however, have shown that this low affinity is compensated for by the high drug levels of RU 34000 in the brain (10 µg/mL) [165]. RU 34000 was an effective antagonist of EtOH responding via the i.p. route. Effects on saccharin responding were seen only with the highest i.p. dose (5 mg/kg). Flumazenil (6 mg/kg, i.p.) completely attenuated the RU 34000 reduction of EtOH responding (data not shown), suggesting that the actions of RU 34000 may be mediated at central BDZ sites. The data with RU 34000 allow several interpretations: First, in addition to the affinity of BDZ ligands at active CNS sites, their bioavailability is an important factor in their capacity to function as EtOH antagonists; second, the capacity of BDZ ligands to function as effective EtOH antagonists is not specific to imidazobenzo-diazepines; and third, it is likely that the DI $GABA_A$ receptors (i.e., those receptors either an α_4 or α_6 subunit) may not be a critical factor regulating EtOH-maintained responding.

Work with several BDZ antagonists has also revealed some interesting findings using operant methodology [166]. Figure 14.11 shows that unlike the prototypic BDZ antagonist RO15-1788 (flumazenil), the pyrazoloquinoline CGS 8216 (1–20 mg) and the β-carboline antagonist ZK 93426 (5–50 mg/kg) produce marked suppressant effects on EtOH responding [166, 167]. Further, 24 h post–drug administration, nonsignificant effects were seen with the lower doses and significant effects with some of the higher doses of these agents [see 161, 168]. It should be noted that, like flumazenil, both ZK 93426 and CGS 8216 are well tolerated in human subjects [169, 170], and it is possible that these agents may have some capacity to reduce EtOH drinking in humans. The exact mechanism by which BDZ antagonists reduce EtOH drinking is not clear. Mild agonist effects for ZK 93426 have also been reported in vivo in rats [171] and humans [172]. In rats, CGS 8216 produces weak to moderate anxiogenic effects, resembling a weak partial inverse agonist [173]. Moderate to strong agonist effects, however, have been consistently reported in vitro in the *Xenous* oocyte assay for ZK 93426 [18, 37] (see below). Thus, one possible interpretation of the antagonism of EtOH drinking by ZK 93426 and CGS 8216 is that a "BDZ agonist–like ligand" substitutes for the reinforcing actions of EtOH [78], as has been reported with DA agonists in blocking the reinforcing properties of EtOH (cf. [17]). Nevertheless, because of the potential clinical applications of BDZ antagonists,

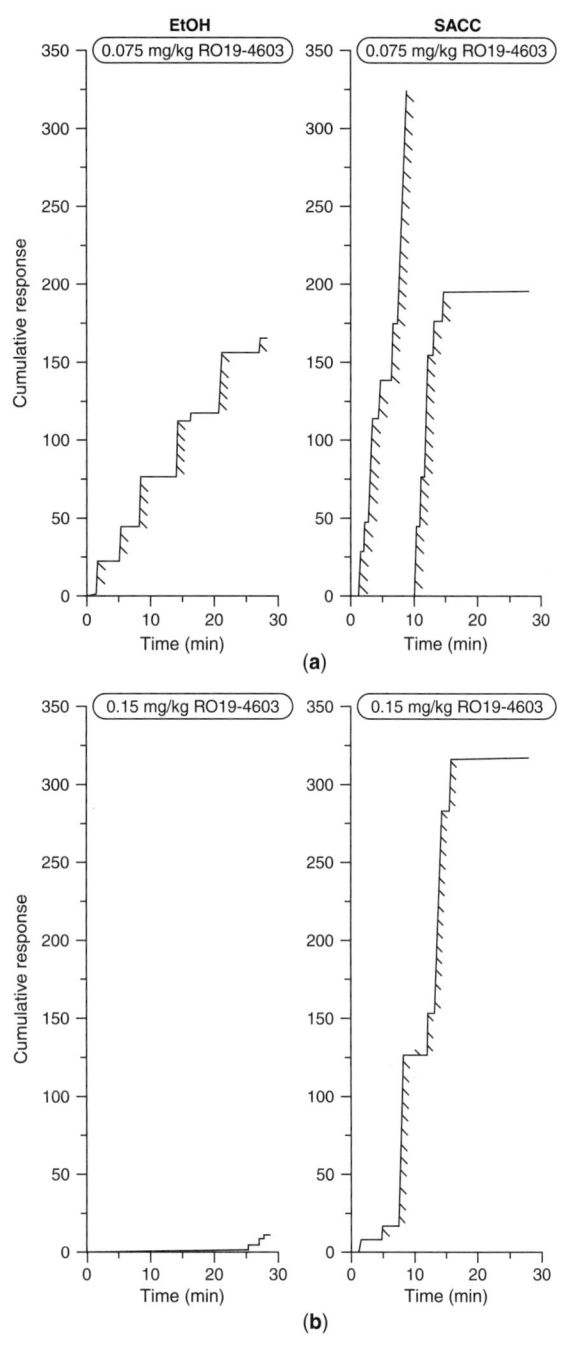

Figure 14.10 Sample cumulative dose–response records for EtOH (10% v/v) and saccharin (0.05% g/v) responding in two additional P rats during a concurrent schedule (FR4–FR4) following 0.075 mg/kg of RO19-4603 (a) (upper panel) or 0.15 mg/kg of RO19-4603 (b) (lower panel). Cross-hatch equals delivery of reinforcer, while the slope of lines indicate response per rate per minute. Adapted from June et al., 1998.

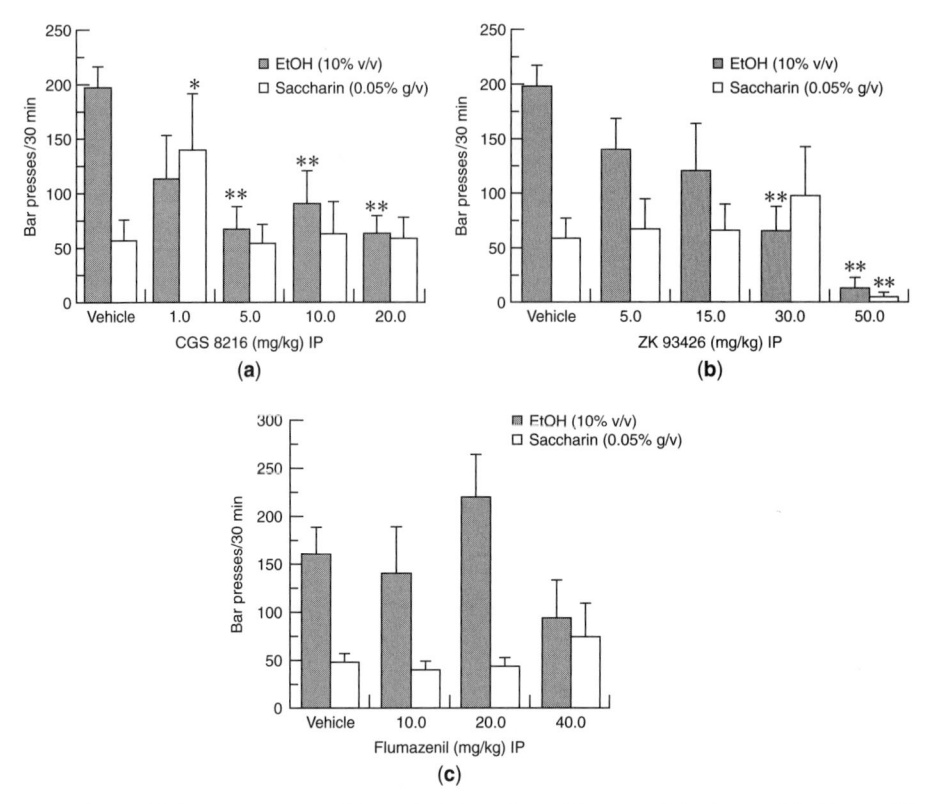

Figure 14.11 (a) Dose–response of i.p. administration of flumazenil in doses of 0 (Tween-80), 10, 20, and 40 mg/kg on responding maintained by EtOH (10% v/v) and saccharin (0.05% g/v) (FR4-FR4). The flumazenil injections were given 20 min before the test sessions ($n = 10$). (b) Dose–response and time course of i.p. administration of CGS 8216 (1, 5, 10, and 20 mg/kg) and vehicle on responding maintained by EtOH (10% v/v) and saccharin (0.05% g/v) (FR4-FR4). The CGS 8216 injections were administered 20 min before the test session. (c) Dose–response and time course of i.p. administration of ZK 93426 (5, 15, 30, and 50 mg/kg) and vehicle on responding maintained by EtOH (10% v/v) and saccharin (0.05% g/v) (FR4-FR4). The ZK 93426 injections were administered 20 min before the test session. (*) $p < 0.05$ and (**) $p < 0.01$ vs. control vehicle values by ANOVA and post hoc Newman–Keuls testing at a corresponding day ($n = 10$). Adapted from June et al., 1998.

additional studies are warranted to further understand the mechanism by which they decrease EtOH reinforcement. Another hypothesis regarding the capacity of BDZ antagonists to attenuate alcohol intake is that because they "generally" do not result in a functional increase or decrease in GABAergic activity, it is possible that their effects on EtOH responding are likely due to their binding at various $GABA_A$-containing receptor subunits [19, 166].

14.6.2.1 Significance of Systemic Studies. Systemic administration of RO19-4603 produced clear dose-related reductions on EtOH-maintained responding. Compared with other inverse agonists [e.g., RU 34000, Samazenil, ethyl beta-carboline-3 carboxylate (βCCE), RO15-4513], RO19-4603 was considerably more potent, selective, and long lasting in reducing EtOH-maintained responding. Cumulative dose-response profiles revealed that RO19-4603's actions on EtOH responding appear to be mediated via recognition sites on the $GABA_A$/BDZ receptor complex which regulate EtOH reinforcement, and not via mechanisms regulating ingestive behaviors in general (see Fig. 14.9). Moreover, the prolonged effects of RO19-4603 on EtOH self-administration was also observed in outbred rats for at least 48 h after a single administration [174], suggesting that these effects are not specific to the P rat line. Attenuation of the RO19-4603-induced suppression on days 1 and 2 by a high-affinity, competitive BDZ antagonist suggests that this effect on EtOH-maintained responding is mediated at the BDZ component of the $GABA_A$/BDZ receptor complex. Thus, RO19-4603 may be the ideal pharmacological tool to microinject into novel CNS sites to evaluate the role of GABAergic neurotransmission in EtOH reinforcement.

The demonstration that selected BDZ antagonists can blunt the reinforcing properties of EtOH suggests a direct role for the BDZ binding site on the $GABA_A$ BDZ receptor complex in EtOH-seeking behavior. The precise mechanisms by which BDZ antagonists reduce EtOH drinking, however, are not clear, primarily because these studies employed systemic injections. Using the microinjection technique, however, it may be possible to more precisely delineate the neurobiological mechanism(s) in regulating EtOH reinforcement, particularly in a well-characterized model of EtOH-seeking behavior (e.g., P and HAD rats). Finally, because "neutral competitive" BDZ ligands produce few untoward effects in animals and humans ([169, 170] see [166]), they represent excellent pharmacological tools to explore the neurobiology of alcohol reinforcement. A review of the literature on BDZ competitive ligands (see [169, 170]) also shows that neither ZK 93426 nor CGS 8216 produces untoward effects in humans, further supporting the utility of its use in alcohol drinking studies.

14.6.3 Site-Specific Microinjection Studies: Manipulation of $GABA_A$ BDZ Receptor Complex in Modifying EtOH Self-Administration

Little is known about the neurochemical and neuroanatomical substrates via which manipulation of the $GABA_A$ BDZ receptor complex can modify EtOH self-administration within the mesolimbic/mesoaccumbens system. The initial paper to appear in the published literature [55] examined the role of $GABA_A$ receptors in the extended amygdala on EtOH-reinforced responding in outbred rats. As noted previously, the extended amygdala comprises the central nucleus of the amygdala, the bed nucleus of the stria terminalis and the shell of the NAcc, and the sublenticular SI [175]. Animals were trained to initiate EtOH intake using the saccharin-fading procedure. The effects of bilateral microinjections of the competitive $GABA_A$ receptor antagonist SR 95531 were evaluated in three of these brain loci. SR 95531 injected in the bed nucleus of the stria terminalis reduced responding for EtOH with the 8- and 16-ng doses, while only a 16-ng dose produced a significant effect in the shell of the NAcc. However, injections into the bed nucleus of the stria terminalis and the NAcc suppressed both EtOH and water responding at the highest doses during the initial part of the drinking session. Intra-amygdaloid injections did not disrupt the initiation of responding. These findings suggested that the $GABA_A$ receptors in the extended amygdala may be involved in the mediation of some aspects of EtOH reinforcement. Hyytiä and Koob [55] contend the differential sensitivity of the central amygdala, bed nucleus, and shell of the NAcc may result from differences in density of GABAergic neurons. Indeed, the NAcc contains fewer GABAergic neurons than the bed nucleus of the stria terminalis or the central amygdala [88]. It is important to note, however, that reinforcer specificity could not accurately be determined in that study because rats responded for a (nonpalatable) water solution and responding for the water solution was so low as to confound ready interpretation.

GABAergic manipulations within the mesocorticolimbic DA systems have been investigated primarily with the $GABA_A$ agonist muscimol and the $GABA_A$ antagonist bicuculline. Hodge et al. [176] hypothesized that since local infusions of muscimol into the VTA had been previously shown to increase DA in the NAcc [177], it was possible that such interactions could modulate (directly or indirectly) EtOH-reinforced responding. Hodge et al. [176] evaluated the effects of bilateral microinjections of muscimol (1–30 ng) and bicuculline (1–10 ng) in the NAcc of outbred rats after they were trained under the sucrose-fading procedure. The 10- and 30-ng doses of muscimol significantly decreased EtOH responding. Similarly, the 3- and 10-ng doses of bicuculline also reduced responding. When a dose of bicuculline (1 ng, a dose that had no effect on EtOH given alone) was coadministered with muscimol, it attenuated the muscimol-induced decrease in EtOH responding. Together, these findings suggested that the effects seen with muscimol were mediated by activity at $GABA_A$ receptors and that GABAergic transmission in the NAcc is involved in EtOH reinforcement, possibly via inhibition of DA function [176]. In a subsequent study, these same researchers [178], employing similar methods, evaluated in the VTA the effects of bilateral infusions of higher doses of muscimol (10, 30, and 100 ng) on EtOH (10%, v/v) and sucrose (75%, w/v) responding in separate groups of rats. The results showed that muscimol (10 ng) increased the number of sucrose responses but had no effect on the total number of EtOH responses. However, the 30-ng dose shifted the response pattern of both groups from high initial rates with early termination to slow initial rates with delayed termination, suggesting nonspecific effects. Nevertheless, taken together, these data suggest that muscimol differentially alters EtOH and sucrose responding via GABAergic mechanisms within the VTA, in that EtOH reinforcement is less sensitive to GABAergic manipulation compared with sucrose responding. These investigators employed a very high sucrose concentration in the VTA study; hence, the efficacy of the alcohol and sucrose is very difficult to equate, particularly in outbred rats (see [4]).

To further investigate the role of the GABA system in the mesoaccumbens system, June and colleagues [161, 179] conducted several studies with RO19-4603. The main objectives of these studies were to evaluate, first, its prolonged time course of alcohol reduction in the operant chamber and, second, the substrate by which it exerted its effects. Figure 14.12 shows data for P rats trained to bar press for EtOH under the saccharin-fading procedure following unilateral intra-acumbens infusions of RO19-4603 (2–100 ng). Similar to the systemic study (see above), infusions were performed *only* on day 1. Microinjections of RO19-4603 (20 and 100 ng) into the NAcc suppressed EtOH responding on day 1 by as much as 53% of control, and responding continued to be suppressed on day 2, with the 100-ng dose reducing responding to 73% of control. Thus, similar to systemic injection, prolonged effects were observed with RO19-4603. Cason et al. [180] examined outbred Wistar rats following unilateral injections of *tert*-butyl-8-acetylene-5,6-dihydro-5-methyl-6-oxo-4*H*-imidazo-[1,5a] [1,4]-benzodiazepine-3 carboxylate (TG) on day 1 and 24 h post–drug administration. Note that RO19-4603 is also a *t*-butyl ligand; however, TG

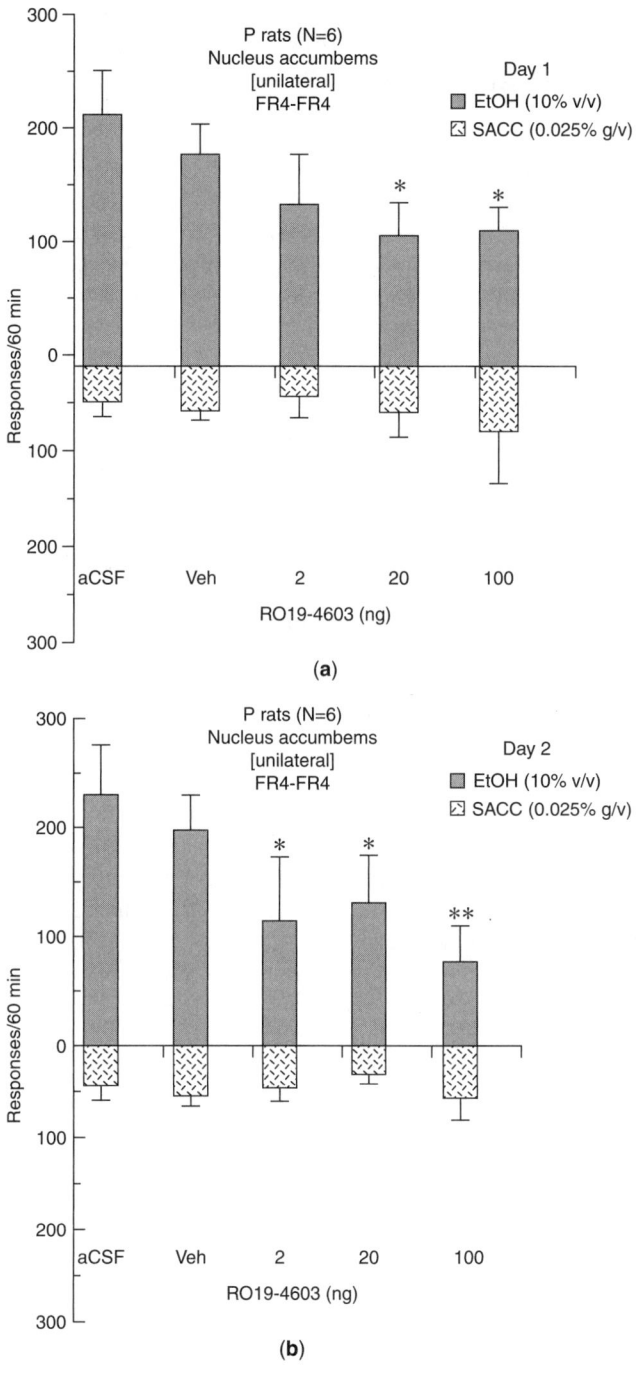

Figure 14.12 Time course of intra-accumbens infusion of RO19-4603 [aCSF (0.0), 2, 20, 100 ng] given acutely on day 1 (a) and 24 h post–drug administration day 2 (b) on EtOH (10% v/v) and saccharin-reinforced (0.05% g/v) responding. (*) $p < 0.05$ and (**) $p < 0.01$ vs. aCSF and vehicle control condition values by ANOVA and post hoc Newman–Keuls test at a corresponding day. Adapted from June et al., 1998.

differs from RO19-4603 in that it is a *t*-butyl acetylene. TG was synthesized by Cook and colleagues for comparison with RO19-403 in our EtOH-maintained responding studies. Following unilateral infusions of TG into the accumbens, the lower dose of TG (200 ng) selectively reduced responding on day 1, but the higher dose (500 ng) nonselectively reduced both EtOH and sacccharin responding. On day 2 (24 h postdrug), TG continued to selectively reduce EtOH responding without altering saccharin-maintained responding. The 24-h post–drug administration results with TG replicate the long time course effects on EtOH-maintained responding seen with RO19-4603 in P rats. It should be noted that both EtOH and saccharin response rates were similar at basal levels in the Wistar rats. However, unlike the RO19-4603 study, rate dependency effects cannot adequately explain the efficacy of TG as an EtOH antagonist [180]. These data suggest [168] that the pharmacokinetics of such ligands may be important in their long duration of action since typical ester-derived agents (e.g., RO15-4513, RY 008) are short-lived in vivo since they are readily deactivated by esterase enzymes. This is not the case with the *t*-butyl analogs since they cannot readily be deactivated by such enzymes. Consequently, *t*-butyl agents may exhibit a more prolonged duration of action in vivo [181]. These data are interesting insofar as modification of such agents to eliminate their negative efficacy could result in prototypes which may reduce alcohol consumption over a long time course.

P rats were administered bilateral microinjections into the VTA using the inverse agonist RU 34000. The purpose of this experiment was to determine if a non-imidazobenzodiazepine inverse agonist could also attenuate EtOH responding via the GABAergic DA reward circuitry. Clear, dose-dependent suppressant effects were observed on EtOH responding following RU 34000 (50–200 ng) in the absence of any effects on saccharin responding. Similar to the systemic studies (see [168]), no effects of RU 34000 were observed on day 2. These data suggest that RU 34000 may be a useful tool to further investigate the effects of the $GABA_A$ BDZ systems in mediating EtOH reward in the VTA and that an imidazobenzodiazepine structure may not be critical to observe reduction on alcohol intake within the mesolimbic circuitry.

These findings allow for several interpretations: (1) GABAergic transmission through $GABA_A$ BDZ receptors contributes to the mediation of EtOH reinforcement in the messoaccumbens limbic circuitry; (2) in rodents, high voluntary EtOH consumption does not appear to be linked to the reinforcing properties of EtOH in a manner that would permit GABAmimetics or BDZ agonists to substitute for EtOH; and (3) the specific neuroanatomical circuits participating in GABAergic modulation of EtOH self-administration cannot be determined from systemic studies, primarily because of the widespread distribution of $GABA_A$ receptors located in the CNS. Hence, additional microinjection studies are needed to further identify central GABAergic mediation of EtOH reward sites.

14.6.4 Studies Supporting Hypothesis That GABA–DA Interactions Regulate Alcohol-Motivated Behaviors: GABAergic Modulation of DA Function

The VTA receives GABAergic inputs from the medial prefrontal cortex (MPC), VP, and NAcc [182]. In addition, it is well established that substantial GABAergic interneurons exist within the VTA [64]. These GABAergic projections appear to modulate activity of DAergic neurons with cell bodies localized within the VTA. Ikemoto et al. [183] demonstrated that microinjections of picrotoxin (a nonselective

GABA antagonist) into the anterior VTA markedly increased extracellular DA in the NAcc. In anesthetized rats, Yim and Mongenson [184] reported that GABA inhibited the discharge rate of DAergic neurons in the VTA, while application of picrotoxin increased the discharge rate of DAergic neurons. Hence, converging evidence suggests that $GABA_A$ receptors in the VTA mediate tonic inhibition over DAergic neurons. In addition, VTA DAergic neurons that project to the NAcc appear to be activated by blockade of $GABA_A$ receptors. Thus, since the projection from the VTA to the NAcc (mesoaccumbens DA system) has been implicated in reward-related processes [185, 186], one possible mechanism that underlies the blockade of EtOH-reinforcing effects by BDZ inverse agonists and specific $GABA_A$ receptor antagonists may be activation of the mesoaccumbens DA system and, thereby, enhanced reinforcing effects.

While a vast and mature literature exists on the interactions between brain GABA and DA systems (see [187] for a review), the modulation of this interaction by BDZ ligands and, more specifically, inverse agonists is not as extensive (for a review see [188]). In general, these data suggest that inverse agonists can mimic the enhancing effects of stress on DA transmission in the prefrontal cortex. Specifically, systemically administered β-carbolines [e.g., beta-carboline-3-carboxylate methyl ester (βCCM), βCCE, FG 7142] have been shown to selectively increase DOPAC, or DOPAC–DA ratios [189, 190]. This increase in DA transmission has been more directly measured as an increase in cortical DA efflux using microdialysis techniques [191]. It is also worth noting that the EtOH antagonist RO15-4513 also increases prefrontal DOPAC [190]. The precise neuronal circuits underlying the BDZ modulation of cortical DA transmission, however, remains unclear because the vast majority of the studies have employed systemic drug injections (for a review see [188]). The effects of inverse agonists on subcortical DA neurotransmission have also been investigated. McCullough and Salamone [192] demonstrated that the inverse agonists FG 7142 (10–30 mg/kg) or βCCE (1.25–2.5 mg/kg) led to dose- and time-dependent increases in DA efflux. Coco et al. [193] examined BDZ ligand modulation in stress-induced DA transmission in the mesoamygdaloid system. Conditioned footshock increased homovanillic acid content in several regions of the amygdaloid and septal nuclei in the absence of any effects in cortical areas. Moreover, these effects were antagonized by diazepam. Collectively, these studies demonstrate the capacity of GABA antagonists and BDZ inverse agonists to modulate cortical and subcortical DA systems and provide support for proposing to use these agents as neuropharmacological tools to investigate GABAergic modulation of DA function.

14.6.5 Conceptual Framework for Hypothesis Generation and Interpretation of GABA–DA Interaction in Alcohol Drinking Behavior

It has become increasingly clear that alcohol-motivated behaviors in selected and outbred rat lines are regulated by multiple neurotransmitter systems [1, 9]. As stated previously in this review, a major task for alcohol self-administration investigators will be to determine the extent to which these neuronal systems singly and collectively regulate alcohol-seeking behaviors. We propose that GABAergic neurons may regulate alcohol's euphoric properties via the involvement of GABA within (in the VP) mesolimbic DA or opioid systems [1, 194]. The topography of the VP [64, 195] places it in a unique position to serve as a pivotal regulator of dopaminergic, opioidergic, and GABAergic inputs that could control EtOH-motivated behaviors. However, the close proximity and coexistence of GABA and DA within this reward cicuitry [177, 196, 197] makes DA a more likely candidate to interact with the GABA system. Previously, Legault et al. [198] have established a DA link between the ventral hippocampus (i.e., subiculum) NAcc and VTA, with DA activation being dependent on initial stimulation of the hippocampus and integrity of the NMDA receptor. We will argue (and present indirect evidence from the literature) that a negative GABA modulator, in particular one selective for the hippocampus, may augment DA to regulate reward-related behavior. In addition, VP GABAergic neurons have been shown to mediate the major DA output neurons of the VP [199]. Thus, we hypothesize in this review that both the VP and hippocampus, because of their high preponderance of GABA α_1 and α_5 receptor subunits, respectively, represent unique substrates to begin systematically testing a GABA–DA interaction hypothesis of alcohol-motivated behaviors. Finally, we will argue that an attempt to understand the GABA–DA interaction in the VP alone would be a gross oversimplification of how this complex interactional pathway functions to mediate alcohol-rewarded behavior.

14.6.6 Novel CNS GABAergic Substrates Regulating Alcohol-Motivated Behaviors

Despite the growing body of evidence for the GABA system in regulating EtOH reinforcement, much remains unknown about the role of specific $GABA_A$ receptor subtypes. This primarily reflects (1) the paucity of high-affinity and selective ligands capable of discriminating among $GABA_A$ receptors and (2) the heterogeneity of various subunits within the known alcohol reward circuitry [141, 143]. Figure 14.13 depicts this heterogeneity of the α subunits (the principal determinant of BDZ ligand affinity) within the alcohol reward loci using in situ hybridization and immunocytochemistry findings [141–143]. However, despite the remarkable heterogeneity within and among the brain reward loci, several substrates exhibit a preponderance of a single α subunit. These structures can be exploited for investigation of alcohol's rewarding effects. The probability of accurately delineating such structures in alcohol reward is markedly enhanced when a selective (albeit low- to moderate-selectivity) $GABA_A$ receptor subtype ligand is employed.

14.6.7 Ligands with Preferential Selectivities for $GABA_A$ Receptors Containing α_1 Subunit ($GABA_{A1}$ Receptors)

β-Carboline-3-carboxylate-t-butyl ester (βCCt) and 3-propoxy-β-carboline hydrochloride (3PBC) were initially synthesized as "neutral" β-carboline antagonists [122, 200–202] with selectivity at the α_1-containing $GABA_A$ receptors (also known to as the BDZ1 receptor). Behavioral studies in several species (e.g., rats, mice, primates) show that both ligands can function as BDZ antagonists, exhibiting competitive binding site interaction with BDZ agonists over a broad range of doses [201–208]. Other studies have shown that both ligands produce anxiolytic effects in rodents [203], while βCCt potentiates the anticonflict response induced by α_1 subunit ligands in primates [205]. Thus, both βCCt and 3PBC are capable of displaying an agonist or antagonist profile depending on the behavioral task, species, and dose employed.

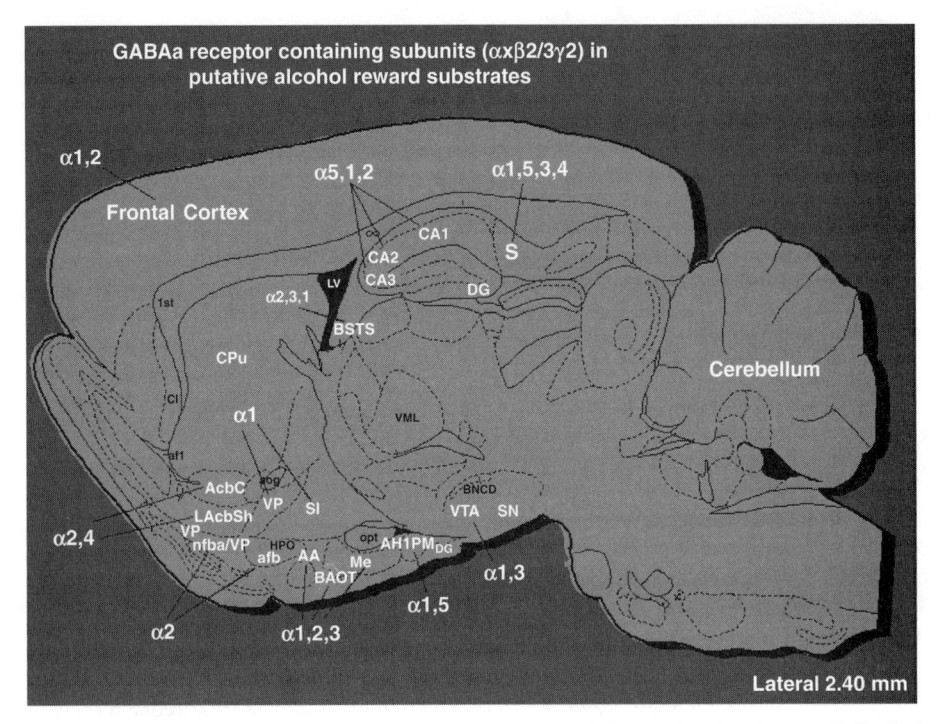

Figure 14.13 Distribution of $GABA_A$ receptor containing subunits (e.g., $\alpha x\beta 2/3\gamma 2$) in putative alcohol reward substrates based on in vitro immunocytochemistry [141, 142, 146], in situ hybridization [143, 146, 213, 214], and in vivo neurobehavioral [18, 19, 30, 37, 123, 125] studies. (See color insert.)

Hence, their behavioral pharmacological profile can best be described as that of "a partial agonist–antagonist" [19, 37].

Until recently, zolpidem and CL 218, 872 were the most selective ligands for the α_1 subunit (see [200]). Studies of recombinant receptors show βCCt exhibits greater than 10-fold selectivity for the α_1 over the α_2 and α_3 subunits and more than 110-fold selectivity for the α_1 over the α_5 subunit [19, 200] (see Table 14.1). Zolpidem has only a 5- and 15-fold greater selectivity at the α_1 subunit compared with α_2 and α_3 subunits, respectively. Neither βCCt nor zolpidem have significant affinities at the α_5 and α_6 subunits. 3PBC also displays a moderate level of selectivity for the α_1 subunit, exhibiting 9.8-, 13-, and 111-fold selectivity relative to the α_2, α_3, and α_5 subunits, respectively [37] (Table 14.1). Hence, βCCt and 3PBC exhibit the greatest binding selectivity of the currently available α_1-subunit ligands reported to date [201, 209, 210].

14.6.8 Efficacies of βCCt and 3PBC in Modulating GABA Responses in Recombinant $GABA_{A1,2,3,5}$ Receptors

Unlike the pharmacological profile of many other neuronal system ligands, the selectivity of GABA BDZ site ligands can also be described in relation to pharmacological efficacy. This efficacy is based on the capacity of a ligand to modulate GABAergic function [137]. As discussed below, there is some debate

TABLE 14.1 Affinity of α_1 (Top) and α_5 (Bottom) Selective Ligands

Compound	α_1	α_2	α_3	α_5	α_6 (DI), nM
βCCT	0.7	15	18.9	111	>5,000
3PBC	5.3	52.3	68.8	591	>1,000
3EBC	6.4	25.1	28.2	826	>1,000
Zolpidem	27	156	383	10,000	>10,000
CL 218, 872	57	1960	1160	561	>10,000
Diazepam	14	20	15	11	>3,000
ZK 93426	11	31	24	3	1,600
L-838,417	0.79	0.67	0.67	267	2.25
RO15-4513	3.3	2.6	2.5	0.26	3.8
RY023	197	143	255	2.61	58.6
RY024	27	26.3	18.7	0.4	5.1
RO15-1788	0.8	0.9	1.05	0.6	148

Note: In vitro **recombinant binding assay**. The affinity of compounds at GABA$_A$/BDZ receptor, subtypes was measured by competition for [^{3}H]RO15-1788 (83 Ci/mmol; NEN) binding to Ltk cells expressing human receptors of composition $\alpha_1\beta_3\gamma_2$, $\alpha_2\beta_3\gamma_2$, $\alpha_3\beta_3\gamma_2$, $\alpha_5\beta_3\gamma_2$, and $\alpha_6\beta_3\gamma_2$. Cells were removed from culture by scraping into phosphate-buffered saline, centrifuged at 3000 g and resuspended in 10 mL of phosphate buffer (10 nM KH$_2$PO$_4$, 100 nM KCl, pH 7.4 at 4°C) for each tray (25 cm^2) of cells. Radioligand binding assays were carried out in a volume of 500 μL which contained 100 μL of cells, [^{3}H]RO15-1788 at a concentration of 1–2 nM and test compound in the range of 10^{-9}–10^{-5} M. Nonspecific binding was defined by 10^{-5} M diazepam and typically represented less than 5% of the total binding. K_I values were calculated using the least-squares iterative fitting routine of RS/1 analysis software (BBN Research Systems, Cambridge, MA) and are either mean±SEM (standard error of the mean) or the means of two determinations which differed by less than 10%. Recombinant receptors expressed with either a β$_3$ or β$_2$ subunit have been shown to exhibit the same benzodiazepine receptor ligand affinities [37, 146, 246, 247].

in the literature as to whether a ligand's affinity or efficacy selectivity is the more salient factor in determining a ligand's capacity to function as an alcohol antagonist [4, 18, 123]. Hence, knowing the efficacy of putative anti–alcohol reward ligands across GABA$_A$ receptors is indeed critical to knowledge of their neuromechanism of action. This is particularly the case with BDZs, insofar as ligands may have a different efficacies depending on their activity at a particular subunit. Hence, the efficacy of βCCt and 3PBC's has been investigated across all "diazepam-sensitive" receptors (i.e., receptors bearing α_1, α_2, α_3, or α_5 subunits) and the α_4 subunit in the *Xenopus* oocyte assay [4, 37]. For comparison, the activities of the prototypical antagonists ZK 93426 and flumazenil were also evaluated. Figure 14.14 shows that βCCt exhibited either a neutral or low-efficacy agonist response at GABA α_1 (96±7%), α_2 (99±10%), α_3 (108+6%), and α_4 (107±5%) subunits compared to a normalized GABA response of 100% in its absence. However, a low-efficacy partial inverse agonist response was observed at the α_5 subunit (88±7% of the GABA response). Flumazenil exhibited an efficacy profile that was qualitatively similar to βCCt at the α_1 (99±5%), α_3 (118±7%), and α_5 (96±6%) subunits. At the α_2 subunit, flumazenil produced a low-efficacy agonist response (115±4%) while βCCt was GABA neutral (98+10%). Flumazenil also produced a qualitatively similar response to βCCt at the α_4 subunit, albeit the magnitude of GABA potentiation by flumazenil far exceeded that of βCCt (132±6% vs. 108±6%, respectively). In contrast, ZK 93426 produced a clear agonist profile, potentiating GABAergic activity (see below).

3PBC acted as a modest positive modulator at α_1-, α_2-, α_3-, and α_4-containing receptors (113±4%, 116±7%, 119±6%, 129±3% of GABA response, respectively). At the α_1 through α_5 subunits, flumazenil exhibited an efficacy profile statistically similar to 3PBC ($p > 0.05$). At the α_1 through α_4 subunits, ZK 93426 exhibited a full agonist profile (146±11%, 140±13%, 147±10%, 137±8%, respectively). These effects were statistically greater than 3PBC and flumazenil at the α_1 through α_3 subunits ($p < 0.05$). By comparison [211, 212], flunitrazepam, the full agonist, markedly enhanced GABAergic activity (152±8% to 164±3%) across the α receptor subunits (data not shown). At the α_5 subunit, each of the three antagonists exhibited a very weak negative profile which was indistinguishable from each other ($p > 0.05$).

In summary, the efficacy data suggest a qualitatively similar profile for βCCt and flumazenil across recombinant $GABA_A$ receptors bearing the α_1 to α_5 subunits. However, βCCt did not significantly affect GABA currents at the α_1, α_2, α_3, or α_4 (Fig. 14.14) subunits; in contrast, flumazenil increased GABA currents at the α_2 ($p < 0.09$), α_3 ($p < 0.05$), and α_4 ($p < 0.01$) subunits relative to the control condition. The effects of 3PBC mirrored that of flumazenil at the α_2, α_3, α_4, and α_5 subunits compared with the control condition (i.e., GABA alone) ($p < 0.01$) [37]. Hence, while βCCt is relatively GABA neutral (i.e., only a minute GABA potentiation) across all receptor subunits studied, 3PBC and flumazenil are partial agonists at some subunits (α_2, α_3, and α_4) and relatively GABA neutral at others (α_1 and α_5). In contrast, however, ZK 93426 produces full agonism at the α_1 to α_4 subunits and GABA-neutral activity at the α_5 subunit. It is possible that the low-efficacy agonist activity across multiple receptor subunits could account for the behavioral pharmacological profile observed with both βCCt and 3PBC in the in vivo behavioral studies noted above.

14.7 EMPLOYING LIGANDS WITH PREFERENTIAL SELECTIVITIES FOR α_1 SUBUNIT CONTAINING $GABA_A$ RECEPTOR AS PHARMACOLOGICAL PROBES TO INVESTIGATE NOVEL ALCOHOL REWARD SUBSTRATES

14.7.1 Ventral Pallidum

Of the potential $GABA_A$ receptors involved in the reinforcing properties of alcohol, evidence suggests the $GABA_{A1}$ subtype within the VP may play an important role in regulating alcohol-seeking behaviors. First, the VP contains one of the highest densities of α_1 subunits in the mesolimbic system [142, 143, 213, 214] (see Fig. 14.15). Second, while a number of unilateral GABAergic projections exist across the reward circuitry from various brain substrates, dense reciprocal GABAergic projections exist from the VP to the NAcc [64, 215–217] (see Fig. 14.16). Third, acute EtOH administration has been reported to selectively enhance the effects of iontophoretically applied GABA in the VP, and these effects are highly correlated with [^{3}H]zolpidem binding (an α_1 subunit selective agonist) [218, 219]. Finally, prior reports have demonstrated that the VP plays a role in regulating the rewarding properties of psychostimulants and opioids [43, 194, 220]. Together, the above findings suggest a possible role for the VP $GABA_{A1}$ receptors in the euphoric properties of alcohol. We hypothesize that the VP might be functionally relevant in regulating alcohol-motivated behaviors.

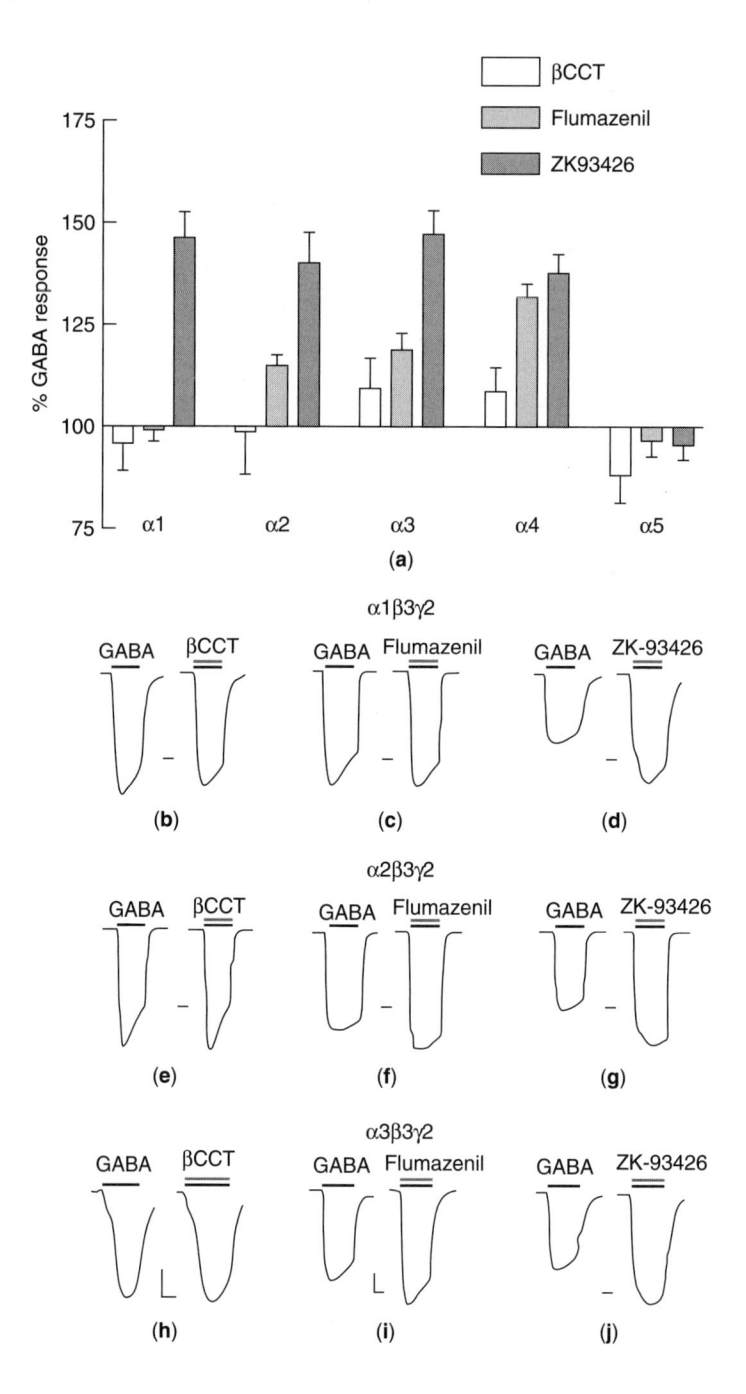

14.7.2 Systemic Studies

The initial objective of these studies was to evaluate the selectivity of systemically administered βCCt and 3PBC to decrease responding maintained by EtOH presentation in P and HAD rats. Figure 14.17a shows the effects of βCCt (5–40 mg/kg) in P rats ($N=10$) on a concurrent schedule presentation of EtOH and saccharin when response rates are equated at basal levels [19]. All tested doses of βCCt significantly suppressed EtOH responding. Twenty-four hours post–drug administration the 40-mg/kg dose continued to suppress EtOH responding by 75% of control levels. Further, similar to the effects observed with ZK 93426 and CGS 8216 [166] (nonselective BDZ antagonists), no significant suppression occurred on saccharin responding on day 1 or 24 h post–drug administration (bottom portion

Figure 14.14 Modulation of GABA$_A$ $\alpha_1\beta_3\gamma_2$, $\alpha_2\beta_3\gamma_2$, $\alpha_3\beta_3\gamma_2$, $\alpha_4\beta_3\gamma_2$, and $\alpha_5\beta_3\gamma_2$ receptor subunit combinations expressed in Ltk cells by βCCt (open bars), flumazenil (shaded bars), and ZK 93426 (black bars). A saturating concentration (1–10 µM) was coapplied over voltage-clamped oocytes along with an EC$_{50}$ of GABA. (a) Each value is the mean % GABA response $\pm$SD of at least four separate oocytes. Actions of βCCt, flumazenil, and ZK 93426 on recombinant GABA$_A$ receptor subtypes. Top, current responses of voltage-clamped oocytes expressing GABA$_A$ $\alpha_1\beta_3\gamma_2$ receptors (b) during application of 50 µM (EC$_{50}$) GABA alone for the duration indicated by the black bar (left trace). Current response from the same oocyte subsequently coapplied with 50 µM GABA along with 10 µM βCCt for the duration indicated by the open bar (right trace). (c) Current response of a voltage-clamped oocyte during application of 50 µM GABA for the duration indicated by the black bar (left trace). Current response from same oocyte subsequently coapplied with 50 µM GABA along with 1 µM flumazenil for the duration indicated by the open bar (right trace). (d) Current response of a voltage-clamped oocyte during application of 50 µM GABA for the duration indicated by the black bar (left trace). Current response from the same oocyte subsequently coapplied with 50 µM GABA along with 10 µM ZK 93426 for the duration indicated by the open bar (right trace). Center, current responses of voltage-clamped oocytes expressing GABA$_A$ $\alpha_2\beta_3\gamma_2$ receptors (e) during application of 50 µM (EC$_{50}$) GABA for the duration indicated by the black bar (left trace). Current response from the same oocyte subsequently coapplied with 50 µM GABA along with 10 µM βCCt for the duration indicated by the open bar (right trace). (f) Current response of a voltage-clamped oocyte during application of 50 µM GABA for the duration indicated by the black bar (left trace). Current response from the same oocyte subsequently coapplied with 50 µM GABA along with 10 µM flumazenil for the duration indicated by the open bar (right trace). (g) Current response of a voltage-clamped oocyte during application of 50 µM GABA for the duration indicated by the black bar (left trace). Current response from the same oocyte subsequently coapplied with 50 µM GABA along with 10 µM ZK 93426 for the duration indicated by the open bar (right trace). Bottom, current responses of voltage-clamped oocytes expressing GABA$_A$ $\alpha_3\beta_3\gamma_2$ receptors (h) during application of 30 µM (EC$_{50}$) GABA for the duration indicated by the black bar (left trace). Current response from the same oocyte subsequently coapplied with 30 µM GABA along with 10 µM βCCt for the duration indicated by the open bar (right trace). (i) Current response of a voltage-clamped oocyte during application of 30 µM GABA for the duration indicated by the black bar (left trace). Current response from the same oocyte subsequently coapplied with 30 µM GABA along with 1 µM flumazenil for the duration indicated by the open bar (right trace). (j) Current response of a voltage-clamped oocyte during application of 30 µM GABA for the duration indicated by the black bar (left trace). Current response from the same oocyte subsequently coapplied with 30 µM GABA along with 10 µM ZK 93426 for the duration indicated by the open bar (right trace). Scale bars: 5 nA, 10 s. Adapted from June et al., 2003.

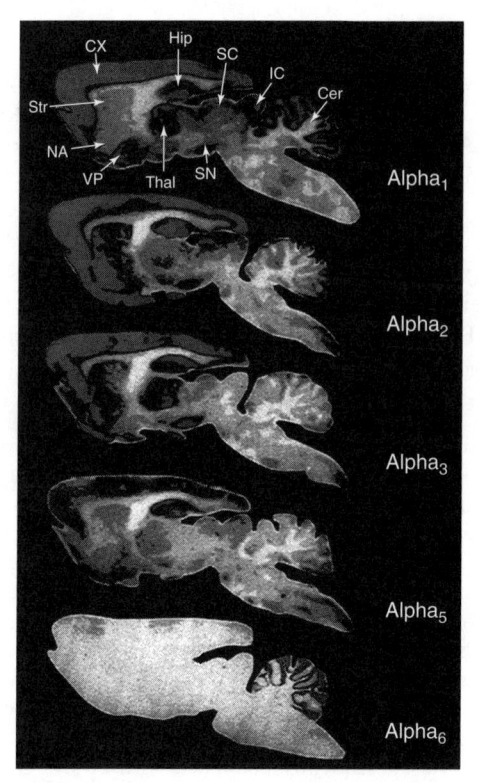

Figure 14.15 Distribution of $GABA_A$ receptor containing subunits α_1-$\alpha_6\beta_2\gamma_2$ in rat CNS based on immunocytochemistry studies by Turner and colleagues [142]. (See color insert.)

of Fig. 14.17a). Figure 14.17a shows basal operant response rates for EtOH and sucrose were very similar in the HAD rats. The 1- to 10-mg/kg βCCt injections dose dependently suppressed responding maintained by alcohol. The bottom portion of Figure 14.17b shows that βCCt suppressed responding maintained by sucrose only with the 10-mg/kg dose.

Figure 14.18 shows data for P rats following i.p. administration of 1–20 mg/kg of 3PBC. Prior to 3PBC administration the no-injection control (EtOH 201 ± 51 responses; saccharin 153 ± 23 responses) and the Tween-20 vehicle (EtOH 191 ± 42; saccharin 161 ± 41) conditions were similar. Hence, these data were pooled and used to compare against the drug treatment. The black bars of Figure 14.18 show that 3PBC produced a significant dose-related reduction on EtOH-maintained responding, reducing responding by as much as 35–84% of control levels. The hashed bars of Figure 14.18 show that, in contrast to the effects observed on alcohol responding, the lower 3PBC doses (1–10 mg/kg) markedly and significantly elevated responding maintained by saccharin, while the 20-mg/kg dose markedly and significantly suppressed responding. Together, these data show that, given systemically, βCCt and 3PBC are capable of selectively reducing EtOH-maintained responding. The data also demonstrated that across two alcohol-selected rat lines, βCCt can function as an antagonist of EtOH-seeking behaviors and not suppress responding for a palatable noncaloric or caloric solution given concurrently with EtOH.

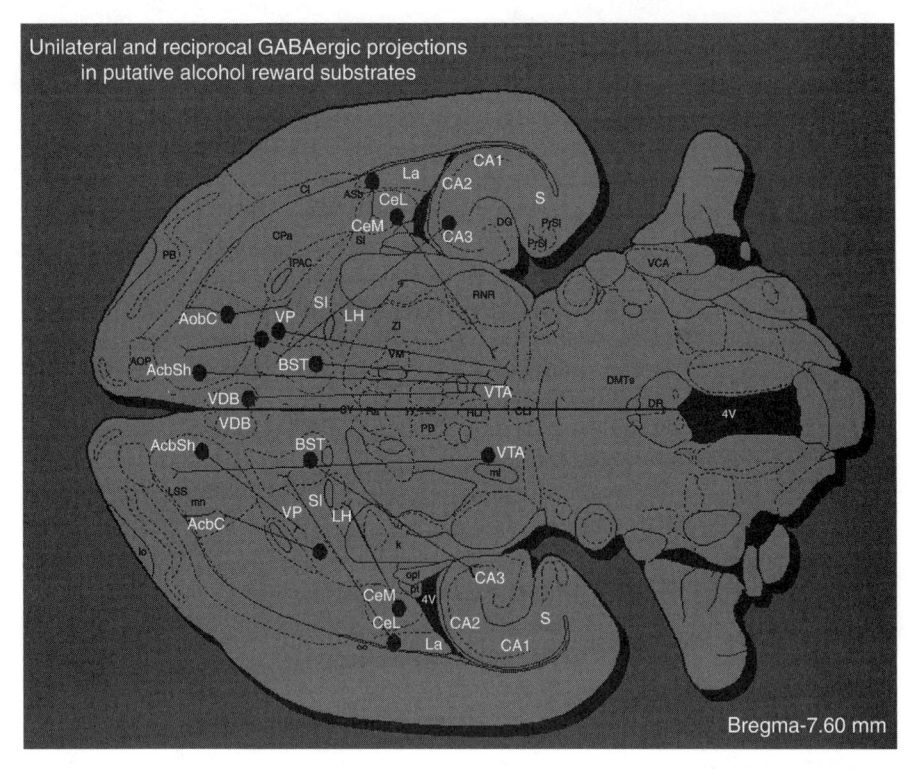

EMPLOYING LIGANDS WITH PREFERENTIAL SELECTIVITIES 505

Figure 14.16 Illustration of both unilateral and reciprocal GABAergic projections in putative alcohol reward substrates based on histological mapping studies [64, 87, 88, 94, 95, 215–217]. (See color insert.)

14.7.3 Microinjection Studies

The second objective employing βCCt and 3PBC was to *directly* test the hypothesis that the $GABA_{A1}$ receptor within the VP plays an important role in regulating alcohol-seeking behaviors. It should be recalled that a substantial number of α_1-subunit-containing $GABA_A$ receptors exist within the VP, while exceedingly low or nondectable levels of the other α subunits (e.g., α_2, α_3, α_4, α_5, and α_6) are found within the VP [142, 143, 213, 214]. Figure 14.19a shows behavioral data for P rats bilaterally infused with βCCt (5–40 μg) in the VP compared with the no-injection baseline (i.e., BL) and the artificial cerebral spinal fluid (aCSF) control conditions. βCCt dose dependently reduced EtOH-maintained responding relative to control conditions. In contrast, βCCt was without effect on responding maintained by saccharin (Fig. 14.19a). Finally, βCCt failed to alter responding maintained by EtOH or saccharin following infusion into the NAcc or caudate putamen (CPu) area (Fig. 14.19b). Hence, βCCt displayed both reinforcer and neuroanatomical specificity.

Figures 14.19c–e show data for HAD rats following administration of βCCt (5–40 μg). The HAD rats were trained to lever press for alcohol only; HAD rats do not lever press for alcohol in significant quantities when concurrently presented with highly palatable reinforcers [4]. To further substantiate the neuroanatomical specificity of the $GABA_{A1}$ receptor in alcohol-related behaviors, HAD rats received a unilateral implant in the VP and a second implant in either the CPu or NAcc.

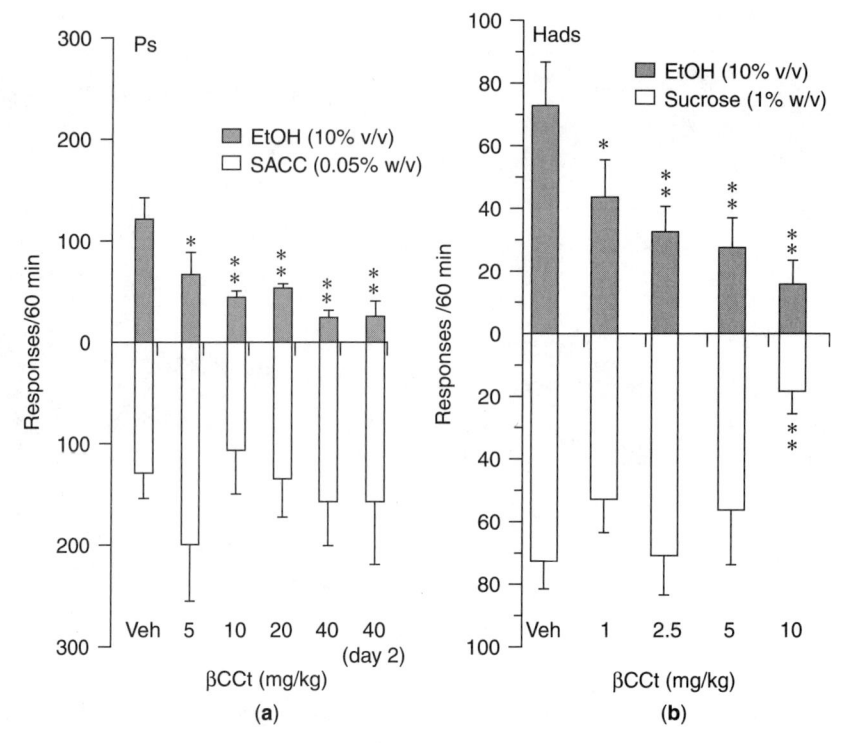

Figure 14.17 Dose–response of systemic βCCt injections (i.p.) in (a) P (Ps) (5–40 mg/kg) and (b) HAD-1 (Hads) (1–10 mg/kg) rats. P rats ($N=11$) performed under a concurrent FR4 schedule for EtOH (10% v/v) and saccharin (0.05% w/v). HAD-1 rats ($N=11$) performed under an alternate-day access paradigm, wherein they received EtOH (10% v/v) on day 1 and sucrose (1% w/v) on day 2. At 15 min after the i.p. injections, rats were placed in the operant chamber to lever press for a 60-min session. (**) $p<0.01$ and (*) $p<0.05$ vs the control condition values by ANOVA and post hoc Newman–Keuls test. Bars represent means ± SEM. Adapted from June et al., 2003.

Figures 14.19c–e show rates of responding maintained by EtOH following unilateral microinjection of the 0.5- to 7.5-µg doses of βCCt into the VP of HAD rats. Compared with the aCSF control condition, βCCt dose dependently reduced EtOH responding. In addition, 24 h post–drug administration the 2.5- to 7.5-µg doses continued to reduce responding by as much as 54–63% of control levels. In contrast, unilateral infusions of βCCt into the CPu/NAcc areas were completely ineffective in altering alcohol-maintained responding (Figs. 14.19d,e).

A study by Harvey et al. [37] evaluated the efficacy of bilaterally administered 3PBC in the VP or NAcc/CPu employing a similar experimental design as June et al. [19]. 3PBC (0.5–40 µg) was found to dose dependently and selectively reduce alcohol-maintained responding relative to the control condition (see Fig. 14.20). Only the 40-µg dose nonsignificantly reduced saccharin responding. To determine the neuroanatomical specificity of the VP α_1 subunit modulation of alcohol-maintained responding, Harvey et al. [37] evaluated the capacity of 3PBC to reduce alcohol-motivated behaviors in the NAcc/striatum, a locus reported to be devoid of the α_1 receptor

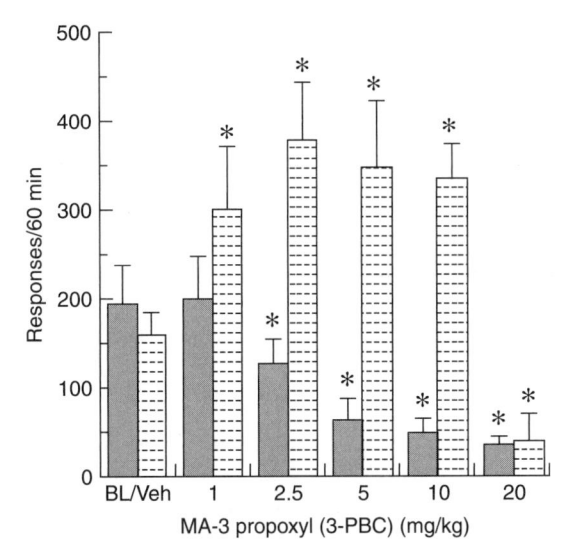

Figure 14.18 Dose–response of systemic (0.0–20 mg/kg; $n=13$) injections of 3PBC on a concurrent FR4 schedule for EtOH (10% v/v) and saccharin (0.05% w/v) responding during the 1-h operant session. (*) $p<0.05$ versus the control condition values by ANOVA and post hoc Newman–Keuls test. Error bars indicate means $\pm$ SEM. The two control conditions were pooled in the systemic group and compared against the drug treatment conditions. BL, Baseline; Veh, vehicle control. Adapted from Harvey et al., 2002.

subunit [141–143, 214]. Similar to the βCCt treatments, responding maintained by EtOH and saccharin (Fig. 14.20b) following 3PBC in the NAcc/CPu locus was not altered. Hence, these data indirectly confirm the significant topography of the $GABA_{A1}$ receptor in the pallidal area of the P rats for EtOH-maintained responding [213, 214].

Taken together, these data show that βCCt and 3PBC in the VP are capable of selectively reducing EtOH-maintained responding with little if any effect on responding for a palatable saccharin/sucrose reinforcer. Since both βCCt and 3PBC are moderately selective for the $GABA_{A1}$ and a high density of these receptors are located in the VP, it is reasonable to hypothesize that the attenuation seen by these agents are mediated at least in part via the $GABA_{A1}$ receptors. Further, some degree of neuroanatomical specificity was also observed since neither βCCt nor 3PBC altered EtOH responding when infused into the NAcc or CPu.

14.8 ORAL ADMINISTRATION OF βCCT OR 3PBC PRODUCES PROLONGED REDUCTION ON ALCOHOL SELF-ADMINISTRATION: DIRECT COMPARISON WITH OPIOID RECEPTOR ANTAGONIST NALTREXONE

To evaluate potential pharmacotherapies for alcohol dependence in rodents, it is necessary to determine their capacity to reduce alcohol drinking via the oral route. Employing the oral gavage route of administration, June et al. (unpublished)

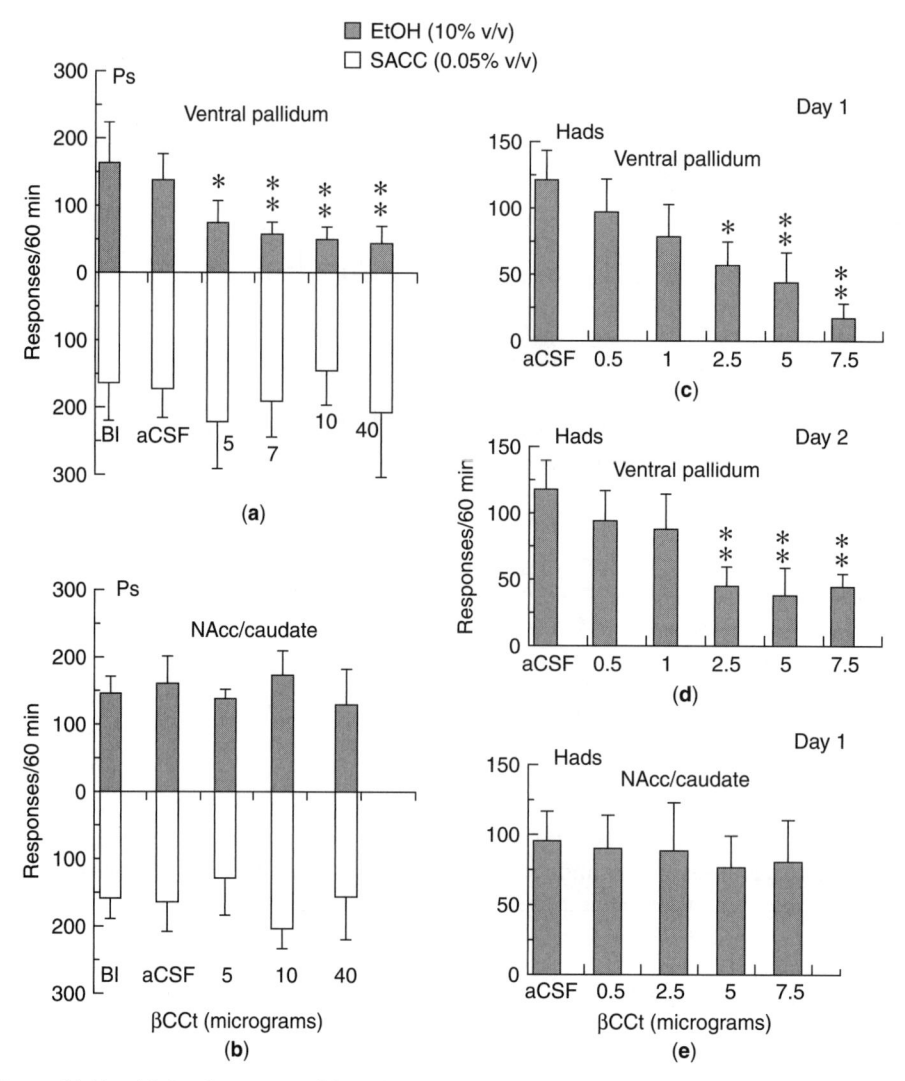

Figure 14.19 (a) Performance of female P rats ($n = 11$) on a concurrent FR4 schedule for EtOH (10% v/v) and saccharin (0.05% w/v) following bilateral infusions of βCCt (0.0–40 mg) in the VP. (b) Performance of control female P rats ($n = 7$) on a concurrent FR4 schedule for EtOH (10% v/v) and saccharin (0.05% w/v) following bilateral infusions of βCCt (0.0–40 mg) in the NAcc/CPu areas. (c, d) Performance of female Had rats ($n = 9$) on an FR4 schedule for EtOH (10% v/v) following unilateral infusions of βCCt (0.0–7.5 mg) in the VP on the first day of infusion and 24 h post–drug administration. (e) Performance of the same female Had rats in (c) ($n = 9$) on an FR4 schedule for EtOH (10% v/v) following unilateral infusions of βCCt (0.0–7.5 mg) in the NAcc/CPu areas on the first day of infusion. (**) $p < 0.01$ and (*) $p < 0.05$ compared with the baseline (BL) and aCSF conditions using post hoc Newman–Keuls tests. Error bars indicate means ± SEM. Adapted from June et al., 2003.

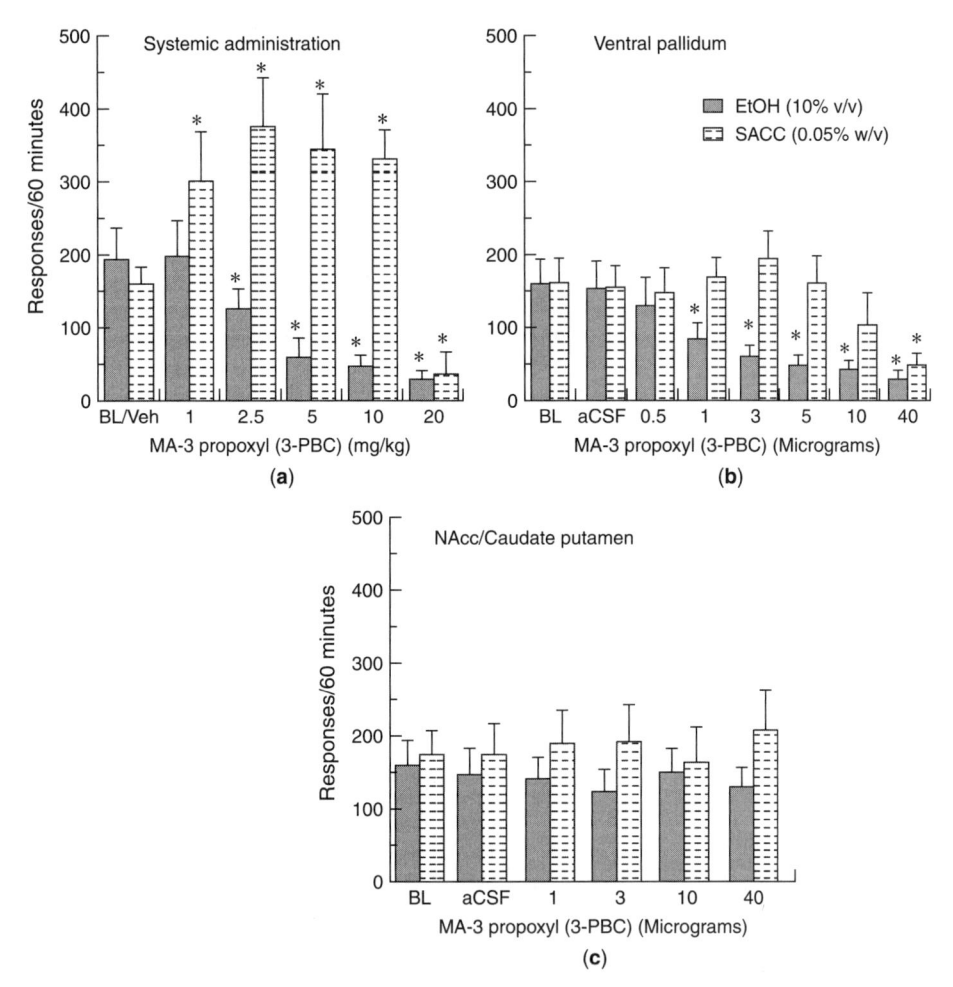

Figure 14.20 Dose–response bilateral infusions of 3PBC (0.5–40 μg) in the VP (a; $n = 12$) and NAcc/CPu (neuroanatomical control loci) (b; $n = 7$) on a concurrent FR4 schedule for EtOH (10% v/v) and saccharin (0.05% w/v) responding during the 1-h operant session. (*) $p < 0.05$ versus the control conditions values by ANOVA and post hoc Newman–Keuls test. Error bars indicate means ± SEM. BL, Baseline; Veh, vehicle control. Adapted from Harvey et al., 2002.

evaluated the actions of βCCt and 3PBC (0–75 mg/kg) on alcohol-motivated responding. The nonselective opioid antagonist naltrexone was used as a reference agent, since it is well established as an alcohol antagonist that reduces both alcohol cravings and intake [221]. Figure 14.21 shows data for naltrexone on day 1, 30 min after drug administration. Naltrexone produces clear dose-dependent reduction on alcohol responding on day 1; however, no effects on alcohol responding were observed on day 2. Figure 14.22 shows that, similar to naltrexone, dose-dependent reductions were observed on alcohol responding on day 1, 30 min following βCCt administration; however, in contrast to naltrexone, marked reductions on alcohol drinking were still detectable 24 h postdrug. 3PBC also produces dose-dependent reductions on alcohol responding on day 1, and similar to βCCt, the marked reductions on alcohol drinking were still apparent 24 h later (Fig. 14.23). At the

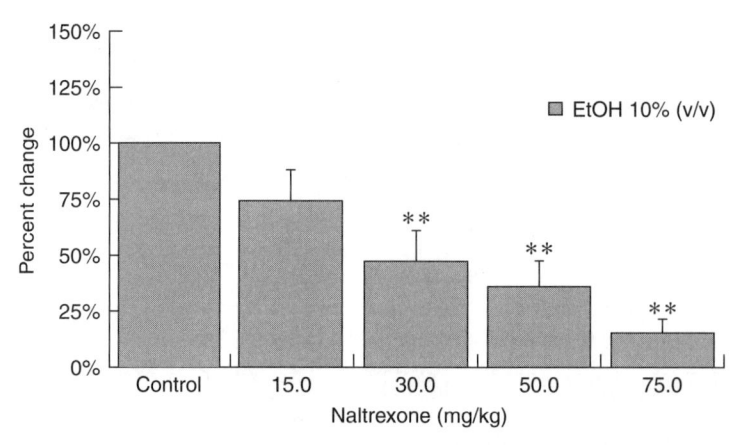

Figure 14.21 Responding for 10% EtOH (v/v) expressed as a percent of baseline line following oral administration of naltrexone (15, 30, 50, 75 mg/kg); **, $p < 0.01$.

highest tested dose (e.g., 75 mg/kg) neither βCCt nor 3PBC altered responding maintained by sucrose; however, naltrexone profoundly reduced sucrose responding. Together, these data show that both βCCt and 3PBC are as effective as naltrexone in reducing alcohol drinking following acute administration. However, βCCt and 3PBC are far superior to naltrexone in their duration of action on alcohol responding, with suppression observed for at least 24 h postadministration. In addition, unlike naltrexone, neither βCCt nor 3PBC reduced sucrose (a highly palatable caloric reinforcer) responding. These findings suggest that βCCt and 3PBC are excellent candidates for reducing alcohol intake and cravings in humans and are not likely to nonselectively reduce other consummatory behaviors such as feeding and drinking.

14.8.1 Oral Efficacy of βCCt and 3PBC in Reducing Anxiety in Alcohol-Preferring Rats

The in vitro data presented above suggest that both βCCt and 3PBC produce agonist activity at some $GABA_A$ receptors while exerting GABA neutral/antagonist activity at others. In many instances, in vitro pharmacology does not extrapolate to whole-animal pharmacology. However, given that βCCt and 3PBC produced a sustained reduction in alcohol drinking behavior, an added advantage of these agents would be a demonstrated effectiveness in reducing anxiety. It is well established in addiction psychiatry that anxiety and alcohol abuse are comorbid disorders [222]. Furthermore, it is possible that anxiety may predispose subjects to initiate alcohol drinking behaviors [223, 224]. Hence, the oral effectiveness of βCCt and 3PBC was evaluated in reducing anxiety (assessed using the elevated-plus maze) in alcohol-preferring rats. Gavage of βCCt and 3PBC was indeed effective in reducing the anxiety in P rats (Fig. 14.24) with βCCt also effective in reducing anxiety in HAD rats. Compared with the NP rat, the P rat is more "anxious" in the plus maze assay [224]. Thus, this behavioral assay is well suited for the assessment of novel anxiolytics in P rats. Taken together, the oral effectiveness of βCCt and 3PBC as anxiolytics combined with their oral efficacy in reducing alcohol drinking behavior makes both of these compounds

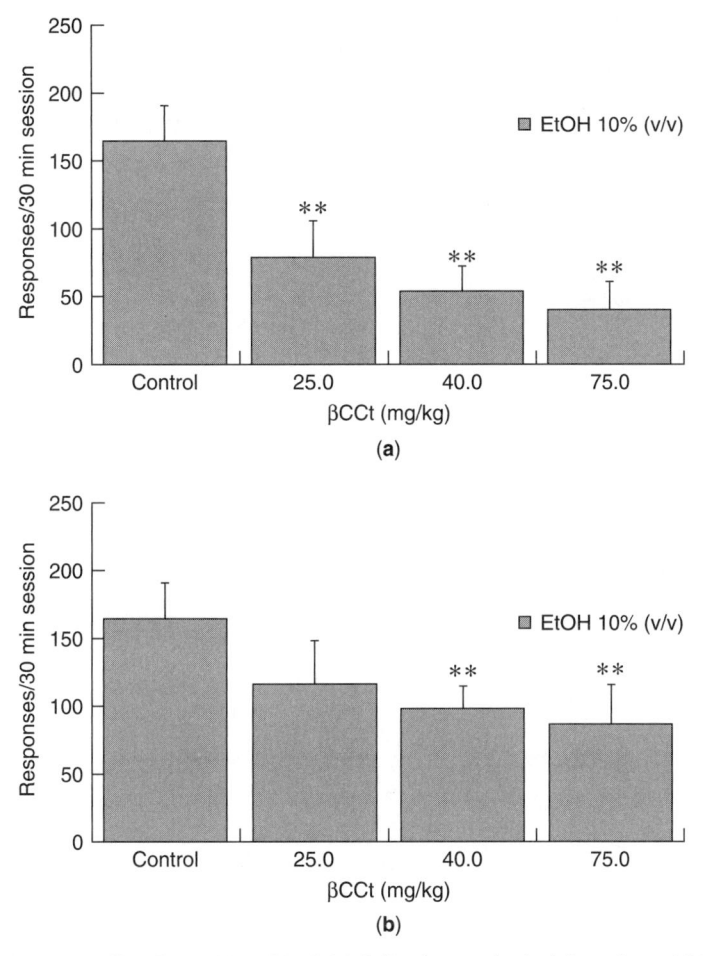

Figure 14.22 Responding for 10% EtOH (v/v) following oral administration of βCCt (25, 40, 75 mg/kg) (a) and 24 h postadministration (b); **, $p<0.01$.

ideal as prototype pharmacotherapeutic agents in reducing alcohol drinking behaviors in humans.

14.9 EMPLOYING LIGANDS WITH PREFERENTIAL SELECTIVITIES FOR α_5-SUBUNIT-CONTAINING GABA$_A$ RECEPTORS AS PHARMACOLOGICAL PROBES TO INVESTIGATE NOVEL ALCOHOL REWARD SUBSTRATES: CA1 AND CA3 HIPPOCAMPUS

While GABA$_{A5}$ receptors are minor constituents of the total GABA$_A$ receptor pool, immunocytochemical, in situ hybridization, and radioligand binding studies show that the CA1, CA2, and CA3 fields are enriched in this subunit compared with other brain areas [141, 143, 225]. Only, low or nondetectable levels of other subunits can be localized within the hippocampus. The CA1 and CA3 hippocampal fields are

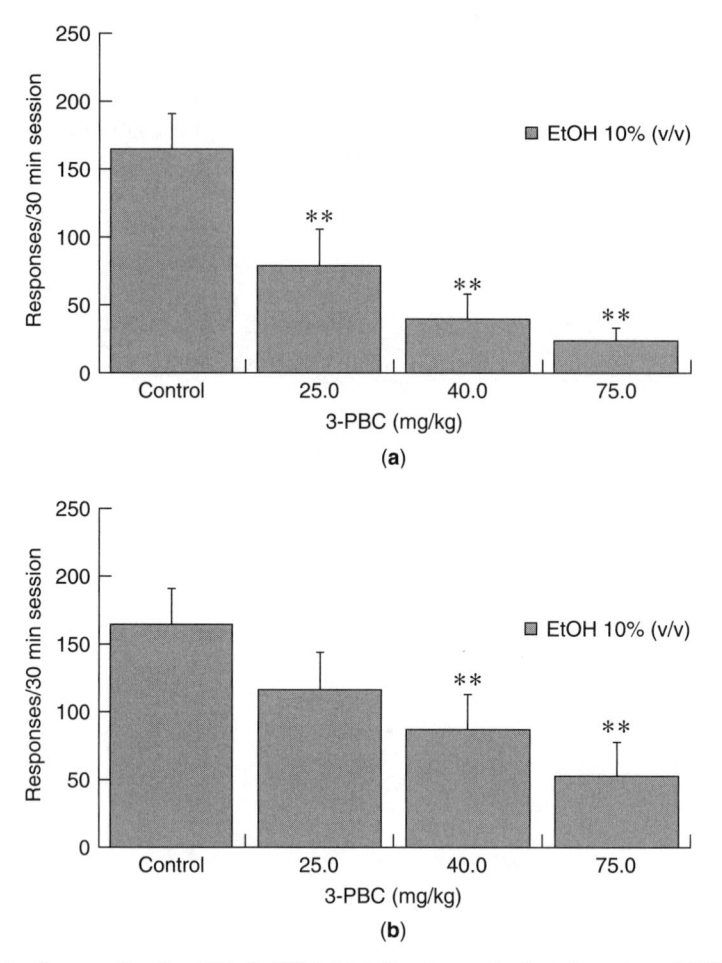

Figure 14.23 Responding for 10% EtOH (v/v) following oral administration of 3PBC (25, 40, 75 mg/kg) (a) and 24 h postadministration (b); **, $p < 0.01$.

particularly interesting candidate sites for the study of alcohol-motivated behaviors since projections from the CA1 and CA3 fields, via the subiculum, innervate several putative EtOH reward substrates [e.g., NAcc, amygdala, bed nucleus of the stria terminalis (BNST), hypothalamus, olfactory tubercle] [215, 226, 227].

RY 023 (*tert*-butyl-8-(trimethylsilyl) acetylene-5,6-dihydro-5-methyl-6-oxo-4*H*-imidazo-[1,5a] [1,4]-benzodiazepine-3-carboxylate) (Table 14.2) is one of a series of 8-substituted imidazobenzodiazepine inverse agonists [145, 228, 229] developed from the anti-EtOH agent RO 15-4513 [132]. RY 023 exhibits both high binding affinity ($K_i \sim 2.7$ nM) and selectivity (~ 75-fold) at recombinant GABA$_A$ receptors composed of $\alpha_5\beta_2\gamma_2$ subunits [229] (see Table 14.1). RY 023 acts as a negative modulator at the $\alpha_1\beta_3\gamma_2$, $\alpha_2\beta_3\gamma_2$, and $\alpha_5\beta_3\gamma_2$ receptor subunits, inhibiting GABA-evoked current responses of voltage-clamped *Xenopus* oocytes by approximately 40–55%. The efficacy of the imidazobenzodiazepines RO 15-4513 and RO 15-1788 (flumazenil) were also examined at the α_1, α_2 and α_5 subunits. These parent compounds were

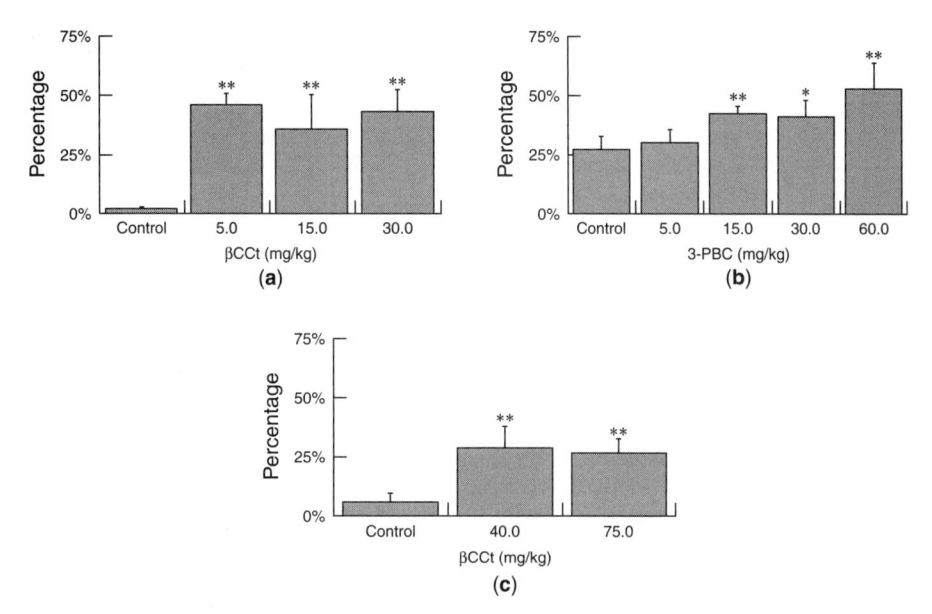

Figure 14.24 Percent of total time spent in open arms of an elevated-plus maze following oral administration of βCCt (5, 15, 30 mg/kg) (a) and 3PBC (5, 15, 30, 60 mg/kg) (b) in P rats and (40 and 75 mg/kg) in HAD rats (c); (*) $p < 0.05$ and ** $p < 0.01$.

selected since June et al. [18] were interested in evaluating the degree to which modification at position 8 (which produced the α_5 selectivity) [18, 228, 229] would change the imidazobenzodiazepine's capacity to modulate GABA at specific receptor subtypes. RO 15-4513 was also selected to compare the intrinsic activity of a reference alcohol antagonist (see [132, 230, 231]) with RY 023. RO 15-4513 produced a very modest inhibition of GABA current at the α_1 and α_2 subunits ($86 \pm 3\%$ and $93 \pm 1\%$ control response, respectively), while exhibiting no efficacy at the α_5 subunit ($99.5 \pm 4.1\%$ control response). RO 15-1788 (flumazenil), the competitive antagonist [232–234], acted as a modest positive modulator at the α_2 subunit ($115 + 4\%$ control response) and exhibited no efficacy at either the α_1 or α_5 subunit.

Taken together, these data reveal several important potency and efficacy differences between RY 023 and the alcohol antagonist RO 15-4513. First, the selectivity of RY 023 for the α_5 receptor subunit is higher than RO 15-4513 (see Table 14.1). Second, the magnitude of GABAergic reduction with RY 023 is far greater than that of RO 15-4513 at the α_1, α_2 and α_5 receptor subunits [18]. Third, RO 15-4513 exhibits an efficacy profile similar to that of RO 15-1788 at the α_2 and α_5 subunits [18]. Hence, it is possible that the antialcohol properties of the two inverse agonists may be differentially regulated (see [123, 125]).

June and colleagues [18] tested the hypothesis that α_5 subunits of the CA1 and CA3 hippocampal fields would regulate EtOH-motivated behaviors in the P rat (also see [123, 125]). To accomplish this, the actions of bilateral and unilateral microinjections of RY 023 in the CA1 and CA3 hippocampal fields were evaluated for their capacity to reduce EtOH-maintained responding. The degree of neuroanatomical specificity was examined using both bilateral and unilateral control injections into the

TABLE 14.2 Affinities of 5,6-Dihydro-5-methyl-6-oxo-4H-imidazo [1,5a] [1,4]-benzodiazepine-3-carboxylic acid *tert*-Butyl Esters for $\alpha_x\beta_3\gamma_2$ (x = 1–3, 5, 6) Benzodiazepine Receptor Isoforms

		K_i (nM)[a]					
Ligand	R_8[b]	α_1	α_2	α_3	α_5	α_6	α_1/α_5
14	Cl	17.3	21.6	29.1	0.65	4	26.6
15	Br	11.4	10.7	9.2	0.47	9.4	24.3
16	I	9.7	11.2	10.9	0.38	4.6	25.5
17	OH	1.50	NA	0.53	0.14	6.89	10.7
18	OCH$_3$	6.74	NA	7.42	0.293	8.28	23.0
19	N(CH$_3$)$_2$	13.1	NA	38.1	0.78	118	16.8
20	X	5.8	NA	169	9.25	325	0.63
21	Y	6.44	NA	148	4.23	247	1.5
22	N=N$^+$=N$^-$	7.25	NA	5.66	0.3	5.25	24.3
23	NCS	17.1	33.7	50	2.5	30.7	6.8
24	NO$_2$	12.8	49.8	30.2	3.5	22.5	3.7
25	Et	14.8	56	25.3	1.72	22.9	8.6
26	C≡C–H	26.9	26.3	18.7	0.4	5.1	67.3
27	C≡C–Si(CH$_3$)$_3$	197	143	255	2.61	58.6	75.5
28	C≡CCH$_2$Si(CH$_3$)$_3$	275.0	387.0	337.0	23.0	301.0	12.0

Source: Adapted from Huang et al., 1998.
[a]Data shown here the means of two determinations which differed by less than 10%. NA, data not available.
[b]X, *N*-tetrahydropyrrole; Y, *N*-hexahydropyridine.

NAcc and VTA. Unlike the hippocampal fields, these brain areas possess higher levels of α_2- and α_1-subunit expression, respectively [141–143]. The specificity of RY 023 on consummatory responding was evaluated by determining the effects of RY 023 in P rats whose response rates for EtOH (10% v/v) and saccharin solutions (0.05% w/v) were similar at basal levels.

Figure 14.25a shows rates of responding maintained by EtOH (upper panel) following microinjection of the 1.5- to 20-μg doses of RY 023 into the CA1 (dorsal and CA3 (ventral) hippocampus. RY 023 produced a dose-related suppression on EtOH-maintained responding. The lower panel shows that RY 023 selectively reduced EtOH responding, reducing saccharin responding only at the highest tested dose (20 μg). When ZK 93426 was administered immediatedly prior to RY 023, it attenuated the RY 023-induced suppression on EtOH-maintained responding, suggesting the suppression was mediated via actions at the BDZ site of the GABA

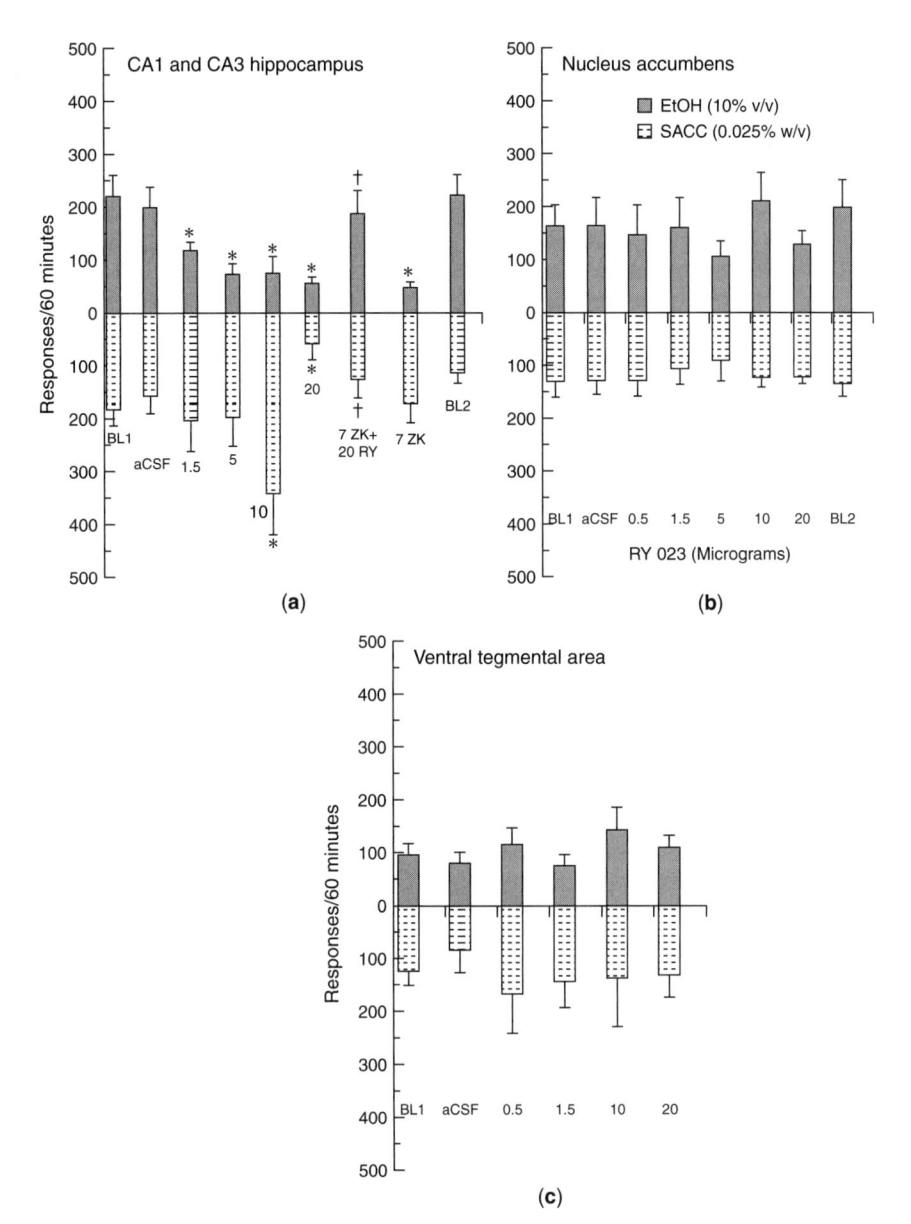

Figure 14.25 Dose–response of bilateral infusions of RY (0.0–20 μg) in the hippocampus ($n = 9$) (a), NAcc ($n = 9$) (b), and VTA ($n = 10$) (c) on a concurrent FR4 schedule for EtOH (10% v/v) and saccharinmaintained (0.025% w/v) (SACC) responding. Immediately after the microinfusions, rats were placed in the operant chamber to lever press for a 60-min session. (*) $p < 0.05$ versus the no-injection control conditions (BL1 and BL2) and aCSF control condition values by ANOVA and post hoc Newman–Keuls test ($n = 9$). Error bars represent ±SEM. (†) $p < 0.01$ versus the 20 μg RY alone condition by ANOVA and post hoc Newman–Keuls test ($n = 9$). ZK, the competitive BDZ antagonist, completely reverses the suppression by RY on EtOH and saccharin-motivated responding. RY was without effect on EtOH or saccharin-maintained responding in the NAcc and VTA. Adapted from June et al., 2001.

receptor complex Figures 14.25b,c show that, in addition to reinforcer selectivity, RY 023 was anatomically selective. Specifically, bilateral infusion into the NAcc or VTA was without effect on responding maintained by EtOH (upper panel) and saccharin (lower panel). Unilateral infusions of RY 023 produced a clear dose-dependent suppression on EtOH-maintained responding. With the exception of the highest tested dose (40 μg), reinforcer selectivity was also observed, as was neuroanatomical selectivity, with no effects on EtOH-maintained responding observed in the NAcc or VTA. RY 023 also failed to alter saccharin-motivated behaviors in the NAcc and VTA.

The above findings provide the *first* demonstration that $GABA_A$ receptors containings α_5 subunits in the hippocampus play a critical role in regulating alcohol-seeking behavior [18]. The findings are supported by recent research with outbred rats [125] and a related α_5 subunit selective ligand, RY 024, in P rats [123]. Finally, previous work has shown that an α_5 agonist substitutes for alcohol in primate drug discrimination studies [235]. Thus, these findings suggest that the hippocampus/hippocampal projection sites may be functionally relevant in regulating EtOH-motivated behaviors.

The precise GABA–hippocampal pathway(s) in which the $GABA_{A5}$ selective ligands modify EtOH reinforcement/related responding is unknown; it has been hypothesized that $GABA_A$ BDZ neuroanatomical circuits within the hippocampus may initiate activation of underlying DA substrates in the mesoaccumbens circuitry to contribute to the reinforcing properties of EtOH [18]. The functional role of conditioning stimuli in the onset and maintenance phases of alcohol-motivated drinking may also be important. It should be recalled that BDZs have long been proposed to modulate learning and memory processes via the hippocampus [236]. We conclude that the GABA–hippocampal pathway may represent an "extension" of the mesolimbic EtOH reward circuitry as has been proposed by Koob and colleagues [52]. Thus, the hippocampus may be an important *target* in the development of potential pharmacotherapies for alcohol addiction and dependence. The *Xenopus* oocyte studies demonstrated that the capacity of BDZs to attenuate EtOH-motivated responding was not directly related to their intrinsic efficacy; rather, their selectivity and differential potency to attenuate EtOH-seeking behaviors appear to be more related to their affinity and selectivity at different $GABA_A$-containing receptor subunits. However, it is possible that the in vitro efficacy observed in the *Xenopus* oocyte assay may not reflect the in vivo efficacy in an animal model of alcoholism following BDZ administration.

14.10 SUBUNIT SELECTIVITY VERSUS INTRINSIC EFFICACY

The rank-order potencies of BDZ site ligands to attenuate EtOH intake are not correlated with either rank-order potencies to inhibit GABA $^{36}Cl^-$ conductance or enhance ^{35}S-*t*-butylbicyclophosphorothionate (TBPS) binding [237]. While the ^{36}Cl flux and TBPS binding assays in brain tissues employ heterogenous subunit populations, with the resulting value obtained representing an "average efficacy," the *Xenopus* oocyte system permits efficacy to be determined at any different subunit–complementary DNA (cDNA) combinations [140, 211, 212]. In the *Xenopus* system RO 15-4513 was essentially GABA neutral at the α_2- and α_5-subunit-containing receptors and slightly GABA negative at the GABA$_{A1}$ receptor. These data are in agreement with previous oocyte studies [29, 211, 212] and work by Wong and Skolnick [238] employing the "GABA shift" assay. The findings with RO 15-4513, however, contrast those with RY 023 and ZK 93426, where the GABA-evoked current is negatively and positively modulated, respectively, at the α_1 and α_2 receptor subunits. Nevertheless, despite the three different intrinsic activity profiles, each ligand was highly effective in attenuating EtOH-motivated behaviors [78, 156, 161, 166, 237]. Thus, while both efficacy and subunit selectivity may interact to effectively alter EtOH-motivated behaviors, the evidence in this review strongly suggests that subunit selectivity may be the critical factor in determining the capacity of a ligand to function as an effective alcohol antagonist. Several investigators suggest that efficacy not only is dependent on subunit composition but also is actually defined by it [145, 162a, 238, 239].

14.11 CONCLUSIONS

Research on the substrates and circuitry regulating alcohol self-administration has experienced enormous growth over the past decade. The primary purpose of this review was to provide the reader with relatively new research findings that have been critical in the delineation of novel brain reward substrates that can be targeted in the potential development of pharmacotherapeutic prototypes for alcohol addiction and dependence in humans. Alcohol–dependent individuals represent a heterogeneous group [19, 240–242]. Hence, it is unlikely that a single pharmacological treatment will be effective for all alcoholics. To this end, a better understanding of the neuromechanisms which regulate alcohol-seeking behaviors and the design of clinically safe and effective drugs that reduce alcohol addiction and dependence remain a high priority in alcoholism research [243–245].

In this review, we presented data implicating novel substrates and circuitry within the dopaminergic and GABAergic systems in alcohol reward. Prior to presenting these data, however, the significance of an optimal animal model of alcoholism and its integration with appropriate behavioral and neuroanatomical paradigms to accurately interpret findings obtained from alcohol self-administration studies were discussed. Relatively new data that implicated brain loci such as the VP, BST, and LH in regulating alcohol-motivated behaviors within the DA systems were also presented. Our conceptual framework was based on the premise that GABA mediates its actions on alcohol self-administration via interaction with the DA system [19, 37]. Indeed, current studies are underway in our laboratory showing that in many cases this DAergic regulation of alcohol intake can in fact be modulated via GABA receptors in other mesolimbic brain reward areas [104]. Finally, June et al. presented compelling data showing that, using a multidiciplinary approach (e.g., medicinal chemistry, molecular biology, behavioral pharmacology, neuroanatomy), it was indeed feasible to exploit the GABAergic system in the potential development of pharmacotherapies for alcohol addiction and dependence in humans (but see [245]). The primary GABA$_A$ receptor candidates in these efforts were the α_1 and α_5 receptor subunits. However, the research efforts exploiting the α_1 receptor subunit demonstrating the oral effectiveness of βCCt and 3PBC as anxiolytics, combined with their oral efficacy in reducing alcohol drinking behavior, are compelling. This seminal research on βCCt and 3 PBC should set the stage for further investigation in the coming years for evaluation of these agents as prototype pharmacotherapeutic agents in reducing alcohol drinking behaviors in human alcoholics.

REFERENCES

1. McBride, W. J., and Li, T.-K. (1998). Animal models of alcoholism: Neurobiology of high alcohol-drinking behavior in rodents. *Crit. Rev. Neurobiol.* 12(4), 339–369.
2. Chick, J. (1996). The efficacy of treatments in reducing alcohol consumption: A meta-analysis. *Subst. Use Misuse* 31(9), 1081.
3. Froehlich, J. C., and Li, T. K. (1991). Animal models for the study of alcoholism: Utility of selected lines. *J. Addict. Dis.* 10(1/2), 61–71.
4. June, H. L. (2002). Alcohol initiation procedures in rats: Methods used in evaluating potential pharmacotherapeutic agents. In *Current Protocols in Neuroscience*, Vol. 9, J. Crawley, C. Gerfen, R. McKay, M. Rogawski, D. Sibley, and P. Skolnick, Eds. Wiley and Sons, New York, pp. 1–23.
5. June, H. L., Cummings, R., Eiler, W. J., II, Foster, K. L., McKay, P. F., Seyoum, R., Garcia, M., McCane, S., Grey, C., Hawkins, S. E., and Mason, D. (2004). Central opioid receptors differentially regulate the nalmefene-induced suppression of ethanol- and saccharin-reinforced behaviors in alcohol-preferring (P) rats. *Neuropsychopharmacology* 29(2), 285–299.
6. Koob, G. F., Roberts, A. J., Kieffer, B. L., Heyser, C. J., Katner, S. N., Ciccocioppo, R., and Weiss, F. (2003). Animal models of motivation for drinking in rodents with a focus on opioid receptor neuropharmacology. *Rec. Dev. Alcohol* 16, 263–281.
7. McBride, W. J., Murphy, J. M., Lumeng, L., and Li, T.-K. (1988). Effects of RO15-4513, fluoxetine, desipramine on the intake of ethanol, water and food by the alcohol-preferring (p) and nonpreferring (np) lines of rats. *Pharmacol. Biochem. Behav.* 30, 1045–1050.
8. Murphy, J. M., Stewart, R. B., Bell, R. L., Badia-Elder, N. E., Carr, L. G., McBride, W. J., Lumeng, L., and Li, T. K. (2002). Phenotypic and genotypic characterization of the Indiana University rat lines selectively bred for high and low alcohol preference. *Behav. Genet.* 32(5), 363–388.
9. Samson, H. H., and Hodge, C. W. (1996). Neurobehavioral regulation of ethanol intake. In *Pharmacological Effects of Ethanol on the Nervous System*, R. A. Deitrich and V. G. Erwin, Eds. CRC Press, New York, pp. 203–226.
10. Cicero, T. J. (1979). A critique of animal analogues of alcoholism. In *Biochemistry and Pharmacology of Ethanol*, Vol. 2, E. Majchrowicz and E. P. Noble, Eds. Plenum, New York, pp. 533–560.
11. Ritz, M. C., Garcia, J. M., Protz, D., Rael, A. M., and George, F. R. (1994). Ethanol-reinforced behavior in P, NP, HAD and LAD rats: Differential genetic regulation of reinforcement and motivation. *Behav. Pharmacol.* 5(4/5), 521–531.
12. Samson, H. H., Files, F. J., Denning, C., and Marvin, S. (1998). Comparison of alcohol-preferring and nonpreferring selectively bred rat lines. I. Ethanol initiation and limited access operant self-administration. *Alcohol Clin. Exp. Res.* 22(9), 2133–2146.
13. Lumeng, L., Murphy, J. M., McBride, W. J., and Li, T.-K. (1995). Genetic influences on alcohol preference in animals. In *The Genetics of Alcoholism*, H. Begleiter and B. Kissin, Eds. Oxford University Press, New York, pp. 165–201.
14. Samson, H. H. (1986). Initiation of ethanol reinforcement using a sucrose-substitution procedure in food- and water-sated rats. *Alcohol. Clin. Exp. Res.* 10(4), 436–442.

15. Samson, H. H., and Pfeffer, A. O. (1987). Initiation of ethanol-maintained responding using a schedule-induction procedure in free feeding rats. *Alcohol Drug Res.* 7(5/6), 461–469.
16. Petry, N. M., and Heyman, G. M. (1995). Behavioral economics of concurrent ethanol-sucrose and sucrose reinforcement in the rat: Effects of altering variable-ratio requirements. *J. Exp. Anal. Behav.* 64(3), 331–359.
17. Koob, G. F., and Weiss, F. (1990). Pharmacology of drug self-administration. *Alcohol* 7(3), 193–197.
18. June, H. L., Harvey, S. C., Foster, K. L., McKay, P. F., Cummings, R., Garcia, M., Mason, D., Grey, C., McCane, S., Williams, L. S., Johnson, T. B., He, X., Rock, S., and Cook, J. M. (2001). GABA(A) receptors containing (alpha)5 subunits in the CA1 and CA3 hippocampal fields regulate ethanol-motivated behaviors: An extended ethanol reward circuitry. *J. Neurosci.* 21(6), 2166–2177.
19. June, H. L., Foster, K. L., McKay, P. F., Seyoum, R., Woods, J. E., Harvey, S. C., Eiler, W. J., Grey, C., Carroll, M. R., McCane, S., Jones, C. M., Yin, W., Mason, D., Cummings, R., Garcia, M., Ma, C., Sarma, P. V., Cook, J. M., and Skolnick, P. (2003). The reinforcing properties of alcohol are mediated by GABA(A1) receptors in the ventral pallidum. *Neuropsychopharmacology* 28(12), 2124–2127.
20. June, H. L., Murphy, J. M., Mellor-Burke, J. J., Lumeng, L., and Li, T. K. (1994). The benzodiazepine inverse agonist RO19-4603 exerts prolonged and selective suppression of ethanol intake in alcohol-preferring (P) rats. *Psychopharmacology (Berl.)* 15(3), 325–331.
21. Linseman, M. A. (1987). Alcohol consumption in free-feeding rats: Procedural, genetic and pharmacokinetic factors. *Psychopharmacology (Berl.)* 92(2), 254–261.
22. Wild, K. D., and Reid, L. D. (1990). Modulation of ethanol-intake by morphine: Evidence for a central site of action. *Life Sci.* 47(14), PL49–54.
23. Froehlich, J. C., Harts, J., Lumeng, L., and Li, T. K. (1987). Naloxone attenuation of voluntary alcohol consumption. *Alcohol Alcohol Suppl.* 1, 333–337.
24. Krishnan-Sarin, S., Jing, S. L., Kurtz, D. L., Zweifel, M., Portoghese, P. S., Li, T. K., and Froehlich, J. C. (1995). The delta opioid receptor antagonist naltrindole attenuates both alcohol and saccharin intake in rats selectively bred for alcohol preference. *Psychopharmacology (Berl.)* 120(2), 177–185.
25. Krishnan-Sarin, S., Wand, G. S., Li, X. W., Portoghese, P. S., and Froehlich, J. C. (1998). Effect of mu opioid receptor blockade on alcohol intake in rats bred for high alcohol drinking. *Pharmacol. Biochem. Behav.* 59(3), 627–635.
26. Melendez, R. I., Rodd, Z. A., McBride, W. J., and Murphy, J. M. (2005). Dopamine receptor regulation of ethanol intake and extracellular dopamine levels in the ventral pallidum of alcohol preferring (P) rats. *Drug Alcohol Depend.* 77(3), 293–301.
27. Roberts, A. J., McDonald, J. S., Heyser, C. J., Kieffer, B. L., Matthes, H. W., Koob, G. F., and Gold, L. H. (2000). Mu-opioid receptor knockout mice do not self-administer alcohol. *J. Pharmacol. Exp. Ther.* 293(3), 1002–1008.
28. June, H. L., Eggers, M. W., Warren-Reese, C., Ricks, A., and Cason, C. R. (1998). The effects of the novel benzodiazepine receptor inverse agonist Ru 34000 on ethanol-maintained responding. *Eur. J. Pharmacol.* 350, 151–158.
29. June, H. L., Cason, C. R., Cheatham, G., Ruiyan, L., Gan, T., and Cook, J. M. (1998). $GABA_A$-benzodiazepine receptors in the striatum are involved in the sedation produced by a moderate, but not an intoxicating ethanol dose in outbred Wistar rats. *Brain Res.* 794, 103–118.

30. Foster, K. L., McKay, P. F., Seyoum, R., Milbourne, D., Yin, W., Sarma, P. V., Cook, J. M., and June, H. L. (2004). GABA(A) and opioid receptors of the central nucleus of the amygdala selectively regulate ethanol-maintained behaviors. *Neuropsychopharmacology* 29(2), 269–284.
31. June, H. L., McCane, S. R., Zink, R. W., Portoghese, P. S., Li, T. K., and Froehlich, J. C. (1999). The delta 2-opioid receptor antagonist naltriben reduces motivated responding for ethanol. *Psychopharmacology (Berl.)* 147(1), 81–89.
32. Petry, N. M., and Heyman, G. M. (1997). Bidirectional modulation of sweet and bitter taste by chlordiazepoxide and Ro 15-4513: Lack of effect with GABA drugs. *Physiol. Behav.* 61(1), 119–126.
33. Samson, H. H., and Grant, K. A. (1985). Chlordiazepoxide effects on ethanol self-administration: Dependence on concurrent conditions. *J. Exp. Anal. Behav.* 43, 353–364.
34. Crabbe, J. C., Janowsky, J. S., Young, E. R., Kosobud, A., Stack, J., and Rigter, H. (1982). Tolerance to ethanol hypothermia in inbred mice: Genotypic correlations with behavioral responses. *Alcohol Clin. Exp. Res.* 6(4), 446–458.
35. Frye, G. D., and Breese, G. R. (1982). GABAergic modulation of ethanol-induced motor impairment. *J. Pharmacol. Exp. Ther.* 223(3), 750–756.
36. Lister, R. G. (1987). The benzodiazepine receptor inverse agonists FG 7142 and RO 15-4513 both reverse some of the behavioral effects of ethanol in a holeboard test. *Life Sci.* 41(12), 1481–1489.
37. Harvey, S. C., Foster, K. L., McKay, P. F., Carroll, M. R., Seyoum, R., Woods, J. E., II, Grey, C., Jones, C. M., McCane, S., Cummings, R., Mason, D., Ma, C., Cook, J. M., and June, H. L. (2002). The GABA(A) receptor alpha1 subtype in the ventral pallidum regulates alcohol-seeking behaviors. *J. Neurosci.* 22(9), 3765–3775.
38. Bodnar, R. J., Glass, M. J., Ragnauth, A., and Cooper, M. L. (1995). General, mu and kappa opioid antagonists in the nucleus accumbens alter food intake under deprivation, glucoprivic and palatable conditions. *Brain Res.* 700(1/2), 205–212.
39. Ragnauth, A., Ruegg, H., and Bodnar, R. J. (1997). Evaluation of opioid receptor subtype antagonist effects in the ventral tegmental area upon food intake under deprivation, glucoprivic and palatable conditions. *Brain Res.* 767(1), 8–16.
40. Heyman, G. M., and Oldfather, C. M. (1992). Inelastic preference for ethanol in rats: Analysis of ethanol's reinforcing effects. *Psychol. Sci.* 3, 122–130.
41. Nowak, K. L., McBride, W. J., Lumeng, L., Li, T. K., and Murphy, J. M. (2000). Involvement of dopamine D2 autoreceptors in the ventral tegmental area on alcohol and saccharin intake of the alcohol-preferring P rat. *Alcohol Clin. Exp. Res.* 24, 476–483.
42. Eiler, W. J., II, Seyoum, R., Foster, K. L., Mailey, C., and June, H. L. (2003). D1 dopamine receptor regulates alcohol-motivated behaviors in the bed nucleus of the stria terminalis in alcohol-preferring (P) rats. *Synapse* 48(1), 45–56.
43. Hubner, C. B., and Koob, G. F. (1990). Bromocriptine produces decreases in cocaine self-administration in the rat. *Neuropsychopharmacology* 3(2), 101–108.
44. Lovinger, D. M., and Crabbe, J. C. (2005). Laboratory models of alcoholism: Treatment target identification and insight into mechanisms. *Nat. Neurosci.* 8(11), 1471–1480.
45. Diamond, I., and Gordon, A. S. (1997). Cellular and molecular neuroscience of alcoholism. *Physiol. Rev.* 77(1), 1–20.
46. Koob, G. F., and Le Moal, M. (2001). Drug addiction, dysregulation of reward, and allostasis. *Neuropsychopharmacology* 24(2), 97–129.

47. Krystal, J. H., Petrakis, I. L., Mason, G., Trevisan, L., and D'Souza, D. C. (2003). N-Methyl-D-aspartate glutamate receptors and alcoholism: Reward, dependence, treatment, and vulnerability. *Pharmacol. Ther.* 99(1), 79–94.

48. Carboni, E., Silvagni, A., Rolando, M. T. P., and Di Chiara, G. (2000). Stimulation of *in vivo* dopamine transmission in the bed nucleus of the stria terminalis by reinforcing drugs. *J. Neurol.* 20, RC102.

49. Volkow, N. D., Fowler, J. S., Wang, G. J., and Swanson, J. M. (2004). Dopamine in drug abuse and addiction: Results from imaging studies and treatment implications. *Mol. Psychiatry* 9(6), 557–569.

50. Nestler, E. J. (2005). Is there a common molecular pathway for addiction? *Nat. Neurosci.* 8(11), 1445–1449.

51. Gonzales, R. A., Job, M. O., and Doyon, W. M. (2004). The role of mesolimbic dopamine in the development and maintenance of ethanol reinforcement. *Pharmacol. Ther.* 103(2), 121–146.

52. Koob, G. F., Roberts, A. J., Schulteis, G., Parsons, L. H., Heyser, C. J., Hyytia, P., Merlo-Pich, E., and Weiss, F. (1998). Neurocircuitry targets in ethanol reward and dependence. *Alcohol Clin. Exp. Res.* 22(1), 3–9.

53. Alheid, G. F., and Heimer, L. (1988). New perspectives in basal forebrain organization of special relevance for neuropsychiatric disorders: The striatopallidal, amygdaloid, and corticopetal components of substantia innominata. *Neuroscience* 27(1), 1–39.

54. Oades, R. D., and Halliday, G. M. (1987). Ventral tegmental (A10) system: Neurobiology. 1. Anatomy and connectivity. *Brain Res.* 434(2), 117–165.

55. Hyytiä, P., and Koob, G. F. (1995). $GABA_A$ receptor antagonism in the extended amygdala decreases ethanol self-administration in rats. *Eur. J. Pharmacol.* 283, 151–159.

56. Melendez, R. I., Rodd-Henricks, Z. A., McBride, W. J., and Murphy, J. M. (2004). Involvement of the mesopallidal dopamine system in ethanol reinforcement. *Alcohol* 32, 137–144.

57. Kelley, A. E., and Berridge, K. C. (2002). The neuroscience of natural rewards: Relevance to addictive drugs. *J. Neurosci.* 22(9), 3306–3311.

58. Tobler, P. N., Fiorillo, C. D., and Schultz, W. (2005). Adaptive coding of reward value by dopamine neurons. *Science* 307(5715), 1642–1645.

59. Weiss, F., and Porrino, L. J. (2002). Behavioral neurobiology of alcohol addiction: Recent advances and challenges. *J. Neurosci.* 22(9), 3332–3337.

60. Badia-Elder, N. E., Stewart, R. B., Powrozek, T. A., Murphy, J. M., and Li, T. K. (2003). Effects of neuropeptide Y on sucrose and ethanol intake and on anxiety-like behavior in high alcohol drinking (HAD) and low alcohol drinking (LAD) rats. *Alcohol Clin. Exp. Res.* 27(6), 894–899.

61. Bell, S. M., Reynolds, J. G., Thiele, T. E., Gan, J., Figlewicz, D. P., and Woods, S. C. (1998). Effects of third intracerebroventricular injections of corticotropin-releasing factor (CRF) on ethanol drinking and food intake. *Psychopharmacology (Berl.)* 139 (1/2), 128–135.

62. Hayes, D. M., Knapp, D. J., Breese, G. R., and Thiele, T. E. (2005). Comparison of basal neuropeptide Y and corticotropin releasing factor levels between the high ethanol drinking C57BL/6J and low ethanol drinking DBA/2J inbred mouse strains. *Alcohol Clin. Exp. Res.* 29(5), 721–729.

63. Thiele, T. E., Marsh, D. J., Ste Marie, L., Bernstein, I. L., and Palmiter, R. D. (1998). Ethanol consumption and resistance are inversely related to neuropeptide Y levels. *Nature* 396(6709), 366–369.

64. Kalivas, P. W., Churchill, L., and Klitenick, M. A. (1993). The circuitry mediating the translation of motivational stimuli into adaptive motor responses. In *Limbic Motor Circuits and Neuropsychiatry*, P. W. Kalavis and C. D. Barnes, Eds. CRC Press, Boca Raton, pp. 237–287.

65. Levy, A. D., Murphy, J. M., McBride, W. J., Lumeng, L., and Li, T. K. (1991). Microinjection of sulpiride into the nucleus accumbens increases ethanol drinking in alcohol-preferring (P) rats. *Alcohol Alcohol Suppl.* 1, 417–420.

66. Hodge, C. W., Samson, H. H., and Haraguchi, M. (1992). Microinjections of dopamine agonists in the nucleus accumbens increase ethanol-reinforced responding. *Pharmacol. Biochem. Behav.* 43(1), 249–254.

67. Samson, H. H., Hodge, C. W., Tolliver, G. A., and Haraguchi, M. (1993). Effect of dopamine agonists and antagonists on ethanol-reinforced behavior: The involvement of the nucleus accumbens. *Brain Res. Bull.* 30(1/2), 133–141.

68. Jeziorski, M., and White, F. J. (1989). Dopamine agonists at repeated "autoreceptor-selective" doses: Effects upon the sensitivity of A10 dopamine autoreceptors. *Synapse* 4(4), 267–280.

69. Pfeffer, A. O., and Samson, H. H. (1988). Haloperidol and apomorphine effects on ethanol reinforcement in free feeding rats. *Pharmacol. Biochem. Behav.* 29(2), 343–350.

70. Weiss, F., Mitchiner, M., Bloom, F. E., and Koob, G. F. (1990). Free-choice responding for ethanol versus water in alcohol preferring (P) and unselected Wistar rats is differentially modified by naloxone, bromocriptine, and methysergide. *Psychopharmacology (Berl.)* 101(2), 178–186.

71. Katner, S. N., and Weiss, F. (2001). Ethanol anticipation enhances dopamine efflux in the nucleus accumbens of alcohol-preferring (P) but not Wistar rats. *Behav. Pharmacol.* 7(7), 669–674.

72. Melendez, R. I., Rodd-Henricks, Z. A., Engleman, E. A., Li, T. K., McBride, W. J., and Murphy, J. M. (2002). Microdialysis of dopamine in the nucleus accumbens of alcohol-preferring (P) rats during anticipation and operant self-administration of ethanol. *Alcohol Clin. Exp. Res.* 26(3), 318–325.

73. Weiss, F., Lorang, M. T., Bloom, F. E., and Koob, G. F. (1993). Oral alcohol self-administration stimulates dopamine release in the rat nucleus accumbens: Genetic and motivational determinants. *J. Pharmacol. Exp. Ther.* 267(1), 250–258.

74. Amit, Z., Levitan, D. E., Brown, Z. E., and Sutherland, E. A. (1977). Catecholaminergic involvement in alcohol's rewarding properties: Implications for a treatment model for alcoholics. *Adv. Exp. Med. Biol.* 85A, 485–494.

75. Kiianmaa, K., and Attila, L. M. (1979). Alcohol intake, ethanol-induced narcosis and intoxication in rats following neonatal 6-hydroxydopamine or 5,7-dihydroxytryptamine treatment. *Naunyn Schmiedebergs Arch. Pharmacol.* 308(2), 165–170.

76. Myers, R. D., and Melchior, C. L. (1975). Alcohol drinking in the rat after destruction of serotonergic and catecholaminergic neurons in the brain. *Res. Commun. Chem. Pathol. Pharmacol.* 10(2), 363–378.

77. Linseman, M. A. (1990). Effects of dopaminergic agents on alcohol consumption by rats in a limited access paradigm. *Psychopharmacology (Berl.)* 100(2), 195–200.

78. Rassnick, S., D'Amico, E., Riley, E., and Koob, G. F. (1993). GABA antagonist and benzodiazepine partial inverse agonist reduce motivated responding for ethanol. *Alcoholism: Clin. Exp. Res.* 17, 124–130.

79. Leshner, A. I., and Koob, G. F. (1999). Drugs of abuse and the brain. *Neuropharmacol. Substance Abuse* 111, 99–108.

80. Freedman, L. J., and Cassell, M. D. (1994). Distribution of dopaminergic fibers in the central division of the extended amygdala of the rat. *Brain Res.* 633, 243–252.
81. Napier, T. C., Muench, M. B., Maslowski, R. J., and Battaglia, G. (1991). Is dopamine a neurotransmitter within the ventral pallidum/substantia innominata. *Adv. Exp. Med. Biol.* 295, 183–195.
82. Napier, T. C., and Maslowski-Cobuzzi, R. J. (1994). Electrophysiological verification of the presence of D1 and D2 dopamine receptors within the ventral pallidum. *Synapse* 3, 160–166.
83. Hernandez, L., and Hoebel, B. G. (1988). Feeding and hypothalamic stimulation increase dopamine turnover in the accumbens. *Physiol. Behav.* 44, 599–606.
84. Leibowitz, S. F., and Rossakis, C. (1979). Mapping study of brain dopamine- and epinephrine-sensitive sites which cause feeding suppression in the rat. *Brain Res.* 172, 101–113.
85. Leibowitz, S. F., and Rossakis, C. (1979). Pharmacological characterization of perifornical hypothalamic dopamine receptors mediating feeding inhibition in the rat. *Brain Res.* 172, 115–130.
86. Leibowitz, S. F., and Brown, L. L. (1980). Histochemical and pharmacological analysis of catecholaminergic projections to the perifornical hypothalamus in relation to feeding inhibition. *Brain Res.* 201, 289–314.
87. McDonald, A. J. (1991). Topographical organization of amygdaloid projections to the caudatoputamen, nucleus accumbens, and related striatal-like areas of the rat brain. *Neuroscience* 44, 15–33.
88. Sun, N., and Cassell, M. D. (1993). Intrinsic GABAergic neurons in the rat central extended amygdala. *J. Comp. Neurol.* 330, 381–404.
89. Mengod, G., Villaro, M. T., Landwehrmeyer, G. B., Martinez-Mir, M. I., Niznik, H. B., Sunahara, R. K., Seeman, P., O'Dowd, B. F., Probst, A., and Palacios, J. M. (1992). Visualization of dopamine D1, D2, and D3 receptor mRNA's in human and rat brain. *Neurochem. Int.* 20(Suppl.), 33S–43S.
90. Scibilia, R. J., Lachowicz, J. E., and Kilts, C. D. (1992). Topographic nonoverlapping distribution of D1 and D2 dopamine receptors in the amygdaloid nuclear complex of the rat brain. *Synapse* 11, 146–154.
91. Georges, F., and Aston-Jones, G. (2002). Activation of ventral tegmental area cells by the bed nucleus of the stria terminalis: A novel excitatory amino acid input to midbrain dopamine neurons. *J. Neurosci.* 22(12), 5173–5187.
92. Veinante, P., and Freund-Mercier, M. J. (1998). Intrinsic and extrinsic connections of the rat central extended amygdala: An in vivo electrophysiological study of the central amygdaloid nucleus. *Brain Res.* 794(2), 188–198.
93. Walker, J. R., Ahmed, S. H., Gracy, K. N., and Koob, G. F. (2000). Microinjections of an opiate receptor antagonist into the bed nucleus of the stria terminalis suppress heroin self-administration in dependent rats. *Brain Res.* 854, 85–92.
94. Canteras, N. S., Simerly, R. B., and Swanson, L. W. (1995). Organization of projections from the medial nucleus of the amygdala: A PHAL study in the rat. *J. Comp. Neurol.* 360, 213–245.
95. Holstege, G., Meiners, L., and Tan, K. (1985). Projections of the bed nucleus of the stria terminalis to the mesencephalon, pons, and medulla oblongata in the cat. *Exp. Brain Res.* 58, 379–391.
96. Lewis, M. J., and June, H. L. (1990). Neurobehavioral studies of ethanol reward and activation. *Alcohol* 7, 213–219.

97. Phillips, T. J., and Shen, E. H. (1996). Neurochemical bases of locomotion and ethanol stimulant effects. *Int. Rev. Neurobiol.* 39, 243–282.

98. Amass, L., Lukas, S. E., and Mendelson, J. H. (1991). Auditory evoked response brain potentials in individuals at risk for alcoholism: Influence of task demands and motivational factors. *NIDA Res. Monogr.* 105, 610–611.

99. Gong, W., Neill, D., and Justice, J. B., Jr., (1996). Conditioned place preference and locomotor activation produced by injection of psychostimulants into ventral pallidum. *Brain Res.* 745, 64–74.

100. Gong, W., Neill, D., and Justice, J. B., Jr., (1997). 6-Hydroxydopamine lesion of ventral pallidum blocks acquisition of place preference conditioning to cocaine. *Brain Res.* 754, 103–112.

101. Sizemore, G. M., Co, C., and Smith, J. E. (2000). Ventral pallidal extracellular fluid levels of dopamine, serotonin, gamma amino butyric acid, and glutamate during cocaine self-administration in rats. *Psychopharmacology (Berl.)* 150(4), 391–398.

102. Melendez, R. I., Rodd-Henricks, Z. A., McBride, W. J., and Murphy, J. M. (2003). Alcohol stimulates the release of dopamine in the ventral pallidum but not in the globus pallidus: A dual-probe microdialysis study. *Neuropsychopharmacology* 28, 939–946.

103. Lu, X. Y., Churchill, L., and Kalivas, P. W. (1997). Expression of D1 receptor mRNA in projections from the forebrain to the ventral tegmental area. *Synapse* 25, 205–214.

104. Foster, K. L., Seyoum, R., Goergen, J., Mensah-Zoe, B., and June, H. L. (2002). GABA/dopamine interaction in the central amygdala (CeA) regulate ethanol-maintained responding. Paper presented at the Annual Meeting of the Society for Neurosciences, Orlando, FL, November 2002.

105. Gessa, G. L., Muntoni, F., Collu, M., Vargiu, L., and Mereu, G. (1985). Low doses of ethanol activate dopaminergic neurons in the ventral tegmental area. *Brain Res.* 348, 201–203.

106. Gong, W., Neill, D. B., and Justice, J. B., Jr. (1988). GABAergic modulation of ventral pallidal dopamine release studied by in vivo microdialysis in the freely moving rat. *Synapse* 9, 406–412.

107. Yokel, R. A., and Wise, R. A. (1976). Attenuation of intravenous amphetamine reinforcement by central dopamine blockade in rats. *Psychopharmacology (Berl.)* 48, 311–318.

108. Roberts, D. C., and Vickers, G. (1987). The effect of haloperidol on cocaine self-administration is augmented with repeated administrations. *Psychopharmacology* 93, 526–528.

109. Engleman, E. A., McBride, W. J., Wilber, A. A., Shaikh, S. R., Eha, R. D., Lumeng, L., Li, T. K., and Murphy, J. M. (2000). Reverse microdialysis of a dopamine uptake inhibitor in the nucleus accumbens of alcohol preferring rats: Effects on dialysate dopamine levels and ethanol intake. *Alcohol Clin. Exp. Res.* 24, 795–801.

110. Fallon, J. H., and Moore, R. Y. (1978). Catecholaminergic innervation of the basal forebrain. IV: Topography of the dopamine projection to basal forebrain and neostriatum. *J. Comp. Neural.* 182, 545–580.

111. Kizer, J. S., Palkovits, M., and Brownstein, M. J. (1976). The projection of the A8, A9, and A10 dopaminergic cell bodies: Evidence for a nigral-hypothalamic-median eminence dopaminergic pathway. *Brain Res.* 108, 363–370.

112. Wamsley, J. K., Gehlert, D. R., Filloux, F. M., and Dawson, T. M. (1989). Comparison of the distribution of D-1 and D-2 dopamine receptors in the rat brain. *J. Chem. Neuroanat.* 2(3), 119–137.

113. Leibowitz, S. F. (1975). Catecholaminergic mechanisms of the lateral hypothalamus: Their role in the mediation of amphetamine anorexia. *Brain Res.* 98, 529–545.

114. Parada, M. A., Hernandez, L., and Santiago, C. (1988). An improved circular tilt-cage shows that intrahypothalamic injections of sulpiride increase locomotion. *Brain Res. Bull.* 21, 873–880.

115. Parada, M. A., Hernandez, L., Puig de Parada, M., Paez, X., and Hoebel, B. G. (1990). Dopamine in the lateral hypothalamus may be involved in the inhibition of locomotion related to food and water seeking. *Brain Res. Bull.* 25, 961–968.

116. Parada, M. A., Hernandez, L., Schwartz, D., and Hoebel, B. G. (1988). Hypothalamic infusion of amphetamine increases serotonin, dopamine and norepinephrine. *Physiol. Behav.* 44, 607–610.

117. Wise, R. A., and Bozarth, M. A. (1987). A psychomotor stimulant theory of addiction. *Psychol. Rev.* 94, 469–492.

118. Parada, M. A., Puig de Parada, M., and Hoebel, B. G. (1995). Rats self-inject a dopamine antagonist in the lateral hypothalamus where it acts to increase extracellular dopamine in the nucleus accumbens. *Pharmacol. Biochem. Behav.* 52(1), 179–187.

119. Goergen, J., Mensa-Zoe, B., and June, H. L. (2003). The D2 dopamine receptor regulates ethanol-motivated behaviors in the lateral hypothalamus of alcohol-preferring (P) rats. *Alcohol Clin. Exp. Res.* 27, 92A (Abstract No. 519).

120. Myers, R. D., and Quarfordt, S. D. (1991). Alcohol drinking attenuated by sertraline in rats with 6-OHDA or 5,7-DHT lesions of *N. accumbens*: A caloric response? *Pharmacol. Biochem. Behav.* 40(4), 923–928.

121. Koob, G. F. (1996). Drug addiction: The yin and yang of hedonic homeostasis. *Neuron* 16(5), 893–896.

122. Huang, Q., He, X., Ma, C., Liu, R., Yu, S., Dayer, C. A., Wenger, G. R., McKernan, R., and Cook, J. M. (2000). Pharmacophore/receptor models for GABA(A)/BzR subtypes (alpha1beta3gamma2, alpha5beta3gamma2, and alpha6beta3gamma2) via a comprehensive ligand-mapping approach. *J. Med. Chem.* 43(1), 71–95.

123. Cook, J. B., Foster, K. L., Eiler, W. J., II, McKay, P. F., Woods, J., II, Harvey, S. C., Garcia, M., Grey, C., McCane, S., Mason, D., Cummings, R., Li, X., Cook, J. M., and June, H. L. (2005). Selective GABAA alpha5 benzodiazepine inverse agonist antagonizes the neurobehavioral actions of alcohol. *Alcohol Clin. Exp. Res.* 29(8), 1390–1401.

124. Draski, L. J., Deitrich, R. A., and Menez, J. F. (1997). Phenobarbital sensitivity in HAS and LAS rats before and after chronic administration of ethanol. *Pharmacol. Biochem. Behav.* 57(4), 651–657.

125. McKay, P. F., Foster, K. L., Mason, D., Cummings, R., Garcia, M., Williams, L. S., Grey, C., McCane, S., He, X., Cook, J. M., and June, H. L. (2004). A high affinity ligand for GABAA-receptor containing alpha5 subunit antagonizes ethanol's neurobehavioral effects in Long-Evans rats. *Psychopharmacology (Berl.)* 172(4), 455–462.

126. Liljequist, S., and Engel, J. (1982). Effects of GABAergic agonists and antagonists on various ethanol-induced behavioral changes. *Psychopharmacology (Berl.)* 78(1), 71–75.

127. Roberts, A. J., Cole, M., and Koob, G. F. (1996). Intra-amygdala muscimol decreases operant ethanol self-administration in dependent rats. *Alcohol Clin. Exp. Res.* 20(7), 1289–1298.

128. Boehm, S. L., II, Ponomarev, I., Jennings, A. W., Whiting, P. J., Rosahl, T. W., Garrett, E. M., Blednov, Y. A., and Harris, R. A. (2004). Gamma-aminobutyric acid A receptor subunit mutant mice: New perspectives on alcohol actions. *Biochem. Pharmacol.* 68(8), 1581–1602.

129. Morrow, A. L., Montpied, P., and Paul, S. (1991). Ethanol and the GABA$_A$ receptor-gated chloride ion channel. In *Neuropharmacology of Ethanol*, R. E. Myers, G. F. Koob, M. J. Lewis, and S. M. Paul, Eds. Birkhauser, Boston, pp. 49–76.

130. Allan, A. M., and Harris, R. A. (1986). Gamma-aminobutyric acid and alcohol actions: Neurochemical studies of long sleep and short sleep mice. *Life Sci.* 39(21), 2005–2015.

131. Mehta, A. K., and Ticku, M. K. (1988). Ethanol potentiation of GABAergic transmission in cultured spinal cord neurons involves gamma-aminobutyric acid$_A$-gated chloride channels. *J. Pharmacol. Exp. Ther.* 246, 558–564.

132. Suzdak, P., Glowa, J. R., Crawley, J. N., Schwartz, R. D., Skolnick, P., and Paul, S. M. (1986). A selective imidazodiazepine antagonist of ethanol in the rat. *Science* 234, 1243–1247.

133. Leidenheimer, N. J., and Harris, R. A. (1992). Acute effects of ethanol on GABAA receptor function: Molecular and physiological determinants. *Adv. Biochem. Psychopharmacol.* 47, 269–279.

134. Rees, D. C., and Balster, R. L. (1988). Attenuation of the discriminative stimulus properties of ethanol and oxazepam, but not of pentobarbital, by Ro 15-4513 in mice. *J. Pharmacol. Exp. Ther.* 244(2), 592–598.

135. Ticku, M. K., and Kulkarni, S. K. (1988). Molecular interactions of ethanol with GABAergic system and potential of RO15-4513 as an ethanol antagonist. *Pharmacol. Biochem. Behav.* 30(2), 501–510.

136. Samson, H. H., and Harris, R. A. (1992). Neurobiology of alcohol abuse. *Trends Pharmacol. Sci.* 13(5), 206–211.

137. Barnard, E. A., Skolnick, P., Olsen, R. W., Mohler, H., Sieghart, W., Biggio, G., Braestrup, C., Bateson, A. N., and Langer, S. Z. (1998). International Union of Pharmacology. XV. Subtypes of gamma-aminobutyric acidA receptors: Classification on the basis of subunit structure and receptor function. *Pharmacol. Rev.* 50(2), 291–313.

138. Burt, D. R. (2005). Reducing GABA receptors. *Life Sci.* 73(14), 1741–1758.

139. Lüddens, H., Seeburg, P. H., and Korpi, E. R. (1994). Impact of beta and gamma variants on ligand-binding properties of gamma-aminobutyric acid type A receptors. *Mol. Pharmacol.* 45(5), 810–814.

140. Pritchett, D. B., Lüddens, H., and Seeburg, P. H. (1989). Type I and type II GABA$_A$-benzodiazepine receptors produced in transfected cells. *Science* 245, 1389–1392.

141. Fritschy, J. M., and Mohler, H. (1995). GABA$_A$-receptor heterogenetity in the adult rat brain. Differential regional and cellular distribution of seven major subunits. *J. Comp. Neurol.* 359, 154–194.

142. Turner, J. D., Bodewitz, G., Thompson, C. L., and Stephenson, F. A. (1993). Immunohistochemical mapping of gamma-aminobutyric acid type-A receptor alpha subunits in rat central nervous system. *Psychopharmacol. Ser.* 11, 29–49.

143. Wisden, W., Laurie, D. J., Monyer, H., and Seeburg, P. H. (1992). The distribution of 13 GABAA receptor subunit mRNAs in the rat brain. I. Telencephalon, diencephalon, mesencephalon. *J. Neurosci.* 12(3), 1040–1062.

144. Lüddens, H., Pritchett, D. B., Kohler, M., Killisch, I., Keinanen, K., Monyer, H., Sprengel, R., and Seeburg, P. H. (1990). Cerebellar GABA$_A$ receptor selective for a behavioral alcohol antagonist. *Nature* 346, 648–651.

145. Skolnick, P., Hu, R. J., Cook, C. M., Hurt, S. D., Trometer, J. D., Liu, R., Huang, Q., and Cook, J. M. (1997). [3H]RY 80: A high-affinity, selective ligand for gamma-aminobutyric acidA receptors containing alpha-5 subunits. *J. Pharmacol. Exp. Ther.* 283(2), 488–493.

146. Hadingham, K. L., Wingrove, P., Le Bourdelles, B., Palmer, K. J., Ragan, C. I., and Whiting, P. J. (1993). Cloning of cDNA sequences encoding human alpha 2 and alpha 3 gamma-aminobutyric acidA receptor subunits and characterization of the benzodiazepine pharmacology of recombinant alpha 1-, alpha 2-, alpha 3-, and alpha 5-containing human gamma-aminobutyric acidA receptors. *Mol. Pharmacol.* 43(6), 970–975.

147. Boismare, F., Daoust, M., Moore, N., Saligaut, C., Lhuintre, J. P., Chretien, P., and Durlach, J. (1984). A homotaurine derivative reduces the voluntary intake of ethanol by rats: Are cerebral GABA receptors involved?. *Pharmacol. Biochem. Behav.* 21(5), 787–789.

148. Fadda, F., Argiolas, A., Melis, M. R., De Montis, G., and Gessa, G. L. (1983). Suppression of voluntary ethanol consumption in rats by gamma-butyrolactone. *Life Sci.* 32(13), 1471–1477.

149. Fuchs, V., Burbes, E., and Cooper, H. (1984). Influence of haloperidol, and aminooxyacetic acid on etonitazene, alcohol, diazepam and barbital consumption. *Drug Alcohol Depend.* 14, 178–186.

150. Mudar, P. J., LeCann, N. C., Czirr, S. A., Hubbell, C. L., and Reid, R. L. (1986). Methadone, pentobarbital, pimozide, and ethanol intake. *Alcohol* 3, 303–308.

151. Duetsh, J. A., and Watson, N. Y. (1997). Diazepam maintenance of ethanol preference during ethanol withdrawal. *Science* 198, 307–309.

152. Boyle, A. E., Smith, B. R., and Amit, Z. (1992). Microstructural analysis of the effects of THIP, a GABA agonist on voluntary ethanol intake in laboratory rats. *Phamacol. Biochem. Behav.* 43, 1121–1127.

153. Smith, B. R., Robidoux, J., and Amit, Z. (1992). GABAergic involvement in the acquisition of voluntary ethanol intake in laboratory rats. *Alcohol Alcohol* 27(3), 227–231.

154. Wegelius, K., Honkanen, A., and Korpi, E. S. (1994). Benzodiazepine receptor ligands modulate ethanol drinking in alcohol-preferring rats. *Eur. J. Pharmacol.* 263, 141–147.

155. Petry, N. M. (1995). Ro 15-4513 selectively attenuates ethanol, but not sucrose, reinforced responding in a concurrent access procedure; comparison to other drugs. *Psychopharmacology (Berl.)* 121(2), 192–203.

156. June, H. L., Hughes, R. W., Spurlock, H. L., and Lewis, M. J. (1994). Ethanol self-administration in freely feeding and drinking rats: Effects of RO15-4513 alone, and in combination with Ro15-1788 (flumazenil). *Psychopharmacology* 115, 332–339.

157. June, H. L., Murphy, J. M., Hewitt, R. L., Greene, T. L., Lin, M., Mellor-Burke, J., Lumeng, L., and Li, T.-K. (1996). Benzodiazepine receptor ligands with different intrinsic efficacies alter ethanol intake in alcohol-nonpreferring (NP) rats. *Neuropsychopharmacology* 14, 55–66.

158. June, H. L., Colker, R. E., Domangue, K. R., Perry, L. E., Hicks, L. H., June, P. L., and Lewis, M. J. (1992). Ethanol self-administration in deprived rats: Effects of RO15-4513 alone, and in combination with flumazenil (Ro15-1788). *Alcoholism: Clin. Exp. Res.* 16, 11–16.

159. Petry, N. M. (1997). Benzodiazepine-GABA modulation of concurrent ethanol and sucrose reinforcement in the rat. *Exp. Clin. Psychopharmacol.* 5(3), 183–194.

160. Samson, H. H., Haraguchi, M., Tolliver, G. A., and Sadeghi, K. G. (1989). Antagonism of ethanol-reinforced behavior by the benzodiazepine inverse agonists RO15-4513 and FG 7142: Relationship to sucrose reinforcement. *Pharmacol. Biochem. Behav.* 33, 601–608.

161. June, H. L., Torres, L., Cason, C. R., Hwang, B. H., Braun, M. R., and Murphy, J. M. (1998). The novel benzodiazepine inverse agonist RO19-4603 antagonizes ethanol motivated behaviors: Neuropharmacological studies. *Brain Res.* 784, 256–275.

162. Mandema, J. W., Kuck, M. T., and Danhof, M. (1992). Differences in intrinsic efficacy of benzodiazepines are reflected in their concentration-EEG effect relationship. *Br. J. Pharmacol.* 105(1), 164–170.

162a. Wong, G., and Skolnick, P. (1992). High affinity ligands for "diazepam" sensitive benzodiazepine receptors. *Eur. J. Pharmacol.* 225, 63–68.

163. Gardner, C. R., Deacon, R., James, V., Parker, F., Budhram, P. (1987). Agonist and antagonist activities at benzodiazepine receptors of novel series of quinoline derivatives. *Eur. J. Pharmacol.* 142, 285–295.

164. Korpi, E. R., Uusi-Oukari, M., and Wegelius, K. (1992). Substrate specificity of diazepam-insensitive cerebellar w3Hx RO15-4513 binding sites. *Eur. J. Pharmacol.* 213, 323–329.

165. Ager, I. R., Doyle, A. B., Hairsine, P. W., McDonald, K. P., Miller, P., and Parker, F. L. (1991). Animal pharmacokinetics of selected imidazopyrimidine ligands for benzodiazepine receptors. *Drug Dev. Res.* 22, 349–361.

166. June, H. L., Zucarelli, D., Craig, K. S., DeLong, J., Cason, C. R., Torres, L., and Murphy, J. M. (1998). High affinity benzodiazepine antagonists reduce responding maintained by EtOH presentation in ethanol-preferring (p) rats. *J. Pharmacol. Exp. Ther.* 284, 1006–1014.

167. Zuccarelli, D., June, H. L., Durr, L. F., and Murphy, J. M. (1996). Benzodiazepine receptor ligands with different intrinsic efficacies modulate EtOH-reinforced responding in alcohol-preferring (P) rats. *Alcoholism: Clin. Exp. Res.* 20, 12A.

168. June, H. L., Dejaravu, S. L., Williams, J., Cason, C. R., Eggers, M. W., Greene, T. L., Leviege, T., Torres, L., Braun, M. R., and Murphy, J. M. (1998). GABAergic modulation of the behavioral actions of ethanol in alcohol-preferring (P) and nonpreferring (NP) rats. *Eur. J. Pharmacol.* 342, 139–151.

169. Duka, T., and Dorow, R. (1995). Human experimental psychopharmacology of benzodiazepine inverse agonists and antagonists. In *Benzodiazepine Receptor Inverse Agonists*, M. Sarter, D. J. Nutt, and R. G. Lister, Eds. Wiley-Liss, New York, pp. 243–270.

170. Reimann, I. W., Jedrychowski, M., Schulz, R., Antonin, K.-H., Roth, A., and Bieck, P. R. (1987). Pharmacokinetic and pharmacodynamic effects of the novel benzodiazepine antagonist 2-phenylpyrazolo(4,3-c)quinolin-one in humans. *Arzneim-Forsch/Drug Res.* 37, 1174–1178.

171. Jensen, L. H., Petersen, E. N., Braestrup, C., Honore, T., Kehr, W., Stephens, D. N., Schneider, H., Seidelmann, D., and Schmiechen, R. (1984). Evaluation of the beta-carboline ZK93 426 as a benzodiazepine receptor antagonist. *Psychopharmacology* 83, 249–256.

172. Duka, T., Goerke, D., Dorow, R., Holler, L., and Fichte, K. (1988). Human studies on the benzodiazepine receptor antagonist beta-carboline ZK 93 426: Antagonism of lormetazepam's psychotropic effects. *Psychopharmacology (Berl.)* 95(4), 463–471.

173. File, S. E., and Pellow, S. (1986). Intrinsic actions of the benzodiazepine receptor antagonist RO 15-1788. *Psychopharmacology* 88, 1–11.

174. Paterson, M. E., Blakley, G. G., and Lewis, M. J. (1996). RO19-4603 produces attenuation of oral self-administration of ethanol for up to 48 h in randomly bred rats. *Alcohol Clin. Exp. Res.* 20, 52 (abstract).

175. Heimer, L., and Alheid, G. F. (1991). Piecing together the puzzle of basal forebrain anatomy. *Adv. Exp. Med. Biol.* 295, 1–42.

176. Hodge, C. W., Chappelle, A. N., and Samson, H. H. (1995). GABAergic transmission in the nucleus accumbens is involved in the termination of ethanol self-administration in rats. *Alcohol Clin. Exp. Res.* 19, 1486–1493.

177. Kalivas, P. W., Duffy, P., and Eberhardt, H. (1990). Modulation of AlO dopamine neurons by gamma-aminobutyric acid agonists. *J. Pharmacol. Exp. Ther.* 253, 858–866.

178. Hodge, C. W., Haraguchi, M., Chappelle, A. M., and Samson, H. H. (1996). Effects of ventral tegmental microinjections of the GABAA agonist muscimol on self-administration of ethanol and sucrose. *Pharmacol. Biochem. Behav.* 53(4), 971–977.

179. June, H. L., Hwang, B. H., and Murphy, J. M. (1997). GABAergic transmission in the meso-accumbens is involved in alcohol motivated behaviors in alcohol-preferring (P) and outbred Wistar rats. Paper presented at the Annual European Society for Biomedical Research on Alcoholism in a symposium entitled "Neurobiology of Alcohol Reinforcement," sponsored by the sixth Congress and Karolinska Institute, Stockholm, Sweden, June 28–July 1, 1997.

180. Cason, C. R., June, H. L., Fredericks, M., Cheatham, G., Chen, A., Cook, J., Gan, T., and Murphy, J. M. (1997). GABAergic regulation of the reinforcing properties of alcohol in Wistar rats. *Soc. Neurosci. Abstr.* 23, 959.

181. Cook, J. M., and Skolnick, P. Personal communication.

182. Haber, S. N., Groenewegen, H. J., Grove, E. A., and Nauta, W. J. (1985). Efferent connections of the ventral pallidum: Evidence of a dual striato pallidofugal pathway. *J. Comp. Neurol.* 235(3), 322–335.

183. Ikemoto, S., Kohl, R. R., and McBride, W. J. (1997). GABA(A) receptor blockade in the anterior ventral tegmental area increases extracellular levels of dopamine in the nucleus accumbens of rats. *J. Neurochem.* 69(1), 137–143.

184. Yim, C. Y., and Mogenson, G. J. (1980). Effect of picrotoxin and nipecotic acid on inhibitory response of dopaminergic neurons in the ventral tegmental area to stimulation of the nucleus aceumbens. *Brain Res.* 199, 466–472.

185. Fibiger, H. C., and Phillips, A. G. (1986). Reward, motivation, cognition: Psychobiology of mesotelencephalic dopamine systems. In *Handbook of Physiology: The Nervous System*, Vol. 4, V. B. Mountcastle, F. F. Bloom, and S. R. Geiger, Eds. American Physiological Society, Bethesda, MD, pp. 647–675.

186. Koob, G. F., and Bloom, F. E. (1988). Cellular and molecular mechanisms of drug dependence. *Science* 242, 715–723.

187. Scheel-Kruger, J. (1986). Dopamine-GABA interactions: Evidence that GABA transmits, modulates and mediates dopaminergic functions in the basal ganglia and the limbic system. *Acta Neurol. Scand. Suppl.* 107, 1–54.

188. Bruno, J. P., and Miller, J. E. (1995). Inhibition of GABAergic transmission: Interactions with other transmitter systems. In *Benzodiazepine Receptor Inverse Agonists*, M. Sarter, D. J. Nutt, and R. G. Lister, Eds. Wiley, New York, pp. 41–81.

189. Claustre, Y., Rivy, J. P., Dennis, T., and Scatton, B. (1986). Pharmacological studies on stress-induced increase in frontal cortical dopamine metabolism in the rat. *J. Pharmacol. Exp. Ther.* 238(2), 693–700.

190. Giorgi, O., Corda, M. G., and Biggio, G. (1988). Ro 15-4513, like anxiogenic beta-carbolines, increases dopamine metabolism in the prefrontal cortex of the rat. *Eur. J. Pharmacol.* 156(1), 71–75.

191. Bradberry, C. W., Lory, J. D., and Roth, R. H. (1991). The anxiogenic beta-carboline FG 7142 selectively increases dopamine release in rat prefrontal cortex as measured by microdialysis. *J. Neurochem.* 56(3), 748–752.

192. McCullough, L. D., and Salamone, J. D. (1992). Anxiogenic drugs beta-CCE and FG 7142 increase extracellular dopamine levels in nucleus accumbens. *Psychopharmacology (Berl.)* 109(3), 379–382.

193. Coco, M. L., Kuhn, C. M., Ely, T. D., and Kilts, C. D. (1992). Selective activation of mesoamygdaloid dopamine neurons by conditioned stress: Attenuation by diazepam. *Brain Res.* 590(1/2), 39–47.

194. Austin, M. C., and Kalivas, P. W. (1990). Enkephalinergic and GABAergic modulation of motor activity in the ventral pallidum. *J. Pharmacol. Exp. Ther.* 252(3), 1370–1377.

195. Phillips, A. G., and Fibiger, H. C. (1991). Dopamine and motivated behavior: Insights provided by *in vivo* analyses. In *The Mesolimbic Dopamine System: From Motivation to Action*, P. Willner and J. Scheel-Kuger, Eds. Wiley, New York, pp. 119–224.

196. Churchill, L., Austin, M. C., and Kalivas, P. W. (1992). Dopamine and endogenous opioid regulation of picrotoxin-induced locomotion in the ventral pallidum after dopamine depletion in the nucleus accumbens. *Psychopharmacology (Berl.)* 108(1/2), 141–146.

197. Kosaka, K., Hama, K., Nagatsu, I., Wu, J. Y., Ottersen, O. P., Storm-Mathisen, J., and Kosaka, T. (1987). Postnatal development of neurons containing both catecholaminergic and GABAergic traits in the rat main olfactory bulb. *Brain Res.* 403(2), 355–360.

198. Legault, M., Rompre, P. P., and Wise, R. A. (2000). Chemical stimulation of the ventral hippocampus elevates nucleus accumbens dopamine by activating dopaminergic neurons of the ventral tegmental area. *J. Neurosci.* 20(4), 1635–1642.

199. Gong, W., Neill, D. B., and Justice, J. B., Jr. (1998). GABAergic modulation of ventral pallidal dopamine release studied by in vivo microdialysis in the freely moving rat. *Synapse* 29(4), 406–412.

200. Cox, E. D., Hagen, T. J., McKernan, R. M., and Cook, J. M. (1995). BZ1 receptor specific ligands. Synthesis and biological properties of BCCt, a BZ1 receptor subtype specific antagonist. *Med. Chem. Res.* 5, 710–718.

201. Cox, E. D., Diaz-Arauzo, H., Huang, Q., Reddy, M. S., Ma, C., Harris, B., McKernan, R. M., Skolnick, P., and Cook, J. M. (1998). Synthesis and evaluation of analogues of the partial agonist 6-(propyloxy)-4-(methoxymethyl)-β-carboline-3-carboxylic acid ethyl ester (6-PBC) and the full agonist 6-(benzyloxy)-4-(methoxymethyl)-β-carboline-3-carboxylic acid ethyl ester (ZK 93423) at wild type and recombinant $GABA_A$ receptors. *J. Med. Chem.* 41, 2537–2552.

202. Shannon, H. E., Guzman, F., and Cook, J. M. (1984). Beta-carboline-3-carboxylate-*t*-butyl ester: A selective BZ1 benzodiazepine receptor antagonist. *Life Sci.* 35(22), 2227–2236.

203. Carroll, M. R., Woods, J., Seyoum, R. A., Cook, J. M., and June, H. L. (2001). The role of the $GABA_A$ α1 subtype in mediating the sedative and anxiolytic properties of benzodiazepines in high and low alcohol drinking rats. Paper presented at the annual meeting of the Research Society on Alcoholism in Montreal, Canada, June 2001.

204. Griebel, G., Perrault, G., Letang, V., Grainger, P., Avenet, P., Schoemaker, H., and Sanger, D. J. (1999). New evidence that the pharmacological effects of benzodiazepine receptor ligands can be associated with activities at different BZ (α) receptor subtypes. *Psychopharmacology (Berl.)* 146, 205–213.

205. Paronis, C. A., Cox, E. D., Cook, J. M., and Bergman, J. (2001). Different types of GABA(A) receptors may mediate the anticonflict and response rate-decreasing effects of zaleplon, zolpidem, and midazolam in squirrel monkeys. *Psychopharmacology (Berl.)* 156(4), 461–468.

206. Rowlett, J. K., Tornatzky, W., Cook, J. M., Chunrong, M., and Miczek, K. A. (2001). Zolpidem, triazolam, and diazepam decrease distress vocalizations in mouse pups: Differential antagonism by flumazenil and the β-carboline-3-carbozylate-*t*-butyl ester (βCCt). *J. Pharmacol. Exp. Ther.* 297, 247–253.

207. Rowlett, J. K., Platt, D. M., Lelas, S., Atack, J. R., and Dawson, G. R. (2005). Different GABAA receptor subtypes mediate the anxiolytic, abuse-related, and motor effects of benzodiazepine-like drugs in primates. *Proc. Natl. Acad. Sci. USA* 102(3), 915–920.

208. Rowlett, J. K., Cook, J. M., Duke, A. N., and Platt, D. M. (2005). Selective antagonism of GABAA receptor subtypes: An in vivo approach to exploring the therapeutic and side effects of benzodiazepine-type drugs. *CNS Spectr.* 10(1), 40–48.

209. McKernan, R. M., Rosh, T. W., Reynolds, D. S., Sure, C., Wafford, K. A., Attack, J. R., Farrar, S., Myers, J., Cook, G., Ferris, P., Garrett, L., Bristow, L., Marshall, G., Macula, N., Brown, N., Howell, O., Moore, K. W., Carling, R. W., Street, L. J., Castro, J. L., Ragan, C. I., Dawson, G. R., and Whiting, P. J. (2000). Sedative but not anxiolytic properties of benzodiazepines are mediated by the GABA$_A$ receptor α_1 subtype. *Nat. Neurosci.* 3, 587–592.

210. Sanger, D. J., Benavides, J., Perrault, G., Morel, E., Cohen, C., Joly, D., and Zivkovic, B. (1994). Recent developments in the behavioral pharmacology of benzodiazepine (omega) receptors: Evidence for the functional significance of receptor subtypes. *Neurosci. Biobehav. Rev.* 18, 355–372.

211. Wafford, K. A., Whiting, P. J., and Kemp, J. A. (1993). Differences in affinity of benzodiazepine receptor ligands at recombinant γ-aminobutyric acid$_A$ receptors subtypes. *Mol. Pharmacol.* 43, 240–244.

212. Wafford, K. A., Bain, C. J., Whiting, P. J., and Kemp, J. A. (1993). Functional comparison of the role of γ subunits in recombinant human γ-aminobutyric acid$_A$/benzodiazepine receptors. *Mol. Pharmacol.* 44, 437–442.

213. Churchill, L., Bourdelais, A., Austin, S., Lolait, S. J., Mahan, L. C., O'Carroll, A. M., and Kalivas, P. W. (1991). GABA$_A$ receptors containing α1 and β2 subunits are mainly localized on neurons in the ventral pallidum. *Synapse* 8, 75–85.

214. Duncan, G. E., Breese, G. R., Criswell, H. E., McCown, T. J., Herbert, J. S., Devaud, L. L., and Morrow, A. L. (1995). Distribution of {^{3}H}zolpidem binding sites in relation to messenger RNA encoding the α1, β2 and γ2 subunits of GABA$_A$ receptors in rat brain. *Neuroscience* 64, 1113–1128.

215. Groenewegen, H. J., Vermeulen-Van Der Zee, E., Te Kortschot, A., and Witter, M. P. (1987). Organization of the projections to the ventral striatum in the rat. A study using anterograde transport of *phaseolus vulgaris leucoagglutinin*. *Neuroscience* 23, 103–120.

216. Nauta, W. J., Smith, G. P., Faull, R. L., and Domesick, V. B. (1978). Efferent connections and nigral afferents of the nucleus accumbens septi in the rat. *Neuroscience* 3(4/5), 385–401.

217. Zahm, D. S., and Heimer, L. (1988). Ventral striatopallidal parts of the basal ganglia in the rat: I. Neurochemical compartmentation as reflected by the distributions of neurotensin and substance P immunoreactivity. *J. Comp. Neurol.* 272(4), 516–535.

218. Criswell, H. E., Simson, P. E., Duncan, G. E., Mc Cown, T. J., Herbert, J. S., and Morrow, A. L., et al. (1993). Molecular basis for regionally specific action of ethanol on

γ-aminobutyric acidA receptors: Generalization to other ligand-gated ion channels. *J. Pharmacol. Exp. Ther.* 267, 522–527.

219. Criswell, H. E., Simson, P. E., Knapp, D. J., Devaud, L. L., Mc Cown, T. J., and Duncan, G. E., et al. (1995). Effect of zolpidem on γ-aminobutyric acid (GABA)-induced inhibition predicts the interaction of ethanol with GABA on individual neurons in several rat brains. *J. Pharmacol. Exp. Ther.* 73, 526–536.

220. Hiroi, N., and White, N. M. (1993). The ventral pallidum area is involved in the acquisition but not expression of the amphetamine conditioned place preference. *Neurosci. Lett.* 156(1/2), 9–12.

221. O'Malley, S. S., Jaffe, A. J., Chang, G., Schottenfeld, R. S., Meyer, R. E., and Rounsaville, B. (1992). Naltrexone and coping skills therapy for alcohol dependence. A controlled study. *Arch. Gen. Psychiatry* 49(11), 881–887.

222. Baldwin, H. A., Wall, T. L., Schuckit, M. A., and Koob, G. F. (1991). Differential effects of ethanol on punished responding in the P and NP rats. *Alcohol Clin. Exp. Res.* 15(4), 700–704.

223. Schuckit, M. A., Irwin, M., and Brown, S. A. (1990). The history of anxiety symptoms among 171 primary alcoholics. *J. Stud. Alcohol* 51, 34–41.

224. Stewart, R. B., Gatto, G. J., Lumeng, L., Li, T. K., and Murphy, J. M. (1993). Comparison of alcohol-preferring (P) and nonpreferring (NP) rats on tests of anxiety and for the anxiolytic effects of ethanol. *Alcohol* 10(1), 1–10.

225. Sur, C., Fresu, L., Howell, O., McKernan, R. M., and Atack, J. R. (1999). Autoradiographic localization of the a5 subunit-containing $GABA_A$ receptor in rat brain. *Brain Res.* 822, 265–270.

226. Amaral, D. G., and Witter, M. P. (1995). Hippocampal formation. In *The Rat Central Nervous System*, G. Paxinos, Ed. Academic, San Diego, pp. 449–492.

227. Kelley, A., and Domesick, V. B. (1982). The distribution of the projection from the hippocampal formation to the nucleus accumbens in the rat: An anterograde- and retrograde-horseradish peroxidase study. *Neuroscience* 7, 2321–2335.

228. Lui, R. Y., Zhang, P. W., McKernan, R., Wafford, K., and Cook, J. M. (1995). Synthesis of a novel imidazobenzodiazepine ligands for the α5β2γ2 Bz5 GABAA receptor subtype. *Med. Chem. Res.* 5, 700–709.

229. Lui, R. Y., Hu, R. J., Zhang, P. W., Skolnick, P., and Cook, J. M. (1996). Synthesis and pharmacological properties of novel 8-substituted midazobenzodiazepines: High affinity, selective probes for α5 containing GABAA receptors. *J. Med.* 39, 1928–1934.

230. Harris, C. M., and Lal, H. (1988). Central nervous system effects of RO15–4513. *Drug Dev. Res.* 13, 187–203.

231. Jackson, H. C., and Nutt, D. J. (1995). Inverse agonist and alcohol. In *Benzodiazepine Receptor Inverse Agonists*, M. Sarter, D. J. Nutt, and R. G. Lister, Eds. Wiley, New York, pp. 243–270.

232. Haefely, W. (1983). Antagonists of benzodiazepine: Functional aspects. In *Benzodiazepine Recognition. Site Ligands Biochemistry and Pharmacology*, G. Biggio and E. Costa, Eds. Raven, New York, pp. 73.

233. Haefely, W. (1985). Pharmacology of benzodiazepine antagonists. *Pharmacopsychiatry* 18, 163–166.

234. Haefely, W. (1990). The GABAA-benzodiazepine receptor: Biology and pharmacology. In *Handbook of Anxiety*, G. D. Burrows, M. Roth, and R. Noyes, Jr., Eds. Elsevier Science, Amsterdam, pp. 165–188.

235. Lelas, S., Rowlett, J. K., Spealman, R. D., Cook, J. M., Ma, C., Li, X., and Yin, W. (2002). Differential role of $GABA_A$ benzodiazepine receptors containing α1 and α5

subunits in the discriminative stimulus effects of triazolam in squirrel monkeys. *Psychopharmacology (Berl.)* 161, 180–188.
236. Izquierdo, I., and Medina, J. H. (1991). GABAA receptor modulation of memory: The role of endogenous benzodiazepines. *Trends Pharmacol. Sci.* 12, 260–265.
237. June, H. L., Duemler, S. E., Greene, T. L., Williams, J. A., Lin, M., Devaraju, S. L., Chen, S. H., Lewis, M. J., and Murphy, J. M. (1995). Effects of the benzodiazepine inverse agonist RO19-4603 on the maintenance of tolerance to a single dose of ethanol. *J. Pharmacol. Exp. Ther.* 274(3), 1105–1112.
238. Graham, D., Faure, C., Besnard, F., and Langer, S. Z. (1996). Pharmacological profile of benzodiazepine site ligands with recombinant $GABA_A$ receptor subtypes. *Eur. Neuropsychopharm.* 6, 119–125.
239. von Blankenfeld, G., Ymer, S., and Pritchett, D. (1990). Differential pharmacology of recombinant $GABA_A$ receptors. *Neurosci. Lett.* 115, 269–273.
240. Cloninger, R. (1987). Neurogenetic adaptive mechanisms in alcoholism. *Science* 236, 410–416.
241. Li, T.-K. (2000). Pharmacogenetics of responses to alcohol and genes that influence alcohol drinking. *J. Stud. Alcohol* 61, 5–12.
242. Li, T.-K., Crabb, D. W., and Lumeng, L. (1991). Molecular and genetic approaches to understanding alcohol-seeking behavior. In *Neuropharmacology of Ethanol*, R. E. Meyer, G. F. Koob, M. J. Lewis, and S. P. Paul, Eds. Birkhauser, Boston, pp. 107–124.
243. Johnson, B. A., and Ait-Daoud, N. (2000). Neuropharmacological treatments for alcoholism: Scientific basis and clinical findings. *Psychopharmacology (Berl.)* 149, 327–344.
244. Kranzler, H. R. (2000). Pharmacotherapy of alcoholism: Gaps in knowledge ad opportunities for research. *Alcohol Alcoholism* 35, 537–547.
245. National Institute on Alcohol Abuse and Alcoholism (NIAAA) (2004). Neuroscience research and therapeutic targets. Alcohol Alert No. 61. NIAAA, Rockville, MD.
246. Lui, R. Y., Zhang P. W., McKernan R., Wafford K., and Cook, J. M. (1995). Synthesis of a novel imidazobenzodiazepine ligands for the $\alpha5\beta2\gamma2$ Bz5 $GABA_A$ receptor subtype. *Med. Chem. Res.* 5, 700–709.
247. Lui, R. Y., Hu R. J., Zhang P. W., Skolnick P., and Cook, J. M. (1996). Synthesis and pharmacological properties of novel 8-substituted imidazobenzodiazepines: High affinity, selective probes for eg. $\alpha5$ containing $GABA_A$ receptors. *J. Med. Med.* 39, 1928–1934.

15

NICOTINE

AUGUST R. BUCHHALTER[1], REGINALD V. FANT[1] AND
JACK E. HENNINGFIELD[1,2]

[1]*Pinney Associates, Bethesda, Maryland; and* [2]*The Johns Hopkins University School of Medicine, Baltimore, Maryland*

15.1	Overview	535
15.2	Pharmacology of Nicotine	536
	15.2.1 Overview	536
	15.2.2 Nicotinic Acetylcholine Receptors	537
	15.2.3 Nicotine Reinforcement Neurosubstrates	537
	15.2.4 nAChR Functional Adaptations	540
	15.2.5 Nicotine Withdrawal Neurosubstrates	541
	15.2.6 Pharmacokinetics	543
	15.2.6.1 Absorption	544
	15.2.6.2 Distribution	544
	15.2.6.3 Metabolism and Elimination	545
15.3	Pharmacological Treatment of Nicotine Dependence and Withdrawal	545
	15.3.1 Overview	545
	15.3.2 Nicotine Replacement Medications	546
	15.3.2.1 Transdermal Nicotine Patch	546
	15.3.2.2 Acute Delivery Systems	547
	15.3.3 Nicotinic Pharmacotherapies	548
	15.3.3.1 Nicotinic Partial Agonists	548
	15.3.3.2 Nicotinic Antagonists	549
	15.3.4 Nonnicotinic Pharmacotherapies	549
	15.3.4.1 Bupropion	549
	15.3.4.2 Tricyclic Antidepressants	550
	15.3.4.3 Cannabinoid Antagonists	550
	15.3.4.4 Opioid Antagonists	550
	15.3.5 Nicotine Pharmacology Implications for Public Health Policy	551
Acknowledgments		552
Disclosures		552
References		552

15.1 OVERVIEW

Nicotine is the drug delivered upon tobacco use that defines the dependence and withdrawal syndromes as recognized by the World Health Organization (WHO) and

---

Handbook of Contemporary Neuropharmacology, Edited by David R. Sibley, Israel Hanin, Michael Kuhar, and Phil Skolnick. Copyright © 2007 John Wiley & Sons, Inc.

American Psychiatric Association (APA) [1, 2]. Many other potentially psychoactive substances are present in tobacco and/or the smoke of burned tobacco [3], but as concluded by Lewin in the 1920s, "the decisive factor in the [psychic] effects of tobacco, desired or undesired, is nicotine" [4, p. 256]. As a pharmacological agent with diverse and powerful neuronal effects and an important historical role in the development of neuroscience research strategies even before the term *neuroscience* was used, nicotine is fascinating to study.

Nicotine itself is not without toxicity, but at doses typically ingested by tobacco users, its direct contribution to disease is comparatively small relative to the more than 60 carcinogens, carbon monoxide, and many lung and cardiovascular toxins produced by tobacco cigarette smoking. Its role in tobacco-caused disease is primarily to sustain high and persistent levels of toxic tobacco smoke exposure. Thus, most tobacco-caused disease may be considered side effects of nicotine dependence. From a public health perspective, then, nicotine is critical in the scope and persistence of a global tobacco epidemic that is so devastating that it led to the first-ever international treaty negotiated by the WHO, put into force in 2005 [5]. This treaty, in turn, has already begun to drive additional research on nicotine and tobacco as part of its strong advocacy of a public health–driven demand reduction approach to controlling tobacco-caused disease.

Nationally, cigarette smoking has been cited as "the leading cause of preventable death in the United States" and is associated with profound health-related and financial costs [6, 7]. In terms of health costs, cigarette smoking causes approximately 442, 398 premature deaths yearly [7]. Projections based on current smoking prevalence rates predict that, among persons who are currently younger than 18, approximately 6.4 million will die prematurely from a tobacco-related illness [7]. Financially, smoking costs approximately $157 billion in annual health-related economic losses [6].

This chapter is intended to provide a state-of-the-art review of the pharmacology of nicotine to lay the foundation for furthering the understanding of nicotine's role in tobacco use and its potential use as a treatment for tobacco use disorders. Research in recent decades involving the understanding, prevention, and treatment of tobacco dependence has already led to breakthroughs that are saving lives, but much has yet to be done. Based on the current course, if stronger actions are not developed and implemented, more than 1 million people will die prematurely every 2.5 years in the United States for decades to come, and approximately one-half billion of current smokers will perish globally. As recognized by the WHO, in its treaty, research is vital to guide public health policy [5]. We begin the chapter with a review of nicotine pharmacology (Section 15.2), followed by a review of pharmacologically based treatments for tobacco dependence (Section 15.3), and conclude with a section on public health policy implications.

15.2 PHARMACOLOGY OF NICOTINE

15.2.1 Overview

This section focuses on nicotine pharmacology (Section 15.2.2), namely nicotinic acetylcholine receptors (nAChRs), the neurobiological mechanisms and/or functional adaptations associated with nicotine reinforcement (Section 15.2.3), dependence and tolerance (Section 15.2.4), withdrawal (Section 15.2.5), and nicotine pharmacokinetics (Section 15.2.6). The content (e.g., selection and order of topics) presented in Sections 15.2.2–15.2.5 has been adapted from Markou, Koob, and Henningfield (2003) [8].

15.2.2 Nicotinic Acetylcholine Receptors

Nicotine was first isolated from the leaves of tobacco, *Nicotiana tabacum*, in 1828 by Posselt and Reiman. It is a natural liquid alkaloid structurally similar to acetylcholine (ACh) that interacts with specific nAChRs in the central and peripheral nervous systems [9–11]. Nicotine and other nicotinic acting agents were used by Langely and colleagues in the 1890s and early twentieth century to explore the function and structure of the nervous system. They employed pharmacological tools, including the study of dose–response relationships, temporal and dose-related aspects of tolerance development and loss, and interactions among agonists and antagonists. This work led Langley (1905) to postulate the existence of some "receptive substance" which mediated the effects of nicotine and other agents and which would explain the selective action of differing chemicals on the same muscular and organ systems.

It is now known that nicotine produces its varied effects by binding to nAChRs, of which there are two categories, muscular and neuronal [12]. These receptors vary in their expression and function. For instance, muscular nAChRs are expressed in mature skeletal neuromuscular junctions while neuronal nAChRs are expressed in the autonomic ganglia and the central nervous system (CNS) [12, 13]. In the context of nicotine addiction and its neurobiological mechanisms, the nAChRs of most relevance are those expressed in the brain, attributable to their proposed role in the neuromodulation of several CNS transmitters [14], as described below.

Nicotinic acetylcholine receptors in the brain, located primarily on presynaptic terminals [14] and to a lesser extent at somatodendritic, axonal, and postsynaptic locations (for review, see [15]), are diverse members of the neurotransmitter-gated ion channel superfamily [16] comprised of five nAChR subunits (i.e., α and β subunits combined or α subunits alone) that combine to form a functional receptor [8, 16–18]. The nAChRs expressed most widely in the brain are comprised of α_4, β_2, or α_7 subunits [11, 17]; nicotine-induced dopamine release is dependent on the β_2 subunit [19]. Importantly, the way in which individual subunits (α_1 to α_{10}; β_1 to β_4 [11, 18, 20]) combine to form a nAChR influences its affinity for nicotine binding [11, 16]. For instance, nAChRs formed in a heteropentameric configuration comprised of α and β subunits, which contain β_2 subunits, have a high affinity while nAChRs formed in a homopentameric configuration comprised only of α_7 subunits have a low affinity [16]; among nAChR subunits, β_2 has the highest affinity for nicotine [21].

Activation of nAChRs in the brain releases multiple neurotransmitters, including dopamine (DA), serotonin (5-HT), glutamate (Glu), γ-aminobutyric acid (GABA), and endogenous opioid peptides (EOPs) [16]. These neurotransmitters are associated with nicotine's reinforcement, dependence and tolerance, and withdrawal, as described below.

15.2.3 Nicotine Reinforcement Neurosubstrates

In the context of substance abuse, nicotine has been known for decades to be dependence producing [22]; nicotine dependence diagnostic criteria have been defined elsewhere [2]. Nicotine's dependence-producing properties are, in part, due to its pharmacodynamic profile. Nicotine serves as an effective reinforcer in humans and in several species of animals, including rats, mice, and nonhuman primates, as demonstrated by self-administration studies [23, 24]. In humans, nicotine's reinforcing effects include mild euphoria [25], increased energy and arousal, and decreased stress and anxiety and appetite [26]. Recent studies of the trajectory of patterns of acquisition of nicotine self-administration in rats may serve as a bridge to human longitudinal work. For instance, studies by Lanza et al. [27] and Donny et al. [28] demonstrate that individual differences appearing early in the acquisition process affect resulting patterns of nicotine self-administration, which is consistent with findings that individual differences in early tobacco use may influence differentially the development of regular tobacco use and the emergence of dependence in humans [29].

Neurosubstrates involved in nicotine reinforcement include the mesolimbic dopaminergic system (for reviews, see [11, 30]) and the following neurotransmitters: DA, Glu, and GABA [8]. Other neurosubstrates involved include corticotropin-releasing factor (CRF) and opioid receptors [8]. The role(s) of each neurosubstrate in the modulation of nicotine reinforcement has been provided below.

Acute nicotine administration, possibly by activating nAChRs on mesolimbic dopaminergic neurons at the ventral tegmental area (VTA) and nucleus accumbens [31], increases the firing rate of VTA dopaminergic neurons [32] and elevates dialysate DA levels specifically in the nucleus accumbens shell [33–36]. A series of studies by Nisell et al. [36–38] have demonstrated that nAChRs in the VTA, compared to those in the nucleus accumbens, have a more salient role in mediating the effects of nicotine on DA release. Further evidence of the role of nAChRs on VTA dopaminergic neurons in nicotine reinforcement has been provided by findings that injections of dihydro-β-erythroidine, a nicotinic antagonist, into the VTA [39], microfusion of 6-hydroxydopamine into the nucleus accumbens, producing mesolimbic dopamine system lesions [40], and administration of DA receptor antagonists (SCH23390 and spiperone) [41] decrease nicotine self-administration. These findings are specific to nicotine's reinforcing effects, as opposed to other potential nicotine-induced effects (cognitive improvement) [42].

Another neurosubstrate that may mediate nicotine reinforcement is the Glu neurotransmitter system [8]. Nicotine may elevate striatal DA levels either directly, by glutamatergic stimulation of the ventral striatum, and/or indirectly, by glutamatergic stimulation of VTA dopaminergic neurons projecting to the striatum [8]. By activating excitatory presynaptic nAChRs on glutamatergic terminals, nicotine increases glutamate release [43, 44]. As in other brain sites, acute nicotine administration increases Glu release in the VTA [45]. Within the VTA, nicotine is thought to act at presynaptic α_7 nAChRs located on Glu afferents [45], whereby increasing Glu release, which in turn stimulates DA release in the nucleus accumbens [45–47]; multiple studies suggest α_7 nAChR subunits and/or $\alpha_4\beta_2$ nAChR subtypes have a role in nicotine reinforcement, DA release, and the anxiolytic effects [19–50] that contribute to continued tobacco use [22] (alternatively, see [51]). As an intermediary step, the enhanced Glu release acts at N-methyl-D-aspartate (NMDA) and non-NMDA receptor sites on postsynaptic dopamingeric neurons, which increases their firing rate [8]. Blockade of metabotropic glutamate receptor 5, using the mGluR5 antagonist 2-methyl-6(phenylethynyl)-pyridine, decreases nicotine self-administration in rats and mice, potentially by decreasing nicotine-stimulated DA release in the mesolimbic system [52].

Another neurosubstrate that may mediate nicotine reinforcement is the GABA neurotransmitter system [8]. Dopaminergic neurons projecting from the VTA to the nucleus accumbens [53] receive descending GABAergic input from the ventral pallidum and the nucleus accumbens [54, 55]. Dopaminergic tone in the VTA and nucleus accumbens is inhibited by these GABAergic neurons [11, 56]. At the VTA, DA inhibition involves GABAergic inhibitory afferents to dopaminergic ventral tegmental neurons [54, 57] and interneurons within the VTA [58]. In the nucleus accumbens, DA inhibition involves medium spiny GABA neurons [58]. Demonstrative of GABA's neuromodulation effects, administration of γ-vinyl-GABA (GVG, or vigabatrin), an irreversible GABA transaminase inhibitor [59], abolishes expression and acquisition of conditioned place preference, nicotine-induced increases in synaptic DA [60], and dose dependently decreases nicotine self-administration in rats [59]. Additionally, administration of baclofen or CGP44532, selective $GABA_B$ agonists, decreases nicotine self-administration [61–63], suggesting that enhancement of GABA transmission via $GABA_B$ receptors may antagonize nicotine's reinforcing effects. Baclofen's effects on tobacco smoking has been examined in only one clinical study [64]. Acute administration of baclofen was not demonstrably efficacious in reducing cigarette smoking or nicotine-craving ratings.

Other neurosubstrates that may mediate nicotine reinforcement involve the hypothalamic–pituitary–adrenal (HPA) axis and corticotropin-releasing factor [8] (CRF; also abbreviated CRH, for corticotropin-releasing hormone [65]), a neuropeptide neurotransmitter involved in stress responses [65]. Corticotropin-releasing factor transmission in the paraventricular nucleus of the hypothalamus (PVN) has been hypothesized to mediate the effects of acute nicotine exposure on the HPA in rodents and humans [8]. In rats, injection of nicotine or exposure to cigarette smoke increases corticosterone and adrenocorticotropic hormone (ACTH) levels [66, 67]. A series of studies by Matta et al. (1987) [68] suggest these effects are mediated by central nicotinic cholinergic receptors. Several findings indicate that CRF in the paraventricular nucleus mediates the effects of nicotine on the HPA stress response system. First, nicotine stimulates CRF release in vitro from the rat hypothalamus [69]. Second, nicotine produces concentration- and time-dependent increases in CRF messenger RNA expression in the AR-5 immortalized amygdalar cell line [70]. Third, CRF-containing synaptic vesicles are located in axon terminals with nAChRs in the rat hypothalamus (i.e., median eminence), indicating that nicotine may act on nAChRs in axon terminals to release CRF [71]. Lastly, nicotine administration induces dose-dependent cFOS expression in CRH-containing regions of the PVN [72], bed nucleus of the stria terminalis and central nucleus of the amygdala, and dorsal raphe [73].

In humans, cigarette smoking or nicotine infusions (i.e., intravenous administration), under limited conditions, increases cortisol and ACTH levels [74–78]. One study [77] demonstrates that within a 10-min smoking period smoking two conventional (2-mg nicotine) cigarettes compared to two very low nicotine (0.2-mg nicotine) cigarettes increases cortisol levels. Another study [78], using controlled smoking procedures (e.g., interpuff interval of 25 s), demonstrates that within a 12-min smoking period 24 puffs (equivalent of two cigarettes, approximately) of high-nicotine (15.48 mg nicotine; [79]) cigarettes, but not low-nicotine (1.1-mg nicotine, as determined by the manufacturer, Murty Pharmaceuticals Inc.) cigarettes, increases ACTH levels. A third study [75], having similar design features as those above, reveals a comparable pattern of results for both cortisol and ACTH levels. Like findings have been reported elsewhere [80]. In nonsmoking, nicotine-naïve subjects receiving intravenous nicotine bitartrate (0.25 and 0.5 µg/kg/min), only infusions of the 0.5-µg dose increase cortisol and ACTH levels [76].

Overall, the relationship between the HPA axis/hormones and abuse-related effects of drugs is not understood fully [78]. However, HPA axis activation is believed to be involved in several phases of the addiction process [78]. Multiple hypotheses regarding the involvement of the HPA axis/hormones have been raised. One hypothesis, using cocaine as a comparator, posits that ACTH and cortisol may contribute to nicotine's reinforcing effects [78]. Another hypothesis proposes that CRH may play a role in mediating nicotine's effects on behaviors pertaining to stress and anxiety [8], generally, and the anxiety and irritability often associated with nicotine withdrawal, specifically [11, 78], as described below (Section 15.2.5).

The final neurosubstrate presented in this chapter that may mediate nicotine reinforcement involves opioid receptors. Two primary lines of evidence suggest opioid receptors at least partially mediate nicotine reinforcement. First, nicotine influences the release of EOPs [81, 82], both within and outside the mesolimbic DA system [11]. Within the mesolimbic DA system, nicotine increases tissue levels of opioid peptides in the nucleus accumbens [83, 84], which contain a high density of µ-opioid receptors [85]. These receptors have been hypothesized to be occupied by endogenous opioid ligands released by nicotine [86]. Outside the mesolimbic DA system, nicotine induces the release of the pro-opiomelanocortin peptide group by stimulating nAChRs within the hypothalamus; the pro-opiomelanocortin peptide group includes the precursor β-endorphin [11, 87] which, while undetermined, may be involved in mediating nicotine's positive reinforcing effects [11]. Taken together, nicotine's positive reinforcing effects may be mediated by activation of enkephalin neurons (i.e., dopamine-independent reward systems) [11]. Second, opioid receptor antagonists such as naloxone and naltrexone have demonstrable efficacy in decreasing cigarette consumption and self-reported smoking satisfaction and increasing smoking cessation rates [88–91], suggesting that opioid receptors may modulate nicotine's reinforcing effects [8] (alternatively see [92, 93]).

15.2.4 nAChR Functional Adaptations

Features common among drugs of abuse are their ability to produce and maintain dependence and tolerance [2]. For nicotine, both dependence and tolerance may involve functional adaptations of nAChRs [8, 11, 18, 94], as described below. Contrary to most agonists, which downregulate receptors with chronic drug exposure [94], chronic nicotine administration desensitizes and inactivates nAChRs, which leads paradoxically to an upregulation of nAChR sites [8, 94, 95]. This nicotine-induced, paradoxical upregulation of nAChRs has been observed in the rodent brain [96, 97], human brain [98–100], and human blood leukocytes [101] and is dose dependent [99, 101].

The role of nAChR desensitization and upregulation in the subjective effects of acute nicotine exposure and in the development and maintenance of nicotine dependence has undergone much speculation [102, 103]. Experimental findings pertaining to the effects of chronic nicotine exposure on nAChRs in animals have been mixed. For instance, there is some evidence that chronic nicotine exposure increases nAChR numbers [104, 105] and function [106]. Conversely, there is some evidence that chronic nicotine exposure decreases nAChR numbers [107] and function [108]. Behaviorally, as a means of counteracting the continuous agonist actions of nicotine on the receptors, nicotine dependence is related to the decrease in nAChR numbers and/or function [8, 109]. In turn, the prolonged functional desensitization or inactivation of nAChRs associated with chronic nicotine administration has been hypothesized to lead to receptor upregulation [107, 110, 111] (alternatively, see [112]). Importantly, because the majority of studies indicating nAChR changes have been conducted in vitro, the functional significance of these changes in vivo is unknown [103] and thus requires further study [113]. Also worth noting, particularly when interpreting seemingly opposite effects, is that different nAChR subtypes vary in their sensitivity to nicotine, as evidenced by differential degrees and rates of desensitization and upregulation [8, 11]. For instance, nAChRs composed of $\alpha_4\beta_2$ subunits desensitize slowly [18] while α_7 receptors desensitize rapidly [18]. Thus behavioral observations may reflect the combined effects of complex adaptations of different nAChR types [8].

It appears plausible that initial discomfort associated with smoking cessation reflects the 300 to 400% increase in nicotine receptors [100], many of which are abruptly unoccupied. In turn, nicotine replacement therapy (NRT) may provide its benefits, in part, by occupying these receptors, thus contributing to stable physiological functioning while the person behaviorally adapts to living without smoking. The therapy, in turn, provides a means to reduce gradually daily nicotine over several weeks or months, potentially, allowing receptor levels to achieve an appropriate balance. The question of returning to "baseline" or "normal" receptor levels may not be meaningful for tobacco users because they typically began smoking during adolescence with long term cessation achieved (if it is achieved) after several decades of tobacco use. The possibility that some tobacco users will require long-term NRT use (or other therapeutic measures) to sustain tobacco-delivered nicotine abstinence is then not surprising.

The aforementioned nAChR adaptations likely are involved in producing tolerance to some of nicotine's acute effects [114]. Tolerance to nicotine's acute effects is gained throughout the day, with repeated acute nicotine exposure, and lost throughout the night, due to overnight abstinence while the smoker sleeps [115]. The time course of tolerance, whether a gain or loss, varies across nicotine-induced responses [114, 116, 117]. For instance, smokers develop a large degree of tolerance to nicotine's acute subjective and cardiovascular effects [114, 118–120].

15.2.5 Nicotine Withdrawal Neurosubstrates

As with many other drugs of abuse, nicotine, upon abrupt cessation (i.e., smoking abstinence in humans), can produce an aversive withdrawal syndrome in humans [121, 122] and rodents, though observed less reliably in mice [109, 123–127]. The nicotine withdrawal syndrome, as defined by the APA [2], consists of subjective, cognitive, and physiological components and has been cited by many smokers as a reason for failed quit attempts [128], which results in continued tobacco use. Common subjective effects include restlessness, impatience, irritability, depressed mood, dysphoria, craving, and anxiety [2, 121, 129]. A common cognitive effect includes difficulty concentrating [2, 121, 129]. Common physiological effects include decreases in heart rate and adrenaline and noradrenaline excretion and increases in skin temperature, electroencephalographic theta power, and weight [130–133]. In rats, the most prominent signs of withdrawal include abdominal constrictions (writhes), gasps, ptosis, facial fasciculation, and eyeblinks [124, 134, 135]. These withdrawal signs are mediated both centrally and peripherally [11, 124, 136]. Other withdrawal signs observed in rodents include disruptions of food-maintained learned behaviors in rats [137], increases in the acoustic startle response in rats [138], decreases in prepulse inhibition in mice [127], and elevations in brain reward thresholds [109, 135, 139]. Several dissociations between threshold elevations and somatic signs [134, 139] suggest that the various components of nicotine withdrawal are mediated by different substrates [8]. Neurosubstrates involved in nicotine withdrawal, comprised of many of the same substrates involved in nicotine reinforcement, include the mesolimbic dopaminergic system and the following neurotransmitters: DA, 5-HT, and Glu [8]. Other neurosubstrates involved include CRF and opioid receptors [8]. The role(s) of each neurosubstrate in nicotine withdrawal has been provided below.

Precipitated nicotine withdrawal, as induced by systemic or intra-VTA mecamylamine (nAChR antagonist) administration, decreases DA dialysate levels in the nucleus accumbens [140, 141] and the central nucleus of the amygdala [142] in nicotine-treated rats. Additionally, mecamylamine injections into the VTA dose dependently precipitates a constellation of somatic withdrawal signs [143], suggesting possibly that nAChR transmission in the VTA has a role in the expression of nicotine withdrawal's somatic signs [8]. Similar decreases in DA levels in the nucleus accumbens have been observed with withdrawal from other drugs of abuse, including ethanol, morphine, cocaine, and amphetamine [144, 145]. Further demonstrative of the involvement of DA in nicotine withdrawal is the finding that bupropion (Zyban), a smoking cessation aid that acts, in part, by inhibiting neuronal reuptake of DA, enhances DA transmission [146, 147]. Moreover, while its effects on nicotine self-administration have been varied [148–150], bupropion has been shown to reverse threshold elevations and somatic signs associated with nicotine withdrawal [135, 151].

Because administration of nAChR antagonists into the VTA decreases nucleus accumbens dialysate levels, as described above, suggests that reductions in endogenous cholinergic tone may cause nicotine withdrawal. The receptors involved most likely are α_4-containing high-affinity nAChRs [152].

Another neurosubstrate that may mediate nicotine withdrawal involves the 5-HT neurotransmitter, generally, and the $5-HT_{1A}$ receptor, specifically [153, 154]. Pretreatment with 8-OH-DPAT and LY274600, $5-HT_{1A}$ receptor agonists, enhance the auditory startle response observed during nicotine withdrawal, whereas NAN-190, WAY-100635, or LY206130, $5-HT_{1A}$ receptor antagonists, blocks the increase in startle response [155]. Additionally, during nicotine withdrawal, the sensitivity of dorsal raphe nucleus neurons to 8-OH-DPAT increases [156]. Therefore, nicotine withdrawal, by increasing potentially the inhibitory influence of somatodendritic $5-HT_{1A}$ autoreceptors located within the raphe nuclei, may decrease 5-HT release into forebrain and limbic brain sites [157, 158]. Evidence of this is provided by the finding that, in rats undergoing nicotine withdrawal, coadministration of fluoxetine, a serotonin-selective reuptake inhibitor, and p-MPPI, a $5-HT_{1A}$ receptor antagonist, reverses elevation of brain reward thresholds but not somatic signs [139], lending further support that nicotine withdrawal's affective and somatic components are not mediated by the same mechanism [8]. Consistent with the overall findings above, buspirone, a partial 5-HT$_{1A}$ agonist, demonstrates efficacy in smoking cessation trials and may alleviate withdrawal severity, at least among short-term symptoms, in abstinent smokers [159–161] (alternatively, see [162]).

Another neurosubstrate that may mediate nicotine withdrawal [8], particularly in light of its role in nicotine reinforcement (Section 15.2.3), is the Glu neurotransmitter system. Because Glu neurotransmission stimulates DA release [45, 47], there is reason to believe that decreases in Glu transmission may have a role in mediating nicotine withdrawal. Contrary to expectation, this hypothesis is not supported empirically. For instance, LY354740, a Glu analog with agonist activity at Group II metabotropic glutamate receptors (mGluRs), dose dependently attenuates enhanced auditory startle responding in rats undergoing nicotine withdrawal [138], suggesting that enhanced Glu transmission is involved, at least with this aspect of nicotine withdrawal [8]. Further investigation in different brain sites is necessary to determine the role of Glu in nicotine withdrawal [8].

Other neurosubstrates that may mediate nicotine withdrawal involve the CRF system and the HPA axis [8]. Cigarette smoking elevates salivary cortisol levels in habitual smokers [163]. During short-term tobacco abstinence, cortisol levels remain virtually unchanged [164]. However, during long-term tobacco abstinence, cortisol levels decrease [165, 166]. There is rapid tolerance to nicotine's effects on plasma corticosterone [158]. The effects of nicotine withdrawal on corticosterone levels are mixed. There is evidence that nicotine withdrawal increases, decreases, or has no effect on corticosterone levels [157, 167, 168]. Further study is necessary to characterize more fully the effects of nicotine withdrawal on CRF transmission and HPA axis function [8].

The final neurosubstrate presented in this chapter that may mediate nicotine withdrawal involves opioid receptors [8]. There is evidence that naloxone, an opiate antagonist, precipitates an abstinence syndrome in nicotine-dependent rats [169]. In a related experiment, morphine, an opioid receptor agonist, reverses signs of spontaneous nicotine withdrawal [169]. Another study demonstrates that nicotine attenuates naloxone-induced jumping behavior in morphine-dependent rats [170]. Taken together, these findings suggest that common neurobiological substrates may mediate nicotine and opiate withdrawal. Findings from another study [134] reveal that, while only high naloxone doses precipitate threshold elevations and somatic signs in nicotine-treated rats, comparably lower doses induce conditioned place aversions. These results indicate that, while brain reward thresholds and somatic withdrawal signs may not be sensitive to alterations in opioid transmission, conditioned motivational states may be [8]. Moreover, findings that naltrexone and naloxone antagonize nAChRs suggest that opioid receptor antagonists may precipitate nicotine withdrawal [171], at least in part, by blocking nAChRs directly [8].

15.2.6 Pharmacokinetics

Pharmacokinetics concerns the absorption, distribution, and metabolism and elimination of a drug. This section addresses each of these areas as it pertains to nicotine, covering a range of nicotine-delivering tobacco products, as described below.

15.2.6.1 Absorption. When delivered by tobacco smoke inhalation, nicotine is carried on tar droplets as part of a complex aerosol that is inhaled into the lung. There, particles are deposited in small airways and alveoli, where nicotine is rapidly absorbed. Venous blood concentrations of nicotine rise rapidly during cigarette smoking and peak at its completion [172]. During smoking, levels of nicotine in arterial blood can more than double the levels observed in venous blood [173]. Presumably, the rapid absorption of nicotine from cigarette smoke through the lung is the result of the huge surface area of the alveoli and the dissolution of nicotine into fluid of physiological pH, which facilitates transfer across cell membranes [174].

Nicotine from chewing tobacco, snuff, and oral nicotine replacement medications (i.e., gum, lozenge, and inhaler) is absorbed through the oral mucosa. The absorption of nicotine across biological membranes depends upon the pH. The pK_a of nicotine is about 8, meaning that 50% of the nicotine is absorbed in a solution with a pH of 8. The pH of smoke from flue-cured tobaccos found in most cigarettes is acidic; thus very little of the nicotine from tobacco smoke is absorbed in the mouth. In contrast, chewing tobacco and snuff are buffered to an alkaline pH to facilitate the absorption of nicotine through the mucosal membranes [175]. Venous plasma nicotine concentrations rise fairly rapidly and reach concentrations comparable to those seen during cigarette smoking or even higher, peaking about 10–20 min after the product is removed from the mouth [176].

The pH of smoke from large cigars and pipes is somewhat alkaline; thus nicotine in the smoke of these products can be absorbed through the oral mucosa or the lung [177]. In addition, the whole tobacco aqueous pH in large cigars is alkaline, suggesting that nicotine can be absorbed into the oral mucosa directly from the cigar when the cigar is held in the mouth [177]. In contrast, the pH of the whole tobacco aqueous pH of small cigars is acidic, like a cigarette [177]. Thus, little nicotine from small cigars would be absorbed through the oral mucosa; however, like a cigarette, nicotine would readily be absorbed into the lung if the smoker inhales.

15.2.6.2 Distribution. After absorption into the blood, nicotine is distributed extensively to body tissues with a steady-state volume of distribution averaging 180 L. Based upon animal research at steady-state nicotine concentrations, spleen, liver, lungs, and brain have a high affinity for nicotine, whereas the affinity of adipose tissue is relatively low [119]. After rapid intravenous injection, concentrations of nicotine decline rapidly because of tissue uptake of the drug. Shortly after injection, concentrations in arterial blood, lung, and brain are high, while concentrations in muscle and adipose tissues are low [119]. Uptake into the brain occurs within 1–2 min, and blood levels fall because of peripheral tissue uptake for 20 or 30 min after administration. Thereafter, blood concentrations decline more slowly, as determined by rates of elimination and rates of distribution out of storage tissues [119].

Nicotine inhaled in tobacco smoke enters the brain almost as quickly as after rapid intravenous injection. Because of the delivery into the lung, peak nicotine levels in the brain may be higher, and the lag time between smoking and entry into the brain shorter than after intravenous injection [119]. The distribution half-life, which describes the movement of nicotine from the blood and other rapidly perfused tissues, such as the brain and other body tissues, is about 9 min [178], whereas the elimination half-life of nicotine is about 2 h. Distribution kinetics determine the time course of CNS actions of nicotine after smoking a single cigarette.

15.2.6.3 Metabolism and Elimination. Nicotine is rapidly and extensively metabolized, primarily in the liver but also to a small extent in the lung [119]. Nicotine's primary metabolites are cotinine and nicotine-*N*-oxide, neither of which appears to be pharmacologically active [174]. The half-life of nicotine averages about 2 h, although there is considerable variability, generally ranging from 1 to 4 h [179]. The half-life of cotinine is much longer (16–20 h), making it a much better marker of nicotine intake than nicotine itself [180]. There is evidence that mentholated cigarette smoking significantly inhibits the metabolism of nicotine, suggesting that mentholated cigarette smoking enhances systemic nicotine exposure [181]. Inhibition of nicotine metabolism occurs both by slower oxidative metabolism to cotinine and by slower glucuronide conjugation. The level of renal excretion depends on urinary pH and urine flow and accounts for 2–35% of total elimination [182].

As reviewed by Henningfield and Benowitz [3], genetic variations can affect nicotine metabolism. Specifically, the cytochrome CYP2A6 enzyme is the liver enzyme largely responsible for the metabolism of nicotine to cotinine, and difference in the expression of this enzyme can have dramatic effects on metabolism. For example, in a study of human liver microsomes, pretreatment with coumarin, a specific and selective CYP2A6 substrate, competitively inhibited cotinine formation by 85% [183]. Genetic variations that alter nicotine metabolism can affect smoking behavior. Tyndale and Sellers [184] found that there was an underrepresentation of individuals carrying defective *CYP2A6* alleles in a tobacco-dependent population and that, among smokers, those with deficient nicotine metabolism smoked fewer cigarettes. Further, inhibition of the CYP2A6 enzyme increases nicotine bioavailability by decreasing first-pass metabolism and decreases smoking [185].

15.3 PHARMACOLOGICAL TREATMENT OF NICOTINE DEPENDENCE AND WITHDRAWAL

15.3.1 Overview

Knowing that cigarette smoking has a pathophysiological basis, as evidenced by the role neurobiological mechanisms have in nicotine reinforcement and dependence, tolerance, and withdrawal, as discussed above, underscores the importance of understanding better nicotine pharmacology and the pharmacotherapies used in the treatment of nicotine dependence (i.e., known vernacularly as nicotine addiction), the foci of the chapter.

As discussed elsewhere, two distinct but typically interrelated disorders comprise what is commonly referred to as nicotine addiction: nicotine dependence and nicotine withdrawal [186]. Nicotine dependence refers to the chronic, relapsing pattern of tobacco use driven strongly by nicotine administration, whereas nicotine withdrawal is the syndrome of signs and symptoms that begin to emerge within a few hours of discontinuation of nicotine intake. Diagnostic criteria for each are provided by the APA [2] and WHO [1]. The most widely recognized goal of therapy is to help the tobacco user achieve and sustain abstinence by treatment of dependence and withdrawal [187–189]. In principle, other goals, such as temporary reduction of withdrawal symptoms to sustain temporary abstinence (e.g., in smoke-free settings) and partial nicotine replacement to enable sustained smoking reduction (i.e., "harm reduction"), are viable and have been discussed elsewhere more recently [190, 191].

As noted in Section 15.2, there are a number of neural mechanisms by which a medication may alleviate withdrawal symptoms, simulate some of nicotine's reinforcing effects, or block nicotine's reinforcing effects. These have led to the postulation of a variety of potential medications for treating tobacco dependence and/or withdrawal, as have been discussed elsewhere [187, 192]. However, the most effective and widely used medications are nicotine replacement medications and other medications that alter the reinforcing effects of nicotine.

As reviewed in Section 15.2, many of the effects of nicotine in the brain are likely to be mediated through neuromodulation in which nicotine potentiates the release of neurotransmitters, including DA, Glu, GABA, and 5-HT. By selectively activating or blocking these neurotransmitters, one might be able to mimic or block some of the reinforcing effects of nicotine.

The following sections review the available pharmacological therapies for smoking cessation and discuss potential targets for the development of new medications.

15.3.2 Nicotine Replacement Medications

The most direct way to help people manage the symptoms of nicotine dependence and withdrawal is therapeutic use of nicotine replacement medications (NRTs) [193–195] to at least partially substitute for the effects of tobacco self-administration. Nicotine medications make it easier to abstain from tobacco by replacing, at least partially, the nicotine formerly obtained from tobacco, thereby providing nicotine-mediated neuropharmacological effects. These neuropharmacological effects include increased expression and reduced turnover of nicotine receptors in the brain and other parts of the body, alteration of brain electroencephalography and regional cerebral glucose metabolism, and activation of dopaminergic reinforcement systems in the brain [196]. Nicotine is the most important substance in tobacco in that it causes and sustains addiction to tobacco. However, a variety of other substances with their own direct pharmacological actions, in interaction with nicotine, and by modulation of sensory effects undoubtedly contribute to the overall addicting effects of tobacco smoke [119, 197–200]. The importance of other substances has not been fully elucidated, but their role may be one factor limiting the effectiveness of NRT.

Laboratory research has demonstrated that animals [201] and humans [202] who have been chronically exposed to nicotine or tobacco smoke will self-administer nicotine infusions. Nicotine administration has been shown to reverse the nicotine withdrawal seen upon discontinuation of chronic nicotine exposure in rats [123] and humans [203, 204].

Currently approved NRT products include the transdermal nicotine patch and several acute NRT products, including nicotine gum, lozenge, sublingual tablet, vapor inhaler, and nasal spray. The differences in the pharmacokinetic profile of these products are illustrated in Figure 15.1.

15.3.2.1 Transdermal Nicotine Patch. Nicotine patches are applied to the skin once a day and deliver nicotine through the skin at a relatively steady rate. Use of transdermal nicotine reduces the symptoms of nicotine withdrawal, including tobacco craving [187, 194]. The nicotine patch has been shown to reduce background craving compared to placebo; however, in contrast to acute NRT formulations, the

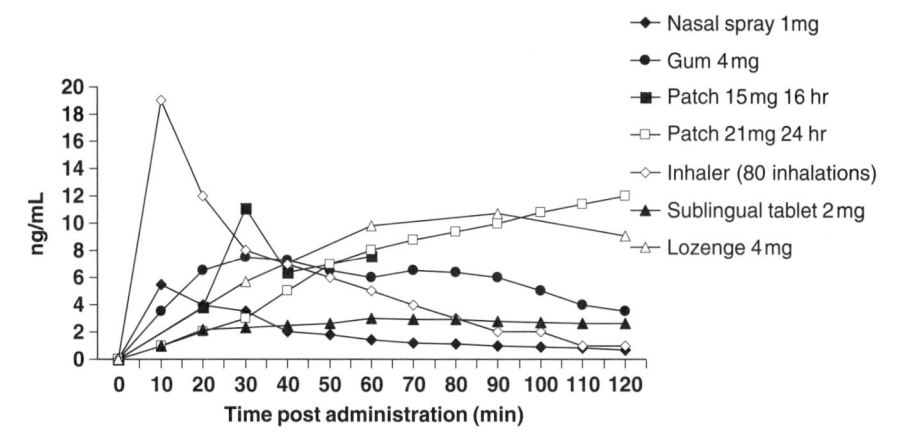

Figure 15.1 Venous blood concentrations in nanograms of nicotine per millimeter of blood as a function of time for various nicotine delivery systems. Data on nasal spray are from Schneider et al. [215]; data on gum are from Benowitz et al. [172]; data on patch are from Benowitz [204a]; data on sublingual tablet are from Molander and Lunell [212]; data on lozenge are from Choi et al. [211]; data on inhaler are from Schneider et al. [204b]; and are based on 80 puffs in 20 min, a dosing regimen not typical of clinical use.

nicotine patch has a weaker effect on craving associated with exposure to a provocative stimulus [205, 206].

Chronic nicotine also may reduce the effects of subsequent nicotine delivery, which might decrease the likelihood that a lapse will result in a complete return to smoking (relapse). For example, a study of cigarette smoking stimulant abusers indicates that nicotine patches produce tolerance to the effects of intravenous nicotine [207]. Under a placebo maintenance condition, intravenous nicotine produces robust dose-related subjective effects, with maximal increases similar to the high dose of cocaine; however, nicotine maintenance significantly decreases the subjective and reinforcing effects of intravenous nicotine. Nicotine patches do not alter responses to cocaine or caffeine.

There are currently four patch formulations on the market, varying widely in their design, pharmacokinetics, and duration of wear (i.e., 24- and 16-h wear). The diversity in patch systems has been described in reviews [194, 208], and the differences in pharmacokinetics have been illustrated in a head-to-head clinical trial [209]. All of the patch types are available in a range of dosages, and progressively lower doses are used to provide weaning over a period of several weeks or longer to enable gradual adjustment of their bodies to lower nicotine levels and ultimately to a nicotine-free state. Some formulations and indications also provide for less dependent smokers to use a lower dose.

15.3.2.2 Acute Delivery Systems. There are several options available to smokers that, unlike the nicotine patch, allow them to self-administer a dose of nicotine on an "as-needed" basis. These include nicotine gum, lozenge, sublingual tablet, oral inhaler, and nasal spray. All of these products except the nasal spray deliver nicotine through the oral mucosa. Acute-dosing products have the benefit that both the amount and timing of doses can be titrated by the user. Thus, smokers with more nicotine tolerance or greater need can get a higher nicotine dose, and smokers who are experiencing acute adverse effects can scale back their intake.

Nicotine gum is available in two doses: 2 and 4 mg, delivering approximately 1 and 2 mg, respectively [210]. A 1-mg lozenge has been available in some European countries for some time; however, no efficacy data are available, and the efficacy of this low dose is in question. A newer nicotine lozenge, available in 2- and 4-mg formulations, has been approved in the United States, Europe, and Australia. Single-dose studies demonstrate 8–10% higher maximum concentration (C_{max}) and 25–27% higher area-under-the-curve ($AUC_{0-\infty}$) values from lozenges compared to gums at both 2- and 4-mg dose levels, which is probably due to the residual nicotine retained in the gum [211]. A small sublingual nicotine tablet has been developed and is currently being marketed in many European countries but is not yet available in the United States. The product is designed to be held under the tongue, where the nicotine is absorbed sublingually over about 30 min. The product that is currently available contains 2 mg nicotine, and the levels of nicotine obtained by use of the 2-mg tablet and 2-mg nicotine gum are similar [212]. The nicotine vapor inhaler consists of a mouthpiece and a plastic cartridge containing nicotine. When the inhaler is "puffed," nicotine is drawn through the mouthpiece into the mouth of the smoker. Each inhaler cartridge contains 10 mg nicotine, of which 4 mg can be delivered and 2 mg is absorbed with intensive use [213]. The product does not deliver nicotine to the bronchi or lungs, but rather its nicotine is deposited and absorbed primarily in the mouth, much like nicotine gum [214]. The nasal spray was designed to deliver doses of nicotine to the smoker more rapidly than other NRT products. The device is a multidose bottle with a pump that delivers 0.5 mg of nicotine per 50-µL squirt. Each dose consists of two squirts, one to each nostril. Nicotine from the nasal spray is absorbed into the blood more rapidly than from gum [215].

As shown in Figure 15.1, nicotine delivery from these acute NRT formulations is faster than transdermal delivery. However, there remains a vast difference in the pharmacokinetic profiles of cigarettes and NRT products. Even nicotine nasal spray, which produces measurably faster increases in venous blood nicotine levels compared to other oral NRT formulations, does not equal the venous levels produced by cigarettes. Even more importantly, none of the currently available formulations produces the spikes in arterial blood, the blood levels that actually enter the brain. A study by Henningfield et al. (1993) demonstrates that the arterial levels achieved by smoking are much higher than levels seen in venous blood, and the nicotine may reach the brain even faster after smoking than after intravenous dosing [173]. Speed of delivery has been shown to influence nicotine's effects in both animals and humans [173, 216].

15.3.3 Nicotinic Pharmacotherapies

15.3.3.1 Nicotinic Partial Agonists. A partial agonist is a compound that, even at high doses, does not produce the same response as a full agonist. Because there is a ceiling on the effects of a partial agonist, it is plausible that a partial nicotine agonist would have a lower risk of adverse events and have a lower abuse potential than a medication containing nicotine. A variety of nAChR subtypes have been identified with distinct structural and functional properties. The subtype that has generally been identified as being associated with the addictive effects of nicotine is the $\alpha_4\beta_2$. It is plausible that a compound that binds with a high degree of specificity or with a greater affinity to this subtype relative to nicotine will have a higher level of safety and possibly a higher level of efficacy. However, to the extent that other subtypes might be associated with these effects, the efficacy could be muted compared to nicotine, which is less specific.

One such compound that received FDA approval in 2006 and is available as a prescription smoking cessation and is varenicline, a nicotine partial agonist that is specific to the $\alpha_4\beta_2$ (nicotinic) receptor. Clinical trials of varenicline suggest that the medication is efficacious for smoking cessation and is safe.

15.3.3.2 Nicotinic Antagonists. In theory, a nicotinic antagonist would block the effects of cigarette smoking, which would subsequently decrease the reinforcing value of smoking, which in turn would lead to extinction of the behavior. Mecamylamine is a noncompetitive antagonist at the nAChR site. Mecamylamine increases ad libitum smoking behavior when administered alone and also attenuates smoking satisfaction as well as many of the physiological, behavioral, and reinforcing effects of nicotine [217]. There is some evidence that mecamylamine may be useful for some recalcitrant smokers as a smoking cessation aid [218]. However, the side effects of the medication (hypotension and constipation) may limit its utility.

Mecamylamine in combination with nicotine transdermal medication may produce better cessation outcomes than nicotine alone. For example, a randomized, double-blind, placebo-controlled clinical trial reveals that a combination of the nicotine patch plus mecamylamine produces abstinence rates three times higher than those for nicotine patch alone [219]. Mecamylamine also significantly reduces cigarette craving, negative affect, and appetite. Side effects such as constipation and dizziness, however, remain common. These results suggest that mecamylamine combined with nicotine replacement may ultimately prove to be a useful aid in smoking cessation.

15.3.4 Nonnicotinic Pharmacotherapies

Nonnicotine pharmacotherapies for smoking cessation have been extensively reviewed elsewhere [192, 220]. As previously mentioned, many of the effects of nicotine in the brain are likely to be mediated through neuromodulation in which nicotine potentiates the release of DA and 5-HT [221]. By selectively activating these neurotransmitters, one might be able to mimic some of the reinforcing effects of nicotine.

15.3.4.1 Bupropion. Bupropion is an atypical antidepressant drug that is the only non-nicotine-based prescription medicine approved for smoking cessation by the Food and Drug Administration (FDA). Its mechanism of action is presumed to be mediated by its capacity to block neuronal reuptake of DA and/or norepinephrine [187]. Relative to other antidepressants, bupropion has a relatively high affinity for the DA transporter [222].

Animal studies demonstrate that bupropion alters the reinforcing and withdrawal effects of nicotine. One study indicates that low doses of bupropion reduce the rewarding effects of nicotine and the affective and somatic symptoms of withdrawal [135]. Another study examined the effects of bupropion (5–40 mg/kg) on the reinforcing properties of nicotine and food in rats under two different schedules of reinforcement [150]. The authors report that pretreatment with the highest dose of bupropion (40 mg/kg) results in a 50% reduction of nicotine intake in rats self-administering 0.03 mg/kg/infusion of nicotine under a fixed-ratio (FR) schedule. However, pretreatment with bupropion does not affect the self-administration of nicotine under a progressive-ratio (PR) schedule. These findings are challenging to interpret but may indicate that a high dose of bupropion decreases the reinforcing properties of nicotine under conditions where doses can be obtained at regular and relatively short intervals, while leaving intact the motivation to work for nicotine when doses are more widely spaced. Taken together, these results suggest that bupropion has several actions demonstrated in animals that could explain its ability to increase rates of cessation in humans.

15.3.4.2 Tricyclic Antidepressants. Tricyclic antidepressants have a relatively high affinity for both 5-HT and 5-HT transporters and some affinity for the DA transporter [222]. Several clinical trials have demonstrated the potential efficacy of nortriptyline for smoking cessation in smokers without history of major depression [223] or with such history [224], and nortriptyline has been listed by the Agency for Health Research Quality as a second-line therapy [187]. The tricyclic antidepressant doxepin has also been shown in a small human study to improve cessation rates [225]; however, larger studies are clearly needed to verify these findings. Other studies have shown that doxepin significantly reduces postcessation tobacco withdrawal symptoms and cigarette craving [226, 227].

15.3.4.3 Cannabinoid Antagonists. The cannabinoid-1 (CB1) receptor plays a role in the regulation of appetitive behavior. For example, exogenously administered cannabinoid receptor agonists stimulate food consumption in animals and humans [228]. The endocannabinoid system appears to mediate the effects of nicotine in rodents. For example, rimonabant, a CB1 receptor antagonist, appears to decrease the motivational effects of nicotine in the rat [229]. Administration of rimonabant (0.3 and 1 mg/kg) decreases nicotine self-administration (0.03 mg/kg/injection). Rimonabant (0.3–3 mg/kg) neither substitutes for nor antagonizes the nicotine cue in a nicotine discrimination procedure. In addition, using brain microdialysis, rimonabant (1–3 mg/kg) blocks nicotine-induced DA release in the shell of the nucleus accumbens and the bed nucleus of the stria terminalis. These results suggest that activation of the endogenous cannabinoid system may participate in the motivational and DA-releasing effects of nicotine.

Rimonabant is one such cannabinoid antagonist that has been recently tested in clinical trials which were reported in the news media. The study reveals that the medication was efficacious for smoking cessation. Also, smokers who quit in the rimonabant group gain less weight than those that quit in the placebo group. Many smokers report weight gain to be one of the factors associated with relapse [230]; thus a medication that reduces the weight gain associated with cessation may decrease the likelihood of relapse during a quit attempt.

15.3.4.4 Opioid Antagonists. As reviewed by Pomerleau [231], opiate agonists such as heroin or methadone have been found to increase cigarette smoking reliably in humans, and morphine has been shown to increase the potency and efficacy of nicotine in rats. There is also an extensive literature documenting the nicotine-stimulated release of endogenous opioids in various brain regions involved in the mediation of opiate reinforcement. In addition, the opioid system may be involved in the reinforcing properties of several drugs of abuse and may be involved in nicotine's reinforcing properties. This may imply that opioid antagonists may attenuate the reinforcing value of cigarette smoking. Naltrexone is an opioid antagonist that has been shown to be effective for the treatment of alcohol dependence and has recently been approved for this indication by the FDA [232]. Two studies have examined the effects of naltrexone during smoking abstinence [92, 233]. These studies generally demonstrate little effect of naltrexone on tobacco withdrawal, smoking behavior, or satisfaction from smoking. Currently available data provide little support for the use of naltrexone for the treatment of tobacco dependence or withdrawal.

15.3.5 Nicotine Pharmacology Implications for Public Health Policy

The importance of the emerging understanding of nicotine as an addictive or dependence-producing drug over the twentieth century has had profound implications for public health policy, is the foundation for efforts by the FDA to regulate tobacco products, and was the cornerstone of the WHO Framework Convention on Tobacco Control (FCTC) [5, 234, 235]. Succinctly stated, regulatory efforts in the United States and many other countries are endeavoring to address tobacco through a combination of demand reduction and supply control efforts that recognize that tobacco use is driven and sustained critically by the pharmacological effects of nicotine.

As is evident from the preceding section of this review, many effective pharmacological treatment strategies have emerged and many more are in various stages of the drug development pipeline. The U.S. Public Health Service advocates that all cigarette smokers be offered treatment, so favorable is the benefit-to-risk ratio [187]. Globally, the WHO [189] and World Bank [236] both recommend that expanded treatment access and utilization are vital to the health, well-being, and economic development of all nations.

In the decades to come, treatment access will be vital to global health. In the very long range, however, reducing demand by more effective tobacco use prevention efforts and the prevention of escalation to dependence will be equally vital. Here, as well, nicotine pharmacology plays a potentially vital role in the needed partnership between prevention and treatment researchers. The rapid development of nicotine tolerance, dependence, and altered brain structure that contribute to persistent tobacco use are factors to be considered in public health efforts to reduce exposure to tobacco, erect barriers to reduce the conversion from any use to dependence, and develop more effective early interventions to steer the trajectory of tobacco use from addiction to abstinence. Animal and human research with nicotine and other addictive drugs has shown the importance of drug-associated stimuli in persistent use and relapse, the importance of efforts to reduce opportunities for use, and reducing overall use through increased cost. These findings are being adapted to public health policy through actions including the following: laws reducing access of youth to tobacco, increasing taxes and hence cost of tobacco products, and efforts to reduce the ubiquity of tobacco dependence–associated stimuli [5, 236, 237]. Additional approaches under consideration are parallel to those taken with medications with abuse potential, namely, to reduce the abuse liability to the greatest degree possible without rendering the product so unacceptable that the effort would simply drive people to other forms of tobacco. Although we do not intend to over represent the importance of behavioral and pharmacological sciences in public health efforts to control one of the world's greatest public health disasters, it is clear that scientific investigation in this area has been vital to global health. As evidenced by this review, research advances have been rapid. The rapidity of these advances implies that future decades will witness even more powerful tools to bring tobacco addiction and associated disease under control. Taken together, in the decades to come, former Surgeon General C. E. Koop's vision that the end of the twenty-first century will be a time when tobacco-associated death will be as rare as it was at the end of the nineteenth century [238] eventually may be realized.

ACKNOWLEDGMENTS

The authors acknowledge the work of A. Markou, G. F. Koob, and J. E. Henningfield (2003) as a model for Section 15.2.

DISCLOSURES

A. R. Buchhalter, R. V. Fant, and J. E. Henningfield serve as consultants to GlaxoSmithKline Consumer Healthcare regarding matters relating to smoking cessation. J. E. Henningfield also has a financial interest in a new nicotine replacement product.

REFERENCES

1. World Health Organization (WHO) (1992). *The ICD-10 Classification of Mental Behavioural Disorders.* WHO, Geneva.
2. American Psychiatric Association (APA) (1994). *Diagnostic and Statistical Manual of Mental Disorders,* 4th ed., APA, Washington, DC.
3. Henningfield, J. E., and Benowitz, N. L. (2004). Pharmacology and nicotine addiction. In *Tobacco and Public Health: Science and Policy,* P. Boyle, N. Gray, J. E. Henningfield, J. Seffrin, and W. Zatonski, Eds. Oxford University Press, Oxford, pp. 129–147.
4. Lewin, L. (1998). *Phantastica: A classic survey on the use and abuse of mind-altering plants.* Park Street Press, Rochester, VT, p. 256.
5. WHO Framework Convention on Tobacco Control (2005). Available at *http://www.who.int/tobacco/framework/en,* June 14, 2005. Presented in Sydney, Australia.
6. Centers for Disease Control and Prevention (2002). Annual smoking-attributable mortality, years of potential life lost, and economic costs—United States, 1995–1999. *MMWR* 51, 300–303.
7. Centers for Disease Control and Prevention (CDC) (2005). *Targeting Tobacco Use: The Nation's Leading Cause of Death.* WHO, Atlanta.
8. Markou, A., Koob, G. F., and Henningfield, J. E. (2003). Background paper on the neurobiology of nicotine addiction. Unpublished work.

9. Taylor, P. (2001). Agents acting at the neuromuscular junction and autonomic ganglia. In *Goodman & Gilman's the Pharmacological Basis of Therapeutics*, 10th ed., J. G. Hardman and L. E. Limbird, Eds. McGraw-Hill, New York, pp. 193–213.

10. Institute of Medicine (2001). Principles of harm reduction. In *Clearing the Smoke: Assessing the Science Base for Tobacco Harm Reduction*, K. Stratton, P. Shetty, R. Wallace, and S. Bondurant, Eds. National Academy Press, Washington, DC, pp. 38–59.

11. Watkins, S. S., Koob, G. F., and Markou, A. (2000). Neural mechanisms underlying nicotine addiction: Acute positive reinforcement and withdrawal. *Nicotine Tobacco Res.* 2, 19–37.

12. Pappano, A. J. (1998). Cholinoceptor-activating and cholinesterase-inhibiting drugs. In *Basic and Clinical Pharmacology*, B. G. Katzung, Ed. Appleton and Lange, Stamford, CT, pp. 90–104.

13. Holladay, M. W., Dart, M. J., and Lynch, J. K. (1997). Neuronal nicotinic acetylcholine receptors as targets for drug discovery. *J. Med. Chem.* 40, 4169–4194.

14. Wonnacott, S. (1997). Presynaptic nicotinic ACh receptors. *Trends Neurosci.* 20, 92–98.

15. Sargent, P. B. (1993). The diversity of neuronal nicotinic acetylcholine receptors. *Annu. Rev. Neurosci.* 16, 403–443.

16. George, T. P., and O'Malley, S. S. (2004). Current pharmacological treatments for nicotine dependence. *Trends Pharmacol. Sci.* 25, 42–48.

17. Picciotto, M. R., Caldarone, B. J., King, S. L., and Zachariou, V. (2000). Nicotinic receptors in the brain. Links between molecular biology and behavior. *Neuropsychopharmacology* 22, 451–465.

18. Leonard, S., and Bertrand, D. (2001). Neuronal nicotine receptors: From structure to function. *Nicotine Tobacco Res.* 3, 203–223.

19. Picciotto, M. R., Zoli, M., Rimondini, R., Lena, C., Marubio, L. M., Pich, E. M., et al. (1998). Acetylcholine receptors containing the beta2 subunit are involved in the reinforcing properties of nicotine. *Nature* 391, 173–177.

20. Elgoyhen, A. B., Vetter, D. E., Katz, E., Rothlin, C. V., Heinemann, S. F., and Boulter, J. (2001). Alpha10: A determinant of nicotinic cholinergic receptor function in mammalian vestibular and cochlear mechanosensory hair cells. *Proc. Natl. Acad. Sci. USA* 98, 3501–3506.

21. Picciotto, M. R., Zoli, M., Lena, C., Bessis, A., Lallemand, Y., Le Novere, N., et al. (1995). Abnormal avoidance learning in mice lacking functional high-affinity nicotine receptor in the brain. *Nature* 374, 65–67.

22. Centers for Disease Control and Prevention (CDC) (1988). *Nicotine Addiction: A Report of the Surgeon General. The Health Consequences of Smoking.* CDC, Atlanta, GA, pp. 241–375.

23. Goldberg, S. R., and Spealman, R. D. (1982). Maintenance and suppression of behavior by intravenous nicotine injections in squirrel monkeys. *Fed. Proc.* 41, 216–220.

24. Henningfield, J. E., and Goldberg, S. R. (1983). Control of behavior by intravenous nicotine injections in human subjects. *Pharmacol. Biochem. Behav.* 19, 1021–1026.

25. Pomerleau, C. S., and Pomerleau, O. F. (1992). Euphoriant effects of nicotine in smokers. *Psychopharmacology (Berl.)* 108, 460–465.

26. Benowitz, N. L. (1996). Pharmacology of nicotine: Addiction and therapeutics. *Annu. Rev. Pharmacol. Toxicol.* 36, 597–613.

27. Lanza, S. T., Donny, E. C., Collins, L. M., and Balster, R. L. (2004). Analyzing the acquisition of drug self-administration using growth curve models. *Drug Alcohol Depend.* 75, 11–21.
28. Donny, E. C., Lanza, S. T., Balster, R. L., Collins, L. M., Caggiula, A., and Rowell, P. P. (2004). Using growth models to relate acquisition of nicotine self-administration to break point and nicotinic receptor binding. *Drug Alcohol Depend.* 75, 23–35.
29. Eissenberg, T., and Balster, R. L. (2000). Initial tobacco use episodes in children and adolescents: Current knowledge, future directions. *Drug Alcohol Depend.* 59, (Suppl. 1), S41–S60.
30. Picciotto, M. R., and Corrigall, W. A. (2002). Neuronal systems underlying behaviors related to nicotine addiction: Neural circuits and molecular genetics. *J. Neurosci.* 22, 3338–3341.
31. Nisell, M., Nomikos, G. G., and Svensson, T. H. (1995). Nicotine dependence, midbrain dopamine systems and psychiatric disorders. *Pharmacol. Toxicol.* 76, 157–162.
32. Grenhoff, J., Aston-Jones, G., and Svensson, T. H. (1986). Nicotinic effects on the firing pattern of midbrain dopamine neurons. *Acta Physiol. Scand.* 128, 351–358.
33. Damsma, G., Day, J., and Fibiger, H. C. (1989). Lack of tolerance to nicotine-induced dopamine release in the nucleus accumbens. *Eur. J. Pharmacol.* 168, 363–368.
34. Mifsud, J. C., Hernandez, L., and Hoebel, B. G. (1989). Nicotine infused into the nucleus accumbens increases synaptic dopamine as measured by in vivo microdialysis. *Brain Res.* 478, 365–367.
35. Pontieri, F. E., Tanda, G., Orzi, F., and Di Chiara, G. (1996). Effects of nicotine on the nucleus accumbens and similarity to those of addictive drugs. *Nature* 382, 255–257.
36. Nisell, M., Marcus, M., Nomikos, G. G., and Svensson, T. H. (1997). Differential effects of acute and chronic nicotine on dopamine output in the core and shell of the rat nucleus accumbens. *J. Neural Transm.* 104, 1–10.
37. Nisell, M., Nomikos, G. G., and Svensson, T. H. (1994). Infusion of nicotine in the ventral tegmental area or the nucleus accumbens of the rat differentially affects accumbal dopamine release. *Pharmacol. Toxicol.* 75, 348–352.
38. Nisell, M., Nomikos, G. G., and Svensson, T. H. (1994). Systemic nicotine-induced dopamine release in the rat nucleus accumbens is regulated by nicotinic receptors in the ventral tegmental area. *Synapse* 16, 36–44.
39. Corrigall, W. A., Coen, K. M., and Adamson, K. L. (1994). Self-administered nicotine activates the mesolimbic dopamine system through the ventral tegmental area. *Brain Res.* 653, 278–284.
40. Corrigall, W. A., Franklin, K. B., Coen, K. M., and Clarke, P. B. (1992). The mesolimbic dopaminergic system is implicated in the reinforcing effects of nicotine. *Psychopharmacology (Berl.)* 107, 285–289.
41. Corrigall, W. A., and Coen, K. M. (1991). Selective dopamine antagonists reduce nicotine self-administration. *Psychopharmacology (Berl.)* 104, 171–176.
42. Levin, E. D. (1997). Chronic haloperidol administration does not block acute nicotine-induced improvements in radial-arm maze performance in the rat. *Pharmacol. Biochem. Behav.* 58, 899–902.
43. Vidal, C., and Changeux, J. P. (1993). Nicotinic and muscarinic modulations of excitatory synaptic transmission in the rat prefrontal cortex in vitro. *Neuroscience* 56, 23–32.
44. Radcliffe, K. A., and Dani, J. A. (1998). Nicotinic stimulation produces multiple forms of increased glutamatergic synaptic transmission. *J. Neurosci.* 18, 7075–7083.

45. Mansvelder, H. D., and McGehee, D. S. (2000). Long-term potentiation of excitatory inputs to brain reward areas by nicotine. *Neuron* 27, 349–357.
46. Schilstrom, B., Svensson, H. M., Svensson, T. H., and Nomikos, G. G. (1998). Nicotine and food induced dopamine release in the nucleus accumbens of the rat: Putative role of alpha7 nicotinic receptors in the ventral tegmental area. *Neuroscience* 85, 1005–1009.
47. Schilstrom, B., Nomikos, G. G., Nisell, M., Hertel, P., and Svensson, T. H. (1998). *N*-Methyl-D-aspartate receptor antagonism in the ventral tegmental area diminishes the systemic nicotine-induced dopamine release in the nucleus accumbens. *Neuroscience* 82, 781–789.
48. Sharples, C. G., Kaiser, S., Soliakov, L., Marks, M. J., Collins, A. C., Washburn, M., et al. (2000). UB-165: A novel nicotinic agonist with subtype selectivity implicates the alpha4beta2* subtype in the modulation of dopamine release from rat striatal synaptosomes. *J. Neurosci.* 20, 2783–2791.
49. Markou, A., and Paterson, N. E. (2001). The nicotinic antagonist methyllycaconitine has differential effects on nicotine self-administration and nicotine withdrawal in the rat. *Nicotine Tobacco Res.* 3, 361–373.
50. Cheeta, S., Tucci, S., and File, S. E. (2001). Antagonism of the anxiolytic effect of nicotine in the dorsal raphe nucleus by dihydro-beta-erythroidine. *Pharmacol. Biochem. Behav.* 70, 491–496.
51. Grottick, A. J., Trube, G., Corrigall, W. A., Huwyler, J., Malherbe, P., and Wyler, R., et al. (2000). Evidence that nicotinic alpha(7) receptors are not involved in the hyperlocomotor and rewarding effects of nicotine. *J. Pharmacol. Exp. Ther.* 294, 1112–1119.
52. Paterson, N. E., Semenova, S., Gasparini, F., and Markou, A. (2003). The mGluR5 antagonist MPEP decreased nicotine self-administration in rats and mice. *Psychopharmacology (Berl.)* 167, 257–264.
53. Fallon, J. H., and Moore, R. Y. (1978). Catecholamine innervation of the basal forebrain. IV. Topography of the dopamine projection to the basal forebrain and neostriatum. *J. Comp. Neurol.* 180, 545–580.
54. Walaas, I., and Fonnum, F. (1979). The distribution and origin of glutamate decarboxylase and choline acetyltransferase in ventral pallidum and other basal forebrain regions. *Brain Res.* 177, 325–336.
55. Sugita, S., Johnson, S. W., and North, R. A. (1992). Synaptic inputs to $GABA_A$ and $GABA_B$ receptors originate from discrete afferent neurons. *Neurosci. Lett.* 134, 207–211.
56. Klitenick, M. A., DeWitte, P., and Kalivas, P. W. (1992). Regulation of somatodendritic dopamine release in the ventral tegmental area by opioids and GABA: An in vivo microdialysis study. *J. Neurosci.* 12, 2623–2632.
57. Yim, C. Y., and Mogenson, G. J. (1980). Electrophysiological studies of neurons in the ventral tegmental area of Tsai. *Brain Res.* 181, 301–313.
58. Kalivas, P. W., Churchill, L., and Klitenick, M. A. (1993). GABA and enkephalin projection from the nucleus accumbens and ventral pallidum to the ventral tegmental area. *Neuroscience* 57, 1047–1060.
59. Markou, A., Paterson, N. E., and Semenova, S. (2004). Role of gamma-aminobutyric acid (GABA) and metabotropic glutamate receptors in nicotine reinforcement: Potential pharmacotherapies for smoking cessation. *Ann. NY Acad. Sci.* 1025, 491–503.

60. Dewey, S. L., Brodie, J. D., Gerasimov, M., Horan, B., Gardner, E. L., and Ashby, C. R., Jr. (1993). A pharmacologic strategy for the treatment of nicotine addiction. *Synapse* 31, 76–86.
61. Fattore, L., Cossu, G., Martellotta, M. C., and Fratta, W. (2002). Baclofen antagonizes intravenous self-administration of nicotine in mice and rats. *Alcohol Alcohol* 37, 495–498.
62. Paterson, N. E., Froestl, W., and Markou, A. (2004). The GABAB receptor agonists baclofen and CGP44532 decreased nicotine self-administration in the rat. *Psychopharmacology (Berl.)* 172, 179–186.
63. Paterson, N. E., Froestl, W., and Markou, A. (2005). Repeated administration of the GABAB receptor agonist CGP44532 decreased nicotine self-administration, and acute administration decreased cue-induced reinstatement of nicotine-seeking in rats. *Neuropsychopharmacology* 30, 119–128.
64. Cousins, M. S., Stamat, H. M., and De Wit, H. (2001). Effects of a single dose of baclofen on self-reported subjective effects and tobacco smoking. *Nicotine Tobacco Res.* 3, 123–129.
65. Sarnyai, Z., Shaham, Y., and Heinrichs, S. C. (2001). The role of corticotropin-releasing factor in drug addiction. *Pharmacol. Rev.* 53, 209–243.
66. Cam, G. R., Bassett, J. R., and Cairncross, K. D. (1979). The action of nicotine on the pituitary-adrenal cortical axis. *Arch. Int. Pharmacodyn. Ther.* 237, 49–66.
67. Andersson, K., Fuxe, K., Eneroth, P., Agnati, L. F., and Harfstrand, A. (1987). Effects of acute continuous exposure of the rat to cigarette smoke on amine levels and utilization in discrete hypothalamic catecholamine nerve terminal systems and on neuroendocrine function. *Naunyn Schmiedebergs Arch. Pharmacol.* 335, 521–528.
68. Matta, S. G., Beyer, H. S., McAllen, K. M., and Sharp, B. M. (1987). Nicotine elevates rat plasma ACTH by a central mechanism. *J. Pharmacol. Exp. Ther.* 243, 217–226.
69. Hillhouse, E. W., and Milton, N. G. (1989). Effect of acetylcholine and 5-hydroxytryptamine on the secretion of corticotrophin-releasing factor-41 and arginine vasopressin from the rat hypothalamus in vitro. *J. Endocrinol.* 122, 713–718.
70. Kasckow, J. W., Regmi, A., Sheriff, S., Mulchahey, J., and Geracioti, T. D., Jr. (1999). Regulation of corticotropin-releasing factor messenger RNA by nicotine in an immortalized amygdalar cell line. *Life Sci.* 65, 2709–2714.
71. Okuda, H., Shioda, S., Nakai, Y., Nakayama, H., Okamoto, M., and Nakashima, T. (1993). The presence of corticotropin-releasing factor-like immunoreactive synaptic vesicles in axon terminals with nicotinic acetylcholine receptor-like immunoreactivity in the median eminence of the rat. *Neurosci. Lett.* 161, 183–186.
72. Valentine, J. D., Matta, S. G., and Sharp, B. M. (1996). Nicotine-induced cFos expression in the hypothalamic paraventricular nucleus is dependent on brainstem effects: Correlations with cFos in catecholaminergic and noncatecholaminergic neurons in the nucleus tractus solitarius. *Endocrinology* 137, 622–630.
73. Matta, S. G., Valentine, J. D., and Sharp, B. M. (1997). Nicotinic activation of CRH neurons in extrahypothalamic regions of the rat brain. *Endocrine* 7, 245–253.
74. Stalke, J., Hader, O., Bahr, V., Hensen, J., Scherer, G., and Oelkers, W. (1992). The role of vasopressin in the nicotine-induced stimulation of ACTH and cortisol in men. *Clin. Investigator.* 70, 218–223.
75. Seyler, L. E., Jr., Fertig, J., Pomerleau, O., Hunt, D., and Parker, K. (1984). The effects of smoking on ACTH and cortisol secretion. *Life Sci.* 34, 57–65.
76. Newhouse, P. A., Sunderland, T., Narang, P. K., Mellow, A. M., Fertig, J. B., Lawlor, B. A., et al. (1990). Neuroendocrine, physiologic, and behavioral responses following

intravenous nicotine in nonsmoking healthy volunteers and in patients with Alzheimer's disease. *Psychoneuroendocrinology* 15, 471–484.

77. Wilkins, J. N., Carlson, H. E., Van Vunakis, H., Hill, M. A., Gritz, E., and Jarvik, M. E. (1982). Nicotine from cigarette smoking increases circulating levels of cortisol, growth hormone, and prolactin in male chronic smokers. *Psychopharmacology (Berl.)* 78, 305–308.

78. Mendelson, J. H., Sholar, M. B., Goletiani, N., Siegel, A. J., and Mello, N. K. (2005). Effects of low- and high-nicotine cigarette smoking on mood states and the HPA axis in men. *Neuropsychopharmacology*. 30, 1751–1763.

79. Koh, H. K. (2002). Accomplishments of the Massachusetts Tobacco Control Program. *Tobacco Control* 11(Suppl. 2ii1–ii3).

80. Gilbert, D. G., Meliska, C. J., Williams, C. L., and Jensen, R. A. (1992). Subjective correlates of cigarette-smoking-induced elevations of peripheral beta-endorphin and cortisol. *Psychopharmacology* 106, 275–281.

81. Boyadjieva, N. I., and Sarkar, D. K. (1997). The secretory response of hypothalamic beta-endorphin neurons to acute and chronic nicotine treatments and following nicotine withdrawal. *Life Sci.* 61, L59–L66.

82. Pomerleau, O. F., and Pomerleau, C. S. (1984). Neuroregulators and the reinforcement of smoking: Towards a biobehavioral explanation. *Neurosci. Biobehav. Rev.* 8, 503–513.

83. Houdi, A. A., Pierzchala, K., Marson, L., Palkovits, M., and Van Loon, G. R. (1991). Nicotine-induced alteration in Tyr-Gly Gly and Met-enkephalin in discrete brain nuclei reflects altered enkephalin neuron activity. *Peptides* 12, 161–166.

84. Pierzchala, K., Houdi, A. A., and Van Loon, G. R. (1987). Nicotine-induced alterations in brain regional concentrations of native and cryptic Met- and Leu-enkephalin. *Peptides* 8, 1035–1043.

85. Tempel, A., and Zukin, R. S. (1987). Neuroanatomical patterns of the mu, delta, and kappa opioid receptors of rat brain as determined by quantitative in vitro autoradiography. *Proc. Natl. Acad. Sci. USA* 84, 4308–4312.

86. Davenport, K. E., Houdi, A. A., and Van Loon, G. R. (1990). Nicotine protects against mu-opioid receptor antagonism by beta-funaltrexamine: Evidence for nicotine-induced release of endogenous opioids in brain. *Neurosci. Lett.* 113, 40–46.

87. Pomerleau, O. F. (1998). Endogenous opioids and smoking: A review of progress and problems. *Psychoneuroendocrinology* 23, 115–130.

88. Gorelick, D. A., Rose, J., and Jarvik, M. E. (1988). Effect of naloxone on cigarette smoking. *J. Subst. Abuse.*, 1, 153–159.

89. Karras, A., and Kane, J. M. (1980). Naloxone reduces cigarette smoking. *Life Sci.* 27, 1541–1545.

90. Wewers, M. E., Dhatt, R., and Tejwani, G. A. (1998). Naltrexone administration affects ad libitum smoking behavior. *Psychopharmacology (Berl.)* 140, 185–190.

91. Covey, L. S., Glassman, A. H., and Stetner, F. (1999). Naltrexone effects on short-term and long-term smoking cessation. *J. Addict. Dis.* 18, 31–40.

92. Sutherland, G., Stapleton, J. A., Russell, M. A., and Feyerabend, C. (1995). Naltrexone, smoking behaviour and cigarette withdrawal. *Psychopharmacology (Berl.)* 120, 418–425.

93. Nemeth-Coslett, R., and Griffiths, R. R. (1986). Naloxone does not affect cigarette smoking. *Psychopharmacology (Berl.)* 89, 261–264.

94. George, T. P., and O'Malley, S. S. (2004). Current pharmacological treatments for nicotine dependence. *Trends Pharmacol. Sci.* 25, 42–48.

95. Mansvelder, H. D., Keath, J. R., and McGehee, D. S. (2002). Synaptic mechanisms underlie nicotine-induced excitability of brain reward areas. *Neuron* 33, 905–919.
96. Flores, C. M., Davila-Garcia, M. I., Ulrich, Y. M., and Kellar, K. J. (1997). Differential regulation of neuronal nicotinic receptor binding sites following chronic nicotine administration. *J. Neurochem.* 69, 2216–2219.
97. Sanderson, E. M., Drasdo, A. L., McCrea, K., and Wonnacott, S. (1993). Upregulation of nicotinic receptors following continuous infusion of nicotine is brain-region-specific. *Brain Res.* 617, 349–352.
98. Benwell, M. E., Balfour, D. J., and Anderson, J. M. (1988). Evidence that tobacco smoking increases the density of (−)-[3 H]nicotine binding sites in human brain. *J. Neurochem.* 50, 1243–1247.
99. Breese, C. R., Marks, M. J., Logel, J., Adams, C. E., Sullivan, B., Collins, A. C., et al. (1997). Effect of smoking history on [3 H]nicotine binding in human postmortem brain. *J. Pharmacol. Exp. Ther.* 282, 7–13.
100. Perry, D. C., Davila-Garcia, M. I., Stockmeier, C. A., and Kellar, K. J. (1999). Increased nicotinic receptors in brains from smokers: Membrane binding and autoradiography studies. *J. Pharmacol. Exp. Ther.* 289, 1545–1552.
101. Benhammou, K., Lee, M., Strook, M., Sullivan, B., Logel, J., Raschen, K., et al. (2000). [(3)H]Nicotine binding in peripheral blood cells of smokers is correlated with the number of cigarettes smoked per day. *Neuropharmacology* 39, 2818–2829.
102. Quick, M. W., and Lester, R. A. (2002). Desensitization of neuronal nicotinic receptors. *J. Neurobiol.* 53, 457–478.
103. Buisson, B., and Bertrand, D. (2002). Nicotine addiction: The possible role of functional upregulation. *Trends Pharmacol. Sci.* 23, 130–136.
104. Buisson, B., and Bertrand, D. (2001). Chronic exposure to nicotine upregulates the human (alpha)4((beta)2 nicotinic acetylcholine receptor function. *J. Neurosci.* 21, 1819–1829.
105. Marks, M. J., Pauly, J. R., Gross, S. D., Deneris, E. S., Hermans-Borgmeyer, I., Heinemann, S. F., et al. (1992). Nicotine binding and nicotinic receptor subunit RNA after chronic nicotine treatment. *J. Neurosci.* 12, 2765–2784.
106. Rowell, P. P., and Wonnacott, S. (1990). Evidence for functional activity of up-regulated nicotine binding sites in rat striatal synaptosomes. *J. Neurochem.* 55, 2105–2110.
107. Marks, M. J., Grady, S. R., and Collins, A. C. (1993). Downregulation of nicotinic receptor function after chronic nicotine infusion. *J. Pharmacol. Exp. Ther.* 266, 1268–1276.
108. Gentry, C. L., Wilkins, L. H., and Lukas, R. J. (2003). Effects of prolonged nicotinic ligand exposure on function of heterologously expressed, human alpha4beta2- and alpha4beta4-nicotinic acetylcholine receptors. *J. Pharmacol. Exp. Ther.* 304, 206–216.
109. Epping-Jordan, M. P., Watkins, S. S., Koob, G. F., and Markou, A. (1998). Dramatic decreases in brain reward function during nicotine withdrawal. *Nature* 393, 76–79.
110. Schwartz, R. D., and Kellar, K. J. (1985). In vivo regulation of [3 H] acetylcholine recognition sites in brain by nicotinic cholinergic drugs. *J. Neurochem.* 45, 427–433.
111. Hulihan-Giblin, B. A., Lumpkin, M. D., and Kellar, K. J. (1990). Effects of chronic administration of nicotine on prolactin release in the rat: Inactivation of prolactin response by repeated injections of nicotine. *J. Pharmacol. Exp. Ther.* 252, 21–25.
112. el Bizri, H., and Clarke, P. B. (1994). Regulation of nicotinic receptors in rat brain following quasi-irreversible nicotinic blockade by chlorisondamine and chronic treatment with nicotine. *Br. J. Pharmacol.* 113, 917–925.

113. Kellar, K. J., Davila-Garcia, M. I., and Xiao, Y. (1999). Pharmacology of neuronal nicotinic acetylcholine recceptors: Effects of acute and chronic nicotine. *Nicotine Tobacco Res.* 1(Suppl. 2), S117–S120.

114. Royal College of Physicians (2000). *Nicotine Addiction In Britain: A Report of the Tobacco Advisory Group of the Royal College of Physicians.* Royal College of Physicians of London, London.

115. Swedberg, M. D. B., Henningfield, J. E., and Goldberg, S. R. (1990). Nicotine dependency: Animal studies. In *Nicotine Psychopharmacology: Molecular, Cellular, and Behavioural Aspects,* S. Wonnacott, M. A. H. Russell, and I. P. Stolerman, Eds. Oxford University Press, Oxford, pp. 38–76.

116. Collins, A. C., and Marks, M. J. (1989). Chronic nicotine exposure and brain nicotinic receptors—influence of genetic factors. *Prog. Brain Res.* 79, 137–146.

117. Balfour, D. J., and Fagerstrom, K. O. (1996). Pharmacology of nicotine and its therapeutic use in smoking cessation and neurodegenerative disorders. *Pharmacol. Ther.* 72, 51–81.

118. Soria, R., Stapleton, J. M., Gilson, S. F., Sampson-Cone, A., Henningfield, J. E., and London, E. D. (1996). Subjective and cardiovascular effects of intravenous nicotine in smokers and non-smokers. *Psychopharmacology (Berl.)* 128, 221–226.

119. U.S. Department of Health and Human Services (1998). *The Health Consequences of Smoking: Nicotine Addiction, a Report of the Surgeon General.* U.S. Government Printing Office, Washington, DC.

120. Heishman, S. J., and Henningfield, J. E. (2000). Tolerance to repeated nicotine administration on performance, subjective, and physiological responses in nonsmokers. *Psychopharmacology* 152, 321–333.

121. Hughes, J. R., and Hatsukami, D. (1986). Signs and symptoms of tobacco withdrawal. *Arch. Gen. Psychiatry* 43, 289–294.

122. Shiffman, S. M., and Jarvik, M. E. (1976). Smoking withdrawal symptoms in two weeks of abstinence. *Psychopharmacology (Berl.)* 50, 35–39.

123. Malin, D. H., Lake, J. R., Newlin-Maultsby, P., Roberts, L. K., Lanier, J. G., Carter, V. A., et al. (1992). Rodent model of nicotine abstinence syndrome. *Pharmacol. Biochem. Behav.* 43, 779–784.

124. Hildebrand, B. E., Nomikos, G. G., Bondjers, C., Nisell, M., and Svensson, T. H. (1997). Behavioral manifestations of the nicotine abstinence syndrome in the rat: Peripheral versus central mechanisms. *Psychopharmacology* 129, 348–356.

125. Isola, R., Vogelsberg, V., Wemlinger, T. A., Neff, N. H., and Hadjiconstantinou, M. (1999). Nicotine abstinence in the mouse. *Brain Res.* 850, 189–196.

126. Carboni, E., Bortone, L., Giua, C., and DiChiara, G. (2000). Dissociation of physical abstinence signs from changes in extracellular dopamine in the nucleus accumbens and in the prefontal cortex of nicotine dependent rats. *Drug Alcohol Depend.* 58, 93–102.

127. Semenova, S., Bespalov, A., and Markou, A. (2003). Decreased prepulse inhibition during nicotine withdrawal in DBA/2J mice is reversed by nicotine self-administration. *Eur. J. Pharmacol.* 472, 99–110.

128. Droungas, A., Ehrman, R. N., Childress, A. R., and O'Brien, C. P. (1995). Effect of smoking cues and cigarette availability on craving and smoking behavior. *Addict. Behav.* 20, 657–673.

129. Buchhalter, A. R., Acosta, M. C., Evans, S. E., Breland, A. B., and Eissenberg, T. (2005). Tobacco abstinence symptom suppression: The role played by the smoking-related stimuli that are delivered by denicotinized cigarettes. *Addiction* 100, 550–559.

130. Hatsukami, D. K., Hughes, J. R., Pickens, R. W., and Svikis, D. (1984). Tobacco withdrawal symptoms: An experimental analysis. *Psychopharmacology (Berl.)* 84, 231–236.
131. Myrsten, A. L., Elgerot, A., and Edgren, B. (1977). Effects of abstinence from tobacco smoking on physiological and psychological arousal levels in habitual smokers. *Psychosom. Med.* 39, 25–38.
132. Pickworth, W. B., Fant, R. V., Butschky, M. F., and Henningfield, J. E. (1996). Effects of transdermal nicotine delivery on measures of acute nicotine withdrawal. *J. Pharmacol. Exp. Ther.* 279, 450–456.
133. Shiffman, S. M. (1979). The tobacco withdrawal syndrome. *NIDA Res. Monogr.* 23, 158–184.
134. Watkins, S. S., Stinus, L., Koob, G. F., and Markou, A. (2000). Reward and somatic changes during precipitated nicotine withdrawal in rats: Centrally and peripherally mediated effects. *J. Pharmacol. Exp. Ther.* 292, 1053–1064.
135. Cryan, J. F., Bruijnzeel, A. W., Skjei, K. L., and Markou, A. (2003). Bupropion enhances brain reward function and reverses the affective and somatic aspects of nicotine withdrawal in the rat. *Psychopharmacology* 168, 347–358.
136. Tloczynski, J., Malinowski, A., and Lamorte, R. (1997). Rediscovering and reapplying contingent informal medication. *Psychologia* 40, 14–21.
137. Carroll, M. E., Lac, S. T., Asencio, M., and Keenan, R. M. (1989). Nicotine dependence in rats. *Life Sci.* 45, 1381–1388.
138. Helton, D. R., Tizzano, J. P., Monn, J. A., Schoepp, D. D., and Kallman, M. J. (1997). LY354740: A metabotropic glutamate receptor agonist which ameliorates symptoms of nicotine withdrawal in rats. *Neuropharmacology* 36, 1511–1516.
139. Harrison, A. A., Liem, Y. T., and Markou, A. (2001). Fluoxetine combined with a serotonin-1A receptor antagonist reversed reward deficits observed during nicotine and amphetamine withdrawal in rats. *Neuropsychopharmacology* 25, 55–71.
140. Fung, Y. K., Schmid, M. J., Anderson, T. M., and Yuen-Sum, L. (1996). Effects of nicotine withdrawal on central dopaminergic systems. *Pharmacol. Biochem. Behav.* 53, 635–640.
141. Hildebrand, B. E., Nomikos, G. G., Hertel, P., Schilstrom, B., and Svensson, T. H. (1998). Reduced dopamine output in the nucleus accumbens but not in the medial prefrontal cortex in rats displaying a mecamylamine-precipitated nicotine withdrawal syndrome. *Brain Res.* 779, 214–225.
142. Panagis, G., Hildebrand, B. E., Svensson, T. H., and Nomikos, G. G. (2003). Selective c-fos induction and decreased dopamine release in the central nucleus of amygdala in rats displaying a mecamylamine-precipitated nicotine withdrawal syndrome. *Synapse* 35, 15–25.
143. Hildebrand, B. E., Panagis, G., Svensson, T. H., and Nomikos, G. G. (1999). Behavioral and biochemical manifestations of mecamylamine-precipitated nicotine withdrawal in the rat: Role of nicotinic receptors in the ventral tegmental area. *Neuropsychopharmacology* 21, 560–574.
144. Rossetti, Z. L., Melis, F., Carboni, S., Diana, M., and Gessa, G. L. (1992). Alcohol withdrawal in rats is associated with a marked fall in extraneuronal dopamine. *Alcoholism: Clin. Exper. Res.* 16, 529–532.
145. Weiss, F., Markou, A., Lorang, M. T., and Koob, G. F. (1992). Basal extracellular dopamine levels in the nucleus accumbens are decreased during cocaine withdrawal after unlimited-access self-administration. *Brain Res.* 593, 314–318.

146. Terry, P., and Katz, J. L. (1997). Dopaminergic mediation of the discriminative stimulus effects of bupropion in rats. *Psychopharmacology* 134, 201–212.

147. Nomikos, G. G., Damsma, G., Wenkstern, D., and Fibiger, H. C. (1992). Effects of chronic bupropion on interstitial concentrations of dopamine in rat nucleus accumbens and striatum. *Neuropsychopharmacology* 7, 7–14.

148. Shoaib, M., Sidhpura, N., and Shafait, S. (2003). Investigating the actions of bupropion on dependence-related effects of nicotine in rats. *Psychopharmacology* 165, 405–412.

149. Glick, S. D., Maisonneuve, I. M., and Kitchen, B. A. (2002). Modulation of nicotine self-administration in rats by combination therapy with agents blocking alpha 3 beta 4 nicotinic receptors. *Eur. J. Pharmacol.* 448, 185–191.

150. Bruijnzeel, A. W., and Markou, A. (2003). Characterization of the effects of bupropion on the reinforcing properties of nicotine and food in rats. *Synapse* 50, 20–28.

151. Malin, D. H. (2001). Nicotine dependence: Studies with a laboratory model. *Pharmacol. Biochem. Behav.* 70, 551–559.

152. Harvey, S. C., and Luetje, C. W. (1996). Determinants of competitive antagonist sensitivity on neuronal nicotinic receptor beta subunits. *J. Neurosci.* 16, 3798–3806.

153. Benwell, M. E. M., Balfour, D. J. K., and Anderson, J. M. (1990). Smoking-associated changes in the serotonergic systems of discrete regions of human brain. *Psychopharmacology* 102, 68–72.

154. Kenny, P. J., File, S. E., and Rattray, M. (2001). Nicotine regulates 5-HT(1A) receptor gene expression in the cerebral cortex and dorsal hippocampus. *Eur. J. Neurosci.* 13, 1267–1271.

155. Rasmussen, K., Kallman, M. J., and Helton, D. R. (1997). Serotonin-1A antagonists attenuate the effects of nicotine withdrawal on the auditory startle response. *Synapse* 27, 145–152.

156. Rasmussen, K., and Czachura, J. F. (1997). Nicotine withdrawal leads to increased sensitivity of serotonergic neurons to the 5-HT1A agonist 8-OH-DPAT. *Psychopharmacology (Berl.)* 133, 343–346.

157. Benwell, M. E., and Balfour, D. J. (1982). Effects of chronic nicotine administration on the response and adaptation to stress. *Psychopharmacology (Berl.)* 76, 160–162.

158. Benwell, M. E., and Balfour, D. J. (1979). Effects of nicotine administration and its withdrawal on plasma corticosterone and brain 5-hydroxyindoles. *Psychopharmacology (Berl.)* 63, 7–11.

159. Hilleman, D. E., Mohiuddin, S. M., and Delcore, M. G. (1994). Comparison of fixed-dose transdermal nicotine, tapered-dose transdermal nicotine, and buspirone in smoking cessation. *J. Clin. Pharmacol.* 34, 222–224.

160. Hilleman, D. E., Mohiuddin, S. M., Del Core, M. G., and Sketch, M. H. (1992). Effect of buspirone on withdrawal symptoms associated with smoking cessation. *Arch. Intern. Med.* 152, 350–352.

161. West, R., Hajek, P., and McNeill, A. (1991). Effect of buspirone on cigarette withdrawal symptoms and short-term abstinence rates in a smokers clinic. *Psychopharmacology (Berl.)* 104, 91–96.

162. Schneider, N. G., Olmstead, R. E., Steinberg, C., Sloan, K., Daims, R. M., and Brown, H. V. (1996). Efficacy of buspirone in smoking cessation: A placebo-controlled trial. *Clin. Pharmacol. Ther.* 60, 568–575.

163. Kirschbaum, C., Wust, S., and Strasburger, C. J. (1992). 'Normal' cigarette smoking increases free cortisol in habitual smokers. *Life Sci.* 50, 435–442.

164. Pickworth, W. B., Baumann, M. H., Fant, R. V., Rothman, R. B., and Henningfield, J. E. (1996). Endocrine responses during acute nicotine withdrawal. *Pharmacol. Biochem. Behav.* 55, 433–437.

165. Puddey, I. B., Vandongen, R., Beilin, L. J., and English, D. (1984). Haemodynamic and neuroendocrine consequences of stopping smoking—a controlled study. *Clin. Exp. Pharmacol. Physiol.* 11, 423–426.

166. Frederick, S. L., Reus, V. I., Ginsberg, D., Hall, S. M., Munoz, R. F., and Ellman, G. (1998). Cortisol and response to dexamethasone as predictors of withdrawal distress and abstinence success in smokers. *Biol. Psychiatry* 43, 525–530.

167. Rasmussen, D. D. (1998). Effects of chronic nicotine treatment and withdrawal on hypothalamic proopiomelanocortin gene expression and neuroendocrine regulation. *Psychoneuroendocrinology* 23, 245–259.

168. Andersson, K., Fuxe, K., Eneroth, P., Jansson, A., and Harfstrand, A. (1989). Effects of withdrawal from chronic exposure to cigarette smoke on hypothalamic and preoptic catecholamine nerve terminal systems and on the secretion of pituitary hormones in the male rat. *Naunyn Schmiedebergs Arch. Pharmacol.* 339, 387–396.

169. Malin, D. H., Lake, J. R., Carter, V. A., Cunningham, J. S., and Wilson, O. B. (1993). Naloxone precipitates nicotine abstinence syndrome in the rat. *Psychopharmacology (Berl.)* 112, 339–342.

170. Zarrindast, M. R., and Farzin, D. (1996). Nicotine attenuates naloxone-induced jumping behaviour in morphine-dependent mice. *Eur. J. Pharmacol.* 298, 1–6.

171. Tome, A. R., Izaguirre, V., Rosario, L. M., Cena, V., and Gonzalez-Garcia, C. (2001). Naloxone inhibits nicotine-induced receptor current and catecholamine secretion in bovine chromaffin cells. *Brain Res.* 903, 62–65.

172. Benowitz, N. L., Porchet, H., Sheiner, L., and Jacob, P., III. (1988). Nicotine absorption and cardiovascular effects with smokeless tobacco use: Comparison with cigarettes and nicotine gum. *Clin. Pharmacol. Ther.* 44, 23–28.

173. Henningfield, J. E., Stapleton, J. M., Benowitz, N. L., Grayson, R. F., and London, E. D. (1993). Higher levels of nicotine in arterial than in venous blood after cigarette smoking. *Drug Alchohol Depend.* 33, 23–29.

174. Benowitz, N. L. (1988). Pharmacologic aspects of cigarette smoking and nicotine addiction. *New Engl. J. Med.* 319, 1318–1330.

175. Tomar, S. L., and Henningfield, J. E. (1997). Review of the evidence that pH is a determinant of nicotine dosage from oral use of smokeless tobacco. *Tobacco Control* 6, 219–225.

176. Fant, R. V., Henningfield, J. E., Nelson, R. A., and Pickworth, W. B. (1999). Pharmacokinetics and pharmacodynamics of moist snuff in humans. *Tobacco Control* 8, 387–392.

177. Henningfield, J. E., Fant, R. V., Radzius, A., and Frost, S. (1999). Nicotine concentration, smoke pH and whole tobacco aqueous pH of some cigar brands and types popular in the United States. *Nicotine Tobacco Res.* 1, 163–168.

178. Feyerabend, C., Ings, R. M. J., and Russell, M. A. H. (1985). Nicotine pharmacokinetics and its application to intake from smoking. *Br. J. Clin. Pharmacol.* 19, 239–247.

179. Benowitz, N. L., Jacob, P., III, Jones, R. T., and Rosenberg, J. (1982). Interindividual variability in the metabolism and cardiovascular effects of nicotine in man. *J. Pharmacol. Exp. Ther.* 221, 368–372.

180. Benowitz, N. L., Kuyt, F., Jacob, P., III, Jones, R. T., and Osman, A. L. (1983). Cotinine disposition and effects. *Clin. Pharmacol. Ther.* 34, 604–611.

181. Benowitz, N. L., Herrera, B., and Jacob, P., III (2004). Mentholated cigarette smoking inhibits nicotine metabolism. *J. Pharmacol. Exp. Ther.* 310, 1208–1215.
182. Benowitz, N. L., and Jacob, P., III. (1985). Nicotine renal excretion rate influences nicotine intake during cigarette smoking. *J. Pharmacol. Exp. Ther.* 234, 153–155.
183. Messina, E. S., Tyndale, R. F., and Sellers, E. M. (1997). A major role for CYP2A6 in nicotine C-oxidation by human liver microsomes. *J. Pharmacol. Exp. Ther.* 282, 1608–1614.
184. Tyndale, R. F., and Sellers, E. M. (2001). Variable CYP2A6-mediated nicotine metabolism alters smoking behavior and risk. *Drug Metab. Disposition* 29, 548–552.
185. Sellers, E. M., Kaplan, H. L., and Tyndale, R. F. (2000). Inhibition of cytochrome P450 2A6 increases nicotine's oral bioavailability and decreases smoking. *Clin. Pharmacol. Ther.* 68, 35–43.
186. Henningfield, J. E., and McLellan, A. T. (2005). Medications work for severely addicted smokers: Implications for addiction therapists and primary care physicians. *J. Substance Abuse Treatment* 28, 1–2.
187. Fiore, M. C., Bailey, W. C., Cohen, S. J., Dorfman, S. F., Goldstein, M. G., Gritz, E. R., et al. (2000). *Treating Tobacco Use and Dependence. Clinical Practice Guideline.* U.S. Department of Health and Human Services, Public Health Service, Rockville, MD.
188. U.S. Department of Health and Human Services (DHHS) (2000). *Reducing Tobacco Use: A Report of the Surgeon General.* DHHS, Centers for Disease Control and Prevention, National Center for Chronic Disease Prevention and Health Promotion, Office on Smoking and Health, Atlanta, GA.
189. World Health Organization (WHO) (2004). *Policy Recommendations for Smoking Cessation and Treatment of Tobacco Dependence.* WHO, Geneva.
190. Henningfield, J. E., and Slade, J. (1998). Tobacco dependence medications: Public health and regulatory issues. *Food Drug Law J.* 53, 75–114.
191. Shiffman, S., Mason, K. M., and Henningfield, J. E. (1998). Tobacco dependence treatments: Review and prospectus. *Annu. Rev. Public Health* 19, 335–358.
192. Henningfield, J. E., Fant, R. V., and Gopalan, L. (1998). Non-nicotine medications for smoking cessation. *J. Respir. Dis.* 19, S33–S42.
193. Fiore, M. C. (2000). A clinical practice guideline for treating tobacco use and dependence. *JAMA* 283, 3244–3254.
194. Henningfield, J. E. (1995). Nicotine medications for smoking cessation. *New Engl. J. Med.* 333, 1196–1203.
195. American Psychiatric Association (1996). Practice guideline for the treatment of patients with nicotine dependence. *Am. J. Pyschiatry* 153, 1–31.
196. U.S. Department of Health and Human Services (DHHS) (1988). *The Health Consequences of Smoking.* DHHS, Washington, DC, pp. 3–20.
197. Henningfield, J. E., Benowitz, N. L., Ahijevych, K., Garrett, B. E., Connolly, G. N., and Wayne, G. F. (2003). Does menthol enhance the addictiveness of cigarettes? An agenda for research. *Nicotine Tobacco Res.* 5, 9–11.
198. Henningfield, J., Pankow, J., and Garrett, B. (2004). Ammonia and other chemical base tobacco additives and cigarette nicotine delivery: Issues and research needs. *Nicotine Tobacco Res.* 6, 199–205.
199. Henningfield, J. E., Benowitz, N. L., Connolly, G. N., Davis, R. M., Gray, N., Myers, M. L., et al. (2004). Reducing tobacco addiction through tobacco product regulation. *Tobbaco Control* 13, 132–135.

200. Henningfield, J. E., Fant, R. V., Gitchell, J., and Shiffman, S. (2000). Tobacco dependence. Global public health potential for new medications development and indications. *Ann. NY Acad. Sci.* 909, 247–256.

201. Goldberg, S. R., Spealman, R. D., Risner, M. E., and Henningfield, J. E. (1983). Control of behavior by intravenous nicotine injections in laboratory animals. *Pharmacol. Biochem. Behav.* 19, 1011–1020.

202. Henningfield, J. E., Miyasato, K., and Jasinski, D. R. (1983). Cigarette smokers self-administer intravenous nicotine. *Pharmacol. Biochem. Behav.* 19, 887–890.

203. West, R. J., Jarvis, M. J., Russell, M. A., Carruthers, M. E., and Feyerabend, C. (1984). Effect of nicotine replacement on the cigarette withdrawal syndrome. *Br. J. Addiction* 79, 215–219.

204. Henningfield, J. E., Goldberg, S. R., Herning, R. I., Jasinski, D. R., Lukas, S. E., Miyasato, K. M., et al., (1986). Human studies of the behavioral pharmacological determinants of nicotine dependence. In *Problems of Drug Dependence, (NIDA Research Monograph # 67)*. L. S. Harris, Ed. National Institute on Drug Abuse, Rockville, MD, pp. 54–65.

204a. Benowitz, N. L. (1993). Nicotine replacement therapy. What has been accomplished—Can we do better? *Drugs* 45, 157–170.

204b. Schneider, N. G., Olmstead, R. E., Franzon, M. A., and Lunell, E. (2001). The nicotine inhaler: Clinical pharmacokinetics and comparison with other nicotine treatments. *Clin. Pharmacokinet.* 40, 661–684.

205. Tiffany, S. T., Cox, L. S., and Elash, C. A. (2000). Effects of transdermal nicotine patches on abstinence-induced and cue-elicited craving in cigarette smokers. *J. Consult. Clin. Psychol.* 68, 233–240.

206. Waters, A. J., Shiffman, S., Sayette, M. A., Paty, J. A., Gwaltney, C. J., and Balabanis, M. H. (2004). Cue-provoked craving and nicotine replacement therapy in smoking cessation. *J. Consult. Clin. Psychol.* 72, 1136–1143.

207. Sobel, B. F., Sigmon, S. C., and Griffiths, R. R. (2004). Transdermal nicotine maintenance attenuates the subjective and reinforcing effects of intravenous nicotine, but not cocaine or caffeine, in cigarette-smoking stimulant abusers. *Neuropsychopharmacology* 29, 991–1003.

208. Gorsline, J. (1993). Nicotine pharmacokinetics of four nicotine transdermal systems. *Health Values* 17, 20–24.

209. Fant, R. V., Henningfield, J. E., Shiffman, S., Strahs, K. R., and Reitberg, D. P. (2000). A pharmacokinetic crossover study to compare the absorption characteristics of three transdermal nicotine patches. *Pharmacol. Biochem. Behav.* 67, 479–482.

210. Benowitz, N. L., Jacob, P., III., and Savanapridi, C. (1987). Determinants of nicotine intake while chewing nicotine polacrilex gum. *Clin. Pharmacol. Ther.* 41, 467–473.

211. Choi, J. H., Dresler, C. M., Norton, M. R., and Strahs, K. R. (2003). Pharmacokinetics of a nicotine polacrilex lozenge. *Nicotine Tobacco Res.* 5, 635–644.

212. Molander, L., and Lunell, E. (2001). Pharmacokinetic investigation of a nicotine sublingual tablet. *Eur. J. Clin. Pharmacol.* 56, 813–819.

213. Molander, L., Lunell, E., Andersson, S. B., and Kuylenstierna, F. (1996). Dose released and absolute bioavailability of nicotine from a nicotine vapor inhaler. *Clin. Pharmacol. Ther.* 59, 394–400.

214. Bergstrom, M., Nordberg, A., Lunell, E., Antoni, G., and Langstrom, B. (1995). Regional deposition of inhaled ^{11}C-nicotine vapor in the human airway as visualized by positron emission tomography. *Clin. Pharmacol. Ther.* 57, 309–317.

215. Schneider, N. G., Lunell, E., Olmstead, R. E., and Fagerstrom, K. O. (1996). Clinical pharmacokinetics of nasal nicotine delivery. A review and comparison to other nicotine systems. *Clin. Pharmacokinet.* 31, 65–80.

216. Samaha, A. N., Yau, W. Y., Yang, P., and Robinson, T. E. (2005). Rapid delivery of nicotine promotes behavioral sensitization and alters its neurobiological impact. *Biol. Psychiatry* 57, 351–360.

217. Nemeth-Coslett, R., Henningfield, J. E., O'Keeffe, M. K., and Griffiths, R. R. (1986). Effects of Mecamylamine on human cigarette smoking and subjective ratings. *Psychopharmacology* 88, 420–425.

218. Tennant, F. S., Tarver, A. L., and Rawason, R. A., (1984). Clinical evaluation of mecamylamine for withdrawal from nicotine dependence. In *Problems of Drug Dependence* (NIDA Research Monograph # 49), L. S. Harris, Ed. Health and Human Services National Institute on Drug Abuse, Rockville, MD, pp. 239–246.

219. Rose, J. E., Behm, F. M., Westman, E. C., Levin, E. D., Stein, R. M., and Ripka, G. V. (1994). Mecamylamine combined with nicotine skin patch facilitates smoking cessation beyond nicotine patch treatment alone. *Clin. Pharmacol. Ther.* 56, 86–99.

220. Hurt, R. D. (1999). New medications for nicotine dependence treatment. *Nicotine Tobacco Res.* 1(Suppl. 2), S175–S179.

221. Picciotto, M. R. (1998). Common aspects of the action of nicotine and other drugs of abuse. *Drug Alcohol Depend.* 51, 165–172.

222. Baldessarini, R. (2001). Drugs and the treatment of psychiatric disorders: Depression and anxiety disorders. In *Goodman & Gilman's the Pharmacological Basis of Therapeutics*, 10th ed., J. G. Hardman and L. E. Limbird, Eds. McGraw-Hill, New York, pp. 447–483.

223. Prochazka, A. V., Weaver, M. J., Keller, R. T., Fryer, G. E., Licari, P. A., and Lofaso, D. (1998). A randomized trial of nortriptyline for smoking cessation. *Arch. Intern. Med.* 158, 2035–2039.

224. Hall, S. M., Reus, V. I., Munoz, R. F., Sees, K. L., Humfleet, G., Hartz, D. T., et al. (1998). Nortriptyline and cognitive-behavioral therapy in the treatment of cigarette smoking. *Arch. Gen. Psychiatry* 55, 683–689.

225. Edwards, N. B., Murphy, J. K., Downs, A. D., Ackerman, B. J., and Rosenthal, T. L. (1989). Doxepin as an adjunct to smoking cessation: A double-blind pilot study. *Am. J. Psychiatry* 146, 373–376.

226. Edwards, N. B., Simmons, R. C., Rosenthal, T. L., Hoon, P. W., and Downs, J. M. (1988). Doxepin in the treatment of nicotine withdrawal. *psychomatics* 29, 203–206.

227. Murphy, J. K., Edwards, N. B., Downs, A. D., Ackerman, B. J., and Rosenthal, T. L. (1990). Effects of doxepin on withdrawal symptoms in smoking cessation. *Am. J. Psychiatry* 147, 1353–1357.

228. Black, S. C. (2004). Cannabinoid receptor antagonists and obesity. *Curr. Opin. Investig. Drugs* 5, 389–394.

229. Cohen, C., Perrault, G., Voltz, C., Steinberg, R., and Soubrie, P. (2002). SR141716, A central cannabinoid (CB(1)) receptor antagonist, blocks the motivational and dopamine-releasing effects of nicotine in rats. *Behav. Pharmacol.* 13, 451–463.

230. Klesges, R. C., Meyers, A. W., Klesges, L. M., and La Vasque, M. E. (1989). Smoking, body weight, and their effects on smoking behavior: A comprehensive review of the literature. *Psychol. Bull.* 106, 204–230.

231. Pomerleau, O. F. (1998). Endogenous opioids and smoking: A review of progress and problems. *Psychoneuroendocrinology* 23, 115–130.

232. Volpicelli, J. R., Alterman, A. I., Hayashida, M., and O'Brien, C. P. (1992). Naltrexone in the treatment of alcohol dependence. *Arch. Gen. Psychiatry* 49, 876–880.
233. Houtsmuller, E. J., Clemmey, P. A., Sigler, L. A., and Stitzer, M. L. (1996). Effects of naltrexone on smoking and abstinence. In *Problems of Drug Dependence 1996: Proceedings of the 58th Annual Scientific Meeting of the College on Problems of Drug Dependence*, L. S. Harris, Ed. U.S. Department of Health and Human Services, National Institutes of Health, Rockville, MD, p. 68.
234. Kessler, D. (2001). *A Question of Intent: A Great American Battle with a Deadly Industry*. PublicAffairs, New York.
235. World Health Organization (WHO) (2001). *Advancing Knowledge on Regulating Tobacco Products*. WHO, Geneva.
236. World Bank (1999). *Curbing the Epidemic: Governments and the Economics of Tobacco Control*. World Bank, Washington, DC.
237. Food and Drug Administration (1996). Regulations restricting the sale and distribution of cigarettes and smokeless tobacco to protect children and adolescents; final rule. *Federal Register* 61, 44396–45318.
238. Koop, C. E., Richmond, J., and Steinfeld, J. (2004). America's choice: Reducing tobacco addiction and disease. *Am. J. Public Health* 94, 174–176.

16

PSYCHOSTIMULANTS

LEONARD L. HOWELL AND HEATHER L. KIMMEL
Emory University, Atlanta, Georgia

16.1 Introduction 567
16.2 Neuropharmacology Related to Psychostimulant Abuse 569
    16.2.1 Monoamines 570
    16.2.2 Glutamate 575
    16.2.3 γ-Aminobutyric Acid 576
    16.2.4 Hypothalamic–Pituitary–Adrenal Axis 577
    16.2.5 Neuropeptides 578
16.3 Neurobiology of Chronic Psychostimulant Exposure 579
    16.3.1 Neurotransmitter and Neuroendocrine Systems 580
    16.3.2 Signal Transduction Mechanisms and Gene Expression 584
16.4 Medication Development 585
16.5 Summary 588
References 589

16.1 INTRODUCTION

Psychostimulants are a broadly defined class of drugs that stimulate the central and sympathetic peripheral nervous systems as their primary pharmacological effect. In humans, psychostimulants reliably elevate mood and promote wakefulness. In animals, psychostimulants increase locomotor activity and reliably maintain self-administration behavior indicative of robust reinforcing effects. The abuse liability of psychostimulants is well established and represents a significant public health concern. Cocaine is widely recognized as one of the most addictive and dangerous illicit drugs in use today. The most recent proceedings of the National Institute on Drug Abuse (NIDA) Community Epidemiology Work Group (CEWG), published in 2003, reported that cocaine and crack abuse was endemic in almost all 21 major U.S. metropolitan areas surveyed. Rates of emergency department visits per 100,000 population were higher for cocaine than for any other illicit drug in 17 areas, and trends in treatment admissions from 2000 to 2002 showed little change in most areas

Handbook of Contemporary Neuropharmacology, Edited by David R. Sibley, Israel Hanin, Michael Kuhar, and Phil Skolnick. Copyright © 2007 John Wiley & Sons, Inc.

surveyed. Drug abuse–related emergency department visits involving amphetamine or methamphetamine increased 54% in the United States between 1995 and 2002. Currently, no effective pharmacotherapy for psychostimulant abuse has demonstrated efficacy for long-term use. Clearly, a better understanding of the neuropharmacological effects of cocaine and related psychostimulants will support efforts to develop and improve useful pharmacotherapies for psychostimulant abuse.

It is important to emphasize that a number of synthetic stimulants, including amphetamines, are useful medications in the treatment of attention-deficit hyperactivity disorder (ADHD), narcolepsy, excessive daytime sleepiness, and obesity. Cocaine is still used clinically as a local anesthetic, primarily for eye, ear, nose, or throat procedures. Some examples of stimulant medications legally available in the United States and their medical indications are provided in Table 16.1. Most of these drugs are analogs of the basic phenethylamine chemical structure closely related to the catecholamine neurotransmitters norepinephrine and dopamine (Fig. 16.1). The present chapter will focus on the neuropharmacology of cocaine, amphetamine, and methamphetamine due to their high abuse potential as reflected in their categorization as Schedule II drugs (Federal Controlled Substances Act). Other stimulants have potential for abuse and dependence due to their similar profile of pharmacological effects. For example, it is well established that methylphenidate is diverted from legitimate sources, such as Ritalin, and is misused or abused by a segment of the U.S. population [1]. However, the neuropharmacology of methylphenidate will be reviewed in a separate chapter on ADHD and stimulants. Also, there are a number of illicit amphetamine derivatives, including 3,4-methylenedioxymethamphetamine (MDMA, "Ecstasy"), that have prominent stimulant and hallucinogenic properties. The latter drugs will be reviewed in Chapter 17 focused on MDMA and other "club drugs". Recently, neurotoxicity associated with the use of amphetamine derivatives has been an area of intense investigation.

TABLE 16.1 Examples of Psychostimulants Used as Therapeutics in the United States

Drug	Trade Names	Medical Indications
Amphetamine	Adderall@ Dexedrine@ Dextrostat@	ADHD, narcolepsy, weight control
Diethylpropion	Tenuate@	Weight control
Methamphetamine	Adipex@ Desoxyn@ Methedrine@	ADHD, weight control
Methylphenidate	Ritalin@	ADHD, narcolepsy
Phentermine	Adipex-P@ Fastin@ Ionamin@	Weight control

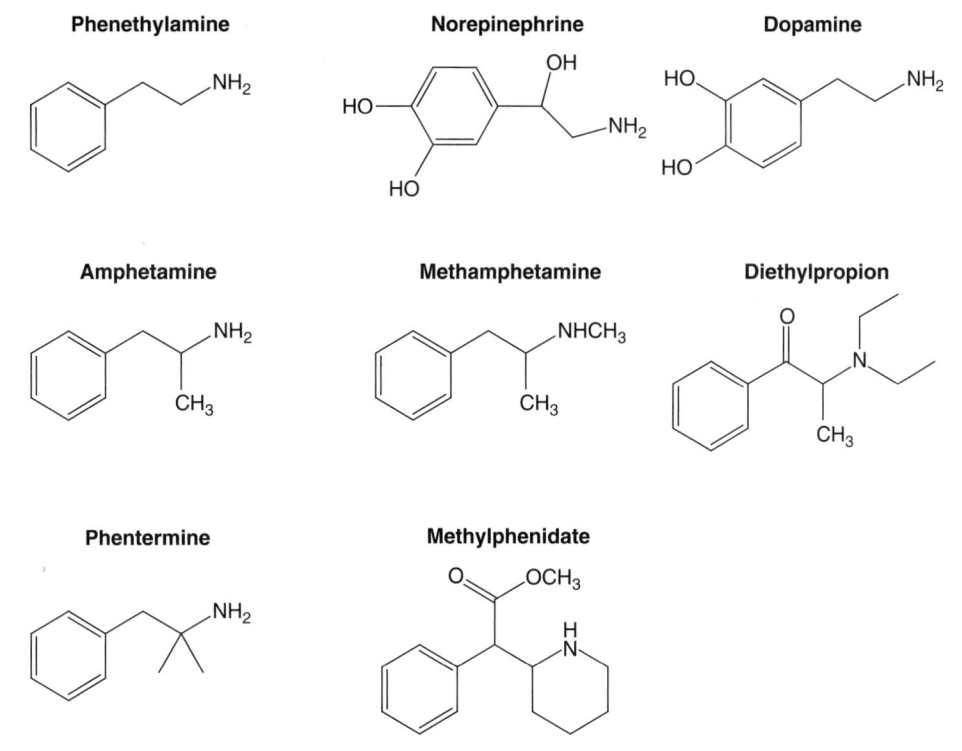

Figure 16.1 Chemical structures of endogenous and exogenous ligands for dopamine receptor. Dopamine and norepinephrine are both endogenous catecholamine neurotransmitters, sharing several chemical features, notably a catechol ring and an amine group. Exogenous ligands for the dopamine transporter, including amphetamine, methamphetamine, diethylpropion, phentermine, and methylphenidate, also share these chemical characteristics and act as psychomotor stimulants.

16.2 NEUROPHARMACOLOGY RELATED TO PSYCHOSTIMULANT ABUSE

Extensive literature documents the critical importance of monoamines (dopamine, serotonin, and norepinephrine) in the behavioral pharmacology and addictive properties of psychostimulants. In particular, dopamine plays a primary role in the reinforcing effects of psychostimulants in animals and humans. However, there is a growing body of evidence that highlights complex interactions among additional neurotransmitter, neuroendocrine, and neuropeptide systems. Cortical glutamatergic systems provide important regulation of dopamine function. Similarly, γ-aminobutyric acid (GABA) systems provide inhibitory neuromodulation of monoaminergic and glutamatergic function. Psychostimulants also activate the hypothalamic–pituitary axis and thereby engage neuroendocrine systems linked to stress reactivity. Alternatively, environmental stressors can alter the neurochemical and behavioral effects of psychostimulants. Finally, endogenous neuropeptide systems, including opioids and neurotensin, appear to play an important role in the neuropharmacology and addictive properties of psychostimulants. Drug abuse and addiction comprise a highly complex behavioral disorder. It is not surprising that the neurobiological substrates underlying psychostimulant abuse and dependence involve a complex interplay among multiple neurochemical systems.

16.2.1 Monoamines

The primary mechanism for inactivation of monoamine signaling is transporter-mediated uptake of released monoamine neurotransmitters. Psychostimulants enhance monoamine signaling by interfering with transporter function (Fig. 16.2). However, psychostimulants differ in their relative affinity for dopamine, serotonin, and norepinephrine transporters. For example, cocaine has approximately equal

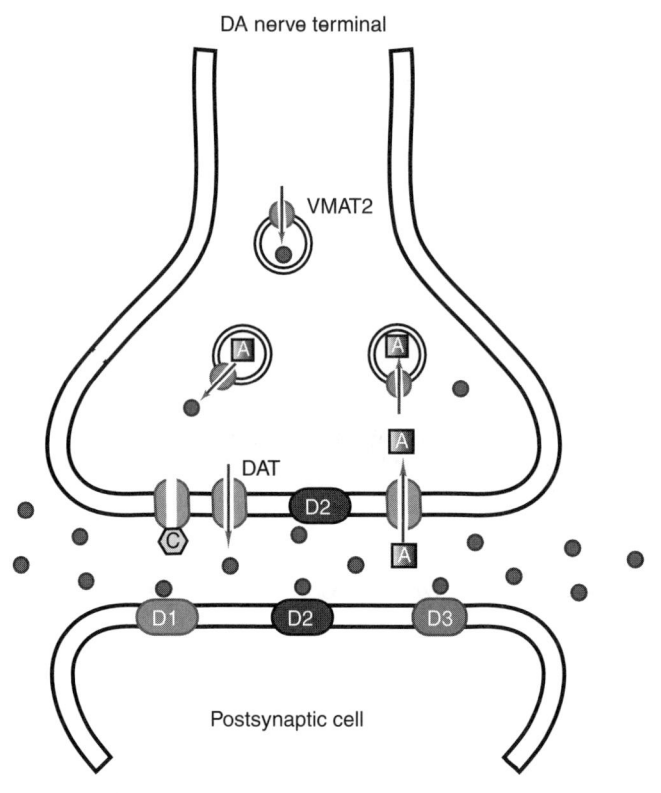

Figure 16.2 Representative dopaminergic nerve terminal and synapse. Dopamine is packaged into vesicles in the presynaptic neuron via VMAT2. Once dopamine is released into the synapse, this neurotransmitter can bind to postsynaptic dopamine receptors, including the D_1, D_2, and D_3 dopamine receptors. Dopamine D_2 receptors are also localized at the presynaptic terminal, acting as a feedback mechanism to regulate dopamine release. The DAT is also located at the presynaptic terminal and functions to remove dopamine from the synapse. Psychostimulants act at the DAT to alter normal dopamine receptor functions. Cocaine blocks the DAT, inhibiting uptake of dopamine into the presynaptic nerve terminal. Amphetamine also blocks the DAT and inhibits dopamine uptake, but also acts to release dopamine from intracellular vesicles. Abbreviations: A, amphetamine; C, cocaine; DAT, dopamine transporter; VMAT2, vesicular monoamine transporter 2.

TABLE 16.2 Drug Affinities at Monoamine Transporters

Drug	Dopamine	Serotonin	Norepinephrine
Cocaine	478[a]	304[a]	777[b]
(+) Amphetamine	34[b]	3830[b]	39[b]
(+) Methamphetamine	114[c]	2137[c]	48[c]
Methylphenidate	82[d]	7600[d]	440[d]

[a]IC_{50} (nM) Matecka et al. (1996) *J. Med. Chem.* 39: 4704–4716.
[b]K_i (nM) Rothman et al. (2001) *Synapse* 39: 32–41.
[c]K_i (nM) Rothman et al. (2000) *Synapse* 35: 222–227.
[d]IC_{50} (nM) Pan et al. (1994) *Eur. J. Pharmacol.* 264: 177–182.

affinity for these three transporters (Table 16.2). In contrast, amphetamine, methamphetamine, and methylphenidate all have relatively lower affinity for serotonin transporters compared to their affinity for dopamine and norepinephrine transporters. In addition, psychostimulants differ in their actions as reuptake inhibitors versus substrate-type releasers [2, 3]. Reuptake inhibitors bind to transporter proteins and interfere with transporter function but are not transported into the nerve terminal. Cocaine is an example of a reuptake inhibitor. In contrast, substrate-type releasers bind to transporter proteins and are subsequently transported into the cytoplasm of the nerve terminal. Releasers elevate extracellular monoamine levels by reversing the process of transporter-mediated exchange, thereby enhancing monoamine efflux. They also increase cytoplasmic levels of monoamines by interfering with vesicular storage [4, 5]. Amphetamine and methamphetamine are examples of substrate-type releasers. Typically, releasers are more effective than reuptake inhibitors in increasing extracellular monoamines because the former increase the pool of neurotransmitters available for release by transporter-mediated exchange. Moreover, the effectiveness of releasers in increasing extracellular monoamines is not dependent upon the basal rate of neurotransmitter release. In contrast, the effectiveness of reuptake inhibitors is impulse dependent and, therefore, limited by the tone of presynaptic activity.

In vivo studies have demonstrated that psychostimulants can interact with multiple monoamine transporters. However, the behavioral effects of psychostimulants associated with their addictive properties have been linked most closely to enhanced dopaminergic activity. The mesocorticolimbic dopamine system comprises dopamine neurons originating in the ventral tegmental area (VTA) of the midbrain that project to several limbic and cortical structures, including the nucleus accumbens, amygdala, and prefrontal cortex [6, 7] (Fig. 16.3). Drug-induced increases in extracellular dopamine in the mesocorticolimbic dopamine system are critical in mediating the behavioral effects of psychostimulants. Two families of dopamine receptors termed D_1-like (D_1 and D_5 receptors) and D_2-like (D_2, D_3, and D_4 receptors) have been described [8, 9], and both have been implicated in the abuse-related effects of cocaine [10–12]. Evidence to support this conclusion is derived from a variety of behavioral studies characterizing the acute effects of direct-acting dopamine agonists, dopamine uptake inhibitors, and dopamine antagonists administered alone or in combination with cocaine and related psychostimulants. Operant-conditioning procedures have been implemented to characterize drug effects on behavior, including schedule-controlled behavior (model of stimulant effects),

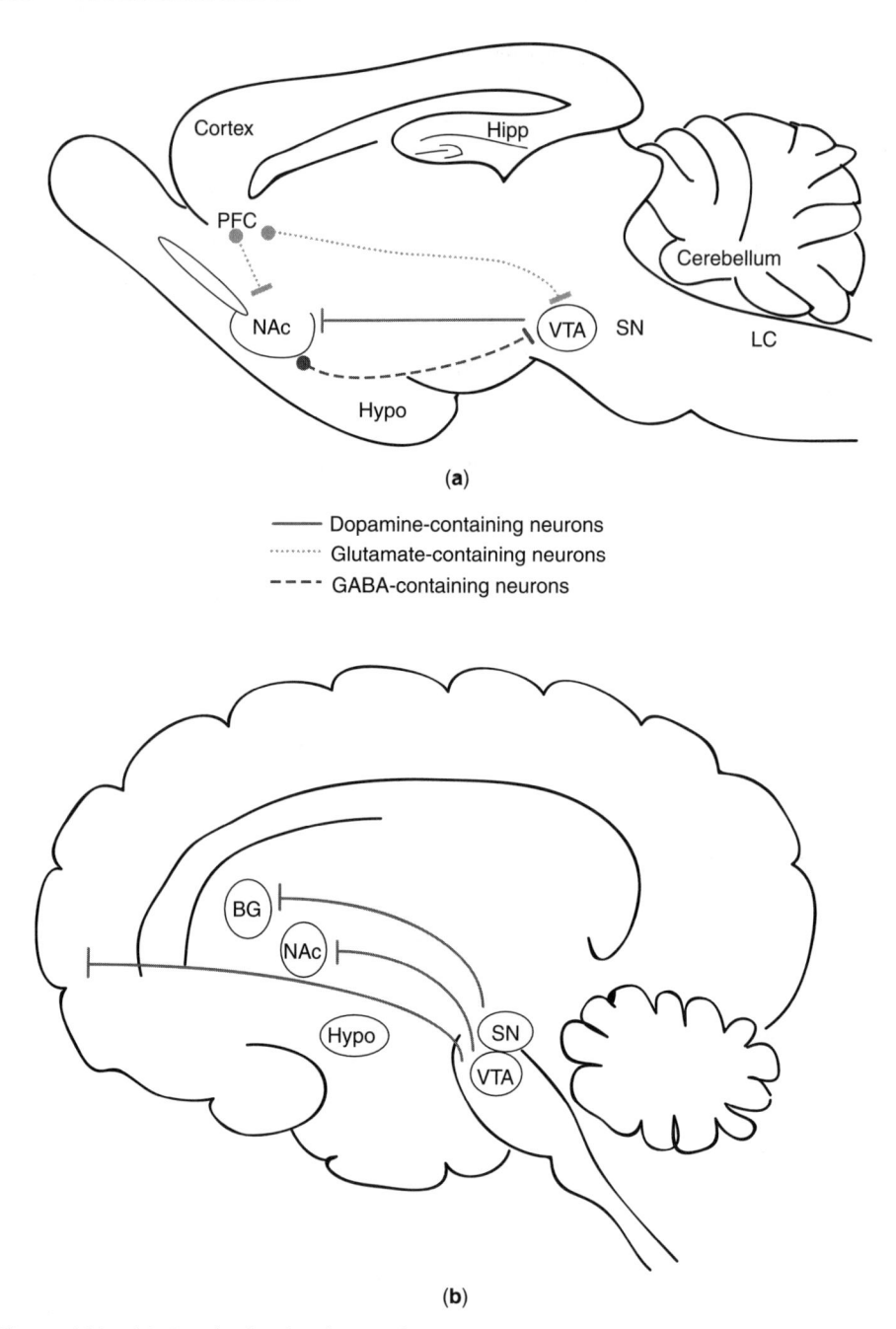

Figure 16.3 (a) Rat brain showing major components of mesolimbic system. Dopamine neurons project from the VTA and terminate in the NAc. Inhibitory GABA neurons project from the NAc and terminate in the VTA. Excitatory glutamatergic neurons project from the PFC to the NAc and to the VTA. (b) Human brain showing major dopaminergic projections. Abbreviations: BG, basal ganglia; LC, locus ceruleus; Hipp, hippocampus; Hypo, hypothalamus; NAc, nucleus accumbens; PFC, prefrontal cortex; SN, substantia nigra; VTA, ventral tegmental area.

drug self-administration (model of reinforcing effects), reinstatement (model of relapse), and drug discrimination (model of subjective effects) [13].

In a series of comprehensive studies, a significant correlation was obtained between dopamine transporter occupancy in vitro and the locomotor stimulant effects of cocaine analogs [14, 15]. In addition, the inhibition constants of 19 different dopamine transporter inhibitors were highly and positively correlated with their discriminative stimulus effects in rodents trained to discriminate cocaine from saline [16]. Similarly, a high correlation was found between the ability of cocaine analogs to displace [^{3}H]cocaine in the caudate and the ability of those compounds to produce cocaine like behavioral effects in squirrel monkeys [17–19]. Cocaine and selective dopamine uptake inhibitors exert similar effects on schedule-controlled behavior and are reliably self-administered in monkeys [17, 20–23]. Moreover, some direct-acting dopamine agonists maintain self-administration in rodents [24] and monkeys [25, 26]. Lastly, dopamine antagonists can attenuate specific behavioral effects of cocaine, including its reinforcing effects [27], its discriminative stimulus effects [28–30], and its stimulant effects on schedule-controlled behavior [20, 31–33]. The results obtained in behavioral studies provide compelling evidence that dopamine plays a major role in the neuropharmacology of cocaine.

The relevance of the dopamine transporter in the reinforcing effects of cocaine is supported further by human and nonhuman primate neuroimaging studies. In human cocaine users, a significant correlation was observed between dopamine transporter occupancy and the subjective high reported following administration of cocaine [34] or the behavioral stimulant methylphenidate [35]. Doses of cocaine within the range used by humans resulted in dopamine transporter occupancy between 67 and 69% in baboons [36]. Moreover, doses of cocaine that maintained peak response rates in drug self-administration studies resulted in dopamine transporter occupancy between 65 and 76% in rhesus monkeys [37, 38]. In addition, dopamine transporter occupancy has been determined for dopamine transporter inhibitors shown to be effective in reducing cocaine self-administration. Doses of GBR 12909 that decreased cocaine self-administration in rhesus monkeys resulted in dopamine transporter occupancy greater than 50% in baboons [39] and rhesus monkeys [38]. Similarly, doses of phenyltropane derivatives of cocaine with selectivity for the dopamine transporter decreased cocaine self-administration in rhesus monkeys at dopamine transporter occupancies between 72 and 84% [37, 38]. Collectively, these results indicate that dopamine transporter occupancy is an important determinant of the reinforcing effects of cocaine and of the effectiveness of dopamine transporter inhibitors to reduce cocaine self-administration.

The dopaminergic system is clearly an important site of action for psychostimulants, but preclinical studies have indicated that the serotonergic system can effectively modulate the behavioral effects of cocaine and amphetamine. Although compounds that selectively increase serotonin (5–HT) neurotransmission lack behavioral stimulant effects and do not reliably maintain self-administration behavior [40, 41], a negative relationship was observed between the potencies of several cocaine- and amphetamine-like drugs in self-administration studies and their binding affinities for 5-HT uptake sites [42, 43]. Coadministration of agents that induce robust increases in both dopamine and 5-HT produces minimal behavioral stimulant effects [44] and does not maintain self-administration behavior [45] in rodents. Similarly, monoamine-releasing agents have decreased reinforcing efficacy in rhesus monkeys when 5-HT-releasing potency is increased relative to dopamine [46]. The behavioral and neurochemical profile of dopamine transporter inhibitors is also influenced by their actions at multiple monoamine transporters in squirrel monkeys [47]. Consistent with these results, administration of the 5-HT uptake inhibitor fluoxetine decreased self-administration of cocaine [48] and amphetamine [49] in rodents and self-administration of cocaine in rhesus monkeys [50]. In nonhuman primate studies, the 5-HT uptake inhibitors citalopram, fluoxetine, and alaproclate attenuated the behavioral stimulant effects of cocaine on schedule-controlled behavior [41, 51]. The 5-HT direct agonist quipazine also attenuated the behavioral stimulant effects of cocaine, whereas the 5-HT antagonists ritanserin and ketanserin enhanced the behavioral stimulant effects of cocaine [41]. Lastly, the 5-HT uptake inhibitor alaproclate attenuated cocaine self-administration and cocaine-induced increases in extracellular dopamine in squirrel monkeys [52] and cocaine-induced activation of prefrontal activity in rhesus monkeys [53]. Collectively, there is a growing body of evidence to suggest that increasing brain 5-HT activity can attenuate the behavioral stimulant and reinforcing effects of psychostimulants.

Brain 5-HT systems are ideally situated to modulate the activity of dopamine neurons and the behavioral effects of dopamine uptake inhibitors such as cocaine. Serotonin neurons from the dorsal and median raphe nuclei innervate the dopaminergic cell bodies and terminal regions of the nigrostriatal and mesolimbic dopamine systems, and the convergence of 5-HT terminals and dopamine neurons has been visualized in the VTA and nucleus accumbens at the light and electron microscopic levels [54, 55]. Serotonin can act on cell bodies to decrease the firing rate of dopamine neurons or at terminals to decrease dopamine release. In either case, the ability of 5-HT to attenuate the behavioral effects of cocaine may result from an attenuation of cocaine-induced elevation of extracellular dopamine. Alternatively, 5-HT may act postsynaptically to dopamine neurons, attenuating the effects of cocaine-induced increases of extracellular dopamine on a downstream component of the pathway.

There is a growing consensus that stimulation of 5-HT_{2C} receptors inhibits the function of the mesolimbic dopamine system [56]. Firing rates of dopamine neurons in the VTA are decreased by 5-HT uptake inhibitors [57] and selective 5-HT_{2C} agonists [58], resulting in a decrease in nucleus accumbens dopamine levels [59]. Conversely, selective 5-HT_{2C} antagonists increase the activity of these neurons [60], leading to increased dopamine release in the nucleus accumbens [61]. Since 5-HT_{2c} receptors appear to be located exclusively on GABA neurons [62], the effects of 5-HT_{2C} receptor stimulation are likely to be indirectly mediated by an enhancement of GABA-mediated inhibition of VTA dopamine neurons. Localization of 5-HT_{2C} receptors on GABAergic terminals may also explain the conflicting results which have been obtained in previous electrophysiological, neurochemical, and behavioral studies. Some studies investigating interactions between 5-HT and dopamine have concluded that 5-HT can exert an excitatory influence on dopamine activity [63] and release [64, 65]. Stimulation of 5-HT_{1B} receptors can enhance cocaine reinforcement [66], likely by decreasing GABA-mediated inhibition in the VTA [63]. The 5-HT_3 receptors also appear to play a facilitatory role in the behavioral effects of dopamine agonists [67, 68]. These seemingly disparate results likely reflect the complexity of interactions between 5-HT and dopamine systems and the 5-HT receptor subtypes influenced by drug administration.

The norepinephrine system has considerable anatomical and functional connectivity to the mesolimbic dopamine system. There is significant noradrenergic innervation of the shell subregion of the nucleus accumbens [69, 70]. The locus ceruleus, the primary norepinephrine nucleus in the brain, projects directly to the VTA and influences neuronal firing of dopamine neurons [71]. Stimulation of the locus ceruleus can increase the activity of VTA dopamine neurons, and this effect is blocked by an α_1 adrenoreceptor antagonist [72]. In addition, lesions of the locus ceruleus can decrease basal release of dopamine in the nucleus accumbens [73]. It appears that interactions between norepinephrine and dopamine may play an important role in the behavioral pharmacology of psychostimulants. For example, amphetamine-induced release of dopamine in the nucleus accumbens and conditioned place preference to amphetamine are attenuated following depletion of norepinephrine in the prefrontal cortex of rodents [74]. Lesion of the locus ceruleus or inactivation of α_1 adrenoreceptors can also attenuate amphetamine- and cocaine-induced locomotion and sensitization in rodents [75–77]. Similarly, α_2 adrenoreceptor agonists which decrease norepinephrine release via autoreceptor activation block stress-induced reinstatement of extinguished cocaine self-administration behavior in rodents [78]. Studies in nonhuman primates also support a role for norepinephrine uptake and α_1 adrenoreceptor mechanisms in the discriminative stimulus effects of cocaine [79]. There is also a significant positive correlation between potency of norepinephrine release in vitro and the oral stimulant dose that produces stimulant-like subjective effects in humans [80]. However, it should be noted that there is little evidence that norepinephrine plays a primary role in the reinforcing properties of psychomotor stimulants in rodents [81] or nonhuman primates [41, 82–84].

16.2.2 Glutamate

The interaction between glutamatergic and dopaminergic systems has been an area of increasing interest in drug abuse and mental health research. Anatomical substrates for glutamate–dopamine interactions have been well characterized in rodents [85]. Dopaminergic afferents from the VTA to the dorsal striatum, nucleus accumbens, and prefrontal cortex are positioned to modulate glutamate function. Conversely, the VTA, dorsal striatum, and nucleus accumbens receive significant glutamatergic innervation from a variety of brain regions, including the prefrontal cortex, hippocampus, basolateral amygdala, and thalamus. Electrophysiological studies have documented complex functional interactions between glutamatergic and dopaminergic systems that play a primary role in frontal–subcortical circuits involved in motor and cognitive function [86]. Behavioral studies have documented that interactions between dopaminergic and glutamatergic inputs in the dorsal striatum and nucleus accumbens contribute to the expression of a variety of psychomotor behaviors in rodents relevant to drug addiction [87]. Importantly, a substantial literature derived from rodent studies has documented that glutamate receptor function plays a major role in the behavioral pharmacology of cocaine and other psychomotor stimulants. In particular, glutamatergic systems have been implicated in the development of locomotor sensitization, conditioned place preference, drug self-administration, and reinstatement of extinguished drug self-administration behavior [88–92].

The excitatory effects of glutamate can be mediated by ionotropic and metabotropic receptors, and localization of both receptor families in the VTA has been documented [93]. Recent evidence indicates that metabotropic glutamate receptors (mGluRs) play an important role in the behavioral effects of cocaine associated with its abuse liability. mGluRs can be divided into three groups based on sequence homology, receptor pharmacology, and signal transduction mechanisms [94]. Group 1 consists of mGluR1 and mGluR5 and is linked to phospholipase C and phosphoinositide hydrolysis. Group II consists of mGluR2 and mGluR3, while group III consists of mGluR4, 6, 7, and 8. Both groups II and III are negatively coupled to adenylyl cyclase. Group II mGluRs function as autoreceptors to regulate presynaptic glutamate release [94] and as heteroreceptors to regulate release of other neurotransmitters, including dopamine [95]. Administration of an mGluR2/3 agonist decreased dopamine and glutamate release in the nucleus accumbens, striatum, and prefrontal cortex [95–98], suggesting that glutamatergic tone on mGluR2/3 suppresses extracellular levels of dopamine and glutamate. The primary origin of extrasynaptic glutamate appears to be nonvesicular glutamate regulated by cystine/glutamate transporters [98, 99]. Withdrawal from repeated exposure to cocaine in rodents led to reduced levels of extracellular glutamate in the nucleus accumbens due to reductions in cystine/glutamate exchange [100, 101]. Restoration of cystine/glutamate exchange by systemically administered N-acetylcysteine (NAC) normalized glutamate levels in cocaine-treated rats. Importantly, cocaine-induced reinstatement of extinguished self-administration behavior was prevented by NAC-induced restoration of extracellular glutamate. Overall, a growing body of evidence derived from rodent studies indicates that glutamate plays a fundamental role in the maintenance and reinstatement of stimulant self-administration behavior [102–104]. Lastly the mGluR5 subtype has also been implicated in cocaine self-administration. mGluR5-deficient mice did not acquire intravenous (i.v.) self-administration of cocaine, and pretreatment with the mGluR5 antagonist MPEP decreased cocaine self-administration without affecting food-maintained behavior under similar schedules of reinforcement in rats [105]. Similarly, MPEP dose dependently attenuated the development of conditioned place preference in mice [106] and suppressed cocaine self-administration behavior in squirrel monkeys [107].

16.2.3 γ-Aminobutyric Acid

The inhibitory amino acid GABA is widely distributed in the central nervous system (CNS) and can modulate basal dopamine and glutamate release [108]. The VTA contains GABAergic inhibitory interneurons that function to control the firing rate of VTA dopamine neurons [109–111]. Moreover, the majority of projection neurons in the nucleus accumbens are GABAergic neurons, some of which project to the VTA and regulate the activity of dopamine neurons [112]. Several studies have indicated that GABAergic compounds can reliably modulate the neurochemical and behavioral effects of cocaine [113, 114]. Allosteric $GABA_A$ agonists, such as benzodiazepines and barbiturates, can inhibit dopamine and glutamate activity but have prominent sedative and hypnotic effects. However, there is considerable interest in $GABA_B$ agents, such as baclofen, due to their attenuation of glutamate and dopamine release [108, 115, 116] and their suppression of cocaine self-administration behavior across a wide range of schedules of reinforcement and access conditions

[114, 117–119]. In addition, pharmacological inhibition of GABA transaminase, the major enzyme involved in the metabolism of GABA, can lead to a rapid increase in extracellular GABA and a corresponding attenuation of cocaine self-administration behavior at doses that do not influence locomotor activity [120, 121]. Inhibition of GABA transaminase activity with γ-vinyl GABA can also block cocaine-induced lowering of brain stimulation reward thresholds [122]. Although psychostimulants do not have direct pharmacological effects on GABAergic systems, there is convincing evidence that GABA can modulate the neurochemical and behavioral effects of psychostimulants.

16.2.4 Hypothalamic–Pituitary–Adrenal Axis

The hypothalamic–pituitary–adrenal (HPA) axis is a neuroendocrine system that responds to stress, resulting in the release of glucocorticoids from the adrenal cortex. The mature HPA axis exhibits a circadian rhythmicity with a peak around the time of waking and a trough during the quiescent time of the activity cycle. Superimposed upon this diurnal pattern is activation of stressor-specific pathways that converge in the hypothalamus, where information is integrated in the paraventricular nucleus by parvocellular neurons expressing corticotropin-releasing factor (CRF). CRF is released from nerve endings in the median eminence in response to metabolic, psychological, or physical threats and stimulates the release of adrenocorticotropic hormone (ACTH) from the anterior pituitary. ACTH, in turn, stimulates the release of glucocorticoids (cortisol in primates, corticosterone in rats) from the adrenal cortex. These steroid hormones mobilize energy substrates during stress and regulate activity of the HPA axis via negative feedback at different levels via two types of corticosteroid receptors: (a) mineralocorticoid receptors involved in the modulation of the circadian HPA rhythm and (b) glucocorticoid receptors primarily responsible for reactive negative feedback during the circadian peak and following an acute stressor. In addition to its endocrine effects, CRF has a broad extrahypothalamic distribution in the CNS [123], and its synthesis and function are affected by stress [124].

Glucocortical hormones have a faciltory role in behavioral responses to psychostimulants, including locomotor activity, self-administration, and reinstatement of extinguished self-administration behavior. These interactions appear to involve glucocorticoid effects on the mesolimbic dopamine system [125, 126]. Suppression of glucocorticoids by adrenalectomy reduces the psychomotor stimulant effects of cocaine [127] and amphetamine [128, 129], and this effect is reversed by corticosterone administration [128]. Although psychostimulants increase corticosterone secretion [130], there is no correlation between drug-induced locomotion and drug-induced corticosterone increase [131, 132]. Similarly, reductions in circulating corticosterone attenuate the reinforcing effects of psychostimulants [133, 134]. However, blocking psychostimulant-induced elevations in glucocorticoid secretion does not affect cocaine self-administration [135–138]. Finally, corticosterone appears to play an important role in cue- and stress-induced reinstatement of extinguished self-administration behavior but not drug-induced reinstatement. Ketoconazole, which decreases glucocorticoid levels, prevents reinstatement induced by drug-paired environmental stimuli [138, 139]. Similarly, basal levels of corticosterone are necessary for stress-induced reinstatement even though stress-induced increases in corticosterone are not required [140, 141]. Moreover, stress-induced reinstatement can be blocked by corticotropin-releasing hormone (CRH) antagonists, suggesting that extra-hypothalamic CRH plays a role in stress-induced reinstatement [140, 142]. In contrast, cocaine-induced reinstatement is minimally influenced by adrenalectomy [140] and is not affected by ketoconazole administration [143].

16.2.5 Neuropeptides

All three opioid receptor subtypes (μ, κ, and δ) have been localized within dopamine systems in rodents [144–147]. Accordingly, it is not surprising to find interactions between the effects of drugs that primarily target these systems. As discussed earlier in this chapter, psychomotor stimulants interact directly with the dopamine system, either by blocking the dopamine transporter (as in the case of cocaine) or by stimulating dopamine release (as in the case of amphetamine). In contrast, opioid interactions with the dopamine systems are indirect. The μ- and δ-opioid receptors are located on GABAergic cells, which normally inhibit dopamine neurons. Activation of these receptors suppresses the activity of these inhibitory GABAergic interneurons, releasing the inhibition of dopamine cells, thereby increasing dopamine release from terminals [148–151]. In contrast, κ-opioid receptors are found on dopamine nerve terminals [152, 153], directly inhibiting dopamine release [145, 148, 154, 155].

Cocaine and heroin are often abused together in a "speedball" combination, resulting in euphoric effects that are greater than those of either drug alone [156, 157]. Preclinical research indicates that the combined administration of psychomotor stimulants and opiates enhances the effects of the individual drugs in several different behavioral assays. In rodent locomotor assays, μ-opioid receptor agonists potentiated the stimulant effects of cocaine and amphetamine [158–160]. The μ–opioid receptor agonists also potentiated the discriminative stimulus effects of cocaine in squirrel monkeys [161, 162]. However, drug self-administration studies in both rats [163] and rhesus monkeys [164] indicated that the combination of cocaine and heroin was not more reinforcing than cocaine alone. In contrast to the μ-opioid receptor agonists, the κ-opioid receptor agonist U-69593 attenuated cocaine- [165] and amphetamine-[166, 167] induced activity in rodents. Similarly, the κ-opioid receptor agonist U50488 attenuated the discriminative stimulus effects of low doses of cocaine in squirrel monkeys [168]. The results of stimulation of δ-opioid receptors on the behavioral effects of cocaine have been inconsistent [169]. The δ-opioid receptor agonist DPDPE potentiated cocaine-induced increases in locomotor activity in rodents [170]. However, the δ-opioid receptor antagonist naltrindole did not alter cocaine self-administration or cocaine-induced conditioned place preference in rodents [171]. The effects of the δ-opioid receptor agonist BW 373U86 did not alter the discriminative stimulus effects of cocaine in squirrel monkeys in one study [168], but in another study, the high-efficacy δ-opioid receptor agonist SNC80 potentiated the discriminative stimulus effects of cocaine [162].

Opiates not only influence psychomotor stimulant-induced changes in behavior but also alter psychomotor stimulant-induced changes in extracellular dopamine in the striatum and nucleus accumbens. When given in combination with cocaine, μ-opioid receptor agonists enhanced cocaine-induced increases in extracellular dopamine in rats [172, 173]. In contrast, κ-opioid receptor agonists attenuated cocaine- and amphetamine-induced increases in extracellular dopamine [167, 174].

Neurotensin is colocalized in tyrosine hydroxylase–containing dopamine neurons in the rat VTA and prefrontal cortex [175, 176]. Direct injections of neurotensin into selected brain regions results in changes in neurochemistry and behavior that are similar to those observed after administration of psychomotor stimulants. In vitro and in vivo studies show that neurotensin increases the firing of dopamine neurons in several brain regions, including the VTA [176, 177]. Intracerebroventricular administration of neurotensin increased levels of dopamine and its metabolites in several brain areas, including the striatum and nucleus accumbens [178, 179]. Infusion of neurotensin into the striatum or the VTA, but not into the nucleus accumbens, increased extracellular dopamine levels in rats [180, 181]. Repeated infusion of neurotensin into the VTA resulted in an enhanced dopamine response compared to an acute injection [180]. Locomotor activity was increased following infusion of neurotensin into the VTA of rats [180, 182] and sensitization to this behavioral effect was apparent after repeated neurotensin treatment [183]. Although rats self-administered neurotensin directly to the VTA [184], the neurotensin receptor agonist NT69L was not self-administered by rhesus monkeys [185].

Changes in dopamine neurotransmission following neurotensin administration are also reflected in alterations of psychostimulant-induced changes in neurochemistry and behavior. Direct neurotensin infusion to the striatum attenuated increases in dopamine induced by low, but not high, cocaine doses in rats [181]. In contrast, neurotensin did not block amphetamine-induced increases in dopamine in the nucleus accumbens [186]. Intravenous or intra-accumbal injections of neurotensin attenuated cocaine- and amphetamine-induced increases in locomotor activity in the rat [187–189]. Similarly, systemic administration of the neurotensin receptor agonist NT69L blocked the acute locomotor effects of cocaine and amphetamine in rats [190, 191]. Repeated, but not acute, administration of the selective neurotensin antagonist SR48692 decreased cocaine-induced increases in locomotor activity in rats [192]. Although neurotensin can alter the neurochemical and behavioral stimulant effects of psychostimulants, it may not play an important role in the reinforcing effects of these drugs. Direct application of neurotensin into the nucleus accumbens did not alter cocaine self-administration in rats [189], and the neurotensin receptor agonist NT69L did not alter the reinforcing effects of cocaine in rhesus monkeys [185].

16.3 NEUROBIOLOGY OF CHRONIC PSYCHOSTIMULANT EXPOSURE

Repeated exposure to psychostimulants can lead to robust and enduring changes in neurobiological substrates and corresponding changes in sensitivity to acute drug effects on neurochemistry and behavior. Diminished sensitivity to the effects of a drug during repeated exposure is indicative of tolerance, whereas enhanced sensitivity is indicative of sensitization. Both tolerance and sensitization have been reported to develop during repeated administration of stimulants in animal studies [193]. However, the outcome depends upon a variety of procedural variables, including the drug effect under investigation, the dosing regimen, the environmental context associated with drug administration, and the animal species. The vast majority of studies have focused on sensitization to locomotor stimulant effects in rodent models. Stimulants including cocaine and amphetamines can produce robust sensitization in rodents, usually identified as a progressive increase in locomotor activity or stereotyped behavior with repeated drug dosing [194]. In fact, sensitization has been proposed as a general model of neural plasticity whereby drug-induced changes in behavior can be linked to concomitant changes in molecular mechanisms. It is important to emphasize that some neurobiological changes are not evident when drug administration is terminated but actually emerge during the period of drug withdrawal.

16.3.1 Neurotransmitter and Neuroendocrine Systems

There is substantial evidence that the mesocorticolimbic dopamine system and its excitatory glutamatergic inputs are critical for the development of sensitization to the behavioral effects of psychostimulants [91, 195]. Studies involving microinjection of drugs into discrete brain regions have indicated that the VTA, a region rich in dopamine cell bodies, plays a critical role in the development of sensitization. In contrast, the nucleus accumbens, a major dopamine projection area from the VTA, appears to be more closely linked to the expression of sensitization. For example, microinjections of dopamine D_1 receptor antagonists [196, 197] or glutamate N-methyl-D-aspartate (NMDA) receptor antagonist [198] into the VTA can disrupt the development of sensitization. However, glutamate NMDA antagonists do not block the expression of sensitization [199]. Similarly, dopamine antagonists can block the development of sensitization to psychostimulants without blocking its expression [200]. Glutamatergic afferents from the prefrontal cortex to the VTA and the nucleus accumbens have been implicated in both the development and expression of sensitization to cocaine and amphetamine [201]. Sensitized animals also reliably show an augmented response to drug-induced increases in extracellular glutamate and dopamine in the nucleus accumbens [88, 202]. Collectively, there is convincing evidence to suggest that glutamatergic afferents from the prefrontal cortex produce adaptations in the VTA that mediate the development of sensitization to psychostimulants and that secondary adaptations within the nucleus accumbens are necessary for the expression of sensitization.

Behavioral sensitization to stimulants, including cocaine, amphetamine, and methylphenidate, also involves neuroadaptation of stress-responsive systems, in particular the HPA axis and CRF pathways. In fact, there is a dynamic crosstalk between these systems. Stimulants affect HPA axis function, but there is also evidence that exposure to stress or stress hormones increases sensitivity to stimulants [136, 203]. The latter effect has been linked to glucocorticoid effects on dopaminergic neurotransmission [203, 204]. Repeated exposure to stimulants in adult rodents produces long-term increases in HPA axis activity, resulting in enhanced ACTH and corticosterone secretion [204–206]. Studies of chronic administration of methylphenidate in periadolescent rats have found similar long-term effects in adulthood, such as increased HPA axis and behavioral (anxiety-like) stress reactivity [207]. Another long-term effect of stimulants on the central components of the HPA axis of the rat includes the downregulation of hippocampal and cerebral cortex glucocorticoids that could affect glucocorticoid-induced negative feedback on HPA axis activity [208, 209]. Stimulants also induce alterations of extrahypothalamic CRF pathways [210], which could mediate the reported anxiogenic effects of chronic psychostimulant administration [204, 207, 211]. There is abundant evidence of bidirectional interactions between sleep–wake and HPA axis activity rhythms. Sleep disturbances have been reported in adults with ADHD and include poorer sleep quality and higher nocturnal motor activity that improve after treatment with methylphenidate [212]. In healthy volunteers, stimulants seem to impair subjective ratings of sleep and increase early morning alertness [213, 214]. Although stimulants improve sleep–wake deficits in children with ADHD, the long-term consequence of chronic stimulant treatment on sleep–wake rhythms has not been established.

Sensitization to psychostimulants has been demonstrated in nonhuman primates, but studies to demonstrate sensitization in humans have yielded equivocal results. Rhesus monkeys trained to self-administer cocaine showed an augmented response to cocaine-induced elevations in striatal extracellular dopamine that emerged over a two-year period of drug exposure [215]. Chronic amphetamine exposure in nonhuman primates also induced a pattern of behavioral response that resembled the positive-like symptoms of schizophrenic humans [216]. Negative-like symptoms have also been observed in nonhuman primates following chronic amphetamine treatment [217]. More recently, a longitudinal study in rhesus monkeys exposed to repeated, escalating doses of amphetamine documented enhanced behavioral responses to subsequent acute low-dose amphetamine challenges [218]. Moreover, the enhanced behavioral responses to amphetamine challenge were evident up to 28 months postwithdrawal from chronic treatment. Several human studies in normal volunteers with no history of prior stimulant use reported evidence of sensitization to psychological (energy level and mood) and physiological (eye-blink rates) measures following two or three daily doses of amphetamine [219–221]. The outcome measures demonstrated enhanced increases following the last amphetamine dose compared to the first dose, suggesting that behavioral sensitization can be documented in human subjects. However, studies conducted in experienced stimulant users have not found evidence of sensitization. Experienced cocaine users failed to show sensitization after one or four prior cocaine exposures [222, 223]. Similarly, subjects with histories of stimulant use failed to show sensitization to oral amphetamine or methamphetamine [224, 225]. Repeated amphetamine challenges in patients with first-episode manic or schizophrenic psychosis also failed to induce sensitization [226].

There is legitimate concern that stimulant treatment during adolescence could have significant and enduring effects on reward processes relevant to mood regulation and risk for drug abuse. Preclinical studies have clearly documented that stimulants can have profound and long-lasting behavioral and neurobiological effects [91, 227]. Repeated exposure to stimulants in rodents reliably produces sensitization to their locomotor stimulant effects [228, 229] and can induce cross-sensitization with different classes of stimulant drugs [230]. Locomotor sensitization has been reported for low-dose stimulant administration intended to model therapeutic dosing [229]. Importantly, repeated dosing protocols that produce locomotor sensitization in rats can enhance the reinforcing properties of stimulants [231–234]. Once established, these behavioral and associated neurobiological changes can be remarkably stable and enduring [91, 235, 236]. Collectively, the results of laboratory studies in rodents raise significant concerns that prior exposure to stimulants, including those prescribed for the treatment of ADHD, may increase vulnerability to drug abuse in humans [237]. However, this area of investigation has received inadequate attention in human subjects and has not been approached with the experimental control and rigor afforded in animal studies. While ADHD is prevalent in treatment-seeking substance abusers [238], clinical studies have not provided direct support for concerns that have emerged from preclinical studies. On the contrary, recent reports suggest the possibility of reduced risk for substance disorders in children with ADHD who received therapeutic administration of stimulants such as methylphenidate [239, 240]. There is an obvious need to develop clinically relevant animal models that effectively extrapolate to the human condition.

Efforts to define the long-term neurobiological consequence of psychostimulant administration have focused primarily on the dopaminergic system and have yielded inconsistent results. For example, cocaine exposure has been reported to increase, decrease, or have no effect on dopamine transporter density in rodents [241–247]. Similarly, chronic cocaine administration in rodents has been reported to increase, decrease, or have no effect on dopamine D_1 or D_2 receptor density [248–251]. The equivocal results likely reflect different dosing regimens and withdrawal periods as well as the use of noncontingent drug administration protocols that do not model voluntary drug use. Active drug self-administration protocols and periods of drug abstinence can have profound influences on neuroadaptive changes in dopamine systems [252]. Accordingly, a more consistent picture has emerged from nonhuman primate studies of cocaine self-administration. For example, in rhesus monkeys trained to self-administer cocaine intravenous for 5 days, 3.3 months, or 1.5 years, initial exposure leads to moderate decreases in dopamine transporter density in the striatum, as determined postmortem with quantitative autoradiography [253]. However, longer exposure resulted in increased striatal dopamine transporter density that was most pronounced in the ventral striatum at the level of the nucleus accumbens. Importantly, the increases in dopamine transporter binding observed after long-term cocaine self-administration in nonhuman primates correspond closely to increases observed in postmortem tissue of human cocaine addicts [254, 255]. In related studies, rhesus monkeys trained to self-administer cocaine on a daily basis over 18–22 months showed lower dopamine D_1 binding density as determined postmortem with quantitative autoradiography [256]. The effects were most pronounced in regions of the striatum where the nucleus accumbens is most fully developed. In parallel studies using the same dosing schedule and quantitative autoradiography, dopamine D_2 binding density was lower in all regions of the striatum rostral to the anterior commissure [257]. Collectively, these drug-induced changes in the status of the dopamine system may contribute to the development of dependence associated with long-term psychostimulant use.

Functional neuroimaging techniques have been used effectively in humans to characterize the long-term consequences of stimulant exposure in the context of drug abuse. Compared to controls, detoxified cocaine abusers had a marked decrease in dopamine release as measured by methylphenidate-induced decreases in striatal [^{11}C]raclopride binding [34]. The self-reports of a "high" induced by methylphenidate were also less intense in cocaine abusers. The decrease in dopamine release in the striatum has been hypothesized to underlie the decrease in sensitivity to natural reinforcers in drug abusers [258, 259]. The density of the dopamine transporter and receptors in humans has also been evaluated with positron emission tomography (PET) imaging studies. In cocaine abusers, dopamine transporter density appears to be elevated shortly after cocaine abstinence but then to normalize with long-term detoxification [260]. In contrast, PET studies characterizing dopamine D_2 receptors have reliably documented long-lasting decreases in D_2 receptor density in stimulant abusers [261]. The reduction in D_2 receptor function coupled with dysfunctional dopamine release may further decrease sensitivity of reward circuits to stimulation by natural rewards and increase the risk for drug taking [262]. Lastly, regional brain glucose metabolism measured by FDG uptake has been characterized in conjunction with dopamine D_2 receptors [263, 264]. Reductions in striatal D_2 receptors were associated with decreased metabolic activity in the orbital frontal cortex and anterior cingulate cortex in detoxified individuals. In contrast, the orbital frontal cortex was hypermetabolic in active cocaine abusers [265]. Collectively, these findings observed in stimulant abusers document significant dysregulation of dopamine systems that are reflected in brain metabolic changes in areas involved in reward circuitry. Unfortunately, such well-designed clinical studies have not been conducted in the context of stimulant use for therapeutic purposes. However, therapeutic doses of methylphenidate block dopamine transporter function and increase extracellular dopamine [266, 267]. There is also a positive correlation between clinical improvement and reduction in dopamine transporter density in the basal ganglia following methylphenidate treatment [268]. Functional magnetic resonance imaging studies suggest that methylphenidate increases frontal cortical activity in children with ADHD [269], while PET imaging studies suggest that methylphenidate modulates brain regions associated with motor function in adults with ADHD [270]. Earlier PET studies using FDG in adults with ADHD found more limited brain metabolic effects following acute administration of *d*-amphetamine [271] and following chronic administration of *d*-amphetamine or methylphenidate [272]. Clearly, there is a need to conduct well-controlled laboratory studies to document the long-term consequences of low-dose stimulant exposure on dopaminergic function and brain metabolism.

Although significant attention has been focused on the dysregulation of the dopaminergic system, it should be emphasized that chronic exposure to stimulants can have long-term neurobiological effects on numerous neurotransmitter systems. Notably, enduring changes in glutamatergic function have been associated with repeated administration of psychostimulants. For example, basal extracellular levels of glutamate in the nucleus accumbens are decreased in rats with a history of repeated cocaine exposure [88] and there is a corresponding augmentation of cocaine-induced increases in glutamate [88, 273]. Others have reported a reduction in signaling through group I and group II metabotropic glutamate receptors [101, 274] and a reduction in sensitivity of α-amino-3-hydroxy-5-methylisoxazole-4-propionic acid (AMPA) glutamate receptors to electrical stimulation of the prefrontal cortex [275]. An enhanced inhibitory effect of dopamine on excitatory AMPA currents has also been reported [276]. The apparent downregulation of presynaptic and postsynaptic glutamate transmission following repeated cocaine exposure has been linked to cocaine-induced reinstatement of extinguished self-administration behavior and may have direct relevance toward understanding relapse to stimulant use in humans [99, 104].

There is evidence that GABAergic function is altered following chronic cocaine administration. An increase in benzodiazepine receptor binding was observed in the striatum and amygdala of rats up to 40 days after repeated cocaine administration was discontinued [277]. A sensitized behavioral response to systemically administered diazepam was also observed following the same dosing regimen [278]. These findings suggest that chronic cocaine exposure can produce alterations in GABAergic mechanisms that may mediate aspects of drug withdrawal. Long-term alterations in the 5-HT system have also been reported. Chronic exposure to cocaine enhanced sensitivity of 5-HT_{1A} receptors to inhibit GABAergic medium spiny neurons of the striatum [279] and reduced 5-HT concentrations in the frontal cortex [280] in rats. However, a postmortem study of human cocaine users documented higher 5-HT levels in the frontal cortex compared to matched controls [281]. Dysregulation of the noradrenergic systems may also be associated with chronic cocaine exposure. Altered noradrenergic tone was observed during cocaine withdrawal in human cocaine abusers [282], and chronic cocaine self-administration in nonhuman primates upregulated the norepinephrine transporter and decreased cerebral metabolism in the bed nucleus stria terminalis, a brain region that plays a key role in cocaine withdrawal and stress-induced reinstatement of extinguished self-administration behavior [283]. Although psychostimulants do not directly interact with opiate receptors, chronic psychostimulant exposure can influence endogenous opiate systems. For example, chronic cocaine administration increased μ- and δ-opioid receptors in several rat brain regions [284]. Downregulation of κ-opioid receptors in both the nucleus accumbens and the striatum was observed after chronic administration of cocaine and amphetamine in one study [285], but no changes in κ-opioid receptors were observed after chronic administration of cocaine in another study [284]. However, postmortem brains from fatal cocaine overdose victims showed increased κ-opioid receptor binding in limbic areas [286]. Similarly, PET neuroimaging in human cocaine users showed increased μ-opioid receptor binding that correlated with self-reported cocaine craving [287].

16.3.2 Signal Transduction Mechanisms and Gene Expression

In addition to regulation of ion channels, neurotransmitters regulate virtually all progresses that occur in neurons, including gene expression. Most of the effects of neurotransmitters on target neurons are achieved through biochemical cascades of intracellular messengers. Intracellular messengers are comprised of G proteins [guanosine triphosphate (GTP) binding membrane proteins], second messengers [such as cyclic adenosine monophosphate (cAMP) and Ca^{2+}], and protein phosphoregulators [288, 289]. Monoamine receptors are coupled to G proteins which regulate adenylyl cyclase activity to modulate the second messenger cAMP. The function of cAMP is to regulate the activity of protein kinases, phospholipases, and other intracellular enzymes. In turn, the enzymes regulate a variety of intracellular processes, including gene transcription that is regulated by transcription factors. Thus, the regulation of neurotransmitter signal transduction mechanisms and changes in gene transcription and protein synthesis can alter the number and type of receptors in target neurons as well as the functional activity of intracellular systems [290]. In recent years, significant advances in molecular biology have identified important drug-induced changes in neurobiology that may play a fundamental role in the transition to addiction.

The most extensively characterized signal transduction pathways activated by psychostimulants are those associated with dopamine receptor activation. The majority of research to date has focused on the VTA and nucleus accumbens [291]. Chronic administration of cocaine upregulates the cAMP pathway in the nucleus accumbens [292]. Cocaine and amphetamine also upregulate the transcription factor cAMP response element binding (CREB) protein in the nucleus accumbens [293, 294]. Convincing evidence suggests that these neuroadaptations can decrease sensitivity to the rewarding effects of psychostimulants and may impair the general reward system resulting in an amotivational, depressed-like state [293, 295, 296].

Acute administration of psychostimulants rapidly activates several immediate early genes in the rat brain, including c-*fos* and c-*jun* [236, 297]. The protein products of these genes function as nuclear transcription factors that regulate gene expression. Chronic exposure to stimulant can lead to tolerance of the gene activation effect and a downregulation of gene products. For example, chronic administration of cocaine significantly reduced the activity of subsequent drug exposure to induce c-*fos* and other *fos* proteins in rats [298]. Moreover, there was an accumulation of *fos*-related antigens, including the transcription factor ΔFosB [299]. Importantly, enhanced ΔFosB expression in the nucleus accumbens and dorsal striatum is associated with sensitization to the locomotor and reinforcing effects of cocaine. Overexpression of ΔFosB increased sensitivity to the locomotor stimulant and rewarding effects of cocaine and increased cocaine self-administration [300, 301]. Due to the extraordinary stability of ΔFosB, it could conceivably sustain these types of behavioral changes for weeks or months after the last drug exposure. Hence, it may serve as a molecular switch to support the initiation and maintenance of drug dependence [291].

Finally, acute administration of psychostimulants in rodents rapidly induces cocaine- and amphetamine-regulated transcript (CART) peptides in brain regions associated with reward systems, including the VTA, ventral pallidum, amygdala, lateral hypothalamus, and nucleus accumbens [302, 303]. Hence, CART is anatomically positioned to regulate mesolimbic dopamine function, and there is evidence that CART may play a role in the behavioral effects of psychostimulants. For example, administration of CART into mesolimbic regions can induce behavioral effects similar to those observed for psychostimulants. Direct injection of CART into the VTA of rats produced modest increases in locomotor activity and promoted conditioned place preference [304]. Intra-VTA injection of CART also induced modest but significant elevations in extracellular dopamine [302]. However, when coadministered with cocaine or amphetamine, CART attenuated drug-induced increases in locomotor activity [305, 306]. This functional antagonism suggests that CART peptides may be considered as potential targets for medication development to treat psychostimulant abuse [302]. It is interesting to note that CART messenger RNA (mRNA) levels were increased in the VTA of cocaine overdose victims [307, 308].

16.4 MEDICATION DEVELOPMENT

There is a growing appreciation that drug addiction is a chronic relapsing disorder with a biological basis. Significant advances in the understanding of neurobiological mechanisms underlying drug abuse and dependence have guided pharmacological treatment strategies to improve clinical outcome. Considerable effort has been directed toward the development of effective medications for substance abuse disorders and has led to useful pharmacological interventions. Notably, methadone has been an effective medication and adjunct in the treatment of heroin abuse for many years [309, 310], nicotine replacement has been effective in smoking cessation [311], and naltrexone has documented efficacy in the treatment of alcoholism [312,

313]. During the past two decades, psychostimulant addiction has been a major focus of multidisciplinary research efforts, including molecular approaches, preclinical behavioral studies, and clinical trials. However, no suitable medication has been approved for the treatment of stimulant use disorders [314, 315]. It should be noted that the vast majority of clinical research has focused on cocaine rather than other psychostimulants such as amphetamines and methylphenidate. The extent to which outcomes related to cocaine addiction can be extended to other psychostimulants remains unclear [316]. There are multiple pharmacological approaches in the treatment of cocaine abuse and dependence, including (1) functional antagonist treatments which block the euphoric effects of cocaine and extinguish illicit drug use; (2) functional agonist treatments which replace some of the pharmacological effects of cocaine, thereby stabilizing neurochemistry and behavior; and (3) treatments that attenuate symptoms of cocaine toxicity or withdrawal [314, 316]. Numerous medications have been evaluated for treatment of cocaine dependence that include a wide range of pharmacological targets. Reviews of the clinical literature have reported no significant benefit from antidepressants or dopamine agonists for cocaine dependence [317, 318]. Antagonist strategies designed to block the euphoric or positive effects of psychostimulants with antipsychotic medications have included risperidone [319], flupenthixol [320], and olanzapine [321] and have yielded negative clinical outcome largely due to poor compliance and treatment retention. Several novel approaches that have shown some clinical promise include disulfiram, a well-established medication for treatment of alcoholism [322–324], and $GABA_B$ receptor agonists [114]. A recent review also reported promising results for agonist-like stimulant medications in the treatment of cocaine and amphetamine dependence [314].

Tricyclic antidepressants are the best-characterized class of medications for the treatment of cocaine dependence. Desipramine was the first medication reported to be effective in an outpatient, controlled clinical trial. An initial meta-analysis found desipramine to be effective in reducing relapse to cocaine use [325], but subsequent clinical trials did not confirm its effectiveness [326, 327] or found it effective only for limited periods [328]. Based on pharmacological mechanisms, there is no convincing rationale for selecting desipramine over other tricyclic antidepressants [316]. Initial human laboratory studies with the selective serotonin reuptake inhibitor fluoxetine were encouraging. A four-week inpatient study in healthy volunteers found that fluoxetine significantly decreased subjective ratings of cocaine-induced positive mood effects [329]. However, controlled clinical trials with fluoxetine have not documented significant advantages over placebo [330, 331]. Similarly, clinical effectiveness has not been documented for the antidepressants bupropion [332] and nefazodone [333].

Agonist medications share pharmacological mechanisms of action with the abused drug, thereby producing some common neurochemical effects. Agonist medications for treatment of cocaine dependence have included direct dopamine receptor agonists and indirect dopamine receptor agonists. Preclinical studies in nonhuman primates involving chronic treatment with direct dopamine receptor agonists on cocaine self-administration have not yielded encouraging results. For example, chronic treatments with full and partial dopamine D_1 receptor agonists produced nonselective decreases in cocaine- and food-maintained responding in squirrel monkeys [334] or moderately selective decreases in cocaine-maintained responding in rhesus monkeys [335]. The D_2/D_3 receptor agonist quinpirole failed to reliably suppress cocaine self-administration at doses that produced overt toxicity in squirrel monkeys

[336]. Clinical studies with dopamine receptor agonists have also been disappointing. For example, bromocriptine is a D_2-like receptor agonists and a partial D_1-like receptor agonist used mainly in the treatment of Parkinson's disease. In a human laboratory study, pretreatment with bromocriptine prior to cocaine administration had no effect on cocaine-induced euphoria [337]. Moreover, the results of outpatient clinical trials with bromocriptine were inconclusive [316]. A recent eight-week open-label study with combined bupropion and bromocriptine in cocaine-dependent subjects did not find improvement based on cocaine-positive urine screens [338]. Collectively, these findings do not support the use of bromocriptine as a pharmacotherapy for cocaine dependence.

Studies evaluating the effects of indirect dopamine agonists have yielded mixed but more encouraging results. Mazindol, a dopamine and norepinephrine reuptake inhibitor used in the treatment of obesity, did not alter the subjective effects of cocaine in a human laboratory study [339]. Moreover, in a six-week, placebo-controlled study in cocaine-dependent subjects, mazindol did not differ from placebo in reducing cocaine use and mazindol treatment was not well tolerated [340]. Methylphenidate, a dopamine and norepinephrine reuptake inhibitor used in the treatment of ADHD and narcolepsy, was well tolerated and led to better retention than placebo but was not effective in reducing cocaine use in cocaine-dependent subjects [341]. In a separate study in cocaine-dependent subjects with ADHD, there was no significant reduction in cocaine use [342]. However, clinical studies with the indirect dopamine agonist disulfiram have been more encouraging. Disulfiram blocks the conversion of dopamine to norepinephrine by inhibiting the enzyme dopamine β-hydroxylase, thereby increasing brain dopamine concentrations. Two controlled clinical trials in cocaine addicts that were not alcoholics found disulfiram to be significantly better than placebo in promoting cocaine abstinence [322, 323]. A recent outpatient study in cocaine-dependent subjects replicated these earlier findings, showing that disulfiram reduced cocaine use more than placebo did [324]. Collectively the results suggest that disulfiram may be effective in treating cocaine addicts, including those who are not alcoholic.

There is growing support from preclinical studies in nonhuman primates and recent clinical studies for the use of stimulant medications in the treatment of cocaine dependence [341, 343–346]. A number of studies in nonhuman primates provide evidence that dopamine transporter inhibitors can effectively attenuate cocaine self-administration [21, 23, 37, 38, 347]. Hence, the development of compounds that target the dopamine transporter represents a logical approach for the pharmacological treatment of cocaine dependence. Similarly, chronic treatment with the nonselective monoamine releaser dextroamphetamine produced sustained and selective decreases in cocaine self-administration in rhesus monkeys [344, 345]. A possible limitation to the use of dopamine transport inhibitors and monoamine releasers as medications for the treatment of cocaine dependence is their potential for abuse, given their documented reinforcing effects. However, recent evidence suggests that the reinforcing effectiveness of dopamine transporter inhibitors may be limited by dual actions at the dopamine and serotonin transporters. For example, a cocaine analog with high affinity at dopamine and serotonin transporters was not reliably self-administered when substituted for cocaine, yet suppressed cocaine self-administered at low levels of dopamine transporter occupancy [38]. Similarly, monoamine-releasing agents exhibited decreasing reinforcing efficacy when the serotonin-releasing potency was increased relative to the dopamine-releasing potency [46]. Accordingly, combined actions at dopamine and serotonin transporters may enhance effectiveness in reducing cocaine use and limit the abuse liability of the medication. Importantly, compelling data have emerged from clinical research supporting indirect agonist pharmacotherapy for stimulant abuse and dependence. Well-designed, placebo-controlled clinical trials in cocaine-dependent subjects found that sustained-released dextroamphetamine was better than placebo at reducing cocaine intake [314].

Medications that target glutamatergic function are reasonable candidates given the involvement of glutamatergic circuits in reward-related brain regions and evidence of cocaine-induced dysregulation of glutamate function [348]. Modafinil, recently approved for the treatment of narcolepsy, enhances glutamate function via unidentified mechanisms that induce increases in glutamate synthesis and striatal glutamate brain levels [349]. Interestingly, modafinil has clinical effects in nondependent subjects that are opposite to the cocaine withdrawal syndrome [350]. In patients with severe cocaine withdrawal symptoms, modafinil treatment resulted in higher rates of cocaine abstinence and treatment retention. In a separate study, the subjective effects of cocaine administration in cocaine-dependent subjects were significantly reduced [351]. Modafinil was well tolerated in both studies and is currently being investigated for treatment of cocaine dependence in large, controlled clinical studies.

Recently, the GABAergic system has received significant attention as a potential target for the pharmacological treatment of cocaine dependence [315]. For example, baclofen is an antispasticity agent that is a nonselective $GABA_B$ agonist. In a placebo-controlled study in cocaine-dependent subjects, baclofen treatment enhanced cocaine abstinence compared to placebo [352]. Tiagabine is an antiepileptic medication that increases synaptic levels of GABA by inhibiting GABA transporters. A placebo-controlled pilot study in opioid-dependent patients maintained on methadone reported that tiagabine attenuated cocaine use [353]. Topiramate is another antiepileptic medication that potentiates GABAergic transmission, but it has a complex pharmacology that includes antagonism of AMPA/kainate glutamate receptors [354]. In a recent placebo-controlled pilot study in cocaine-dependent subjects, topiramate treatment enhanced cocaine abstinence [355]. Collectively, these initial studies suggest that the GABAergic systems may be a useful pharmacological target for cocaine medication development, although additional, larger scale clinical trials are clearly warranted.

16.5 SUMMARY

The abuse liability of psychostimulants is well established and represents a significant public health concern. Currently, no effective pharmacotherapy for psychostimulant abuse has demonstrated efficacy for long-term use. A better understanding of the neuropharmacological effects of cocaine and related psychostimulants has supported efforts to develop and improve useful pharmacotherapies for psychostimulant use and dependence. An extensive literature documents the critical importance of the monoamines in the behavioral pharmacology and addictive properties of psychostimulants. In particular, dopamine plays a primary role in their reinforcing effects and abuse liability. The relevance of the dopamine transporter in the reinforcing effects of cocaine is supported by numerous preclinical studies of drug self-administration and, more recently, by nonhuman primate and human neuroimaging studies. Also, a growing literature indicates that the serotonergic and noradrenergic systems can effectively modulate the neurochemical and behavioral effects of cocaine and amphetamine. Similarly, cortical glutamatergic systems provide important regulation of dopamine function, and GABAergic systems provide inhibitory neuromodulation of monoaminergic and glutamatergic function. Psychostimulants also activate the HPA axis and thereby engage neuroendocrine systems linked to stress reactivity. Lastly, endogenous neuropeptide systems appear to play an important role in the neuropharmacology and addictive properties of psychostimulants. Repeated exposure to psychostimulants can lead to robust and enduring changes in all of these neurobiological substrates, resulting in altered sensitivity to acute drug effects on neurochemistry and behavior as well as dysregulation of brain function linked to dependence and addiction. Recent approaches in medication development to treat psychostimulant abuse and dependence have focused largely on these well-established neurobiological mechanisms with some degree of success. In particular, functional agonist treatments may be used effectively to stabilize neurochemistry and behavior. Similarly, medications that target glutamatergic and GABAergic function are reasonable candidates that have received significant attention, and some have demonstrated effectiveness in attenuating cocaine use and enhancing cocaine abstinence. However, these encouraging results will require additional clinical studies in order to identify safe and efficacious pharmacotherapies.

REFERENCES

1. Williams, R. J., Goodale, L. A., Shay-Fiddler, M. A., Gloster, S. P., and Chang, S. Y. (2004). Methylphenidate and dextroamphetamine abuse in substance-abusing adolescents. *Am. J. Addict.* 13(4), 381–389.
2. Fleckenstein, A. E., Gibb, J. W., and Hanson, G. R. (2000). Differential effects of stimulants on monoaminergic transporters: Pharmacological consequences and implications for neurotoxicity. *Eur. J. Pharmacol.* 406(1), 1–13.
3. Rothman, R. B., and Baumann, M. H. (2003). Monoamine transporters and psychostimulant drugs. *Eur. J. Pharmacol.* 479(1–3), 23–40.
4. Rudnick, G., and Clark, J. (1993). From synapse to vesicle: The reuptake and storage of biogenic amine neurotransmitters. *Biochim. Biophys. Acta* 1144(3), 249–263.
5. Rudnick, G. (1997). Mechanisms of biogenic amine transporters. In *Neurotransmitter Transporters: Structure, Function, and Regulation*, M. Reith, Ed. Totowa, NY, Humana, pp. 73–100.
6. Tzschentke, T. M., and Schmidt, W. J. (2000). Functional relationship among medial prefrontal cortex, nucleus accumbens, and ventral tegmental area in locomotion and reward. *Crit. Rev. Neurobiol.* 14(2), 131–142.
7. Tzschentke, T. M. (2001). Pharmacology and behavioral pharmacology of the mesocortical dopamine system. *Prog. Neurobiol.* 63(3), 241–320.
8. Civelli, O., Bunzow, J. R., Grandy, D. K., Zhou, Q. Y., and Van Tol, H. H. (1991). Molecular biology of the dopamine receptors. *Eur. J. Pharmacol.* 207(4), 277–286.
9. Schwartz, J., Giros, B., Martres, M., and Sokoloff, P. (1992). The dopamine receptor family: Molecular biology and pharmacology. *Neurosciences* 4, 99–108.

10. Spealman, R. D., Bergman, J., Madras, B. K., Kamien, J. B., and Melia, K. F. (1992). Role of D1 and D2 dopamine receptors in the behavioral effects of cocaine. *Neurochem. Int.* 20(Suppl.), 147S–152S.

11. Woolverton, W. L., and Johnson, K. M. (1992). Neurobiology of cocaine abuse. *Trends Pharmacol. Sci.* 13(5), 193–200.

12. Mello, N. K., and Negus, S. S. (1996). Preclinical evaluation of pharmacotherapies for treatment of cocaine and opioid abuse using drug self-administration procedures. *Neuropsychopharmacology* 14(6), 375–424.

13. Platt, D. M., Rowlett, J. K., and Spealman, R. D. (2002). Behavioral effects of cocaine and dopaminergic strategies for preclinical medication development. *Psychopharmacology (Berl.)* 163(3/4), 265–282.

14. Cline, E. J., Scheffel, U., Boja, J. W., Carroll, F. I., Katz, J. L., and Kuhar, M. J. (1992). Behavioral effects of novel cocaine analogs: A comparison with in vivo receptor binding potency. *J. Pharmacol. Exp. Ther.* 260(3), 1174–1179.

15. Kuhar, M. J. (1993). Neurotransmitter transporters as drug targets: Recent research with a focus on the dopamine transporter. *Pharmacologist* 35, 28–33.

16. Katz, J. L., Izenwasser, S., and Terry, P. (2000). Relationships among dopamine transporter affinities and cocaine-like discriminative-stimulus effects. *Psychopharmacology* 148, 90–98.

17. Bergman, J., Madras, B. K., Johnson, S. E., and Spealman, R. D. (1989). Effects of cocaine and related drugs in nonhuman primates. III. Self-administration by squirrel monkeys. *J. Pharmacol. Exp. Ther.* 251, 150–155.

18. Madras, B. K., Fahey, M. A., Bergman, J., Canfield, D. R., and Spealman, R. D. (1989). Effects of cocaine and related drugs in nonhuman primates. I. [3H]cocaine binding sites in caudate-putamen. *J. Pharmacol. Exp. Ther.* 251(1), 131–141.

19. Spealman, R. D., Madras, B. K., and Bergman, J. (1989). Effects of cocaine and related drugs in nonhuman primates. II. Stimulant effects on scheduled-controlled behavior. *J. Pharmacol. Exp. Ther.* 251(1), 142–149.

20. Howell, L. L., and Byrd, L. D. (1991). Characterization of the effects of cocaine and GBR 12909, a dopamine uptake inhibitor, on behavior in the squirrel monkey. *J. Pharmacol. Exp. Ther.* 258(1), 178–185.

21. Nader, M. A., Grant, K. A., Davies, H. M., Mach, R. H., and Childers, S. R. (1997). The reinforcing and discriminative stimulus effects of the novel cocaine analog 2beta-propanoyl-3beta-(4-tolyl)-tropane in rhesus monkeys. *J. Pharmacol. Exp. Ther.* 280(2), 541–550.

22. Howell, L. L., Czoty, P. W., and Byrd, L. D. (1997). Pharmacological interactions between serotonin and dopamine on behavior in the squirrel monkey. *Psychopharmacology (Berl.)* 131(1), 40–48.

23. Howell, L. L., Czoty, P. W., Kuhar, M.J., and Carroll, F. I. (2000). Comparative behavioral pharmacology of cocaine and the selective dopamine uptake inhibitor RTI-113 in the squirrel monkey. *J. Pharmacol. Exp. Ther.* 292(2), 521–529.

24. Self, D.W., and Stein, L. (1992). The D1 agonists SKF 82958 and SKF 77434 are self-administered by rats. *Brain Res.* 582(2), 349–352.

25. Woolverton, W. L., Goldberg, L. I., and Ginos, J. Z. (1984). Intravenous self-administration of dopamine receptor agonists by rhesus monkeys. *Psychopharmacology* 123, 34–41.

26. Weed, M. R., and Woolverton, W. L. (1995). The reinforcing effects of dopamine D1 receptor agonists in rhesus monkeys. *J. Pharmacol. Exp. Ther.* 275(3), 1367–1374.

27. Woolverton, W. L. (1986). Effects of a D1 and a D2 dopamine antagonist on the self-administration of cocaine and piribedil by rhesus monkeys. *Pharmacol. Biochem. Behav.* 24(3), 531–535.

28. Barrett, R. L., and Appel, J. B. (1989). Effects of stimulation and blockade of dopamine receptor subtypes on the discriminative stimulus properties of cocaine. *Psychopharmacology (Berl.)* 99(1), 13–16.

29. Callahan, P. M., Appel, J. B., and Cunningham, K. A. (1991). Dopamine D1 and D2 mediation of the discriminative stimulus properties of *d*-amphetamine and cocaine. *Psychopharmacology* 103(1), 50–55.

30. Kleven, M. S., Anthony, E. W., Goldberg, L. I., and Woolverton, W. L. (1988). Blockade of the discriminative stimulus effects of cocaine in rhesus monkeys with the D1 dopamine antagonist SCH 23390. *Psychopharmacology (Berl.)* 95(3), 427–429.

31. Bergman, J., and Spealman, R. D. (1988). Behavioral effects of histamine H1 antagonists: Comparison with other drugs and modification by haloperidol. *J. Pharmacol. Exp. Ther.* 245(2), 471–478.

32. Howell, L. L., and Byrd, L. D. (1992). Enhanced sensitivity to the behavioral effects of cocaine after chronic administration of D2-selective dopamine antagonists in the squirrel monkey. *J. Pharmacol. Exp. Ther.* 262(3), 907–915.

33. Spealman, R. D. (1990). Antagonism of behavioral effects of cocaine by selective dopamine receptor blockers. *Psychopharmacology (Berl.)* 101(1), 142–145.

34. Volkow, N. D., Wang, G. J., Fischman, M. W., Foltin, R. W., Fowler, J. S., Abumrad, N. N., Vitkun, S., Logan, J., Gatley, S. J., Pappas, N., Hitezmann, R., and Shea, C. E. (1997). Relationship between subjective effects of cocaine and dopamine transporter occupancy. *Nature* 386(6627), 827–830.

35. Volkow, N. D., Wang, G. J., Fowler, J. S., Gatley, S. J., Logan, J., Ding, Y. S., Dewey, S. L., Hitzemann, R., Gifford, A. N., and Pappas, N. R. (1999). Blockade of striatal dopamine transporters by intravenous methylphenidate is not sufficient to induce self-reports of "high."*J. Pharmacol. Exp. Ther.* 288(1), 14–20.

36. Volkow, N. D., Gatley, S. J., Fowler, J. S., Logan, J., Fischman, M., Gifford, A. N., Pappas, N., King, P., Vitkun, S., Ding, Y. S., and Wang, G. J. (1996). Cocaine doses equivalent to those abused by humans occupy most of the dopamine transporters. *Synapse* 24(4), 399–402.

37. Wilcox, K. M., Lindsey, K. P., Votaw, J. R., Goodman, M. M., Martarello, L., Carroll, F. I., and Howell, L. L. (2002). Self-administration of cocaine and the cocaine analog RTI-113: Relationship to dopamine transporter occupancy determined by PET neuroimaging in rhesus monkeys. *Synapse* 43(1), 78–85.

38. Lindsey, K. P., Wilcox, K. M., Votaw, J. R., Goodman, M. M., Plisson, C., Carroll, F.I., Rice, K. C., and Howell, L. L. (2004). Effects of dopamine transporter inhibitors on cocaine self-administration in rhesus monkeys: Relationship to transporter occupancy determined by positron emission tomography neuroimaging. *J. Pharmacol. Exp. Ther.* 309(3), 959–969.

39. Villemagne, V. L., Rothman, R. B., Yokoi, F., Rice, K. C., Matecka, D., Dannals, R. F., and Wong, D. F. (1999). Doses of GBR12909 that suppress cocaine self-administration in non-human primates substantially occupy dopamine transporters as measured by [11C] WIN35,428 PET scans. *Synapse* 32(1), 44–50.

40. Vanover, K. E., Nader, M. A., and Woolverton, W. L. (1992). Evaluation of the discriminative stimulus and reinforcing effects of sertraline in rhesus monkeys. *Pharmacol. Biochem. Behav.* 41(4), 789–793.

41. Howell, L. L., and Byrd, L. D. (1995). Serotonergic modulation of the behavioral effects of cocaine in the squirrel monkey. *J. Pharmacol. Exp. Ther.* 275(3), 1551–1559.
42. Ritz, M. C., Lamb, R. J., Goldberg, S. R., and Kuhar, M. J. (1987). Cocaine receptors on dopamine transporters are related to self-administration of cocaine. *Science* 237, 1219–1223.
43. Ritz, M. C., and Kuhar, M. J. (1989). Relationship between self-administration of amphetamine and monoamine receptors in brain: Comparison with cocaine. *J. Pharmacol. Exp. Ther.* 248, 1010–1017.
44. Baumann, M. H., Ayestas, M. A., Dersch, C. M., Brockington, A., Rice, K. C., and Rothman, R. B. (2000). Effects of phentermine and fenfluramine on extracellular dopamine and serotonin in rat nucleus accumbens: Therapeutic implications. *Synapse* 36(2), 102–113.
45. Glatz, A. C., Ehrlich, M., Bae, R. S., Clarke, M. J., Quinlan, P. A., Brown, E. C., Rada, P., and Hoebel, B. G. (2002). Inhibition of cocaine self-administration by fluoxetine or D-fenfluramine combined with phentermine. *Pharmacol. Biochem. Behav.* 71(1/2), 197–204.
46. Wee, S., Anderson, K. G., Baumann, M. H., Rothman, R. B., Blough, B. E., and Woolverton, W. L. (2005). Relationship between the serotonergic activity and reinforcing effects of a series of amphetamine analogs. *J. Pharmacol. Exp. Ther.* 313(2), 848–854.
47. Ginsburg, B. C., Kimmel, H. L., Carroll, F. I., Goodman, M. M., and Howell, L. L. (2005). Interaction of cocaine and dopamine transporter inhibitors on behavior and neurochemistry in monkeys. *Pharmacol. Biochem. Behav.* 80(3), 481–491.
48. Carroll, M. E., Lac, S. T., Asencio, M., and Kragh, R. (1990). Fluoxetine reduces intravenous cocaine self-administration in rats. *Pharmacol. Biochem. Behav.* 35(1), 237–244.
49. Porrino, L. J., Ritz, M. C., Goodman, N. L., Sharpe, L. G., Kuhar, M. J., and Goldberg, S. R. (1989). Differential effects of the pharmacological manipulation of serotonin systems on cocaine and amphetamine self-administration in rats. *Life Sci.* 45, 1529–1535.
50. Kleven, M. S., and Woolverton, W. L. (1993). Effects of three monoamine uptake inhibitors on behavior maintained by cocaine or food presentation in rhesus monkeys. *Drug Alcohol. Depend.* 31(2), 149–158.
51. Spealman, R. D. (1993). Modification of behavioral effects of cocaine by selective serotonin and dopamine uptake inhibitors in squirrel monkeys. *Psychopharmacology (Berl.)* 112(1), 93–99.
52. Czoty, P. W., Ginsburg, B. C., and Howell, L. L. (2002). Serotonergic attenuation of the reinforcing and neurochemical effects of cocaine in squirrel monkeys. *J. Pharmacol. Exp. Ther.* 300(3), 831–837.
53. Howell, L. L., Hoffman, J. M., Votaw, J. R., Landrum, A. M., Wilcox, K. M., and Lindsey, K. P. (2002). Cocaine-induced brain activation determined by positron emission tomography neuroimaging in conscious rhesus monkeys. *Psychopharmacology (Berl.)* 159(2), 154–160.
54. Herve, D., Pickel, V. M., Joh, T. H., and Beaudet, A. (1987). Serotonin axon terminals in the ventral tegmental area of the rat: Fine structure and synaptic input to dopaminergic neurons. *Brain Res.* 435(1/2), 71–83.
55. Phelix, C. F., and Broderick, P. A. (1995). Light microscopic immunocytochemical evidence of converging serotonin and dopamine terminals in ventrolateral nucleus accumbens. *Brain Res. Bull.* 37(1), 37–40.

56. Di Matteo, V., De Blasi, A., Di Giulio, C., and Esposito, E. (2001). Role of 5-HT(2C) receptors in the control of central dopamine function. *Trends Pharmacol. Sci.* 22(5), 229–232.

57. Di Mascio, M., Di Giovanni, G., Di Matteo, V., Prisco, S., and Esposito, E. (1998). Selective serotonin reuptake inhibitors reduce the spontaneous activity of dopaminergic neurons in the ventral tegmental area. *Brain Res. Bull.* 46(6), 547–554.

58. Prisco, S., Pagannone, S., and Esposito, E. (1994). Serotonin-dopamine interaction in the rat ventral tegmental area: An electrophysiological study in vivo. *J. Pharmacol. Exp. Ther.* 271(1), 83–90.

59. Di Matteo, V., Di Giovanni, G., Di Mascio, M., and Esposito, E. (2000). Biochemical and electrophysiological evidence that RO 60-0175 inhibits mesolimbic dopaminergic function through serotonin(2C) receptors. *Brain Res.* 865(1), 85–90.

60. Ashby, C., and Minabe, Y. (1996). Differential effect of the 5-HT2C/2B antagonist SB200646 and the selective 5-HT2A antagonist MDL 100907 on midbrain dopamine neurons in rats: An electrophysiological study. *Soc. Neurosci. Abstr.* 22, 1723.

61. Di Matteo, V., Di Giovanni, G., Di Mascio, M., and Esposito, E. (1999). SB 242084, a selective serotonin2C receptor antagonist, increases dopaminergic transmission in the mesolimbic system. *Neuropharmacology* 38(8), 1195–1205.

62. Eberle-Wang, K., Mikeladze, Z., Uryu, K., and Chesselet, M. F. (1997). Pattern of expression of the serotonin2C receptor messenger RNA in the basal ganglia of adult rats. *J. Comp. Neurol.* 384(2), 233–247.

63. Cameron, D. L., and Williams, J. T. (1994). Cocaine inhibits GABA release in the VTA through endogenous 5-HT. *J. Neurosci.* 14(11, Pt. 1), 6763–6767.

64. Blandina, P., Goldfarb, J., Craddock-Royal, B., and Green, J. P. (1989). Release of endogenous dopamine by stimulation of 5-hydroxytryptamine3 receptors in rat striatum. *J. Pharmacol. Exp. Ther.* 251(3), 803–809.

65. De Deurwaerdere, P., L'Hirondel, M., Bonhomme, N., Lucas, G., Cheramy, A., and Spampinato, U. (1997). Serotonin stimulation of 5-HT4 receptors indirectly enhances in vivo dopamine release in the rat striatum. *J. Neurochem.* 68(1), 195–203.

66. Parsons, L. H., Weiss, J., and Koob, G. F. (1998). Serotonin$_{1B}$ receptor stimulation enhances cocaine reinforcement. *J. Neurosci.* 18(23), 10078–10089.

67. Layer, R. T., Uretsky, N. J., and Wallace, L. J. (1992). Effect of serotonergic agonists in the nucleus accumbens on *d*-amphetamine-stimulated locomotion. *Life Sci.* 50(11), 813–820.

68. Kankaanpaa, A., Lillsunde, P., Ruotsalainen, M., Ahtee, L., and Seppala, T. (1996). 5-HT3 receptor antagonist MDL 72222 dose-dependently attenuates cocaine- and amphetamine-induced elevations of extracellular dopamine in the nucleus accumbens and the dorsal striatum. *Pharmacol. Toxicol.* 78(5), 317–321.

69. Berridge, C. W., Stratford, T. L., Foote, S. L., and Kelley, A. E. (1997). Distribution of dopamine beta-hydroxylase-like immunoreactive fibers within the shell subregion of the nucleus accumbens. *Synapse* 27(3), 230–241.

70. Delfs, J. M., Zhu, Y., Druhan, J. P., and Aston-Jones, G. S. (1998). Origin of noradrenergic afferents to the shell subregion of the nucleus accumbens: Anterograde and retrograde tract-tracing studies in the rat. *Brain Res.* 806(2), 127–140.

71. Liprando, L. A., Miner, L. H., Blakely, R. D., Lewis, D. A., and Sesack, S. R. (2004). Ultrastructural interactions between terminals expressing the norepinephrine transporter and dopamine neurons in the rat and monkey ventral tegmental area. *Synapse* 52(4), 233–244.

72. Grenhoff, J., Nisell, M., Ferre, S., Aston-Jones, G., and Svensson, T. H. (1993). Noradrenergic modulation of midbrain dopamine cell firing elicited by stimulation of the locus coeruleus in the rat. *J. Neural. Transm. Gen. Sect.* 93(1), 11–25.

73. Lategan, A. J., Marien, M. R., and Colpaert, F. C. (1990). Effects of locus coeruleus lesions on the release of endogenous dopamine in the rat nucleus accumbens and caudate nucleus as determined by intracerebral microdialysis. *Brain Res.* 523(1), 134–138.

74. Ventura, R., Cabib, S., Alcaro, A., Orsini, C., and Puglisi-Allegra, S. (2003). Norepinephrine in the prefrontal cortex is critical for amphetamine-induced reward and mesoaccumbens dopamine release. *J. Neurosci.* 23(5), 1879–1885.

75. Drouin, C., Darracq, L., Trovero, F., Blanc, G., Glowinski, J., Cotecchia, S., and Tassin, J. P. (2002). Alpha1b-adrenergic receptors control locomotor and rewarding effects of psychostimulants and opiates. *J. Neurosci.* 22(7), 2873–2884.

76. Drouin, C., Blanc, G., Villegier, A. S., Glowinski, J., and Tassin, J. P. (2002). Critical role of alpha1-adrenergic receptors in acute and sensitized locomotor effects of D-amphetamine, cocaine, and GBR 12783: Influence of preexposure conditions and pharmacological characteristics. *Synapse* 43(1), 51–61.

77. Weinshenker, D., Miller, N. S., Blizinsky, K., Laughlin, M. L., and Palmiter, R. D. (2002). Mice with chronic norepinephrine deficiency resemble amphetamine-sensitized animals. *Proc. Natl. Acad. Sci. USA* 99(21), 13873–13877.

78. Erb, S., Hitchcott, P. K., Rajabi, H., Mueller, D., Shaham, Y., and Stewart, J. (2000). Alpha-2 adrenergic receptor agonists block stress-induced reinstatement of cocaine-seeking. *Neuropsychopharmacology* 23(2), 138–150.

79. Spealman, R. D. (1995). Noradrenergic involvement in the discriminative stimulus effects of cocaine in squirrel monkeys. *J. Pharmacol. Exp. Ther.* 275(1), 53–62.

80. Rothman, R. B., Baumann, M. H., Dersch, C. M., Romero, D. V., Rice, K. C., Carroll, F. I., and Partilla, J. S. (2001). Amphetamine-type central nervous system stimulants release norepinephrine more potently than they release dopamine and serotonin. *Synapse* 39(1), 32–41.

81. Tella, S. R. (1995). Effects of monoamine reuptake inhibitors on cocaine self-administration in rats. *Pharmacol. Biochem. Behav.* 51(4), 687–692.

82. Woolverton, W. L. (1987). Evaluation of the role of norepinephrine in the reinforcing effects of psychomotor stimulants in rhesus monkeys. *Pharmacol. Biochem. Behav.* 26(4), 835–839.

83. Kleven, M. S., and Woolverton, W. L. (1990). Effects of bromocriptine and desipramine on behavior maintained by cocaine or food presentation in rhesus monkeys. *Psychopharmacology (Berl.)* 101(2), 208–213.

84. Mello, N. K., Lukas, S. E., Bree, M. P., and Mendelson, J. H. (1990). Desipramine effects on cocaine self-administration by rhesus monkeys. *Drug Alcohol Depend.* 26(2), 103–116.

85. Sesack, S. R., Carr, D. B., Omelchenko, N., and Pinto, A. (2003). Anatomical substrates for glutamate-dopamine interactions: Evidence for specificity of connections and extrasynaptic actions. *Ann. NY Acad. Sci.* 1003, 36–52.

86. West, A. R., Floresco, S. B., Charara, A., Rosenkranz, J. A., and Grace, A. A. (2003). Electrophysiological interactions between striatal glutamatergic and dopaminergic systems. *Ann. NY Acad. Sci.* 1003, 53–74.

87. Kelley, A. E., and Berridge, K. C. (2002). The neuroscience of natural rewards: Relevance to addictive drugs. *J. Neurosci.* 22(9), 3306–3311.

88. Pierce, R. C., Bell, K., Duffy, P., and Kalivas, P. W. (1996). Repeated cocaine augments excitatory amino acid transmission in the nucleus accumbens only in rats having developed behavioral sensitization. *J. Neurosci.* 16(4), 1550–1560.
89. Cornish, J. L., and Kalivas, P. W. (2000). Glutamate transmission in the nucleus accumbens mediates relapse in cocaine addiction. *J. Neurosci.* 20(15), (online) RC89.
90. Cornish, J. L., and Kalivas, P. W. (2001). Cocaine sensitization and craving: Differing roles for dopamine and glutamate in the nucleus accumbens. *J. Addict. Dis.* 20(3), 43–54.
91. Carlezon, W. A. Jr., and Nestler, E. J. (2002). Elevated levels of GluR1 in the midbrain: A trigger for sensitization to drugs of abuse? *Trends Neurosci.* 25(12), 610–615.
92. Harris, G. C., and Aston-Jones, G. (2003). Critical role for ventral tegmental glutamate in preference for a cocaine-conditioned environment. *Neuropsychopharmacology* 28(1), 73–76.
93. Adell, A., and Artigas, F. (2004). The somatodendritic release of dopamine in the ventral tegmental area and its regulation by afferent transmitter systems. *Neurosci. Biobehav. Rev.* 28(4), 415–431.
94. Conn, P. J., and Pin, J. P. (1997). Pharmacology and functions of metabotropic glutamate receptors. *Annu. Rev. Pharmacol. Toxicol.* 37, 205–237.
95. Hu, G., Duffy, P., Swanson, C., Ghasemzadeh, M. B., and Kalivas, P. W. (1999). The regulation of dopamine transmission by metabotropic glutamate receptors. *J. Pharmacol. Exp. Ther.* 289(1), 412–416.
96. Battaglia, G., Monn, J. A., and Schoepp, D. D. (1997). In vivo inhibition of veratridine-evoked release of striatal excitatory amino acids by the group II metabotropic glutamate receptor agonist LY354740 in rats. *Neurosci. Lett.* 229(3), 161–164.
97. Moghaddam, B., and Adams, B. W. (1998). Reversal of phencyclidine effects by a group II metabotropic glutamate receptor agonist in rats. *Science* 281(5381), 1349–1352.
98. Xi, Z. X., Baker, D. A., Shen, H., Carson, D. S., and Kalivas, P. W. (2002). Group II metabotropic glutamate receptors modulate extracellular glutamate in the nucleus accumbens. *J. Pharmacol. Exp. Ther.* 300(1), 162–171.
99. Baker, D. A., Xi, Z. X., Shen, H., Swanson, C. J., and Kalivas, P. W. (2002). The origin and neuronal function of in vivo nonsynaptic glutamate. *J. Neurosci.* 22(20), 9134–9141.
100. Baker, D. A., McFarland, K., Lake, R. W., Shen, H., Tang, X. C., Toda, S., and Kalivas, P. W. (2003). Neuroadaptations in cystine-glutamate exchange underlie cocaine relapse. *Nat. Neurosci.* 6(7), 743–749.
101. Xi, Z. X., Ramamoorthy, S., Baker, D. A., Shen, H., Samuvel, D. J., and Kalivas, P. W. (2002). Modulation of group II metabotropic glutamate receptor signaling by chronic cocaine. *J. Pharmacol. Exp. Ther.* 303(2), 608–615.
102. Vezina, P., and Suto, N. (2002). Glutamate and the self-administration of psychomotor-stimulant drugs. In *Glutamate and Addiction*, B. H. Herman, Ed. Humana, Totowa, NJ, pp. 183–200.
103. Kalivas, P. W., McFarland, K., Bowers, S., Szumlinski, K., Xi, Z. X., and Baker, D. (2003). Glutamate transmission and addiction to cocaine. *Ann. NY Acad. Sci.* 1003, 169–175.
104. McFarland, K., Lapish, C. C., and Kalivas, P. W. (2003). Prefrontal glutamate release into the core of the nucleus accumbens mediates cocaine-induced reinstatement of drug-seeking behavior. *J. Neurosci.* 23(8), 3531–3537.

105. Tessari, M., Pilla, M., Andreoli, M., Hutcheson, D. M., and Heidbreder, C. A. (2004). Antagonism at metabotropic glutamate 5 receptors inhibits nicotine- and cocaine-taking behaviours and prevents nicotine-triggered relapse to nicotine-seeking. *Eur. J. Pharmacol.* 499(1/2), 121–133.

106. McGeehan, A. J., and Olive, M. F. (2003). The mGluR5 antagonist MPEP reduces the conditioned rewarding effects of cocaine but not other drugs of abuse. *Synapse* 47(3), 240–242.

107. Lee, B., Platt, D. M., Rowlett, J. K., Adewale, A. S., and Spealman, R. D. (2005). Attenuation of behavioral effects of cocaine by the metabotropic glutamate receptor 5 antagonist 2-methyl-6-(phenylethynyl)-pyridine in squirrel monkeys: Comparison with dizocilpine. *J. Pharmacol. Exp. Ther.* 312(3), 1232–1240.

108. Dewey, S. L., Smith, G. S., Logan, J., Brodie, J. D., Yu, D. W., Ferrieri, R. A., King, P. T., MacGregor, R. R., Martin, T. P., Wolf, A. P., et al. (1992). GABAergic inhibition of endogenous dopamine release measured in vivo with 11C-raclopride and positron emission tomography. *J. Neurosci.* 12(10), 3773–3780.

109. Churchill, L., Dilts, R. P., and Kalivas, P. W. (1992). Autoradiographic localization of gamma-aminobutyric acidA receptors within the ventral tegmental area. *Neurochem. Res.* 17(1), 101–106.

110. White, F. J. (1996). Synaptic regulation of mesocorticolimbic dopamine neurons. *Ann. Rev. Neurosci.* 19, 405–436.

111. Steffensen, S. C., Svingos, A. L., Pickel, V. M., and Henriksen, S. J. (1998). Electrophysiological characterization of GABAergic neurons in the ventral tegmental area. *J. Neurosci.* 18(19), 8003–8015.

112. Kita, H., and Kitai, S. T. (1988). Glutamate decarboxylase immunoreactive neurons in rat neostriatum: Their morphological types and populations. *Brain Res.* 447(2), 346–352.

113. Roberts, D. C., and Brebner, K. (2000). GABA modulation of cocaine self-administration. *Ann. NY Acad. Sci.* 909, 145–158.

114. Cousins, M. S., Roberts, D. C., and de Wit, H. (2002). GABA(B) receptor agonists for the treatment of drug addiction: A review of recent findings. *Drug Alcohol Depend.* 65(3), 209–220.

115. Dewey, S. L., Chaurasia, C. S., Chen, C. E., Volkow, N. D., Clarkson, F. A., Porter, S. P., Straughter-Moore, R. M., Alexoff, D. L., Tedeschi, D., Russo, N. B., Fowler, J. S., and Brodie, J. D. (1997). GABAergic attenuation of cocaine-induced dopamine release and locomotor activity. *Synapse* 25(4), 393–398.

116. Morgan, A. E., and Dewey, S. L. (1998). Effects of pharmacologic increases in brain GABA levels on cocaine-induced changes in extracellular dopamine. *Synapse* 28, 60–65.

117. Shoaib, M., Swanner, L. S., Beyer, C. E., Goldberg, S. R., and Schindler, C. W. (1998). The $GABA_B$ agonist baclofen modifies cocaine self-adminstration in rats. *Behav. Pharmacol.* 9, 195–206.

118. Brebner, K., Phelan, R., and Roberts, D. C. S. (2000). Effect of baclofen on cocaine self-administration in rats reinforced under fixed-ratio 1 and progressive-ratio schedules. *Psychopharmacology* 148, 314–321.

119. Campbell, U. C., Lac, S. T., and Carroll, M. E. (1999). Effects of baclofen on maintenance and reinstatement of intravenous cocaine self-administration in rats. *Psychopharmacology (Berl.)* 143(2), 209–214.

120. Dewey, S. L., Morgan, A. E., Ashby, C. R. Jr., Horan, B., Kushner, S. A., Logan, J., Volkow, N. D., Fowler, J. S., Gardner, E. L., and Brodie, J. D. (1998). A novel strategy for the treatment of cocaine addiction. *Synapse* 30(2), 119–129.

121. Kushner, S. A., Dewey, S. L., and Kornetsky, C. (1999). The irreversible gamma-aminobutyric acid (GABA) transaminase inhibitor gamma-vinyl-GABA blocks cocaine self-administration in rats. *J. Pharmacol. Exp. Ther.* 290(2), 797–802.

122. Kushner, S. A., Dewey, S. L., and Kornetsky, C. (1997). Gamma-vinyl GABA attenuates cocaine-induced lowering of brain stimulation reward thresholds. *Psychopharmacology (Berl.)* 133(4), 383–388.

123. Swanson, L. W., Sawchenko, P. E., Rivier, J., and Vale, W. W. (1983). Organization of ovine corticotropin-releasing factor immunoreactive cells and fibers in the rat brain: An immunohistochemical study. *Neuroendocrinology* 36(3), 165–186.

124. Whitnall, M. H. (1993). Regulation of the hypothalamic corticotropin-releasing hormone neurosecretory system. *Prog. Neurobiol.* 40(5), 573–629.

125. Sarnyai, Z., Shaham, Y., and Heinrichs, S. C. (2001). The role of corticotropin-releasing factor in drug addiction. *Pharmacol. Rev.* 53(2), 209–243.

126. Marinelli, M., and Piazza, P. V. (2002). Interaction between glucocorticoid hormones, stress and psychostimulant drugs. *Eur. J. Neurosci.* 16(3), 387–394.

127. Marinelli, M., Piazza, P. V., Deroche, V., Maccari, S., Le Moal, M., and Simon, H. (1994). Corticosterone circadian secretion differentially facilitates dopamine-mediated psychomotor effect of cocaine and morphine. *J. Neurosci.* 14(5, Pt. 1), 2724–2731.

128. Cador, M., Dulluc, J., and Mormede, P. (1993). Modulation of the locomotor response to amphetamine by corticosterone. *Neuroscience* 56(4), 981–988.

129. Mormede, P., Dulluc, J., and Cador, M. (1994). Modulation of the locomotor response to amphetamine by corticosterone. *Ann. NY Acad. Sci.* 746, 394–397.

130. Mello, N. K., and Mendelson, J. H. (1997). Cocaine's effects on neuroendocrine systems: Clinical and preclinical studies. *Pharmacol. Biochem. Behav.* 57(3), 571–599.

131. Spangler, R., Zhou, Y., Schlussman, S. D., Ho, A., and Kreek, M. J. (1997). Behavioral stereotypies induced by "binge" cocaine administration are independent of drug-induced increases in corticosterone levels. *Behav. Brain. Res.* 86(2), 201–204.

132. Schmidt, E. D., Tilders, F. J., Binnekade, R., Schoffelmeer, A. N., and De Vries, T. J. (1999). Stressor- or drug-induced sensitization of the corticosterone response is not critically involved in the long-term expression of behavioural sensitization to amphetamine. *Neuroscience* 92(1), 343–352.

133. Goeders, N. E., and Guerin, G. F. (1996). Effects of surgical and pharmacological adrenalectomy on the initiation and maintenance of intravenous cocaine self-administration in rats. *Brain Res.* 722(1/2), 145–152.

134. Goeders, N. E., and Guerin, G. F. (1996). Role of corticosterone in intravenous cocaine self-administration in rats. *Neuroendocrinology* 64(5), 337–348.

135. Baumann, M. H., Gendron, T. M., Becketts, K. M., Henningfield, J. E., Gorelick, D. A., and Rothman, R. B. (1995). Effects of intravenous cocaine on plasma cortisol and prolactin in human cocaine abusers. *Biol. Psychiatry* 38(11), 751–755.

136. Deroche, V., Marinelli, M., Le Moal, M., and Piazza, P. V. (1997). Glucocorticoids and behavioral effects of psychostimulants. II: Cocaine intravenous self-administration and reinstatement depend on glucocorticoid levels. *J. Pharmacol. Exp. Ther.* 281(3), 1401–1407.

137. Mantsch, J. R., Schlussman, S. D., Ho, A., and Kreek, M. J. (2000). Effects of cocaine self-administration on plasma corticosterone and prolactin in rats. *J. Pharmacol. Exp. Ther.* 294(1), 239–247.

138. Goeders, N. E. (2002). The HPA axis and cocaine reinforcement. *Psychoneuroendocrinology* 27(1/2), 13–33.
139. Goeders, N. E., and Clampitt, D. M. (2002). Potential role for the hypothalamo-pituitary-adrenal axis in the conditioned reinforcer-induced reinstatement of extinguished cocaine seeking in rats. *Psychopharmacology (Berl.)* 161(3), 222–232.
140. Erb, S., Shaham, Y., and Stewart, J. (1998). The role of corticotropin-releasing factor and corticosterone in stress- and cocaine-induced relapse to cocaine seeking in rats. *J. Neurosci.* 18(14), 5529–5536.
141. Mantsch, J. R., and Goeders, N. E. (1999). Ketoconazole blocks the stress-induced reinstatement of cocaine-seeking behavior in rats: Relationship to the discriminative stimulus effects of cocaine. *Psychopharmacology (Berl.)* 142(4), 399–407.
142. Shaham, Y., Erb, S., Leung, S., Buczek, Y., and Stewart, J. (1998). CP-154,526, a selective, non-peptide antagonist of the corticotropin-releasing factor1 receptor attenuates stress-induced relapse to drug seeking in cocaine- and heroin-trained rats. *Psychopharmacology (Berl.)* 137(2), 184–190.
143. Mantsch, J. R., and Goeders, N. E. (1999). Ketoconazole does not block cocaine discrimination or the cocaine-induced reinstatement of cocaine-seeking behavior. *Pharmacol. Biochem. Behav.* 64(1), 65–73.
144. Mansour, A., Khachaturian, H., Lewis, M. E., Akil, H., and Watson, S. J. (1988). Anatomy of CNS opioid receptors. *Trends. Neurosci.* 11(7), 308–314.
145. Wood, P. L., and Iyengar, S. (1988). Central actions of opiates and opioid peptides. In vivo evidence for opioid receptor multiplicity. In *The Opiate Receptors*, G. W. Pasternak, Ed. Humana, Clifton, NY, pp. 307–356.
146. Sharif, N. A., and Hughes, J. (1989). Discrete mapping of brain mu and delta opioid receptors using selective peptides: Quantitative autoradiography, species differences and comparison with kappa receptors. *Peptides* 10(3), 499–522.
147. Goodman, R. R., Aider, B. A., and Pasternak, G. W. (1988). Regional distribution of opioid receptors. In *The Opiate Receptors*, G. W. Pasternak, Ed. Humana, Clifton, NY, pp. 197–228.
148. Jiang, Z. G., and North, R. A. (1992). Pre- and post-synaptic inhibition by opioids in rat striatum. *J. Neurosci.* 12(1), 356–361.
149. Klitenick, M. A., De Witte, P., and Kalivas, P. W. (1992). Regulation of somatodendritic dopamine release in the ventral tegmental area by opioids and GABA: An in vivo microdialysis study. *J. Neurosci.* 12(7), 2623–2632.
150. Joyce, E. M., and Iversen, S. D. (1979). The effect of morphine applied locally to mesencephalic dopamine cell bodies on spontaneous motor activity in the rat. *Neurosci. Lett.* 14(2/3), 207–212.
151. Johnson, S. W., and North, R. A. (1992). Opioids excite dopamine neurons by hyperpolarization of local interneurons. *J. Neurosci.* 12(2), 483–488.
152. Smith, J. A. M., Loughlin, S. E., and Leslie, F. M. (1992). κ-Opioid inhibition of [3H]dopamine release from rat ventral mesencephalic dissociated cell cultures. *Mol. Pharmacol.* 42, 575–583.
153. Meshul, C. K., and McGinty, J. F. (2000). Kappa opioid receptor immunoreactivity in the nucleus accumbens and caudate-putamen is primarily associated with synaptic vesicles in axons. *Neuroscience* 96(1), 91–99.
154. Di Chiara, G., and Imperato, A. (1988). Opposite effects of mu and kappa opiate agonists on dopamine release in the nucleus accumbens and in the dorsal caudate of freely moving rats. *J. Pharmacol. Exp. Ther.* 244(3), 1067–1080.

155. Manzaneres, J., Lookingland, K. J., and Moore, K. E. (1991). Kappa opioid receptor-mediated regulation of dopaminergic neurons in the rat brain. *J. Pharmacol. Exp. Ther.* 256(2), 500–505.

156. Kosten, T. R., Rounsaville, B. J., and Kleber, H. D. (1987). A 2.5-year follow-up of cocaine use among treated opioid addicts. Have our treatments helped? *Arch. Gen. Psychiatry* 44(3), 281–284.

157. Walsh, S. L., Sullivan, J. T., Preston, K. L., Garner, J. E., and Bigelow, G. E. (1996). Effects of naltrexone on response to intravenous cocaine, hydromorphone and their combination in humans. *J. Pharmacol. Exp. Ther.* 279(2), 524–538.

158. Kimmel, H. L., and Holtzman, S. G. (1997). Mu-opioid agonists potentiate amphetamine- and cocaine-induced rotational behavior in the rat. *J. Pharmacol. Exp. Ther.* 282(2), 734–746.

159. Kimmel, H. L., Tallarida, R. J., and Holtzman, S. G. (1997). Synergism between buprenorphine and cocaine on the rotational behavior of the nigrally-lesioned rat. *Psychopharmacology* 133(4), 372–377.

160. Smith, M. A., Gordon, K. A., Craig, C. K., Bryant, P. A., Ferguson, M. E., French, A. M., Gray, J. D., McClean, J. M., and Tetirick, J. C. (2003). Interactions between opioids and cocaine on locomotor activity in rats: Influence of an opioid's relative efficacy at the mu receptor. *Psychopharmacology (Berl.)* 167(3), 265–273.

161. Spealman, R. D., and Bergman, J. (1992). Modulation of the discriminative stimulus effects of cocaine by mu and kappa opioids. *J. Pharmacol. Exp. Ther.* 261(2), 607–615.

162. Rowlett, J. K., and Spealman, R. D. (1998). Opioid enhancement of the discriminative stimulus effects of cocaine: Evidence for involvement of mu and delta opioid receptors. *Psychopharmacology (Berl.)* 140(2), 217–224.

163. Ward, S. J., Morgan, D., and Roberts, D. C. (2005). Comparison of the reinforcing effects of cocaine and cocaine/heroin combinations under progressive ratio and choice schedules in rats. *Neuropsychopharmacology* 30(2), 286–295.

164. Rowlett, J. K., and Woolverton, W. L. (1997). Self-administration of cocaine and heroin combinations by rhesus monkeys responding under a progressive-ratio schedule. *Psychopharmacology (Berl.)* 133(4), 363–371.

165. Collins, S. L., D'Addario, C., and Izenwasser, S. (2001). Effects of kappa-opioid receptor agonists on long-term cocaine use and dopamine neurotransmission. *Eur. J. Pharmacol.* 426(1/2), 25–34.

166. Tzaferis, J. A., and McGinty, J. F. (2001). Kappa opioid receptor stimulation decreases amphetamine-induced behavior and neuropeptide mRNA expression in the striatum. *Brain Res. Mol. Brain Res.* 93(1), 27–35.

167. Gray, A. M., Rawls, S. M., Shippenberg, T. S., and McGinty, J. F. (1999). The kappa-opioid agonist, U-69593, decreases acute amphetamine-evoked behaviors and calcium-dependent dialysate levels of dopamine and glutamate in the ventral striatum. *J. Neurochem.* 73(3), 1066–1074.

168. Spealman, R. D., and Bergman, J. (1994). Opioid modulation of the discriminative stimulus effects of cocaine: Comparison of micro, kappa and delta agonists in squirrel monkeys discriminating low doses of cocaine. *Behav. Pharmacol.* 5(1), 21–31.

169. Negus, S. S., Mello, N. K., Portoghese, P. S., Lukas, S. E., and Mendelson, J. H. (1995). Role of delta opioid receptors in the reinforcing and discriminative stimulus effects of cocaine in rhesus monkeys. *J. Pharmacol. Exp. Ther.* 273(3), 1245–1256.

170. Waddell, A. B., and Holtzman, S. G. (1998). Modulation of cocaine-induced motor activity in the rat by opioid receptor agonists. *Behav. Pharmacol.* 9(5/6), 397–407.

171. de Vries, T. J., Babovic-Vuksanovic, D., Elmer, G., and Shippenberg, T. S. (1995). Lack of involvement of delta-opioid receptors in mediating the rewarding effects of cocaine. *Psychopharmacology (Berl.)* 120(4), 442–448.

172. Hemby, S. E., Co, C., Dworkin, S. I., and Smith, J. E. (1999). Synergistic elevations in nucleus accumbens extracellular dopamine concentrations during self-administration of cocaine/heroin combinations (Speedball) in rats. *J. Pharmacol. Exp. Ther.* 288(1), 274–280.

173. Smith, J. E., Co, C., Coller, M. D., Hemby, S. E., and Martin, T. J. (2006). Self-administered heroin and cocaine combinations in the rat: Additive reinforcing effects-supra-additive effects on nucleus accumbens extracellular dopamine. *Neuropsychopharmacology* 31(1), 139–150.

174. Zhang, Y., Butelman, E. R., Schlussman, S. D., Ho, A., and Kreek, M. J. (2004). Effect of the kappa opioid agonist R-84760 on cocaine-induced increases in striatal dopamine levels and cocaine-induced place preference in C57BL/6J mice. *Psychopharmacology (Berl.)* 173(1–2), 146–152.

175. Studler, J. M., Kitabgi, P., Tramu, G., Herve, D., Glowinski, J., and Tassin, J. P. (1988). Extensive co-localization of neurotensin with dopamine in rat meso-cortico-frontal dopaminergic neurons. *Neuropeptides* 11(3), 95–100.

176. Kalivas, P. W. (1993). Neurotransmitter regulation of dopamine neurons in the ventral tegmental area. *Brain Res. Rev.* 18(1), 75–113.

177. Seutin, V., Massotte, L., and Dresse, A. (1989). Electrophysiological effects of neurotensin on dopaminergic neurones of the ventral tegmental area of the rat in vitro. *Neuropharmacology* 28(9), 949–954.

178. Widerlov, E., Kilts, C. D., Mailman, R. B., Nemeroff, C. B., Mc Cown, T. J., Prange, A. J. Jr., and Breese, G. R. (1982). Increase in dopamine metabolites in rat brain by neurotensin. *J. Pharmacol. Exp. Ther.* 223(1), 1–6.

179. Blaha, C. D., Coury, A., Fibiger, H. C., and Phillips, A. G. (1990). Effects of neurotensin on dopamine release and metabolism in the rat striatum and nucleus accumbens: Cross-validation using in vivo voltammetry and microdialysis. *Neuroscience* 34(3), 699–705.

180. Kalivas, P. W., and Duffy, P. (1990). Effect of acute and daily neurotensin and enkephalin treatments on extracellular dopamine in the nucleus accumbens. *J. Neurosci.* 10(9), 2940–2949.

181. Chapman, M. A., See, R. E., and Bissette, G. (1992). Neurotensin increases extracellular striatal dopamine levels in vivo. *Neuropeptides* 22(3), 175–183.

182. Kalivas, P. W. (1994). Blockade of neurotensin-induced motor activity by inhibition of protein kinase. *Psychopharmacology (Berl.)* 114(1), 175–180.

183. Kalivas, P. W., and Taylor, S. (1985). Behavioral and neurochemical effect of daily injection with neurotensin into the ventral tegmental area. *Brain Res.* 358(1/2), 70–76.

184. Glimcher, P. W., Giovino, A. A., and Hoebel, B. G. (1987). Neurotensin self-injection in the ventral tegmental area. *Brain Res.* 403(1), 147–150.

185. Fantegrossi, W. E., Ko, M. C., Woods, J. H., and Richelson, E. (2005). Antinociceptive, hypothermic, hypotensive, and reinforcing effects of a novel neurotensin receptor agonist, NT69L, in rhesus monkeys. *Pharmacol. Biochem. Behav.* 80(2), 341–349.

186. Blaha, C. D., and Phillips, A. G. (1992). Pharmacological evidence for common mechanisms underlying the effects of neurotensin and neuroleptics on in vivo dopamine efflux in the rat nucleus accumbens. *Neuroscience* 49(4), 867–877.

187. Ervin, G. N., Birkemo, L. S., Nemeroff, C. B., and Prange, A. J., Jr. (1981). Neurotensin blocks certain amphetamine-induced behaviours. *Nature* 291(5810), 73–76.
188. Jolicoeur, F. B., De Michele, G., Barbeau, A., and St-Pierre, S. (1983). Neurotensin affects hyperactivity but not stereotypy induced by pre and post synaptic dopaminergic stimulation. *Neurosci. Biobehav. Rev.* 7(3), 385–390.
189. Robledo, P., Maldonado, R., and Koob, G. F. (1993). Neurotensin injected into the nucleus accumbens blocks the psychostimulant effects of cocaine but does not attenuate cocaine self-administration in the rat. *Brain Res.* 622(1/2), 105–112.
190. Boules, M., Warrington, L., Fauq, A., McCormick, D., and Richelson, E. (2001). A novel neurotensin analog blocks cocaine- and D-amphetamine-induced hyperactivity. *Eur. J. Pharmacol.* 426(1/2), 73–76.
191. Boules, M., Warrington, L., Fauq, A., McCormick, D., and Richelson, E. (2001). Antiparkinson-like effects of a novel neurotensin analog in unilaterally 6-hydroxydopamine lesioned rats. *Eur. J. Pharmacol.* 428(2), 227–233.
192. Betancur, C., Cabrera, R., de Kloet, E. R., Pelaprat, D., and Rostene, W. (1998). Role of endogenous neurotensin in the behavioral and neuroendocrine effects of cocaine. *Neuropsychopharmacology* 19(4), 322–332.
193. Woolverton, W. L., and Weiss, S. R. B. (1998). Tolerance and sensitization to cocaine: An integrated view. In *Cocaine Abuse: Behavior, Pharmacology, and Clinical Applications*, S. T. Higgins and J. L. Katz, Ed. Academic, San Diego, pp. 107–134.
194. Robinson, T. E., and Berridge, K. C. (2000). The psychology and neurobiology of addiction: An incentive-sensitization view. *Addiction* 95(Suppl. 2), S91–117.
195. Wolf, M. E., Sun, X., Mangiavacchi, S., and Chao, S. Z. (2004). Psychomotor stimulants and neuronal plasticity. *Neuropharmacology* 47(Suppl. 1), 61–79.
196. Stewart, J., and Vezina, P. (1989). Microinjections of SCH-23390 into the ventral tegmental area and substantia nigra pars reticulata attenuate the development of sensitization to the locomotor activating effects of systemic amphetamine. *Brain Res* 495(2), 401–406.
197. Vezina, P. (1996). D1 dopamine receptor activation is necessary for the induction of sensitization by amphetamine in the ventral tegmental area. *J. Neurosci.* 16(7), 2411–2420.
198. Kalivas, P. W., and Alesdatter, J. E. (1993). Involvement of N-methyl-D-aspartate receptor stimulation in the ventral tegmental area and amygdala in behavioral sensitization to cocaine. *J. Pharmacol. Exp. Ther.* 267(1), 486–495.
199. Wolf, M. E., and Jeziorski, M. (1993). Coadministration of MK-801 with amphetamine, cocaine or morphine prevents rather than transiently masks the development of behavioral sensitization. *Brain Res.* 613, 291–294.
200. Weiss, S. R., Post, R. M., Pert, A., Woodward, R., and Murman, D. (1989). Context-dependent cocaine sensitization: Differential effect of haloperidol on development versus expression. *Pharmacol. Biochem. Behav.* 34(3), 655–661.
201. Wolf, M. E., Dahlin, S. L., Hu, X. T., Xue, C. J., and White, K. (1995). Effects of lesions of prefrontal cortex, amygdala, or fornix on behavioral sensitization to amphetamine: Comparison with N-methyl-D-aspartate antagonists. *Neuroscience* 69(2), 417–439.
202. Kalivas, P. W., and Duffy, P. (1993). Time course of extracellular dopamine and behavioral sensitization to cocaine. I. Dopamine axon terminals. *J. Neurosci.* 13(1), 266–275.

203. Czyrak, A., Mackowiak, M., Chocyk, A., Fijal, K., and Wedzony, K. (2003). Role of glucocorticoids in the regulation of dopaminergic neurotransmission. *Pol. J. Pharmacol.* 55(5), 667–674.

204. Goeders, N. E. (1997). A neuroendocrine role in cocaine reinforcement. *Psychoneuroendocrinology* 22(4), 237–259.

205. Budziszewska, B., Jaworska-Feil, L., and Lason, W. (1996). The effect of repeated amphetamine and cocaine administration on adrenal, gonadal and thyroid hormone levels in the rat plasma. *Exp. Clin. Endocrinol. Diabetes* 104(4), 334–338.

206. Laviola, G., Adriani, W., Morley-Fletcher, S., and Terranova, M. L. (2002). Peculiar response of adolescent mice to acute and chronic stress and to amphetamine: Evidence of sex differences. *Behav. Brain Res.* 130(1/2), 117–125.

207. Bolanos, C. A., Barrot, M., Berton, O., Wallace-Black, D., and Nestler, E. J. (2003). Methylphenidate treatment during pre- and periadolescence alters behavioral responses to emotional stimuli at adulthood. *Biol. Psychiatry* 54(12), 1317–1329.

208. Budziszewska, B., Leskiewicz, M., Jaworska-Feil, L., and Lason, W. (1996). Repeated cocaine administration down-regulates glucocorticoid receptors in the rat brain cortex and hippocampus. *Pol. J. Pharmacol.* 48(6), 575–581.

209. Shilling, P. D., Kelsoe, J. R., and Segal, D. S. (1996). Hippocampal glucocorticoid receptor mRNA is up-regulated by acute and down-regulated by chronic amphetamine treatment. *Brain Res. Mol. Brain Res.* 38(1), 156–160.

210. Koob, G. F. (1999). Stress, corticotropin-releasing factor, and drug addiction. *Ann. NY Acad. Sci.* 897, 27–45.

211. Cancela, L. M., Basso, A. M., Martijena, I. D., Capriles, N. R., and Molina, V. A. (2001). A dopaminergic mechanism is involved in the "anxiogenic-like" response induced by chronic amphetamine treatment: A behavioral and neurochemical study. *Brain Res.* 909(1/2), 179–186.

212. Kooij, J. J., Middelkoop, H. A., van Gils, K., and Buitelaar, J. K. (2001). The effect of stimulants on nocturnal motor activity and sleep quality in adults with ADHD: An open-label case-control study. *J. Clin. Psychiatry* 62(12), 952–956.

213. Chapotot, F., Pigeau, R., Canini, F., Bourdon, L., and Buguet, A. (2003). Distinctive effects of modafinil and *d*-amphetamine on the homeostatic and circadian modulation of the human waking EEG. *Psychopharmacology (Berl.)* 166(2), 127–138.

214. Zisapel, N., and Laudon, M. (2003). Subjective assessment of the effects of CNS-active drugs on sleep by the Leeds sleep evaluation questionnaire: A review. *Hum. Psychopharmacol.* 18(1), 1–20.

215. Bradberry, C. W. (2000). Acute and chronic dopamine dynamics in a nonhuman primate model of recreational cocaine use. *J. Neurosci.* 20(18), 7109–7115.

216. Ellison, G. (1994). Stimulant-induced psychosis, the dopamine theory of schizophrenia, and the habenula. *Brain Res. Brain Res. Rev.* 19(2), 223–239.

217. Schlemmer, R. F., Young, J., and Davis, J. M. (1996). Stimulant-induced disruption of nonhuman primate social behavior and the psychopharmacology of schizophrenia. *J. Psychopharmacol.* 10, 64–76.

218. Castner, S. A., and Goldman-Rakic, P. S. (1999). Long-lasting psychotomimetic consequences of repeated low-dose amphetamine exposure in rhesus monkeys. *Neuropsychopharmacology* 20(1), 10–28.

219. Strakowski, S. M., Sax, K. W., Setters, M. J., and Keck, P. E. Jr. (1996). Enhanced response to repeated *d*-amphetamine challenge: Evidence for behavioral sensitization in humans. *Biol. Psychiatry* 40(9), 872–880.

220. Strakowski, S. M., and Sax, K. W. (1998). Progressive behavioral response to repeated d-amphetamine challenge: Further evidence for sensitization in humans. *Biol. Psychiatry* 44(11), 1171–1177.
221. Strakowski, S. M., Sax, K. W., Rosenberg, H. L., DelBello, M. P., and Adler, C. M. (2001). Human response to repeated low-dose d-amphetamine: Evidence for behavioral enhancement and tolerance. *Neuropsychopharmacology* 25(4), 548–554.
222. Gorelick, D. A., and Rothman, R. B. (1997). Stimulant sensitization in humans. *Biol. Psychiatry* 42(3), 230–231.
223. Walsh, S. L., Haberny, K. A., and Bigelow, G. E. (2000). Modulation of intravenous cocaine effects by chronic oral cocaine in humans. *Psychopharmacology (Berl.)* 150(4), 361–373.
224. Wachtel, S. R., and de Wit, H. (1999). Subjective and behavioral effects of repeated d-amphetamine in humans. *Behav. Pharmacol.* 10(3), 271–281.
225. Comer, S. D., Hart, C. L., Ward, A. S., Haney, M., Foltin, R. W., and Fischman, M. W. (2001). Effects of repeated oral methamphetamine administration in humans. *Psychopharmacology (Berl.)* 155(4), 397–404.
226. Strakowski, S. M., Sax, K. W., Setters, M. J., Stanton, S. P., and Keck, P. E. Jr. (1997). Lack of enhanced response to repeated D-amphetamine challenge in first-episode psychosis: Implications for a sensitization model of psychosis in humans. *Biol. Psychiatry* 42(9), 749–755.
227. Carlezon, W. A. Jr., and Konradi, C. (2004). Understanding the neurobiological consequences of early exposure to psychotropic drugs: Linking behavior with molecules. *Neuropharmacology* 47(Suppl. 1), 47–60.
228. Kalivas, P. W., Duffy, P., DuMars, L. A., and Skinner, C. (1988). Behavioral and neurochemical effects of acute and daily cocaine administration in rats. *J. Pharmacol. Exp. Ther.* 245(2), 485–491.
229. Kuczenski, R., and Segal, D. S. (2001). Locomotor effects of acute and repeated threshold doses of amphetamine and methylphenidate: Relative roles of dopamine and norepinephrine. *J. Pharmacol. Exp. Ther.* 296(3), 876–883.
230. Kalivas, P. W., and Stewart, J. (1991). Dopamine transmission in the initiation and expression of drug- and stress-induced sensitization of motor activity. *Brain Res. Rev.* 16, 223–244.
231. Piazza, P. V., Deminiere, J. M., Le Moal, M., and Simon, H. (1989). Factors that predict individual vulnerability to amphetamine self-administration. *Science* 245(4925), 1511–1513.
232. Horger, B. A., Giles, M. K., and Schenk, S. (1992). Preexposure to amphetamine and nicotine predisposes rats to self-administer a low dose of cocaine. *Psychopharmacology (Berl.)* 107(2/3), 271–276.
233. Vezina, P., Pierre, P. J., and Lorrain, D. S. (1999). The effect of previous exposure to amphetamine on drug-induced locomotion and self-administration of a low dose of the drug. *Psychopharmacology (Berl.)* 147(2), 125–134.
234. Morgan, D., and Roberts, D. C. (2004). Sensitization to the reinforcing effects of cocaine following binge-abstinent self-administration. *Neurosci. Biobehav. Rev.* 27(8), 803–812.
235. Vanderschuren, L. J., and Kalivas, P. W. (2000). Alterations in dopaminergic and glutamatergic transmission in the induction and expression of behavioral sensitization: A critical review of preclinical studies. *Psychopharmacology (Berl.)* 151(2/3), 99–120.
236. Nestler, E. J. (2001). Molecular neurobiology of addiction. *Am. J. Addict.* 10(3), 201–217.

237. Robinson, T. E., and Berridge, K. C. (2001). Incentive-sensitization and addiction. *Addiction* 96(1), 103–114.
238. Clure, C., Brady, K. T., Saladin, M. E., Johnson, D., Waid, R., and Rittenbury, M. (1999). Attention-deficit/hyperactivity disorder and substance use: Symptom pattern and drug choice. *Am. J. Drug Alcohol Abuse* 25(3), 441–448.
239. Biederman, J., Wilens, T., Mick, E., Spencer, T., and Faraone, S. V. (1999). Pharmacotherapy of attention-deficit/hyperactivity disorder reduces risk for substance use disorder. *Pediatrics* 104(2), e20.
240. Wilens, T. E., Faraone, S. V., Biederman, J., and Gunawardene, S. (2003). Does stimulant therapy of attention-deficit/hyperactivity disorder beget later substance abuse? A meta-analytic review of the literature. *Pediatrics* 111(1), 179–185.
241. Pilotte, N. S., Sharpe, L. G., and Kuhar, M. J. (1994). Withdrawal of repeated intravenous infusions of cocaine persistently reduces binding to dopamine transporters in the nucleus accumbens of Lewis rats. *J. Pharmacol. Exp. Ther.* 269, 963–969.
242. Wilson, J. M., Nobrega, J. N., Corrigall, W. A., Coen, K. M., Shannak, K., and Kish, S. J. (1994). Amygdala dopamine levels are markedly elevated after self- but not passive-administration of cocaine. *Brain Res.* 668(1/2), 39–45.
243. Claye, L. H., Akunne, H. C., Davis, M. D., DeMattos, S., and Soliman, K. F. A. (1995). Behavioral and neurochemical changes in the dopaminergic system after repeated cocaine administration. *Mol. Neurobiol.* 11, 55–66.
244. Boulay, D., Duterte-Boucher, D., Leroux-Nicollet, I., Naudon, L., and Costenin, J. (1996). Locomotor sensitization and decrease in [3H]mazindol binding to the dopamine transporter in the nucleus accumbens are delayed after chronic treatments by GBR12782 or cocaine. *J. Pharmacol. Exp. Ther.* 278(1), 330–337.
245. Tella, S. R., Ladenheim, B., Andrews, A. M., Goldberg, S. R., and Cadet, J. L. (1996). Differential reinforcing effects of cocaine and GBR-12909: Biochemical evidence for divergent neuroadaptive changes in the mesolimbic dopaminergic system. *J. Neurosci.* 16(23), 7416–7427.
246. Letchworth, S. R., Daunais, J. B., Hedgecock, A. A., and Porrino, L. J. (1997). Effects of chronic cocaine administration on dopamine transporter mRNA and protein in the rat. *Brain Res.* 750(1/2), 214–222.
247. Letchworth, S. R., Sexton, T., Childers, S. R., Vrana, K. E., Vaughan, R. A., Davies, H. M. L., and Porrino, L. J. (1999). Regulation of rat dopamine transporter mRNA and protein by chronic cocaine administration. *J. Neurochem.* 73, 1982–1989.
248. Goeders, N. E., and Kuhar, M. J. (1987). Chronic cocaine administration induces opposite changes in dopamine receptors in the striatum and nucleus accumbens. *Alcohol Drug Res.* 7(4), 207–216.
249. Dwoskin, L. P., Peris, J., Yasuda, R. P., Philpott, K., and Zahniser, N. R. (1988). Repeated cocaine administration results in supersensitivity of striatal D-2 dopamine autoreceptors to pergolide. *Life Sci.* 42(3), 255–262.
250. Kleven, M. S., Perry, B. D., Woolverton, W. L., and Seiden, L. S. (1990). Effects of repeated injections of cocaine on D1 and D2 dopamine receptors in rat brain. *Brain Res.* 532, 265–270.
251. Kuhar, M. J., and Pilotte, N. S. (1996). Neurochemical changes in cocaine withdrawal. *Trends Pharmacol. Sci.* 17(7), 260–264.
252. Mateo, Y., Lack, C. M., Morgan, D., Roberts, D. C., and Jones, S. R. (2005). Reduced dopamine terminal function and insensitivity to cocaine following cocaine binge self-administration and deprivation. *Neuropsychopharmacology* 30(8), 1455–1463.

253. Letchworth, S. R., Nader, M. A., Smith, H. R., Friedman, D. P., and Porrino, L. J. (2001). Progression of changes in dopamine transporter binding site density as a result of cocaine self-administration in rhesus monkeys. *J. Neurosci.* 21(8), 2799–2807.
254. Little, K. Y., Kirkman, J. A., Carroll, F. I., Clark, T. B., and Duncan, G. E. (1993). Cocaine use increases [3H]WIN 35428 binding sites in human striatum. *Brain Res.* 628(1/2), 17–25.
255. Staley, J. K., Hearn, W. L., Ruttenber, A. J., Wetli, C. V., and Mash, D. C. (1994). High affinity cocaine recognition sites on the dopamine transporter are elevated in fatal cocaine overdose victims. *J. Pharmacol. Exp. Ther.* 271(3), 1678–1685.
256. Moore, R. J., Vinsant, S. L., Nader, M. A., Porrino, L. J., and Friedman, D. P. (1998). Effect of cocaine self-administration on striatal dopamine D1 receptors in rhesus monkeys. *Synapse* 28(1), 1–9.
257. Moore, R. J., Vinsant, S. L., Nader, M. A., Porrino, L. J., and Friedman, D. P. (1998). Effect of cocaine self-administration on dopamine D2 receptors in rhesus monkeys. *Synapse* 30(1), 88–96.
258. Garavan, H., Pankiewicz, J., Bloom, A., Cho, J. K., Sperry, L., Ross, T. J., Salmeron, B. J., Risinger, R., Kelley, D., and Stein, E. A. (2000). Cue-induced cocaine craving: Neuroanatomical specificity for drug users and drug stimuli. *Am. J. Psychiatry* 157(11), 1789–1798.
259. Martin-Soelch, C., Leenders, K. L., Chevalley, A. F., Missimer, J., Kunig, G., Magyar, S., Mino, A., and Schultz, W. (2001). Reward mechanisms in the brain and their role in dependence: Evidence from neurophysiological and neuroimaging studies. *Brain Res. Brain Res. Rev.* 36(2/3), 139–149.
260. Malison, R. T., Best, S. E., van Dyck, C. H., McCance, E. F., Wallace, E. A., Laruelle, M., Baldwin, R. M., Seibyl, J. P., Price, L. H., Kosten, T. R., and Innis, R. B. (1998). Elevated striatal dopamine transporters during acute cocaine abstinence as measured by [123I] beta-CIT SPECT. *Am. J. Psychiatry* 155(6), 832–834.
261. Volkow, N. D., and Fowler, J. S. (2000). Addiction, a disease of compulsion and drive: Involvement of the orbitofrontal cortex. *Cereb. Cortex* 10(3), 318–325.
262. Volkow, N. D., Fowler, J. S., and Wang, G. J. (2004). The addicted human brain viewed in the light of imaging studies: Brain circuits and treatment strategies. *Neuropharmacology* 47(Suppl. 1), 3–13.
263. Volkow, N. D., Fowler, J. S., Wang, G. J., Hitzemann, R., Logan, J., Schlyer, D. J., Dewey, S. L., and Wolf, A. P. (1993). Decreased dopamine D2 receptor availability is associated with reduced frontal metabolism in cocaine abusers. *Synapse* 14(2), 169–177.
264. Volkow, N. D., Chang, L., Wang, G. J., Fowler, J. S., Ding, Y. S., Sedler, M., Logan, J., Franceschi, D., Gatley, J., Hitzemann, R., Gifford, A., Wong, C., and Pappas, N. (2001). Low level of brain dopamine D2 receptors in methamphetamine abusers: Association with metabolism in the orbitofrontal cortex. *Am. J. Psychiatry* 158(12), 2015–2021.
265. Volkow, N. D., Fowler, J. S., Wolf, A. P., Hitzemann, R., Dewey, S., Bendriem, B., Alpert, R., and Hoff, A. (1991). Changes in brain glucose metabolism in cocaine dependence and withdrawal. *Am. J. Psychiatry* 148(5), 621–626.
266. Volkow, N. D., Wang, G. J., Fowler, J. S., Gatley, S. J., Logan, J., Ding, Y. S., Hitzemann, R., and Pappas, N. (1998). Dopamine transporter occupancies in the human brain induced by therapeutic doses of oral methylphenidate. *Am. J. Psychiatry* 155(10), 1325–1331.
267. Volkow, N. D., Wang, G., Fowler, J. S., Logan, J., Gerasimov, M., Maynard, L., Ding, Y., Gatley, S. J., Gifford, A., and Franceschi, D. (2001). Therapeutic doses of oral

methylphenidate significantly increase extracellular dopamine in the human brain. *J. Neurosci.* 21(2), RC121.

268. Laruelle, M. (2000). Imaging synaptic neurotransmission with in vivo binding competition techniques: A critical review. *J. Cereb. Blood Flow Metab.* 20, 423–451.

269. Vaidya, C. J., Austin, G., Kirkorian, G., Ridlehuber, H. W., Desmond, J. E., Glover, G. H., and Gabrieli, J. D. (1998). Selective effects of methylphenidate in attention deficit hyperactivity disorder: A functional magnetic resonance study. *Proc. Natl. Acad. Sci. USA* 95(24), 14494–14499.

270. Schweitzer, J. B., Lee, D. O., Hanford, R. B., Tagamets, M. A., Hoffman, J. M., Grafton, S. T., and Kilts, C. D. (2003). A positron emission tomography study of methylphenidate in adults with ADHD: Alterations in resting blood flow and predicting treatment response. *Neuropsychopharmacology* 28(5), 967–973.

271. Ernst, M., Zametkin, A. J., Matochik, J. A., Liebenauer, L., Fitzgerald, G. A., and Cohen, R. M. (1994). Effects of intravenous dextroamphetamine on brain metabolism in adults with attention-deficit hyperactivity disorder (ADHD). Preliminary findings. *Psychopharmacol. Bull.* 30(2), 219–225.

272. Matochik, J. A., Liebenauer, L. L., King, A. C., Szymanski, H. V., Cohen, R. M., and Zametkin, A. J. (1994). Cerebral glucose metabolism in adults with attention deficit hyperactivity disorder after chronic stimulant treatment. *Am. J. Psychiatry* 151(5), 658–664.

273. Reid, M. S., and Berger, S. P. (1996). Evidence for sensitization of cocaine-induced nucleus accumbens glutamate release. *Neuroreport* 7(7), 1325–1329.

274. Swanson, C. J., Baker, D. A., Carson, D., Worley, P. F., and Kalivas, P. W. (2001). Repeated cocaine administration attenuates group I metabotropic glutamate receptor-mediated glutamate release and behavioral activation: A potential role for Homer. *J. Neurosci.* 21(22), 9043–9052.

275. Thomas, M. J., Beurrier, C., Bonci, A., and Malenka, R. C. (2001). Long-term depression in the nucleus accumbens: A neural correlate of behavioral sensitization to cocaine. *Nat. Neurosci.* 4(12), 1217–1223.

276. Beurrier, C., and Malenka, R. C. (2002). Enhanced inhibition of synaptic transmission by dopamine in the nucleus accumbens during behavioral sensitization to cocaine. *J. Neurosci.* 22(14), 5817–5822.

277. Zeigler, S., Lipton, J., Toga, A., and Ellison, G. (1991). Continuous cocaine administration produces persisting changes in brain neurochemistry and behavior. *Brain Res.* 552(1), 27–35.

278. Lipton, J. W., and Ellison, G. D. (1992). Continuous cocaine induces persisting changes in behavioral responsivity to both scopolamine and diazepam. *Neuropsychopharmacology* 7(2), 143–148.

279. Pierce, R. C., and Kalivas, P. W. (1997). A circuitry model of the expression of behavioral sensitization to amphetamine-like psychostimulants. *Brain Res. Brain Res. Rev.* 25(2), 192–216.

280. Egan, M. F., Wing, L., Li, R., Kirch, D. G., and Wyatt, R. J. (1994). Effects of chronic cocaine treatment on rat brain: Long-term reduction in frontal cortical serotonin. *Biol. Psychiatry* 36(9), 637–640.

281. Little, K. Y., Patel, U. N., Clark, T. B., and Butts, J. D. (1996). Alteration of brain dopamine and serotonin levels in cocaine users: A preliminary report. *Am. J. Psychiatry* 153(9), 1216–1218.

282. McDougle, C. J., Black, J. E., Malison, R. T., Zimmermann, R. C., Kosten, T. R., Heninger, G. R., and Price, L. H. (1994). Noradrenergic dysregulation during discontinuation of cocaine use in addicts. *Arch. Gen. Psychiatry* 51(9), 713–719.

283. Macey, D. J., Smith, H. R., Nader, M. A., and Porrino, L. J. (2003). Chronic cocaine self-administration upregulates the norepinephrine transporter and alters functional activity in the bed nucleus of the stria terminalis of the rhesus monkey. *J. Neurosci.* 23(1), 12–16.

284. Unterwald, E. M., Rubenfeld, J. M., and Kreek, M. J. (1994). Repeated cocaine administration upregulates kappa and mu, but not delta, opioid receptors. *Neuroreport* 5(13), 1613–1616.

285. Turchan, J., Przewlocka, B., Lason, W., and Przewlocki, R. (1998). Effects of repeated psychostimulant administration on the prodynorphin system activity and kappa opioid receptor density in the rat brain. *Neuroscience* 85(4), 1051–1059.

286. Staley, J. K., Rothman, R. B., Rice, K. C., Partilla, J., and Mash, D. C. (1997). Kappa2 opioid receptors in limbic areas of the human brain are upregulated by cocaine in fatal overdose victims. *J. Neurosci.* 17(21), 8225–8233.

287. Zubieta, J. K., Gorelick, D. A., Stauffer, R., Ravert, H. T., Dannals, R. F., and Frost, J. J. (1996). Increased mu opioid receptor binding detected by PET in cocaine-dependent men is associated with cocaine craving. *Nat. Med.* 2(11), 1225–1229.

288. Nestler, E. J., and Duman, R. (1994). G-proteins and cyclic nucleotides in the nervous system. In *Basic Neurochemistry: Molecular, Cellular, and Medical Aspects*, G. Siegel, R. Albers, B. Agranoff, and P. Molinoff, Ed. Little, Brown, Boston, 5th ed., pp. 429–448.

289. Nestler, E. J., and Greengard, P. (1994). Protein phosphorylation and the regulation of neuronal function. In *Basic Neurochemistry: Molecular, Cellular, and Medical Aspects*, G. Siegel, R. Albers, B. Agranoff, and P. Molinoff, Ed. Little, Brown, 5th ed., Boston, pp. 449–474.

290. Nestler, E. J. (1994). Molecular neurobiology of drug addiction. *Neuropsychopharmacology* 11(2), 77–87.

291. Nestler, E. J. (2004). Historical review: Molecular and cellular mechanisms of opiate and cocaine addiction. *Trends Pharmacol. Sci.* 25(4), 210–218.

292. Terwilliger, R. Z., Beitner-Johnson, D., Sevarino, K. A., Crain, S. M., and Nestler, E. J. (1991). A general role for adaptations in G-proteins and the cyclic AMP system in mediating the chronic actions of morphine and cocaine on neuronal function. *Brain Res.* 548, 100–110.

293. Self, D. W., Genova, L. M., Hope, B. T., Barnhart, W. J., Spencer, J. J., and Nestler, E. J. (1998). Involvement of cAMP-dependent protein kinase in the nucleus accumbens in cocaine self-administration and relapse of cocaine-seeking behavior. *J. Neurosci.* 18(5), 1848–1859.

294. Shaw-Lutchman, T. Z., Impey, S., Storm, D., and Nestler, E. J. (2003). Regulation of CRE-mediated transcription in mouse brain by amphetamine. *Synapse* 48(1), 10–17.

295. Carlezon, J. W. A., Thome, J., Olson, V. G., Lane-Ladd, S. B., Brodkin, E. S., Hiroi, N., Duman, R. S., Neve, R. L., and Nestler, E. J. (1998). Regulation of cocaine reward by CREB. *Science* 282, 2272–2275.

296. Walters, C. L., and Blendy, J. A. (2001). Different requirements for cAMP response element binding protein in positive and negative reinforcing properties of drugs of abuse. *J. Neurosci.* 21(23), 9438–9444.

297. Kuhar, M. J., Joyce, A., and Dominguez, G. (2001). Genes in drug abuse. *Drug Alcohol Depend.* 62(3), 157–162.

298. Hope, B., Kosofsky, B., Hyman, S. E., and Nestler, E. J. (1992). Regulation of immediate early gene expression and AP-1 binding in the rat nucleus accumbens by chronic cocaine. *Proc. Natl. Acad. Sci. USA* 89(13), 5764–5768.
299. Nestler, E. J., Barrot, M., and Self, D. W. (2001). DeltaFosB: A sustained molecular switch for addiction. *Proc. Natl. Acad. Sci. USA* 98(20), 11042–11046.
300. Colby, C. R., Whisler, K., Steffen, C., Nestler, E. J., and Self, D. W. (2003). Striatal cell type-specific overexpression of DeltaFosB enhances incentive for cocaine. *J. Neurosci.* 23(6), 2488–2493.
301. Kelz, M. B., Chen, J., Carlezon, W. A. Jr., Whisler, K., Gilden, L., Beckmann, A. M., Steffen, C., Zhang, Y. J., Marotti, L., Self, D. W., Tkatch, T., Baranauskas, G., Surmeier, D. J., Neve, R. L., Duman, R. S., Picciotto, M. R., and Nestler, E. J. (1999). Expression of the transcription factor ΔFosB in the brain controls sensitivity to cocaine. *Nature* 401, 272–276.
302. Kuhar, M. J., Jaworski, J. N., Hubert, G. W., Philpot, K. B., and Dominguez, G. (2005). Cocaine- and amphetamine-regulated transcript peptides play a role in drug abuse and are potential therapeutic targets. *AAPS J.* 7(1), E259–E265.
303. Yermolaieva, O., Chen, J., Couceyro, P. R., and Hoshi, T. (2001). Cocaine- and amphetamine-regulated transcript peptide modulation of voltage-gated Ca^{2+} signaling in hippocampal neurons. *J. Neurosci.* 21(19), 7474–7480.
304. Kimmel, H. L., Gong, W., Dall Vechia, S., Hunter, R. G., and Kuhar, M. J. (2000). Intra-VTA injection of rat CART peptide 55-102 induces locomotor activity and promotes conditioned place preference. *J. Pharmacol. Exp. Ther.* 294, 784–792.
305. Jaworski, J. N., Kozel, M. A., Philpot, K. B., and Kuhar, M. J. (2003). Intra-accumbal injection of CART (cocaine-amphetamine regulated transcript) peptide reduces cocaine-induced locomotor activity. *J. Pharmacol. Exp. Ther.* 307(3), 1038–1044.
306. Kim, J. H., Creekmore, E., and Vezina, P. (2003). Microinjection of CART peptide 55-102 into the nucleus accumbens blocks amphetamine-induced locomotion. *Neuropeptides* 37(6), 369–373.
307. Albertson, D. N., Pruetz, B., Schmidt, C. J., Kuhn, D. M., Kapatos, G., and Bannon, M. J. (2004). Gene expression profile of the nucleus accumbens of human cocaine abusers: Evidence for dysregulation of myelin. *J. Neurochem.* 88(5), 1211–1219.
308. Tang, W. X., Fasulo, W. H., Mash, D. C., and Hemby, S. E. (2003). Molecular profiling of midbrain dopamine regions in cocaine overdose victims. *J. Neurochem.* 85(4), 911–924.
309. Dole, V. P., and Nyswander, M. (1965). A medical treatment for diacetylmorphine (heroin) addiction. A clinical trial with methadone hydrochloride. *JAMA* 193, 646–650.
310. Kreek, M. J. (1992). Rationale for maintenance pharmacotherapy of opiate dependence. *Res. Publ. Assoc. Res. Nerv. Ment. Dis.* 70, 205–230.
311. Rose, J. E., Behm, F. M., and Westman, E. C. (1998). Nicotine-mecamylamine treatment for smoking cessation: The role of pre-cessation therapy. *Exp. Clin. Psychopharmacol.* 6(3), 331–343.
312. O'Malley, S. S., Jaffe, A. J., Chang, G., Schottenfeld, R. S., Meyer, R. E., and Rounsaville, B. (1992). Naltrexone and coping skills therapy for alcohol dependence. A controlled study. *Arch. Gen. Psychiatry* 49(11), 881–887.
313. Volpicelli, J. R., Alterman, A. I., Hayashida, M., and O'Brien, C. P. (1992). Naltrexone in the treatment of alcohol dependence. *Arch. Gen. Psychiatry* 49(11), 876–880.
314. Grabowski, J., Shearer, J., Merrill, J., and Negus, S. S. (2004). Agonist-like, replacement pharmacotherapy for stimulant abuse and dependence. *Addict. Behav.* 29(7), 1439–1464.

315. Sofuoglu, M., and Kosten, T. R. (2005). Novel approaches to the treatment of cocaine addiction. *CNS Drugs* 19(1), 13–25.

316. Gorelick, D. A. (2003). Pharmacological intervention for cocaine, crack, and other stimulant addiction. In *Principles of Addiction Medicine*, A. W. Graham, T. K.Schultz, M. F.Mayo-Smith, R. K. Ries, and B. B. Wilford, Ed. American Society of Addiction Medicine, Chevy Chase, MD, pp. 785–800.

317. de Lima, M.S., de Oliveira Soares, B. G., Reisser, A. A., and Farrell, M. (2002). Pharmacological treatment of cocaine dependence: A systematic review. *Addiction* 97(8), 931–949.

318. Soares, B. G., Lima, M. S., Reisser, A. A., and Farrell, M. (2003). Dopamine agonists for cocaine dependence. *Cochrane Database Syst. Rev.* (2), CD003352.

319. Grabowski, J., Rhoades, H., Silverman, P., Schmitz, J. M., Stotts, A., Creson, D., and Bailey, R. (2000). Risperidone for the treatment of cocaine dependence: Randomized, double-blind trial. *J. Clin. Psychopharmacol.* 20(3), 305–310.

320. Evans, S. M., Walsh, S. L., Levin, F. R., Foltin, R. W., Fischman, M. W., and Bigelow, G. E. (2001). Effect of flupenthixol on subjective and cardiovascular responses to intravenous cocaine in humans. *Drug Alcohol Depend* 64(3), 271–283.

321. Kampman, K. M., Pettinati, H., Lynch, K. G., Sparkman, T., and O'Brien, C. P. (2003). A pilot trial of olanzapine for the treatment of cocaine dependence. *Drug Alcohol Depend* 70(3), 265–273.

322. George, T. P., Verrico, C. D., Picciotto, M. R., and Roth, R. H. (2000). Nicotinic modulation of mesoprefrontal dopamine neurons: Pharmacologic and neuroanatomic characterization. *J. Pharmacol Exp. Ther.* 295(1), 58–66.

323. Petrakis, I. L., Carroll, K. M., Nich, C., Gordon, L. T., McCance-Katz, E. F., Frankforter, T., and Rounsaville, B. J. (2000). Disulfiram treatment for cocaine dependence in methadone-maintained opioid addicts. *Addiction* 95(2), 219–228.

324. Carroll, K. M., Fenton, L. R., Ball, S. A., Nich, C., Frankforter, T. L., Shi, J., and Rounsaville, B. J. (2004). Efficacy of disulfiram and cognitive behavior therapy in cocaine-dependent outpatients: A randomized placebo-controlled trial. *Arch. Gen. Psychiatry* 61(3), 264–272.

325. Levin, F. R., and Lehman, A. F. (1991). Meta-analysis of desipramine as an adjunct in the treatment of cocaine addiction. *J. Clin. Psychopharmacol.* 11(6), 374–378.

326. Arndt, I. O., Dorozynsky, L., Woody, G. E., McLellan, A. T., and O'Brien, C. P. (1992). Desipramine treatment of cocaine dependence in methadone-maintained patients. *Arch. Gen. Psychiatry* 49(11), 888–893.

327. Campbell, J. L., Thomas, H. M., Gabrielli, W., Liskow, B. I., and Powell, B. J. (1994). Impact of desipramine or carbamazepine on patient retention in outpatient cocaine treatment: Preliminary findings. *J. Addict. Dis.* 13(4), 191–199.

328. Kosten, T. R., Morgan, C. M., Falcione, J., and Schottenfeld, R. S. (1992). Pharmacotherapy for cocaine-abusing methadone-maintained patients using amantadine or desipramine. *Arch. Gen. Psychiatry* 49(11), 894–898.

329. Walsh, S. L., Preston, K. L., Sullivan, J. T., Fromme, R., and Bigelow, G. E. (1994). Fluoxetine alters the effects of intravenous cocaine in humans. *J. Clin. Psychopharmacol.* 14(6), 396–407.

330. Batki, S. L., Washburn, A. M., Delucchi, K., and Jones, R. T. (1996). A controlled trial of fluoxetine in crack cocaine dependence. *Drug Alcohol Depend.* 41(2), 137–142.

331. Grabowski, J., Rhoades, H., Elk, R., Schmitz, J., Davis, C., Creson, D., and Kirby, K. (1995). Fluoxetine is ineffective for treatment of cocaine dependence or concurrent

opiate and cocaine dependence: Two placebo-controlled double-blind trials. *J. Clin. Psychopharmacol.* 15(3), 163–174.

332. Hollister, L. E., Krajewski, K., Rustin, T., and Gillespie, H. (1992). Drugs for cocaine dependence: Not easy. *Arch. Gen. Psychiatry* 49(11), 905–906.

333. Specker, S., Crosby, R., Borden, J., and Hatsukami, D. (2000). Nefadozone in the treatment of females with cocaine abuse. *Drug Alcohol Depend.* 60(Suppl. 1), S211.

334. Platt, D. M., Rowlett, J. K., and Spealman, R. D. (2001). Modulation of cocaine and food self-administration by low- and high-efficacy d1 agonists in squirrel monkeys. *Psychopharmacology (Berl.)* 157(2), 208–216.

335. Mutschler, N. H., and Bergman, J. (2002). Effects of chronic administration of the D(1) receptor partial agonist SKF 77434 on cocaine self-administration in rhesus monkeys. *Psychopharmacology (Berl.)* 160(4), 362–370.

336. Platt, D. M., Rodefer, J. S., Rowlett, J. K., and Spealman, R. D. (2003). Suppression of cocaine- and food-maintained behavior by the D2-like receptor partial agonist terguride in squirrel monkeys. *Psychopharmacology (Berl.)* 166(3), 298–305.

337. Kumor, K., Sherer, M., and Jaffe, J. (1989). Effects of bromocriptine pretreatment on subjective and physiological responses to i.v. cocaine. *Pharmacol. Biochem. Behav.* 33(4), 829–837.

338. Montoya, I. D., Preston, K. L., Rothman, R., and Gorelick, D. A. (2002). Open-label pilot study of bupropion plus bromocriptine for treatment of cocaine dependence. *Am. J. Drug Alcohol Abuse* 28(1), 189–196.

339. Preston, K., Sullivan, J.T., Strain, E. C., and Bigelow, G. E. (1993). Effects of cocaine alone and in combination with mazindol in human cocaine abusers. *J. Pharmacol. Exp. Ther.* 267, 296–307.

340. Stine, S. M., Krystal, J. H., Kosten, T. R., and Charney, D. S. (1995). Mazindol treatment for cocaine dependence. *Drug Alcohol Depend.* 39, 245–252.

341. Grabowski, J., Roache, J. D., Schmitz, J. M., Rhoades, H., Creson, D., and Korszun, A. (1997). Replacement medication for cocaine dependence: Methylphenidate. *J. Clin. Psychopharmacol.* 17(6), 485–488.

342. Schubiner, H., Saules, K. K., Arfken, C. L., Johanson, C. E., Schuster, C. R., Lockhart, N., Edwards, A., Donlin, J., and Pihlgren, E. (2002). Double-blind placebo-controlled trial of methylphenidate in the treatment of adult ADHD patients with comorbid cocaine dependence. *Exp. Clin. Psychopharmacol.* 10(3), 286–294.

343. Howell, L. L., and Wilcox, K. M. (2001). The dopamine transporter and cocaine medication development: Drug self-administration in nonhuman primates. *J. Pharmacol. Exp. Ther.* 298(1), 1–6.

344. Negus, S. S. (2003). Rapid assessment of choice between cocaine and food in rhesus monkeys: Effects of environmental manipulations and treatment with *d*-amphetamine and flupenthixol. *Neuropsychopharmacology* 28(5), 919–931.

345. Negus, S. S., and Mello, N. K. (2003). Effects of chronic d-amphetamine treatment on cocaine- *d* and food-maintained responding under a second-order schedule in rhesus monkeys. *Drug Alcohol Depend.* 70(1), 39–52.

346. Rothman, R. B., Blough, B. E., Woolverton, W. L., Anderson, K. G., Negus, S. S., Mello, N. K., Roth, B. L., and Baumann, M. H. (2005). Development of a rationally designed, low abuse potential, biogenic amine releaser that suppresses cocaine self-administration. *J. Pharmacol. Exp. Ther.* 313(3), 1361–1369.

347. Glowa, J. R., Wojnicki, F. H. E., Matecka, D., Bacher, J. J., Mansbach, R. S., Balster, R. L., and Rice, K. C. (1995). Effects of dopamine reuptake inhibitors on food- and

cocaine-maintained responding: I. Dependence on unit dose of cocaine. *Exp. Clin. Psychopharmacol.* 3, 219–231.
348. Dackis, C., and O'Brien, C. (2003). Glutamatergic agents for cocaine dependence. *Ann. NY Acad. Sci,* 1003, 328–345.
349. Touret, M., Sallanon-Moulin, M., Fages, C., Roudier, V., Didier-Bazes, M., Roussel, B., Tardy, M., and Jouvet, M. (1994). Effects of modafinil-induced wakefulness on glutamine synthetase regulation in the rat brain. *Brain Res. Mol. Brain Res.* 26(1/2), 123–128.
350. Dackis, C. A., Lynch, K. G., Yu, E., Samaha, F. F., Kampman, K. M., Cornish, J. W., Rowan, A., Poole, S., White, L., and O'Brien, C. P. (2003). Modafinil and cocaine: A double-blind, placebo-controlled drug interaction study. *Drug Alcohol Depend.* 70(1), 29–37.
351. Dackis, C. A., Kampman, K. M., Lynch, K. G., Pettinati, H. M., and O'Brien, C. P. (2005). A double-blind, placebo-controlled trial of modafinil for cocaine dependence. *Neuropsychopharmacology* 30(1), 205–211.
352. Shoptaw, S., Yang, X., Rotheram-Fuller, E. J., Hsieh, Y. C., Kintaudi, P. C., Charuvastra, V. C., and Ling, W. (2003). Randomized placebo-controlled trial of baclofen for cocaine dependence: Preliminary effects for individuals with chronic patterns of cocaine use. *J. Clin. Psychiatry* 64(12), 1440–1448.
353. Gonzalez, G., Sevarino, K., Sofuoglu, M., Poling, J., Oliveto, A., Gonsai, K., George, T. P., and Kosten, T. R. (2003). Tiagabine increases cocaine-free urines in cocaine-dependent methadone-treated patients: Results of a randomized pilot study. *Addiction* 98(11), 1625–1632.
354. Shank, R. P., Gardocki, J. F., Streeter, A. J., and Maryanoff, B. E. (2000). An overview of the preclinical aspects of topiramate: Pharmacology, pharmacokinetics, and mechanism of action. *Epilepsia* 41(Suppl 1), S3–S9.
355. Kampman, K. M., Pettinati, H., Lynch, K. G., Dackis, C., Sparkman, T., Weigley, C., and O'Brien, C. P. (2004). A pilot trial of topiramate for the treatment of cocaine dependence. *Drug Alcohol Depend.* 75(3), 233–240.

17

MDMA AND OTHER "CLUB DRUGS"

M. Isabel Colado[1], Esther O'Shea[1], and A. Richard Green[2]

[1]*Facultad de Medicina, Universidad Complutense, Madrid, Spain and* [2]*Institute of Neuroscience, School of Biomedical Sciences, Queen's Medical Centre, University of Nottingham, Nottingham, United Kingdom*

17.1	MDMA		614
	17.1.1	Introduction	614
	17.1.2	Reinforcing Properties	614
	17.1.3	Acute Biochemical and Behavioral Effects	616
		17.1.3.1 Monoamine Release in Brain	616
		17.1.3.2 Tryptophan Hydroxylase	617
		17.1.3.3 Effect on Neurotransmitter Receptors and Transporters	617
		17.1.3.4 Effect on Body Temperature	617
		17.1.3.5 Neuroendrocrine and Immune Responses following MDMA	618
		17.1.3.6 Effects on Behavior	618
	17.1.4	Long-Lasting Biochemical and Behavioral Effects: Neurotoxicity	619
		17.1.4.1 Long-Term Neurochemical Changes	619
		17.1.4.2 Experimental Studies with Similar Doses to that Consumed by Humans	620
		17.1.4.3 Mechanisms of Neurotoxicity	621
		17.1.4.4 Functional Consequences of Neurotoxic Lesion	629
	17.1.5	Biochemical and Functional Changes in Human Brain	631
17.2	GHB		632
	17.2.1	Pharmacological Effects	633
	17.2.2	Mechanism of Action	634
	17.2.3	GHB and Addiction	635
17.3	Ketamine		636
	17.3.1	Pharmacological Effects	636
17.4	Flunitrazepam (Rohypnol)		637
	17.4.1	Pharmacological Effects	637
17.5	LSD		637
	17.5.1	Pharmacological Effects	638
	17.5.2	Mechanism of Action	638
	17.5.3	Hallucinogens and Addiction	639
17.6	Summary		640
References			640

Handbook of Contemporary Neuropharmacology, Edited by David R. Sibley, Israel Hanin, Michael Kuhar, and Phil Skolnick. Copyright © 2007 John Wiley & Sons, Inc.

17.1 MDMA

17.1.1 Introduction

Gary Henderson, a pharmacist from the University of California, first coined the term "designer drugs" in the 1960s. Its purpose was to encompass substances of synthetic origin which were structurally and pharmacologically similar to existing substances (widely used illegal drugs) but which, due to their chemical novelty, had not been specifically listed and therefore escaped legal control. One group to appear on the scene is the methylenedioxy derivatives of amphetamine and methamphetamine, and of these, perhaps the best known and probably one of the most widely abused member is 3,4-methylenedioxymethamphetamine (MDMA), popularly known as "Ecstasy."

The first recorded mention of the compound is in a German patent filed by E. Merck in 1912 and granted in 1914, where it appears as a possible precursor of pharmacologically active compounds. The 1980s saw the rapid establishment of MDMA as a recreational drug of abuse. It became popular with North American university students among whom it came to be known under a number of different names: XTC, Adam, MDMA, M&M.

Concurrently, low-dose MDMA [75–175 mg, by mouth (p.o.)] was being used as an adjuvant in psychotherapy due to the apparent ability of the drug to reduce anxiety and psychological defense barriers, increase self-confidence, and facilitate communication between therapist and patient.

In 1985, the U.S. Drug Enforcement Administration (DEA) placed MDMA in Schedule I of the Controlled Substances Act due to its high potential for abuse, lack of clinical application, disagreement among experts as to its safety under medical supervision, and evidence that 3,4-methylenedioxyamphetamine (MDA), a related compound and principal metabolite of the drug, produced degeneration of serotonergic terminals in rat brain.

The drug is taken orally in the form of tablets and generally consumed at weekends, often at dance clubs, or "raves." Ecstasy tablets are available in a wide variety of colors, shapes, and sizes, each decorated with a different design or logo. It produces a series of subjective symptoms and sensations among which the most frequent include an increase in empathy, that is, a sense of closeness to other people, an emotional opening up, an increased ability and willingness to communicate, a reduction in negative thoughts and inhibitions, a heightened sense of perception of sound, color, and touch, an increase in locomotor activity, insomnia, and an increase in alertness. These effects appear in the first 20–60 min after a single dose, reaching a maximal effect after 60–90 min and lasting 3–5 h.

17.1.2 Reinforcing Properties

There have been several studies on the rewarding properties of MDMA, and these studies generally implicate dopamine in the actions of the drug. Systemic MDMA administration has been shown to increase extracellular dopamine in the mesolimbic forebrain, namely the nucleus accumbens (NAc) [1–3]. The NAc is responsible for the incentive motivational properties of most drugs of abuse, and the rewarding effects of MDMA have been shown using the appropriate paradigms. Thus, rats treated with MDMA developed a positive and dose-dependent response in the conditioned place preference (CPP) test [2, 4–6]. Since CPP is believed to be a measure of appetitive behavior, where the animal associates contextual cues with either a positive or negative feeling produced by the drug, these results provide direct evidence of the rewarding properties of MDMA in rats. A rewarding effect of MDMA has also been shown in the self-stimulation paradigm in rats [7], where MDMA lowers the reward threshold of electrical stimulation, and in the drug self-administration test in rats [8, 9] and baboons [10]. The locomotor hyperactivity observed after MDMA injection is also consistent with this drug exerting a positive rewarding effect [11, 12]. In order to determine whether dopaminergic mechanisms mediate the reinforcing effects of MDMA, Daniela and coinvestigators [9] have evaluated the effects of the D_1 receptor antagonist 7-chloro-8-hydroxy-3-methyl-1-phenyl-2,3,4,5-tetrahydro-1H-3-benzazepine hydrochloride (SCH 23390) on MDMA self-administration and compared them to the effects on MDMA-induced hyperactivity. SCH 23390 pretreatment produced a dose-dependent decrease in MDMA-induced hyperactivity and a rightward shift in the dose–response curve for MDMA self-administration. These data indicate that dopamine plays a key role in the hyperactivity that follows MDMA injection and suggest that MDMA self-administration, like the self-administration of other drugs of abuse, is dependent on the activation of dopaminergic substrates.

Recently, it has been suggested that the rewarding effects of MDMA are more pronounced at high ambient temperature and that the enthusiasm of recreational users for consuming the drug in hot environments might not be coincidental. It has been shown that an elevation of ambient room temperature enhanced the prosocial effects of MDMA and the number of MDMA infusions self-administered by rats [13]. In addition, the neurochemical changes related to rewarding effects of MDMA are more pronounced when the drug is given at high ambient room temperature [14]. By means of in vivo microdialysis, it has been shown that elevation of ambient temperature enhances the effect induced by low and medium doses of MDMA on dopamine release in the shell of the NAc, but not the striatum, of freely moving rats. The output of serotonin (5-HT) is also enhanced in the NAc, but not the striatum, by high ambient temperature conditions. Taken together, it seems reasonable to propose that the enhanced mesolimbic dopamine release seen at high ambient temperature is responsible for the changes seen by Cornish and coinvestigators [13].

It is also possible that previous exposure to MDMA may increase the reinforcing effects of other psychostimulants such as cocaine and amphetamine. There is strong experimental evidence indicating that rats treated with MDMA subsequently develop enhanced behavioral and biochemical responses to psychomotor stimulants. Studies have shown that in animals pretreated with MDMA cocaine produces a greater increase in the extracellular levels of dopamine in the NAc than that seen in control rats [15]. If the reinforcing effect of cocaine is dependent, in part, upon increased dopamine release in the NAc, these data suggest that MDMA may increase vulnerability to cocaine abuse. Subsequently, using the appropriate paradigms, it has been shown that rats pretreated with MDMA show a significantly greater CPP response to cocaine than vehicle-treated animals [16] although this may depend on the protocol of MDMA administration since another study failed to confirm this [17]. In mice, adolescent exposure to MDMA increased hyperlocomotion and facilitated the reinstatement of cocaine-seeking behavior, as assessed by CPP after a 14-day drug-free period [18]. These results provide direct evidence of an increase in the rewarding properties of cocaine in rats preexposed to MDMA and suggest that MDMA abuse leads to increased vulnerability to cocaine addiction and dependence. In fact, preexposure to a high dose of MDMA facilitates acquisition of cocaine self-administration in rats [19], which again confirms that MDMA preexposure sensitizes rats to the reinforcing effects of cocaine.

The effect of MDMA on the acquisition of intravenous amphetamine self-administration and the reinstatement of amphetamine-seeking behavior by either MDMA or amphetamine has been recently evaluated [20]. Preexposure to a 5-HT-depleting regimen of MDMA slows the acquisition of amphetamine self-administration but may sensitize animals to the locomotor stimulating and priming effects of MDMA on drug-seeking behavior. Therefore, it seems likely that MDMA exposure may result in an enhanced sensitivity to psychostimulants and that this is a vulnerability to relapse that may be rather long-lasting.

Consequently, and although we must be extremely cautious when extrapolating results from animals to humans, it would be reasonable to propose that MDMA users may be at greater risk of developing addiction and dependence to other psychomotor stimulants.

17.1.3 Acute Biochemical and Behavioral Effects

17.1.3.1 Monoamine Release in Brain. MDMA is an amphetamine compound, and therefore, like other compounds of this class, its primary property is the release of monoamines in the brain.

MDMA administration produces an acute rapid release of 5-HT in the rat brain. This has been demonstrated both by in vivo microdialysis [21–23] and the decreased concentration of 5-HT in cerebral tissue taken from treated animals [24–26]. These references reflect only a few of the many studies that have reported these changes. The release occurs in all the major forebrain regions [27] and is inhibited by prior administration of 5-HT selective uptake blockers such as fluoxetine [23]. MDMA-induced 5-HT release can also be demonstrated in vitro by using brain slices [28] or synaptosomal preparations [29].

MDMA is also a potent compound in inducing dopamine release, and again this has been demonstrated using in vivo microdialysis [1, 30, 31] and in vitro using cerebral tissue slices [28].

The role of the dopamine uptake site in MDMA-induced dopamine release is controversial [32], and Mechan and coinvestigators [23] have suggested that MDMA may enter the dopamine terminal primarily by diffusion rather than via the uptake carrier site.

The role of 5-HT release in inducing dopamine efflux is indicated by the fact that pretreatment with fluoxetine attenuates MDMA-induced dopamine release in the striatum [33] and administration of a 5-HT agonist will enhance dopamine release [30]. Since ritanserin attenuates MDMA-induced dopamine release [22], it is reasonable to propose that MDMA can modify dopamine release by enhancing the efflux of 5-HT, which then acts on 5-HT$_{2A/2C}$ receptors.

While in vitro evidence suggests that MDMA can enhance norepinephrine release from brain tissue [34] and from synaptosomes [35], in vivo microdialysis data are presently lacking.

17.1.3.2 Tryptophan Hydroxylase. MDMA administration inhibits the activity of tryptophan hydroxylase in the brain [36–38] and this effect is very rapid [37]. Inhibition is still observable two weeks after a single dose of MDMA [39]. Since tryptophan hydroxylase is the rate-limiting enzyme involved in 5-HT synthesis, this indicates that a proportion of the 5-HT loss seen soon after MDMA administration may be due to hydroxylase inhibition rather than release, while the long-term decrease in cerebral 5-HT content following MDMA may be due in part to inhibition of the enzyme rather than neurotoxicity (see later).

Since MDMA has no direct inhibitory action on the enzyme in vitro [39], it is possible that the inhibition seen in vivo results from the action of an MDMA metabolite, an hypothesis supported by the finding that the MDMA quinone derivative can inactivate the enzyme [40].

17.1.3.3 Effect on Neurotransmitter Receptors and Transporters. MDMA binds to the 5-HT, dopamine, and norepinephrine transporters, although its affinity for the 5-HT site is at least 10 times higher than for the other monoamine transporter sites [41, 42].

MDMA binds with a 1–10 µM affinity for $5-HT_2$, α-adrenergic, M_1 muscarinic, and H_1 histaminic sites. Other sites (including $5-HT_1$) are in the 10–100 µM range while dopamine D_1 and D_2 sites are >100 µM [42].

17.1.3.4 Effect on Body Temperature. The effect of MDMA on body temperature has been investigated extensively in experimental animals, partly because there is a clear clinical correlate.

MDMA produces a rapid hyperthermic response in rats housed in normal or warm room conditions ($\leq 20°C$) with a peak of 1–2°C above normal rectal temperature [43–46]. The response is dose dependent [47]. When the rats are present in a cool ambient room temperature ($<19°C$), the effect of MDMA is to produce a hypothermic response [45, 48, 49].

If the rats are in a warm environment, the MDMA-induced hyperthermia is greater than in a normal environment [48, 50] (Fig. 17.1). Furthermore, giving divided doses over several hours to mimic "binge dosing" (but with the same total dose administered) results in a greater peak response than after a single dose [50] (Fig. 17.1).

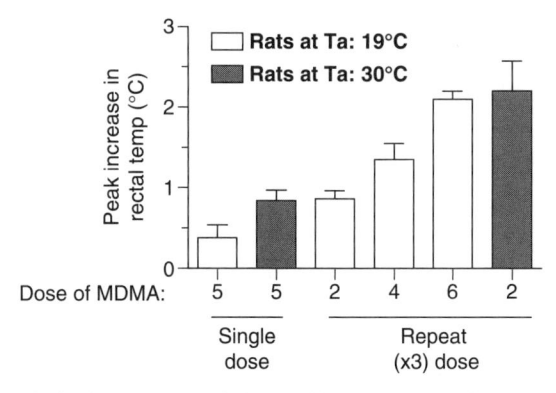

Figure 17.1 Effect of single or repeated doses (binge dosing) of MDMA (mg/kg) on peak rectal temperature increase in Dark Agouti rats housed at ambient temperature (T_a) of either 19 or 30°C. Doses of MDMA are shown.

The rise in rectal temperature appears to result from the action of the dopamine released by MDMA, on dopamine D_1 receptors, since the effect was antagonized by the D_1 antagonist SCH 23390, but not the D_2 antagonist remoxipride [23]. However, the hypothermia seen after MDMA is given to rats in a cool environment is dopamine D_2 receptor mediated, since remoxipride blocks the effect while SCH 23390 is without effect (Green and coinvestigators, unpublished).

Gordon and coinvestigators [51] found that the metabolic rate increased when MDMA was given to rats housed at 20°C, together with an increase in evaporative water loss. This suggests increased thermogenesis. This interpretation is supported by the fact that there is an involvement of the hypothalamic–pituitary–thyroid axis in the response [52] and crucially that β_3 adrenoceptors are involved, which indicates an action in brown adipose tissue [53]. Heat loss mechanisms do not appear to be activated immediately to compensate for the thermogenesis, since the tail temperature does not rise following MDMA [23] (the tail is a major heat loss organ in the rat [54]).

It has been known for many years that grouping mice increases the hyperthermic effect of amphetamine and increases its toxicity compared to the effect of the drug when given to individually housed animals [55]. Recently, Fantegrossi and coinvestigators [56] observed that the same phenomenon occurred when MDMA was examined in both singly housed and grouped mice. This has implications for the recreational use of MDMA in humans since the drug is primarily used in hot, crowded club conditions.

17.1.3.5 Neuroendrocrine and Immune Responses following MDMA. The monoamine release by MDMA initiates neuroendocrine changes. In rats both serum corticosterone and prolactin concentrations increase after MDMA [43], with the corticosterone response lasting over 4 h and the prolactin more than 1 h. The corticosterone response was dose dependent and blocked by ketanserin, suggesting an involvement of 5-HT.

Both aldosterone and renin also increase after MDMA administration to rats, and again, the aldosterone rise appears to be induced through increased 5-HT release [57]. In vitro studies have also demonstrated MDMA-induced oxytocin and vasopressin release in hypothalamic tissue [58, 59].

Several studies have demonstrated that MDMA can alter the immune function of the rat. Leucocyte counts are reduced for several hours after MDMA, as is concanavalin A–induced lymphocyte proliferation. This suggests that the drug produces a sustained suppression of mitogen-stimulated lymphocyte proliferation as well as leucocyte count and indicates a suppression of immune function [60].

17.1.3.6 Effects on Behavior. Since MDMA releases 5-HT from the nerve ending, it is not surprising that it can produce aspects of the *serotonin behavioral syndrome* [44, 61–63]. This syndrome was first described by Grahame-Smith [64] and consists of head weaving, reciprocal forepaw treading, proptosis, piloerection, and salivation. MDMA also produces a dose-dependent increase in locomotor activity [65], which can be antagonized by N-[4-methoxy-3-(4-methyl-1-piperazinyl)]-2'-methyl-4'-(5-methyl-1,2,4-oxadiazol-3-yl) [1,1-biphenyl]-4 carboxamide hydrochloride monohydrate (GR127935), a 5-$HT_{1B/1D}$ antagonist, but not by N-(2-[4-(2-methoxy-phenyl)-1-piperazinyl] ethyl)-N-(2-pyridinyl) cyclohexane trihydrochloride (WAY100635), a 5-HT_{1A}

antagonist. However, the work of Bankson and Cunningham [66] has emphasized the complexity of the hyperactivity response by showing the possible involvement of 5-HT$_{2B/2C}$ receptor function. Acute MDMA administration has been examined in various tests of anxiety-like behavior and data still remain somewhat conflicting. In the elevated-plus maze test Morley and McGregor [67] found the drug to produce an anxiogenic-like effect in rats. However, in the social interaction test an anxiolytic-like effect was seen. In contrast, Bhattacharya and coinvestigators [68] observed an anxiogenic effect in both tests. Lin and coinvestigators [69] saw an anxiogenic effect in mice exposed to the elevated-plus maze following low doses of the drug but an anxiolytic effect following high-dose administration. An anxiogenic effect was also reported to occur following MDMA administration to mice when the social interaction test was used [70].

17.1.4 Long-Lasting Biochemical and Behavioral Effects: Neurotoxicity

MDMA produces a characteristic biphasic neurochemical response which can be divided into acute effects, consisting of changes in cerebral biochemistry which are reversible, and long-term effects, including biochemical and structural changes in the brain which are persistent and are considered to reflect neurotoxicity.

MDMA administration produces a marked and rapid (3–4-h) depletion of 5-HT in several brain regions [71]. There is a recovery of brain 5-HT concentration within 24 h, but this is followed within three to four days by a long-term decrease which is unequivocal and which lasts for several months [71, 72]. This second phase of monoamine loss reflects neurodegenerative changes in serotonergic nerve terminals that have occurred, and it has been demonstrated in rats, guinea pigs, and several species of nonhuman primates. In mice the response is quite different, for while MDMA also behaves as a neurotoxin, it produces a reduction in the number of dopaminergic nerve terminals in striatum but leaves 5-HT-containing neurons intact. It is worth emphasizing that neurotoxicity in mice requires repeated injection of MDMA and also higher doses than those used in rats.

17.1.4.1 Long-Term Neurochemical Changes. There is clear and unequivocal evidence for a substantial and sustained long-term neurotoxic loss of 5-HT nerve terminals in several regions of the rat brain [31, 71, 73–77]. The degeneration has been demonstrated histologically [78, 79] and biochemically and is reflected in a substantial decrease in tryptophan hydroxylase activity; a reduction in the concentration of 5-HT and its metabolite, 5-hydroxyindoleacetic acid (5-HIAA); a decrease in the density of 5-HT uptake sites labeled with [^{3}H]paroxetine [77, 80–82]; and a reduction in the immunoreactivity of fine 5-HT axons in the neocortex, striatum, and hippocampus [78]. The dose required to induce neurotoxicity in rats is strain dependent. For example, Dark Agouti rats require a single dose (10–15 mg/kg) of MDMA to produce a clear 30–50% or greater loss in cerebral 5-HT content [47, 83] while strains such as Sprague–Dawley, Hooded-Lister, and Wistar require repeated and higher doses of MDMA (often 20 mg/kg or more) [44, 63, 84].

Although the neurotoxic potential of MDMA is well established, there is relatively little information on the fate of lesioned 5-HT neurons. Some authors have suggested that there is a substantial recovery of 5-HT function after MDMA-induced lesions in rodents [85–90]. While rats exposed to repeated administration of MDMA (10 mg/kg) show a marked reduction (60–80%) of 5-HT transporters in the hippocampus, striatum, and cerebral cortex 2 weeks after dosing, some signs of recovery are observed in all brain areas at 16 weeks, and by 32 weeks the recovery is complete in the striatum and cerebral cortex [88]. Immunohistochemical data confirm these biochemical results and show that the recovery of 5-HT presynaptic markers is due to the regeneration of 5-HT-containing axons [79, 88]. Axonal reinnervation refers to fine 5-HT axons coming from the dorsal raphe nucleus, which are the axons selectively lesioned by MDMA [78, 91], while thicker and varicose axons coming from medial raphe nucleus are not affected by MDMA [78, 91] and do not show any evidence of collateral ramification [79]. Nevertheless, the pattern of reinnervation is anomalous, since distal brain areas such as the neocortex remain denervated while proximal areas such as the hypothalamus appear either reinnervated or hyperinnervated [92]. Together, these results confirm the plasticity of central 5-HT neurons [93, 94] and indicate that under specific conditions 5-HT neurons have recovered from the MDMA-induced damage. Nevertheless, although the effects of MDMA in rodents seem to be partially reversible, they are probably permanent in primates. Insel and coinvestigators [95] observed significant 5-HT deficits in the hippocampus, striatum, and cortex of the *Maccacus rhesus* 14 weeks after repeated administration of MDMA. Similar results have been found in the hippocampus, caudate nucleus, and frontal cortex of squirrel monkeys 18 months after dosing [96]. In a study carried out seven years after MDMA dosing, Hatzidimitriou and coinvestigators [97] found that 5-HT axon density is only 50–65% of control values in neocortical regions. These data suggest that the 5-HT axons in nonhuman primates do not recover from MDMA-induced damage, and this information is particularly significant since it could be indicative of what happens in human beings, considering that the dose given to nonhuman primates is similar to that taken by humans.

17.1.4.2 Experimental Studies with Similar Doses to that Consumed by Humans. Recreational Ecstasy users tend to believe that the doses administered to experimental animals to induce toxicity are much higher than those that they use and that the data obtained are not relevant to human use. They therefore conclude that MDMA is a safe drug. Ecstasy tablets have been reported to contain generally between 70 and 150 mg [98], which is equivalent to 1–2 mg/kg of MDMA in a 70-kg human. However, Ecstasy is often ingested repeatedly in such a way that it is frequent for an individual to consume several tablets during a weekend [99]. What is perhaps most important is the *exposure* to the drug, and measurement of plasma levels is particularly important for that assessment. However, this measurement is rarely made in experimental animals. Nevertheless, the study of Colado and coinvestigators [83] did show that a single dose of MDMA of 10 mg/kg administered to Dark Agouti rats produced a plasma level of MDMA of near 10 nmol/mL 45 min later. Similar values have been observed clinically in overdose cases. This therefore suggests that dosing schedules in rats are often producing exposure that is not markedly different from those experienced by recreational users.

Several studies have been performed modeling the doses and dosing schedules of MDMA often used by human recreational users. O'Shea and coinvestigators [47] administered MDMA to Dark Agouti rats at the dose of 4 mg/kg once or twice daily for four consecutive days. The rats were killed seven days after dosing. Once-daily injection had no effect on regional brain concentration of 5-HT and 5-HIAA, while twice-daily administration resulted in a substantial depletion in all brain areas examined. These data thus indicate that high or frequent doses of MDMA are required to produce neurotoxic damage.

Studies giving low and repeated doses of MDMA have also been performed in nonhuman primates, and these showed that neurotoxic effects are more pronounced than those observed in rodents [100]. For example, administration of 2.5 mg/kg MDMA twice daily for four consecutive days produced 44% depletion of 5-HT in the somatosensory cortex of the monkey [101], while to obtain similar depletion in the brain of Dark Agouti rats, it is necessary to administer 4 mg/kg MDMA when following the same dosing protocol [47].

The degree of 5-HT depletion may also be dependent upon the route of administration, although data on this point are conflicting. While similar neurotoxic effects were observed in rats following oral or subcutaneous dosing [102], oral administration in monkeys seemed to be less effective than subcutaneous injection [103]. In contrast, Kleven and coinvestigators [104] obtained a more marked effect of the drug when it was given to rhesus monkeys by the intragastric route rather than subcutaneously.

A practice sometimes employed by recreational users of Ecstasy is "binge" dosing, comprising the ingestion of several doses on a single occasion [105, 106]. This type of dosing has been recently modeled by administering three doses of MDMA (2, 4, or 6 mg/kg) 3 h apart and evaluating its consequences on the long-term neurotoxic effects of MDMA when administered to rats housed either at 19°C or in a room kept at 30°C to simulate the way in which the drug is sometimes taken by human beings in a hot, dance club environment [107]. At 19°C MDMA produced a dose-dependent long-term loss of 5-HT in several brain regions with an approximate 50% loss following 3 × 4 mg/kg and a 65% decrease following 3 × 6 mg/kg. When MDMA at the dose of 4 mg/kg was injected repeatedly to rats housed at 30°C, a larger long-term 5-HT depletion (65%) than that found in rats treated at 19°C was observed, the effect being similar to that produced by the dose of 6 mg/kg given at 19°C ambient temperature.

17.1.4.3 *Mechanisms of Neurotoxicity.*

17.1.4.3.1 Neurotoxic Metabolite. The toxicity induced by MDMA in both rat and mouse is mediated by one or more metabolites of the drug that have been formed peripherally. Evidence for this in rats stems from the fact that central administration of MDMA does not produce reductions in the concentrations of 5-HT in various terminal fields [108–110] in spite of brain concentrations being greater than those following systemic administration of a neurotoxic dose of the drug [110]. Central administration of the MDMA did, however, produce an increase in 5-HT release in the hippocampus, and dopamine release in the striatum, similar to that produced by systemic administration [31, 110], suggesting that whereas the neurotoxic effects of the drug are produced by a peripherally formed metabolite, the acute effects are induced by the parent compound.

In contrast to that which occurs in the rat, recent studies indicate that in mice MDMA is responsible for neither the acute nor the long-term effects of the drug [111]. Intrastriatal administration of MDMA does not reproduce the reduction in dopamine and the changes in 3,4-dihydroxyphenylacetic acid (DOPAC) and homovanillic acid (HVA) observed following systemic administration.

The lack of neurotoxicity following the central administration of the drug has led to numerous studies on the peripheral metabolism of MDMA, mostly in the rat. One of the principal metabolites of MDMA in this species is MDA, the product of N demethylation via the CYP1A2 isoform of the cytochrome P450 monooxygenase system. This compound exhibits a similar profile but higher potency as a serotonergic neurotoxicant than MDMA and, like MDMA, is not toxic when injected directly into the brain [108]. Thus, MDA may be an intermediate product but is not the final neurotoxic metabolite.

The drug can undergo various other routes of metabolism (O demethylenation, deamination, and hydroxylation) and conjugation (O methylation, O glucuronidation, and O sulfation), giving rise to 17 in vivo metabolites [112–114], several of which have been tested in vivo. None, however, has been found to produce the same pattern of toxicity as that produced by systemic MDMA. Thus, aromatic hydroxylation gives rise to 6-hydroxy-MDMA [114, 115], which is demethylated by CYP2D1 to yield 2,4, 5-trihydroxymethamphetamine [112, 113], both of which have been shown to produce a different profile of toxicity to MDMA—either lack of toxic effect or toxicity of both the 5-HT and dopamine neurotransmitter systems, respectively [116, 117].

Direct demethylation of MDMA or MDA by CYP2D1 gives rise to 3,4-dihydroxymethamphetamine (HHMA; N-methyl-α-methyldopamine, N-Me-α-Me DA) and its demethylated equivalent, 3,4-dihydroxyamphetamine (HHA; α-methyldopamine, α-Me DA), which are unstable reactive catechol derivatives that may in turn form quinones that can auto-oxidize and produce free radicals. Alternatively, these catechols can undergo O methylation at position 3 or 4 of the aromatic ring to form 3-hydroxy-4-methoxy(meth)amphetamine [4-O-methyl-α-(methyl)dopamine, 4-O-Me-α-(Me) DA] or 4-hydroxy-3-methoxy(meth)amphetamine [3-O-methyl-α-(methyl)dopamine, 3-O-Me-α-(Me) DA]. Neither α-Me DA nor 3-O-Me-α-Me DA produce serotonergic toxicity [118].

In recent years, the glutathione-formed conjugates of the quinones that are discussed above have been suggested as possible neurotoxic metabolites of the drug [119, 120]. Thus, a putative metabolite adduct, 5-(glutathion-S-yl)-α-Me DA, crosses the blood–brain barrier by means of the glutathione carrier [121] and is neurotoxic to 5-HT terminals following repeated intracerebral injection [119]. Addition of a further glutathione molecule to 5-(glutathion-S-yl)-α-Me DA yields 2,5-(glutathion-S-yl)-α-Me DA, which is a more potent neurotoxin [119]. Once in the brain these compounds can be further metabolized to cysteine or acetylcysteine adducts which are more potent toxins [119, 120, 122]. Jones and coinvestigators [122] recently identified glutathione and N-acetyl cysteine conjugates of N-Me-α-Me DA in rat striatal dialysate after subcutaneous MDMA administration. Furthermore, inhibition of γ-glutamyl transpeptidase increases the toxicity produced by MDMA and MDA and the levels of the N-acetyl cysteine adducts in brain by increasing the pool of the thioether compounds available for transport by the glutathione carrier [121, 122].

In the mouse, no studies have been carried out on products of metabolism, although Escobedo and coinvestigators [111] found that the major compound in brain following peripheral MDMA administration is MDMA itself. This is in sharp contrast to what is observed in rats, where MDA is the major metabolite at low doses, and in humans, where HHMA predominates [123]. Further studies on the different profiles of metabolism in the rat and mouse are required in order to evaluate if these differences could account for the neurotoxic selectivity of the drug in the different animal species.

17.1.4.3.2 Oxidative Stress. There is much experimental evidence indicating that a major mechanism by which MDMA induces damage to 5-HT-containing neurons in the rat brain is by inducing an oxidative stress process [77, 124] which is ultimately reflected by an increase in lipid peroxidation in several brain areas [125]. Two factors contribute to this process, a decrease in the antioxidant capacity of the brain reflected as a reduction in vitamin E and ascorbate levels [126] and an increase in the formation of hydroxyl-free radicals [77, 127]. The use of intracerebral microdialysis has demonstrated that systemic administration of MDMA increases the formation of 2,3-dihydroxybenzoic acid (2,3-DHBA) from salicylate in hippocampal and striatal dialysates of rats and mice [77, 128–130], a conversion that only occurs in the presence of a high concentration of hydroxyl-free radicals. Administration of the hydroxyl radical scavenger α-phenyl-*N*-*tert*-butyl nitrone (PBN) abolished the MDMA-induced rise in 2,3-DHBA and attenuated neurotoxic damage and did so without altering MDMA-induced hyperthermia [77, 127]. Other free-radical scavenging drugs have also been found to protect against MDMA-induced damage. Thus, administration of large doses of sodium ascorbate or L-cysteine 30 min prior to and 5 h following MDMA injection prevented the long-term depletion of 5-HT induced by MDMA [131]. Ascorbic acid administration also suppressed hydroxyl radical formation in the striatum [126]. The metabolic antioxidant α-lipoic acid injected repeatedly (up to two days after MDMA) also totally prevented the reduction in the number of 5-HT transporters observed seven days after MDMA dosing [132]. In addition to hydroxyl radicals, nitrogen-reactive species are also involved in MDMA-induced neurotoxicity. Gudelsky's team [133] found evidence for the involvement of nitric oxide in MDMA-induced serotonergic neurotoxicity. A multiple-dose regimen of MDMA produced a significant increase in levels of nitrotyrosine and nitric oxide in the striatum. Pretreatment with the neuronal nitric oxide synthase (NOS) inhibitor *S*-methyl-L-thiocitrulline (*S*-MTC) afforded neuroprotection against MDMA-induced 5-HT depletion without attenuating MDMA-induced hyperthermia. In addition, administration of NOS inhibitors, as well as a peroxynitrite decomposition catalyst, attenuated the long-term depletion of striatal 5-HT and dopamine depletion produced by the local perfusion of MDMA and malonate.

In mice there is also evidence for a key role of oxygen- and nitrogen-reactive species in the MDMA-induced neurotoxicity on dopamine neurons. Pretreatment with either of the NOS inhibitors *S*-MTC and N-(4-(2-((3-chlorophenyl methyl)amino)-ethyl)-phenyl) 2-thiopene carboxamidine hydrochloride (AR-R17477AR) provided significant neuroprotection against the long-lasting MDMA-induced dopamine depletion, and AR-R17477AR prevented the rise in 2,3-DHBA levels in striatal dialysates of the mice [129]. Also supporting the suggestion that free-radical formation is responsible for MDMA-induced neurotoxicity is the study in which mice fed a selenium-deficient diet showed an enhancement of the long-term dopamine depletion and, strikingly, also a long-term loss of 5-HT content in several brain areas, an effect not observed in mice maintained with a standard diet [134]. This effect is due to an impairment of the antioxidant detoxification system mediated by glutathione, as these animals also show a decrease in the activity of glutathione peroxidase and an increase in the degree of lipid peroxidation [134]. In fact, MDMA administration to mice maintained with a standard diet caused a decrease in glutathione peroxidase and superoxide dismutase activities and an increase in lipid peroxidation in several regions of mouse brain [135]. Finally, transgenic mice overexpressing CuZn superoxide dismutase have been shown to be resistant to the neurotoxic action of MDMA [136]. A recent study by Fornai and coinvestigators [137] reported DNA oxidation and DNA single-strand breaks accompanied by increased clustering of heat shock protein-70 (HSP-70) in the nucleus close to chromatin filaments in the substantia nigra and striatum of mice seven days following repeated MDMA administration. The presence of ubiquitin-positive inclusion bodies has also been reported. These findings suggest that MDMA-induced oxidation involves neuronal cell bodies and extends to the nucleus of neurons.

The source of free-radical formation is controversial. There are data supporting a role for extracellular dopamine in producing free radicals and neurotoxic damage. However, other data fail to support this contention. According to the first hypothesis, dopamine, released massively after MDMA administration, is transported into the 5-HT-depleted terminals and deaminated by monoamine oxidase type B (MAO_B), resulting in the production of hydrogen peroxide and hydroxyl free radicals [128, 138]. This hypothesis fails to demonstrate why MDMA produces damage in brain areas with little dopaminergic innervation such as the hippocampus, where the reduction in several serotonergic parameters is even more pronounced and persistent than that detected in striatum. In addition, there are data indicating that administration of dopamine precursor 3,4-dihydroxy-L-phenylalanine (L-DOPA), while enhancing the MDMA-induced dopamine release in the striatal dialysate, nevertheless fails to alter the subsequent neurodegeneration in this region [31].

Free-radical formation is increased by the acute hyperthermia produced by MDMA administration, and the rise in 2,3-DHBA levels in cerebral dialysate was markedly inhibited when the hyperthermic response was prevented. This result provides a plausible explanation as to why hypothermia or normothermia is neuroprotective against MDMA-induced damage and why hypothermia is neuroprotective against other forms of neurodegeneration such as that produced by transitory cerebral ischemia [139, 140]. However, although hyperthermia markedly enhances free-radical production, neurodegeneration can occur in normothermic animals [47], so hyperthermia is not an absolute requirement for the expression of the neurotoxic damage.

The 5-HT nerve endings are the site of the enhanced free-radical formation since a prior 5-HT lesion (produced by pretreatment with fenfluramine) prevented the MDMA-induced rise in free-radical formation [77]. This proposal was supported by the subsequent study by Shankaran and coinvestigators [141], who found that fluoxetine attenuated the MDMA-induced free-radical production. This indicates that free-radical production occurs following the transport of MDMA or a neurotoxic metabolite into the 5-HT nerve terminal by activation of the 5-HT transporter.

17.1.4.3.3 Hyperthermia. In addition to being an immediate risk factor of exposure to MDMA, the drug-induced hyperthermia plays an important role in the development of neurotoxicity in experimental animals, and numerous studies have shown that the hyperthermic reaction following MDMA, although not essential, does modulate the degree of long-term damage. Thus, a close correlation has been found between the hyperthermic response and the degree of neurotoxicity in rats [48]. Animals maintained at an elevated room temperature (26–33°C) have an augmented hyperthermic response and show a greater degree of neurotoxicity [107, 142, 143]. In contrast, physical and pharmacological modifications that either attenuate or prevent the hyperthermic reaction induced by the drug attenuate or prevent the neurotoxic effect. Thus, the administration of MDMA to rats maintained at low ambient temperature (10°C) prevents the hyperthermic response and either attenuates or eliminates the long-term serotonergic toxicity [142, 144].

A similar observation has been made in the mouse where administration of the drug to mice at an ambient temperature of 15°C reduced body temperature by approximately 2°C and blocked the long-term dopaminergic damage [145]. Furthermore, restraint, which protects mice from the neurotoxic effects of MDMA, is thought to mediate its effect by lowering body temperature [146].

Further evidence for the importance of the hyperthermic response in the degree of neurotoxicity derives from neuroprotection studies. A number of compounds, including haloperidol, pentobarbital, reserpine, α-methyl dopamine, dizocilpine, and ketanserin, have been shown to be protective against the neurotoxic effects of MDMA in the rat because they prevent the hyperthermic response to the drug or produce hypothermia [31, 46, 143, 147, 148]. The protective effect of these compounds disappears when the temperature of the animals is kept similar to that in animals treated with just MDMA. Clomethiazole appears to possess a partial protective action which is independent of its temperature-lowering effects [149].

Despite the preceding evidence on the correlation between the magnitude of the acute hyperthermia and the degree of neurotoxic damage, MDMA may also cause neurotoxic damage in the absence of a hyperthermic response. The repeated administration of low-dose MDMA (4 mg/kg twice daily for four days) produced a substantial neurotoxic effect in Dark Agouti rats but caused only a slight increase in temperature above saline-treated controls after the first dose. This increase in temperature after the initial dose was not sufficient in itself to produce a neurotoxic effect [47]. In addition, high doses of MDMA have also been reported to produce serotonergic toxicity in the absence of a hyperthermic response [142].

Taken together, this evidence indicates that hyperthermia has an important modulatory role but is not an essential factor in the neurotoxicity induced by the drug. Other factors such as high doses or increased frequency of dosing are also important factors and may overcome a lack of hyperthermic response to produce neurotoxicity.

17.1.4.3.4 Monoaminergic Transporter. Evidence indicating a role of the 5-HT transporter in the long-term damage on 5-HT nerve terminals induced by MDMA is based on the findings that 5-HT transporter inhibitors prevent the long-lasting loss of 5-HT brain concentration. The first study showing the neuroprotective effect of fluoxetine against MDMA neurotoxicity is the report of Schmidt [71]. This study shows that coadministration of this selective 5-HT uptake inhibitor completely blocked the reduction in cortical 5-HT concentrations one week after MDMA. Administration of fluoxetine at various times after MDMA revealed that the long-term effects of the drug could be partially blocked by the uptake inhibitor as long as 6 h after drug administration. The neuroprotective effect of fluoxetine administered concurrently with MDMA was confirmed subsequently [46, 82, 141] and extended to fluvoxamine [82] (Fig. 17.2). Neither fluoxetine nor fluvoxamine altered MDMA-induced acute hyperthermic response [46, 82]. Fluoxetine continued to provide total protection when given up to four days before MDMA (Fig. 17.2), but fluvoxamine only produced neuroprotection when coadministered with MDMA (Fig. 17.2). This longer-lasting neuroprotective effect of fluoxetine might be due to the persistent

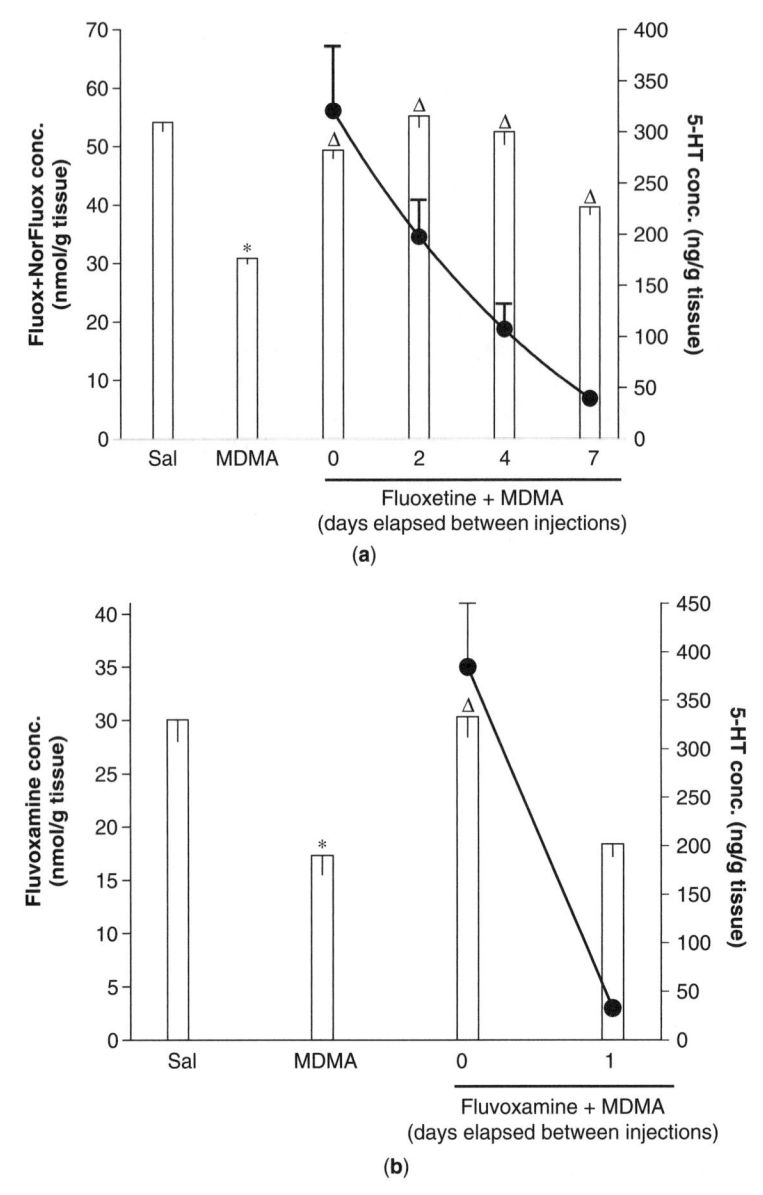

Figure 17.2 Effect of (a) fluoxetine and (b) fluvoxamine on MDMA-induced decrease in cortical 5-HT concentration 1 week after injection. Two injections of fluoxetine (10 mg/kg, i.p) with an interval of 60 min were given 2, 4, or 7 days before MDMA (15 mg/kg, i.p.). Two injections of fluvoxamine (15 mg/kg, i.p.) with an interval of 60 min were given 1 day before MDMA. A group of animals received fluoxetine or fluvoxamine 5 min before and 55 min after MDMA. Results are shown as mean ± standard error of the mean (SEM) ($n = 6$–16). Different from saline: ($*$) $p < 0.001$. Different from MDMA: (Δ) $p < 0.001$. Curves show the corresponding time course of fluoxetine plus norfluoxetine (a) and fluvoxamine (b) concentrations in cortex after administration of two doses of fluoxetine (10 mg/kg, i.p) or fluvoxamine (15 mg/kg, i.p.) with an interval of 60 min. Levels were measured at 0.5 h and 2, 4, and 7 days after the last dose of fluoxetine and at 0.5 h and 1 day after the last dose of fluvoxamine. Results are shown as mean ± SEM ($n = 5$ at each time point).

presence of fluoxetine and its main active metabolite norfluoxetine in the brain (Fig. 17.2). Both compounds inhibit the 5-HT transporter and could be blocking the entry of a toxic metabolite of MDMA into 5-HT nerve terminal [82]. In contrast to fluoxetine, fluvoxamine generates several metabolites, none of which appears to be pharmacologically active. Moreover, the parent compound undergoes a rapid plasma clearance in such a way that fluvoxamine brain concentrations are practically undetectable 24 h after injection (Fig. 17.2).

It has been reported that fluoxetine not only prevents MDMA-induced neurotoxicity but also inhibits hydroxyl radical formation [141]. Fluoxetine administration 1 h prior to or 4 h following MDMA administration reduced the MDMA-induced formation of 2,3-DHBA and also attenuated the MDMA-induced depletion of 5-HT in the striatum. As fluoxetine does not modify the in vitro generation of 2,3-DHBA, authors indicate that a potential mechanism by which fluoxetine attenuates the MDMA-induced formation of hydroxyl radicals is by preventing the entry into the 5-HT terminal of reactive substances that are capable of generating free radicals.

Not only is the long-term depletion of 5-HT dependent on the activation of the 5-HT transporter but, since fluoxetine is able to attenuate the immediate 5-HT release induced by MDMA in both the striatum [27] and hippocampus [23], it appears that acute MDMA-induced 5-HT release also involves a carrier-mediated mechanism.

Monoaminergic transporters also appear to be involved in MDMA-induced neurotoxicity in mice. MDMA induces a long-lasting depletion of dopamine concentration in the striatal neurons of the mouse, and administration of the dopamine uptake inhibitor GBR 12909 provides substantial protection [150]. Using in vivo microdialysis it has been shown that N-[4-methoxy-3-(4-methyl-1-piperazinyl)phenyl]-2′-methyl-4′-(5-methyl-1,2,4-oxadiazol-3-yl) [1,1-biphenyl]-4-carboxamide hydrochloride monohydrate (GBR 12909) inhibited the MDMA-induced increase in free-radical formation in the striatum and enhanced the acute release of dopamine induced by MDMA [130]. Altogether these data suggest that, in mice, (1) dopamine release does not involve a transporter-mediated mechanism, (2) MDMA probably enters into the dopamine nerve terminal by passive diffusion, (3) free-radical formation is not associated with dopamine release, and (4) free-radical-producing neurotoxic metabolites may enter the dopamine nerve ending via the dopamine uptake site.

17.1.4.3.5 Cytokines and Microglia. It is well established that cytokines such as interleukin-1β, interleukin-6, and tumor necrosis factor-α increase body temperature by acting through direct or indirect mechanisms on the brain. In particular, interleukin-1β has been shown to be involved in the development of the hyperthermic response induced by exogenous pyrogens such as lipopolysaccharide [151], turpentine [152], and leptin [153]. Administration of interleukin-1β antibodies or an interleukin-1 receptor antagonist to experimental animals inhibits the rise in temperature induced by these external inflammatory stimuli.

Recently, it has been shown that immediately following MDMA administration to rats there is an acute and dramatic increase in interleukin-1β concentration in the hypothalamus that appears at an early time point after MDMA administration and is of short duration, levels returning to basal values 12 h after drug injection [154]. A similar but less pronounced effect was observed in cortex. It is worth mentioning that under physiological conditions the hypothalamus produces significantly greater amounts of pro-interleukin-1β than frontal cortex and that this precursor is converted to its bioactive form and released in a more efficient way in the hypothalamus than in frontal cortex. Thus, pro-interleukin-1β immunoreactivity, caspase-1-like protease activity, and interleukin-1β levels are higher in the hypothalamus than in the frontal cortex [154, 155].

Interestingly, there was a clear dissociation in the time course of the changes induced by MDMA on body temperature and interleukin-1β release. While a marked hyperthermia was evident within the first 20 min of MDMA administration [44], with rectal temperature peaking 60 min after treatment and remaining elevated for over 12 h, the increase in levels of interleukin-1β peaked at 3 h [154]. These data, and the more definitive observation that intracerebroventricular administration of interleukin-1 receptor antibody did not modify the peak hyperthermic response immediately following MDMA, indicate that interleukin-1β production could be a consequence, rather than the cause, of hyperthermia and that hyperthermia could represent a signal generated by MDMA which occurs early enough to allow secretion of interleukin-1β and probably a host of other soluble factors from the microglia. In line with these results, when animals are kept at an ambient temperature of 4°C during MDMA treatment, the hyperthermic response is totally abolished and there is a significant reduction in interleukin-1β production. These data all indicate that release of interleukin-1β is, in part, a consequence of the hyperthermia [154].

The rise in interleukin-1β release following MDMA is accompanied by an enhancement of pro-interleukin-1β production and/or an increase in caspase-1-like protease activity, the enzyme required for maturation of interleukin-1β, in the frontal cortex but not in the hypothalamus [155]. Interleukin-1β is generated as an inactive 31-kDa precursor protein (pro-interleukin-1β) [156] which is proteolytically processed into the 17-kDa mature interleukin-1β by a specific intracellular cysteine protease, the interleukin-1β converting enzyme (ICE), also termed caspase-1 [156]. MDMA increased the immunoreactivity of pro-interleukin-1β in frontal cortex, not in hypothalamus, 3 and 6 h after administration. Caspase-1-like protease activity was increased in frontal cortex 3 h after MDMA injection compared with saline-treated animals. No change in caspase-1-like protease activity was observed in hypothalamus. Altogether these data indicate that MDMA alters, in a region-specific manner, the mechanisms which regulate interleukin-1β production in the brain of Dark Agouti rats and suggest that the release of interleukin-1β in hypothalamus may be regulated independently of caspase-1 activation.

In addition to increasing interleukin-1β release, MDMA also induced an increase in the density of peripheral benzodiazepine receptor binding sites, labeled with [^{3}H]PK 11195 [(1-(2-chlorophenyl)-*N*-methyl-*N*-(1-methylpropyl)3-isoquinolinecarboxamide)], in both the hypothalamus and cortex of the rat. This increase could be reflecting an activation of microglia as revealed by immunohistochemical studies in the anterior hypothalamus. However, and in contrast to the increase in interleukin-1β release, neither the upregulation of peripheral benzodiazepine receptor binding sites nor the staining for OX-42 (monoclonal antibody directed toward complement receptor 3), which stains activated microglia, was significantly modified when the hyperthermic response to MDMA was abolished. These results, together with the fact that the maximal microglial activation occurs 24 h after MDMA (when the hyperthermia induced by MDMA has disappeared), indicate that a hyperthermic response may not be necessary for the morphological changes that occur in the microglia.

17.1.4.4 Functional Consequences of Neurotoxic Lesion.

17.1.4.4.1 On Thermoregulation. While an MDMA-induced neurotoxic lesion does not alter the hyperthermic temperature response of rats to a further challenge dose of MDMA when the animals are housed in normal room temperature conditions (20°C), it does modify the response in rats housed in a warm (30°C) room. In such conditions, the hyperthermic response is prolonged compared to nonlesioned animals [50]. This prolongation appears to be due to the MDMA-induced loss of cerebral 5-HT since a prolonged response is also seen in rats pretreated with the 5-HT synthesis inhibitor *p*-chlorophenylalanine (PCPA) or either of the 5-HT antagonists methysergide and WAY 100635 [157]. The data suggest that a decrease in 5-HT function impairs heat loss in rats housed in warm conditions and is supported by the fact that PCPA pretreatment increases heat-induced mortality in rats housed at high ambient temperature [158, 159].

Other evidence indicates an MDMA-induced neurotoxic lesion can impair heat loss. When lesioned rats are placed in a warm environment and then returned to normal temperature conditions, their rectal temperature remains elevated for longer than control rats [49, 160]. Again normal heat loss mechanisms appear to have been impaired by the neurotoxic lesion. The experiment with WAY 100635 indicates the involvement of the $5-HT_{1A}$ receptor and it can be proposed that the lesion impairs 5-HT release onto $5-HT_{1A}$ receptors, thereby producing this defect in thermoregulation. No clinical studies have been performed, but the results suggest that heavy users of MDMA should exercise caution in using the drug in hot room conditions in order to avoid possible problems with hyperthermia.

17.1.4.4.2 On Behavior. Most experimental studies on MDMA have mainly focused on the behavioral changes associated with the immediate neurochemical effects induced by MDMA. There is relatively little information on the consequences of the long-lasting depletion of brain 5-HT induced by MDMA on behavioral and cognitive functions.

Marston and coinvestigators [161] performed a study to explore the posttreatment consequences of a 3-day neurotoxic exposure to MDMA in the rat using a variety of behavioral paradigms. Male Lister Hooded rats were injected twice daily with ascending doses of MDMA (10, 15, and 20 mg/kg) over 3 days and behavior was analyzed over the following 16 days. Three weeks after the period of exposure to MDMA, rats showed a persistent depletion of 5-HT (40–60%) in cortex, hippocampus, and striatum and no change in dopamine levels. MDMA exposure resulted in a lasting cognitive impairment as it was found that the MDMA-treated group did not show the progressive improvement in performance of the delayed nonmatched-to-place procedure seen in the control group. Delay-dependent impairments in accuracy are often attributed to perturbations in short-term memory and related systems. The level of locomotor activity of the MDMA-treated rats was significantly greater than the saline controls during the MDMA dosing period and 3 days later but thereafter was indistinguishable from control values. Different results have been reported by Wallace and coinvestigators [162] following administration of 10 mg/kg of MDMA four times 2 h apart to Sprague–Dawley rats and subsequent testing of diurnal and nocturnal spontaneous locomotor activity. Two weeks after dosing rats showed a depletion of striatal 5-HT content of approximately 50% and also exhibited significant reductions in both diurnal and nocturnal locomotor activity. This effect may be due to the reported regulatory actions of 5-HT on the sleep–wake cycle [163, 164]. In fact, rats with a significant reduction in the neocortical density of 5-HT transporter 3 weeks after exposure to a single 15-mg/kg dose of MDMA show long-term changes in regulation of circadian rhythms and sleep generation [165].

Prior MDMA exposure also alters anxiety-related behaviors, but results have been conflicting and may be dependent on the basal anxiety level of the rat strain being investigated [166]. Using the same paradigm for behavioral testing (elevated-plus maze), obtaining a similar decrease in cerebral 5-HT concentration (30–40% loss), and considering a similar delay for testing animals following MDMA administration (70–90 days posttreatment), Morley and coinvestigators [167] reported anxiety-like behaviors in Wistar rats while Mechan and coinvestigators [168] described an apparent anxiolytic response in Dark Agouti rats. It thus appears that a 5-HT lesion may produce an anxiolytic response in an anxious strain (Dark Agouti) but an anxiogenic response in strains displaying low endogenous anxiety (Wistar rats) [166].

Acute exposure of young Lister Hooded rats to MDMA produces a long-term anxiety-like behavioral response in the social interaction paradigm, even though there were only modest reductions in indole brain concentrations and no change in the density of cortical 5-HT transporters [167]. Similar results were obtained following exposure of young Wistar rats to low and repeated doses of MDMA, the anxiety-related behavior being accompanied by changes in 5-HT$_{2A}$ receptor function [169].

Recently McGregor's team [170] has performed a study to investigate the long-lasting behavioral and neurochemical effects of combined MDMA and methamphetamine administration in the rat. Animals received four injections, one every 2 h, of MDMA (2.5 or 5 mg/kg per injection) or methamphetamine (2.5 or 5 mg/kg per injection) given alone or in combined low doses (1.25 + 1.25 mg/kg per injection or 2 + 2 mg/kg per injection). Several weeks after drug administration, both MDMA + methamphetamine groups, both metamphetamine groups, and the higher dose MDMA group showed decreased social interaction relative to controls while both MDMA + methamphetamine groups and the lower dose MDMA group showed increased anxiety-like behavior on the emergence test. MDMA treatment caused 5-HT and 5-HIAA depletion in several brain regions, while methamphetamine treatment reduced dopamine in the prefrontal cortex. Combined MDMA + methamphetamine treatment caused 5-HT and 5-HIAA depletion in several brain regions and a unique depletion of dopamine and DOPAC in the striatum. These data have potentially important implications for public awareness as they demonstrate specific adverse behavioral and neurochemical effects of MDMA and methamphetamine given alone at relatively low doses in a novel one-day regimen. Results also show that coadministration of MDMA and methamphetamine leads to adverse effects that may be more pronounced and consistent than those observed with similar doses of MDMA or methamphetamine administered alone.

As mentioned above, the study of Marston and coinvestigators [161] was the first to report that administration of ascending doses of MDMA for three days resulted in an impaired cognitive behavior and a pronounced depletion of 5-HT brain concentration. Subsequently, Broening and coinvestigators [171] reported that exposure to MDMA in rats during stages analogous to early and late third-trimester human fetal brain development induces specific types of long-term learning and memory impairments. MDMA exposure on post natal days P11–P20 resulted in dose-related impairments of sequential learning and spatial learning and memory. These learning deficits reflect a developmentally specific vulnerability in that they were selective, affecting only those animals treated on P11–P20 and not those treated on P1–P10. The effects were also long term in that they were seen in the offspring as adults and not related to any long-term changes in 5-HT, dopamine, or noradrenaline.

An impairment of nonspatial working memory has also been reported in rats exposed to intermittent administration of MDMA every fifth day from P35 to P60 trying to model the typical intermittent MDMA human use pattern in adolescent Sprague–Dawley rats. Five days after dosing animals showed a significant reduction of about 25% in the density of 5-HT transporters in cerebral cortex, not in hippocampus [172].

In nonhuman primates there have been few studies performed to evaluate cognitive functions such as learning and memory. Frederick and coinvestigators [173–175] did not find any long-term alteration in performance on a number of operant tasks in rhesus monkeys exposed to neurotoxic doses of MDMA. Thus, repeated exposure to doses of MDMA sufficient to produce long-lasting changes in brain neurotransmitter systems results in residual effects (e.g., tolerance, sensitivity) on behavioral task performance when subjects are subsequently challenged with acute MDMA, whereas baseline (nonchallenged) performance of these tasks after such exposure generally remains unchanged. Similarly, Taffe and coinvestigators [176] found no apparent lasting effect induced by MDMA on a battery of cognitive/behavioral measures in rhesus monkeys with cerebrospinal fluid (CSF) 5-HIAA concentration reduced by 40–50%. Winsauer and coinvestigators [177] showed that neurotoxic doses of MDMA failed to disrupt learning in squirrel monkeys in spite of impairment being demonstrated following administration of fenfluramine. Nevertheless, although cognitive/behavioral measures performed in nonhuman primates following neurotoxic doses of MDMA are normal, brain stem auditory-evoked potentials are abnormal for a period of at least three months after MDMA dosing [176]. This long-lasting effect is consistent with a loss of 5-HT innervation of brain stem auditory nuclei and suggests that auditory pathways are much more sensitive to the deleterious effect of MDMA. It is interesting to note that studies which have failed to show memory impairment in human beings employed nonauditory tasks [178] while those reporting memory disruption showed some auditory memory task [179, 180].

17.1.5 Biochemical and Functional Changes in Human Brain

Neuroimaging studies performed on recreational users of MDMA have shown sustained reductions in brain 5-HT transporter density [181–183] which positively correlated with the extent of previous MDMA use [183] and duration of abstinence [182]. The effect might be more pronounced in women and reversible after prolonged abstinence [184, 185]. A reduction in the CSF 5-HIAA concentration has also been observed in recreational users of MDMA, the reduction being greater in females (46%) than in males (20%) [186, 187]. MDMA users show a downregulation of 5-HT$_{2A}$ receptors in the cerebral cortex while in the abstinent MDMA user group there is an upregulation of 5-HT$_{2A}$ receptors. The combined results of this study suggest a compensatory upregulation of postsynaptic 5-HT$_{2A}$ receptors in the occipital cortex of ex-MDMA users due to low synaptic 5-HT levels [188]. MDMA users do not appear to suffer any reduction in nigrostriatal dopamine neurons. However, subjects regularly using amphetamine in addition to MDMA did display a 20% loss in the density of striatal dopamine transporters [189].

Neuroendocrine tests have shown that abstinent MDMA users exhibit blunted cortisol and prolactin responses to fenfluramine challenge compared to controls, the prolactin response still being observed after one year of abstinence [190]. The presence of a long-lasting impairment of brain serotonergic function in recreational users of MDMA could potentially account for the reported cognitive and mood impairments, particularly when there is a relationship between the extent of lifetime consumption of MDMA and the severity of cognitive deficits [191–193].

Long-term MDMA use impairs performance in a multitude of cognitive abilities (most notably memory, learning, attention, executive function). Deficits in verbal and visual memory have been most frequently observed [180, 185, 193–195]. Users also show impaired verbal learning, are more easily distracted, and are less efficient at focusing attention on complex tasks [196–198].

Cognitive impairments have also been detected in a recent pilot study focused on adolescent MDMA users [199]. It appears that many of the neuropsychological performance problems reported to occur in MDMA users are not reversed by prolonged abstinence, suggesting the existence of a selective neurotoxic lesion [200]. It is essential to mention that many subjects are polydrug users; therefore, it cannot be stated unequivocally that any effect seen results solely from MDMA use. Cannabis users, whether or not they also used MDMA, showed significantly impaired memory function on word free recall and on immediate and delayed story recall compared to nonusers. The findings highlight the importance of controlling other drug use (particularly cannabis) when investigating persistent effects of MDMA in humans [201]. Gouzoulis-Mayfrank and coinvestigators [202] performed a comprehensive cognitive test battery on 28 recreational Ecstasy users with concomitant use of cannabis only and two equal-size matched groups of cannabis users and nonusers. The test battery included tests of attention, memory and learning, frontal lobe function, and general intelligence. Ecstasy users performed worse than one or both control groups in the more complex tests of attention, in memory and learning tasks, and in the tasks reflecting aspects of general intelligence. Poorer performance scores or longer reaction times in the working memory, verbal memory, and divided attention tasks were associated with heavier Ecstasy and heavier cannabis use. These results raise the concern that Ecstasy use, even in typical moderate recreational doses and possibly in conjunction with cannabis use, may lead to a subclinical cognitive decline in otherwise healthy young people.

Alternatively the problem may relate to the combination of MDMA with another recreational compound; a significant percentage of Ecstasy tablets contain psychoactive compounds other than MDMA. Therefore, although only MDMA and other amphetamine derivatives have been clearly demonstrated to produce neurotoxicity, the possibility cannot be ruled out that neurotoxicity is due to a combination of MDMA and other compounds ingested.

17.2 GHB

In recent years, γ-hydroxybutyric acid (GHB) has grown in popularity as a drug of abuse, due mainly to its ability to produce euphoria and promote relaxation, increase sociability, and produce a heightened sense of sexuality and an increased disinhibition similar to that produced by ethanol [203]. The drug is most commonly referred to on the street as "liquid Ecstasy" but also goes under the names "liquid X," "liquid E," "Grievous Bodily Harm" (a play-on-words with the initials), and "Salty Water" due to the slightly salty taste of its preparations. GHB is usually found as a clear, colorless liquid, almost tasteless with a slight salty taste which is easily masked in alcoholic drinks. These characteristics together with its amnesic and hypotonic effects have led to its use in some cases of "date rape."

The drug was first synthesized in 1960 [204] as an orally active analog of the neurotransmitter γ-aminobutyric acid (GABA), with the capacity to cross the blood–brain barrier [205]. Due to its ability to induce sleep and coma, its potential use as an anesthetic was explored, but its lack of sufficient analgesia and high incidence of vomiting as well as ability to cause convulsions limited its use.

The drug was first introduced into the North American market in the early 1990s as a dietary supplement available in health food shops for the treatment of anxiety and insomnia and to increase body mass in athletes and body builders. There have been reports of the therapeutic potential of GHB in the treatment of alcohol and opioid withdrawal, but such studies are far from conclusive [206–208].

Reports of its adverse effects followed soon after the introduction of GHB into the market [209], and this led to its prohibition, by the Food and Drug Administration (FDA), for use in humans except under medical prescription. In March 2000, the FDA reclassified GHB as a Schedule I controlled substance. In 2002, the FDA approved the use of GHB in patients suffering form narcolepsy with cataplexy. For this condition only, Xyrem was included in Schedule III of the Controlled Substances Act for medicinal use. Meanwhile the illegal use of GHB remains under the control of Schedule I [210].

GHB is a short-chain fatty acid found in mammalian brain [211] and was first identified in human brain in 1963 [212]. GHB is synthesized during the metabolism of the neurotransmitter GABA via an intermediate product, succinic semialdehyde, by means of the enzyme succinic semialdehyde reductase [213]. However, controversy exists as to whether GABA is the principal endogenous source of GHB. A marked reduction in GABA levels in the brain due to the administration of a glutamate decarboxylase inhibitor does not modify GHB levels [214]. In addition, GHB is found in peripheral tissues such as heart, kidney, and muscle at a higher concentration than that of GABA, suggesting an extraneuronal origin [215, 216]. It has been suggested that another compound in the brain, 1,4-butanediol, could also give rise to GHB by the action of alcohol dehydrogenase and aldehyde dehydrogenase [214, 217].

GHB is rapidly absorbed by oral administration [218], and its effects are evident after 15 min with peak plasma levels being reached between 30 and 60 min after consumption, depending on the dose [205, 219]. It does not bind significantly to plasma proteins [219]. Within the therapeutic range, GHB follows nonlinear pharmacokinetics. At low doses of 12.5 mg/kg the half-life is estimated at 20 min whereas higher doses exhibit longer half-lives. It is mainly eliminated by metabolism to carbon dioxide with only 2–5% being eliminated in urine [220].

17.2.1 Pharmacological Effects

GHB exhibits a steep dose–response curve leading to the appearance of adverse effects with a small increase in dose. The principal effects are those relating to the central nervous system (CNS) and cardiovascular and respiratory systems; GHB does not appear to affect the hepatic or renal systems [220]. For the most part, the adverse effects are acute in nature, appearing in the first 15 min and disappearing after 7 h.

Adverse effects on the CNS constitute the majority of GHB acute toxic reaction reports. They appear even at intermediate doses (25–50 mg/kg) and consist of sleepiness, dizziness, vertigo, and headaches [218, 219]. At higher doses it can cause the rapid onset of a state of coma (with no participation of the reticular activating system) which is short-lived and apparently fully reversible [221].

With regard to the cardiovascular system, GHB produces bradycardia both as an anesthesia inducer as well as in overdose with cardiac rhythms of fewer than 55 beats per minute having been recorded. Hypotension often accompanies the reduced heart rate.

Respiratory depression, difficulty breathing, and apnea have all been reported following GHB consumption [209, 220].

All the effects listed above are enhanced by ethanol such that the ingestion of both drugs together produces greater toxic effects than those produced by each drug taken alone [222]. In fact, 64% of the emergency room visits due to GHB involve the use of ethanol as well [223].

GHB also produces effects on the visual system, such as myopia and pupils unreactive to light, and the gastrointestinal system, such as nausea and vomiting, as well as motor effects such as clonic movements and uncontrollable shaking and slight hypothermia [209, 220, 224].

On occasion GHB has been associated with psychopathological symptoms such as hostile behavior, belligerence, and agitation. Other psychiatric symptoms such as delirium, paranoia, depression, and hallucinations have also been described [225].

Studies in humans, reports from emergency room admittances, as well as surveys and statements, all point toward a withdrawal syndrome of the characteristics produced by ethanol or benzodiazepine withdrawal. The syndrome appears 1–6 h after the last dose [226] and can last up to 15 days. Initial symptoms include insomnia, anxiety, agitation, tremors, nausea, and vomiting. This is followed by autonomic nervous system instability which manifests itself with diaphoresis, hypertension, shaking, and tachycardia. Following withdrawal after chronic or high-dose use, psychotic symptoms, hallucinations, and delirium have been described [227]. A prolonged abstinence syndrome period has been described which lasts between three and six months and is characterized by dysphoria, anxiety, memory problems, and insomnia. During this time the risk of relapse or development of ethanol or benzodiazepine dependence is high [228].

17.2.2 Mechanism of Action

The mechanism of action of GHB has not been completely elucidated. Although it was first synthesized as a GABA analog, early experimental evidence showed it to have different biochemical and behavioral effects.

There is a large body of evidence indicating that GHB produces many of its effects by means of interaction with the GABAergic system. GHB has no affinity for the $GABA_A$ receptor [229] but acts as a partial agonist at the $GABA_B$ receptor [230], although at concentrations higher than those normally found in the brain. In

GABA$_B$ ($-/-$) knockout mice, GHB does not produce hyperlocomotion, hypothermia, increases in dopamine synthesis, or increases in delta waves as measured by EEG, effects which are observed in wild-type mice [231]. Therefore, it appears that at least some of the effects produced by GHB are mediated by the GABA$_B$ receptor.

However, GHB does not consistently exhibit a GABA agonist profile, suggesting that it must act, at least in part, through some other mechanism. This naturally occurring compound has been proposed as a neurotransmitter or neuromodulator in its own right. GHB is found in high concentrations in the substantia nigra and hypothalamus [215, 232]. It is released from neurons in a calcium-dependent manner in response to potassium, and these neurons contain highly specific sodium-dependent uptake sites [233, 234]. In addition, G-protein-coupled GHB receptors have been located in dopaminergic areas on GABAergic and/or enkephalinergic neurons [235].

Regardless of the exact mechanism of action, exogenous administration of GHB has been shown to modulate various neurotransmitter systems, including the dopaminergic system. GHB inhibits the release of dopamine [236], and animals show sedation and a dose-dependent reduction in locomotor activity [231, 237]. The reduction in dopamine is inhibited by GABA$_B$ antagonists [238]. At high doses the rapid reduction in dopamine release is followed by an accumulation of tissue dopamine in the frontal cortex [239], most likely due to an increase in the activity of tyrosine hydroxylase, and an increase in its release in the striatum and various areas of the corticolimbic system [240].

GHB does not bind to opioid receptors [241], although some of its effects can be reproduced by opioid agonists. Local administration of GHB produces an increase in the release of endogenous opioids which appears to be mediated by the decrease in dopaminergic function [241].

GHB increases 5-HT turnover [242] and synthesis through a modulatory effect on GABA release [213].

17.2.3 GHB and Addiction

In drug discrimination studies in rats, GHB has been shown to be partially substituted for by morphine, lysergic acid diethylamide (LSD), d-amphetamine, GABA agonists (baclofen), and chlordiazepoxide [243]. These effects appear to be mediated, in part, by the GABA system since 3-Aminopropyl (diethoxymethyl) phosphinic acid (CGP35348), a GABA$_B$ receptor antagonist, blocked discrimination both at low and especially at high doses of GHB [244]. In addition, GHB has been shown to substitute for intermediate doses of ethanol [245].

In reinforcement studies, after repeated GHB administration, animals showed a place preference suggesting that the reinforcing effects of the drug are weaker than those produced by cocaine or opiates, which require only single exposure [246].

Self-administration studies indicate that rats trained to drink GHB prefer GHB in a subsequent two-drinking-bottle paradigm [247]. Furthermore, rats receiving GHB in response to nose-pokes will respond with more nose-pokes than those animals who are yoked to passively receive the same dose of GHB and who receive a vehicle in response to nose-pokes [248].

There is some evidence of tolerance to the motor dysfunction effects in mice and there is cross-tolerance with ethanol [249]. A withdrawal syndrome has been described using the same scale as is used to evaluate ethanol intoxication withdrawal following repeated daily administration for three to six days [250].

17.3 KETAMINE

Another popular club drug is ketamine, a phencyclidine derivative, first introduced into clinical practice in the 1960s as a dissociative anesthetic [251]. Its clinical use has diminished, but it is still used in circumstances where its dissociative/analgesic effects are advantageous, such as in patients with burns. It is administered by the intravenous or intramuscular routes, and drugs such as diazepam are often coadministered in order to reduce the incidence of hallucinations and/or psychosis symptoms. These symptoms appear to be less common in children. Ketamine is still quite widely used in veterinary practice for the sedation of animals for surgery, transport, or euthanasia [252].

It is thought that ketamine first entered the club scene as an adulterant of MDMA (Ecstasy), but it is now consumed in its own right [253]. On the street it is known by a number of names, including "K," "Special K," "Vitamin K," or "Kit-kat." Supply of ketamine originates mainly from the diversion of prescription products. The drug can be injected either intravenously or intramuscularly [254], taken orally either as a powder or liquid, snorted as a powder, or smoked [255]. Orally it is less well absorbed and undergoes extensive first-pass metabolism [254]. The drug is tasteless, odorless, and colorless, which makes it suitable for its secret addition to drinks in order to facilitate sexual assault. This property, as well as its ability to cause anterograde amnesia and hallucinations making the victims unreliable as witnesses, has led to its use in cases of date rape [256].

17.3.1 Pharmacological Effects

Ketamine has a rapid onset of action, lasting approximately 30–45 min. Low doses produce a dreamlike dissociative effect with analgesia and can lead to involuntary lesions. Higher doses can lead to hallucinations and vivid dreams as well as to amnesia. Users describe an "out-of-body" experience where the mind is taken to "K-land" or "K-hole," an experience that can be either spiritual or unpleasant depending on the individual [257]. Neurological toxicity may manifest itself as nystagmus, mydriasis, agitation, slurred speech, confusion, delirium, floating sensation, hypertonus, rigidity, anxiety, vivid dreams, hallucinations, hostility, and seizures [255]. Cardiovascular toxicity includes hypertension, tachycardia, and palpitations, and respiratory toxicity may appear in the form of depression and apnea [252]. Rhabdomyolysis has also been reported [258]. Its effects can be potentiated by ethanol, GHB, or benzodiazepine ingestion.

Ketamine is an N-methyl-D-aspartate (NMDA) agonist that also acts at non-NMDA–glutamate receptors, nicotinic and muscarinic cholinergic receptors, σ receptors, monoaminergic receptors, opioid receptors, and sodium and calcium channels. At the NMDA channels, ketamine binds noncompetitively to the phencyclidine site and inhibits glutamate activation of the channel. The drug also stimulates nitric oxide synthesis and acts as an inhibitor of norepinephrine, dopamine, and 5-HT uptake [251, 259, 260]. In addition, it produces dopamine release in the nucleus accumbens [261], and there are reports of the induction of dependence in rats [262]. Therefore, it appears that ketamine has the potential to be an addictive drug of abuse.

17.4 FLUNITRAZEPAM (ROHYPNOL)

Flunitrazepam is a fast-acting potent hypnotic/sedative benzodiazepine which, although never approved for use in the United States, has been widely used in Europe and some Latin American countries under the brand name Rohypnol for the treatment of insomnia, sedation, and preanesthesia [252]. The drug has become increasingly popular among teenagers and young adults and is often consumed in combination with alcohol and/or other illicit drugs. Reports suggest that it is the preferred benzodiazepine of heroin addicts and has also been identified in numerous cases of drug-facilitated sexual assault due to its induction of anterograde amnesia.

The drug is generally taken orally as the commercially available pill or dissolved in a drink. The drug has good bioavailability, is rapidly distributed from plasma into tissue, and is metabolized by the liver into two active compounds [263]. The effects appear after approximately 20–30 min and last 4–6 h, although residual effects can be observed at much later time points. The half-life of the drug is approximately 20 h and the metabolites are excreted renally.

17.4.1 Pharmacological Effects

As with other benzodiazepines, flunitrazepam produces a reduction in anxiety, muscle relaxation, and sedation. In addition, the drug produces amnesia which is enhanced by the concurrent ingestion of alcohol.

At higher doses, flunitrazepam can cause lack of muscle control and loss of consciousness. The drug can produce hypotension, dizziness, confusion, visual disturbances, urinary retention, and, occasionally, aggression [263].

As with other benzodiazepines, flunitrazepam can cause dependence and a withdrawal syndrome, although due to its long half-life this may take several days to appear and persists for weeks after the last dose. The symptoms include headache, tension, anxiety, restlessness, insomnia, loss of appetite, tremor, and perceptual disturbances.

17.5 LSD

LSD belongs to the hallucinogenic class of drugs. Hallucinogens are defined as pharmacologically active substances which alter consciousness, often in a dramatic and unpredictable manner, and which at high doses can produce delirium, hallucinations, separation from reality, and in some cases death, which is not due to overdose. These substances are also referred to as psychomimetics since they alter cognitive functions and personality and mimic psychosis.

The hallucinogens are included in Schedule I of the Controlled Substances Act and are traditionally classified into one of two groups: phenylalkylamines (mescaline, DOB, DOI) and the indolealkylamines (DMT, 5-MeO-DMT, psilocybin, LSD, harmaline, bufotenine) (Table 17.1).

TABLE 17.1 Hallucinogens: Dose, Duration of Effects, and Route of Administration in Humans

Hallucinogen	Dose (mg)	Duration of Effects	Route of Administration
DMT	60–100	1 h	Smoked, inhaled, nasal, injection
5-MeO-DMT	6–20	20–30 min	Smoked, inhaled, nasal, injection
Psilocybin	6–20	4–6 h	Oral
LSD	0.06–20	10–12 h	Oral
Mescaline	200–400	10–12 h	Oral
DOB	1–3		Oral
DOI	1.5–3		

DMT: N,N-dimethyltryptamine; 5-MeO-DMT: 5-methoxy-dimethyltryptamine; DOB: 2,5-dimethoxy-4-bromoamphetamine; DOI: 2,5-dimethoxy-4-iodoamphetamine

LSD is a prototypical hallucinogen which was first introduced to Europe and North America in 1949 [264]. It is a semisynthetic molecule derived from lysergic acid, which is produced by a fungus which grows on rye. Its effects were first identified by a chemist, A. Hoffman, working for Sandoz Pharmaceuticals, who experienced the mental effects of the drug after working with the compound [265]. The drug, as with most hallucinogens, is orally active and is the most potent of all hallucinogens [266]. At the other end of the spectrum is mescaline, which is the least potent of the classical hallucinogens (Table 17.1).

17.5.1 Pharmacological Effects

The main effects of LSD, which are common to most of the hallucinogens, are listed in Table 17.2. It is generally considered safe from a physiological standpoint since it alters consciousness at low doses which are not toxic to the cardiovascular, renal, or hepatic systems. At lower doses (25–50 μg) the drug produces mild visual effects which are not considered hallucinations or distortions of perception. At higher doses (250 μg) the drug produces sympathetic arousal characterized by increased pulse and blood pressure, dilated pupils causing blurred vision, hyperreflexia, and slight pyrexia [264]. In one reported case of multiple overdose, hemorrhage occurred which may have been mediated by LSD antagonism of platelet 5-HT function [267].

17.5.2 Mechanism of Action

LSD appears to mediate most its hallucinogenic effects by its action at the 5-HT$_{2A}$ receptor. Studies carried out in experimental animals reveal that 5-HT$_{2A}$ receptor antagonists such as ketanserin and pirenperone block the discriminative effects of both classes of hallucinogens in rats trained to discriminate between the effects of saline and the training drug [268, 269]. In addition, other studies with more highly selective antagonists of the 2A receptor over the 2C receptor have confirmed the 5-HT$_{2A}$ receptor as the target [270]. Similar observations have been made in humans

TABLE 17.2 Pharmacological Effects and Adverse Reactions of Hallucinogens

Somatic Alterations	Alterations of Perception	Mental Alterations	Adverse Reactions
Dizziness, weakness, shaking, nausea, sleepiness, paresthesias, blurred vision	Distortion of shapes and colors, difficulty in focusing, heightened sense of hearing, synesthesias (unusual)	Mood changes (happiness, sadness, or irritability), tension, distorted perception of the passage of time, difficulty in expressing thoughts, depersonalization, dream-like state, and visual hallucinations	Anxiety, agitation (bad trips), flashbacks, precipitation of psychosis and depression (in susceptible individuals), suicide

[271, 272]. The development of tolerance, as seen in both animals and humans, appears to be related to the selective downregulation of the 5-HT$_{2A}$ receptor following daily administration [273].

Hallucinogen-induced activation of 5-HT$_{2A}$ receptors located on neocortical pyramidal neurons leads to an increase in glutamate levels in the prefrontal cortex [274] presumably through an action mediated by the presynaptic receptors of thalamic afferents. This release of glutamate is thought to contribute to the behavioral effects produced by the hallucinogens since antagonism of the metabotropic glutamate mGlu2/3 receptor, a putative presynaptic autoreceptor on glutamatergic neurons [275], increases appropriate responding in rats trained to discriminate LSD [276]. Opposite effects were observed with an mGlu2/3 agonist. Agonists and antagonists of the mGlu2/3 receptor have been observed to decrease and increase glutamate release, respectively [277, 278].

Although activation of 5-HT$_{2A}$ receptors is accepted to be an essential component for the acute behavioral effects of the hallucinogens, it is possible that interaction with other receptors in the CNS may modulate their overall psychopharmacological effect. The hallucinogens, with the exception of LSD, have no affinity for dopaminergic receptors or for the dopamine transporter and therefore do not directly alter dopaminergic neurotransmission. However, systemic administration of DOI produces a 5-HT$_{2A}$-mediated increase in dopamine release in the prefrontal cortex [279], and local infusion of DOI in the nucleus accumbens also increases dopamine release [280]. Therefore it is possible that dopamine may participate in some of the behavioral effects of these drugs. In fact, it is thought that later onset behavioral effects of LSD appear to be mediated by dopamine pathways [281].

17.5.3 Hallucinogens and Addiction

In contrast to other drugs of abuse, the hallucinogens do not produce dependence or addiction and are not considered to be reinforcing substances [282] in spite of producing alterations in dopamine neurotransmission either directly or indirectly (see above). In fact, in the rhesus monkey LSD produces negative reinforcement [283], although in the rat the drug appears to have weak reinforcing properties [284] which may be related to the drug's direct action on dopamine receptors. This lack of addictive properties is interesting to note in light of the fact that modifications of dopamine neurotransmission, in particular dopamine release in the mesolimbic pathways, seem to be involved in the mechanism of action of drugs of abuse which cause dependence.

Studies designed to train animals to self-administer classical hallucinogens have failed, indicating that these substances do not possess the pharmacological properties necessary to establish and maintain a state of dependency. The drugs are generally consumed sporadically in a noncompulsive manner, and the majority of experimental first-time consumers do not go on to establishing a pattern of regular consumption. This pattern of consumption contrasts with the compulsive nature of amphetamine, cocaine, and opiate abuse which alter the pathways of reward and produce craving.

Tolerance to the behavioral effects of LSD occurs after daily administration for four to seven days and lasts for approximately three days [285]. Cross-tolerance occurs between LSD and other hallucinogens such as psilocybin and mescaline [286, 287].

17.6 SUMMARY

This chapter summarizes the latest literature on MDMA (Ecstasy), the most popular drug used by teens and adults in raves and other dance parties, and other compounds also categorized as club drugs—GHB, ketamine, Rohypnol, and LSD. Consumption, in general, appears to have increased in Western countries over the last 20 years, although trends show a variety of users and settings. Each drug produces diverse characteristic acute behavioral and biochemical effects which require different specific acute-care protocols. However, all of them share the common property of producing rewarding effects probably by activation of the mesolimbic system and the release of dopamine in the nucleus accumbens. MDMA induces long-lasting neurochemical changes reflected by a loss of 5-HT nerve terminals in the brain of rats, guinea pigs, and nonhuman primates. An increasing number of neuroimaging studies indicate that damage might also appear in human beings. The fact that the doses of MDMA that produce damage in experimental animals are similar to that used by humans places consumers in an area of high risk even after relatively short-time exposures to Ecstasy.

REFERENCES

1. Yamamoto, B. K., and Spanos, L. J. (1988). The acute effects of methylenedioxymethamphetamine on dopamine release in the awake-behaving rat. *Eur. J. Pharmacol.* 148, 195–203.
2. Marona-Lewicka, D., Rhee, G. S., Sprague, J. E., and Nichols, D. E. (1996). Reinforcing effects of certain serotonin-releasing amphetamine derivatives. *Pharmacol. Biochem. Behav.* 53, 99–105.
3. Kankaanpaa, A., Meririnne, E., Lillsunde, P., and Seppala, T. (1998). The acute effects of amphetamine derivatives on extracellular serotonin and dopamine levels in rat nucleus accumbens. *Pharmacol. Biochem. Behav.* 59, 1003–1009.

4. Bilsky, E. J., Hubbell, C. L., Delconte, J. D., and Reid, L. D. (1991). MDMA produces a conditioned place preference and elicits ejaculation in male rats: A modulatory role for the endogenous opioids. *Pharmacol. Biochem. Behav.* 40, 443–447.
5. Bilsky, E. J., and Reid, L. D. (1991). MDL72222, a serotonin 5-HT3 receptor antagonist, blocks MDMA's ability to establish a conditioned place preference. *Pharmacol. Biochem. Behav.* 39, 509–512.
6. Schechter, M. D. (1991). Effect of MDMA neurotoxicity upon its conditioned place preference and discrimination. *Pharmacol. Biochem. Behav.* 38, 539–544.
7. Hubner, C. B., Bird, M., Rassnick, S., and Kornetsky, C. (1988). The threshold lowering effects of MDMA (ecstasy) on brain-stimulation reward. *Psychopharmacology* 95, 49–51.
8. Schenk, S., Gittings, D., Johnstone, M., and Daniela, E. (2003). Development, maintenance and temporal pattern of self-administration maintained by ecstasy (MDMA) in rats. *Psychopharmacology* 169, 21–27.
9. Daniela, E., Brennan, K., Gittings, D., Hely, L., and Schenk, S. (2004). Effect of SCH 23390 on (+/−)-3,4-methylenedioxymethamphetamine hyperactivity and self-administration in rats. *Pharmacol. Biochem. Behav.* 77, 745–750.
10. Lamb, R. J., and Griffiths, R. R. (1987). Self-injection of d,1-3,4-methylenedioxymethamphetamine (MDMA) in the baboon. *Psychopharmacology* 91, 268–272.
11. Gold, L. H., and Koob, G. F. (1988). Methysergide potentiates the hyperactivity produced by MDMA in rats. *Pharmacol. Biochem. Behav.* 29, 645–648.
12. Gold, L. H., Geyer, M. A., and Koob, G. F. (1989a). Neurochemical mechanisms involved in behavioral effects of amphetamines and related designer drugs. *NIDA Res. Monogr.* 94, 101–126.
13. Cornish, J. L., Shahnawaz, Z., Thompson, M. R., Wong, S., Morley, K. C., Hunt, G. E., and McGregor, I. S. (2003). Heat increases 3,4-methylenedioxymethamphetamine self-administration and social effects in rats. *Eur. J. Pharmacol.* 482, 339–341.
14. O'Shea, E., Escobedo, I., Orio, L., Sanchez, V., Navarro, M., Green, A. R., and Colado, M. I. (2005). Elevation of ambient room temperature has differential effects on MDMA-induced 5-HT and dopamine release in striatum and nucleus accumbens of rats. *Neuropsychopharmacology.* 30, 1312–1323.
15. Morgan, A. E., Horan, B., Dewey, S. L., and Ashby, C. R. Jr. (1997). Repeated administration of 3,4-methylenedioxymethamphetamine augments cocaine's action on dopamine in the nucleus accumbens: A microdialysis study. *Eur. J. Pharmacol.* 331, R1–R3.
16. Horan, B., Gardner, E. L., and Ashby, C. R. Jr. (2000). Enhancement of conditioned place preference response to cocaine in rats following subchronic administration of 3,4-methylenedioxymethamphetamine (MDMA). *Synapse* 35, 160–162.
17. Cole, J. C., Sumnall, H. R., O'Shea, E., and Marsden, C. A. (2003). Effects of MDMA exposure on the conditioned place preference produced by other drugs of abuse. *Psychopharmacology* 166, 383–390.
18. Achat-Mendes, C., Anderson, K. L., and Itzhak, Y. (2003). Methylphenidate and MDMA adolescent exposure in mice: Long-lasting consequences on cocaine-induced reward and psychomotor stimulation in adulthood. *Neuropharmacology* 45, 106–115.
19. Fletcher, P. J., Robinson, S. R., and Slippoy, D. L. (2001). Pre-exposure to (±)3,4-methylenedioxymethamphetamine (MDMA) facilitates acquisition of intravenous cocaine self-administration. *Neuropsychopharmacology* 25, 195–203.
20. Morley, K. C., Cornish, J. L., Li, K. M., and McGregor, I. S. (2004). Preexposure to MDMA ("ecstasy") delays acquisition but facilitates MDMA-induced reinstatement of

amphetamine self-administration behavior in rats. *Pharmacol. Biochem. Behav.* 79, 331–342.

21. Gough, B., Ali, S. F., Slikker Jr., W., and Holson, R. R. (1991). Acute effects of 3,4-methylenedioxymethamphetamine (MDMA) on monoamines in rat caudate. *Pharmacol. Biochem. Behav.* 39, 619–623.

22. Yamamoto, B. K., Nash, J. F., and Gudelsky, G. A. (1995). Modulation of methylenedioxymethamphetamine-induced striatal dopamine release by the interaction between serotonin and γ-aminobutyric acid in the substantia nigra. *J. Pharmacol. Exp. Ther.* 273, 1063–1070.

23. Mechan, A. O., Esteban, B., O'Shea, E., Elliott, J. M., Colado, M. I., and Green, A. R. (2002). The pharmacology of the acute hyperthermic response that follows administration of 3,4-methylenedioxymethamphetamine (MDMA, "ecstasy") to rats. *Br. J. Pharmacol.* 135, 170–180.

24. Schmidt, C. J., Wu, L., and Lovenberg, W. (1986). Methylenedioxymethamphetamine: A potentially neurotoxic amphetamine analogue. *Eur. J. Pharmacol.* 124, 175–178.

25. Logan, B. J., Laverty, R., Sanderson, W. D., and Yee, Y. B. (1988). Differences between rats and mice in MDMA (methylenedioxymethamphetamine) neurotoxicity. *Eur. J. Pharmacol.* 152, 227–234.

26. Colado, M. I., and Green, A. R. (1994). A study of the mechanism of MDMA ("Ecstasy")-induced neurotoxicity of 5-HT neurones using chlormethiazole, dizocilpine and other protective compounds. *Br. J. Pharmacol.* 111, 131–136.

27. Gudelsky, G. A., and Nash, J. F. (1996). Carrier-mediated release of serotonin by 3,4-methylenedioxymethamphetamine: Implications for serotonin-dopamine interactions. *J. Neurochem.* 66, 243–249.

28. Crespi, D., Mennini, T., and Gobbi, M. (1997). Carrier-dependent and Ca^{2+}-dependent 5-HT and dopamine release induced by (+)-amphetamine, 3,4-methylenedioxymethamphetamine, *p*-chloroamphetamine and (+)-fenfluramine. *Br. J. Pharmacol.* 121, 1735–1743.

29. Berger, U. V., Gu, X. F., and Azmitia, E. C. (1992). The substituted amphetamines 3,4-methylenedioxymethamphetamine, methamphetamine, *p*-chloroamphetamine and fenfluramine induce 5-hydroxytryptamine release via a common mechanism blocked by fluoxetine and cocaine. *Eur. J. Pharmacol.* 215, 153–160.

30. Gudelsky, G. A., Yamamoto, B. K., and Nash, J. F. (1994). Potentiation of 3,4-methylenedioxymethamphetamine-induced dopamine release and serotonin neurotoxicity by 5-HT2 receptor agonists. *Eur. J. Pharmacol.* 264, 325–330.

31. Colado, M. I., O'Shea, E., Granados, R., Esteban, B., Martín, A. B., and Green, A. R. (1999). Studies on the role of dopamine in the degeneration of 5-HT nerve endings in the brain of Dark Agouti rats following 3,4-methylenedioxymethamphetamine (MDMA or "ecstasy") administration. *Br. J. Pharmacol.* 126, 911–924.

32. Green, A. R., Mechan, A. O., Elliott, J. M., O'Shea, E., and Colado, M. I. (2003). The pharmacology and clinical pharmacology of 3,4-methylenedioxymethamphetamine (MDMA, "Ecstasy"). *Pharmacol. Rev.* 55, 463–509.

33. Koch, S., and Galloway, M. P. (1997). MDMA induced dopamine release in vivo: Role of endogenous serotonin. *J. Neural Transm.* 104, 135–146.

34. Fitzgerald, J. L., and Reid, J. J. (1990). Effects of methylenedioxymethamphetamine on the release of monoamines from rat brain slices. *Eur. J. Pharmacol.* 191, 217–220.

35. Rothman, R. B., Baumann, M. H., Dersch, C. M., Romero, D. V., Rice, K. C., Carroll, F. I., and Partilla, J. S. (2001). Amphetamine-type central nervous system stimulants

release norepinephrine more potently than they release dopamine and serotonin. *Synapse* 39, 32–41.

36. Stone, D. M., Hanson, G. R., and Gibb, J. W. (1987). Differences in the central serotonergic effects of methylenedioxymethamphetamine (MDMA) in mice and rats. *Neuropharmacology* 26, 1657–1661.
37. Stone, D. M., Merchant, K. M., Hanson, G. R., and Gibb, J. W. (1987). Immediate and long-term effects of 3,4-methylenedioxymethamphetamine on serotonin pathways in brain of rat. *Neuropharmacology* 26, 1677–1683.
38. Che, S., Johnson, M., Hanson, G. R., and Gibb, J. W. (1995). Body temperature effect on methylenedioxymethamphetamine-induced acute decrease in tryptophan hydroxylase activity. *Eur. J. Pharmacol.* 293, 447–453.
39. Schmidt, C. J., and Taylor, V. L. (1987). Depression of rat brain tryptophan hydroxylase following the acute administration of methylenedioxymethamphetamine. *Biochem. Pharmacol.* 36, 4095–4102.
40. Rattray, M. (1991). Ecstasy: Towards an understanding of the biochemical basis of the actions of MDMA. *Essays Biochem.* 26, 77–87.
41. Steele, T. D., Nichols, D. E., and Yim, G. K. (1987). Stereochemical effects of 3,4-methylenedioxymethamphetamine (MDMA) and related amphetamine derivatives on inhibition of uptake of [^{3}H]monoamines into synaptosomes from different regions of rat brain. *Biochem. Pharmacol.* 36, 2297–2303.
42. Battaglia, G., Brooks, B. P., Kulsakdinun, C., and De Souza, E. B. (1988). Pharmacologic profile of MDMA (3,4-methylenedioxymethamphetamine) at various brain recognition sites. *Eur. J. Pharmacol.* 149, 159–163.
43. Nash, J. F., Meltzer, H. Y., and Gudelsky, G. A. (1988). Elevation of serum prolactin and corticosterone concentrations in the rat after the administration of 3,4-methylenedioxymethamphetamine. *J. Pharmacol. Exp. Ther.* 245, 873–879.
44. Colado, M. I., Murray, T. K., and Green, A. R. (1993). 5-HT loss in rat brain following 3,4-methylenedioxymethamphetamine (MDMA), *p*-chloroamphetamine and fenfluramine administration and effects of chlormethiazole and dizocilpine. *Br. J. Pharmacol.* 108, 583–589.
45. Dafters, R. I. (1994). Effect of ambient temperature on hyperthermia and hyperkinesis induced by 3,4-methylenedioxymethamphetamine (MDMA or "ecstasy") in rats. *Psychopharmacology* 114, 505–508.
46. Malberg, J. E., Sabol, K. E., and Seiden, L. S. (1996). Co-administration of MDMA with drugs that protect against MDMA neurotoxicity produces different effects on body temperature in the rat. *J. Pharmacol. Exp. Ther.* 278, 258–267.
47. O'Shea, E., Granados, R., Esteban, B., Colado, M. I., and Green, A. R. (1998). The relationship between the degree of neurodegeneration of rat brain 5-HT nerve terminals and the dose and frequency of administration of MDMA ("ecstasy"). *Neuropharmacology* 37, 919–926.
48. Malberg, J. E., and Seiden, L. S. (1998). Small changes in ambient temperature cause large changes in 3,4-methylenedioxymethamphetamine (MDMA)-induced serotonin neurotoxicity and core body temperature in the rat. *J. Neurosci.* 18, 5086–5094.
49. Dafters, R. I., and Lynch, E. (1998). Persistent loss of thermoregulation in the rat induced by 3,4-methylenedioxymethamphetamine (MDMA or "Ecstasy") but not by fenfluramine. *Psychopharmacology* 138, 207–212.
50. Green, A. R., O'Shea, E., and Colado, M. I. (2004). A review of the mechanisms involved in the acute MDMA (ecstasy)-induced hyperthermic response. *Eur. J. Pharmacol.* 500, 3–13.

51. Gordon, C. J., Watkinson, W. P., O'Callaghan, J. P., and Miller, D. B. (1991). Effects of 3,4-methylenedioxymethamphetamine on autonomic thermoregulatory responses of the rat. *Pharmacol. Biochem. Behav.* 38, 339–344.

52. Sprague, J. E., Banks, M. L., Cook, E. J., and Mills, E. M. (2003). Hypothalamic-pituitary-thyroid axis and sympathetic nervous system involvement in the hyperthermia induced by 3,4-methylenedioxymethamphetamine (MDMA, Ecstasy). *J. Pharmacol. Exp. Ther.* 305, 159–166.

53. Sprague, J. E., Brutcher, R. E., Mills, E. M., Caden, D., and Rusynaik, D. E. (2004). Attenuation of 3,4-methylenedioxymethamphetamine (MDMA, Ecstasy)-induced rhabdomyolysis with α_1- plus β_3-adrenoreceptor antagonists. *Br. J. Pharmacol.* 142, 667–670.

54. Grant, R. T. (1963). Vasodilatation and body warming in the rat. *J. Physiol.* 157, 311–317.

55. Gunn, J. A., and Gurd, M. R. (1940). The action of some amines related to adrenaline. Cyclohexylalkylamines. *J. Physiol.* 97, 435–470.

56. Fantegrossi, W. E., Godlewski, T., Karabenick, R. L., Stephens, J. M., Ullrich, T., Rice, K. C., and Woods, J. H. (2003). Pharmacological characterization of the effects of 3,4-methylenedioxymethamphetamine ("ecstasy") and its enantiomers on lethality, core temperature and locomotor activity in singly housed and crowded mice. *Psychopharmacology* 166, 202–211.

57. Burns, N., Olverman, H. J., Kelly, P. A., and Williams, B. C. (1996). Effects of ecstasy on aldosterone secretion in the rat in vivo and in vitro. *Endocr. Res.* 2, 601–601.

58. Forsling, M., Fallon, J. K., Kicman, A. T., Hutt, A. J., Cowan, A. D., and Henry, J. A. (2001). Arginine vasopressin release in response to the administration of 3,4-methylenedioxymethamphetamine ("ecstasy"): Is metabolism a contributory factor? *J. Pharmacol. Pharmacol.* 53 1357–1363.

59. Forsling, M. L., Fallon, J. K., Shah, D., Tilbrook, G. S., Cowan, D. A., Kicman, A. T., and Hutt, A. J. (2002). The effect of 3,4-methylenedioxymethamphetamine (MDMA, "ecstasy") and its metabolites on neurohypophysial hormone release from the isolated rat hypothalamus. *Br. J. Pharmacol.* 135, 649–656.

60. Connor, T. J., McNamara, M. G., Finn, D., Currid, A., O'Malley, M., Redmond, A. M., Kelly, J. P., and Leonard, B. E. (1998). Acute 3,4-methylenedioxymethamphetamine (MDMA) administration produces a rapid and sustained suppression of immune function in the rat. *Immunopharmacology* 38, 253–260.

61. Slikker, W., Jr., Holson, R. R., Ali, S. F., Kolta, M. G., Paule, M. G., Scallet, A. C., McMillan, D. E., Bailey, J. R., Hong, J. S., and Scalzo, F. M. (1989). Behavioral and neurochemical effects of orally administered MDMA in the rodent and nonhuman primate. *Neurotoxicology* 10, 529–542.

62. Spanos, L. J., and Yamamoto, B. K. (1989). Acute and subchronic effects of methylenedioxymethamphetamine [($\pm$)MDMA] on locomotion and serotonin syndrome behavior in the rat. *Pharmacol. Biochem. Behav.* 32, 835–840.

63. Shankaran, M., and Gudelsky, G. A. (1999). A neurotoxic regimen of MDMA suppresses behavioral, thermal and neurochemical responses to subsequent MDMA administration. *Psychopharmacology* 147, 66–72.

64. Grahame-Smith, D. G. (1971). Studies in vivo on the relationship between brain tryptophan, brain 5-HT synthesis and hyperactivity in rats treated with a monoamine oxidase inhibitor and L-tryptophan. *J. Neurochem.* 18, 1053–1066.

65. Callaway, C. W., Wing, L. L., and Geyer, M. A. (1990). Serotonin release contributes to the locomotor stimulant effects of 3,4-methylenedioxymethamphetamine in rats. *J. Pharmacol. Exp. Ther.* 254, 456–464.

66. Bankson, M. G., and Cunningham, K. A. (2002). Pharmacological studies of the acute effects of (+)-3,4-methylenedioxymethamphetamine on locomotor activity: Role of 5-$HT_{1B/1D}$ and 5-HT_2 receptors. *Neuropsychopharmacology* 26, 40–52.

67. Morley, K. C., and McGregor, I. S. (2000). (±)-3,4-Methylenedioxymethamphetamine (MDMA, "Ecstasy") increases social interaction in rats. *Eur. J. Pharmacol.* 408, 41–49.

68. Bhattacharya, S. K., Bhattacharya, A., and Ghosal, S. (1998). Anxiogenic activity of methylenedioxymethamphetamine (ecstasy)—An experimental study. *Biogenic Amines* 14, 217–237.

69. Lin, H. Q., Burden, P. M., Christie, M. J., and Johnston, G. A. R. (1999). The anxiogenic-like and anxiolytic-like effects of MDMA on mice in the elevated plus-maze: A comparison with amphetamine. *Pharmacol. Biochem. Behav.* 62, 403–408.

70. Maldonado, E., and Navarro, J. F. (2001). MDMA ("ecstasy") exhibits an anxiogenic-like activity in social encounters between male mice. *Pharmacol. Res.* 44, 27–31.

71. Schmidt, C. J. (1987). Neurotoxicity of the psychedelic amphetamine, methylenedioxymethamphetamine. *J. Pharmacol. Exp. Ther.* 240, 1–7.

72. McKenna, D. J., and Peroutka, S. J. (1990). Neurochemistry and neurotoxicity of 3,4-methylenedioxymethamphetamine (MDMA; "Ecstasy"). *J. Neurochem.* 54, 14–22.

73. Stone, D. M., Stahl, D. C., Hanson, G. R., and Gibb, J. W. (1986). The effects of 3,4-methylenedioxymethamphetamine (MDMA) and 3,4-methylenedioxyamphetamine (MDA) on monoaminergic systems in the rat brain. *Eur. J. Pharmacol.* 128, 41–48.

74. Schmidt, C. J., and Kehne, J. H. (1990). Neurotoxicity of MDMA: Neurochemical effects. *Ann. NY Acad. Sci.* 600, 665–681.

75. Steele, T. D., McCann, U. D., and Ricaurte, G. A. (1994). 3,4-Methylenedioxymethamphetamine (MDMA, "Ecstasy"): Pharmacology and toxicology in animals and humans. *Addiction* 89, 539–551.

76. Green, A. R., Cross, A. J., and Goodwin, G. M. (1995). Review of the pharmacology and clinical pharmacology of 3,4-methylenedioxymethamphetamine (MDMA or "ecstasy"). *Psychopharmacology* 119, 247–260.

77. Colado, M. I., O'Shea, E., Granados, R., Murray, T. K., and Green, A. R. (1997). In vivo evidence for free radical involvement in 5-HT following administration of MDMA ("ecstasy") and p-chloroamphetamine but not the degeneration following fenfluramine. *Br. J. Pharmacol.* 121, 889–900.

78. O'Hearn, E., Battaglia, G., De Souza, E. B., Kuhar, M. J., and Molliver, M. E. (1988). Methylenedioxyamphetamine (MDA) and methylenedioxymethamphetamine (MDMA) cause selective ablation of serotonergic axon terminals in forebrain: Immunocytochemical evidence for neurotoxicity. *J. Neurosci.* 8, 2788–2803.

79. Molliver, M. E., Berger, U. V., Mamounas, L. A., Molliver, D. C., O'Hearn, E., and Wilson, M. A. (1990). Neurotoxicity of MDMA and related compounds: Anatomic studies. *Ann. NY Acad. Sci.* 600, 640–661.

80. Sharkey, J., McBean, D. E., and Kelly, P. A. (1991). Alterations in hippocampal function following repeated exposure to the amphetamine derivative methylenedioxymethamphetamine ("Ecstasy"). *Psychopharmacology* 105, 113–118.

81. Hewitt, K. E., and Green, A. R. (1994). Chlormethiazole, dizocilpine and haloperidol prevent the degeneration of serotonergic nerve terminals induced by administration of MDMA ("Ecstasy") to rats. *Neuropharmacology* 33, 1589–1595.

82. Sanchez, V., Camarero, J., Esteban, B., Peter, M. J., Green, A. R., and Colado, M. I. (2001). The mechanisms involved in the long-lasting neuroprotective effect of fluoxetine against MDMA ("ecstasy")-induced degeneration of 5-HT nerve endings in rat brain. *Br. J. Pharmacol.* 134, 46–57.

83. Colado, M. I., Williams, J. L., and Green, A. R. (1995). The hyperthermic and neurotoxic effects of "Ecstasy" (MDMA) and 3,4 methylenedioxyamphetamine (MDA) in the Dark Agouti (DA) rat, a model of the CYP2D6 poor metabolizer phenotype. *Br. J. Pharmacol.* 115, 1281–1289.

84. Aguirre, N., Ballaz, S., Lasheras, B., and Del Río, J. (1998). MDMA ("Ecstasy") enhances 5-HT$_{1A}$ receptor density and 8-OH-DPAT-induced hypothermia: Blockade by drugs preventing 5-hydroxytryptamine depletion. *Eur. J. Pharmacol.* 346, 181–188.

85. Battaglia, G., Zaczek, R., and De Souza, E. B. (1990). MDMA effects in brain: Pharmacologic profile and evidence of neurotoxicity from neurochemical and autoradiographic studies. In *Ecstasy: The Clinical, Pharmacological and Neurotoxicological Effects of the Drug MDMA*, S. J. Peroutka Ed. Kluwer, Boston, pp. 171–190.

86. De Souza, E. B., and Battaglia, G. (1989). Effects of MDMA and MDA on brain serotonin neurons: Evidence from neurochemical and autoradiographic studies. In *Pharmacology and Toxicology of Amphetamine and Related Drugs*, K. Ashgar and E. B. Souza, Eds. National Institute on Drug Abuse, Rockville pp. 196–222.

87. De Souza, E. B., Battaglia, G., and Insel, T. (1990). Neurotoxic effects of MDMA on brain serotonin neurons: Evidence from neurochemical and radioligand binding studies. *Ann. NY Acad. Sci.* 600, 682–698.

88. Scanzello, C. R., Hatzidimitriou, G., Martello, A. L., Katz, J. L., and Ricaurte, G. A. (1993). Serotonergic recovery after ($\pm$)3,4-(methylenedioxy) methamphetamine injury: Observations in rats. *J. Pharmacol. Exp. Ther.* 264, 1484–1491.

89. Sabol, K. E., Lew, R., Richards, J. B., Vosmer, G. L., and Seiden, L. S. (1996). Methylenedioxymethamphetamine-induced serotonin deficits are followed by partial recovery over a 52-week period. Part I: Synaptosomal uptake and tissue concentrations. *J. Pharmacol. Exp. Ther.* 276, 846–854.

90. Lew, R., Sabol, K. E., Chou, C., Vosmer, G. L., Richards, J., and Seiden, L. S. (1996). Methylenedioxymethamphetamine-induced serotonin deficits are followed by partial recovery over a 52-week period. Part II: Radioligand binding and autoradiography studies. *J. Pharmacol. Exp. Ther.* 276, 855–865.

91. Wilson, M. A., Ricaurte, G. A., and Molliver, M. E. (1989). Distinct morphologic classes of serotonergic axons in primates exhibit differential vulnerability to the psychotropic drug 3,4-methylenedioxymethamphetamine. *Neuroscience* 28, 121–137.

92. Fischer, C., Hatzidimitriou, G., Wlos, J., Katz, J., and Ricaurte, G. (1995). Reorganization of ascending 5-HT axon projections in animals previously exposed to the recreational drug ($\pm$)-3,4-methylenedioxymethamphetamine (MDMA, "Ecstasy"). *J. Neurosci.* 15, 5476–5485.

93. Bjorklund, A., Wiklund, L., and Descarries, L. (1981). Regeneration and plasticity of central serotoninergic neurons: A review. *J. Physiol. (Paris)* 77, 247–255.

94. Jacobs, B. L., and Azmitia, E. C. (1992). Structure and function of the brain serotonin system. *Physiol. Rev.* 72, 165–229.

95. Insel, T. R., Battaglia, G., Johannessen, J. N., Marra, S., and De Souza, E. B. (1989). 3,4-Methylenedioxymethamphetamine ("ecstasy") selectively destroys brain serotonin terminals in rhesus monkeys. *J. Pharmacol. Exp. Ther.* 249, 713–720.

96. Ricaurte, G. A., Martello, A. L., Katz, J. L., and Martello, M. B. (1992). Lasting effects of ($\pm$)-3,4-methylenedioxymethamphetamine (MDMA) on central serotonergic

neurons in nonhuman primates: Neurochemical observations. *J. Pharmacol. Exp. Ther.* 261, 616–622.

97. Hatzidimitriou, G., McCann, U. D., and Ricaurte, G. A. (1999). Altered serotonin innervation patterns in the forebrain of monkeys treated with ($\pm$)3,4-methylenedioxymethamphetamine seven years previously: Factors influencing abnormal recovery. *J. Neurosci.* 19, 5096–5107.

98. Parrott, A. C. (2004). Is ecstasy MDMA? A review of the proportion of ecstasy tablets containing MDMA, their dosage levels and changing perceptions of purity. *Psychopharmacology* 173, 234–241.

99. Parrott, A. C. (2005). Chronic tolerance to recreational MDMA (3,4-methylenedioxymethamphetamine) or Ecstasy. *J. Psychopharmacol.* 19, 71–83.

100. Slikker, W., Jr., Ali, S. F., Scallet, A. C., Frith, C. H., Newport, G. D., and Bailey, J. R. (1988). Neurochemical and neurohistological alterations in the rat and monkey produced by orally administered methylenedioxymethamphetamine (MDMA). *Toxicol. App. Pharmacol.* 96, 448–457.

101. Ricaurte, G. A., Forno, L. S., Wilson, M. A., DeLanney, L. E., Irwin, I., Molliver, M. E., and Langston, J. W. (1988). ($\pm$)-3,4-Methylenedioxymethamphetamine selectively damages central serotonergic neurons in nonhuman primates. *JAMA* 260, 51–55.

102. Finnegan, K. T., Ricaurte, G. A., Ritchie, L. D., Irwin, I., Peroutka, S. J., and Langston, J. W. (1988). Orally administered MDMA causes a long-term depletion of serotonin in rat brain. *Brain Res.* 447, 141–144.

103. Ricaurte, G. A., DeLanney, L. E., Irwin, I., and Langston, J. W. (1988). Toxic effects of MDMA on central serotonergic neurons in the primate: Importance of route and frequency of drug administration. *Brain Res.* 446, 165–168.

104. Kleven, M. S., Woolverton, W. L., and Seiden, L. S. (1989). Evidence that both intragastric and subcutaneous administration of methylenedioxymethylamphetamine (MDMA) produce serotonin neurotoxicity in rhesus monkeys. *Brain Res.* 488, 121–125.

105. Parrott, A. C. (2002). Recreational Ecstasy/MDMA, the serotonin syndrome, and serotonergic neurotoxicity. *Pharmacol. Biochem. Behav.* 71, 837–844.

106. Weir, E. (2000). Raves: A review of the culture, the drugs and the prevention of harm. *Can. Med. Assoc. J.* 162, 1843–1848.

107. Sanchez, V., O'Shea, E., Saadat, K. S., Elliott, J. M., Colado, M. I., and Green, A.R. (2004). Effect of repeated ("binge") dosing of MDMA to rats housed at normal and high temperature on neurotoxic damage to cerebral 5-HT and dopamine neurones. *J. Psychopharmacol.* 18, 412–416.

108. Molliver, M. E., O'Hearn, E., Battaglia, G., and De Souza, E. R. (1986). Direct intracerebral administration of MDMA and MDA does not produce serotonin neurotoxicity. *Soc. Neurosci. Abstr.* 12, 1234.

109. Paris, J. M., and Cunningham, K. A. (1992). Lack of serotonin neurotoxicity after intraraphe microinjection of (+)-3,4-methylenedioxymethamphetamine (MDMA). *Brain Res. Bull.* 28, 115–119.

110. Esteban, B., O'Shea, E., Camarero, J., Sanchez, V., Green, A. R., and Colado, M. I. (2001). 3,4-Methylenedioxymethamphetamine induces monoamine release, but not toxicity, when administered centrally at a concentration occurring following a peripherally injected neurotoxic dose. *Psychopharmacology* 154, 251–260.

111. Escobedo, I., O'Shea, E., Orio, L., Sanchez, V., Segura, M., de la Torre, R., Farre, M., Green, A. R., and Colado, M. I. (2005). A comparative study on the acute and long-term effects of MDMA and 3,4-dihydroxymethamphetamine (HHMA) on brain

monoamine levels after i.p. or striatal administration in mice. *Br. J. Pharmacol.* 144, 231–241.

112. Lim, H. K., and Foltz, R. L. (1988). In vivo and in vitro metabolism of 3,4-(methylenedioxy)methamphetamine in the rat: Identification of metabolites using an ion trap detector. *Chem. Res. Toxicol.* 1, 370–378.

113. Lim, H. K., and Foltz, R. L. (1991). Ion trap tandem mass spectrometric evidence for the metabolism of 3,4-(methylenedioxy)methamphetamine to the potent neurotoxins 2,4,5-trihydroxymethamphetamine and 2,4,5-trihydroxyamphetamine. *Chem. Res. Toxicol.* 4, 626–632.

114. Lim, H. K., and Foltz, R. L. (1991). In vivo formation of aromatic hydroxylated metabolites of 3,4-(methylenedioxy)methamphetamine in the rat: Identification by ion trap tandem mass spectrometric (MS/MS and MS/MS/MS) techniques. *Biol. Mass Spectrom.* 20, 677–686.

115. Chu, T., Kumagai, Y., DiStefano, E. W., and Cho, A. K. (1996). Disposition of methylenedioxymethamphetamine and three metabolites in the brains of different rat strains and their possible roles in acute serotonin depletion. *Biochem. Pharmacol.* 51, 789–796.

116. Johnson, M., Elayan, I., Hanson, G. R., Foltz, R. L., Gibb, J. W., and Lim, H. K. (1992). Effects of 3,4-dihydroxymethamphetamine and 2,4,5-trihydroxymethamphetamine, two metabolites of 3,4-methylenedioxymethamphetamine, on central serotonergic and dopaminergic systems. *J. Pharmacol. Exp. Ther.* 261, 447–453.

117. Zhao, Z. Y., Castagnoli, N., Ricaurte, G. A., Steele, T., and Martello, M. (1992). Synthesis and neurotoxicological evaluation of putative metabolites of the serotonergic neurotoxin 2-(methylamino)-1-[3,4-(methylenedioxy)phenyl] propane. *Chem. Res. Toxicol.* 5, 89–94.

118. McCann, U. D., and Ricaurte, G. A. (1991). Major metabolites of (+/−)3,4-methylenedioxyamphetamine (MDA) do not mediate its toxic effects on brain serotonin neurons. *Brain Res.* 545, 279–282.

119. Miller, R. T., Lau, S. S., and Monks, T. J. (1997). 2,5-Bis-(glutathion-S-yl)-alpha-methyldopamine, a putative metabolite of (+/−)-3,4-methylenedioxyamphetamine, decreases brain serotonin concentrations. *Eur. J. Pharmacol.* 323, 173–180.

120. Bai, F., Lau, S. S., and Monks, T. J. (1999). Glutathione and N-acetylcysteine conjugates of alpha-methyldopamine produce serotonergic neurotoxicity: Possible role in methylenedioxyamphetamine-mediated neurotoxicity. *Chem. Res. Toxicol.* 12, 1150–1157.

121. Bai, F., Jones, D. C., Lau, S. S., and Monks, T. J. (2001). Serotonergic neurotoxicity of 3,4-(+/−)-methylenedioxyamphetamine and 3,4-(+/−)-methylenedioxymethamphetamine (ecstasy) is potentiated by inhibition of gamma-glutamyl transpeptidase. *Chem. Res. Toxicol.* 14, 863–870.

122. Jones, D. C., Duvauchelle, C., Ikegami, A., Olsen, C. M., Lau, S. S., de la Torre, R., and Monks, T. J., (2005). Serotonergic neurotoxic metabolites of ecstasy identified in rat brain. *J. Pharmacol. Exp. Ther.* 313, 422–431.

123. De la Torre, R., Farre, M., Roset, P. N., Pizarro, N., Abanades, S., Segura, M., Segura, J., and Cami, J. (2004). Human pharmacology of MDMA: Pharmacokinetics, metabolism, and disposition. *Ther. Drug Monitoring* 26, 137–144.

124. Sprague, J. E., and Nichols, D. E. (1995). The monoamine oxidase-B inhibitor L-deprenyl protects against 3,4-methylenedioxymethamphetamine-induced lipid peroxidation and long-term serotonergic deficits. *J. Pharmacol. Exp. Ther.* 273, 667–673.

125. Colado, M. I., O'Shea, E., Granados, R., Misra, A., Murray, T. K., and Green, A.R. (1997). A study of the neurotoxic effect of MDMA ("ecstasy") on 5-HT neurons in the brains of mothers and neonates following administration of the drug during pregnancy. *Br. J. Pharmacol.* 121, 827–833.

126. Shankaran, M., Yamamoto, B. K., and Gudelsky, G. A. (2001). Ascorbic acid prevents 3,4-methylenedioxymethamphetamine (MDMA)-induced hydroxyl radical formation and the behavioral and neurochemical consequences of the depletion of brain 5-HT. *Synapse* 40, 55–64.

127. Yeh, S. Y. (1999). *N-tert*-Butyl-alpha-phenylnitrone protects against 3,4-methylene-dioxymethamphetamine-induced depletion of serotonin in rats. *Synapse* 31, 169–177.

128. Shankaran, M., Yamamoto, B. K., and Gudelsky, G. A. (1999). Mazindol attenuates the 3,4-methylenedioxymethamphetamine-induced formation of hydroxyl radicals and long-term depletion of serotonin in the striatum. *J. Neurochem.* 72, 2516–2522.

129. Colado, M. I., Camarero, J., Mechan, A. O., Sanchez, V., Esteban, B., Elliott, J. M., and Green, A. R. (2001). A study of the mechanisms involved in the neurotoxic action of 3,4-methylenedioxymethamphetamine (MDMA, "ecstasy") on dopamine neurones in mouse brain. *Br. J. Pharmacol.* 134, 1711–1723.

130. Camarero, J., Sanchez, V., O'Shea, E., Green, A. R., and Colado, M. I. (2002). Studies, using *in vivo* microdialysis, on the effect of the dopamine uptake inhibitor GBR 12909 on 3,4-methylenedioxymethamphetamine (MDMA, "ecstasy")-induced dopamine release and free radical formation in the mouse striatum. *J. Neurochem.* 81, 961–972.

131. Gudelsky, G. A. (1996). Effect of ascorbate and cysteine on the 3,4-methylenediox-ymethamphetamine-induced depletion of brain serotonin. *J. Neural Transm.* 102, 1397–1404.

132. Aguirre, N., Barrionuevo, M., Ramirez, M. J., Del Rio, J., and Lasheras, B. (1999). Alpha-lipoic acid prevents 3,4-methylenedioxy-methamphetamine (MDMA)-induced neurotoxicity. *Neuroreport* 10, 3675–3680.

133. Darvesh, A. S., Yamamoto, B. K., and Gudelsky, G. A. (2005). Evidence for the involvement of nitric oxide in 3,4-methylenedioxymethamphetamine-induced serotonin depletion in the rat brain. *J. Pharmacol. Exp. Ther.* 312, 694–701.

134. Sanchez, V., Camarero, J., O'Shea, E., Green, A. R., and Colado, M. I. (2003). Differential effect of dietary selenium on the long term neurotoxicity induced by MDMA in mice and rats. *Neuropharmacology* 44, 449–461.

135. Jayanthi, S., Ladenheim, B., Andrews, A. M., and Cadet, J. L. (1999). Overexpression of human copper/zinc superoxide dismutase in transgenic mice attenuates oxidative stress caused by methylenedioxymethamphetamine (Ecstasy). *Neuroscience* 91, 1379–1387.

136. Cadet, J. L., Ladenheim, B., Hirata, H., Rothman, R. B., Ali, S., Carlson, E., Epstein, C., and Moran, T. H. (1995). Superoxide radicals mediate the biochemical effects of methylenedioxymethamphetamine (MDMA): Evidence from using CuZn-superoxide dismutase transgenic mice. *Synapse* 21, 169–176.

137. Fornai, F., Lenzi, P., Frenzilli, G., Gesi, M., Ferrucci, M., Lazzeri, G., Biagioni, F., Nigro, M., Falleni, A., Giusiani, M., Pellegrini, A., Blandini, F., Ruggieri, S., and Paparelli, A. (2004). DNA damage and ubiquitinated neuronal inclusions in the substantia nigra and striatum of mice following MDMA (ecstasy). *Psychopharmacology* 173, 353–363.

138. Hrometz, S. L., Brown, A. W., Nichols, D. E., and Sprague, J. E. (2004). 3,4-Methylenedioxymethamphetamine (MDMA, ecstasy)-mediated production of hydrogen

peroxide in an in vitro model: The role of dopamine, the serotonin-reuptake transporter, and monoamine oxidase-B. *Neurosci. Lett.* 367, 56–59.

139. Globus, M. Y.-T., Busto, R., Lin, B., Schnippering, H., and Ginsberg, M. D. (1995). Detection of free radical formation during transient global ischemia and recirculation: Effects of intraischemic brain temperature modulation. *J. Neurochem.* 65, 1250–1256.

140. Kil, H. Y., Zhang, J., and Piantadosi, L. A. (1996). Brain temperature alters hydroxyl radical production during cerebral ischaemia/reperfusion in rats. *J. Cereb. Blood Flow Metabol.* 16, 100–106.

141. Shankaran, M., Yamamoto, B. K., and Gudelsky, G. A. (1999). Involvement of the serotonin transporter in the formation of hydroxyl radicals induced by 3,4-methylenedioxymethamphetamine. *Eur. J. Pharmacol.* 385, 103–110.

142. Broening, H. W., Bowyer, J. F., and Slikker, W., Jr. (1995). Age-dependent sensitivity of rats to the long-term effects of the serotonergic neurotoxicant $(+/-)$-3,4-methylenedioxymethamphetamine (MDMA) correlates with the magnitude of the MDMA-induced thermal response. *J. Pharmacol. Exp. Ther.* 275, 325–333.

143. Yuan, J., Cord, B. J., McCann, U. D., Callahan, B. T., and Ricaurte, G. A. (2002). Effect of glucoprivation on serotonin neurotoxicity induced by substituted amphetamines. *J. Pharmacol. Exp. Ther.* 303, 831–839.

144. Schmidt, C. J., Black, C. K., Abbate, G. M., and Taylor, V. L. (1990). Methylenedioxymethamphetamine-induced hyperthermia and neurotoxicity are independently mediated by 5-HT$_2$ receptors. *Brain Res.* 529, 85–90.

145. Miller, D. B., and O'Callaghan, J. P. (1995). The role of temperature, stress, and other factors in the neurotoxicity of the substituted amphetamines 3,4-methylenedioxymethamphetamine and fenfluramine. *Mol. Neurobiol.* 11, 177–192.

146. Johnson, E. A., Sharp, D. S., and Miller, D. B. (2000). Restraint as a stressor in mice: Against the dopaminergic neurotoxicity of D-MDMA, low body weight mitigates restraint-induced hypothermia and consequent neuroprotection. *Brain Res.* 875, 107–118.

147. Farfel, G. M., and Seiden, L. S. (1995). Role of hypothermia in the mechanism of protection against serotonergic toxicity. I. Experiments using 3,4-methylenedioxymethamphetamine, dizocilpine, CGS 19755 and NBQX. *J. Pharmacol. Exp. Ther.* 272, 860–867.

148. Colado, M. I., O'Shea, E., Esteban, B., Granados, R., and Green, A. R. (1999). In vivo evidence against chlomethiazole being neuroprotective against MDMA ("ecstasy")-induced degeneration of rat brain 5-HT nerve terminals by a free radical scavenging mechanism. *Neuropharmacology* 38, 307–314.

149. Colado, M. I., Esteban, B., O'Shea, E., Granados, R., and Green, A. R. (1999). Studies on the neuroprotective effect of pentobarbitone on MDMA-induced neurodegeneration. *Psychopharmacology* 142, 421–425.

150. O'Shea, E., Esteban, B., Camarero, J., Green, A. R., and Colado, M. I. (2001). Effect of GBR 12909 and fluoxetine on the acute and long term changes induced by MDMA ("ecstasy") on the 5-HT and dopamine concentrations in mouse brain. *Neuropharmacology* 40, 65–74.

151. Klir, J. J., McClellan, J. L., and Kluger, M. J. (1994). Interleukin-1 beta causes the increase in anterior hypothalamic interleukin-6 during LPS-induced fever in rats. *Am. J. Physiol.* 266, R1845–R1848.

152. Luheshi, G. N., Stefferl, A., Turnbull, A. V., Dascombe, M. J., Brouwer, S., Hopkins, S. J., and Rothwell, N. J. (1997). Febrile response to tissue inflammation involves both peripheral and brain IL-1 and TNF-alpha in the rat. *Am. J. Physiol.* 272, R862–R868.

153. Luheshi, G. N., Gardner, J. D., Rushforth, D. A., Loudon, A. S., and Rothwell, N. J. (1999). Leptin actions on food intake and body temperature are mediated by IL-1. *Proc. Nat. Acad. Sci. USA* 96, 7047–7052.
154. Orio, L., O'Shea, E., Sanchez, V., Pradillo, J. M., Escobedo, I., Camarero, J., Moro, M. A., Green, A. R., and Colado, M. I. (2004). 3,4-Methylenedioxymethamphetamine increases interleukin-1beta levels and activates microglia in rat brain: Studies on the relationship with acute hyperthermia and 5-HT depletion. *J. Neurochem.* 89, 1445–1453.
155. Sanchez, V., Orio, L., O'Shea, E., Escobedo, I., Green, A. R., and Colado, M. I. (2005). 3,4-Methylenedioxymethamphetamine increases pro-IL-1β production and caspase-1 protease activity in frontal cortex, but not in hypothalamus, of Dark Agouti rats. *Neuroscience* 135, 1095–1105.
156. March, C. J., Mosley, B., Larsen, A., Cerretti, D. P., Braedt, G., Price, V., Gillis, S., Henney, C. S., Kronheim, S. R., and Grabstein, K., et al. (1985). Cloning, sequence and expression of two distinct human interleukin-1 complementary DNAs. *Nature* 315, 641–647.
157. Saadat, K. S., O'Shea, E., Colado, M. I., Elliott, J. M., and Green, A. R. (2005). The role of 5-HT in the impairment of thermoregulation observed in rats administered MDMA ("ecstasy")-when housed at high ambient temperature. *Psychopharmacology*. 179, 884–890.
158. Read, W. D., Volicer, L., Smookler, H., Beaven, M. A., and Brodie, B.B. (1968). Brain amines and temperature regulation. *Pharmacology* 1, 329–344.
159. Cronin, M. J. (1976). *p*-Chlorophenylalanine hyperthermia in a warm environment: Reversal with 5-hydroxytryptophan. *Brain Res.* 112, 194–199.
160. Mechan, A. O., O'Shea, E., Elliott, J. M., Colado, M. I., and Green, A. R. (2001). A neurotoxic dose of 3,4-methylenedioxymethamphetamine (MDMA; ecstasy) to rats results in a long term defect in thermoregulation. *Psychopharmacology* 155, 413–418.
161. Marston, H. M., Reid, M. E., Lawrence, J. A., Olverman, H. J., and Butcher, S. P. (1999). Behavioural analysis of the acute and chronic effects of MDMA treatment in the rat. *Psychopharmacology* 144, 67–76.
162. Wallace, T. L., Gudelsky, G. A., and Vorhees, C. V. (2001). Alterations in diurnal and nocturnal locomotor activity in rats treated with a monoamine-depleting regimen of methamphetamine or 3,4-methylenedioxymethamphetamine. *Psychopharmacology* 153, 321–326.
163. Williams, J. H., and Azmitia, E. C. (1981). Hippocampal serotonin re-uptake and nocturnal locomotor activity after microinjections of 5,7-DHT in the fornix-fimbria. *Brain Res.* 207, 95–107.
164. Portas, C. M., Bjorvatn, B., and Ursin, R. (2000). Serotonin and the sleep/wake cycle: Special emphasis on microdialysis studies. *Prog. Neurobiol.* 60, 13–35.
165. Balogh, B., Molnar, E., Jakus, R., Quate, L., Olverman, H. J., Kelly, P. A., Kantor, S., and Bagdy, G. (2004). Effects of a single dose of 3,4-methylenedioxymethamphetamine on circadian patterns, motor activity and sleep in drug-naive rats and rats previously exposed to MDMA. *Psychopharmacology* 173, 296–309.
166. Green, A. R., and McGregor, I. S. (2002). On the anxiogenic and anxiolytic nature of long-term cerebral 5-HT depletion following MDMA. *Psychopharmacology* 164, 448–450.
167. Morley, K. C., Gallate, J. E., Hunt, G. E., Mallet, P. E., and McGregor, I. S. (2001). Increased anxiety and impaired memory in rats 3 months after administration of 3,4-methylenedioxymethamphetamine ("ecstasy"). *Eur. J. Pharmacol.* 433, 91–99.

168. Mechan, A. O., Moran, P. M., Elliott, J. M., Young, A. M. J., Joseph, M. H., and Green, A. R. (2002). A study of the effect of a single neurotoxic dose of 3,4-methylenedioxymethamphetamine (MDMA: "ecstasy") on the subsequent long-term behaviour of rats in the plus maze and open field. *Psychopharmacology* 159, 167–175.

169. Bull, E. J., Hutson, P. H., and Fone, K. C. (2004). Decreased social behaviour following 3,4-methylenedioxymethamphetamine (MDMA) is accompanied by changes in 5-HT2A receptor responsivity. *Neuropharmacology* 46, 202–210.

170. Clemens, K. J., Van Nieuwenhuyzen, P. S., Li, K. M., Cornish, J. L., Hunt, G. E., and McGregor, I. S. (2004). MDMA ("ecstasy"), methamphetamine and their combination: Long-term changes in social interaction and neurochemistry in the rat. *Psychopharmacology* 173, 318–325.

171. Broening, H. W., Morford, L. L., Inman-Wood, S. L., Fukumura, M., and Vorhees, C. V. (2001). 3,4-Methylenedioxymethamphetamine (ecstasy)-induced learning and memory impairments depend on the age of exposure during early development. *J. Neurosci.* 21, 3228–3235.

172. Piper, B. J., and Meyer, J. S. (2004). Memory deficit and reduced anxiety in young adult rats given repeated intermittent MDMA treatment during the periadolescent period. *Pharmacol. Biochem. Behav.* 79, 723–731.

173. Frederick, D. L., Ali, S. F., Slikker, W., Jr., Gilliam, M. P., Allen, R. R., and Paule, M. G. (1995). Behavioral and neurochemical effects of chronic methylenedioxymethamphetamine (MDMA) treatments in rhesus monkeys. *Neurotoxicol. Teratol.* 17, 531–541.

174. Frederick, D. L., Ali, S. F., Gillam, M. P., Gossett, J., Slikker, W., and Paule, M. G. (1998). Acute effects of dexfenfluramine (d-FEN) and methylenedioxymethamphetamine (MDMA) before and after short-course, high-dose treatment. *Ann. NY Acad. Sci.* 44, 183–190.

175. Frederick, D. L., and Paule, M. G. (1997). Effects of MDMA on complex brain function in laboratory animals. *Neurosci. Biobehav. Rev.* 21, 67–78.

176. Taffe, M. A., Weed, M. R., David, S., Huitrón-Resendiz, S., Schroeder, R., Parsons, L. H., Henriksen, S. J., and Gold, L. H. (2001). Functional consequences of repeated (±)3,4-methylenedioxymethamphetamine (MDMA) treatment in rhesus monkeys. *Neuropsychopharmacology* 24, 230–239.

177. Winsauer, P. J., McCann, U. D., Yuan, J., Delatte, M. S., Stevenson, M. W., Ricaurte, G. A., and Moerschbaecher, J. M. (2002). Effects of fenfluramine, m-CPP and triazolam on repeated-acquisition in squirrel monkeys before and after neurotoxic MDMA administration. *Psychopharmacology* 159, 388–396.

178. Morgan, M. J. (1998). Recreational use of "ecstasy" (MDMA) is associated with elevated impulsivity. *Neuropsychopharmacology* 19, 252–264.

179. Bolla, K. I., McCann, U. D., and Ricaurte, G. A. (1998). Memory impairment in abstinent MDMA ("Ecstasy") users. *Neurology* 51, 1532–1537.

180. Morgan, M. J. (1999). Memory deficits associated with recreational use of "ecstasy" (MDMA). *Psychopharmacology* 141, 30–36.

181. McCann, U. D., Szabo, Z., Scheffel, U., Dannals, R. F., and Ricaurte, G. A. (1998). Positron emission tomographic evidence of toxic effect of MDMA ("Ecstasy") on brain serotonin neurons in human beings. *Lancet* 352, 1433–1437.

182. Semple, D. M., Ebmeier, K. P., Glabus, M. F., O'Carroll, R. E., and Johnstone, E. C. (1999). Reduced in vivo binding to the serotonin transporter in the cerebral cortex of MDMA ("ecstasy") users. *Br. J. Psychiatry* 175, 63–69.

183. Ricaurte, G. A., McCann, U. D., Szabo, Z., and Scheffel, U. (2000). Toxicodynamics and long-term toxicity of the recreational drug, 3,4-methylenedioxymethamphetamine (MDMA, "Ecstasy"). *Toxicol. Lett.* 112/113, 143–146.

184. Reneman, L., Booij, J., de Bruin, K., Reitsma, J. B., de Wolff, F. A., Gunning, W. B., den Heeten, G. J., and van den Brink, W. (2001). Effects of dose, sex, and long-term abstention from use on toxic effects of MDMA (ecstasy) on brain serotonin neurons. *Lancet* 358, 1864–1869.

185. Reneman, L., Lavalaye, J., Schmand, B., de Wolff, F. A., van den Brink, W., den Heeten, G. J., and Booij, J. (2001). Cortical serotonin transporter density and verbal memory in individuals who stopped using 3,4-methylenedioxymethamphetamine (MDMA or "ecstasy"): Preliminary findings. *Arch. Gen. Psychiatry* 58, 901–906.

186. McCann, U. D., Ridenour, A., Shaham, Y., and Ricaurte, G. A. (1994). Serotonin neurotoxicity after ($\pm$)3,4-methylenedioxymethamphetamine (MDMA; "Ecstasy"): A controlled study in humans. *Neuropsychopharmacology* 10, 129–138.

187. McCann, U. D., Mertl, M., Eligulashvili, V., and Ricaurte, G. A. (1999). Cognitive performance in ($\pm$)3,4-methylenedioxymethamphetamine (MDMA, "ecstasy") users: A controlled study. *Psychopharmacology* 143, 417–425.

188. Reneman, L., Endert, E., de Bruin, K., Lavalaye, J., Feenstra, M. G., de Wolff, F. A., and Booij, J. (2002). The acute and chronic effects of MDMA ("ecstasy") on cortical 5-HT2A receptors in rat and human brain. *Neuropsychopharmacology* 26, 387–396.

189. Reneman, L., Booij, J., Lavalaye, J., de Bruin, K., Reitsma, J. B., Gunning, B., den Heeten, G. J., and van Den Brink, W. (2002). Use of amphetamine by recreational users of ecstasy (MDMA) is associated with reduced striatal dopamine transporter densities: A [123I]beta-CIT SPECT study—Preliminary report. *Psychopharmacology* 159, 335–340.

190. Gerra, G., Zaimovic, A., Ferri, M., Zambelli, U., Timpano, M., Neri, E., Marzocchi, G. F., Delsignore, R., and Brambilla, F. (2000). Long-lasting effects of ($+/-$)3, 4-methylenedioxymethamphetamine (ecstasy) on serotonin system function in humans. *Biol. Psychiatry* 47, 127–136.

191. Bhattachary, S., and Powell, J. H. (2001). Recreational use of 3,4-methylenedioxymethamphetamine (MDMA) or "ecstasy": Evidence for cognitive impairment. *Psychol. Med.* 31, 647–658.

192. Croft, R. J., Klugman, A., Baldeweg, T., and Gruzelier, J. H. (2001). Electrophysiological evidence of serotonergic impairment in long-term MDMA ("ecstasy") users. *Am. J. Psychiatry* 158, 1687–1692.

193. Verkes, R. J., Gijsman, H. J., Pieters, M. S., Schoemaker, R. C., de Visser, S., Kuijpers, M., Pennings, E. J., de Bruin, D., Van de Wijngaart, G., Van Gerven, J. M., and Cohen, A. F. (2001). Cognitive performance and serotonergic function in users of ecstasy. *Psychopharmacology* 153, 196–202.

194. Parrott, A. C., and Lasky, J. (1998). Ecstasy (MDMA) effects upon mood and cognition: Before, during and after a Saturday night dance. *Psychopharmacology* 139, 261–268.

195. Gouzoulis-Mayfrank, E., Thimm, B., Rezk, M., Hensen, G., and Daumann, J. (2003). Memory impairment suggests hippocampal dysfunction in abstinent ecstasy users. *Prog. Neuro-psychopharmacol. Biol. Psychiatry* 27, 819–827.

196. Wareing, M., Fisk, J. E., and Murphy, P. N. (2000). Working memory deficits in current and previous users of MDMA ("ecstasy"). *Br. J. Psychol.* 91, 181–188.

197. Daumann, J., Fimm, B., Willmes, K., Thron, A., and Gouzoulis-Mayfrank, E. (2003). Cerebral activation in abstinent ecstasy (MDMA) users during a working memory

task: A functional magnetic resonance imaging (fMRI) study. *Brain Res. Cognitive Brain Res.* 16, 479–487.
198. McCardle, K., Luebbers, S., Carter, J. D., Croft, R. J., and Stough, C. (2004). Chronic MDMA (ecstasy) use, cognition and mood. *Psychopharmacology* 173, 434–439.
199. Jacobsen, L. K., Mencl, W. E., Pugh, K. R., Skudlarski, P., and Krystal, J. H. (2004). Preliminary evidence of hippocampal dysfunction in adolescent MDMA ("ecstasy") users: Possible relationship to neurotoxic effects. *Psychopharmacology* 173, 383–390.
200. Morgan, M. J., McFie, L., Fleetwood, H., and Robinson, J. A. (2002). Ecstasy (MDMA): Are the psychological problems associated with its use reversed by prolonged abstinence? *Psychopharmacology* 159, 294–303.
201. Dafters, R. I., Hoshi, R., and Talbot, A. C. (2004). Contribution of cannabis and MDMA ("ecstasy") to cognitive changes in long-term polydrug users. *Psychopharmacology* 173, 405–410.
202. Gouzoulis-Mayfrank, E., Daumann, J., Tuchtenhagen, F., Pelz, S., Becker, S., Kunert, H. J., Fimm, B., and Sass, H. (2000). Impaired cognitive performance in drug free users of recreational ecstasy (MDMA). *J. Neurol. Neurosurg. Psychiatry* 68, 719–725.
203. Gonzales, A., and Nutt, D. J. (2005). Gamma hydroxyl butyrate abuse and dependency. *J. Psychopharmacol.* 19, 195–204.
204. Laborit, H. (1964). Sodium 4-hydroxybutyrate. *Int. J. Neuropharmacol.* 32, 433–451.
205. Galloway, G. P., Frederick, S. L., Staggers, F. E., Gonzales, M., Stalcup, S. A., and Smith, D. E. (1997). Gamma-hydroxybutyrate: An emerging drug of abuse that causes physical dependence. *Addiction* 92, 89–96.
206. Gallimberti, L., Ferri, M., Ferrara, S. D., Fadda, F., and Gessa, G. L. (1992). Gamma-hydroxybutyric acid in the treatment of alcohol dependence: A double-blind study. *Alcohol Clin. Exp. Res.* 16, 673–676.
207. Gallimberti, L., Schifano, F., Forza, G., Miconi, L., and Ferrara, S. D. (1994). Clinical efficacy of gamma-hydroxybutyric acid in treatment of opiate withdrawal. *Eur. Arch. Psychiatry Clin. Neurosci.* 244, 113–114.
208. Maldonado, C., Rodriguez-Arias, M., Aguilar, M. A., and Minarro, J. (2004). GHB ameliorates naloxone-induced conditioned place aversion and physical aspects of morphine withdrawal in mice. *Psychopharmacology* 177, 130–140.
209. Dyer, J. E. (1991). gamma-hydroxybutyrate: A health-food product producing coma and seizurelike activity. *Am. J. Emerg. Med.* 9, 321–324.
210. U.S. Food and Drug Administration. (2006). FDA approves Xyrem for cataplexy attacks in patients with narcolepsy. FDA Talk Paper. Date accessed November 22, 2006. http://www.fda.gov/bbs/topics/ANSWERS/2002/ANS01157.html.
211. Doherty, J. D., Hattox, S. E., Snead, O. C., and Roth, R. H. (1978). Identification of endogenous gamma-hydroxybutyrate in human and bovine brain and its regional distribution in human, guinea pig and rhesus monkey brain. *J. Pharmacol. Exp. Ther.* 207, 130–139.
212. Bessman, S. P., and Fishbein, W. N. (1963). Gamma-hydoxybutyrate, a normal brain metabolite. *Nature* 200, 1207–1208.
213. Maitre, M. (1997). The gamma-hydroxybutyrate signalling system in brain: Organization and functional implications. *Prog. Neurobiol.* 51, 337–361.
214. Snead, O. C., Liu, C. C., and Bearden, L. J. (1982). Studies on the relation of gamma-hydroxybutyric acid (GHB) to gamma-aminobutyric acid (GABA). Evidence that GABA is not the sole source for GHB in rat brain. *Biochem. Pharmacol.* 31, 3917–3923.

215. Roth, R. H. (1970). Formation and regional distribution of gamma-hydroxybutyric acid in mammalian brain. *Biochem. Pharmacol.* 19, 3013–3019.
216. Nelson, T., Kaufman, E., Kline, J., and Sokoloff, L. (1981). The extraneural distribution of gamma-hydroxybutyrate. *J. Neurochem.* 37, 1345–1348.
217. Feigenbaum, J. J., and Howard, S. G. (1996). Gamma hydroxybutyrate is not a GABA agonist. *Prog. Neurobiol.* 50, 1–7.
218. Hoes, M. J., Vree, T. B., and Guelen, P. J. (1980). Gamma-hydroxybutyric acid as hypnotic. Clinical and pharmacokinetic evaluation of gamma-hydroxybutyric acid as hypnotic in man. *Encephale* 6, 93–99.
219. Palatini, P., Tedeschi, L., Frison, G., Padrini, R., Zordan, R., Orlando, R., Gallimberti, L., Gessa, G. L., and Ferrara, S. D. (1993). Dose-dependent absorption and elimination of gamma-hydroxybutyric acid in healthy volunteers. *Eur. J. Clin. Pharmacol.* 45, 353–356.
220. Vickers, M. D. (1969). Gammahydroxybutyric acid. *Int. Anesthesiol. Clin.* 7, 75–89.
221. Louagie, H. K., Verstraete, A. G., De Soete, C. J., Baetens, D. G., and Calle, P. A. (1997). A sudden awakening from a near coma after combined intake of gamma-hydroxybutyric acid (GHB) and ethanol. *J. Toxicol. Clin. Toxicol.* 35, 591–594.
222. Zvosec, D. L., Smith, S. W., McCutcheon, J. R., Spillane, J., Hall, B. J., and Peacock, E. A. (2001). Adverse events, including death, associated with the use of 1,4-butanediol. *New Engl. J. Med.* 344, 87–94.
223. Drug Abuse Warning Network (2002). *The Dawn Report: Club Drugs, Update.* U.S. Department of Health and Human Services, Washington, DC.
224. Li, J., Stokes, S. A., and Woeckener, A. (1998). A tale of novel intoxication: A review of the effects of gamma-hydroxybutyric acid with recommendations for management. *Ann. Emerg. Med.* 31, 729–736.
225. Sanguineti, V. R., Angelo, A., and Frank, M.R. (1997). GHB: A home brew. *Am. J. Drug Alcohol Abuse* 23, 637–642.
226. Dyer, J. E., Roth, B., and Hyma, B. A. (2001). The gamma-hydroxybutyrate withdrawal syndrome. *Ann. Emerg. Med.* 37, 147–153.
227. Tarabar, A. F., and Nelson, L. S. (2004). The gamma-hydroxybutyrate withdrawal syndrome. *Toxicol. Rev.* 23, 45–49.
228. McDaniel, C. H., and Miotto, K. A. (2001). Gamma hydroxybutyrate (GHB) and gamma butyrolactone (GBL) withdrawal: Five case studies. *J. Psychoactive Drugs* 33, 143–149.
229. Serra, M., Sanna, E., Foddi, C., Concas, A., and Biggio, G. (1991). Failure of gamma-hydroxybutyrate to alter the function of the GABAA receptor complex in the rat cerebral cortex. *Psychopharmacology* 104, 351–355.
230. Lingenhoehl, K., Brom, R., Heid, J., Beck, P., Froestl, W., Kaupmann, K., Bettler, B., and Mosbacher, J. (1999). Gamma-hydroxybutyrate is a weak agonist at recombinant GABA(B) receptors. *Neuropharmacology* 38, 1667–1673.
231. Kaupmann, K., Cryan, J. F., Wellendorph, P., Mombereau, C., Sansig, G., Klebs, K., Schmutz, M., Froestl, W., van der Putten, H., Mosbacher, J., Brauner-Osborne, H., Waldmeier, P., and Bettler, B. (2003). Specific gamma-hydroxybutyrate-binding sites but loss of pharmacological effects of gamma-hydroxybutyrate in GABA(B)(1)-deficient mice. *Eur. J. Neurosci.* 18, 2722–2730.
232. Teter, C. J., and Guthrie, S. K. (2001). A comprehensive review of MDMA and GHB: Two common club drugs. *Pharmacotherapy* 21, 1486–1513.

233. Benavides, J., Rumigny, J. F., Bourguignon, J. J., Wermuth, C. G., Mandel, P., and Maitre, M. (1982). A high-affinity, Na$^+$-dependent uptake system for gamma-hydroxybutyrate in membrane vesicles prepared from rat brain. *J. Neurochem.* 38, 1570–1575.

234. Benavides, J., Rumigny, J. F., Bourguignon, J. J., Cash, C., Wermuth, C. G., Mandel, P., Vincendon, G., and Maitre, M. (1982). High affinity binding sites for gamma-hydroxybutyric acid in rat brain. *Life Sci.* 30, 953–961.

235. Ratomponirina, C., Hode, Y., Hechler, V., and Maitre, M. (1995). Gamma-hydroxybutyrate receptor binding in rat brain is inhibited by guanyl nucleotides and pertussis toxin. *Neurosci. Lett.* 189, 51–53.

236. Feigenbaum, J. J., and Howard, S. G. (1997). Naloxone reverses the inhibitory effect of gamma-hydroxybutyrate on central DA release in vivo in awake animals: A microdialysis study. *Neurosci. Lett.* 224, 71–74.

237. Itzhak, Y., and Ali, S. F. (2002). Repeated administration of gamma-hydroxybutyric acid (GHB) to mice: Assessment of the sedative and rewarding effects of GHB. *Ann. NY Acad. Sci.* 965, 451–460.

238. Nissbrandt, H., Elverfors, A., and Engberg, G. (1994). Pharmacologically induced cessation of burst activity in nigral dopamine neurons: Significance for the terminal dopamine efflux. *Synapse* 17, 217–224.

239. Lundborg, P., Hedner, T., and Engel, J. (1980). Catecholamine concentration in the developing rat brain after gamma-hydroxybutyric acid. *J. Neurochem.* 35, 425–429.

240. Hechler, V., Gobaille, S., Bourguignon, J. J., and Maitre, M. (1991). Extracellular events induced by gamma-hydroxybutyrate in striatum: A microdialysis study. *J. Neurochem.* 56, 938–944.

241. Feigenbaum, J. J., and Simantov, R. (1996). Lack of effect of gamma-hydroxybutyrate on mu, delta and kappa opioid receptor binding. *Neurosci. Lett.* 212, 5–8.

242. Miguez, I., Aldegunde, M., Duran, R., and Veira, J. A. (1988). Effect of low doses of gamma-hydroxybutyric acid on serotonin, noradrenaline, and dopamine concentrations in rat brain areas. *Neurochem. Res.* 13, 531–533.

243. Winter, J. C. (1981). The stimulus properties of gamma-hydroxybutyrate. *Psychopharmacology* 73, 372–375.

244. Lobina, C., Agabio, R., Reali, R., Gessa, G. L., and Colombo, G. (1999). Contribution of GABA(A) and GABA(B) receptors to the discriminative stimulus produced by gamma-hydroxybutyric acid. *Pharmacol. Biochem. Behav.* 64, 363–365.

245. Colombo, G., Agabio, R., Lobina, C., Reali, R., Fadda, F., and Gessa, G.L. (1995). Symmetrical generalization between the discriminative stimulus effects of gamma-hydroxybutyric acid and ethanol: Occurrence within narrow dose ranges. *Physiol. Behav.* 57, 105–111.

246. Martellotta, M. C., Fattore, L., Cossu, G., and Fratta, W. (1997). Rewarding properties of gamma-hydroxybutyric acid: An evaluation through place preference paradigm. *Psychopharmacology* 132, 1–5.

247. Colombo, G., Agabio, R., Balaklievskaia, N., Diaz, G., Lobina, C., Reali, R., and Gessa, G. L. (1995). Oral self-administration of gamma-hydroxybutyric acid in the rat. *Eur. J. Pharmacol.* 285, 103–107.

248. Martellotta, M. C., Balducci, C., Fattore, L., Cossu, G., Gessa, G. L., Pulvirenti, L., and Fratta, W. (1998). Gamma-hydroxybutyric acid decreases intravenous cocaine self-administration in rats. *Pharmacol. Biochem. Behav.* 59, 697–702.

249. Colombo, G., Agabio, R., Lobina, C., Reali, R., Fadda, F., and Gessa, G. L. (1995). Cross-tolerance to ethanol and gamma-hydroxybutyric acid. *Eur. J. Pharmacol.* 273, 235–238.

250. Bania, T. C., Ashar, T., Press, G., and Carey, P. M. (2003). Gamma-hydroxybutyric acid tolerance and withdrawal in a rat model. *Academic Emerg. Med.* 10, 697–704.

251. Kohrs, R., and Durieux, M. E. (1998). Ketamine: Teaching an old drug new tricks. *Anesthesie et Analgesie* 87, 1186–1193.

252. Smith, K. M., Larive, L. L., and Romanelli, F. (2002). Club drugs: Methylenedioxymethamphetamine, flunitrazepam, ketamine hydrochloride, and gamma-hydroxybutyrate. *Am. J. Health Syst. Pharm.* 59, 1067–1076.

253. Jansen, K. L. (1993). Non-medical use of ketamine. *Br. Med. J.* 306, 601–602.

254. Reich, D. L., and Silvay, G. (1989). Ketamine: An update on the first twenty-five years of clinical experience. *Can. J. Anaesth.* 36, 186–197.

255. Graeme, K. A. (2000). New drugs of abuse. *Emerg. Med. Clin. North Am.* 18, 625–636.

256. Smith, K. M. (1999). Drugs used in acquaintance rape. *J. Am. Pharmacol. Assoc. (Wash.)* 39, 519–525.

257. Ayesta, F.J., and Cami, J. (2003). Farmacodependencias In *Farmacologia Humana*, J. Florez, Ed. Masson, Barcelona, pp. 595–621.

258. Weiner, A. L., Vieira, L., McKay, C. A., and Bayer, M. J. (2000). Ketamine abusers presenting to the emergency department: A case series. *J. Emerg. Med.* 18, 447–451.

259. Martin, D. C., Watkins, C. A., Adams, R. J., and Nason, L. A. (1988). Anesthetic effects on 5-hydroxytryptamine uptake by rat brain synaptosomes. *Brain Res.* 455, 360–365.

260. Tso, M. M., Blatchford, K. L., Callado, L. F., McLaughlin, D. P., and Stamford, J. A. (2004). Stereoselective effects of ketamine on dopamine, serotonin and noradrenaline release and uptake in rat brain slices. *Neurochem. Int.* 44, 1–7.

261. Masuzawa, M., Nakao, S., Miyamoto, E., Yamada, M., Murao, K., Nishi, K., and Shingu, K. (2003). Pentobarbital inhibits ketamine-induced dopamine release in the rat nucleus accumbens: A microdialysis study. *Anesthesie et Analgesie* 96, 148–152.

262. Beardsley, P. M., and Balster, R. L. (1987). Behavioral dependence upon phencyclidine and ketamine in the rat. *J. Pharmacol. Exp. Ther.* 242, 203–211.

263. Schwartz, R. H., and Weaver, A. B. (1998). Rohypnol, the date rape drug. *Clin. Pediatr. (Phila.)* 37, 321.

264. Abraham, H. D., Aldridge, A. M., and Gogia, P. (1996). The psychopharmacology of hallucinogens. *Neuropsychopharmacology* 14, 285–298.

265. Hofmann, A. (1979). How LSD originated. *J. Psychedelic Drugs* 11, 53–60.

266. Nichols, D. E. (2004). Hallucinogens. *Pharmacol. Ther.* 101, 131–181.

267. Klock, J. C., Boerner, U., and Becker, C. E. (1975). Coma, hyperthermia, and bleeding associated with massive LSD overdose, a report of eight cases. *Clin. Toxicol.* 8, 191–203.

268. Winter, J. C. (1975). Blockade of the stimulus properties of mescaline by a serotonin antagonist. *Arch. Int. Pharmacodyn. Ther.* 214, 250–253.

269. Colpaert, F. C., Niemegeers, C. J., and Janssen, P. A. (1982). A drug discrimination analysis of lysergic acid diethylamide (LSD): In vivo agonist and antagonist effects of purported 5-hydroxytryptamine antagonists and of pirenperone, an LSD-antagonist. *J. Pharmacol. Exp. Ther.* 221, 206–214.

270. Schreiber, R., Brocco, M., and Millan, M.J. (1994). Blockade of the discriminative stimulus effects of DOI by MDL 100,907 and the "atypical" antipsychotics, clozapine and risperidone. *Eur. J. Pharmacol.* 264, 99–102.
271. Meltzer, H. Y., Wiita, B., Tricou, B. J., Simonovic, M., Fang, V., and Manov, G. (1982). Effect of serotonin precursors and serotonin agonists on plasma hormone levels. *Adv. Biochem. Psychopharmacol.* 34, 117–139.
272. Vollenweider, F. X., Vollenweider-Scherpenhuyzen, M. F., Babler, A., Vogel, H., and Hell, D. (1998). Psilocybin induces schizophrenia-like psychosis in humans via a serotonin-2 agonist action. *Neuroreport* 9, 3897–3902.
273. Buckholtz, N. S., Zhou, D. F., Freedman, D. X., and Potter, W. Z. (1990). Lysergic acid diethylamide (LSD) administration selectively downregulates serotonin2 receptors in rat brain. *Neuropsychopharmacology* 3, 137–148.
274. Muschamp, J. W., Regina, M. J., Hull, E. M., Winter, J. C., and Rabin, R. A. (2004). Lysergic acid diethylamide and [−]-2,5-dimethoxy-4-methylamphetamine increase extracellular glutamate in rat prefrontal cortex. *Brain Res.* 1023, 134–140.
275. Conn, P. J., and Pin, J. P. (1997). Pharmacology and functions of metabotropic glutamate receptors. *Ann. Rev. Pharmacol. Toxicol.* 37, 205–237.
276. Winter, J. C., Eckler, J. R., and Rabin, R. A. (2004). Serotonergic/glutamatergic interactions: The effects of mGlu(2/3) receptor ligands in rats trained with LSD and PCP as discriminative stimuli. *Psychopharmacology* 172, 233–240.
277. Lorrain, D. S., Baccei, C. S., Bristow, L. J., Anderson, J. J., and Varney, M. A. (2003). Effects of ketamine and N-methyl-D-aspartate on glutamate and dopamine release in the rat prefrontal cortex: Modulation by a group II selective metabotropic glutamate receptor agonist LY379268. *Neuroscience* 117, 697–706.
278. Xi, Z.-X., Baker, D. A., Shen, H., Carson, D. S., and Kalivas, P. W. (2002). Group II metabotropic glutamate receptors modulate extracellular glutamate in the nucleus accumbens. *J. Pharmacol. Exp. Ther.* 300, 162–171.
279. Pehek, E. A., McFarlane, H. G., Maguschak, K., Price, B., and Pluto, C. P. (2001). M100,907, a selective 5-HT(2A) antagonist, attenuates dopamine release in the rat medial prefrontal cortex. *Brain Res.* 888, 51–59.
280. Yan, Q. S. (2000). Activation of 5-HT2A/2C receptors within the nucleus accumbens increases local dopaminergic transmission. *Brain Res. Bull.* 51, 75–81.
281. Marona-Lewicka, D., Thisted, R. A., and Nichols, D. E. (2005). Distinct temporal phases in the behavioral pharmacology of LSD: Dopamine D(2) receptor-mediated effects in the rat and implications for psychosis. *Psychopharmacology.* 180, 427–435.
282. O'Brien, C. P. (2001). Drug addiction and drug abuse. In *Goodman and Gilman's The Pharmacological Basis of Therapeutics*, J. G. Hardman, L. E. Limbird, P. B. Molinoff, R. W. Ruddon and A. G. Gilman, Eds. McGraw-Hill, New York, pp. 574–639.
283. Hoffmeister, F. (1975). Negative reinforcing properties of some psychotropic drugs in drug-naive rhesus monkeys. *J. Pharmacol. Exp. Ther.* 192, 468–477.
284. Parker, L. A. (1996). LSD produces place preference and flavor avoidance but does not produce flavor aversion in rats. *Behav. Neurosci.* 110, 503–508.
285. Abramson, H. A., Jarvik, M. E., Gorin, M. H., and Hirsch, M. W. (1956). Tolerance development and its relation to the theory of psychosis. *J. Psychol.* 41, 81–105.
286. Balestrieri, A., and Fontanari, D. (1959). Acquired and crossed tolerance to mescaline, LSD-25, and BOL-148. *Arch. Gen. Psychiatry* 1, 279–282.
287. Isbell, H., Wolbach, A. B., Wikler, A., and Miner, E. J. (1961). Cross tolerance between LSD and psilocybin. *Psychopharmacologia* 2, 147–159.

18

MARIJUANA: PHARMACOLOGY AND INTERACTION WITH THE ENDOCANNABINOID SYSTEM

Jenny L. Wiley and Billy R. Martin
Virginia Commonwealth University, Richmond, Virginia

18.1	Introduction	659
18.2	Endocannabinoid System	662
	18.2.1 Cannabinoid Receptors and Signaling	662
	18.2.2 Synthesis and Metabolism of Endocannabinoids	663
	18.2.3 Development	664
18.3	Marijuana Pharmacology: Implications for Physiology of Endocannabinoid System	665
	18.3.1 Pain	666
	18.3.2 Cognition	669
	18.3.3 Appetite Regulation	670
	18.3.4 Neurotoxicity	672
	18.3.5 Emesis	673
18.4	Endocannabinoid Role in Reward, Tolerance, and Dependence	675
18.5	Future Directions	676
Acknowledgments		676
References		677

18.1 INTRODUCTION

Comprised of the dried leaves of the cannabis plant, marijuana (*Cannabis sativa*) is the most commonly abused illicit substance in the United States today, particularly among adolescents. In 2004, nearly half of seniors in high school had tried marijuana at least once and 20% were current users [1]. Further, while the number of regular adult users was approximately the same during the early part of this decade, the prevalence of marijuana abuse and dependence among these users (especially among racial and ethnic minorities) significantly increased, suggesting a combination of causal factors [2]. Yet, marijuana use is not a new phenomenon. Marijuana and other

Handbook of Contemporary Neuropharmacology, Edited by David R. Sibley, Israel Hanin, Michael Kuhar, and Phil Skolnick. Copyright © 2007 John Wiley & Sons, Inc.

constituents of the cannabis plant (e.g., hashish) have a long history of medicinal and religious use which dates back to ancient China. Even in the United States, marijuana was commonly used for medicinal purposes (e.g., nausea, arthritis) and as an intoxicant until after World War I. In the 1930s, however, a concerted effort by the Federal Bureau of Narcotics (a predecessor of the Drug Enforcement Administration) resulted in a change in public attitude toward marijuana. It became to be perceived as a "gateway drug" that led to addiction to "harder drugs" such as heroin. This new perception culminated with the Controlled Substances Act of 1970, in which marijuana was listed as a Schedule I drug with high abuse potential and no accepted medical use. The current debate over medical marijuana highlights this dichotomy between the demonstrated abuse properties of marijuana (as codified by its classification as a Schedule I drug) and growing evidence of its therapeutic potential for a wide variety of medical problems.

Scientific interest in marijuana, although relatively recent, has increased in response to several important discoveries in the field. First, the primary psychoactive constituent of the marijuana plant, Δ^9-tetrahydrocannabinol (Δ^9-THC), was isolated and identified [3]. Identification of this substance (Fig. 18.1) allowed further clinical and preclinical research to characterize its pharmacological effects in the body and on behavior. It also allowed manipulation of dosage so that dose dependence of these effects could be evaluated as well as better determination of the psychoactive potency of marijuana. In recent years, the average Δ^9-THC content of street marijuana in the United States has increased to greater than 4%, although exact concentration in any sample varies considerably depending upon the growing conditions, the plant variety, and the preparation. For example, sinsemilla, the dried flowering tops of unfertilized female plants, may have Δ^9-THC concentrations as high as 20%. Although it is hypothesized that the effects of the numerous other unique chemical constituents of marijuana (cannabinoids) may modulate the primary effects of Δ^9-THC, direct

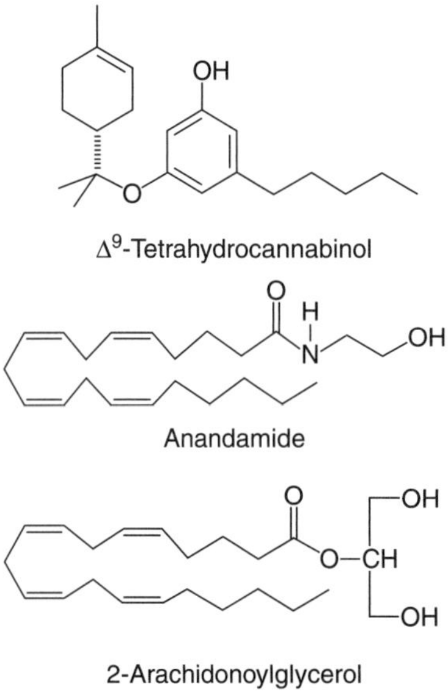

Figure 18.1 Structures of Δ^9-THC, anandamide, and 2-arachidonoylglycerol.

evidence for their role in marijuana's pharmacological effects is lacking. Hence, most of the preclinical mechanistic research on the pharmacological effects of marijuana is actually research on the effects of Δ^9-THC.

A second discovery that increased scientific interest in marijuana was identification of a cannabinoid receptor (CB_1) in the brain [4]. Prior to this discovery, it was theorized that Δ^9-THC and other highly lipophilic cannabinoids produced their effects in the central nervous system by disordering neuronal cell membranes and hence interfering with their normal function. Despite the membrane perturbation theory, however, there was ample evidence for a specific action of cannabinoids. Δ^9-THC is a highly potent drug that produces a distinct profile of pharmacological effects with a strict structure–activity relationship. Each of these factors suggests a selective receptor-mediated action rather than generalized disruption of membranes. In addition, synthetic cannabinoid derivatives were prepared that were extremely potent and enantioselective, thereby enhancing the likelihood of a receptor mechanism. Direct evidence for cannabinoid receptors, however, awaited development of a radiolabeled ligand with which to perform ligand binding studies.

Analysis of binding data with [^{3}H]CP 55,940, the first radiolabeled ligand for CB_1 receptors, revealed a single site that possessed saturable and reversible binding and that displayed selectivity for cannabinoids [4]. Further, the affinity of cannabinoids for this binding site correlated well with their potency in a variety of pharmacological assays, including production of antinociception, catalepsy and hypothermia, and suppression of spontaneous locomotor activity in mice [5]. In addition, a high correlation was found between CB_1 binding affinity and in vivo potency in the rat drug discrimination model (an animal model of the subjective effects of psychoactive drugs) and for marijuana-like psychoactivity in humans [6]. Subsequently, a second cannabinoid receptor (CB_2) was discovered in the periphery. Both CB_1 and CB_2 receptors have been cloned [7, 8].

An interest in the endogenous ligand for these cannabinoid receptors sparked the discovery of arachidonoylethanolamide (anandamide) in porcine brain [9]. Later, a number of other endogenous cannabinoids (or endocannabinoids) were described, including 2-arachidonoylglycerol (2-AG), 2-arachidonylglycerol ether (noladin ether), N-arachidonoyldopamine, and O-arachidonoylethanolamine (virodhamine) [see [10] for a review]. The structures of THC, anandamide, and 2-AG are depicted in Figure 18.1. Although the chemical structure of anandamide does not resemble the structure of classical cannabinoids such as Δ^9-THC or of nonclassical synthetic cannabinoids, such as CP 55,940 [11] and the aminoalkylindoles [12], it shares with these diverse cannabinoids the ability to bind to and activate identified cannabinoid receptors and to produce a similar profile of pharmacological effects, although there are also some differences (see [13] for a review).

Another important tool in cannabinoid pharmacology was development of selective CB_1 and CB_2 cannabinoid receptor antagonists SR141716A (rimonabant, trade name Accomplia) and SR144528, respectively [14, 15]. The initial importance of these antagonists rested with their usefulness as tools in determining receptor mediation of cannabinoid effects. Subsequently, it was reported that SR141716A acted as an inverse agonist in certain in vitro tests, particularly at higher concentrations [16]. In vivo, SR141716A blocks most of the cannabinoid effects of plant-derived and synthetic cannabinoids; however, it also produces locomotor stimulation (opposite of the locomotor suppression produced by active cannabinoids) [17]. Tests with a series of structural analogs of SR141716A indicated that this stimulatory effect did not show a systematic structure–activity relationship; hence, it is probably not CB_1 receptor mediated [18]. Currently, SR141716A has been approved in the United States as an anti craving agent for smoking cessation and is undergoing phase III clinical trials as an appetite suppressant.

While the initial focus of marijuana research was on understanding the abuse potential of this drug, increasing interest has been shown in medical marijuana as well as in the therapeutic implications of pharmacological manipulations of the endocannabinoid system through which marijuana acts. The possible physiological roles of this system are only now starting to be delineated. In the following sections, we describe the endocannabinoid system and its potential physiological roles as well as discuss the ways in which marijuana may interact with this system.

18.2 ENDOCANNABINOID SYSTEM

The endocannabinoid system is one of several lipid signaling systems in the brain and in the body. This system consists of four basic elements: (a) two identified receptors, (b) several derivatives of arachidonic acid that serve as endogenous ligands, (c) synthetic and degradative pathways for these endocannabinoids, and (d) signal transduction pathways. Each of these components contributes to the overall functioning of the signaling system and is discussed in further detail below. In addition, the endocannabinoid system is not static over the course of development. For this reason, a brief description of age-dependent changes that occur during early life is included.

18.2.1 Cannabinoid Receptors and Signaling

To date two cannabinoid receptors, CB_1 and CB_2, have been identified. A splice variant of the CB_1 receptor, CB_{1A}, has also been cloned [19], but its biological significance remains unknown. CB_1 receptors are located primarily in the brain (as discussed in greater detail later). In contrast, CB_2 receptors are located primarily (but not exclusively; see [20]) in the periphery and are involved in the immunoregulatory effects of cannabinoids [21, 22]. Δ^9-THC binds with approximately equal affinity to both subtypes of receptors [23]. Recent research results have raised the possibility that additional non-CB_1, non-CB_2 receptor(s) may exist, although none has been definitively identified (see [24] for a review).

The largest concentration of CB_1 receptors is located in the central nervous system, although their presence has also been noted in other parts of the body. Autoradiograpic studies have shown high levels of CB_1 receptor binding in the basal ganglia (substantia nigra pars reticulata, globus pallidus, entropeduncular nucleus, and lateral caudate putamen) and the molecular layer of the cerebellum [25]. Cannabinoid-induced motor impairment may be related to activation of CB_1 receptors in these regions. Intermediate levels of binding are present in the CA pyramidal cell layers of the hippocampus, the dentate gryus, and layers I and VI of the cortex. These receptors are most likely responsible for cannabinoid effects on memory and cognition. CB_1 receptors are also present in the ventromedial striatum and nucleus accumbens, areas that are associated with dopamine and mediation of brain reward. Localization here is consistent with the observation that most drugs of abuse (including marijuana) directly or indirectly modulate dopamine release in these brain regions. Sparse levels were detected in the brain stem, which likely explains the low respiratory depressant effects of cannabinoids.

The predominant centrally mediated effects of cannabinoids occur through activation of inhibitory G proteins ($G_{i/o}$ and/or G_i) coupled to CB_1 receptors [26], although there was a report that CB_1 receptors can couple to G_s proteins [27]. Binding and activation of CB_1 receptors by Δ^9-THC, anandamide, and other cannabinoid agonists results in a number of intracellular signaling processes, including inhibition of adenylyl cylase, inhibition of calcium channels (N and Q types), and activation of inwardly rectifying potassium channels [28, 29]. In addition, mitogen-activated protein kinases are activated by the CB_1 receptor [30]. Whether all signal transduction systems are activated simultaneously is not known nor is the extent to which they are involved in specific cannabinoid actions. In addition, recent evidence has demonstrated the presence of an allosteric binding site on CB_1 receptors that modulates the affinity and efficacy of exogenous cannabinoids [31]. The effects of binding to this site on modulation of endocannabinoid activity under physiological conditions remain unknown.

In most traditional neurotransmitter systems (e.g., monoamines), receptors may be either pre- or postsynaptic; however, one-to-one correspondence between specific neurons and the neurotransmitter that they release is the general rule. A unique aspect of the endocannabinoid system is that endocannabinoids are released from neurons that are associated with release of many other neurotransmitters, including dopamine, γ-aminobutyric acid (GABA), and glutamate [32]. CB_1 receptors are prevalent on presynaptic terminals of neurons associated with almost all known neurotransmitters. Activation of these receptors is modulatory with respect to release of the primary neurotransmitter. The complexity of cannabinoid modulation of neurotransmitter release is further illustrated by recent findings that endogenous cannabinoids may act in a retrograde signaling fashion [33]. In this process, depolarization of a postsynaptic neuron elicits release of an endocannabinoid such as anandamide from that neuron. Endocannabinoids have a direct inhibitory action on release; however, their presynaptic localization on neurons that release both excitatory and inhibitory neurotransmitters means that the end result of CB_1 receptor activation may be either inhibitory [if release of an excitatory neurotransmitter such as glutamate is inhibited; i.e., depolarization-induced suppression of excitation (DSE)] or excitatory [if release of an inhibitory neurotransmitter such as GABA is inhibited; i.e., depolarization-induced suppression of inhibition (DSI)]. Indeed, inhibition of release of a neurotransmitter that tonically regulates the release of another neurotransmitter can result in increased release of the latter. For example, cannabinoids are also known to stimulate the release of dopamine in the nucleus accumbens by inhibition of glutamate release.

18.2.2 Synthesis and Metabolism of Endocannabinoids

To date, at least three arachidonic acid derivatives that serve as endocannabinoid ligands have been identified: arachidonylethanolamide (anandamide [9]), 2-AG [34], and 2-arachidonoyl-glyceryl ether (noladin ether [35]). Two other endocannabinoid ligands, N-arachidonoyldopamine [36] and O-arachidonoylethanolamine (virodhamine) [37], have also been proposed. Anandamide, by far, is the best characterized.

In the brain, anandamide binds to and activates CB_1 receptors, which, as described above, are G-protein-coupled receptors. Anandamide also interacts with transient receptor potential V1 (TRPV1) receptors and with a number of cation channels [38–40].

Synthetic and degradative pathways for endocannabinoids have been identified. Substantial evidence indicates that anandamide is formed from arachidonic acid that is bound to cell membranes. This process is calcium and energy independent and involves activation of a transacylase that transfers arachidonic acid from the *sn*-1 position of phosphatidylcholine to the amino group in phosphatidylethanolamine, with subsequent hydrolysis by a phospholipase-D-type enzyme [41]. Since anandamide is not stored in vesicles, it is synthesized and released on an "as-needed" basis. Inactivation of anandamide occurs primarily via degradation by fatty acid amide hydrolase (FAAH), an enzyme that also degrades a number of other endogenous fatty acids, including the sleep-inducing lipid oleamide [42]. This enzyme has been cloned [43]. In mice, potentiation of the actions of exogenously administered anandamide is observed with pharmacological blockade of FAAH with a FAAH inhibitor and with deletion of the gene encoding for FAAH [44]. Anandamide may also be inactivated in part through a specific uptake mechanism in which it is transported across cellular membranes by a protein-mediated process that has the characteristics of facilitated diffusion [i.e., bidirectional and sodium and adenosine triphosphate (ATP) independence] [45].

18.2.3 Development

In humans, most of the research into the effects of marijuana on development has concentrated on identification of possible marijuana-induced fetal and birth defects. To this end, epidemiological studies have revealed that the most consistent effect of maternal marijuana use is shortened gestation and reduced birth weights; however, few long-term developmental consequences have been noted in the offspring of mothers who smoked marijuana during pregnancy [46]. By and large, the effects that have been reported are subtle and most appear to be reversible. The major exception appears to be higher cognitive functioning (executive functioning) that is impaired for a sustained period of time in the children who were exposed in utero.

Much of what we know about the acute and long-term effects of marijuana on the developing brain was discovered in the course of preclinical research with Δ^9-THC in rodents. Prenatal exposure studies in rodents have shown that high doses of cannabinoids can produce resorption, growth retardation, and malformations, but only at doses that also produced malnutrition, which has similar consequence [47]. Doses of Δ^9-THC that do not alter maternal body weight produce little effect on fetal development. The results of a number of studies of postnatal exposure to Δ^9-THC in rodents have also been published. Since rats are born at a more immature stage than are humans, the preweanling period of a rat's life most closely corresponds to prenatal development in humans. During the first month or so of a rat's life, the endocannabinoid system in the brain undergoes a number of important changes. CB_1 receptors in the rat brain exhibit a progressive increase in number, but not in affinity, during the preweanling period (i.e., before postnatal day 21) and during early adolescence (females peak at postnatal day 30 and males peak at postnatal day 40). Receptors are pruned and decline to adult levels during later adolescence [48–50]. By postnatal day 60, adult levels of cannabinoid receptors are achieved [48]. Increases in levels of the endogenous cannabinoid anandamide and N-arachidonoyl-phosphatidylethanolamine (an anandamide precursor) accompany these changes in receptor number throughout development [51]. While most brain CB_1 receptors present during development are distributed similarly to adult receptors (e.g., high levels in striatum, cerebellum, and cortex), an early transient atypical localization in presynaptic white matter has also been observed, suggesting a role for the endogenous cannabinoid system in neuronal migration and brain development [52, 53]. In addition, functional brain CB_1 receptors and anandamide also play a crucial role in physical growth and development, as they are necessary for milk suckling [54]. Although similar experiments obviously cannot be performed in human children and adolescents, it has recently been recognized that the human brain also undergoes substantial reorganization during adolescence [55].

18.3 MARIJUANA PHARMACOLOGY: IMPLICATIONS FOR PHYSIOLOGY OF ENDOCANNABINOID SYSTEM

Marijuana is typical of most psychoactive substances in that it produces a broad array of behavioral and pharmacological effects, many of which are subjective and differ among users. Some of the more prevalent effects on the central nervous system include euphoria, sedation, dreamlike state, distorted perceptions of sensory information and time, disrupted cognition, and impairment of fine motor skills [56]. Δ^9-THC produces the subjective "high" associated with smoking marijuana and represents the chemical basis for many of its other effects in the central nervous system.

In rodents, Δ^9-THC, other plant-derived cannabinoids, and synthetic cannabinoids that bind to CB_1 receptors with reasonable affinity produce a characteristic tetrad of pharmacological effects in mice, including suppression of locomotor activity, hypothermia, antinociception, and catalepsy [57]. These psychoactive cannabinoids also produce Δ^9-THC-like discriminative stimulus effects in rats and rhesus monkeys (for a review, see [58]). Among this group of cannabinoids, potencies for producing these effects are highly correlated with affinities for the CB_1 receptor [5], suggesting that these effects are mediated via interaction with this receptor. Further evidence for CB_1 receptor mediation of these pharmacological properties is seen in blockade of the effects by SR141716A [17, 59], but not by administration of the CB_2 antagonist SR144528 [60].

Anandamide and structural analogs of anandamide produce a profile of pharmacological effects in mice that resemble those produced by Δ^9-THC; however, anandamide-like cannabinoids have lower efficacies for effecting hypothermia: Body temperature decreases are about half that of traditional cannabinoids [61–63]. Further, correlations between in vitro affinities of anandamide analogs for CB_1 receptors and their in vivo potencies were not as strong as for other classes of cannabinoids [64, 65]. Differences in anandamide pharmacology also have been noted in drug discrimination studies [66] as well as in the mechanism through which anandamide produces spinal antinociception in mice [63, 67, 68]. In addition, it was reported that anandamide's pharmacological effects were not blocked by the CB_1 antagonist SR141716A, although SR141716A blocked the cannabimimetic effects of more stable anandamide analogs, such as 2-methyl-2'-fluoroethylanandamide [69].

An issue of concern with respect to these differences in anandamide's pharmacological effects is the extent to which pharmacokinetics may play a role. As mentioned previously, FAAH rapidly hydrolyzes anandamide to arachidonic acid [70, 71]. In contrast, Δ^9-THC and other plant-derived cannabinoids are metabolized primarily through the hepatic P_{450} system [72], a process which requires much more time. For the most part, studies that have addressed the extent to which the observed differences in anandamide pharmacology might be related to these differences in its biodisposition have suggested that many of the anomalies in anandamide pharmacology (as compared to that of traditional cannabinoids) are not observed when the metabolism of anandamide is slowed, as in FAAH knockout mice [44] or as a result of administration of an agent that inhibits FAAH [73, 74]. Nevertheless, differences in anandamide pharmacology that cannot be explained by its rapid metabolism remain (see [13] for a review), suggesting that the effects of exogenously administered cannabinoids (including marijuana) may not entirely mimic physiological activation of the endocannabinoid system. This caveat should be kept in mind throughout the following descriptions of specific areas in which endocannabinoid involvement is strongly implicated and in which marijuana has prominent pharmacological effects.

18.3.1 Pain

Interest in cannabinoids as analgesic agents began with cannabis before attention turned to Δ^9-THC and finally the endogenous cannabinoid system. Noyes et al. [75] demonstrated that orally administered Δ^9-THC elevated mood, stimulated appetite, and produced some analgesia in cancer patients at doses that also produced dizziness, blurred vision, and impaired thinking. They concluded that Δ^9-THC and codeine had comparable efficacy [76], while other investigators found it to have little analgesic efficacy [77, 78]. There has also been a conscientious effort to develop synthetic cannabinoid derivatives that might be useful as analgesics, but they too have been hampered by their behavioral side effects [79, 80].

Evaluations of cannabinoids in animal models have consistently shown them to be antinociceptive [81]. However, the fact that Δ^9-THC analgesia is also accompanied by other effects, such as motor depression, raised questions regarding the validity of these antinociceptive measures. However, Walker et al. [82] showed that cannabinoids suppress nociceptive neurotransmission at the level of the spinal cord and the thalamus and that the effects were selective for painful as opposed to nonpainful somatic stimuli. Earlier, it had been shown that intrathecal administration of either the α_2-noradrenergic antagonist yohimbine [83] or the κ-opioid antagonist norbinaltorphimine (nor-BNI) [84] blocked cannabinoid-induced antinociception but failed to attenuate cannabinoid-induced motor impairment. Furthermore, intrastriatal administration of cannabinoids into the caudate nucleus produced catalepsy [85] without producing antinociception [86]. Cannabinoids have also been shown to be exhibit antinociception in several chronic-pain models. The synthetic cannabinoid agonist WIN 55,212-2 produced anti-hyperalgesic responses following a chronic constriction injury of the sciatic nerve [87]. Another study that employed an arthritic pain model using Freund's adjuvant found Δ^9-THC to be antinociceptive in both arthritic and nonarthritic rats [88].

With the identification of the endogenous cannabinoid system, it became possible to establish the mechanism of cannabinoid-induced analgesia and to further delineate between direct and indirect effects. Initial studies showed that exogenous administration of anandamide to mice [63, 89] and rats [90] was antinociceptive. This evidence coupled with observations that cannabinoids inhibit nociception [86, 91] when injected into brain areas associated with antinociception [92] and that contain cannabinoid receptors [93] suggested the presence of a cannabinoid system that functioned to modulate pain. Electrical stimulation of periaqueductal gray (PAG) induced CB_1-mediated analgesia and simultaneously released anandamide [94]. Also the injection of formalin into the paw induced a nociceptive response and concomitant release of anandamide from the PAG. In fact, an earlier investigation had suggested that an endocannabinoid tone may downmodulate pain perception via CB_1 receptors in another region of the brain stem, the rostral ventromedial medulla, through the same circuit previously shown to contribute to the pain-suppressing effects of morphine [95]. Calignano et al. [96] suggested an endocannabinoid and CB_1/CB_2-mediated tone controlling pain at the peripheral level, mostly based on the observation that local administration of the antagonist for each receptor subtype led to hyperalgesia, whereas exogenous anandamide blocked the painful response of mice to formalin injection. In a subsequent study, however, no difference with vehicle-treated rat paws was found in the amounts of anandamide and 2-AG in the hind paw of rats after injection of formalin and during the maximal nociceptive response [97]. These studies, taken together with that by Meng et al. [95] and Walker et al. [94], suggest that if endocannabinoids tonically modulate inflammatory pain perception they may do so at sites different from those of inflammation.

It is also well known that stress will induce antinociception. Suplita et al. [98] demonstrated that a descending cannabinergic neural system is activated by stress to modulate pain sensitivity in a CB_1 receptor-dependent manner. Furthermore, this pathway involves both brain stem rostral ventromedial medullar and midbrain dorsolateral PAG. Stress produces an elevation in both anandamide and 2-AG levels in the PAG, and SR141716 blocks the associated stress-induced analgesia [99]. These latter investigators provided further evidence for endocannabinoid involvement by demonstrating that inhibitors of monoacylglycerol lipase (degrades 2-AG) and FAAH (degrades anandamide) also enhance stress-induced antinociception when injected into the PAG. It had been shown previously that FAAH inhibitors greatly elevated anandamide levels in rodent brain and produced CB_1 receptor-dependent antinociception [100]. As mentioned above, it is logical to presume that a CB_1 receptor antagonist might produce hyperalgesia if elevation of anandamide produces antinociception. However, one study reported that SR141716 produced hyperalgesia in the hot-plate test [101], whereas another failed to show hyperalgesia to a mechanical stimulus in either nonarthritic or arthritic rats [88].

The first electrophysiological evidence that cannabinoids can block spinal pain pathways was the intravenous administration of WIN 55,212-2 that selectively suppressed noxious-evoked firing of the wide-dynamic-range (WDR) neurons to a noxious pressure stimulus [102]. Importantly, WIN 55,212-2 did not affect the stimulus-evoked activity of non-nociceptive neurons in the spinal cord. WIN 55,212-2 also inhibited noxious stimulus-evoked activity of neurons in the ventrolateral posterior nucleus of the thalamus [103]. Although these results demonstrated that cannabinoids suppress the ascending nociceptive pathway, they did not address the site of cannabinoid action in the central nervous system (CNS). Experimental evidence indicates that cannabinoids inhibit nociceptive responses at both spinal and supraspinal sites. Intravenous administration of either Δ^9-THC or CP 55,940 to spinally transected rats was found to reduce, but not eliminate, antinociception [104]. Direct injections of cannabinoids into the brain provided evidence for a supraspinal site of action [86, 105]. Direct administration of WIN 55,212-2 into the dorsolateral PAG or dorsal raphe nucleus, but not the ventral PAG, medial septal area, lateral habenula, arcuate nucleus, or perihypothalamic area, produced a partial antinociceptive effect [91]. Similarly, CP 55,940 infused into the posterior ventrolateral area in the region of the dorsal raphe produced antinociception as well as other pharmacological actions [86]. In contrast, drug administration into either dorsolateral or anterior ventrolateral PAG sites or outside of the PAG borders was without effect.

Many antinociceptive drugs acting in the brain activate descending neurochemical systems to inhibit the input of noxious stimuli at the spinal level. Spinal noradrenergic and serotonergic fibers are believed to play a predominant role in the antinociceptive effects of a variety of drugs. There is evidence suggesting the involvement of monoaminergic systems in cannabinoid-induced antinociception. Both 5,7-dihydroxytryptamine [106], a serotonergic neurotoxin, and 6-hydroxydopamine [107], a dopaminergic neurotoxin, reduced the antinociceptive effects of cannabinoids. Other evidence implicating the involvement of norepinephrine in cannabinoid-induced antinociception is that intrathecal (i.t.) administration of the α_2-noradrenergic antagonist yohimbine blocked the antinociceptive effects of intravenous (i.v.)–administered Δ^9-THC [83]. In contrast, i.t. injection of the nonspecific serotonin antagonist methysergide failed to reduce Δ^9-THC-induced antinociception. These findings are consistent with the hypothesis that the supraspinal component of cannabinoid-induced antinociception is mediated through a descending spinal noradrenergic system. There is also evidence that $GABA_B$ receptor agonists produce antinociception through modulation of the endocannabinoid system at the spinal level. SR141716 blocked the antinociceptive effects of baclofen but the, $GABA_B$ antagonist saclofen did not block the analgesic effects of CP55940 [108].

Recently, attention has turned to the CB_2 receptor as an important target for regulation inflammation and the pain associated with it. The CB_2 selective agonist HU-308 reduced formalin-induced pain and arachidonic acid-induced inflammation (ear swelling) [109]. Another CB_2 selective agonist, AM1241, has been reported to be anti-inflammatory and analgesic in several pain models [110]. The nonselective agonist CP 55940 was reported to be effective in a neuropathic pain (spinal nerve ligation) model, and its effects were blocked only by the CB_2 receptor antagonist [111]. Valenzano et al. reported that a selective CB_2 receptor agonist was active in neuropathic, incisional, and chronic inflammatory pain models and was inactive in CB_2 receptor knockout animals [112]. Moreover, CB_2 receptors were upregulated in dorsal root ganglia (DRG) following sciatic nerve section or spinal nerve ligation [113].

TRPV1 represents another possible target for cannabinoid action. Jerman et al. demonstrated that anandamide caused a concentration-dependent increase in intracellular calcium concentrations in VR1-HEK (human embryonic kidney) and DRG cells that was blocked by capsazepine but not by SR141716 [114]. The authors concluded that anandamide analgesic properties are likely to be mediated at least in part through TRPV1 activation. Lam et al. also found that anandamide was a partial agonist in increasing intracellular concentrations in TRPV1-containing HEK cells, but they did not report whether its effects were blocked by capsazepine [115].

Unfortunately, there is little in vivo evidence that anandamide antinociception is mediated through TRPV1, in part because TRPV1 antagonists are typically not very effective when administered to animals. Capsazepine does not attenuate cannabinoid stress-induced analgesia [98]. There are suggestions that hybrid anandamide/capsaicin analogs may produce some of their antinociceptive effects through TRPV1, but direct evidence is lacking [116].

18.3.2 Cognition

One of the most prominent behavioral effects of Δ^9-THC and other psychoactive cannabinoids is disruption of cognition. This effect has been observed in humans and in animal models. In human marijuana users, smoked marijuana interferes with the ability to learn and recall verbal information and it impairs short-term memory [117–119]. In addition, smoked marijuana disrupts timing ability in experiments requiring subjects to estimate elapsed time. Subjects in these experiments responded prior to completion of the specified time interval, suggesting overestimation of elapsed time [120, 121]. Similar impairments of short-term (i.e., working) memory and timing ability have been observed in animal models (see [122] for a review). Rodents injected with an acute dose of a psychoactive cannabinoid exhibited impairments in recognition memory as well as delay-dependent deficits in accuracy in delayed match/nonmatch to sample procedures and in spatial water and land maze tasks [123–126]. CB_1 receptor mediation is indicated, as these effects were reversible upon elimination of the drug or administration of SR141716A and were not evident in CB_1 knockout mice [127]. Interestingly, memory impairment produced by Δ^9-THC in a delayed match-to-sample task was accompanied by decreases in firing rates of hippocampal neurons during the sample, but not the match, phase of the experiment, suggesting that, at least for this task, Δ^9-THC disrupts encoding of memories during the sample phase, but not their retrieval during the match phase [124]. Δ^9-THC-induced dopamine hyperactivity in the prefrontal area also has been implicated in some types of observed memory impairments [128]. While cannabinoids affect acquisition (i.e., learning) to a lesser degree than they do working memory, acquisition of new information *is* impaired. For example, Δ^9-THC increased the number of errors made by rats working in a repeated acquisition task [129]. In contrast, long-term memory is relatively unaffected in both humans [130] and animals [122] following cannabinoid administration, suggesting cannabinoid interference with only certain types of cognition.

In addition to inducing selective cognitive impairments, Δ^9-THC is reported to produce severe disruption of timing and temporal discrimination in rodents. Consistent with results of human studies with smoked marijuana [120], peripherally injected Δ^9-THC impaired performance of rats responding for food reward under differential reinforcement of low rates (DRL) operant schedules [131, 132]. In this type of schedule, an animal is required to wait for a specified length of time since the last response before responding will again be reinforced; that is, the interresponse time (IRT) must be of a specified minimum length. Under conditions in which the specified IRT was short (5 s or less), Δ^9-THC had no effect on the pattern of responding; however, when the target wait time was lengthened to 10–15 s, premature responding was observed. Collectively, the results of both human and rodent studies suggest that Δ^9-THC disrupts timing by making longer delays seem shorter.

Conversely, Han and Robinson [133] found that SR141716A increased estimated time in another type of operant procedure, raising the possibility that it may do so by blocking endogenous anandamide.

Cannabinoid effects on learning, working memory, and temporal discrimination occur within the range of doses that are intoxicating in humans and that produce discriminative stimulus effects in animals, but at doses lower than those required to elicit other characteristic cannabinoid effects (e.g., motor suppression, analgesia, and hypothermia). This separation of effects suggests a degree of selectivity for cannabinoid effects on higher functioning.

Results of studies that involved CB_1 receptor nullification (e.g., pharmacological blockade, genetic manipulation) have suggested a possible physiological role of endocannabinoids in cognition. Selective antagonism of CB_1 receptors with SR141716A delayed extinction in a previously learned water maze task in mice at doses that did not affect swim speeds, and mice lacking CB_1 receptors exhibited a similar delay in extinction in this task [127]. In each case, CB_1 receptor nullification increased perseveration in a previously learned behavior. These findings may result from interference with cognitive processes related to forgetting (e.g., memory duration) and/or to suppression of behavior (i.e., extinction). If increased memory duration were the primary factor effecting perseveration, the delay between acquisition of a behavior and its recall would be most important to performance (i.e., perseveration would occur at short delays and would be independent of number of trials). In contrast, a primary deficit in extinction would evince in less perseveration with increasing number of trials. In a study that varied number and spacing of trials, SR141716A-induced perseveration was most apparent in extinction trials that occurred infrequently (spaced trials) versus those that occurred consecutively on the same day (massed trials) [134]. Although these results seem to suggest that SR141716A's primary effect was on extinction, its effects on forgetting could not be assessed adequately due to the extended duration of memory in the control group. Given that SR141716A produced its pharmacological effects on cognition at doses that have not been associated with inverse agonism at CB_1 receptors, antagonism of endocannabinoid action at these receptors is the most likely mechanism. However, while it is tempting to speculate that endocannabinoids tonically modulate the neural pathways that underlie cognition, empirical results supporting this hypothesis are still inconclusive.

18.3.3 Appetite Regulation

Marijuana increases appetite in humans, which was recognized even in historical accounts. Indeed, this effect serves as the basis for development of oral formulations of Δ^9-THC that are currently in therapeutic use to treat cachexia in cancer and AIDS patients [135, 136]. As in humans, Δ^9-THC and other psychoactive cannabinoids increase food intake in rodent models, as does exogenously administered anandamide [137–139]. This effect is blocked by coadministration of SR141716A (but not SR144528) and is not observed in CB_1 knockout mice [140–142]; hence, it appears to be CB_1 receptor mediated. Further, SR141716A and several of its analogs produce effects on feeding that are opposite those of cannabinoid agonists; that is, they dose-dependently decrease food consumption in rodents [141, 143, 144], and in clinical trials in humans SR141716A produces weight loss [145].

In humans and other mammals, food intake is a complex physiological process that is regulated by both homeostatic mechanisms and the hedonic value of food. Endocannabinoid involvement is implicated in both types of regulation [146], as anandamide levels in both the hypothalamus (associated with homeostatic mechanisms) and limbic forebrain (associated with hedonics of food intake) are increased in hungry rats and return to basal levels when rats are satiated [147]. The hypothalamus is a major player in homeostatic control of appetite, and it is here where endocannabinoids exert their primary central effects on this type of regulation of food intake. Although the hypothalamus does not have many CB_1 receptors as compared to other areas rich in these receptors (e.g., hippocampus), those that it has appear to be very efficient at activating intracellular messenger systems. An increase in hypothalamic anandamide levels, through either endogenous release or exogenous administration directly into the hypothalamus, acts to stimulate eating [148].

Of course, the endocannabinoid system is but one of the many neuromodulatory systems that affect food intake (e.g., [149]). For example, the hormone leptin is a key regulator of feeding behavior that is found mainly in white adipose tissue. Upon feeding, it is released into the circulation. Once leptin reaches the hypothalamus, it initiates a series of signaling events that eventually leads to release of anorexigenic peptides (e.g., pro-opiomelanocortin and cocaine- and amphetamine-regulated transcript) or orexigenic peptides (e.g., neuropeptide Y and agouti-related protein). Leptin also exerts negative control over levels of anandamide and/or 2-AG in the hypothalamus [140]. Further, these investigators found higher levels of hypothalamic endocannabinoids in obese mice and rats with congenitally disrupted leptin signaling.

Endocannabinoids may also play a direct role in lipid metabolism in the periphery via activation of CB_1 receptors in adipocytes [150]. Blockade of these receptors by rimonabant stimulated Acrp30 (adiponectin) messenger RNA (mRNA) expression in adipose tissue and reduced hyperinsulinemia in obese *(fa/fa)* rats [151]. These findings suggest that inactivation of the endocannabinoid system may aid weight loss by altering energy balance and lipid metabolism, an hypothesis that has recently received additional support at the genomic level in a diet-induced obesity model in rats [152].

In addition to their roles in homeostatic control of eating, however, endocannabinoids also may be involved in regulation of the hedonic value of food (via action in brain areas associated with reward; e.g., nucleus accumbens and limbic forebrain). Levels of anandamide and 2-AG in these reward-associated areas were increased during food restriction and returned to baseline when rats were satiated, much as they were in the hypothalamus under similar conditions [147, 153]. Yet, other feeding-induced changes in endocannabinoids in these reward areas were not associated with similar changes in the hypothalamus. Whereas significant decreases in CB_1 receptor density in the hippocampus, cortex, nucleus accumbens, and entopeduncular nucleus were observed in rats fed palatable food to induce obesity, changes in the density of hypothalamic CB_1 receptors were not noted [154]. Downregulation of cannabinoid receptors in reward areas in obese rats were hypothesized to be the result of prolonged elevation of endocannabinoid levels in these areas. The fact that these region-specific differences in CB_1 receptor density were selectively induced in obese rats by a taste-enhanced diet, and not by a normal laboratory rodent diet, suggests a special sensitivity to the hedonic aspects of food in these reward-associated areas. These areas also appear to mediate the hedonic effects of drugs of abuse (including marijuana), although the degree to which the rewarding properties of food and drugs involve similar mechanisms within these areas is still unclear. Nevertheless, it is intriguing that SR141716A, which was originally marketed as a pharmacological aid for smoking cessation, has also been shown to be effective in decreasing intake of palatable food.

18.3.4 Neurotoxicity

There has been considerable interest in the influence of cannabinoids on neuronal excitability and toxicity that may have relevance to several disease states. Δ^9-THC has been shown to have both convulsant and anticonvulsant properties depending upon the model. Δ^9-THC will enhance kindling elicited by either chemical or electrical stimuli [155], whereas it will decrease maximal electroshock-induced tonic–clonic convulsions [156]. The observation that cannabidiol, a structurally related cannabinoid lacking affinity for CB_1 receptors, is also anticonvulsant [157] raises the question of mechanism of action. There are several lines of evidence indicating that the endogenous cannabinoid system is capable of regulating neuronal excitability. The anticonvulsant effects of Δ^9-THC in the maximal electroshock procedure is blocked by the CB_1 receptor antagonist SR141716, while the anticonvulsant effects of cannabidiol are not [158]. Subsequent studies demonstrated that anandamide and one of its stable congeners were also anticonvulsant and that a CB_1 receptor antagonist lowered electroshock seizure threshold [159]. Collectively, these observations suggest disruptions in endogenous cannabinoid tone can result in altered neuroexcitability.

The endocannabinoid system also influences the rat pilocarpine model of epilepsy. Cannabinoid receptor agonists completely blocked spontaneous epileptic seizures in this model, whereas the CB_1 receptor antagonist SR141716A increased both seizure duration and frequency [160]. Furthermore, levels of 2-AG were increased significantly within the hippocampal brain region during seizures, and Western blot and immunohistochemical analyses revealed that CB_1 receptor protein expression was significantly increased throughout the CA regions of the hippocampus of epileptic animals [160]. Similar results were obtained in animals lacking CB_1 receptors in that they exhibited increased kainic acid–induced seizures, and kainic acid increased hippocampal levels of anandamide in wild-type mice [161]. These investigators concluded that the endogenous cannabinoid system provides on-demand protection against acute excitotoxicity in the CNS. One possible explanation for cannabinoid protective effects is the presence of CB_1 receptors on excitatory glutamatergic neurons. Activation of these receptors decreases glutamate release and therefore decreases excitotoxicity [162].

As for a possible explanation for convulsant effects of cannabinoids, it has been suggested that exogenous cannabinoids, such as Δ^9-THC, might also activate CB_1 receptors on inhibitory GABAergic neurons, leading to a decreased release of GABA and a concomitant increase in seizure susceptibility [162]. There is also evidence that anandamide itself can be proconvulsive. FAAH($-/-$) mice exhibit increased sensitivity to kainic acid [163]. Administration of anandamide dramatically augments the severity of kainic acid–induced seizures in FAAH($-/-$) mice but not in wild-type mice and enhanced neuronal damage in the CA1 and CA3 regions of the hippocampus. These findings do not support a general neuroprotective role for endocannabinoids in response to chemical-induced excitotoxicity. On the other hand, inhibition of FAAH by organophosphates did not lead to any overt neurotoxicity or change in behavior despite elevating anandamide levels [164].

A number of in vitro studies support an anticonvulsant mechanism of action for cannabinoids. WIN 55,212-2 attenuated low-magnesium-induced burst firing in hippocampal culture [165], and both anandamide and 2-AG decreased stimulation-induced population spikes and low-magnesium-induced epileptiform discharges in rat hippocampal slice preparations [166]. The mechanism underlying this dampening of excitability is believed to involve inhibition of presynaptic glutamate release [165]. However, in fever-induced seizures, there is an increase in the number of CB_1 receptors associated with cholecystokinin-containing perisomatic inhibitory inputs, no effect on glutamate release, and enhanced retrograde inhibition of GABA release [167]. These results suggest that inhibition of GABA rather than glutamate release is important for febrile seizures. In vitro, there is evidence that endocannabinoids act in a retrograde manner to produce depolarization-induced suppression of inhibition by suppressing GABA release and thus disinhibiting pyramidal neuronal activity [168]. As such it would be expected that endocannabinoids would be excitotoxic.

As for general neurotoxicity, Chan et al. reported that Δ^9-THC caused shrinkage of neuronal cell bodies and nuclei and genomic DNA strand breaks [169]. Δ^9-THC also stimulated release of anrachidonic acid leading to speculation that Δ^9-THC's mechanism for neurotoxicity involves arachidonic acid metabolism to prostanoid synthesis and generation of free radicals by cyclooxygenase. Δ^9-THC induces apoptosis in cultured cortical neurons through activation of both c-Jun N-terminal protein kinase isoforms JNK1 and JNK2 [170].

On the other hand, endocannabinoids inhibit Aβ toxicity, and this protective effect was prevented by the CB_1 receptor antagonist [171]. Anandamide's effects appear to be mediated through the mitogen-activated protein kinase pathway. The observation that cannabinoids retained their antioxidative properties in cultured cerebellar granule cells derived from either CB_1 receptor knockout mice or control wild-type littermates suggests that the CB_1 receptor is not involved in the cellular antioxidant neuroprotective effects of cannabinoids [172]. The specificity of cannabinoid neuroprotection is subject to further question when non-CB_1 receptor cannabinoids such as cannabidiol also produce neuroprotection. Cannabidiol protects against hippocampal and entorhinal cortical neurodegeneration in a dose-dependent manner [173]. Earlier studies had also found Δ^9-THC and cannabidiol to be equally effective in preventing hydroperoxide-induced oxidation [174].

The role of the endogenous cannabinoid system in neuronal excitation and toxicity remains to be resolved. It appears that the endocannabinoids are capable of exerting both protection and causation of toxicity depending upon the neuronal insult. This possible dual action may arise from the ability of endocannabinoids to alter the release of both excitatory and inhibitory neurotransmitters.

18.3.5 Emesis

Several animal studies indicate a direct role for endocannabinoid modulation of emesis. Darmani et al. [175] showed that CB_1 receptor agonists reduced cisplatin-induced emesis in the least shrew while the antagonist rimonabant produced the opposite effects. Similar findings were reported with cannabinoid agonists that attenuated lithium-induced vomiting in the musk shrew [176, 177]. In addition, combinations of inactive doses of Δ^9-THC and ondansetron were effective in blocking vomiting in the musk shrew [177]. The musk shrew has also been used to study conditioned retching, an animal model of anticipatory nausea and vomiting. Δ^9-THC completely suppressed conditioned retching in this model [178]. In addition, cannabinoid agonists suppressed lithium-induced conditioned rejection, a model of nausea in rats [179]. Opioids are known to be powerful emetogenic agents. Activation of the cannabinoid system was also effective in blocking opioid-induced vomiting in ferrets [180]. CB_1 receptors were strongly implicated in that rimonabant blocked the action of cannabinoid agonists in this model. Importantly, Darmani et al. [181] found prominent CB_1 receptor binding in the nucleus tractus solartius of the shrew. Van Sickle et al. demonstrated that cannabinoid agonists inhibited emesis and retching in ferrets whereas CB_1 receptor antagonists potentiated emetic responses [182]. Moreover, these investigators found both CB_1 receptors and FAAH in dorsal vagal complex consisting of the area postrema, nucleus of the solitary tract, and dorsal motor nucleus of the vagus in the brain stem. In addition, the CB_1 receptor was also found in the myenteric plexus of the stomach and duodenum. The antiemetic effects of Δ^9-THC in ferrets were reported to be mediated selectively via the CB_1 receptor [183]. Evidence in the shrew suggests that cannabinoids act both presynaptically and postsynaptically in both central and peripheral serotonergic neurons to block emesis [184] as well as at D_2/D_3 dopaminergic receptors [185].

The recent discovery of CB_2 receptors in the dorsal motor nucleus of the vagus led to speculation that they may be involved in emesis [20]. However, CB_2 selective agonists failed to inhibit emesis in ferrets. On the other hand, 2-AG reduced emesis in ferrets, an effect that was attenuated by administration of both CB_1 and CB_2 antagonists, leading the authors to conclude that if CB_2 receptors are indeed involved in emesis, they require the presence of CB_1 receptors. Finally, a metabolically stable analog of anandamide blocked vomiting, whereas another endocannabinoid, 2-AG, was emetogenic in shrew [181], suggesting possible species differences in the effects of endocannabinoids on emesis.

As for clinical evidence, anecdotal reports of patients smoking marijuana to control chemotherapy-induced nausea and vomiting provided the initial clues. These reports led to clinical studies with Δ^9-THC in which it was found to be useful in patients whose chemotherapy-induced nausea and vomiting were refractory to other standard antiemetics available at that time [186]. Plasse et al. [187] reported that combinations of Δ^9-THC and prochlorperazine resulted in enhancement of efficacy as measured by duration of episodes of nausea and vomiting and by severity of nausea. In addition, the incidence of psychotropic effects from Δ^9-THC appeared to be decreased by concomitant administration of prochlorperazine. The combination was significantly more effective than was either single agent in controlling chemotherapy-induced nausea and vomiting [188]. Nabilone, a synthetic derivative of Δ^9-THC, was also reported to be an effective oral antiemetic drug for moderately toxic chemotherapy [189]. Cannabinoids have also been found to be effective in treating nausea and vomiting in children undergoing chemotherapy [190, 191]. As for the current status of antiemetics, serotonergic anatagonists such as ondansetron have become the standards for managing emesis. These agents have proven to be effective in preventing chemotherapy-induced nausea and vomiting in most patients. However, delayed nausea and vomiting are less well controlled. Therefore, the search for more effective agents continues. Combination therapy with ondansetron and

Δ^9-THC has not been fully explored. In addition, there is a need for a higher efficacy CB_1 receptor agonist with fewer side effects.

18.4 ENDOCANNABINOID ROLE IN REWARD, TOLERANCE, AND DEPENDENCE

With the exception of medical marijuana use, most people who have experienced the psychoactive effects of cannabinoids did so through voluntary self-administration of smoked or oral marijuana for the sole purpose of becoming intoxicated. Laboratory animals (including rats, mice, pigeons, and monkeys) can also detect the distinctive psychoactive effects of cannabinoids in drug discrimination, an animal model of these subjective effects [6, 58]. Moreover, monkeys and rats find cannabinoids reinforcing and will self-administer them under appropriate experimental conditions [192–194]. SR141716A blockade of the discriminative stimulus and reinforcing properties of cannabinoids in both humans and animals implicates direct CB_1 receptor mediation in cannabinoid intoxication and reward [194–196]; however, as with most other abused substances, indirect alteration of dopamine neurotransmission in brain reward areas [e.g., ventral tegmental area (VTA) and nucleus accumbens (NAc)] is also involved (for a review, see [197]).

Several mechanisms through which neural functioning in reward-related areas is affected by cannabinoids have been identified. First, peripherally administered Δ^9-THC directly increased dopamine levels in the NAc in a calcium-dependent manner, an effect that was blocked by SR141716A as well as by preventing generation of action potential by administration of the sodium channel blocker tetrodotoxin [198, 199]. Second, Δ^9-THC preferentially increased burst activity of dopamine neurons in the VTA [200, 201]. Since CB_1 receptors are not localized in the VTA, this increase is probably mediated via disinhibition of local GABA circuitry [202, 203], perhaps by a mechanism similar to that responsible for depolarization-induced suppression of inhibition. Third, although the exact mechanism is unclear, opioid mechanisms also play a role in cannabinoid modulation of reward pathways, as indicated by reversal of cannabinoid effects by administration of the opioid antagonists naloxone and naloxonazine [198, 204]. Interestingly, regulation of dopamine activity in reward-associated brain areas by cannabinoids may be bidirectional. Whereas research has shown that exogenous cannabinoids increase dopamine activity via several mechanisms (as described above), there is also evidence that dopamine activity affects endocannabinoid levels (anandamide and/or 2-AG) in limbic forebrain and prefrontal areas through intermediate glutamatergic mechanisms [205]. Further research is needed to elucidate completely all of the various mechanisms through which endocannabinoids play a role in the regulation of neural transmission in reward-related areas.

Although initial exposure to marijuana may be unpleasant, individuals who continue to use typically find the acute effects of marijuana rewarding, at least in the short term (most likely due to its effects on dopamine neurotransmission; see above). By definition, however, abuse involves repeated or chronic administration. Repeated administration of Δ^9-THC and other psychoactive cannabinoids results in the development of profound tolerance (up to 100-fold) and cross tolerance to most cannabinoid effects in a number of animal species, including pigeons, rodents, dogs, monkeys, and rabbits (see [206] for a review). Pharmacodynamic events appear to play the primary role in cannabinoid tolerance, as pharmacokinetic parameters (absorption, distribution, metabolism, and excretion) are relatively unaltered by chronic administration. Further, cross tolerance between Δ^9-THC and anandamide-like cannabinoids has been reported to develop under certain circumstances, even though the primary metabolic pathways for these two classes of cannabinoids differ dramatically [207–209]. Pharmacodynamic tolerance is also indicated by the fact that the brains of cannabinoid-tolerant animals show profound CB_1 receptor down-regulation and reduced second-messenger signaling [210, 211].

Dependence also occurs with chronic exposure to cannabinoids, albeit it is somewhat more difficult to measure than for some other drugs of abuse (e.g., opioids). Dependence implies the presence of symptoms of withdrawal with abrupt termination following a period of chronic administration. Although a few reports have noted behavioral changes indicative of spontaneous withdrawal upon abrupt cessation of cannabinoids, heroic doses or continuous-infusion methods are typically required [212]. Most studies assessing cannabinoid dependence have used precipitated withdrawal. In this approach, dependent animals that have been chronically treated with a psychoactive cannabinoid are administered an antagonist such as SR141716A. Symptoms of precipitated withdrawal in rats and mice chronically infused with Δ^9-THC and then administered SR141716A included head shakes, facial tremors, tongue rolling, biting, wet-dog shakes, eyelid ptosis, facial rubbing, paw treading, retropulsion, immobility, ear twitch, chewing, licking, stretching, and arched back [213–215]. This syndrome was reversed by readministration of Δ^9-THC [216]. These studies provide convincing evidence that cannabinoids can produce dependence and are consistent with clinical observations of marijuana dependence [217]. Nevertheless, the marijuana dependence syndrome is milder than that typically reported for opioids and psychomotor stimulants.

18.5 FUTURE DIRECTIONS

The discovery of the endogenous cannabinoid system makes it possible to conduct a systematic evaluation of the effects of marijuana and its constituents in order to discern their direct and indirect effects. It appears that most of the recreational and medicinal effects of marijuana are produced through the endogenous cannabinoid system. However, the discovery of this system has provided an exciting new avenue for exploring a wide range of physiological functions and new development strategies for treating disease. The endocannabinoid system is best described as a modulator of other systems, thereby adding to the complexity of defining its physiological roles. In the future, it is likely that our knowledge of the endocannabinoid system will expand with the identification of additional receptor subtypes and endogenous ligands and with a better understanding of how it modulates other biological systems.

ACKNOWLEDGMENTS

Preparation of this manuscript was supported by National Institute on Drug Abuse grants DA-09789, DA-03672, and DA-016644.

REFERENCES

1. Johnston, L. D., O'Malley, P. M., Bachman, J. G., and Schulenberg, J. E. (2004). *Monitoring the future: National results on adolescent drug use, overview and key findings.* (NIH Pub. No. 05-5506). Bethesda, MD: National Institute of Drug Abuse.

2. Compton, W. M., Grant, B. F., Colliver, J. D., Glantz, M. D., and Stinson, F. S. (2004). Prevalence of marijuana use disorders in the United States: 1991–1992 and 2001–2002. *JAMA* 291, 2114–2121.

3. Gaoni, Y., and Mechoulam, R. (1964). Isolation, structure, and partial synthesis of an active constituent of hashish. *J. Am. Chem. Soc.* 86, 1646–1647.

4. Devane, W. A., Dysarz, F. A., Johnson, M. R., Melvin, L. S., and Howlett, A. C. (1988). Determination and characterization of a cannabinoid receptor in rat brain. *Mol. Pharmacol.* 34, 605–613.

5. Compton, D. R., Rice, K. C., De Costa, B. R., Razdan, R. K., Melvin, L. S., Johnson, M. R., and Martin, B. R. (1993). Cannabinoid structure-activity relationships: Correlation of receptor binding and in vivo activities. *J. Pharmacol. Exp. Ther.* 265, 218–226.

6. Balster, R. L., and Prescott, W. R. (1992). Δ9-Tetrahydrocannabinol discrimination in rats as a model for cannabis intoxication. *Neurosci. Biochem. Rev.* 16, 55–62.

7. Matsuda, L. A., Lolait, S. J., Brownstein, M. J., Young, A. C., and Bonner, T. I. (1990). Structure of a cannabinoid receptor and functional expression of the cloned cDNA. *Nature* 346, 561–564.

8. Munro, S., Thomas, K. L., and Abu-Shaar, M. (1993). Molecular characterization of a peripheral receptor for cannabinoids. *Nature* 365, 61–64.

9. Devane, W. A., Hanus, L., Breuer, A., Pertwee, R. G., Stevenson, L. A., Griffin, G., Gibson, D., Mandelbaum, A., Etinger, A., and Mechoulam, R. (1992). Isolation and structure of a brain constituent that binds to the cannabinoid receptor. *Science* 258, 1946–1949.

10. Bisogno, T., Ligresti, A., and Di Marzo, V. (2005). The endocannabinoid signalling system: Biochemical aspects. *Pharmacol. Biochem. Behav.* 81, 224–238.

11. Johnson, M. R., and Melvin, L. S. (1986). The discovery of nonclassical cannabinoid analgetics. In *Cannabinoids as Therapeutic Agents*, R. Mechoulam, Ed. CRC Press, Boca Raton, FL, pp. 121–144.

12. Ward, S. J., Childers, S. R., and Pacheco, M. (1989). Pravadoline and aminoalkylindole (AAI) analogues: Actions which suggest a receptor interaction. *Br. J. Pharmacol.* 98(Supp.1), 831P.

13. Wiley, J. L., and Martin, B. R. (2002). Cannabinoid pharmacology: Implications for additional cannabinoid receptor subtypes. *Chem. Phys. Lipids* 121, 57–63.

14. Rinaldi-Carmona, M., Barth, F., Héaulme, M., Shire, D., Calandra, B., Congy, C., Martinez, S., Maruani, J., Néliat, G., Caput, D., Ferrara, P., Soubrié, P., Brelière, J. C., and Le Fur, G. (1994). SR141716A, a potent and selective antagonist of the brain cannabinoid receptor. *FEBS Lett.* 350, 240–244.

15. Rinaldi-Carmona, M., Barth, F., Millan, J., Defrocq, J., Casellas, P., Congy, C., Oustric, D., Sarran, M., Bouaboula, M., Calandra, B., Portier, M., Shire, D., Breliere, J., and Le Fur, G. (1998). SR 144528, the first potent and selective antagonist of the CB2 cannabinoid receptor. *J. Pharmacol. Exp. Ther.* 284, 644–650.

16. Pertwee, R. G. (2005). Inverse agonism and neutral antagonism at cannabinoid CB1 receptors. *Life Sci.* 76, 1307–1324.

17. Compton, D., Aceto, M., Lowe, J., and Martin, B. (1996). In vivo characterization of a specific cannabinoid receptor antagonist (SR141716A): Inhibition of Δ^9-tetrahydrocannabinol-induced responses and apparent agonist activity. *J. Pharmacol. Exp. Ther.* 277, 586–594.
18. Bass, C., Griffin, G., Grier, M., Mahadevan, A., Razdan, R., and Martin, B. (2002). SR-141716A-induced stimulation of locomotor activity. A structure-activity relationship study. *Pharmacol. Biochem. Behav.* 74, 31.
19. Shire, D., Carillon, C., Kaghad, M., Calandra, B., Rinaldi-Carmona, M., Le Fur, G., Caput, D., and Ferrara, P. (1995). An amino-terminal variant of the central cannabinoid receptor resulting from alternative splicing. *J. Biol. Chem.* 270, 3730–3731.
20. Van Sickle, M. D., Duncan, M., Kingsley, P. J., Mouihate, A., Urbani, P., Mackie, K., Stella, N., Makriyannis, A., Piomelli, D., Davison, J. S., Marnett, L. J., Di Marzo, V., Pittman, Q. J., Patel, K. D., and Sharkey, K. A. (2005). Identification and functional characterization of brainstem cannabinoid CB2 receptors. *Science* 310, 329–332.
21. Galiegue, S., Mary, S., Marchand, J., Dussossoy, D., Carriere, D., Carayon, P., Boulaboula, M., Shire, D., Le Fur, G., and Casellas, P. (1995). Expression of central and peripheral cannabinoid receptors in human immune tissues and leukocyte subpopulations. *Eur. J. Biochem.* 232, 54–61.
22. Kaminski, N. E. (1996). Immune regulation by cannabinoid compounds through the inhibition of the cyclic AMP signaling cascade and altered gene expression. *Biochem. Pharmacol.* 52, 1133–1140.
23. Showalter, V., Compton, D. R., Martin, B. R., and Abood, M. E. (1996). Evaluation of binding in a transfected cell line expressing a peripheral cannabinoid receptor (CB_2): Identification of cannabinoid receptor subtype selective ligands. *J. Pharmacol. Exp. Ther.* 278, 989–999.
24. Begg, M., Pacher, P., Batkai, S., Osei-Hyiaman, D., Offertaler, L., Mo, F. M., Liu, J., and Kunos, G. (2005). Evidence for novel cannabinoid receptors. *Pharmacol. Ther.* 106, 133–145.
25. Herkenham, M., Lynn, A. B., Little, M. D., Johnson, M. R., Melvin, L. S., DeCosta, B. R., and Rice, K. C. (1990). Cannabinoid receptor localization in the brain. *Proc. Natl. Acad. Sci. USA* 87, 1932–1936.
26. Prather, P. L., Martin, N. A., Breivogel, C. S., and Childers, S. R. (2000). Activation of cannabinoid receptors in rat brain by WIN 55212-2 produces coupling to multiple G protein alpha-subunits with different potencies. *Mol. Pharmacol.* 57, 1000–1010.
27. Glass, M., and Felder, C. C. (1997). Concurrent stimulation of cannabinoid CB1 and dopamine D2 receptors augments cAMP accumulation in striatal neurons: Evidence for a G_s linkage to the CB1 receptor. *J. Neurosci.* 17, 5327–5333.
28. Mackie, K., and Hille, B. (1992). Cannabinoids inhibit N-type calcium channels in neuroblastoma-glioma cells. *Proc. Natl. Acad. Sci. USA* 89, 3825–3829.
29. Mackie, K., Lai, Y., Westenbroek, R., and Mitchell, R. (1995). Cannabinoids activate an inwardly rectifying potassium conductance and inhibit Q-type calcium currents in AtT20 cells transfected with rat brain cannabinoid receptor. *J. Neurosci.* 15, 6552–6561.
30. Bouaboula, M., Bourrié, B., Rinaldi-Carmona, M., Shire, D., Le Fur, G., and Casellas, P. (1995). Stimulation of cannabinoid receptor CB1 induces *krox*-24 expression in human astrocytoma cells. *J. Biol. Chem.* 270, 13973–13980.
31. Price, M. R., Baillie, G. L., Thomas, A., Stevenson, L. A., Easson, M., Goodwin, R., McLean, A., McIntosh, L., Goodwin, G., Walker, G., Westwood, P., Marrs, J., Thomson, F., Cowley, P., Christopoulos, A., Pertwee, R. G., and Ross, R. A. (2005). Allosteric modulation of the cannabinoid CB1 receptor. *Mol. Pharmacol.* 68, 1484–1495.

32. Howlett, A. C., Barth, F., Bonner, T. I., Cabral, G., Casellas, P., Devane, W. A., Felder, C. C., Herkenham, M., Mackie, K., Martin, B. R., Mechoulam, R., and Pertwee, R. G. (2002). International Union of Pharmacology. XXVII. Classification of cannabinoid receptors. *Pharmacol. Rev.* 54, 161–202.

33. Wilson, R. I., and Nicoll, R. A. (2001). Endogenous cannabinoids mediate retrograde signalling at hippocampal synapses. *Nature* 410, 588–592.

34. Mechoulam, R., Ben-Shabat, S., Hanus, L., Ligumsky, M., Kaminski, N., Schatz, A., Gopher, A., Almog, S., Martin, B., Compton, D., Pertwee, R., Griffin, G., Bayewitch, M., Barg, J., and Vogel, Z. (1995). Identification of an endogenous 2-monoglyceride, present in canine gut, that binds to cannabinoid receptors. *Biochem. Pharmacol.* 50, 83–90.

35. Hanus, L., Abu-Lafi, S., Fride, E., Breuer, A., Vogel, Z., Shalev, D. E., Kustanovich, I., and Mechoulam, R. (2001). 2-Arachidonyl glyceryl ether, an endogenous agonist of the cannabinoid CB1 receptor. *Proc. Natl. Acad. Sci. USA* 98, 3662–3665.

36. Huang, S. M., Bisogno, T., Trevisani, M., Al-Hayani, A., De Petrocellis, L., Fezza, F., Tognetto, M., Petros, T. J., Krey, J. F., Chu, C. J., Miller, J. D., Davies, S. N., Geppetti, P., Walker, J. M., and Di Marzo, V. (2002). An endogenous capsaicin-like substance with high potency at recombinant and native vanilloid VR1 receptors. *Proc. Natl. Acad. Sci. USA* 99, 8400–8405.

37. Porter, A. C., Sauer, J. M., Knierman, M. D., Becker, G. W., Berna, M. J., Bao, J., Nomikos, G. G., Carter, P., Bymaster, F. P., Leese, A. B., and Felder, C. C. (2002). Characterization of a novel endocannabinoid, virodhamine, with antagonist activity at the CB1 receptor. *J. Pharmacol. Exp. Ther.* 301, 1020–1024.

38. Howlett, A. C., and Mukhopadhyay, S. (2000). Cellular signal transduction by anandamide and 2-arachidonoylglycerol. *Chem. Phys. Lipids* 108, 53–70.

39. Smart, D., and Jerman, J. C. (2000). Anandamide: An endogenous activator of the vanilloid receptor [letter; comment]. *Trends Pharmacol. Sci.* 21, 134.

40. Zygmunt, P. M., Peterson, J., Andersson, D. A., Chuang, H. H., Sorgard, M., DiMarzo, V., and Julius, D. (1999). Vanilloid receptors on sensory nerves mediate the vasodilator action of anandamide. *Nature* 400, 452–457.

41. Schmid, H. H. (2000). Pathways and mechanisms of N-acylethanolamine biosynthesis: Can anandamide be generated selectively? *Chem. Phys. Lipids* 108, 71–87.

42. Cravatt, B. F., and Lichtman, A. H. (2002). The enzymatic inactivation of the fatty acid amide class of signaling lipids. *Chem. Phys. Lipids* 121, 135–148.

43. Patricelli, M. P., Patterson, J. E., Boger, D. L., and Cravatt, B. F. (1998). An endogenous sleep-inducing compound is a novel competitive inhibitor of fatty acid amide hydrolase. *Bioorg. Med. Chem. Lett.* 8, 613–618.

44. Cravatt, B. F., Demarest, K., Patricelli, M. P., Bracey, M. H., Giang, D. K., Martin, B. R., and Lichtman, A. H. (2001). Supersensitivity to anandamide and enhanced endogenous cannabinoid signaling in mice lacking fatty acid amide hydrolase. *Proc. Natl. Acad. Sci. USA* 98, 9371–9376.

45. Hillard, C. J., and Jarrahian, A. (2000). The movement of N-arachidonoylethanolamine (anandamide) across cellular membranes. *Chem. Phys. Lipids* 108, 123–134.

46. Fried, P. A. (2002). Adolescents prenatally exposed to marijuana: Examination of facets of complex behaviors and comparisons with the influence of in utero cigarettes. *J. Clin. Pharmacol.* 42, 97S–102S.

47. Abel, E. L. (1984). Effects of delta 9-THC on pregnancy and offspring in rats. *Neurobehav. Toxicol. Teratol.* 6, 29–32.

48. Belue, R., Howlett, A., Westlake, T., and Hutchings, D. (1995). The ontogeny of cannabinoid receptors in the brain of postnatal and aging rats. *Neurotoxicol. Teratol.* 17, 25–30.

49. McLaughlin, C. R., Martin, B. R., Compton, D. R., and Abood, M. E. (1994). Cannabinoid receptors in developing rats: Detection of mRNA and receptor binding. *Drug Alcohol Depend.* 36, 27–31.

50. Rodriguez de Fonseca, F., Ramos, J. A., Bonnin, A., and Fernandez, R. J. J. (1993). Presence of cannabinoid binding sites in the brain from early postnatal ages. *Neuroreport* 4, 135–138.

51. Berrendero, F., Sepe, N., Ramos, J. A., Di Marzo, V., and Fernandez-Ruiz, J. J. (1999). Analysis of cannabinoid receptor binding and mRNA expression and endogenous cannabinoid contents in the developing rat brain during late gestation and early postnatal period. *Synapse* 33, 181–191.

52. Berrendero, F., Garcia-Gil, L., Hernandez, M. L., Romero, J., Cebeira, M., de Miguel, R., Ramos, J. A., and Fernandez-Ruiz, J. J. (1998). Localization of mRNA expression and activation of signal transduction mechanisms for cannabinoid receptor in rat brain during fetal development. *Development* 125, 3179–3188.

53. Romero, J., Garcia-Palomero, E., Berrendero, F., Garcia-Gil, L., Hernandez, M. L., Ramos, J. A., and Fernandez-Ruiz, J. J. (1997). Atypical location of cannabinoid receptors in white matter areas during rat brain development. *Synapse* 26, 317–323.

54. Fride, E., Ginzburg, Y., Breuer, A., Bisogno, T., Di Marzo, V., and Mechoulam, R. (2001). Critical role of the endogenous cannabinoid system in mouse pup suckling and growth. *Eur. J. Pharmacol.* 419, 207–214.

55. de Graff-Peters, V. B., and Hadders-Algra, M. (2006). Ontogeny of the human central nervous system: What is happening when? *Early Hum. Dev.* 82, 257–266.

56. Martin, B. R. (1995). Marijuana. In *Psychopharmacology: The Fourth Generation of Progress*, F. E. Bloom and D. J. Kupfer, Eds. Raven, New York, pp. 1757–1765.

57. Martin, B. R., Compton, D. R., Thomas, B. F., Prescott, W. R., Little, P. J., Razdan, R. K., Johnson, M. R., Melvin, L. S., Mechoulam, R., and Ward, S. J. (1991). Behavioral, biochemical, and molecular modeling evaluations of cannabinoid analogs. *Pharmacol. Biochem. Behav.* 40, 471–478.

58. Wiley, J. L. (1999). Cannabis: Discrimination of "internal bliss"? *Pharmacol. Biochem. Behav.* 64, 257–260.

59. Wiley, J., Lowe, J., Balster, R., and Martin, B. (1995). Antagonism of the discriminative stimulus effects of Δ^9-tetrahydrocannabinol in rats and rhesus monkeys. *J. Pharmacol. Exp. Ther.* 275, 1–6.

60. Wiley, J. L., Jefferson, R. G., Griffin, G., Liddle, J., Yu, S., Huffman, J. W., and Martin, B. R. (2002). Paradoxical pharmacological effects of deoxy-tetrahydrocannabinol analogs lacking high CB(1) receptor Affinity. *Pharmacology* 66, 89–99.

61. Ryan, J. W., Banner, W. K., Wiley, J. L., Martin, B. R., and Razdan, R. K. (1997). Potent anandamide analogs: The effect of changing the length and branching of the end pentyl chain. *J. Med. Chem.* 40, 3617–3625.

62. Seltzman, H. H., Fleming, D. N., Thomas, B. F., Gilliam, A. F., McCallion, D. S., Pertwee, R. G., Compton, D. R., and Martin, B. R. (1997). Synthesis and pharmacological comparison of dimethylheptyl and pentyl analogs of anandamide. *J. Med. Chem.* 40, 3626–3634.

63. Smith, P. B., Compton, D. R., Welch, S. P., Razdan, R. K., Mechoulam, R., and Martin, B. R. (1994). The pharmacological activity of anandamide, a putative endogenous cannabinoid, in mice. *J. Pharmacol. Exp. Ther.* 270, 219–227.

64. Adams, I. B., Ryan, W., Singer, M., Thomas, B. F., Compton, D. R., Razdan, R. K., and Martin, B. R. (1995). Evaluation of cannabinoid receptor binding and in vivo activities for anandamide analogs. *J. Pharmacol. Exp. Ther.* 273, 1172–1181.

65. Adams, I. B., Ryan, W., Singer, M., Razdan, R. K., Compton, D. R., and Martin, B. R. (1995). Pharmacological and behavioral evaluation of alkylated anandamide analogs. *Life Sci.* 56, 2041–2048.

66. Wiley, J. L., Golden, K. M., Ryan, W. J., Balster, R. L., Razdan, R. K., and Martin, B. R. (1997). Discriminative stimulus effects of anandamide and methylated fluoro-anandamide in Λ^9-THC-trained rhesus monkeys. *Pharmacol. Biochem. Behav.* 58, 1139–1143.

67. Houser, S. J., Eads, M., Embrey, J. P., and Welch, S. P. (2000). Dynorphin B and spinal analgesia: Induction of antinociception by the cannabinoids CP55,940, Delta(9)-THC and anandamide. *Brain Res.* 857, 337–342.

68. Welch, S. P., and Eads, M. (1999). Synergistic interactions of endogenous opioids and cannabinoid systems. *Brain Res.* 848, 183–190.

69. Adams, I. B., Compton, D. R., and Martin, B. R. (1998). Assessment of anandamide interaction with the cannabinoid brain receptor: SR 141716A antagonism studies in mice and autoradiographic analysis of receptor binding in rat brain. *J. Pharmacol. Exp. Ther.* 284, 1209–1217.

70. Cravatt, B. F., Giang, D. K., Mayfield, S. P., Boger, D. L., Lerner, R. A., and Gilula, N. B. (1996). Molecular characterization of an enzyme that degrades neuromodulatory fatty-acid amides. *Nature* 384, 83–87.

71. Willoughby, K. A., Moore, S. F., Martin, B. R., and Ellis, E. F. (1997). The biodisposition and metabolism of anandamide in mice. *J. Pharmacol. Exp. Ther.* 282, 243–247.

72. Watanabe, K., Narimatsu, S., Matsunaga, T., Yamamoto, I., and Yoshimura, H. (1993). A cytochrome P450 isozyme having aldehyde oxygenase activity plays a major role in metabolizing cannabinoids by mouse hepatic microsomes. *Biochem. Pharmacol.* 46, 405–411.

73. Fegley, D., Gaetani, S., Duranti, A., Tontini, A., Mor, M., Tarzia, G., and Piomelli, D. (2005). Characterization of the fatty acid amide hydrolase inhibitor cyclohexyl carbamic acid 3'-carbamoyl-biphenyl-3-yl ester (URB597): Effects on anandamide and oleoylethanolamide deactivation. *J. Pharmacol. Exp. Ther.* 313, 352–358.

74. Compton, D. R., and Martin, B. R. (1997). The effect of the enzyme inhibitor phenylmethylsulfonyl fluoride on the pharmacological effect of anandamide in the mouse model of cannabimimetic activity. *J. Pharmacol. Exp. Ther.* 283, 1138–1143.

75. Noyes, J. R., Brunk, S. F., Avery, D. H., and Canter, A. (1975). The analgesic properties of Δ^9-tetrahydrocannabinol and codeine. *Clin. Pharmacol. Ther.* 18, 84–89.

76. Noyes, R., Jr., Brunk, S. F., Baram, D. A., and Canter, A. (1975). Analgesic effect of Δ^9-tetrahydrocannabinol. *J. Clin. Pharmacol.* 15, 139–143.

77. Karniol, I. G., Shirakawa, I., Takahashi, R. N., Knobel, E., and Musty, R. E. (1975). Effects of Δ^9-tetrahydrocannabinol and cannabinol in man. *Pharmacology* 13, 502–512.

78. Raft, D., Gregg, J., Ghia, J., and Harris, L. (1977). Effects of intravenous tetrahydrocannabinol on experimental and surgical pain. Psychological correlates of the analgesic response. *Clin. Pharmacol. Ther.* 21, 26–33.

79. Jain, A. K., Ryan, J. E., McMahan, F. G., and Smith, G. (1981). Evaluation of intramuscular levonantradol in acute post-operative pain. *J. Clin. Pharmacol.* 21, 3205–3265.

80. Jochimsen, P. R., Lawton, R. L., VerSteeg, K., and Noyes, J. R. (1978). Effect of benzopyranoperidine, a Δ-9-THC congener, on pain. *Clin. Pharmacol. Ther.* 24, 223–227.

81. Martin, B. R., and Lichtman, A. H. (1998). Cannabinoid transmission and pain perception. *Neurobiol. Dis.* 5, 447–461.
82. Walker, J. M., Hohmann, A. G., Martin, W. J., Strangman, N. M., Huang, S. M., and Tsou, K. (1999). The neurobiology of cannabinoid analgesia. *Life Sci.* 65, 665–673.
83. Lichtman, A. H., and Martin, B. R. (1991). Cannabinoid induced antinociception is mediated by a spinal α_2 noradrenergic mechanism. *Brain Res.* 559, 309–314.
84. Smith, P. B., Welch, S. P., and Martin, B. R. (1993). *nor*-Binaltorphimine specifically inhibits Δ^9-tetrahydrocannabinol-induced antinociception in mice without altering other pharmacological effects. *J. Pharmacol. Exp. Ther.* 268, 1381–1387.
85. Gough, A. L., and Olley, J. E. (1978). Catalepsy induced by intrastriatal injections of Δ^9-THC and 11-OH-Δ^9-THC in the rat. *Neuropharmacology* 17, 137–144.
86. Lichtman, A. H., Cook, S. A., and Martin, B. R. (1996). Investigation of brain sites mediating cannabinoid-induced antinociception in rats: Evidence supporting periaqueductal gray involvement. *J. Pharmacol. Exp. Ther.* 276, 585–593.
87. Herzberg, U., Eliav, E., Bennett, G. J., and Kopin, I. J. (1997). The analgesic effects of $R(+)$ WIN 55,212-2 mesylate, a high affinity cannabinoid agonist, in a rat model of neuropathic pain. *Neurol. Lett.* 221, 157–160.
88. Smith, F. L., Fujimori, K., Lowe, J., and Welch, S. P. (1998). Characterization of delta9-tetrahydrocannabinol and anandamide antinociception in nonarthritic and arthritic rats. *Pharmacol. Biochem. Behav.* 60, 183–191.
89. Fride, E., and Mechoulam, R. (1993). Pharmacological activity of the cannabinoid receptor agonist, anandamide, a brain constituent. *Eur. J. Pharmacol.* 231, 313–314.
90. Stein, E. A., Fuller, S. A., Edgemond, W. S., and Campbell, W. B. (1996). Physiological and behavioural effects of the endogenous cannabinoid, arachidonylethanolamide (anandamide), in the rat. *Br. J. Pharmacol.* 119, 107–114.
91. Martin, W. J., Patrick, S. L., Coffin, P. O., Tsou, K., and Walker, J. M. (1995). An examination of the central sites of action of cannabinoid-induced antinociception in the rat. *Life Sci.* 56, 2103–2109.
92. Basbaum, A. I., and Fields, H. L. (1984). Endogenous pain control systems: Brainstem spinal pathways and endorphin circuitry. *Annu. Rev. Neurosci.* 7, 309–338.
93. Herkenham, M., Lynn, A. B., Johnson, M. R., Melvin, L. S., de Costa, B. R., and Rice, K. C. (1991). Characterization and localization of cannabinoid receptors in rat brain: A quantitative in vitro autoradiographic study. *J. Neurosci.* 11, 563–583.
94. Walker, J. M., Huang, S. M., Strangman, N. M., Tsou, K., and Sanudo-Pena, M. C. (1999). Pain modulation by release of the endogenous cannabinoid anandamide. *Proc. Natl. Acad. Sci. USA* 96, 12198–12203.
95. Meng, I. D., Manning, B. H., Martin, W. J., and Fields, H. L. (1998). An analgesia circuit activated by cannabinoids. *Nature* 395, 381–383.
96. Calignano, A., La Rana, G., Giuffrida, A., and Piomelli, D. (1998). Control of pain initiation by endogenous cannabinoids. *Nature* 394, 277–281.
97. Beaulieu, P., Bisogno, T., Punwar, S., Farquhar-Smith, W. P., Ambrosino, G., Di Marzo, V., and Rice, A. S. (2000). Role of the endogenous cannabinoid system in the formalin test of persistent pain in the rat. *Eur. J. Pharmacol.* 396, 85–92.
98. Suplita, R. L., II, Farthing, J. N., Gutierrez, T., and Hohmann, A. G. (2005). Inhibition of fatty-acid amide hydrolase enhances cannabinoid stress-induced analgesia: Sites of action in the dorsolateral periaqueductal gray and rostral ventromedial medulla. *Neuropharmacology* 49, 1201–1209.

99. Hohmann, A. G., Suplita, R. L., Bolton, N. M., Neely, M. H., Fegley, D., Mangieri, R., Krey, J. F., Walker, J. M., Holmes, P. V., Crystal, J. D., Duranti, A., Tontini, A., Mor, M., Tarzia, G., and Piomelli, D. (2005). An endocannabinoid mechanism for stress-induced analgesia. *Nature* 435, 1108–1112.
100. Lichtman, A. H., Leung, D., Shelton, C. C., Saghatelian, A., Hardouin, C., Boger, D. L., and Cravatt, B. F. (2004). Reversible inhibitors of fatty acid amide hydrolase that promote analgesia: Evidence for an unprecedented combination of potency and selectivity. *J. Pharmacol. Exp. Ther.* 311, 441–448.
101. Richardson, J. D., Aanonsen, L., and Hargreaves, K. M. (1998). Hypoactivity of the spinal cannabinoid system results in NMDA-dependent hyperalgesia. *J. Neurosci.* 18, 451–457.
102. Hohmann, A. G., Martin, W. J., Tsou, K., and Walker, J. M. (1995). Inhibition of noxious stimulus-evoked activity of spinal cord dorsal horn neurons by the cannabinoid WIN 55,212-2. *Life Sci.* 56, 2111–2118.
103. Martin, W. J., Hohmann, A. G., and Walker, J. M. (1996). Suppression of noxious stimulus-evoked activity in the ventral posterolateral nucleus of the thalamus by a cannabinoid agonist: Correlation between electrophysiological and antinociceptive effects. *J. Neurosci.* 16, 6601–6611.
104. Lichtman, A. H., and Martin, B. R. (1991). Spinal and supraspinal mechanisms of cannabinoid-induced antinociception. *J. Pharmacol. Exp. Ther.* 258, 517–523.
105. Martin, W. J., Lai, N. K., Patrick, S. L., Tsou, K., and Walker, J. M. (1993). Antinociceptive actions of cannabinoids following intraventricular administration in rats. *Brain Res.* 629, 300–304.
106. Jacob, J. J., Ramabadran, K., and Campos-Medeiros, M. (1981). A pharmacological analysis of levonantradol antinociception in mice. *J. Clin. Pharmacol.* 21, 327S–333S.
107. Ferri, S., Cavicchini, E., Romualdi, P., Speroni, E., and Murari, G. (1986). Possible mediation of catecholaminergic pathways in the antinociceptive effect of an extract of *Cannabis sativa L. Psychopharmacology* 89, 244–247.
108. Naderi, N., Shafaghi, B., Khodayar, M. J., and Zarindast, M. R. (2005). Interaction between gamma-aminobutyric acid GABAB and cannabinoid CB1 receptors in spinal pain pathways in rat. *Eur. J. Pharmacol.* 514, 159–164.
109. Hanus, L., Breuer, A., Tchilibon, S., Shiloah, S., Goldenberg, D., Horowitz, M., Pertwee, R. G., Ross, R. A., Mechoulam, R., and Fride, E. (1999). HU-308: A specific agonist for CB(2), a peripheral cannabinoid receptor. *Proc. Natl. Acad. Sci. USA* 96, 14228–14233.
110. Quartilho, A., Mata, H. P., Ibrahim, M. M., Vanderah, T. W., Porreca, F., Makriyannis, A., and Malan, T. P., Jr. (2003). Inhibition of inflammatory hyperalgesia by activation of peripheral CB2 cannabinoid receptors. *Anesthesiology* 99, 955–960.
111. Scott, D. A., Wright, C. E., and Angus, J. A. (2004). Evidence that CB-1 and CB-2 cannabinoid receptors mediate antinociception in neuropathic pain in the rat. *Pain* 109, 124–131.
112. Valenzano, K. J., Tafesse, L., Lee, G., Harrison, J. E., Boulet, J. M., Gottshall, S. L., Mark, L., Pearson, M. S., Miller, W., Shan, S., Rabadi, L., Rotshteyn, Y., Chaffer, S. M., Turchin, P. I., Elsemore, D. A., Toth, M., Koetzner, L., and Whiteside, G. T. (2005). Pharmacological and pharmacokinetic characterization of the cannabinoid receptor 2 agonist, GW405833, utilizing rodent models of acute and chronic pain, anxiety, ataxia and catalepsy. *Neuropharmacology* 48, 658–672.
113. Wotherspoon, G., Fox, A., McIntyre, P., Colley, S., Bevan, S., and Winter, J. (2005). Peripheral nerve injury induces cannabinoid receptor 2 protein expression in rat sensory neurons. *Neuroscience* 135, 235–245.

114. Jerman, J. C., Gray, J., Brough, S. J., Ooi, L., Owen, D., Davis, J. B., and Smart, D. (2002). Comparison of effects of anandamide at recombinant and endogenous rat vanilloid receptors. *Br. J. Anaesth.* 89, 882–887.

115. Lam, P. M., McDonald, J., and Lambert, D. G. (2005). Characterization and comparison of recombinant human and rat TRPV1 receptors: Effects of exo- and endocannabinoids. *Br. J. Anaesth.* 94, 649–656.

116. Di Marzo, V., Griffin, G., De Petrocellis, L., Brandi, I., Bisogno, T., Williams, W., Grier, M. C., Kulasegram, S., Mahadevan, A., Razdan, R. K., and Martin, B. R. (2002). A structure/activity relationship study on arvanil, an endocannabinoid and vanilloid hybrid. *J. Pharmacol. Exp. Ther.* 300, 984–991.

117. Curran, H. V., Brignell, C., Fletcher, S., Middleton, P., and Henry, J. (2002). Cognitive and subjective dose-response effects of acute oral delta 9-tetrahydrocannabinol (THC) in infrequent cannabis users. *Psychopharmacology* 164, 61–70.

118. Kurzthaler, I., Hummer, M., Miller, C., Sperner-Unterweger, B., Gunther, V., Wechdorn, H., Battista, H. J., and Fleischhacker, W. W. (1999). Effect of cannabis use on cognitive functions and driving ability. *J. Clin. Psychiatry* 60, 395–399.

119. Pope, H. G., Jr., Gruber, A. J., Hudson, J. I., Huestis, M. A., and Yurgelun-Todd, D. (2001). Neuropsychological performance in long-term cannabis users. *Arch. Gen. Psychiatry* 58, 909–915.

120. Hicks, R. E., Gualtieri, C. T., Mayo, J. P., Jr., and Perez-Reyes, M. (1984). Cannabis, atropine, and temporal information processing. *Neuropsychobiology* 12, 229–237.

121. Vachon, L., Sulkowski, A., and Rich, E. (1974). Marihuana effects on learning, attention and time estimation. *Psychopharmacologia* 39, 1–11.

122. Castellano, C., Rossi-Arnaud, C., Cestari, V., and Costanzi, M. (2003). Cannabinoids and memory: Animal studies. *Curr. Drug. Targets CNS Neurol. Disord.* 2, 389–402.

123. Hampson, R. E., and Deadwyler, S. A. (1998). Role of cannabinoid receptors in memory storage. *Neurobiol. Dis.* 5, 474–482.

124. Heyser, C. J., Hampson, R. E., and Deadwyler, S. A. (1993). Effects of Δ^9-tetrahydrocannabinol on delayed match to sample performance in rats: Alterations in short-term memory associated with changes in task specific firing of hippocampal cells. *J. Pharmacol. Exp. Ther.* 264, 294–307.

125. Lichtman, A. H., and Martin, B. R. (1996). Δ^9-Tetrahydrocannabinol impairs spatial memory through a cannabinoid receptor mechanism. *Psychopharmacology* 126, 125–131.

126. Lichtman, A. H., Dimen, K. R., and Martin, B. R. (1995). Systemic or intrahippocampal cannabinoid administration impairs spatial memory in rats. *Psychopharmacology* 119, 282–290.

127. Varvel, S. A., and Lichtman, A. H. (2002). Evaluation of CB1 receptor knockout mice in the Morris water maze. *J. Pharmacol. Exp. Ther.* 301, 915–924.

128. Jentsch, J., Andrusiak, E., Tran, A., Bowers, M., and Roth, R. (1997). Δ^9-Tetrahydrocannabinol increases prefrontal cortical catecholaminergic utilization and impairs spatial working memory in the rat: Blockade of dopaminergic effects with HA966. *Neuropsychopharmacology* 16, 426–432.

129. Delatte, M. S., Winsauer, P. J., and Moerschbaecher, J. M. (2002). Tolerance to the disruptive effects of delta(9)-THC on learning in rats. *Pharmacol. Biochem. Behav.* 74, 129–140.

130. Miller, L. L., McFarland, D. J., Cornett, T. L., Brightwell, D. R., and Wikler, A. (1977). Marijuana: Effects on free recall and subjective organization of pictures and words. *Psychopharmacology* 55, 257–262.

131. McClure, G. Y., and McMillan, D. E. (1997). Effects of drugs on response duration differentiation. VI: Differential effects under differential reinforcement of low rates of responding schedules. *J. Pharmacol. Exp. Ther.* 281, 1368–1380.
132. Wiley, J. L., Compton, A. D., and Golden, K. M. (2000). Separation of drug effects on timing and behavioral inhibition by increased stimulus control. *Exp. Clin. Psychopharmacol.* 8, 451–461.
133. Han, C. J., and Robinson, J. K. (2001). Cannabinoid modulation of time estimation in the rat. *Behav. Neurosci.* 115, 243–246.
134. Varvel, S. A., Bridgen, D. T., Tao, Q., Thomas, B. F., Martin, B. R., and Lichtman, A. H. (2005). Delta9-tetrahydrocannabinol accounts for the antinociceptive, hypothermic, and cataleptic effects of marijuana in mice. *J. Pharmacol. Exp. Ther.* 314, 329–337.
135. Beal, J. E., Olson, R., Laubenstein, L., MOrales, J. O., Bellman, B., Yangco, B., Lefkowitz, L., Plasse, T. F., and Shepard, K. V. (1995). Dronabinol as a treatment for anorexia associated with weight loss in patients with AIDS. *J. Pain Symptom Manag.* 10, 89–97.
136. Jatoi, A., Windschitl, H. E., Loprinzi, C. L., Sloan, J. A., Dakhil, S. R., Mailliard, J. A., Pundaleeka, S., Kardinal, C. G., Fitch, T. R., Krook, J. E., Novotny, P. J., and Christensen, B. (2002). Dronabinol versus megestrol acetate versus combination therapy for cancer-associated anorexia: A North Central Cancer Treatment Group study. *J. Clin. Oncol.* 20, 567–573.
137. Avraham, Y., Ben-Shushan, D., Breuer, A., Zolotarev, O., Okon, A., Fink, N., Katz, V., and Berry, E. M. (2004). Very low doses of delta 8-THC increase food consumption and alter neurotransmitter levels following weight loss. *Pharmacol. Biochem. Behav.* 77, 675–684.
138. Williams, C. M., and Kirkham, T. C. (2002). Observational analysis of feeding induced by delta9-THC and anandamide. *Physiol. Behav.* 76, 241–250.
139. Williams, C. M., Rogers, P. J., and Kirkham, T. C. (1998). Hyperphagia in pre-fed rats following oral delta9-THC. *Physiol. Behav.* 65, 343–346.
140. Di Marzo, V., Goparaju, S. K., Wang, L., Liu, J., Batkai, S., Jarai, Z., Fezza, F., Miura, G. I., Palmiter, R. D., Sugiura, T., and Kunos, G. (2001). Leptin-regulated endocannabinoids are involved in maintaining food intake. *Nature* 410, 822–825.
141. Wiley, J. L., Burston, J. J., Leggett, D. C., Alekseeva, O. O., Razdan, R. K., Mahadevan, A., and Martin, B. R. (2005). CB1 cannabinoid receptor-mediated modulation of food intake in mice. *Br. J. Pharmacol.* 145, 293–300.
142. Williams, C. M., and Kirkham, T. C. (1999). Anandamide induces overeating: Mediation by central cannabinoid (CB1) receptors. *Psychopharmacology* 143, 315–317.
143. McLaughlin, P. J., Winston, K., Swezey, L., Wisniecki, A., Aberman, J., Tardif, D. J., Betz, A. J., Ishiwari, K., Makriyannis, A., and Salamone, J. D. (2003). The cannabinoid CB1 antagonists SR 141716A and AM 251 suppress food intake and food-reinforced behavior in a variety of tasks in rats. *Behav. Pharmacol.* 14, 583–588.
144. Rowland, N. E., Mukherjee, M., and Robertson, K. (2001). Effects of the cannabinoid receptor antagonist SR 141716, alone and in combination with dexfenfluramine or naloxone, on food intake in rats. *Psychopharmacology* 159, 111–116.
145. Van Gaal, L. F., Rissanen, A. M., Scheen, A. J., Ziegler, O., and Rossner, S. (2005). Effects of the cannabinoid-1 receptor blocker rimonabant on weight reduction and cardiovascular risk factors in overweight patients: 1-year experience from the RIO-Europe study. *Lancet* 365, 1389–1397.
146. Harrold, J. A., and Williams, G. (2003). The cannabinoid system: A role in both the homeostatic and hedonic control of eating?. *Br. J. Nutr.* 90, 729–734.

147. Kirkham, T. C., Williams, C. M., Fezza, F., and Di Marzo, V. (2002). Endocannabinoid levels in rat limbic forebrain and hypothalamus in relation to fasting, feeding and satiation: Stimulation of eating by 2-arachidonoyl glycerol. *Br. J. Pharmacol.* 136, 550–557.

148. Jamshidi, N., and Taylor, D. A. (2001). Anandamide administration into the ventromedial hypothalamus stimulates appetite in rats. *Br. J. Pharmacol.* 134, 1151–1154.

149. Chiesi, M., Huppertz, C., and Hofbauer, K. G. (2001). Pharmacotherapy of obesity: Targets and perspectives. *Trends Pharmacol. Sci.* 22, 247–254.

150. Cota, D., Marsicano, G., Tschop, M., Grubler, Y., Flachskamm, C., Schubert, M., Auer, D., Yassouridis, A., Thone-Reineke, C., Ortmann, S., Tomassoni, F., Cervino, C., Nisoli, E., Linthorst, A. C., Pasquali, R., Lutz, B., Stalla, G. K., and Pagotto, U. (2003). The endogenous cannabinoid system affects energy balance via central orexigenic drive and peripheral lipogenesis. *J. Clin. Invest.* 112, 423–431.

151. Bensaid, M., Gary-Bobo, M., Esclangon, A., Maffrand, J. P., Le Fur, G., Oury-Donat, F., and Soubrie, P. (2003). The cannabinoid CB1 receptor antagonist SR141716 increases Acrp30 mRNA expression in adipose tissue of obese fa/fa rats and in cultured adipocyte cells. *Mol. Pharmacol.* 63, 908–914.

152. Jbilo, O., Ravinet-Trillou, C., Arnone, M., Buisson, I., Bribes, E., Peleraux, A., Penarier, G., Soubrie, P., Le Fur, G., Galiegue, S., and Casellas, P. (2005). The CB1 receptor antagonist rimonabant reverses the diet-induced obesity phenotype through the regulation of lipolysis and energy balance. *FASEB J.* 19, 1567–1569.

153. Hanus, L., Avraham, Y., Ben-Shushan, D., Zolotarev, O., Berry, E. M., and Mechoulam, R. (2003). Short-term fasting and prolonged semistarvation have opposite effects on 2-AG levels in mouse brain. *Brain Res.* 983, 144–151.

154. Harrold, J. A., Elliott, J. C., King, P. J., Widdowson, P. S., and Williams, G. (2002). Down-regulation of cannabinoid-1 (CB-1) receptors in specific extrahypothalamic regions of rats with dietary obesity: A role for endogenous cannabinoids in driving appetite for palatable food? *Brain Res.* 952, 232–238.

155. Karler, R., Calder, L. D., Sangdee, P., and Turkanis, S. A. (1984). Interaction between Δ^9-tetrahydrocannabinol and kindling by electrical and chemical stimuli in mice. *Neuropharmacology* 23, 1315–1320.

156. Karler, R., Cely, W., and Turkanis, S. A. (1974). A study of the relative anticonvulsant and toxic activities of Δ^9-tetrahydrocannabinol and its congeners. *Res. Comm. Chem. Path. Pharm.* 7, 353–358.

157. Karler, R., Cely, W., and Turkanis, S. A. (1973). The anticonvulsant activity of cannabidiol and cannabinol. *Life Sci.* 13, 1527–1531.

158. Wallace, M. J., Wiley, J. L., Martin, B. R., and DeLorenzo, R. J. (2001). Assessment of the role of CB1 receptors in cannabinoid anticonvulsant effects. *Eur. J. Pharmacol.* 428, 51–57.

159. Wallace, M., Martin, B., and DeLorenzo, R. (2002). Evidence for a physiological role of endocannabinoids in the modulation of seizure threshold and severity. *Eur. J. Pharmacol.* 452, 295.

160. Wallace, M. J., Blair, R. E., Falenski, K. W., Martin, B. R., and DeLorenzo, R. J. (2003). The endogenous cannabinoid system regulates seizure frequency and duration in a model of temporal lobe epilepsy. *J. Pharmacol. Exp. Ther.* 307, 129–137.

161. Marsicano, G., Goodenough, S., Monory, K., Hermann, H., Eder, M., Cannich, A., Azad, S. C., Cascio, M. G., Gutierrez, S. O., van der Stelt, M., Lopez-Rodriguez, M. L., Casanova, E., Schutz, G., Zieglgansberger, W., Di Marzo, V., Behl, C., and Lutz, B. (2003). CB1 cannabinoid receptors and on-demand defense against excitotoxicity. *Science* 302, 84–88.

162. Lutz, B. (2004). On-demand activation of the endocannabinoid system in the control of neuronal excitability and epileptiform seizures. *Biochem. Pharmacol.* 68, 1691–1698.
163. Clement, A. B., Hawkins, E. G., Lichtman, A. H., and Cravatt, B. F. (2003). Increased seizure susceptibility and proconvulsant activity of anandamide in mice lacking fatty acid amide hydrolase. *J. Neurosci.* 23, 3916–3923.
164. Quistad, G. B., Sparks, S. E., Segall, Y., Nomura, D. K., and Casida, J. E. (2002). Selective inhibitors of fatty acid amide hydrolase relative to neuropathy target esterase and acetylcholinesterase: Toxicological implications. *Toxicol. Appl. Pharmacol.* 179, 57–63.
165. Shen, M., and Thayer, S. A. (1999). Delta9-tetrahydrocannabinol acts as a partial agonist to modulate glutamatergic synaptic transmission between rat hippocampal neurons in culture. *Mol. Pharmacol.* 55, 8–13.
166. Ameri, A., Wilhelm, A., and Simmet, T. (1999). Effects of the endogeneous cannabinoid, anandamide, on neuronal activity in rat hippocampal slices. *Br. J. Pharmacol.* 126, 1831–1839.
167. Chen, K., Ratzliff, A., Hilgenberg, L., Gulyas, A., Freund, T. F., Smith, M., Dinh, T. P., Piomelli, D., Mackie, K., and Soltesz, I. (2003). Long-term plasticity of endocannabinoid signaling induced by developmental febrile seizures. *Neuron* 39, 599–611.
168. Wilson, R. I., and Nicoll, R. A. (2002). Endocannabinoid signaling in the brain. *Science* 296, 678–682.
169. Chan, G. C., Hinds, T. R., Impey, S., and Storm, D. R. (1998). Hippocampal neurotoxicity of Δ9-tetrahydrocannabinol. *J. Neurosci.* 18, 5322–5332.
170. Downer, E. J., Fogarty, M. P., and Campbell, V. A. (2003). Tetrahydrocannabinol-induced neurotoxicity depends on CB1 receptor-mediated c-Jun N-terminal kinase activation in cultured cortical neurons. *Br. J. Pharmacol.* 140, 547–557.
171. Milton, N. G. (2002). Anandamide and noladin ether prevent neurotoxicity of the human amyloid-beta peptide. *Neurosci. Lett.* 332, 127–130.
172. Marsicano, G., Moosmann, B., Hermann, H., Lutz, B., and Behl, C. (2002). Neuroprotective properties of cannabinoids against oxidative stress: Role of the cannabinoid receptor CB1. *J. Neurochem.* 80, 448–456.
173. Hamelink, C., Hampson, A., Wink, D. A., Eiden, L. E., and Eskay, R. L. (2005). Comparison of cannabidiol, antioxidants, and diuretics in reversing binge ethanol-induced neurotoxicity. *J. Pharmacol. Exp. Ther.* 314, 780–788.
174. Hampson, A. J., Grimaldi, M., Axelrod, J., and Wink, D. (1998). Cannabidiol and (-)delta9-tetrahydrocannabinol are neuroprotective antioxidants. *Proc. Natl. Acad. Sci. USA* 95, 8268–8273.
175. Darmani, N. A. (2001). Delta(9)-tetrahydrocannabinol and synthetic cannabinoids prevent emesis produced by the cannabinoid CB(1) receptor antagonist/inverse agonist SR 141716A. *Neuropsychopharmacology* 24, 198–203.
176. Parker, L. A., Kwiatkowska, M., Burton, P., and Mechoulam, R. (2004). Effect of cannabinoids on lithium-induced vomiting in the *Suncus murinus* (house musk shrew). *Psychopharmacology* 171, 156–161.
177. Kwiatkowska, M., Parker, L. A., Burton, P., and Mechoulam, R. (2004). A comparative analysis of the potential of cannabinoids and ondansetron to suppress cisplatin-induced emesis in the *Suncus murinus* (house musk shrew). *Psychopharmacology* 174, 254–259.
178. Parker, L. A., and Kemp, S. W. (2001). Tetrahydrocannabinol (THC) interferes with conditioned retching in *Suncus murinus*: An animal model of anticipatory nausea and vomiting (ANV). *Neuroreport* 12, 749–751.

179. Parker, L. A., and Mechoulam, R. (2003). Cannabinoid agonists and antagonists modulate lithium-induced conditioned gaping in rats. *Integr. Physiol. Behav. Sci.* 38, 133–145.

180. Simoneau, I. I., Hamza, M. S., Mata, H. P., Siegel, E. M., Vanderah, T. W., Porreca, F., Makriyannis, A., and Malan, T. P., Jr. (2001). The cannabinoid agonist WIN55,212-2 suppresses opioid-induced emesis in ferrets. *Anesthesiology* 94, 882–887.

181. Darmani, N. A., Sim-Selley, L. J., Martin, B. R., Janoyan, J. J., Crim, J. L., Parekh, B., and Breivogel, C. S. (2003). Antiemetic and motor-depressive actions of CP55,940: Cannabinoid CB1 receptor characterization, distribution, and G-protein activation. *Eur. J. Pharmacol.* 459, 83–95.

182. Van Sickle, M. D., Oland, L. D., Ho, W., Hillard, C. J., Mackie, K., Davison, J. S., and Sharkey, K. A. (2001). Cannabinoids inhibit emesis through CB1 receptors in the brainstem of the ferret. *Gastroenterology* 121, 767–774.

183. Van Sickle, M. D., Oland, L. D., Mackie, K., Davison, J. S., and Sharkey, K. A. (2003). Delta9-tetrahydrocannabinol selectively acts on CB1 receptors in specific regions of dorsal vagal complex to inhibit emesis in ferrets. *Am. J. Physiol. Gastrointest. Liver Physiol.* 285, G566–G576.

184. Darmani, N. A., and Johnson, J. C. (2004). Central and peripheral mechanisms contribute to the antiemetic actions of delta-9-tetrahydrocannabinol against 5-hydroxytryptophan-induced emesis. *Eur. J. Pharmacol.* 488, 201–212.

185. Darmani, N. A., and Crim, J. L. (2005). Delta-9-tetrahydrocannabinol differentially suppresses emesis versus enhanced locomotor activity produced by chemically diverse dopamine D2/D3 receptor agonists in the least shrew (*Cryptotis parva*). *Pharmacol. Biochem. Behav.* 80, 35–44.

186. McCabe, M., Smith, F. P., Macdonald, J. S., Woolley, P. V., Goldberg, D., and Schein, P. S. (1988). Efficacy of tetrahydrocannabinol in patients refractory to standard antiemetic therapy. *Invest. New Drugs* 6, 243–246.

187. Plasse, T. F., Gorter, R. W., Krasnow, S. H., Lane, M., Shepard, K. V., and Wadleigh, R. G. (1991). Recent clinical experience with Dronabinol. *Pharmacol. Biochem. Behav.* 40, 695–700.

188. Lane, M., Vogel, C. L., Ferguson, J., Krasnow, S., Saiers, J. L., Hamm, J., Salva, K., Wiernik, P. H., Holroyde, C. P., Hammill, S., et al. 1991). Dronabinol and prochlorperazine in combination for treatment of cancer chemotherapy-induced nausea and vomiting. *J. Pain Symptom Manag.* 6, 352–359.

189. Ahmedzai, S., Carlyle, D. L., Calder, I. T., and Moran, F. (1983). Anti-emetic efficacy and toxicity of nabilone, a synthetic cannabinoid, in lung cancer chemotherapy. *Br. J. Cancer* 48, 657–663.

190. Abrahamov, A., and Mechoulam, R. (1995). An efficient new cannabinoid antiemetic in pediatric oncology. *Life Sci.* 56, 2097–2102.

191. Chan, H. S., Correia, J. A., and MacLeod, S. M. (1987). Nabilone versus prochlorperazine for control of cancer chemotherapy-induced emesis in children: A double-blind, crossover trial. *Pediatrics* 79, 946–952.

192. Fattore, L., Cossu, G., Martellotta, C. M., and Fratta, W. (2001). Intravenous self-administration of the cannabinoid CB1 receptor agonist WIN 55,212-2 in rats. *Psychopharmacology (Berl.)* 156, 410–416.

193. Justinova, Z., Tanda, G., Redhi, G. H., and Goldberg, S. R. (2003). Self-administration of delta9-tetrahydrocannabinol (THC) by drug naive squirrel monkeys. *Psychopharmacology* 169, 135–140.

194. Tanda, G., Munzar, P., and Goldberg, S. R. (2000). Self-administration behavior is maintained by the psychoactive ingredient of marijuana in squirrel monkeys. *Nat. Neurosci.* 3, 1073–1074.

195. Huestis, M. A., Gorelick, D. A., Heishman, S. J., Preston, K. L., Nelson, R. A., Moolchan, E. T., and Frank, R. A. (2001). Blockade of effects of smoked marijuana by the CB1-selective cannabinoid receptor antagonist SR141716. *Arch. Gen. Psychiatry* 58, 322–328.

196. Justinova, Z., Goldberg, S. R., Heishman, S. J., and Tanda, G. (2005). Self-administration of cannabinoids by experimental animals and human marijuana smokers. *Pharmacol. Biochem. Behav.* 81, 285–299.

197. Lupica, C. R., Riegel, A. C., and Hoffman, A. F. (2004). Marijuana and cannabinoid regulation of brain reward circuits. *Br. J. Pharmacol.* 143, 227–234.

198. Chen, J., Paredes, W., Li, J., Smith, D., Lowinson, J., and Gardner, E. (1990). Δ^9-Tetrahydrocannabinol produces naloxone-blockable enhancement of presynaptic basal dopamine efflux in nucleus accumbens of conscious, freely moving rats as measured by intracerebral microdialysis. *Psychopharmacology* 102, 156–162.

199. Chen, J., Paredes, W., Lowinson, J. H., and Gardner, E. L. (1990). Δ^9-Tetrahydrocannabinol enhances presynaptic dopamine efflux in medial prefrontal cortex. *Eur. J. Pharmacol.* 190, 259–262.

200. Diana, M., Melis, M., and Gessa, G. L. (1998). Increase in meso-prefrontal dopaminergic activity after stimulation of CB1 receptors by cannabinoids. *Eur. J. Neurosci.* 10, 2825–2830.

201. French, E. D., Dillon, K., and Wu, X. (1997). Cannabinoids excite dopamine neurons in the ventral tegmentum and substantia nigra. *Neuroreport* 8, 649–652.

202. Cheer, J. F., Marsden, C. A., Kendall, D. A., and Mason, R. (2000). Lack of response suppression follows repeated ventral tegmental cannabinoid administration: An in vitro electrophysiological study. *Neuroscience* 99, 661–667.

203. Szabo, B., Siemes, S., and Wallmichrath, I. (2002). Inhibition of GABAergic neurotransmission in the ventral tegmental area by cannabinoids. *Eur. J. Neurosci.* 15, 2057–2061.

204. Tanda, G., Pontieri, F., and Chiara, G. (1997). Cannabinoid and heroin activation of mesolimbic dopamine transmission by a common μ_1 opioid receptor mechanism. *Science* 276, 2048–2050.

205. Melis, M., Pistis, M., Perra, S., Muntoni, A. L., Pillolla, G., and Gessa, G. L. (2004). Endocannabinoids mediate presynaptic inhibition of glutamatergic transmission in rat ventral tegmental area dopamine neurons through activation of CB1 receptors. *J. Neurosci.* 24, 53–62.

206. Compton, D. R., Dewey, W. L., and Martin, B. R. (1990). Cannabis dependence and tolerance production. In *Addiction Potential of Abused Drugs and Drug Classes*, C. K. Erickson, M. A. Javors, and W. W. Morgan, Eds. Hayworth, Binghampton, NY, pp. 129–147.

207. Lamb, R. J., Jarbe, T. U., Makriyannis, A., Lin, S., and Goutopoulos, A. (2000). Effects of delta9-tetrahydrocannabinol, (*R*)-methanandamide, SR 141716, and *d*-amphetamine before and during daily delta9-tetrahydrocannabinol dosing. *Eur. J. Pharmacol.* 398, 251–258.

208. Welch, S. P., Dunlow, L. D., Patrick, G. S., and Razdan, R. K. (1995). Characterization of anandamide- and fluoroanandamide-induced antinociception and cross-tolerance to Δ^9-THC following intrathecal administration to mice: Blockade of Δ^9-THC-induced antinociception. *J. Pharmacol. Exp. Ther.* 273, 1235–1244.

209. Wiley, J. L., Smith, F. L., Razdan, R. K., and Dewey, W. L. (2005). Task specificity of cross-tolerance between delta9-tetrahydrocannabinol and anandamide analogs in mice. *Eur. J. Pharmacol.* 510, 59–68.

210. Breivogel, C. S., Scates, S. M., Beletskaya, I. O., Lowery, O. B., Aceto, M. D., and Martin, B. R. (2003). The effects of delta9-tetrahydrocannabinol physical dependence on brain cannabinoid receptors. *Eur. J. Pharmacol.* 459, 139–150.

211. Sim-Selley, L. J., and Martin, B. R. (2002). Effect of chronic administration of R-(+)-[2,3-dihydro-5-methyl-3-[(morpholinyl)methyl]pyrrolo[1,2,3-*de*]-1,4-benzoxazinyl]-(1-naphthalenyl)methanone mesylae (WIN55,212-2) or Δ^9-tetrahydrocannabinol on cannabinoid receptor adaptation in mice. *J. Pharmacol. Exp. Ther.* 303, 36–44.

212. Aceto, M. D., Scates, S. M., and Martin, B. B. (2001). Spontaneous and precipitated withdrawal with a synthetic cannabinoid, WIN 55212-2. *Eur. J. Pharmacol.* 416, 75–81.

213. Aceto, M., Scates, S., Lowe, J., and Martin, B. (1996). Dependence on Δ^9-tetrahydrocannabinol: Studies on precipitated and abrupt withdrawal. *J. Pharmacol. Exp. Ther.* 278, 1290–1295.

214. Tsou, K., Patrick, S., and Walker, J. M. (1995). Physical withdrawal in rats tolerant to Δ^9-tetrahydrocannabinol precipated by a cannabinoid receptor antagonist. *Eur. J. Pharmacol.* 280, R13–R15.

215. Hutcheson, D. M., Tzavara, E. T., Smadja, C., Valjent, E., Roques, B. P., Hanoune, J., and Maldonado, R. (1998). Behavioral and biochemical evidence for signs of abstinence in mice chemically treated with Δ9-terahydrocannabinol. *J. Pharmacol.* 125, 1567–1577.

216. Lichtman, A. H., Fisher, J., and Martin, B. R. (2001). Precipitated cannabinoid withdrawal is reversed by delta(9)-tetrahydrocannabinol or clonidine. *Pharmacol. Biochem. Behav.* 69, 181–188.

217. Budney, A. J., and Moore, B. A. (2002). Development and consequences of cannabis dependence. *J. Clin. Pharmacol.* 42, 28S–33S.

19

OPIATES AND ADDICTION

FRANK J. VOCCI

National Institute on Drug Abuse, National Institutes of Health, Bethesda, Maryland

19.1	Incidence and Prevalence of Heroin and Prescription Opiate Abuse	692
19.2	Treatment Statistics	694
19.3	Current Treatment Needs	696
19.4	Buprenorphine Studies	696
	19.4.1 Buprenorphine and Buprenorphine/Naloxone: Studies for Food and Drug Administration Approval	696
	19.4.2 Buprenorphine: Comparative Efficacy Studies	697
	19.4.3 Buprenorphine: Implementation Issues and Pilot Studies	698
19.5	Future Challenges for Opiate Dependence Treatment	698
19.6	Drug Discovery Efforts for Opiate Dependence Treatments	699
19.7	Summary and Conclusions	700
	References	700

The abuse liability of opiates was recognized and written about as early as the sixteenth century. Abuse of and tolerance to opiates were described in manuscripts from Turkey, Egypt, Germany, and England [1]. Abuse of and dependence on opiates continue to represent a worldwide problem that is associated with significant morbidity and mortality. According to the World Health Organization, almost 13 million people abused opiate drugs in the years 1999–2001 [2].

Opiate abuse and dependence are associated with significant morbidity and mortality. Morbidity associated with opiate addiction includes the risk of contracting acquired immunodeficiency syndrome (AIDS) and hepatitis C infections from unsafe injection practices and high-risk sexual practices. The worldwide human immunodeficiency virus (HIV) epidemic continues at a rapid pace. Of the estimated 40 million people infected with HIV, 5 million were infected during 2003. In regions of the world where the infection is spreading the fastest, drug injectors and their sexual partners account for most of the new infections [3]. The U.S. Centers for Disease Control and Prevention (CDC) estimates that 36% of the AIDS cases in the United States are due to injection drug use or sexual activity with an injection drug user. Chitwood et al. [4] compared HIV infection prevalence across new injectors, long-term injectors, and heroin sniffers. The new injectors and the heroin sniffers had

---

Handbook of Contemporary Neuropharmacology, Edited by David R. Sibley, Israel Hanin, Michael Kuhar, and Phil Skolnick. Copyright © 2007 John Wiley & Sons, Inc.

prevalence rates of 13.3 and 12.7%, respectively, whereas the long-term injectors had a 24.7% prevalence rate. The attributable HIV risk from injection was 5.8% for the new injectors versus 55% for the long-term injectors. These data suggest that sexual risk factors play a major role in the spread of HIV into the general population in the new-injector and sniffer groups. The injection drug–using population is a significant contributor to the AIDS epidemic, suggesting that curtailment of the epidemic will not occur until this population is successfully treated for drug use and effectively counseled regarding unsafe sexual practices. Moreover, noninjection heroin users who are HIV positive also can contribute to the HIV epidemic by sexual transmission to their partners [5, 6].

Hepatitis C infections generally have a higher prevalence than HIV in injection drug users. Many infections occur early in the course of injection drug use. Garfein et al. [7] reported a 65% incidence of hepatitis C infection in a population with a one-year or less history of injection drug use. Over 95% of injection heroin users found to have significant liver disease in an early cohort (late 1970s and early 1980s) were later retrospectively found to have hepatitis C infection [8, 9]. Injection drug users infected with hepatitis C in this era will soon be or are already presenting with need for treatment and possible hepatic transplantation since 20% of hepatitis C–infected persons will progress to severe liver disease over a 20-year period of time. Of considerable concern, a very recent study has shown that essentially all of the former heroin addicts in methadone maintenance treatment who are HIV positive, and thus require treatment of AIDS infection, also have markers indicating prior or current hepatitis C infection [10]. Sixty-seven percent of the cohort were hepatitis C positive and 29% were HIV positive. Coinfection rates for the overall study group were 26%. HIV–hepatitis C virus (HCV) coinfection increases the progression of HCV-induced liver disease, resulting in faster progression to cirrhosis and end-stage liver disease [11]. Mortality increases from liver disease in HIV–HCV coinfected patients have been reported [12].

"All-causes mortality" is high in untreated opiate-addicted populations. Desmond and Maddux [13] reported death rates in the illicit opiate–using population not in treatment ranged from 1.65 to 8.3% per year; the median yearly death rate was 3.5%. HIV disease has also impacted mortality and causes of mortality in this population. Quaglio et al. [14], analyzed heroin-related deaths in northeast Italy occurring from 1985 to 1998. Of the 2708 deaths, 37% were due to overdose and 32.5% were AIDS related. The mortality rate among the injection drug users (IDUs) was 13 times that of the general population. The effect of HIV infection on mortality in heroin users was also evaluated in the Vancouver Injection Drug Users Study [15]. Irrespective of HIV status, the leading cause of death was opiate overdose, accounting for 42% of the HIV-negative deaths and 25% of the HIV-positive cohort deaths. Of the 65 deaths among the HIV-positive group, 34% were AIDS related.

19.1 INCIDENCE AND PREVALENCE OF HEROIN AND PRESCRIPTION OPIATE ABUSE

The prevalence of heroin use is greater in developed countries; 2% of youth in western Europe, Canada, and the United States have tried heroin [2]. Moreover, the "purity" of heroin in the United States has increased significantly and the price has fallen in the last 25 years from 7% in 1980 to an average of 51% in 2001 [16]. Heroin purity as high as 72% has been noted in Philadelphia. The change in purity has allowed a shift from intravenous use to intranasal use. The intranasal route is an acceptable route of administration for many heroin initiates. In fact, it is considered the method of choice for American adolescents [17]. Peak blood levels from intranasal use occur in 5 min, essentially equal to that seen with intramuscular injection [18]. The average age at which heroin was first used has dropped from 27 in 1988 to 19 in 1995 [17]. Use by the intranasal route tripled between 1991 and 1995. There is evidence that adolescent admission for heroin abuse and dependence tripled from 1993 to 1998 (see Section 19.2). One report noted that the average age was 17 years old for admission to treatment for heroin abuse [19]. For an overview of adolescent heroin abuse, see the review of Hopfer et al. [20]. There is also evidence that a significant percentage of heroin "snorters" will shift to injection [5, 6, 21].

Global statistics on the abuse of prescription opiates are unavailable. In the United States, incidence and prevalence rates of abuse of prescription opiates were obtained in the 2003 National Survey on Drug Use and Health (NSDUH) [22]. This survey is the primary source of information on illicit drug and alcohol use for the civilian, noninstitutionalized U.S. population aged 12 or older. In 2002, there were 2.5 million new users who endorsed nonmedical use of opiate analgesics. This is approximately a fivefold increase since 1990. (Another database, The Monitoring the Future study, a survey that questions 8th, 10th, and 12th graders about their drug use, has also noted a threefold increase in prescription opiate abuse since 1991 [23]). Fifty-five percent of the new users were females and 56% were age 18 or older. Individuals that were current users of opiate analgesics taken nonmedically totaled 4.7 million. It is doubtful that all of these individuals would meet the criteria of the fourth edition of the *Diagnostic and Statistical Manual of Mental Disorders* (DSM-IV) for an opiate abuse diagnosis. In terms of lifetime prevalence, over 31 million Americans have used opiate analgesics in a nonmedical fashion. Opiate medications used most often in the survey were hydrocodone combinations (15.7 million), oxycodone combinations (10.8 million), hydrocodone (5.7 million), OxyContin (2.8 million), methadone (1.2 million), and Tramadol (186,000). When survey respondents were diagnosed using DSM-IV criteria, 57.4% of the heroin users met criteria for opiate abuse or dependence whereas 12.2% of the prescription opiate users met criteria for opiate abuse or dependence.

These data suggest that although there is a greater prevalence of prescription opiate abuse, the risk of dependence is lower in the population that abuses prescription opiate medications. Moreover, the data suggest an increasing problem with dependence on prescription opiates. Assuming one-eighth of the current nonmedical prescription opiate users meet DSM-IV criteria for abuse or dependence, that would equate to 600,000 people currently in need of treatment. Given the increasing incidence of nonmedical use of prescription opiates, the current situation is likely to worsen before it gets better.

Opiate abusers can be categorized into three groups: those abusing only heroin, those abusing only prescription opiates, and those abusing heroin and prescription opiates. An analysis of heroin, oxycodone, and heroin and oxycodone users was conducted in the 2003 NSDUH. Heroin and heroin-plus-oxycodone users had a 2:1 male–female ratio whereas the oxycodone-only group had more females (57:43). The majority of users of oxycodone, either alone or in combination with heroin, were white (91%). Groups using heroin, either alone or in combination, were older than 35, whereas the majority (56%) of the oxycodone users were younger than 35. Past-year dependence diagnoses were 4, 16, and 7% for heroin, heroin plus oxycodone, and oxycodone alone, respectively.

In 2003, the NSDUH estimated that 19.5 million Americans were current illicit drug users (use within 30 days of the NSDUH survey). Of these, 3.8 million were considered to meet criteria for abuse or dependence and another 3.1 million were diagnosed with abuse or dependence to alcohol and illicit drugs. When alcohol use alone is added to these categories, 21.6 million people aged 12 or older were classified with a substance abuse disorder. Of this group, 3.3 million sought treatment in 2003. In terms of opiate users, 415,000 prescription opiate users and 281,000 heroin users sought treatment.

The treatment of opiate addiction can be conceptualized as occurring in three categories: discovery of new therapies, development of new therapies, and implementation of new therapies. The extant treatment system will be considered first so that the context of discovery, development, and implementation of new pharmacotherapies can be better understood.

19.2 TREATMENT STATISTICS

The Treatment Episode Data Set (TEDS) is another SAMHSA [24] data set that summarizes patient demographics and treatment characteristics of the 1.9 million patients admitted to treatment centers that report to individual state administrative systems. This system is not comprehensive but captures data that can be analyzed for year-to-year changes as well as long-term treatment trends.

As can be seen in Table 19.1, heroin admissions in the TEDS system increased from 1992 to 2002. In fact, heroin admissions accounted for 15% of the treatment admissions, making it the largest illicit drug for which individuals seek treatment. Admissions for adolescent heroin use tripled in the 1990s (TEDS 2000 data not shown). Male heroin users outnumber female users. A plurality of heroin users are white. Subtle shifts in racial composition of patients entering treatment and route of administration differences were also seen. The number of white heroin admissions increased from 1992, whereas the number of African-Americans had a slight drop (data not shown). Moreover, the data show a shift toward less injection use and more inhalation use among African-Americans whereas inhalation and injection use both increased among white heroin users. Additionally, the use of methadone as a treatment in this system appears to be declining for both injectors and inhalers.

In contrast, the overwhelming majority of prescription opiate users admitted into treatment are white. They also abuse the drug by the oral route of administration. The male-to-female ratio appears to be close to 1, suggesting a greater likelihood for females to be prescription opiate abusers. Although the number of treatment admissions represents only a small percentage of the treatment admissions in TEDS, the percentage has increased from 1992 to 2002. An even smaller percentage of these patients received methadone in their treatment.

Methadone was developed by in the 1960s as a treatment for heroin addiction (for a review, see [25]). There is documented evidence that methadone reduces morbidity

TABLE 19.1 Comparison of Treatment Facilities Admissions for Heroin Users and Prescription Opiate Users in 1992 and 2002 from TEDS

Patient Demographics and Use Variables	Heroin Admissions		Prescription Opiate Dependence Admissions	
	1992	2002	1992	2002
Number of admissions	170,370	285,657	13,671	45,605
Male, %	—	69	—	54
White				
Percent	—	48	—	88
Male/female ratio	—	31/17	—	47/41
Hispanic				
Percent	—	25	—	3.5
Male/female ratio[a]	—	17/4	—	1.5/1.0
African-American				
Percent	—	25	—	5
Male/female ratio	—	15.6/8.6	—	2.8/2.6
Median age	—	36	—	35
Injectors, %	77	62	25	13
Inhalation, %	20	33	3	9
Opiate smokers, %	1.4	3		3
Oral ingestion, %	0.7	2	66	75
Daily Opiate Use, %	—	80	—	68
Admissions to TEDS, %	10.9	15.2	0.9	2.4
Methadone therapy for injectors, %	61	38		
Methadone therapy for inhalers, %	44	32		
Methadone therapy, %	—	—	—	19

[a]Mexican and Puerto Rican admissions (excludes Cubans and other Hispanic groups).

and mortality associated with heroin addiction. The death rate falls dramatically for former heroin addicts in methadone maintenance treatment [26–28]. Methadone is primarily dispensed in specialty outpatient clinics [29]. The National Survey of Substance Abuse Treatment Services reported that 1215 of 13,428 facilities dispensed methadone or levomethadyl acetate (LAAM). On the survey reference date of October 1, 2000, 17% of the patients in the survey were reported to be in methadone treatment. There are a number of barriers to obtaining methadone. Patients entering treatment for detoxification from heroin actually receive methadone less often than patients receiving longer treatment (22 vs. 35%) [29]. For prescription opiate-dependent patients entered into the 2000 TEDS data set, those who worked full or parttime were more likely to receive methadone. No sex differences in receipt of methadone were seen in the TEDS system for prescription opiate users. Other potential barriers are lack of treatment facilities in rural areas. For example, admission rates for prescription opiate user treatment increased 155% in the United

States. The greatest increase (269%) was seen in nonmetropolitan areas (without a city population of 10,000 or more).

19.3 CURRENT TREATMENT NEEDS

To address the unmet treatment needs of heroin- and prescription opiate-dependent patients, several changes are needed. The first is a greater test of the concept of medical maintenance with methadone. Initial studies have shown that medical maintenance is not only feasible but can be highly successful with stable patients [30–33]. Expanded research with methadone in this model is necessary to continue the medicalization of the treatment of opiate dependence. Increasing access to the medical care system should have benefits to patients accessing medical care [34].

The second change needed is a greater uptake of opiate pharmacotherapy with buprenorphine (SUBUTEX) and buprenorphine/naloxone (SUBOXONE).

19.4 BUPRENORPHINE STUDIES

19.4.1 Buprenorphine and Buprenorphine/Naloxone: Studies for Food and Drug Administration Approval

Buprenorphine was recognized to possess pharmacological properties that could be utilized for treatment of opiate dependence [35]. Specifically, buprenorphine had an ability to block the effects of administered morphine while it had intrinsic opiatelike effects that would likely ensure better compliance than a nonopiate or narcotic antagonist. Its duration of action implied that it could be administered as a single daily dose. Buprenorphine was classified as a partial agonist of the μ receptor [36]. Its partial agonist properties produce a ceiling effect on respiration [37] that suggests a lower risk of severe respiratory depression or apnea. Moreover, the withdrawal syndrome reported was minimal [35].

Buprenorphine's efficacy was established in three large, prospective studies that formed the basis of its marketing approval. Johnson et al. [38] reported the initial efficacy of buprenorphine in the outpatient setting. In this study, the 8-mg sublingual buprenorphine liquid-per-day group had better retention and lower opiate use than an active control group receiving 20 mg of oral methadone. A second study reported that an 8-mg dose of sublingual buprenorphine liquid produced better retention and less opiate use than a 1-mg buprenorphine active-control group [39].

During the development of buprenorphine, Reckitt-Benckiser decided to market a solid dosage form of different tablet strengths. Moreover, it also agreed with National Institute on Drug Abuse (NIDA) that a second dosage form that contained naloxone would serve as an abuse deterrent. The two decisions to develop solid dosage forms of different tablet strengths and to add naloxone as an abuse deterrent necessitated additional research in the following areas: dosage form development, determination of the ratio of buprenorphine to naloxone, efficacy and safety of the tablet formulations, and bioequivalence of buprenorphine tablets to sublingual liquid. Dosage strengths of 2 and 8 mg were chosen. Several clinical pharmacology studies were conducted in various opiate-dependent populations maintained on morphine [40, 41], methadone [42], or buprenorphine [43] to determine the ratio of buprenorphine to naloxone for the combination tablets. A 4:1 buprenorphine–naloxone ratio was chosen. A randomized, double-blind, placebo-controlled multicenter trial compared the buprenorphine tablet, the buprenorphine–naloxone tablet, and placebo in opiate-dependent patients [44]. Both tablets reduced opiate use in the first month of the study compared to placebo.

The U.S. Food and Drug Administration (FDA) approved buprenorphine (SUBUTEX) and buprenorphine/naloxone (SUBOXONE) in October 2002. These medications are indicated for the management of opiate dependence. As there are other medications used in the management of opiate dependence, the comparative efficacy of buprenorphine will be reviewed before addressing the implementation issues.

19.4.2 Buprenorphine: Comparative Efficacy Studies

The Cochrane Review Group recently reviewed the efficacy of buprenorphine versus placebo or methadone [45]. Thirteen studies were reviewed. Buprenorphine was judged to be superior to placebo in terms of retention at all buprenorphine doses, but high and very high doses were needed to show greater suppression of heroin abuse than placebo. In comparison to methadone, buprenorphine does not retain patients as well as methadone and does not suppress heroin use as well as methadone. Study design issues may confound the conclusion of inferior suppression of heroin use of buprenorphine. For example, there are two randomized, active controlled studies that allow flexible dosing with buprenorphine and methadone. Mattick et al. [46] randomized 405 opiate-dependent patients in three methadone clinics to buprenorphine or methadone in a flexible dosing design. There were no differences in illicit opiate use across groups, although retention in the buprenorphine group (50%) was less than that seen in the methadone group (59%, n.s.). Johnson et al. [47] randomized 220 patients to one of four medications groups: buprenorphine (16–32 mg), methadone low dose (20 mg), methadone high dose (60–100 mg), or levomethadyl acetate (75–115 mg). There were no differences in illicit opiate use in the buprenorphine versus methadone groups. The buprenorphine-treated group had a nonstatistically significantly lower retention (58%) than the high-dose methadone group (73%).

Gowing et al. [48] have recently reviewed the efficacy of buprenorphine for the management of opiate withdrawal. Buprenorphine was compared to methadone (three studies), clonidine (seven studies), or differing rates of dose tapering of buprenorphine. Buprenorphine–treated patients completed treatment more often that clonidine patients and with fewer adverse effects. No differences in completion rate were seen between buprenorphine and methadone, although buprenorphine may provide better symptom management. Gradual dose reduction of buprenorphine may assist patients in completing withdrawal. A recent study evaluated two dose regimens of buprenorphine tablets (2–4–8–4–2 or 8–8–8–4–2 mg/day) versus clonidine in the management of heroin withdrawal [49]. Both dose regimens suppressed withdrawal better than clonidine, but the high-dose buprenorphine group was superior to clonidine on such measures as drug craving.

19.4.3 Buprenorphine: Implementation Issues and Pilot Studies

While the final stages of development of the buprenorphine products were ongoing, the U.S. Congress passed the Drug Abuse Treatment Act (DATA) of 2000. This law allows qualified physicians to prescribe FDA-approved opiate products in Schedules III–V of the Controlled Substances Act (CSA) that are indicated for the treatment of opiate dependence. Both products were scheduled into C. III of the CSA. Qualified physicians can prescribe these products (as defined in the DATA) to 30 opiate-dependent patients in their medical practices. Physicians can be qualified by experience or training. Then they request a waiver to prescribe buprenorphine. To date, over 7000 physicians have received waivers.

Physicians in office-based practice can now prescribe buprenorphine. A consensus statement on office-based treatment of opiate dependence using buprenorphine has now been developed [50]. O'Connor et al. [51] reported that patients randomized to buprenorphine in a primary-care setting had greater retention and less opiate use than those randomized to a methadone clinic. Fiellin et al. [52] treated heroin-dependent patients with thrice-weekly buprenorphine in a primary-care center. Eleven of the 13 patients were retained through the 13-week study period. Nine of the 13 patients achieved at least 3 consecutive weeks of opiate-free urines. Gibson et al. [53] reported that retention and reduction of opiate use were equivalent in patients assigned to buprenorphine in a specialty clinic versus a primary-care setting.

Additional research on buprenorphine products has been conducted. The NIDA's Clinical Trials Network has conducted medically assisted withdrawal studies in clinic settings [54]. In this report, 234 buprenorphine/naloxone-treated patients were followed for 13 days; 68% completed the detoxification. Only 1 of 18 serious adverse events was considered possibly related to buprenorphine. The authors concluded that the use of buprenorphine/naloxone in diverse community settings was practical and safe. Lintzeris et al. [55] reported on an Australian study of the implementation of buprenorphine in community treatment settings by general practitioners and pharmacists. Patients were randomized to either buprenorphine or methadone in this study. Seventy-four percent of the methadone transfer and 46% of the heroin patients treated with buprenorphine were retained for six months in treatment. The authors concluded that buprenorphine could be safely delivered in the community setting.

19.5 FUTURE CHALLENGES FOR OPIATE DEPENDENCE TREATMENT

The NIDA will concentrate on the development of non-opiate-based treatments for opiate dependence. Naltrexone is approved for the prevention of relapse in formerly opiate-dependent patients. Although naltrexone has been shown to be superior to placebo for prevention of relapse in a criminal justice population [56], the major problem with naltrexone is adherence to therapy. One of the naltrexone depot dosage forms has been tested in an outpatient trial [57]. A clinical trial of a depot form of naltrexone in outpatients being treated for alcoholism was recently published [58]. It is anticipated that the development of this dosage form will continue. If and when the depot form of naltrexone is marketed for alcoholism, studies will commence in detoxified formerly opiate-dependent populations. Since adherence is the major problem with the use of naltrexone, it is anticipated that this dosage form would be an advance in treatment.

The management of opiate withdrawal by nonopioid medications is another medications development challenge. For example, lofexidine is a congener of the α_2 agonist clonidine. It has been tested in opiate-dependent populations undergoing withdrawal. The initial double-blind, placebo-controlled multicenter trial of lofexidine was halted due to overwhelming efficacy. Although buprenorphine has been shown to be superior to clonidine, the potential of a medication like lofexidine would be for managing withdrawal in settings where buprenorphine and methadone were not available.

Buspirone has been shown in an initial study to reduce opiate withdrawal symptomatology in patients undergoing detoxification from heroin or medically assisted withdrawal from methadone [59].

19.6 DRUG DISCOVERY EFFORTS FOR OPIATE DEPENDENCE TREATMENTS

The potential success in developing new treatments for opiate dependence will depend on translation of neuroscience-based treatments into new medications. Two of the most promising targets will be highlighted here. One of the most promising therapeutic targets is a corticotropin releasing factor (CRF) receptor antagonist. CRF has been shown to be involved in the mediation of responses involving arousal, affect, and aversion to negative situations (for a review, see [60]). CRF is involved in coordinating responses to internal or external threats to an organism's homeostasis. Drug withdrawal syndromes can be considered an aversive state. Writhing, chewing movements, "wet dog" shakes, salivation, lacrimation, diarrhea, and increased emotionality characterize opiate withdrawal in rats. The CRF-1 antagonist CP-154,526 has been shown to attenuate several signs of naltrexone-precipitated withdrawal in opiate-dependent rats [61]. The CRF-1 antagonist CRA 1000 attenuated naloxone-precipitated withdrawal signs in chronically morphine-treated mice [62]. The CRF-1 antagonist antalarmin reversed naloxone-induced place aversion in morphine-pelleted rats [63]. Lu et al. [64, 65] have reported a role for CRF in morphine relapse in animal models. These investigators reported that CP-154,526 blocked the reinstatement of footshock-induced morphine place preference. Shaham et al. [66] reported that CRF reinstated heroin self-administration and α-helical CRF blocked footshock-induced reinstatement of heroin self-administration. CP-154,526 also attenuated footshock-induced reinstatement of heroin self-administration in rats [67]. The aggregate results suggest that a CRF antagonist would attenuate opiate withdrawal and block conditioned aversion responses and stress-related lapses or relapses to opiates.

The cannabinoid antagonist SR141716A (rimonabant) has also shown promise as a potential medication for the treatment of opiate dependence in preclinical models. Rimonabant has been shown to decrease components of the opiate withdrawal syndrome in rats [68]. Rimonabant blocked morphine-induced place preference in mice [69]. In rats trained to self-administer heroin, rimonabant reduced self-administration in fixed-ratio [69] and fixed- and progressive-ratio conditions [70, 71]. Further, Devries et al. [71] showed rimonabant blockade of heroin-seeking behavior that was provoked by either a priming injection of heroin or heroin-associated cues. These data provide a strong rationale for testing of rimonabant in opiate-dependent patients. For further details, the reader is referred to LeFoll and Goldberg [72].

19.7 SUMMARY AND CONCLUSIONS

Abuse and dependence on opiate drugs are chronic problems. There have been some fundamental changes in abuse patterns in the United States, notably the increase in both heroin use and prescription opiate abuse in the last 10 years. The increase in heroin use has been fueled by the availability of concentrated heroin that can be used for inhalation or smoking. Adolescent heroin use has risen concomitantly with the higher concentration of heroin. The age of first heroin use has dropped by nine years, suggesting that a greater number of young people will become heroin dependent. Treatment for heroin abuse is currently the primary diagnosis of individuals treated for illicit drug use in the TEDS database. The incidence figures noted in adolescents suggest that it will remain so for some time.

An increase in prescription opiate use and treatment for opiate abuse have been recorded in the drug use and treatment system databases. There are more prescription opiate users than heroin users (and more women than men are prescription opiate users who seek treatment). This is reflected in the fact that more opiate users than heroin users reported getting treatment for their dependence [73]. A different locus of use has been noted for prescription opiate users; that is, the greatest increase has been in rural areas.

Consequently, the treatment delivery system for opiate users is undergoing some unique challenges. Even in light of a worsening situation, funding for pharmacotherapy seems to be diminishing in the publicly funded part of the treatment system. This situation needs to be reversed. Additionally, treatment delivery must be given in reasonable proximity to the users' domiciles. This means that the treatment system must undergo a major change to reach the prescription opiate users who are concentrated in rural areas. The current availability of SUBUTEX and SUBOXONE should help to address the problem of treatment delivery outside urban areas by qualified physicians who can now prescribe these medications as part of their primary-care practices. Physicians are currently constrained to a 30-patient limit. This limit can be changed by legislation or administrative action at the level of the secretary of the U.S. Department of Health and Human Services (DHHS).

The use of methadone for "office-based practice" would be another useful tool for physicians to be able to prescribe for patients. This has been evaluated in several studies and is a feasible treatment approach.

The development and marketing of new medications, primarily nonopiate in nature, are feasible, although the time frame is several years away. Multiple medications of diverse mechanisms might be used as stand-alone medications or as combinations. For example, the testing of a CB-1 antagonist or inverse agonist would be a high priority for testing. Nonopiate medications with good efficacy would usher in another change to the management of opiate dependence. Moreover, these medications would likely enjoy broad societal support.

REFERENCES

1. Brownstein, M. J. (1993). A brief history of opiates, opiate peptides, and opioid receptors. *Proc. Natl. Acad. Sci.* 90, 5391–5393.

2. World Health Organization (WHO) (2004). *Neuroscience of Psychoactive Substance Use and Dependence*. WHO, Geneva.
3. United Nations AIDS (UNAIDS) (2004). *Report on the Global AIDS Epidemic*. UNAIDS, Geneva.
4. Chitwood, D. D., Comerford, M., and Sanchez, J. (2003). Prevalence and risk factors for HIV among sniffers, short term injectors, and long-term injectors of heroin. *J. Psychoactive Drugs* 35(4), 445–453.
5. Neaigus, A., Miller, M., Freidman, S. R., and Des Jarlais, D. C. (2001). Sexual transmission risk among noninjecting heroin users infected with human immunodeficiency virus or hepatitis C virus. *J. Infect. Dis.* 184, 359–363.
6. Neaigus, A., Miller, M., Freidman, S. R., Hagan, D. I., Sifaneck, S. J., Ildenfonso, G., and Des Jarlais, D. C. (2001). Potential risk factors for the transition to injecting among non-injecting heroin users: A comparison of former injectors and never injectors. *Addiction* 96, 847–860.
7. Garfein, R. S., Vlahov, D., Galai, N., Doherty, M. C., and Nelson, K. E. (1996). Viral infections in short-term injection drug users: The prevalence of the hepatitis C, hepatitis B, human immunodeficiency, and human T-lymphotropic viruses. *Am. J. Public Health* 86(5), 655–661.
8. Novick, D., Reagan, K., Croxson, T. S., Gelb, A., Stenger, R., and Kreek, M. J. (1997). Hepatitis C virus serology in parenteral drug users with chronic liver disease. *Addiction* 92, 167–171.
9. Novick, D. M. (2000). The impact of hepatitis C virus infection on methadone maintenance treatment. *Mt. Sinai J. Med.* 67, 437–443.
10. Piccolo, P., Borg, L., Linn, A., Melia, D., Ho, A., and Kreek, M. J. (2002). Hepatitis C virus and human immunodeficiency virus-1 co-infection in former heroin addicts in methadone maintenance treatment. *J. Addict. Dis.* 21(4), 55–66.
11. Mathews, G., and Bhagani, S. (2003). The epidemiology and natural history of HIV/HBV and HIV/HCV co-infections. *J. HIV Ther.* 8(4), 77–84.
12. Bonacini, M., Louie, S., Bzowej, N., and Wohl, A. R. (2004). Survival in patients with HIV infection and viral hepatitis B or C: A cohort study. *AIDS* 18, 2039–2045.
13. Desmond, D. P., and Maddux, J. F., (1997). Death rates of heroin users in and out of methadone maintenance treatment. In *Effective Medical Treatment of Heroin Addiction*, NIH Consensus Development Conference, Bethesda, MD, pp. 73–77.
14. Quaglio, G., Talamini, G., Lechi, A., Venturini, L., Lugoboni, F., and Mezzelani, P., Gruppo Intersert di Collaborazione Scientifica (GICS) (2001). Study or 2708 heroin-related deaths in north-eastern Italy 1985–1998 to establish the main causes of death. *Addiction* 96(8), 1127–1137.
15. Tyndall, M. W., Craib, K. J. P., Currie, S., Li, K., O'Shaughnessy, M. V., and Schecter, M. T. (2001). Impact of HIV infection on mortality in a cohort of injection drug users. *J. AIDS* 28(4), 351–357.
16. Drug Enforcement Administration (DEA) (2001). *Drug Trafficking in the United States*. DEA, Washington, DC, September issue.
17. Schwartz, R. H. (1998). Adolescent heroin use: A review. *Pediatrics* 102(6), 1461–1466.
18. Cone, E. J., Holicky, B. A., Grant, T. M., Darwin, W. D., and Goldberger, B. A. (1993). Pharmacokinetics and pharmacodynamics of intranasal "snorted" heroin. *J. Anal. Toxicol.* 17(6), 327–337.

19. Gordon, S. M., Mulvaney, F., and Rowan, A. (2004). Characteristics of adolescents in residential treatment for heroin dependence. *Am. J. Drug Alcohol Abuse* 30(3), 593–603.

20. Hopfer, C. J., Khuri, E., Crowley, T. J., and Hooks, A. (2002). Adolescent heroin use: A review of the descriptive and treatment literature. *J. Subst. Abuse Treat.* 23, 231–237.

21. Griffiths, P., Gossop, M., Powis, B., and Strang, J. (1994). Transitions in patterns of heroin chasers (chasing the dragon) and heroin injectors. *Addiction* 89, 301–309.

22. Substance Abuse and Mental Health Services Administration (SAMHSA) (2004). *Results from the 2003 National Survey on Drug Use and Health: National Findings*, Office of Applied Studies, NSDUH Series H–25, DHHS Publication No. SMA 04–3964. SAMHSA, Rockville, MD.

23. Johnson, L. D., O'Malley, P. M., Bachman, J. G., and Schulenberg, J. E. (2004). Overall teen drug use continues gradual decline but use of inhalants rises. *University of Michigan News and Information Services*, Ann. Arbor, MI.

24. Substance Abuse and Mental Health Services Administration (SAMHSA), Office of Applied Studies (2004). *Treatment Episode Data Set (TEDS): 1992-2002. National Admissions to Substance Abuse Treatment Services*, DASIS Series: S-23, DHHS Publication No. (SMA) 04-3965. SAMSHA, Rockville, MD.

25. Kreek, M. J., and Vocci, F. J. (2002). History and current status of opioid maintenance treatments: Blending conference session. *J. Subst. Abuse Treat.* 23(2), 93–105(review).

26. Gunne, L., and Grönbladh, L. (1984). The Swedish methadone maintenance program. In *The Social and Medical Aspects of Drug Abuse*, Serban, G., Ed. Spectrum Publications, Jamaica, NY, pp. 205–213.

27. Grönbladh, L., and Gunne, L. (1989). Methadone-assisted rehabilitation of Swedish heroin addicts. *Drug Alcohol Depend.* 24, 31–37.

28. Grönbladh, L., Ohlund, L. S., and Gunne, L. M. (1990). Mortality in heroin addiction: Impact of methadone treatment. *Acta Psychiatr. Scand.* 82, 223–227.

29. Substance Abuse and Mental Health Services Administration (SAMHSA), Office of Applied Studies (2002). *National Survey of Substance Abuse Treatment Services (N-SSATS). Data on Substance Abuse Treatment Facilities*, S-16 DHHS Publication no. (SMA) 02-3668. SAMHSA, Rockville, MD.

30. Novick, D. M., Pascarelli, E. F., Joseph, H., Salsitz, E. A., Richman, B. L., Des Jarlais, D. C., Anderson, M., Dole, V. P., and Nyswander, M. E. (1988). Methadone maintenance patients in general medical practice: A preliminary report. *JAMA* 259, 3299–3302.

31. Schwartz, R. P., Brooner, R. K., Montoya, I. D., Currens, M., and Hayes, M. (1999). A 12-year follow-up of a methadone medical maintenance program. *Am. J. Addict.* 8, 293–299.

32. Senay, E. C., Barthwell, A. G., Marks, R., Bokos, P., Gillman, D., and White, R. (1993). Medical maintenance: A pilot study. *J. Addict. Dis.* 12, 59–77.

33. Fiellin, D. A., O'Connor, P. G., Chawarski, M., Pakes, J. P., Pantalon, M. V., and Schottenfeld, R. S. (2001). Methadone maintenance in primary care: A randomized trial. *JAMA* 286, 1724–1731.

34. Lewis, D. C. (1999). Access to narcotic addiction treatment and medical care: Prospects for the expansion of methadone maintenance treatment. *J. Addict. Dis.* 18, 5–21.

35. Jasinski, D. R., Pevnick, J. S., and Griffith, J. D. (1978). Human pharmacology and abuse potential of the analgesic buprenorphine: A potential agent for treating narcotic addiction. *Arch. Gen. Psychiatry* 35(4), 501–516.

36. Martin, W. R., Eades, C. G., Thompson, J. A., Huppler, R. E., and Gilbert, P. E. (1976). The effects of morphine and nalorphine like drugs in the nondependent and morphine-dependent chronic spinal dog. *J. Pharmacol. Exp. Ther.* 197(3), 517–532.

37. Walsh, S.L., Preston, K. L., Stitzer, M. L., Cone, E. J., and Bigelow, G. E. (1994). Clinical pharmacology of buprenorphine: Ceiling effects at high doses. *Clin. Pharmacol. Ther.* 55(5), 569–580.

38. Johnson, R. E., Jaffe, J. H., and Fudala, P. J. (1992). A controlled trial of buprenorphine treatment for opioid dependence. *JAMA* 27; 267(20), 2750–2755.

39. Ling, W., Charuvastra, C., Collins, J. F., Batki, S., Brown, L. S., Jr., Kintaudi, P., Wesson, D. R., McNicholas, L., Tusel, D. J., Malkerneker, U., Renner, J. A., Jr., Santos, E., Casadonte, P., Fye, C., Stine, S., Wang, R. I., and Segal, D. (1998). Buprenorphine maintenance treatment of opiate dependence: A multicenter randomized clinical trial. *Addiction* 93(4), 475–486.

40. Fudala, P. J., Yu, E., Macfadden, W., Boardman, C., and Chiang, C. N., (1998). Effects of buprenorphine and naloxone in morphine-stabilized opioid addicts. *Drug Alcohol Depend.* 1;50(1), 1–8.

41. Mendelson, J., Jones, R. T., Welm, S., Baggott, M., Fernandez, I., Melby, A. K., and Nath, R. P. (1999). Buprenorphine and naloxone combinations: The effects of three dose ratios in morphine-stabilized, opiate-dependent volunteers. *Psychopharmacology (Berl.)* 141(1), 37–46.

42. Mendelson, J., Jones, R. T., Welm, S., Brown, J., and Batki, S. L., (1997). Buprenorphine and naloxone interactions in methadone maintenance patients. *Biol Psychiatry* 1;41(11), 1095–1101.

43. Harris, D., Jones, R. T., Welm, S., Upton, R., Lin, E., and Mendelson, J. (2000). Buprenorphine and naloxone co-administration in opiate-dependent patients stabilized on sublingual buprenorphine. *Drug Alcohol Depend.* 61, 85–94.

44. Fudala, P. J., Bridge, T. P., Herbert, S., Williford, W. O., Chiang, C. N., Jones, K., Collins, J., Raisch, D., Casadonte, P., Goldsmith, R. J., Ling, W., Malkerneker, U., McNicholas, L., Renner, J., Stine, S., and Tusel, D., Buprenorphine/Naloxone Collaborative Study Group (2003). Office-based treatment of opiate addiction with a sublingual-tablet formulation of buprenorphine and naloxone. *N. Engl. J. Med.* 349(10), 949–958.

45. Mattick, R. P., Kimber, J., Breen, C., and Davoli, M. (2004). Buprenorphine maintenance versus placebo or methadone maintenance for opioid dependence. *Cochrane Database Syst. Rev.* 3, CD002207.

46. Mattick, R. P., Ali, R., White, J., O'Brien, S., Wolk, S., and Danz, C. (2003). Buprenorphine versus methadone maintenance therapy: A randomized double blind trial with 405 opioid-dependent patients. *Addiction* 98(4), 441–452.

47. Johnson, R. E., Chutuape, M. A., Strain, E. C., Walsh, S. L., Stitzer, M. L., and Bigelow, G. E. (2000). A comparison of levomethadyl acetate, buprenorphine, and methadone for opioid dependence. *N. Engl. J. Med.* Nov. 2;343(18), 1290–1297.

48. Gowing, L., Ali, R., and White, J. (2004). Buprenorphine for the management of opiate withdrawal. *Cochrane Database Syst. Rev.* 18(4), CD002025.

49. Oreskovitch, M. R., Saxon, A. J., Ellis, M. L. K., Malte, C. A., Reoux, J. P., and Knox, P. C. (2005). A double-blind, double dummy, randomized, prospective pilot study of the partial mu opiate agonist, buprenorphine, for acute detoxification from heroin. *Drug Alcohol Depend.* 77, 71–79.

50. Fiellin, D. A., Kleber, H., Trumble-Hejduk, J. G., MCLellan, A. T., and Kosten, T. R. (2004). Consensus statement on office-based treatment of opioid dependence using buprenorphine. *J. Subst. Abuse Treat.* 27(2), 153–159.
51. O'Connor, P. G., Oliveto, A. H., Shi, J. M., Triffleman, E. G., Carroll, K. M., Kosten, T. R., Rounsaville, B. J., Pakes, J. A., and Schottenfeld, R. S. (1998). A randomized trial of buprenorphine maintenance for heroin dependence in a primary care clinic for substance users versus a methadone clinic. *Am. J. Med.* 105(2), 100–105.
52. Fiellin, D. A., Pantalon, M. V., Pakes, J. P., O'Connor, P. G., Chawarski, M., and Schottenfeld, R. S. (2002). Treatment of heroin dependence with buprenorphine in primary care. *Am. J. Drug Alcohol Abuse* 28(2), 231–241.
53. Gibson, A. E., Doran, C. M., Bell, J. R., Ryan, A., and Lintzeris, N. (2003). A comparison of buprenorphine treatment in clinic and primary care settings: A randomized trial. *Med. J. Australia* 179, 38–42.
54. Amass, L., Ling, W., Freese, T. E., Reiber, C., Annon, J. J., Cohen, A. J., McCarty, D., Reid, M. S., Brown, L. S., Clark, C., Ziedonis, D. M., Krejci, J., Stine, S., Winhusen, T., Brigham, G., Babcock, D., Muir, J. A., Buchan, B. J., and Horton, T. (2004). Bringing buprenorphine-naloxone detoxification to community treatment providers: The NIDA Clinical Trials Network field experience. *Am. J. Addict.* 13(Suppl. 1), S42–S66.
55. Lintzeris, N., Ritter, A., Panjari, M., Clark, N., Kutin, J., and Bammer, G. (2004). Implementing buprenorphine treatment in community settings in Australia: Experiences from the buprenorphine implementation trial. *Am. J. Addict.* 13, S29–S41.
56. Cornish, J. W., Metzger, D., Woody, G. E., Wilson, D., McLellan, A. T., Vandergrift, B., and O'Brien, C. P. (1997). Naltrexone pharmacotherapy for opioid dependent federal probationers. *J. Subst. Abuse Treat.* 14(6), 529–534.
57. Comer, S. D., Collins, E. D., Kleber, H. D., Nuwayser, E. S., Kerrigan, J. H., and Fischman, M. W. (2002). Depot naltrexone: Long-lasting antagonism of the effects of heroin in humans. *Psychopharmacology (Berl.)* 159(4), 351–360.
58. Garbutt, J. C., Kranzler, H. R., O'Malley, S. S., Gastfriend, D. R., Pettinati, H. M., Silverman, B. L., Loewy, J. W., and Ehrich, E. W. (2005). Efficacy and tolerability of long-acting injectable naltrexone for alcohol dependence: A randomized controlled study. *JAMA* 293(13), 1617–1625.
59. Rose, J. S., Branchey, M., Wallach, L., and Buydens-Branchey, L. (2003). Effect of buspirone in withdrawal from opiates. *Am. J. Addict.* 12(3), 253–259.
60. Heinrichs, S. C., and Koob, G. F. (2004). Corticotropin-releasing factor in brain: A role in activation, arousal, and affect regulation. *J. Pharmacol. Exp. Ther.* 311(2), 427–440.
61. Iredale, P. A., Alvaro, J. D., Lee, Y., Terwilliger, R., Chen, Y. L., and Duman, R. S. (2000). Role of corticotropin-releasing factor receptor-1 in opiate withdrawal. *J. Neurochem.* 74(1), 199–208.
62. Funada, M., Hara, C., and Wada, K. (2001). Involvement of corticotropin-releasing factor receptor subtype 1 in morphine withdrawal regulation of the brain noradrenergic system. *Eur. J. Pharmacol.* 430(2/3), 277–281.
63. Stinus, L., Cador, M., Zorrilla, E. P., and Koob, G. F. (2005). Buprenorphine and a CRF1 antagonist block the acquisition of opiate withdrawal-induced conditioned place aversion in rats. *Neuropsychopharmacology* 30(1), 90–98.
64. Lu, L., Ceng, X., and Huang, M. (2000). Corticotropin-releasing factor receptor type I mediates stress-induced relapse to opiate dependence in rats. *Neuroreport* 3;11(11), 2373–2378.

65. Lu, L., Liu, D., Ceng, X., and Ma, L. (2000). Differential roles of corticotropin-releasing factor receptor subtypes 1 and 2 in opiate withdrawal and in relapse to opiate dependence. *Eur. J. Neurosci.* 12(12), 4398–4404.
66. Shaham, Y., Funk, D., Erb, S., Brown, T. J., Walker, C. D., and Stewart, J. (1997). Corticotropin-releasing factor, but not corticosterone, is involved in stress-induced relapse to heroin-seeking in rats. *J. Neurosci.* 17(7), 2605–2614.
67. Shaham, Y., Erb, S., Leung, S., Buczek, Y., and Stewart, J. (1998). CP-154,526, a selective, non-peptide antagonist of the corticotropin-releasing factor1 receptor attenuates stress-induced relapse to drug seeking in cocaine- and heroin-trained rats. *Psychopharmacology (Berl.)* 137(2), 184–190.
68. Rubino, T., Massi, P., Fuzio, D., and Parolaro, D. (2000). Long-term treatment with SR141617A, the CB1 receptor antagonist, influences morphine withdrawal syndrome. *Life Sci.* 66(22), 2213–2219.
69. Navarro, M., Carrera, M. R., Fratta, W., Valverde, O., Cossu, G., Fattore, L., Chowen, J. A., Gomez, R., del Arco, I., Villanua, M. A., Maldonado, R., Koob, G. F., and Rodriguez de Fonseca, F. (2001). Functional interaction between opioid and cannabinoid receptors in drug self-administration. *J. Neurosci.* 21, 5344–5350.
70. Caille, S., and Parsons, L. H. (2003). SR141716A reduces the reinforcing properties of heroin but not heroin-induced increases in nucleus accumbens dopamine in rats. *Eur. J. Neurosci.* 18, 3145–3149.
71. De Vries, T. J., Homberg, J. R., Binnekade, R., Raaso, H., and Schoffelmeer, A. N. (2003). Cannabinoid modulation of the reinforcing and motivational properties of heroin and heroin-associated cues in rats. *Psychopharmacology (Berl.)* 168, 164–169.
72. LeFoll, B., and Goldberg, S. R. (2005). Cannabinoid CB1 receptor antagonists as promising new medications for drug dependence. *J. Pharmacol. Exp. Ther.* 312(3), 875–883.
73. Substance Abuse and Mental Health Services Administration (2005). Results from the 2004 National Survey on Drug Use and Health: National Findings (Office of Applied Studies, NSDUH Series H-28, DHHS Publication No. SMA 05-4062). Rockville, MD.

PART IV

Pain

20

NEURONAL PATHWAYS FOR PAIN PROCESSING

GAVRIL W. PASTERNAK AND YAHONG ZHANG

*Laboratory of Molecular Neuropharmacology, Memorial Sloan-Kettering Cancer Center
New York, New York*

20.1 Introduction 709
20.2 Pain Pathways 711
20.3 Descending Pain Modulatory Pathways 712
20.4 Neuropharmacology of Pain 714
20.5 Localization of Drug Action 718
20.6 Anatomical Drug Interactions and Pain 718
20.7 Conclusion 721
References 721

20.1 INTRODUCTION

Pain remains a prominent factor in all facets of medicine. Pain helps maintain the safety and integrity of subjects by alerting them to potential injury. Pathways that transmit nociceptive stimuli from the periphery to the central nervous system have been studied extensively. However, situations exist where survival may depend upon minimizing or ignoring pain. A major function of the sensory nervous system is its ability to filter sensory input. The vast array of sensation from all modalities makes it essential for the individual to focus upon a selected few and to place others in the background. Thus, it is not surprising that the nervous system has developed a highly complex system to "filter," or modulate, the perception of pain.

Pain is unlike most sensations. The International Association for the Study of Pain defines pain as "an unpleasant sensory and emotional experience associated with actual or potential tissue damage, or described in terms of such damage" [1]. Thus, in addition to the actual perception of the stimulus, pain requires a processing of this input to provoke a sensation that is perceived as unpleasant. This contrasts with traditional sensations that are more easily quantified, such as touch and

Handbook of Contemporary Neuropharmacology, Edited by David R. Sibley, Israel Hanin, Michael Kuhar, and Phil Skolnick. Copyright © 2007 John Wiley & Sons, Inc.

temperature. What makes the understanding of pain particularly difficult is that stimuli that are considered painful in one situation may not be perceived as painful in a different context. Many of us have found bruises after playing a sport without remembering when the injury occurred. Yet, at other times, a less intense injury may be associated with profound pain. The ability to dissociate the stimulus from pain has been observed in patients on opioids, which diminish pain without interfering with more basic sensations. Indeed, patients on opioids may comment, "The pain is still there but it doesn't hurt." Another complexity in understanding pain is its many different types, as illustrated by the wide range of descriptors, such as sharp, dull, aching, shooting, throbbing, and burning.

Clinically, pain has been categorized as somatic, visceral, and neuropathic [1a]. Somatic, or "nociceptive," pain is typically a result of tissue injury. It is common, easily recognized by most people, and typically described as sharp or aching. Of the various types of pain, this is the most sensitive to opioids and the simplest to treat. Visceral pain, as its name implies, involves internal organs. The nature of the pain is dependent upon the structure involved and can feel like cramping, or pressure, such as cholecystitis, panacreatitis, or angina. It can be referred to a different region of the body, such as the shoulder pain seen with diaphragmatic irritation.

Neuropathic pain, on the other hand, is quite novel and unique. It is the most atypical pain and the most difficult to treat. It is usually associated with injury to peripheral nerves, as seen in plexopathies or neuropathies, central pain pathways, as in thalamic pain syndromes, or combinations of both. The pain is typically described as burning, dysesthetic, or shooting, and patients commonly have difficulty describing it. A number of syndromes such as reflex sympathetic dystrophy and causalgia (complex regional pain syndromes) are due to involvement of the sympathetic nervous system. Although traditional analgesics, including the opioids, are used to treat this pain, they often require far higher doses than normal, which in turn can lead to increased side effects and difficulties with the patients tolerating them. Many other classes of drugs are used to manage neuropathic pain, including antidepressants and anticonvulsants. Unfortunately, it is not unusual for these drugs, either alone or in combination, to give only partial relief.

In addition to its quality, pain is also characterized by its duration as either acute or chronic. Once a pain has been present for six months, it is typically considered chronic [1a]. Clinically, acute and chronic pain can be separated by more than their duration. Acute pain is often associated with autonomic effects, such as tachycardia, papillary dilation, and diaphoresis, signs typically associated with pain. However, most of the autonomic signs seen acutely are lost in chronic-pain states, making it more difficult for the clinician to assess the severity of the pain. Indeed, with chronic pain the clinician is left with only the assessment by the patient. Chronic pain is further complicated by a number of factors and can be very difficult to treat. These include sensitization and "wind-up" and the commonly associated depression seen in these patients. Other issues, such as the impact of potential disability and financial issues, also can complicate its diagnosis and treatment.

Thus, pain is not simple. It requires higher integrative processing to define its unpleasant aspects and its perception is highly dependent upon the situation in which it occurs and its meaning. There are three major types of pain that differ in their sensitivities to pharmacological approaches, and most clinical pain is composed of combinations of them.

20.2 PAIN PATHWAYS

Pain pathways are complex. They involve far more than the simple conduction of an impulse from a peripheral nociceptor to the brain. Ascending systems dissociate discriminative aspects of pain from the emotional components (Table 20.1) while descending pathways provide a mechanism for the modulation of nociceptive transmission at all levels of the neuroaxis. Discriminative aspects of pain have been well localized to specific pathways and regions of sensory cortex. In contrast, the affective component is mediated predominantly through subcortical pathways involving limbic circuits, making their mapping difficult.

Nociceptors have a widespread localization peripherally in skin and subcutaneous tissues, joints, muscles, blood vessels, and viscera and are located on neurons whose cell bodies are within the dorsal root or trigeminal ganglia [1a–4]. Myelinated nociceptors respond to either intense mechanical or mechanothermal stimuli whereas unmyelinated nociceptors are polymodal, responding to thermal, mechanical, or chemical stimuli. Certain unmyelinated nociceptors are particularly sensitive to pH and chemical agents, such as histamine and bradykinin, which are released by tissue damage and can be further sensitized by serotonin and prostaglandins in the damaged tissues.

Aδ fibers and C fibers carry pain information from the periphery to the central nervous system. Aδ fibers are myelinated and thicker than the unmyelinated C fibers, explaining their faster transmission of pain impulses (5–30 m/s when compared to C fibers (0.5–2 m/s) and contributing to the phenomenon of "first" and "second" pain.

The primary sensory neuron cell bodies are located in the dorsal root ganglia or cranial nerve ganglia. Axons from dorsal root ganglia enter the spinal cord through the dorsal horn where they ascend or descend for several spinal cord segments before interacting with intrinsic spinal cord neurons. Aδ fibers typically terminate within lamina I (marginal zone) and, to a lesser extent, within lamina V. C fibers tend to

TABLE 20.1 Comparison of Neospinothalamic and Paleospinothalamic Pain Pathways

	Neospinothalamic Tract	Paleospinothalamic Tract
Anatomy		
Thalamic target	VPL	Intralaminar and midline nuclei
Intermediate synapses between dorsal horn and thalamus	None	Periaqueductal gray, reticular formation
Thalamic projections	Somatosensory cortex (parietal lobe)	Subcortical (cingulate gyrus, limbic system, hypothalamus)
Pain sensation	Fast or first pain	Slow or second pain
	Discriminative component (intensity, localization, quality)	Affective component ("hurt")
	Well localized	Poorly localized
Other sensations	Light touch, temperature	

Note: Sensory neurons with their cell bodies in the dorsal root ganglia enter the dorsal horn of the spinal cord where the Aδ fibers synapse in laminae I and V and ascend to the thalamus as the neospinothalamic tract and the C fibers synapse primarily in laminae I and II and ascend as the paleospinothalamic, or spinoreticular, tract.

project to lamina I and lamina II (substantia gelatinosa) where they synapse with interneurons and neurons that project rostrally. Some axons synapse on motor neurons in the ventral horn, completing the pain reflex arc. Trigeminal ganglia axons enter the brain stem and project to the spinal nucleus of the trigeminal tract, which is analogous to the substantia gelatinosa within the spinal cord (Fig. 20.1b).

Nociception is transmitted rostrally through two important pathways: the lateral spinothalamic tract (Fig. 20.1, Table 20.1) and the anterior spinothalamic tract. The lateral spinothalamic tract receives information regarding the location and intensity of the nociceptive stimuli and has a distinct somatotopic organization within the tract as it ascends and comprises the neospinothalamic pathway. Axons in the tract cross to the opposite side of the spinal cord over several spinal segments through the anterior commissure and proceed to ascend to the ventroposterior lateral (VPL) nucleus of the thalamus. Axons in the trigeminal thalamic tract cross the midline and synapse in the ventroposterior medial (VPM) nucleus of the thalamus. From the thalamus, these tracts ascend to primary somatosensory cortex with its well-defined somatotopic organization. Cortical lesions, such as seen in strokes, lead to loss of this well-localized pain sensation. This pathway transmits primarily nociception carried by Aδ fibers and corresponds to first pain, in distinction from second pain, which involves primarily C fibers and the paleospinothalamic tract.

The anterior spinothalamic, which is a component of the paleospinothalamic tract (Fig. 20.2), is involved with the affective, or unpleasant, component of pain. It carries "second" or "slow" pain and it is this component of pain that is sensitive to opioids. Unlike the neospinothalamic tract which ascends directly to the thalamus, the paleospinothalamic tract has numerous interactions with a range of brain stem nuclei (nucleus gigantocellularis and parabrachial region), the reticular formation, and periaqueductal gray before converging on the medial and intralaminar nuclei of the thalamus. From there, the impulses are relayed not to the somatosensory cortex but to limbic structures and association cortex instead, including the anterior cingulate gyrus, amygdala, and hypothalamus. The importance of many of these higher structures in pain clinically has now been supported by positron emission tomography [5, 6]. Nociception carried by this pathway is slower, due to both the slower conduction rate of the C fibers and the multiple synapses within the pathway as it ascends, leading to the description of this pain as second or slow pain. Unlike the rapidly conducted first pain, second pain is poorly localized and more diffuse with a dysethetic quality. The selectivity of opioids for this pathway may help explain the observation by some patients after taking opioids that the they can still feel the pain, but it does not bother them, consistent with a selectivity of the opioid response to the affective component of pain, or "hurt," carried by the paleospinothalamic tract.

20.3 DESCENDING PAIN MODULATORY PATHWAYS

The central nervous system can modulate the perception of pain. This can be observed in a variety of situations, such as athletes who are unaware of an injury until after the game or the lower morphine requirements of wounded soldiers during the stress of battle [7]. Even acupuncture has been proposed to involve the activation of intrinsic antinociceptive pathways [8]. In the 1960s, Wall and Melzack proposed

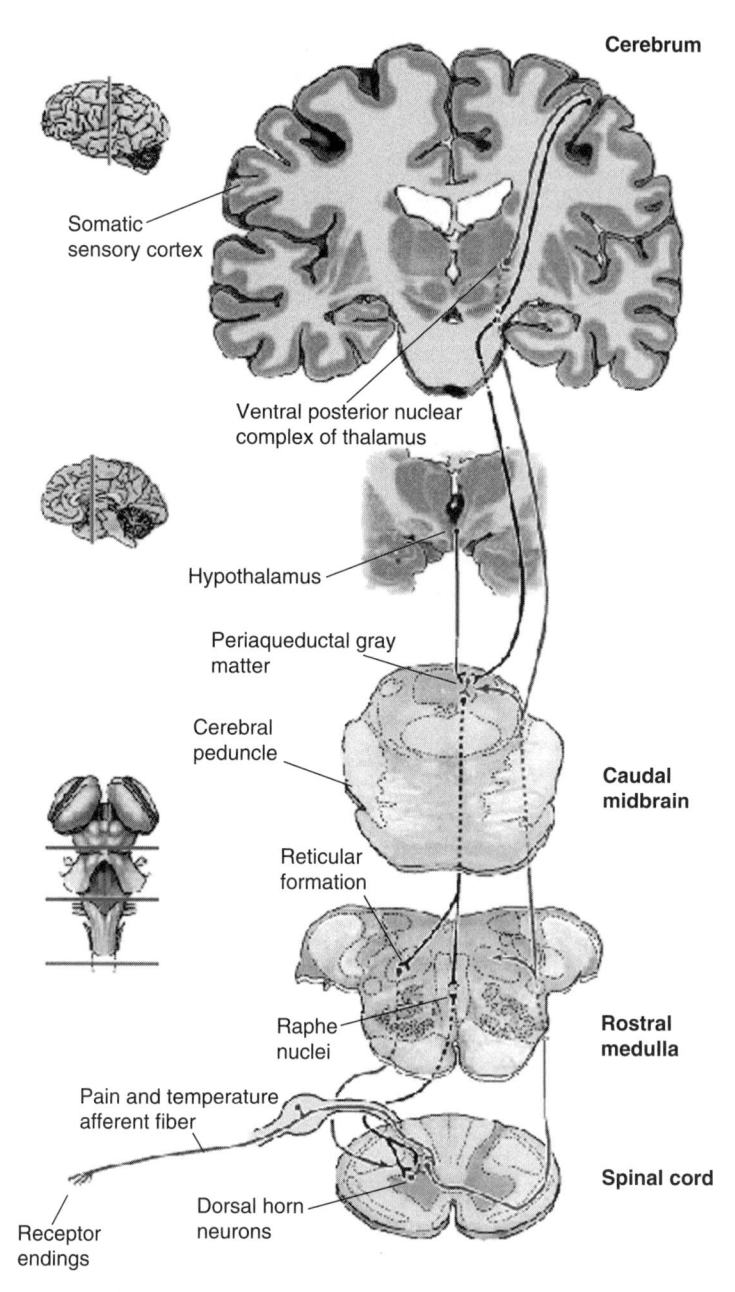

Figure 20.1 Ascending spinothalamic tract. Major pathways for pain (and temperature) sensation. (a) Spinothalamic system. (b) Trigeminal pain and temperature system, which carries information about these sensations from the face. (Reproduced with permission from D. Purues et al. (2001). *NeuroScience*. Sinauer, Sunderland, MA, Fig. 10.3.) (See color insert.)

the "gate control" theory, which has now been much expanded, to explain how central systems can modulate peripheral nociceptive input [9]. Descending pathways from the brain that are heavily influenced by opioids and a number of other selected neurotransmitters are primarily responsible for these actions (Fig. 20.3) [2, 10–12].

Ascending Nociceptive Pathways

```
Neospinothalamic              Paleospinothalamic
     Tract                           Tract

┌─────────────────┐           ┌─────────────────┐
│  Sensory Cortex │           │  Cingulate Gyrus│
│ (Parietal Lobe) │           │    & Limbic     │
│                 │           │   structures    │
└─────────────────┘           └─────────────────┘
         │                             │
┌─────────────────┐           ┌─────────────────┐
│    Thalamus     │           │    Thalamus     │
│     (VPL)       │           │ (Intralaminar and│
│                 │           │  Medial nuclei) │
└─────────────────┘           └─────────────────┘
         │                             │
         │                   ┌─────────────────┐
         │                   │    Reticular    │
         │                   │   Formation,    │
         │                   │  periaqueductal │
         │                   │      Gray       │
         │                   └─────────────────┘
         │                             │
         │      ┌─────────────────────┐
    ─(DRG)──────│  Dorsal Horn of     │
         │      │  the spinal cord    │
                └─────────────────────┘
```

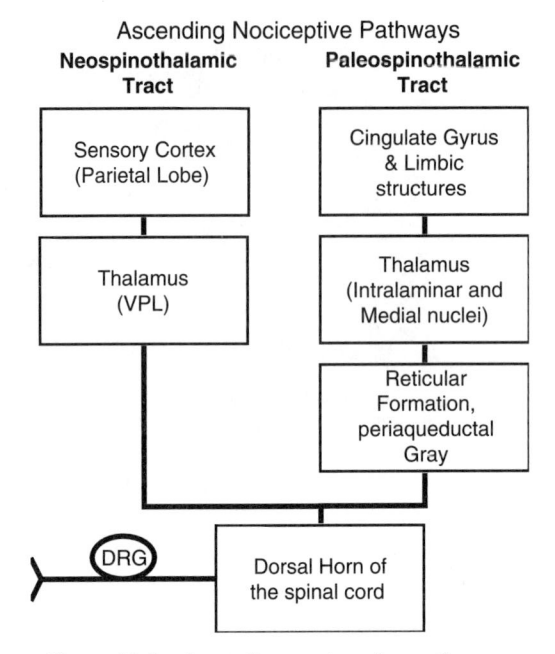

Figure 20.2 Ascending nociceptive pathways.

Pain sensation is modulated by the descending pain modulatory pathways in a balance of excitation and inhibition [2, 3, 13, 14]. The periaqueductal gray (PAG) is particularly important in this system. Early studies showed that morphine was an extremely potent analgesic when microinjected into this site [15]. Additional studies have identified a number of midbrain areas, including the locus ceruleus, nucleus raphe magnus, and nucleus paragigantocellularis [11, 16–18]. Stimulation of the PAG produced analgesia in rodents that was naloxone reversible [19–21], observations similar to those seen clinically [22]. These studies imply that that activation of the PAG would produce an opioidlike analgesia. The PAG receives input from a wide range of structures, including the amygdala, frontal and insular cortex, and hypothalamus. It projects to the nucleus raphe magnus, which then descends to suppress pain transmission in the dorsal horn of the spinal cord. The PAG receives input from a wide range of structures, including the somatosensory cortex, frontal and insular cortex, amygdala, and hypothalamus. The PAG, in turn, projects to neurons in the nucleus raphe magnus and other nuclei in the rostral ventral medulla, the nucleus reticularis paragigantocellularis in particular [6–9]. The medullary nuclei transmit signals in the dorsolateral column down to the same regions of the dorsal horn of the spinal cord in which primary sensory neurons synapse onto secondary sensory neurons. Descending exons from the PAG, raphe nuclei, and locus coruleus also project directly to the spinal cord.

20.4 NEUROPHARMACOLOGY OF PAIN

Many neurotransmitter systems have been implicated in both the transmission of nociception and its modulation. Indeed, few transmitters are not involved. Some

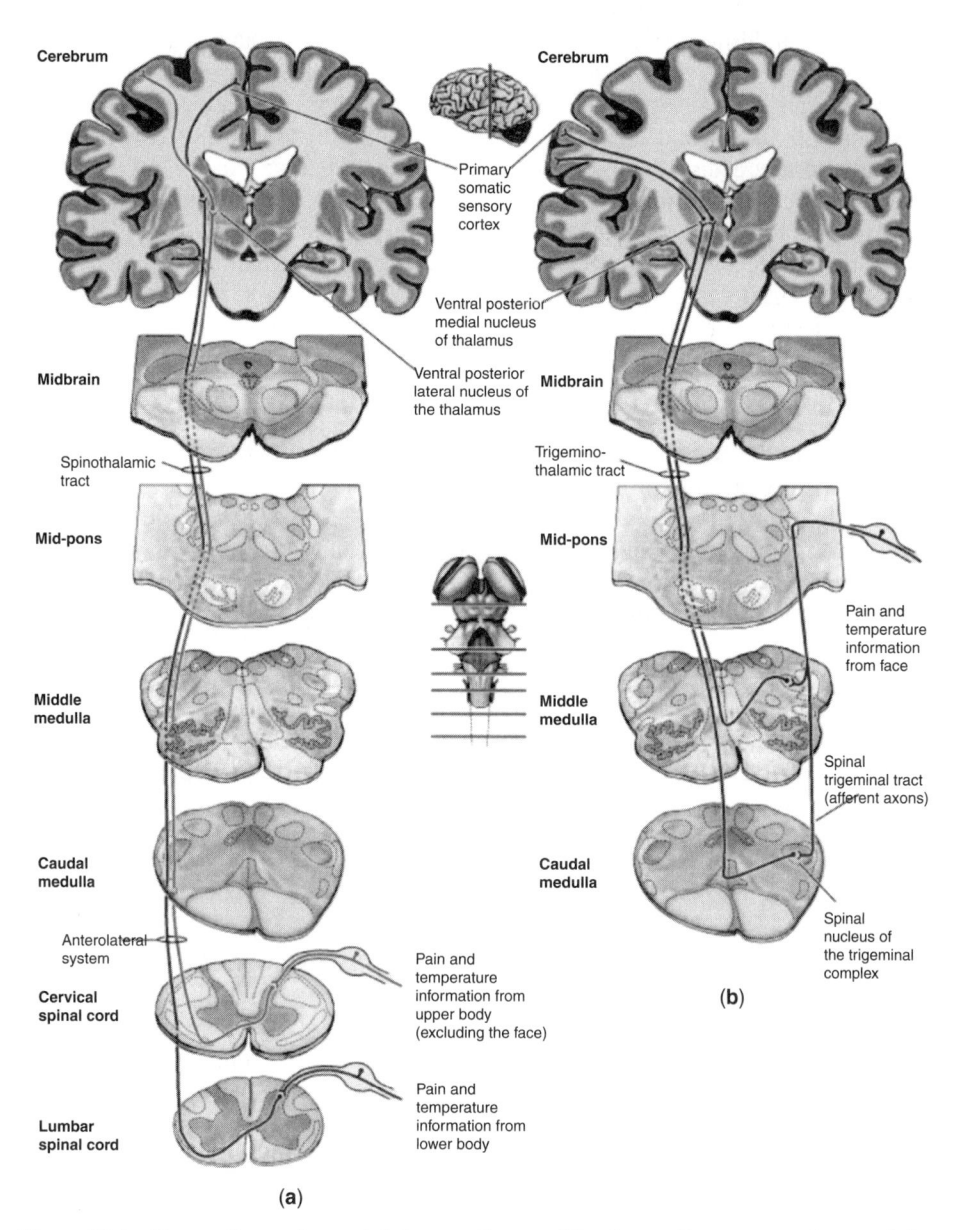

Figure 20.3 Descending pain modulatory pathways. The descending systems that modulate the transmission of ascending pain signals. These modulatory systems originate in the somatic sensory cortex, the hypothalamus, the periaqueductal gray matter of the midbrain, the raphe nuclei, and other nuclei of the rostral ventral medulla. Complex modulatory effects occur at each of these sites, as well as in the dorsal horn. (Reproduced with permission from D. Purues et al. (2001). *NeuroScience*. Sinauer, Sunderland, MA, Fig. 10.5). (See color insert.)

provide potent pain relief, such as the endogenous opioids [1a], nicotinic analogs [23], and cannabinoids [24, 25], while others demonstrate limited activity due to ceiling effects or are restricted to specific pain syndromes. One of the best examples of agents with ceiling effects are the nonsteroidal anti-inflammatory drugs, which are quite effective for mild/moderate pain but lack the efficacy needed for severe pain. Antidepressants and anticonvulsants are typically used for neuropathic pain, such as the peripheral neuropathies and postherpetic neuralgia, or headaches. Trigeminal neuralgia with its lancinating pain is quite unique and the first-line drug to treat this relatively common disorder is the anticonvulsant carbamazepine. Thus, from the clinical perspective, a wide range of drugs are valuable in pain management, with various types of pain responding differently to these agents [1a, 3, 26–28].

The most effective clinical agents in pain management remain the opioids. These drugs mimic the actions of the endogenous opioid peptides and have been classified by their selectivity for the three major classes of receptors: μ, δ, and κ. Although some agents with κ actions are available clinically, most opioid analgesics are morphine-like and are selective for μ-opioid receptors. Extensive structure–activity studies have dissected the structure of morphine and generated a host of drugs with widely dissimilar structures that act through μ receptors (Fig. 20.4). Although δ compounds are effective in animal pain models, none have yet been approved for general clinical use. There are three major families of endogenous opioids, each with its own precursor peptide: enkephalins, dynorphin A, and β-endorphin [29, 30]. The enkephalins and dynorphin A are the endogenous ligands for the δ and $κ_1$ receptors, respectively. The endogenous ligand for the μ receptors is still uncertain. There is evidence implicating endomorphin 1 and endomorphin 2 as well as β-endorphin, but some questions still remain. The complexity of the μ-opioid system is further illustrated by the recent identification of a number of splice variants of the cloned μ-opioid receptor MOR-1 with their distinct regional distributions and pharmacological properties [31–36]. The question that now arises is whether or not the identification of these splice variants of MOR-1 will enable the dissociation of analgesia from its troublesome side effects.

As the number of neurotransmitters involved with pain pathways has expanded, they have raised the possibility of novel approaches toward pain management [37]. Many peptidergic systems were considered "anti-opioid," including cholecystokinin (CCK), neuropeptide FF (NPFF), and melanocyte-inhibiting factor (MIF)–related peptides, although their actions are complex and can inhibit or enhance nociceptive perceptions depending upon the situation [38]. The antio-pioid activity of CCK appears to involve activation of CCK_B receptors, while stimulation of CCK_A receptors can induce an opioid-like activity. The major focus of CCK has been on its modulation of opioid tolerance [39, 40], but this approach has not proven successful clinically. The role of substance P and calcitonin gene–related peptide (CGRP) in nociceptive transmission in the spinal cord has been well established. Opioids inhibit their release at the spinal level and antagonists looked promising in animal models. Yet, substance P antagonists have not proven themselves clinically [41].

More traditional neurotransmitter systems implicated in pain mechanisms that may be of therapeutic importance include the monoamines, acetylcholine, gluatamate, glycine, and both sodium and calcium channels. Almost all the monoamines can be implicated in pain modulation, perhaps explaining the importance of many of the antidepressants in pain management. Both muscarinic and nicotinic acetylcholine systems influence pain. Many of the antidepressants used clinically are effective muscarinic antagonists, which may help explain a portion of their utility. A highly potent nicotinic acetylcholine receptor agonists has been developed [23], but its side effects were too problematic for generalized use.

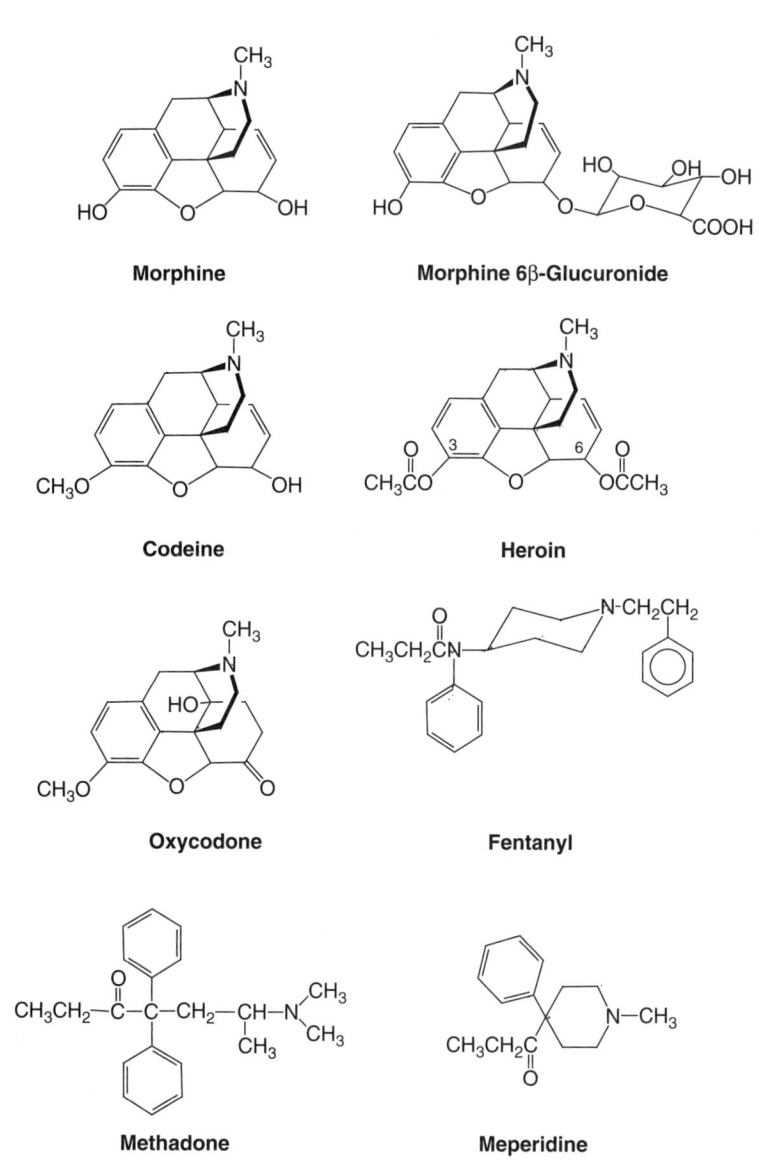

Figure 20.4 Structures of selected opioids.

Glutamate has a special place in pain pharmacology [42–44]. Although *N*-methyl-D-aspartate (NMDA) receptors are involved in the production of opioid tolerance, their role in central sensitization and wind-up may be more important. These systems lead to the facilitation of the transmission of pain impulses and may play a role in the development of chronic pain states, which can be very difficult to treat. This has led some clinicians to use "preemptive analgesia" to prevent sensitization. Unfortunately, the side-effect profile of NMDA antagonists is problematic, making the use of these agents clinically unacceptable with the exception of memantine.

20.5 LOCALIZATION OF DRUG ACTION

Peripheral mechanisms associated with pain have been extensively explored. Local anesthetics, which block sodium channels, effectively prevent pain [4], but they suffer from their lack of selectivity in that they also block other sensory modalities, such as light touch. A variety of transmitter receptors located on peripheral nerves also can modulate pain transmission. For example, opiate receptors have now been identified on sensory dorsal root ganglion neurons both in the periphery and presynaptically in the dorsal horn of the spinal cord [45–49]. Opioids traditionally were thought to act centrally by presynaptic inhibition of the release of nociceptive transmitters, such as substance P or CGRP, as well as on intrinsic spinal neurons. One of the MOR-1 variants, MOR-1C, is colocalized presynaptically on neurons containing CGRP while the predominant MOR-1 is not [51]. The release of CGRP can be blocked by morphine, presumably through these MOR-1C receptors. Substance P neurons terminating within the dorsal horn do appear to be associated with MOR-1 [51]. Opioids inhibit the release of substance P, diminishing nociceptive transmission [52]. Substance P drugs also can modulate pain perception at the spinal cord level, but their utility clinically is not clear [41, 53].

Opioid receptors have been demonstrated on peripheral nerves, explaining the analgesic actions of opioids administered locally to the nerves and without central activity [54–60]. Similarly, other drugs acting through various neurotransmitter systems also can directly influence peripheral nerves, including the antidepressant amitriptyline, the NMDA antagonist ketamine, and a variety of channel blockers, as well as through central sites of action [60].

Within the brain the sites involved with nociception include a broad range of structures, particularly regions within the brain stem and limbic systems. Our understanding of the regions involved initially came from classical studies examining the sensitivity of various brain structures to the microinjection of opioids [15]. The primary sites implicated in morphine analgesia included the PAG, the nucleus raphe magnus, and the locus ceruleus, regions subsequently shown to contain high densities of opioid receptors both autoradiographically [61–64] and immunohistochemically and at the messenger RNA (mRNA) levels [65–67].

Chronic pain is pharmacologically distinct from acute pain and involves plasticity with neurochemical changes. The maintenance of chronic pain has been associated with activation of glutamate receptors. NMDA mechanisms act centrally in sensitization and are involved with plasticity. Indeed, the identification of NMDA receptors in "windup" or central sensitization [68, 69] has led to the concept that early and agressive treatment of pain can help minimize the sensitization process [70].

20.6 ANATOMICAL DRUG INTERACTIONS AND PAIN

Pain pathways have an additional complexity. For example, morphine is a potent analgesic when administered either supraspinally or spinally in the rat. However, administering morphine to both sites simultaneously leads to a profound potentiation of their actions (i.e., synergy) (Table 20.2) [71]. The total dose of morphine required for an analgesic response when it is given both spinally and supraspinally is

TABLE 20.2 Spinal–Supraspinal Morphine Interactions

Site of Drug Administration	Morphine ED$_{50}$ (µg)
Supraspinal	10 (7.23–14.17) i.c.v.
Spinal	4.2 (3.1–5.4) i.t.
Combination ^{a}(supraspinal–spinal)	0.7 (0.38–1.08)
	(0.35 i.c.v. + 0.35 i.t.)

Note: ED$_{50}$ = median effective dose; i.c.v. = intracerebrovascular; i.t. = intrathecal.
^{a}This value corresponds to the ED$_{50}$ for the total dose for the animal using a supraspinal–spinal ratio of 1:1. Thus, the ED$_{50}$ for the combination corresponds to 0.35l µg given in each location. From [71].

at least sixfold lower than if it is given to either location alone. Thus, there are important interactions among the sites along the pain modulatory pathways.

Since then, other examples of site–site synergy have been observed. Morphine is an active analgesic when administered into the PAG, rostroventral medulla (RVM), or locus ceruleus. However, coadministration of low morphine doses which are inactive alone into combinations of these three regions elicits dramatic analgesic responses, implying the existence of synergy. The most effective combination is the PAG–RVM, whereas the PAG–LC and RVM–LC combinations are much less efficacious. Thus, there are important brain stem interactions involved with morphine analgesia.

Peripherally acting opiates also synergize with central sites. Topical morphine is effective in traditional analgesic paradigms in mice and rats [54, 58, 59, 72–74]. Under conditions that are associated with no appreciable systemic absorption, a variety of opioids produce reproducible dose–respose relationships and show the same pharmacological characteristics as seen centrally. However, the combination of topical and spinal morphine is highly synergistic (Fig. 20.5). Thus, morphine shows interactions among a wide range of sites within the central and peripheral nervous systems, adding to the complexity of the system.

These interactions among sites help explain some clinical observations. Epidural opiates are widely used in pain management. The advantage is that there are far fewer side effects, such as nausea, constipation, and respiratory depression, and the drugs can give prolonged pain relief. When given epidurally, morphine concentrations in the cerebrospinal fluid at the spinal level reach levels far beyond those achieved following systemic administration. Equally important, there also is significant systemic absorption through Batson's plexus, leading to blood levels not far below those seen following intramuscular administration. Studies in animals have shown that very low morphine concentrations at the spinal level can markedly potentiate systemic morphine (Table 20.3). Intrathecal doses of morphine that are approximately 10-fold below the ED$_{50}$ of spinal morphine can shift the systemic morphine dose response curve sixfold to the left. Thus, the utility of epidural morphine likely reflects the combined actions of spinal and systemic drug. Since the side affects associated with morphine, such as sedation, nausea, and respiratory depression, are mediated supraspinally, side effects are avoided by the low levels of systemic drug.

The importance of peripheral sites of action have also been established in other situations. When morphine is given centrally into the lateral ventricle, one would

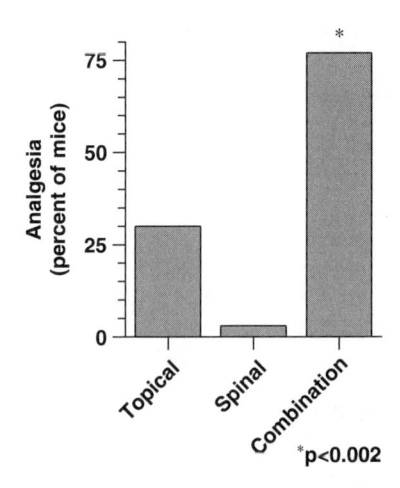

Figure 20.5 Interations between topical and spinal morphine. Groups of mice ($n<10$) received topical morphine (15 mM, 2 min) alone or with spinal (100 ng, i.t.). The spinal morphine dose alone had no observable analgesic action. After 30 min, when the response to topical drug alone was lost, the responses of the combinations were significantly greater ($p<0.002$). From [59].

TABLE 20.3 Peripheral–Central Morphine Interactions

Route of Administration	ED_{50}	Shift
Spinal (i.t.) alone	305 ng, i.t.	
Systemic alone	3.1 mg/kg, s.c.	
+25 ng, i.t.	0.5 mg/kg, s.c.	6
+50 ng, i.t.	0.3 mg/kg, s.c.	10
+200 ng, i.t.	0.04 mg/kg, s.c.	84

Mice received various doses of morphine intrathecally to determine the ED_{50}. Additional groups of mice then received the stated fixed dose of intrathecal morphine and various doses of morphine [subcutaneous (s.c.)]. The ED_{50} for the systemic morphine was then determined. From [54].

have assumed that its actions were restricted to the brain. However, morphine given intrathecally is rapidly secreted from the brain into the periphery by mechanisms involving P glycoprotein and can be detected in the blood [75]. These systemic levels of morphine are relevant, since a topical antagonist limited to the periphery shifts the analgesic response of supraspinal morphine over fourfold, implying that the overall response reflected interactions between central and peripheral sites. Downregulation of P glycoprotein using either an antisense or a knockout approach eliminates the ability of the topical antagonist to shift the supraspinal analgesic response, consistent with the role of P glycoprotein in transporting the drug to the systemic circulation. Thus, site–site interactions are extremely important in understanding the activity of analgesic drugs.

Interactions have also been seen among different groups of drugs working through different mechanisms. This is best illustrated by the interactions between local anesthetics and opioids at the spinal level [76] and peripherally [77, 78]. Similar interactions topically have been observed with combinations of antidepressants, NMDA antagonists, and other classes of drugs [60].

20.7 CONCLUSION

The pathways transmitting nociceptive stimuli and those involved with its modulation are exceedingly complex. Interactions between these counteracting systems occur at multiple levels of the neuraxis, with each influencing the others. While the anatomy of the pathways has been known for many years, understanding their functional and pharmacological significance is more recent. These pathways are not static "transmission lines." Rather, they are interacting pathways providing complex pharmacological interactions that may prove helpful in our continuing efforts in pain management.

REFERENCES

1. Mersky, H. (1986). Classification of chronic pain: Description of chronic pain syndromes and definitions of pain terms. *Pain* 3, S217.
1a. Payne, R., and Pasternak, G. W. (1992). Pharmacology of pain treatment. In *Contemporay Neurolog Series: Scientific Basis of Neurologic Drug Therapy*, M. V. Johnston, R. MacDonald, and A. B. Young, Eds. Davis, Philadelphia, pp. 268–301.
2. Basbaum, A. I., and Fields, H. L. (1984). Endogenous pain control systems: Brainstem spinal pathways and endorphin circuitry. *Ann. Rev. Neurosci.* 7, 309–338.
3. Fields, H. L., and Martin, J. B. (2001). Pain: Pathophysiology and management. In *Harrison's Principles of Internal Medicine*, E. Braunwald, S. L. Hauser, A. S. Fauci, D. L. Longo, D. L. Kasper, and J. L. Jameson, Eds. McGraw-Hill, New York, pp. 55–60.
4. Siddall, P. J., Hudspith, M. J., and Munglani, R. (2000). Sensory systems and pain In *Foundations of Anesthesia: basic and Clinical Sciences.* H. Hemmings, and P. Hopkins, Eds. Mosby, Philadelphia pp. 213–231.
5. Schreckenberger, M., Siessmeier, T., Viertmann, A., Landvogt, C., Buchholz, H. G., Rolke, R., Treede, R. D., Bartenstein, P., and Birklein, F. (2005). The unpleasantness of tonic pain is encoded by the insular cortex. *Neurology* 64, 1175–1183.
6. Jones, A. K., Brown, W. D., Friston, K. J., Qi, L. Y., and Frackowiak, R. S. (1991). Cortical and subcortical localization of response to pain in man using positron emission tomography. *Proc. Biol. Sci.* 244, 39–44.
7. Beecher, H. K. (1963). Pain. *Surg. Clin. North Am.* 43, 609–618.
8. Zhang, A.-Z. (1980). Endorphin and acupuncture analgesia research in the People's Republic of China (1975–1979). *Acupuncture Electro-Therapeut. Res. Int. J.* 5, 131–146.
9. Wolfe, C. J. (1994). The dorsal horn: State-dependent sensory processing and the generation of pain. In *Textbook of Pain*, P. D. Wall and R. Melzak, Eds. Churchil Livingston, Edinburgh, pp. 101–112.
10. Mitchell, J. M., Lowe, D., and Fields, H. L. (1998). The contribution of the rostral ventromedial medulla to the antinociceptive effects of systemic morphine in restrained and unrestrained rats. *Neuroscience* 87, 123–133.
11. Fields, H. L., and Basbaum, A. I. (1978). Brainstem control of spinal pain-transmission neurons. *Ann. Rev. Physiol.* 40, 217–248.

12. Fields, H. L. (2000). Pain modulation: Expectation, opioid analgesia and virtual pain. *Prog. Brain Res.* 122, 245–253.
13. Heinricher, M. M., Morgan, M. M., and Fields, H. L. (1992). Direct and indirect actions of morphine on medullary neurons that modulate nociception. *Neuroscience* 48, 533–543.
14. Morgan, M. M., Heinricher, M. M., and Fields, H. L. (1992). Circuitry linking opioid-sensitive nociceptive modulatory systems in periaqueductal gray and spinal cord with rostral ventromedial medulla. *Neuroscience* 47, 863–871.
15. Pert, A., and Yaksh, T. L. (1974). Sites of morphine induced analgesia in primate brain: Relation to pain pathways. *Brain Res.* 80, 135–140.
16. Fields, H. L., Vanegas, H., Hentall, I. D., and Zorman, G. (1983). Evidence that disinhibition of brain stem neurones contributes to morphine analgesia. *Nature* 306, 684–686.
17. Bodnar, R. J., Williams, C. W., and Pasternak, G .W. (1988). Role of mu_1 opiate receptors in supraspinal opiate analgesia: A microinjection study. *Brain Res.* 447, 45–52.
18. Rossi, G. C., Pasternak, G. W., and Bodnar, R. J. (1993). Synergistic brainstem interactions for morphine analgesia. *Brain Res.* 624, 171–180.
19. Liebeskind, J. C., Guilbaud, G., Besson, J. M., and Oliveras, J. L. (1973). Analgesia from electrical stimulation of the periaqueductal gray matter in the cat: Behavioral observations and inhibitory effects on spinal interneurons. *Brain Res.* 50, 441–446.
20. Mayer, D. J., and Liebeskind, J. C. (1974). Pain reduction by focal electrical stimulation of the brain: An anatomical and behavioral analysis. *Brain Res.* 68, 73–93.
21. Akil, H., Mayer, D. J., and Liebeskind, J. C. (1976). Antagonism of stimulation-produced analgesia by naloxone, a narcotic antagonist. *Science* 191, 961–962.
22. Hosobuchi, Y., and Wemmer, J. (1977). Disulfiram inhibition of development of tolerance to analgesia induced by central gray stimulation in humans. *Eur. J. Pharmacol.* 43, 385–387.
23. Bannon, A. W., Decker, M. W., Holladay, M. W., Curzon, P., Donnelly-Roberts, D., Puttfarcken, P. S., Bitner, R. S., Diaz, A., Dickenson, A. H., Porsolt, R. D., Williams, M., and Arneric, S. P. (1998). Broad-spectrum, non-opioid analgesic activity by selective modulation of neuronal nicotinic acetylcholine receptors. *Science* 279, 77–81.
24. Meng, I. D., Manning, B. H., Martin, W. J., and Fields, H. L. (1998). An analgesia circuit activated by cannabinoids. *Nature* 395, 381–384.
25. Calignano, A., Rana, G. L., Giuffrida, A., and Piomelli, D. (1998). Control of pain initiation by endogenous cannabinoids. *Nature* 394, 277–282.
26. Foley, K. M. (1996). Controlling the pain of cancer. *Sci. Am.* 275, 164–165.
27. Foley, K. M. (1996). Pain syndromes in patients with cancer. In *Pain Management: Theory and Practice*, R. K. Portenoy and R. M. Kanner, Eds. F.A. Davis, Philadelphia, pp. 191–215.
28. Foley, K. M. (1993). Supportive care and the quality of life of the cancer patient. In *Cancer: Principles and Practice of Oncology*, V. T. DeVita, S. Hellman, and S. A. Rosenberg, Eds. Lippincott, Philadelphia, pp. 2417–2448.
29. Reisine, T., and Pasternak, G. W. (1996). Opioid analgesics and antagonists. In *Goodman & Gilman's: The Pharmacological Basis of Therapeutics*, J. G. Hardman and L. E. Limbird, Eds. McGraw-Hill, New York, pp. 521–556.
30. Evans, C. J., Hammond, D. L., and Frederickson, R. C. A. (1998). The opioid peptides. In *The opiate receptors*, G. W. Pasternak, Ed. Humana, Clifton, NJ, pp. 23–74.

31. Pan, L., Xu, J., Yu, R., Xu, M., Pan, Y. X., and Pasternak, G. W. (2005). Identification and characterization of six new alternatively spliced variants of the human mu opioid receptor gene, Oprm. *Neuroscience* 133, 209–220.
32. Pan, Y. -X., Xu, J., Mahurter, L., Bolan, E. A., Xu, M. M., and Pasternak, G. W. (2001). Generation of the mu opioid receptor (MOR-1) protein by three new splice variants of the *Oprm* gene. *Proc. Natl. Acad. Sci. USA* 98, 14084–14089.
33. Pasternak, G. W. (2001). Incomplete cross tolerance and multiple mu opioid peptide receptors. *Trends Pharmacol. Sci.* 22, 67–70.
34. Pasternak, G. W. (2001). Insights into mu opioid pharmacology—The role of mu opioid receptor subtypes. *Life Sci.* 68, 2213–2219.
35. Pasternak, G. W. (2004). Multiple opiate receptors: Deja vu all over again. *Neuropharmacology* 47(Suppl. 1), 312–323.
36. Snyder, S. H., and Pasternak, G. W. (2003). Historical review: Opioid receptors. *Trends Pharmacol. Sci.* 24, 198–205.
37. Fields, H. L., Heinricher, M. M., and Mason, P. (1991). Neurotransmitters in nociceptive modulatory circuits. *Annu. Rev. Neurosci.* 14, 219–245.
38. Cesselin, F. (1995). Opioid and anti-opioid peptides. *Fund. Clin. Pharmacol.* 9, 409–433.
39. Watkins, L. R., Kinscheck, I. B., and Mayer, D. J. (1984). Potentiation of opiate analgesia and apparent reversal of morphine tolerance by proglumide. *Science* 224, 395–396.
40. Ding, X. Z., Fan, S. G., Zhou, J. P., and Han, J. S. (1986). Reversal of tolerance to morphine but no potentiation of morphine-induced analgesia by antiserum against cholecystokinin octapeptide. *Neuropharmacology* 25, 1155–1160.
41. Hill, R. (2000). NK1 (substance P) receptor antagonists—Why are they not analgesic in humans? *Trends Pharmacol. Sci.* 21, 244–246.
42. Furst, S. (1999). Transmitters involved in antinociception in the spinal cord. *Brain Res. Bull.* 48, 129–141.
43. Mao, J. R. (1999). NMDA and opioid receptors: Their interactions in antinociception, tolerance and neuroplasticity. *Brain Res. Rev.* 30, 289–304.
44. Dickenson, A. H. (1995). Central acute pain mechanisms. *Ann. Med.* 27, 223–227.
45. Fields, H. L., Emson, P. C., Leigh, B. K., Gilbert, R. F. T., and Iversen, L. L. (1980). Multiple opiate receptor sites on primary afferent fibres. *Nature* 284, 351–353.
46. Li, J. L., Ding, Y. Q., Li, Y. Q., Li, J. S., Nomura, S., Kaneko, T., and Mizuno, N. (1998). Immunocytochemical localization of mu-opioid receptor in primary afferent neurons containing substance P or calcitonin gene-related peptide. A light and electron microscope study in the rat. *Brain Res.* 794, 347–352.
47. Zhang, X., Bao, L., Arvidsson, U., Elde, R., and Hokfelt, T. (1998). Localization and regulation of the delta-opioid receptor in dorsal root ganglia and spinal cord of the rat and monkey: Evidence for association with the membrane of large dense-core vesicles. *Neuroscience* 82, 1225–1242.
48. Aicher, S. A., Mitchell, J. L., and Mendelowitz, D. (2002). Distribution of mu-opioid receptors in rat visceral premotor neurons. *Neuroscience* 115, 851–860.
49. Wenk, H. N., and Honda, C. N. (1999). Immunohistochemical localization of delta opioid receptors in peripheral tissues. *J. Comp. Neurol.* 408, 567–579.
50. Abbadie, C., Pasternak, G. W., and Aicher, S. A. (2001). Presynaptic localization of the carboxy-terminus epitopes of the mu opioid receptor splice variants MOR-1C and MOR-1D in the superficial laminae of the rat spinal cord. *Neuroscience* 106, 833–842.

51. Aicher, S. A., Sharma, S., Cheng, P. Y., Liu-Chen, L. Y., and Pickel, V. M. (2000). Dual ultrastructural localization of μ-opiate receptors and substance P in the dorsal horn. *Synapse* 36, 12–20.

52. Kuraishi, Y., Hirota, N., Sugimoto, M., Satoh, M., and Takagi, H. (1983). Effects of morphine on noxious stimuli-induced release of substance P from rabbit dorsal horn in vivo. *Life Sci.* 33(Suppl. 1),693–696.

53. Bester, H., De, F. C., and Hunt, S. P. (2001). The NK1 receptor is essential for the full expression of noxious inhibitory controls in the mouse. *J. Neurosci.* 21, 1039–1046.

54. Kolesnikov, Y. A., Jain, S., Wilson, R., and Pasternak, G. W. (1996). Peripheral morphine analgesia: Synergy with central sites and a target of morphine tolerance. *J. Pharmacol. Exp. Ther.* 279, 502–506.

55. Stein, C., Schafer, M., and Machelska, H. (2003). Attacking pain at its source: New perspectives on opioids. *Nat. Med.* 9, 1003–1008.

56. Stein, C. (1995). Mechanisms of disease: The control of pain in peripheral tissue by opioids. *N. Engl. J. Med.* 332, 1685–1690.

57. Stein, C., Schäfer, M., and Hassan, A. H. S. (1995). Peripheral opioid receptors. *Ann. Med.* 27, 219–221.

58. Kolesnikov, Y., Jain, S., Wilson, R., and Pasternak, G. W. (1996). Peripheral kappa 1-opioid receptor-mediated analgesia in mice. *Eur. J. Pharmacol.* 310, 141–143.

59. Kolesnikov, Y., and Pasternak, G. W. (1999). Topical opioids in mice: Analgesia and reversal of tolerance by a topical N-methyl-D-aspartate antagonist. *J. Pharmacol. Exp. Ther.* 290, 247–252.

60. Sawynok, J. (2003). Topical and peripherally acting analgesics. *Pharmacol. Rev.* 55, 1–20.

61. Atweh, S. F., and Kuhar, M. J. (1977). Autoradiographic localization of opiate receptors in rat brain. III. The telencephalon. *Brain Res.* 134, 393–405.

62. Atweh, S. F., and Kuhar, M. J. (1977). Autoradiographic localization of opiate receptors in rat brain. I. Spinal cord and lower medulla. *Brain Res.* 124, 53–67.

63. Atweh, S. F., and Kuhar, M. J. (1977). Autoradiographic localization of opiate receptors in rat brain. II. The brain stem. *Brain Res.* 129, 1–12.

64. Pert, C. B., Kuhar, M. J., and Snyder, S. H. (1975). Autoradiographic localization of the opiate receptor in rat brain. *Life Sci.* 16, 1849–1853.

65. Arvidsson, U., Riedl, M., Chakrabarti, S., Lee, J.-H., Nakano, A. H., Dado, R. J., Loh, H. H., Law, P.-Y., Wessendorf, M. W., and Elde, R. (1995). Distribution and targeting of a μ-opioid receptor (MOR1) in brain and spinal cord. *J. Neurosci.* 15, 3328–3341.

66. Mansour, A., Fox, C. A., Burke, S., Akil, H., and Watson, S. J. (1995). Immunohistochemical localization of the cloned μ opioid receptor in the rat CNS. *J. Chem. Neuroanat.* 8, 283–305.

67. Mansour, A., Fox, C. A., Akil, H., and Watson, S. J. (1995). Opioid-receptor mRNA expression in the rat CNS: Anatomical and functional implications. *Trends Neurosci.* 18, 22–29.

68. Dickenson, A. H. (1990). A cure for wind up: NMDA receptor antagonists as potential analgesics. *Trends Pharmacol. Sci.* 11, 307–309.

69. Price, D. D., Mao, J., Frenk, H., and Mayer, D. J. (1994). The N-methyl-D-aspartate receptor antagonist dextromethorphan selectively reduces temporal summation of second pain in man. *Pain* 59, 165–174.

70. Warncke, T., Stubhaug, A., and Jorum, E. (2000). Preinjury treatment with morphine or ketamine inhibits the development of experimentally induced secondary hyperalgesia in man. *Pain* 86, 293–303.
71. Yeung, J. C., and Rudy, T. A. (1980). Multiplicative interaction between narcotic agonisms expressed at spinal and supraspinal sites of antinociceptive action as revealed by concurrent intrathecal and intracerebroventricular injections of morphine. *J. Pharmacol. Exp. Ther.* 215, 633–642.
72. Kolesnikov, Y., Cristea, M., Oksman, G., Torosjan, A., and Wilson, R. (2004). Evaluation of the tail formalin test in mice as a new model to assess local analgesic effects. *Brain Res.* 1029, 217–223.
73. Kolesnikov, Y. A., and Pasternak, G. W. (1999). Peripheral blockade of topical morphine tolerance by ketamine. *Eur. J. Pharmacol.* 374, R1–R2.
74. Kolesnikov, Y. A., and Pasternak, G. W. (1999). Peripheral orphanin FQ/nociceptin analgesia in the mouse. *Life Sci.* 64, 2021–2028.
75. King, M., Su, W., Chang, A., Zuckerman, A., and Pasternak, G. W. (2001). Transport of opioids from the brain to the periphery by P-glycoprotein: Peripheral actions of central drugs. *Nat. Neurosci.* 4, 268–274.
76. Saito, Y., Kaneko, M., Kirihara, Y., Sakura, S., and Kosaka, Y. (1998). Interaction of intrathecally infused morphine and lidocaine in rats (part I)—Synergistic antinociceptive effects. *Anesthesiology* 89, 1455–1463.
77. Kolesnikov, Y. A., Chereshnev, I., and Pasternak, G. W. (2000). Analgesic synergy between topical lidocaine and topical opioids. *J. Pharmacol. Exp. Ther.* 295, 546–551.
78. Kolesnikov, Y. A., Cristea, M., and Pasternak, G. W. (2003). Analgesic synergy between topical morphine and butamben in mice. *Anesth. Analg.* 97, 1103–1107 (table).
79. Purves, D., Agustine, G.J., Fitzpatrick, D., Katz, L.C., LaMantia, A.S., McNamar, J.O., and Williams, S.M. (2001). *NeuroScience*, Sinauer Assoc., INC, Sunderland, MA.

21

VANILLOID RECEPTOR PATHWAYS

MAKOTO TOMINAGA

Section of Cell Signaling, Okazaki Institute for Integrative Bioscience,
National Institutes of Natural Sciences, Okazaki, Japan

21.1	Cloning of Vanilloid Receptor	727
21.2	TRPV1 Exhibits Highly Specific Expression Pattern	729
21.3	TRPV1 Activation by Capsaicin, Protons, and Heat	730
21.4	Diverse Chemical Activators of TRPV1	732
21.5	Antagonists of TRPV1 and Their Implication in Clinical Settings	733
21.6	Sensitization of TRPV1	733
21.7	Desensitization of TRPV1	735
21.8	Knockout Mouse Study	736
21.9	Other TRPV Channels Involved in Nociception	736
	References	737

21.1 CLONING OF VANILLOID RECEPTOR

Hot chili peppers have been long used in food, and people know well that the peppers produce a burning sensation in the mouth. The structure of capsaicin, a main pungent ingredient of capsicum peppers, was solved as 8-methyl-*N*-vanillyl-6-noneamide in 1928 [1], and several decades later Hungarian researchers revealed that capsaicin could cause pain and desensitize further capsaicin challenge at the same time in rats [2, 3]. Three important findings—(1) that capsaicin and resiniferatoxin (RTX), a pungent substance derived form *Euphorbia* species, share a similar structure, including a vanilloid motif necessary for pungency (Fig. 21.1) [4]; (2) specific bindings of [^{3}H]RTX to the small-diameter sensory neurons [5]; and (3) development of a competitive antagonist of vanilloid action, capsazepine (Fig. 21.1) [6]—resulted in the belief that a receptor protein was responsible for the capsaicin action. Data obtained using electrophysiological methods provided further evidence that vanilloid receptor activation allows cation influx through its ionic pore, leading to the depolarization of the nociceptive neurons, followed by action potential generation. This seems to be one of the mechanisms whereby noxious stimuli are

Handbook of Contemporary Neuropharmacology, Edited by David R. Sibley, Israel Hanin, Michael Kuhar, and Phil Skolnick. Copyright © 2007 John Wiley & Sons, Inc.

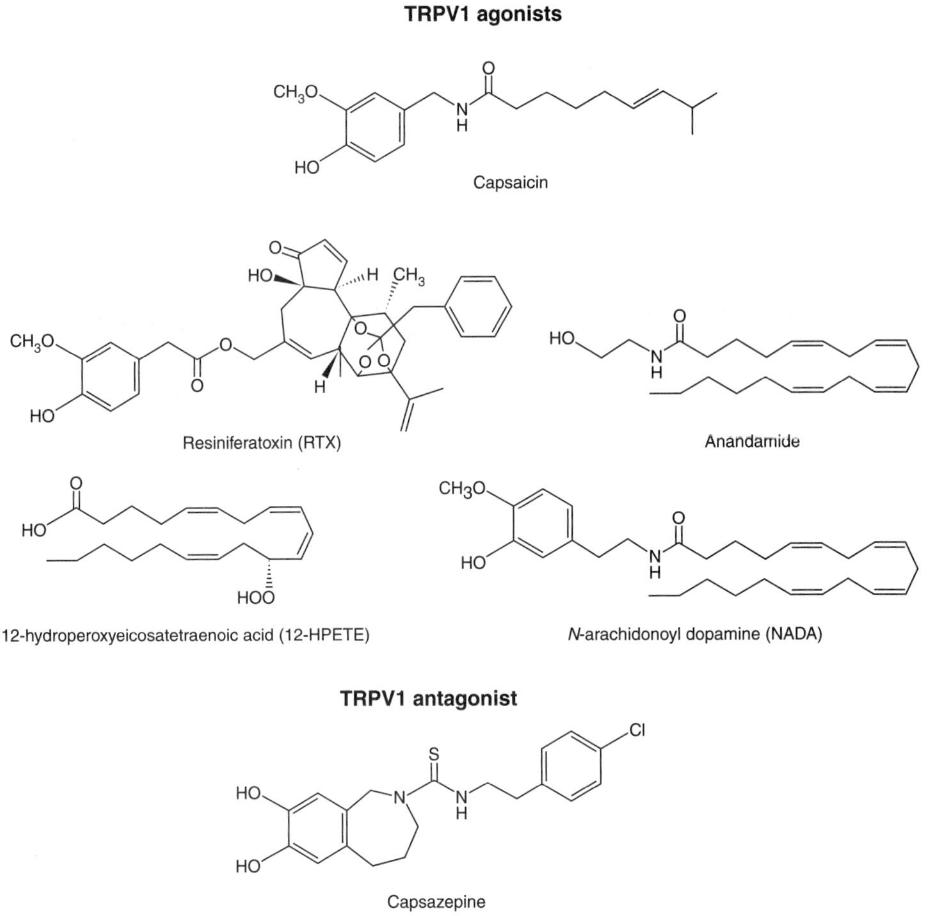

Figure 21.1 Representative chemical agonists and antagonist of TRPV1.

converted to electrical signals which are then transmitted to the brain through the ascending sensory pathways, leading to the perception of pain. At the same time, Ca^{2+} influx through the vanilloid receptor in the nociceptive neuron endings was found to cause the release of some substances, such as substance P (SP) and calcitonin gene–related peptide (CGRP), a phenomenon called *neurogenic inflammation*.

High Ca^{2+} permeability of the vanilloid receptor [7] allowed Julius and colleagues to isolate the gene encoding the capsaicin receptor by using a Ca^{2+} imaging-based expression cloning strategy in 1997, and they found that a single complementary DNA (cDNA) unit from rat sensory ganglia caused capsaicin-induced cytosolic Ca^{2+} increase in nonneuronal cells transfected with the library cDNAs [8]. Accordingly, the 838-amino-acid proteins encoded by the cDNA was designated vanilloid receptor 1 (VR1). From its deduced amino acid sequence, VR1 was predicted to function as an ion channel with six transmembrane (TM) domains, a pore loop domain, and cytosolic amino and carboxyl termini. VR1 turned out to be a member of the transient receptor potential (TRP) superfamily of ion channels and was renamed TRPV1 as the first member of the TRPV (vanilloid) subfamily. A prototypical member of the TRP superfamily of ion channels was reported in 1989 and found to be deficient in a *Drosophila* mutant exhibiting abnormal responsiveness to continuous light [9]. Now, this large TRP superfamily of ion channels is divided into seven subfamilies (TRPC, TRPV, TRPM, TRPP, TRPN, TRPA, and TRPML) [10].

21.2 TRPV1 EXHIBITS HIGHLY SPECIFIC EXPRESSION PATTERN

TRPV1 expression at both messenger RNA (mRNA) and protein levels was extensively examined, and those studies revealed that TRPV1 is highly expressed in dorsal root, trigeminal, and nodose ganglia, specifically within a subset of small- to medium-diameter sensory neurons that project to the superficial layers of the spinal cord (laminae I and II), trigeminal nucleus, and solitary tract nucleus, respectively [8, 11–14]. These observations, plus the fact that the TRPV1 protein is detected in nerve terminals of the bladder [14], indicates that TRPV1 is expressed in both central and peripheral termini of sensory neurons involved in nociception. This expression pattern is consistent with the finding that capsaicin selectively activates unmyelinated C fibers and thinly myelinated Aδ fibers. Although TRPV1 expression is also reported in a number of other neuronal and nonneuronal tissues such as brain, keratinocytes, and urinary epithelial cells [15–17] where nonnociceptive functions are hypothesized, expression level in sensory neurons appears to be much higher than in any other region. Primary afferent nociceptors have been histochemically divided into two distinct classes in the adult rodent: one expresses neuropeptides such as SP and CGRP; the other expresses specific enzyme markers such as fluoride-resistant acid phosphatase and binds the isolectin By (IBy) [18]. These two classes of neurons are sensitive to the neurotrophic nerve growth factor (NGF) and glial cell line–derived neurotrophic factor (GDNF), respectively. Both subpopulations of sensory neurons respond to capsaicin, and colocalization studies of TRPV1 with IB4 and SP probes revealed that many SP immunoreactive cells or IB4-positive cells costained with TRPV1, although $\sim$10% of the TRPV1-positive neurons did not stain with either SP or IB4 [14].

It has been reported that inflammation or tissue injury induced an increase in the number of unmyelinated C fibers expressing TRPV1 [19]. Furthermore, increased TRPV1 expression induced by inflammation was predominantly observed in myelinated Aδ fibers compared to C fibers [20]. NGF induced increase of TRPV1 mRNA and release of CGRP with capsaicin treatment in primary cultured DRG neurons [21]. Activation of p38MAPK (mitogen-activated protein kinase) by NGF was found to enhance the translocation of TRPV1 proteins from cell bodies in DRG to sensory nerve endings [22]. Furthermore, p38MAPK inhibitor reduced inflammatory hyperalgesia. Thus, increase of TRPV1 expression in the sensory nerve endings seems to be involved in the development of hyperalgesia.

In the visceral organs, including intestine, TRPV1 was found to be expressed throughout the sensory neurons, and most apparent expression was observed in nerve fibers that innervated the myenteric plexus of visceral organs [23]. TRPV1-expressing neurons detected with specific anti-TRPV1 antibody seem to be not vagal afferent fibers but spinal in origin.

21.3 TRPV1 ACTIVATION BY CAPSAICIN, PROTONS, AND HEAT

Upon exposure to capsaicin, TRPV1 exhibits an outwardly rectifying, nonselective cation current with high Ca^{2+} permeability [8]. Upon application of capsaicin to membrane patches excised from human embryonic kidney (HEK) cells expressing TRPV1, clear single-channel openings were observed (conductance of ~ 80 pS for Na^+) (Fig. 21.2), indicating that no cytosolic second messengers are necessary for TRPV1 activation. This channel also exhibits a voltage-dependent gating property such that depolarization promotes TRPV1 activation [24]. TRPV1 expressed alone in HEK293 cells or *Xenopus* oocytes can account for the majority of the electrophysiological properties exhibited by native capsaicin receptors in sensory neurons, including ligand affinity, permeability sequence, current–voltage (I–V) relationship, conductance, and open probability at both single-channel and whole-cell levels [8, 14, 24, 25]. These results suggest either that TRPV1 can form homomultimers (probably tetramer) without other subunits or that incorporation of subunits other than TRPV1 does not influence the functional properties.

Because capsaicin and its analogs such as RTX are lipophilic, it is quite possible that they pass through the cell membrane and act on binding sites present in the intracellular surface of TRPV1. An apparent time lag between capsaicin uptake and pungent sensation might be partially explained by such a process. Comparison of rat TRPV1 with its avian ortholog from chicken sensory neurons, which is insensitive to capsaicin, together with mutational analysis revealed that tyrosine 511 and serine 512, located at the transition between the second intracellular loop and the third TM domain, might interact with vanilloid ligands at the intracellular face of the membrane [26].

Tissue acidification is induced in pathological conditions such as ischemia and inflammation. Such acidification exacerbates or causes pain [27, 28]. Acidification of the extracellular milieu has two primary effects on TRPV1 function [14]. First, extracellular protons increase the potency of heat or capsaicin as TRPV1 agonists, in part, by lowering the threshold for channel activation by either stimulus. Second, extracellular protons can, themselves, be viewed as agonists because further acidification (to pH < 6.0) leads to channel opening at room temperature. Acidic solution evoked ionic currents with a mean effective concentration (EC_{50}) of about pH 5.4 at room temperature when applied to outside-out but not inside-out membrane patches

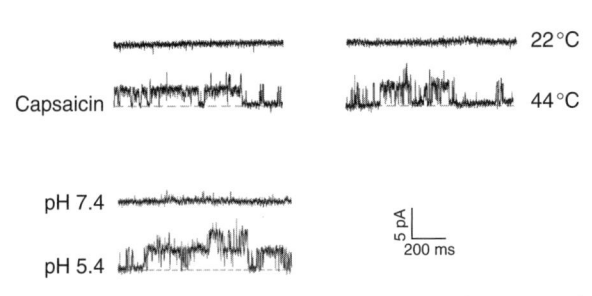

Figure 21.2 Representative single-channel currents in membrane patches excised from HEK293 cells expressing TRPV1 to bath-applied capsaicin (100 µM, inside out), protons (pH 5.4, outside out), or heat (44 °C, inside out). Dotted lines indicate closed level. Holding potential +40 mV.

excised from HEK293 cells expressing TRPV1 (Fig. 21.2), suggesting that protons act on amino acids in the extracellular domain of TRPV1 having side chain pK_a values in the physiologically relevant range. Mutational analyses revealed that glutamate 600, located within a putative extracellular domain, serves as an important regulator site for proton potentiation of TRPV1 activity, whereas glutamate 648 is involved in direct proton-evoked activation of TRPV1 [29]. In sensory neurons, proton-evoked currents consist of two major components: one is rapidly inactivating and Na^+ selective with a linear $I–V$ relation [30]; the other is a more sustained, nonselective cation conductance with an outwardly rectifying $I–V$ profile [31]. The latter is believed to underlie the prolonged sensation of pain, and TRPV1 may represent a responsible molecular entity for this component. In addition to its activating or modulating effects on TRPV1, protons were found to permeate the nonselective TRPV1 pore in acidic extracellular solution, resulting in marked intracellular acidification [32].

The burning quality of capsaicin-induced pain suggests that capsaicin and heat may evoke painful responses through a common molecular pathway. TRPV1 was, in fact, found to be activated by heat at >43 °C (Fig. 21.3), a temperature threshold

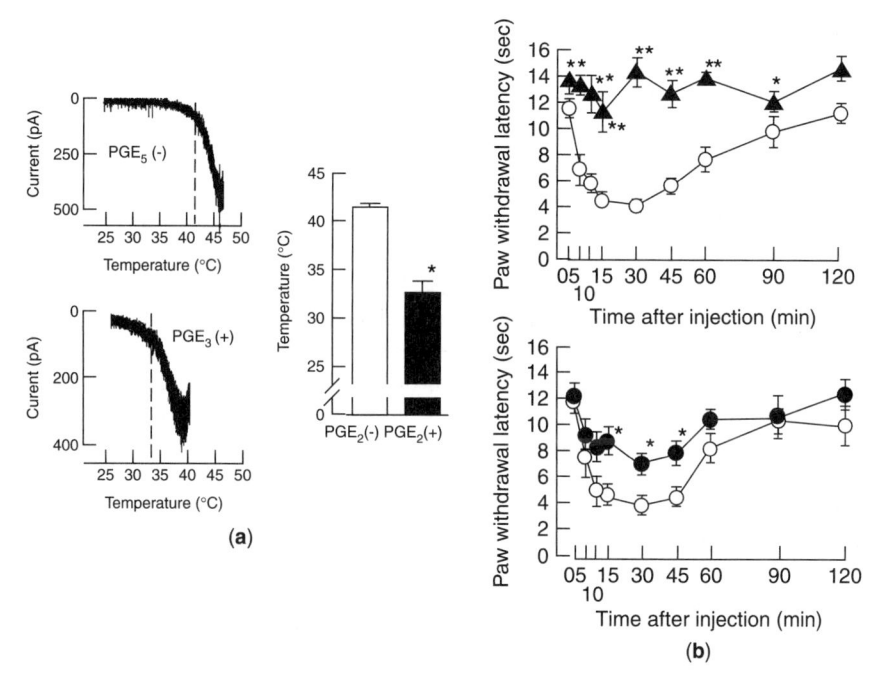

Figure 21.3 Reduction of temperature threshold for TRPV1 activation with PGE_2 (1 μM), and inhibition of PGE_2-induced thermal hyperalgesia in TRPV1- or EP_1-deficient mice. (a) Representative temperature response profiles in the absence (upper) and presence (lower) of PGE_2 (left). Temperature threshold for TRPV1 activation in the presence of PGE_2 (30.6 ± 1.1 °C) was significantly lower than that in the absence of PGE_2 (40.7 ± 0.3 °C) (right). (∗) $p < 0.05$ vs. PGE_2 (−). (b) Paw withdrawal latency after injection of PGE_2 into hind paw in wild-type mice (open circle), TRPV1-deficient mice (closed triangle), or EP_1-deficient mice (closed circle). (∗) $p < 0.05$ and (∗∗) $p < 0.01$ vs. wild-type mice. (From Moriyama et al., *Mol. Pain* 1: 3, 2005).

that is similar to that at which heat evokes pain in vivo, suggesting that TRPV1 is involved in the detection of painful heat by primary sensory neurons [14]. Heat-evoked TRPV1 currents show properties similar to those of capsaicin-evoked currents. However, there are several differences in the properties, including cationic permeability ratio and Ca^{2+}-independent desensitization, suggesting that TRPV1-mediated responses to capsaicin and heat involve distinct but overlapping mechanisms. Heat-evoked single-channel openings were observed in inside-out membrane patches excised from HEK293 cells expressing TRPV1 (Fig. 21.2), suggesting that TRPV1 is, itself, a heat sensor.

21.4 DIVERSE CHEMICAL ACTIVATORS OF TRPV1

Not only capsaicin and RTX but also other chemically related substances such as zingerol and piperin, chemicals responsible for the pungency of ginger and black pepper, respectively, were reported to have the ability to activate TRPV1 [33]. In addition to these vanilloid compounds, allicin, the chemical causing pungency in garlic, was found to activate TRPV1 [34].

Numerous endogenous lipid metabolites of arachidonic acid (AA) in plasma membrane are also capable of activating TRPV1. Palmitoyl ethanolamide (anandamide) (Fig. 21.1), an endocannabinoid, is the first such substance in lipids which might work as an endogenous ligand for TRPV1 [35]. However, anandamide's ability to be a physiologically relevant activator of TRPV1 is controversial because concentrations at which anandamide can activate TRPV1 (micromolars) are higher than those that activate G-protein-coupled cannabinoid CB_1 or CB_2 receptors (nanomolars) and because anandamide exhibits partial agonism [36]. Various oxygenated AA derivatives, including 12- and 15-hydroperoxyeicosatetraenoic acid (12-HPETE and 15-HPETE, respectively) (Fig. 21.1) were also found to activate TRPV1 [37]. These AA metabolites can be produced by lipoxygenases that introduce molecular oxygen in AA released from the membrane by phospholipase A_2 enzymes. Again, reported EC_{50} values for activation of TRPV1 by 12-HPETE or 15-HPETE are relatively high (micromolars), although, to date, no pharmacological study has been performed to examine how much 12-HPETE or 15-HPETE is produced in pathological conditions. However, Shin et al. provided evidence that 12-HPETE is produced endogenously in sensory neurons upon stimulation of sensory nerve endings by the inflammatory mediator bradykinin and activates TRPV1 [38]. This suggests that lipoxygenase products might be important in the development of inflammatory pain. N-Arachidonoyl dopamine (NADA) (Fig. 21.1), originally characterized in the striatum, is a full agonist of TRPV1 and the most potent endogenous lipid ligand discovered to date [39]. N-Oleoildopamine also possesses the ability to activate TRPV1 with the same potency as NADA [40]. However, the distribution of NADA in dorsal root ganglia (DRG) is much lower than in brain regions (striatum, hippocampus, and cerebellum). In addition, as yet, no TRPV1-mediated physiological or pathological conditions have been attributed to endogenously formed NADA, making the concept that NADA can produce pain in vivo obscure. On the other hand, widespread distribution of the compounds, not only in peripheral tissues innervated by TRPV1-expressing afferents, but also in the spinal cord and brain, might explain why TRPV1 is expressed throughout the central nervous system, albeit at levels lower than in nociceptive neurons. To qualify as an endogenous activator of TRPV1, the three classes of lipids described above have to be formed by cells and be released in an activity-dependent manner in sufficient amounts to evoke a TRPV1-mediated response. Further experiments should be done to clarify the importance of the lipids.

21.5 ANTAGONISTS OF TRPV1 AND THEIR IMPLICATION IN CLINICAL SETTINGS

The two antagonists that have been traditionally used to block capsaicin receptors are capsazepine and ruthenium red. Capsazepine shares structure similarity with vanilloid compounds (Fig. 21.1). In vitro, capsazepine competitively antagonizes both vanilloid activation of TRPV1-mediated currents and RTX binding to membranes containing native or recombinant TRPV1. This compound can also block the activation of TRPV1 by protons, anandamide, or heat. However, there are significant species differences in the potency of capsazepine at blocking TRPV1 responses evoked by nonvanilloid stimuli. Furthermore, capsazepine is known to act on other targets, including nicotinic acetylcholine receptors at micromolar concentrations. Capsazepine was reported to inhibit some pain-related behaviors in animal models, although no clinical trials have been carried out partly because of its nonspecificity. Ruthenium red is a highly charged organic cation that acts as a noncompetitive TRPV1 antagonist, apparently by blocking the channel pore. This compound, however, is even more promiscuous than capsazepine, as it blocks a number of nonselective cation channels.

Halogenated vanilloids such as iodinated resiniferatoxin (I-RTX) and N-(3-methoxyphenyl)-4-chlorocinnamide (SB36679) seem to exhibit somewhat better selectivity [41, 42]. However, they have not been employed with much success in vivo. One of the surprising findings arising from the in vivo studies of the TRPV1 antagonists is that some of the antagonists, such as N-(4-tertiarybutylphenyl)-4-(3-cholorophyridine-2-yl) tetrahydropyrazine-1(2H)-carbox-amide (BCTC) and capsazepine, were also effective for mechanical hyperalgesia in a neurpathic pain model [43, 44]. These findings apparently contradict the previous results that normal mechanical nociception was observed in mice lacking TRPV1 and that TRPV1 in a heterologous expression system did not show mechanical sensitivity [45]. The possibility that TRPV1 is involved in mechanosensation in nociceptors, especially in pathological conditions, cannot be excluded. Indeed, mechanical responsiveness in the urinary bladder appears to be diminished in mice lacking TRPV1, and proteinase-activated receptor 2 (PAR 2) agonist-induced mechanical allodynia was significantly reduced in TRPV1-deficient mice. Highly selective TRPV1 antagonists will hopefully be identified through high-throughput screening in the near future, and studies using the new selective TRPV1 antagonists will address the issue of mechanosensitivity of TRPV1.

21.6 SENSITIZATION OF TRPV1

Inflammatory pain is initiated by tissue damage/inflammation and is characterized by hypersensitivity both at the site of damage and in adjacent tissue. Stimuli that normally would not produce pain do so (allodynia), while previously noxious stimuli evoke even greater pain responses (hyperalgesia). One mechanism underlying these phenomena is the sensitization of ion channels such as TRPV1. Sensitization is triggered by extracellular inflammatory mediators that are released in vivo from surrounding damaged or inflamed tissues and from nociceptive neurons themselves (i.e., neurogenic inflammation) [46, 47]. Mediators known to cause sensitization include prostaglandins, adenosine, serotonin, bradykinin, and adenosine triphosphate (ATP) [48]. Tissue acidification is also induced in the context of inflammation as described above. Among the inflammatory mediators, extracellular ATP, bradykinin, prostaglandin E_2, prostaglandin I_2, trypsin, and tryptase have been reported to potentiate TRPV1 responses through metabotropic ATP receptor $(P2Y)_2$, B2, EP_1, IP, and proteinase-activated receptor 2 (PAR2) receptors, respectively, in a protein kinase C (PKC)–dependent manner in both heterologous expression systems and native DRG neurons [49–53]. In addition to potentiating capsaicin- or proton-evoked currents, those mediators also lower the temperature threshold for heat activation of TRPV1 to as low as 30 °C (Fig. 21.3), such that normally nonpainful thermal stimuli (i.e., normal body temperature) are capable of activating TRPV1, thereby leading to the sensation of pain. Under these circumstances, they thus can be viewed as direct activators of TRPV1. This represents a novel mechanism through which the large amounts of mediators released from different cells in inflammation might trigger a sensation of pain. The inflammatory mediator-induced TRPV1-mediated hypersensitivity has been confirmed at the whole-animal level using TRPV1-deficient mice or mice lacking the receptors of the mediators (Fig. 21.3). PKC-dependent phosphorylation of TRPV1 has been reported to be involved in the sensitization of TRPV1 by the mediators, based on the observation that several different PKC inhibitors blocked the inflammatory mediator-induced potentiation or sensitization of TRPV1 activity. Indeed, two serine residues in the cytoplasmic domain of TRPV1 were identified as substrates for PKC-dependent phosphorylation [54, 55]. There has been extensive work demonstrating the activation of a protein kinase A (PKA)–dependent pathway that influences capsaicin- or heat-mediated actions in rat sensory neurons [56–60] as well as interactions between cloned TRPV1 and PKA [61–64]. These results suggest that PKA plays a pivotal role in the development of hyperalgesia and inflammation and that a PKA-dependent pathway is also involved in TRPV1 sensitization, and PKA-dependent phosphorylation of serine residues on TRPV1, S144, S370, and S502 has been reported [64]. Further, both PKA- and PKC-dependent pathways have been reported to function on some ligands, such as serotonin and prostaglandins [50, 65]. The physiological relevance of the two different pathways downstream of serotonin or prostaglandin exposure remains to be elucidated. The fact that only PKC activation leads to the reduction of temperature threshold for TRPV1 activation might be pertinent to this issue [50]. Disruption of interaction between phosphatidylinositol-4,5-bisphosphate (PIP_2) and TRPV1 has also been reported to be involved in the sensitization of TRPV1 downstream of phospholipase C (PLC) activation by, for example, bradykinin or NGF since the amount of PIP_2, a tonic inhibitor of TRPV1, is reduced in its hydrolysis to inositol 1,4,5-trisphosphate (IP_3) and diacyl glycerol (DAG) [66, 67]. It is also known that phospholipase A_2 (PLA_2) is activated downstream of PLC activation, leading to the generation of lipoxygenase products such as 12-HPETE from AA [38]. These facts indicate three different pathways can work to modulate TRPV1 function downstream of PLC activation: a PKC-dependent pathway, a

PIP$_2$-mediated pathway, and a lipoxygenase product–mediated pathway. It is not currently clear which pathway is predominantly functioning in vivo.

In addition to the direct activation of TRPV1, acidification induced in inflammation also shifts the temperature response curve of TRPV1 to the left so that the channel can be activated at lower temperatures (lower than body temperature) and responses to heat are bigger at a given suprathreshold temperature. This phenomenon might also contribute to inflammatory pain. Calmodulin kinase II (CaMKII) was also reported to control TRPV1 activity upon phosphorylation of TRPV1 at S502 and T704 by regulating capsaicin binding [68]. Thus, phosphorylation of TRPV1 by several different kinases seems to control TRPV1 activity through the dynamic balance between phosphorylation and dephosphorylation. Furthermore, NGF activates the phosphatidylinositol 3-kinase (PI3 K) and extracellular signal-regulated protein kinase (ERK), and then PI3K and ERK have been reported to sensitize TRPV1 [69]. Mechanisms underlying TRPV1 sensitization seem to be very complicated.

21.7 DESENSITIZATION OF TRPV1

Capsaicin not only causes pain but also seems to exhibit analgesic properties, particularly when used to treat pain associated with diabetic neuropathies or rheumatoid arthritis [7]. This paradoxical effect may relate to the ability of capsaicin to desensitize nociceptive terminals to capsaicin as well as to other noxious stimuli following prolonged exposure. At the molecular level, an extracellular Ca^{2+}-dependent reduction of TRPV1 responsiveness upon continuous vanilloid exposure (electrophysiological desensitization) may partially underlie this phenomenon [7, 8], although physical damage to the nerve terminal and depletion of SP and CGRP probably contribute to this effect as well. Ca^{2+}- and voltage-dependent desensitization of capsaicin-activated currents has also been observed in rat DRG neurons [70–73]. This inactivation of nociceptive neurons by capsaicin has generated extensive research on the possible therapeutic effectiveness of capsaicin as a clinical analgesic tool [74, 75].

Desensitization to capsaicin is a complex process with varying kinetic components: a fast component that appears to depend on Ca^{2+} influx through TRPV1 [70–73] and a slow component that does not. Calcineurin inhibitors reduce TRPV1 desensitization (the slow component), indicating the involvement of the Ca^{2+}-dependent phophorylation/dephosphorylation process [73]. In agreement with this finding, phosphorylation of TRPV1 by CaMKII was reported to prevent its desensitization [68]. In addition, PKA-dependent phosphorylation of TRPV1 has been reported to mediate the slow component of TRPV1 desensitization [61]. TRPV1 becomes dephosphorylated upon exposure to capsaicin and this phosphorylation can be restored by 8bromo-cyclic adenosine monophosphate (cAMP).

CaM has also been reported to be involved in Ca^{2+}-dependent desensitization of TRPV1. CaM was found to bind to the carboxyl terminus of TRPV1. Disruption of the CaM binding segment prevented extracellular Ca^{2+}-dependent TRPV1 desensitization to brief capsaicin application, although some desensitization was still observed upon more prolonged capsaicin application in cells expressing the mutant [76]. It has also been reported that CaM binds to the first ankyrin repeat in the amino terminus of TRPV1 and to be involved in desensitization [77]. Whether the amino or carboxyl terminus is more predominantly involved in Ca^{2+}-dependent desensitization by CaM is not known. Ca^{2+}-dependent desensitization is a relatively common feature of many cation channels, including cyclic nucleotide–gated channels [78], L-type Ca^{2+} channels [79, 80], P/Q-type Ca^{2+} channels [81], N-methyl-D-aspartate (NMDA) receptor channels [82, 83], and TRP channels [84, 85]. It may represent a physiological safety mechanism against a harmful Ca^{2+} overload in the cell, especially during large Ca^{2+} influx through the channels.

21.8 KNOCKOUT MOUSE STUDY

Electrophysiological analysis in a heterologous expression system revealed the importance of TRPV1 in detecting noxious thermal and chemical stimuli. To determine whether TRPV1 really contributes to the detection of these noxious stimuli in vivo, mice lacking this protein were generated and analyzed for nociceptive function [45, 86]. Sensory neurons from mice lacking TRPV1 were deficient in their responses to each of the reported noxious stimuli: capsaicn, proton, and heat. Consistent with this observation, behavioral responses to capsaicin were absent and responses to acute thermal stimuli were diminished in these mice. Pungency-related behaviors were not observed in the TRPV1-deficient mice when capsaicin was applied to their oral cavity, suggesting the involvement of TRPV1 in detection of pungency. In contrast, TRPV1 knockout mice showed normal physiological and behavioral responses to noxious mechanical stimuli, implying the existence of other mechanisms for the detection of such stimuli. The most prominent feature of the knockout mouse thermosensory phenotype was a virtual absence of thermal hypersensitivity in the setting of inflammation. These findings indicate that TRPV1 is essential for selective modalities of pain sensation and for tissue injury-induced thermal hyperalgesia.

The extent to which TRPV1 underlies the responses to noxious thermal stimuli and the contribution of other heat-sensitive channels remain to be clarified. There was a drastic reduction of heat sensitivity in DRG neurons cultured from TRPV1-deficient mice, but a small yet significant percentage of DRG neurons showed large heat-evoked current responses to heat stimuli over 55 °C. Furthermore, the TRPV1-deficient mice showed impaired responses to noxious thermal stimuli only over 50 °C, and a small but significant amount of heat-evoked c-*fos* induction persisted in spinal cord laminae I and II of TRPV1-deficient mice. These data supported the idea that other heat-sensitive channels contribute to the transmission and perception of high-intensity noxious thermal stimuli.

Recent studies have provided further support for TRPV1 involvement in inflammatory pain and have, in addition, demonstrated that the participation of TRPV1 in pain sensation may also extend to neuropathic pain, mechanical allodynia, and mechanical hyperalgesia. These conclusions are based on enhanced expression of TRPV1 in sensory neurons in the context of these conditions as well as behavioral effects of TRPV1 antagonism with capsazepine [22, 43, 49, 87, 88]

21.9 OTHER TRPV CHANNELS INVOLVED IN NOCICEPTION

TRPV2 (VRL-1) might be a potential candidate for the receptor detecting the high heat stimulus responsible for the residual high temperature-evoked nociceptive responses observed in TRPV1-deficient mice. TRPV2 with about 50% identity to TRPV1 was found to be activated by high temperatures with a threshold of $\sim 52\,°C$ [89]. TRPV2 currents showed similar properties to those of TRPV1 such as an outwardly rectifying I–V relationship, inhibition by ruthenium red, and relatively high Ca^{2+} permeability. Intense TRPV2 immunoreactivity was observed in medium- to large-diameter cells in rat DRG neurons [89–92]. In addition, many of the TRPV2-positive neurons costained with the anti-neurofilament antibody N52, a marker for myelinated neurons. Temperatures activating TRPV2 are more harmful to our body than those activating TRPV1. Therefore, expression of TRPV2 in the myelinated sensory fibers seems reasonable because Aδ fibers can transmit the nociceptive information much faster than C fibers. Aδ mechano- and heat-sensitive (AMH) neurons in monkey are medium- to large-diameter, lightly myelinated neurons that fall into two groups: type I AMHs have a heat threshold of $\sim 53\,°C$, and type II AMHs are activated at $43\,°C$ [93]. TRPV2 expression might account for the high thermal threshold ascribed to type I AMH nociceptors. However, it has very recently been reported that nociceptors lacking TRPV1 and TRPV2 still have normal heat responses [94]. This result suggests the existence of another heat-sensitive mechanism.

Two TRPV channels, TRPV3 and TRPV4, have been found to be activated by warm temperatures, ~ 34–$38\,°C$ for TRPV3 and ~ 27–$35\,°C$ for TRPV4, in heterologous expression systems and to be expressed in multiple tissues, including, among others, sensory and hypothalamic neurons and keratinocytes [95–99]. TRPV4 was originally reported as an osmotically activated channel (VROAC or OTRPC4 from vanilloid receptor–related osmotically activated channel or OSM-9-like TRP channel 4, respectively) [100, 101]. Several approaches, including the knockdown of TRPV4 with gene disruption or antisense oligonucleotides, have led to reports that this protein is involved in mechanical stimulus- and hypotonicity-induced nociception in rodents [102–104]. It remains unclear whether TRPV3 is involved in nociception. However, the data that TRPV1 and TRPV3 were predicted to reside on the same chromosome and that TRPV3 was sensitized upon repeated noxious heat stimuli suggest the involvement of TRPV3 in nociception.

REFERENCES

1. Nelson, E. (1919). The constitution of capsaicin, the pungent principal of capsicum. *J. Am. Chem.* 41, 1115–1151.
2. Jancso, N., Jancso-Gabor, A., and Szolcsanyi, J. (1967). Direct evidence for neurogenic inflammation and its prevention by denervation and by pretreatment with capsaicin. *Br. J. Pharmacol.* 31, 138–151.
3. Jancso, G., Kiraly, E., and Jancso-Gabor, A. (1977). Pharmacologically induced selective degeneration of chemosensitive primary sensory neurones. *Nature* 270, 741–743.
4. Szallasi, A., and Blumberg, P. M. (1989). Resiniferatoxin, a phorbol-related diterpene, acts as an ultrapotent analog of capsaicin, the irritant constituent in red pepper. *Neuroscience* 30, 515–520.
5. Szallasi, A., and Blumberg, P. M. (1990). Specific binding of resiniferatoxin, an ultrapotent capsaicin analog, by dorsal root ganglion membranes. *Brain Res.* 524, 106–111.

6. Bevan, S., Hothi, S., Hughes, G., James, I. F., Rang, H. P., Shah, K., Walpole, C. S., and Yeats, J. C. (1992). Capsazepine: A competitive antagonist of the sensory neurone excitant capsaicin. *Br. J. Pharmacol.* 107, 544–552.
7. Szallasi, A., and Blumberg, P. M. (1999). Vanilloid (capsaicin) receptors and mechanisms. *Pharmacol. Rev.* 51, 159–212.
8. Caterina, M. J., Schumacher, M. A., Tominaga, M., Rosen, T. A., Levine, J. D., and Julius, D. (1997). The capsaicin receptor: A heat-activated ion channel in the pain pathway. *Nature* 389, 816–824.
9. Montell, C., and Rubin, G. M. (1989). Molecular characterization of the *Drosophila* trp locus: A putative integral membrane protein required for phototransduction. *Neuron* 2, 1313–1323.
10. Montell, C. (2005). The TRP superfamily of cation channels. *Sci. STKE.* 272, re3.
11. Ma, Q. P. (2002). Expression of capsaicin receptor (VR1) by myelinated primary afferent neurons in rats. *Neurosci. Lett.* 319, 87–90.
12. Michael, G. J., and Priestley, J. V. (1999). Differential expression of the mRNA for the vanilloid receptor subtype 1 in cells of the adult rat dorsal root and nodose ganglia and its downregulation by axotomy. *J. Neurosci.* 19, 1844–1854.
13. Guo, A., Vulchanova, L., Wang, J., Li, X., and Elde, R. (1999). Immunocytochemical localization of the vanilloid receptor 1 (VR1): Relationship to neuropeptides, the P2X3 purinoceptor and IB4 binding sites. *Eur. J. Neurosci.* 11, 946–958.
14. Tominaga, M., Caterina, M. J., Malmberg, A. B., Rosen, T. A., Gilbert, H., Skinner, K., Raumann, B. E., Basbaum, A. I., and Julius, D. (1998). The cloned capsaicin receptor integrates multiple pain-producing stimuli. *Neuron* 21, 531–543.
15. Birder, L. A., Kanai, A. J., de Groat, W. C., Kiss, S., Nealen, M. L., Burke, N. E., Dineley, K. E., Watkins, S., Reynolds, I. J., and Caterina, M. J. (2001). Vanilloid receptor expression suggests a sensory role for urinary bladder epithelial cells. *Proc. Natl. Acad. Sci. USA* 98, 13396–13401.
16. Denda, M., Fuziwara, S., Inoue, K., Denda, S., Akamatsu, H., Tomitaka, A., and Matsunaga, K. (2001). Immunoreactivity of VR1 on epidermal keratinocyte of human skin. *Biochem. Biophys. Res. Commun.* 285, 1250–1252.
17. Mezey, E., Toth, Z. E., Cortright, D. N., Arzubi, M. K., Krause, J. E., Elde, R., Guo, A., Blumberg, P. M., and Szallasi, A. (2000). Distribution of mRNA for vanilloid receptor subtype 1 (VR1), and VR1-like immunoreactivity, in the central nervous system of the rat and human. *Proc. Natl. Acad. Sci. USA* 97, 3655–3660.
18. Snider, W. D., and McMahon, S. B. (1998). Tackling pain at the source: New ideas about nociceptors. *Neuron* 20, 629–632.
19. Carlton, S. M., and Coggeshall, R. E. (2001). Peripheral capsaicin receptors increase in the inflamed rat hindpaw: A possible mechanism for peripheral sensitization. *Neurosci. Lett.* 310, 53–56.
20. Amaya, F., Oh-hashi, K., Naruse, Y., Iijima, N., Ueda, M., Shimosato, G., Tominaga, M., Tanaka, Y., and Tanaka, M. (2003). Local inflammation increases vanilloid receptor 1 expression within distinct subgroups of DRG neurons. *Brain Res.* 963, 190–196.
21. Winston, J., Toma, H., Shenoy, M., and Pasricha, P. J. (2001). Nerve growth factor regulates VR-1 mRNA levels in cultures of adult dorsal root ganglion neurons. *Pain* 89, 181–186.
22. Ji, R. R., Samad, T. A., Jin, S. X., Schmoll, R., and Woolf, C. J. (2002). p38 MAPK activation by NGF in primary sensory neurons after inflammation increases TRPV1 levels and maintains heat hyperalgesia. *Neuron* 36, 57–68.

23. Ward, S. M., Bayguinov, J., Won, K. J., Grundy, D., and Berthoud, H. R. (2003). Distribution of the vanilloid receptor (VR1) in the gastrointestinal tract. *J. Comp. Neurol.* 465, 121–135.
24. Gunthorpe, M. J., Harries, M. H., Prinjha, R. K., Davis, J. B., and Randall, A. (2000). Voltage- and time-dependent properties of the recombinant rat vanilloid receptor (rVR1). *J. Physiol.* 525(Pt. 3), 747–759.
25. Premkumar, L. S., Agarwal, S., and Steffen, D. (2002). Single-channel properties of native and cloned rat vanilloid receptors. *J. Physiol.* 545, 107–117.
26. Jordt, S. E., and Julius, D. (2002). Molecular basis for species-specific sensitivity to "hot" chili peppers. *Cell* 108, 421–430.
27. Steen, K. H., Reeh, P. W., Anton, F., and Handwerker, H. O. (1992). Protons selectively induce lasting excitation and sensitization to mechanical stimulation of nociceptors in rat skin, in vitro. *J. Neurosci.* 12, 86–95.
28. Bevan, S., and Geppetti, P. (1994). Protons: Small stimulants of capsaicin-sensitive sensory nerves. *Trends Neurosci.* 17, 509–512.
29. Jordt, S. E., Tominaga, M., and Julius, D. (2000). Acid potentiation of the capsaicin receptor determined by a key extracellular site. *Proc. Natl. Acad. Sci. USA* 97, 8134–8139.
30. Krishtal, O. A., and Pidoplichko, V. I. (1980). A receptor for protons in the nerve cell membrane. *Neuroscience* 5, 2325–2327.
31. Bevan, S., and Yeats, J. (1991). Protons activate a cation conductance in a subpopulation of rat dorsal root ganglion neurones. *J. Physiol.* 433, 145–161.
32. Hellwig, N., Plant, T. D., Janson, W., Schafer, M., Schultz, G., and Schaefer, M. (2004). TRPV1 acts as proton channel to induce acidification in nociceptive neurons. *J. Biol. Chem.* 279, 34553–34561.
33. Sterner, O., and Szallasi, A. (1999). Novel natural vanilloid receptor agonists: New therapeutic targets for drug development. *Trends Pharmacol. Sci.* 20, 459–465.
34. Macpherson, L. J., Geierstanger, B. H., Viswanath, V., Bandell, M., Eid, S. R., Hwang, S., and Patapoutian, A. (2005). The pungency of garlic: Activation of TRPA1 and TRPV1 in response to allicin. *Curr. Biol.* 15, 929–934.
35. Zygmunt, P. M., Petersson, J., Andersson, D. A., Chuang, H., Sorgard, M., Di Marzo, V., Julius, D., and Hogestatt, E. D. (1999). Vanilloid receptors on sensory nerves mediate the vasodilator action of anandamide. *Nature* 400, 452–457.
36. Van Der Stelt, M., and Di Marzo, V. (2004). Endovanilloids. Putative endogenous ligands of transient receptor potential vanilloid 1 channels. *Eur. J. Biochem.* 271, 1827–1834.
37. Hwang, S. W., Cho, H., Kwak, J., Lee, S. Y., Kang, C. J., Jung, J., Cho, S., Min, K. H., Suh, Y. G., Kim, D., and Oh, U. (2000). Direct activation of capsaicin receptors by products of lipoxygenases: Endogenous capsaicin-like substances. *Proc. Natl. Acad. Sci. USA* 97, 6155–6160.
38. Shin, J., Cho, H., Hwang, S. W., Jung, J., Shin, C. Y., Lee, S. Y., Kim, S. H., Lee, M. G., Choi, Y. H., Kim, J., Haber, N. A., Reichling, D. B., Khasar, S., Levine, J. D., and Oh, U. (2002). Bradykinin-12-lipoxygenase-VR1 signaling pathway for inflammatory hyperalgesia. *Proc. Natl. Acad. Sci. USA* 99, 10150–10155.
39. Huang, S. M., Bisogno, T., Trevisani, M., Al-Hayani, A., De Petrocellis, L., Fezza, F., Tognetto, M., Petros, T. J., Krey, J. F., Chu, C. J., Miller, J. D., Davies, S. N., Geppetti, P., Walker, J. M., and Di Marzo, V. (2002). An endogenous capsaicin-like substance with high potency at recombinant and native vanilloid VR1 receptors. *Proc. Natl. Acad. Sci. USA* 99, 8400–8405.

40. Chu, C. J., Huang, S. M., De Petrocellis, L., Bisogno, T., Ewing, S. A., Miller, J. D., Zipkin, R. E., Daddario, N., Appendino, G., Di Marzo, V., and Walker, J. M. (2003). N-Oleoyldopamine, a novel endogenous capsaicin-like lipid that produces hyperalgesia. *J. Biol. Chem.* 278, 13633–13639.

41. Gunthorpe, M. J., Rami, H. K., Jerman, J. C., Smart, D., Gill, C. H., Soffin, E. M., Luis Hannan, S., Lappin, S. C., Egerton, J., Smith, G. D., Worby, A., Howett, L., Owen, D., Nasir, S., Davies, C. H., Thompson, M., Wyman, P. A., Randall, A. D., and Davis, J. B. (2004). Identification and characterisation of SB-366791, a potent and selective vanilloid receptor (VR1/TRPV1) antagonist. *Neuropharmacology* 46, 133–149.

42. Wahl, P., Foged, C., Tullin, S., and Thomsen, C. (2001). Iodo-resiniferatoxin, a new potent vanilloid receptor antagonist. *Mol. Pharmacol.* 59, 9–15.

43. Walker, K. M., Urban, L., Medhurst, S. J., Patel, S., Panesar, M., Fox, A. J., and McIntyre, P. (2003). The VR1 antagonist capsazepine reverses mechanical hyperalgesia in models of inflammatory and neuropathic pain. *J. Pharmacol. Exp. Ther.* 304, 56–62.

44. Pomonis, J. D., Harrison, J. E., Mark, L., Bristol, D. R., Valenzano, K. J., and Walker, K. (2003). N-(4-Tertiarybutylphenyl)-4-(3-cholorphyridin-2-yl)tetrahydropyrazine-1(2H)-carbox-amide (BCTC), a novel, orally effective vanilloid receptor antagonist with analgesic properties: II. In vivo characterization in rat models of inflammatory and neuropathic pain. *J. Pharmacol. Exp. Ther.* 306, 387–393.

45. Caterina, M. J., Leffler, A., Malmberg, A. B., Martin, W. J., Trafton, J., Petersen-Zeitz, K. R., Koltzenburg, M., Basbaum, A. I., and Julius, D. (2000). Impaired nociception and pain sensation in mice lacking the capsaicin receptor. *Science* 288, 306–313.

46. Julius, D., and Basbaum, A. I. (2001). Molecular mechanisms of nociception. *Nature* 413, 203–210.

47. Woolf, C. J., and Salter, M. W. (2000). Neuronal plasticity: Increasing the gain in pain. *Science* 288, 1765–1769.

48. Numazaki, M., and Tominaga, M. (2004). Nociception and TRP channels. *Curr. Drug Targets CNS Neurol. Disord.* 3, 479–485.

49. Dai, Y., Moriyama, T., Higashi, T., Togashi, K., Kobayashi, K., Yamanaka, H., Tominaga, M., and Noguchi, K. (2004). Proteinase-activated receptor 2-mediated potentiation of transient receptor potential vanilloid subfamily 1 activity reveals a mechanism for proteinase-induced inflammatory pain. *J. Neurosci.* 24, 4293–4299.

50. Moriyama, T., Higashi, T., Togashi, K., Iida, T., Segi, E., Sugimoto, Y., Tominaga, T., Narumiya, S., and Tominaga, M. (2005). Sensitization of TRPV1 by EP1 and IP reveals peripheral nociceptive mechanism of prostaglandins. *Mol. Pain* 1, 3–12.

51. Moriyama, T., Iida, T., Kobayashi, K., Higashi, T., Fukuoka, T., Tsumura, H., Leon, C., Suzuki, N., Inoue, K., Gachet, C., Noguchi, K., and Tominaga, M. (2003). Possible involvement of P2Y2 metabotropic receptors in ATP-induced transient receptor potential vanilloid receptor 1-mediated thermal hypersensitivity. *J. Neurosci.* 23, 6058–6062.

52. Sugiura, T., Tominaga, M., Katsuya, H., and Mizumura, K. (2002). Bradykinin lowers the threshold temperature for heat activation of vanilloid receptor 1. *J. Neurophysiol.* 88, 544–548.

53. Tominaga, M., Wada, M., and Masu, M. (2001). Potentiation of capsaicin receptor activity by metabotropic ATP receptors as a possible mechanism for ATP-evoked pain and hyperalgesia. *Proc. Natl. Acad. Sci. USA* 98, 6951–6956.

54. Bhave, G., Hu, H. J., Glauner, K. S., Zhu, W., Wang, H., Brasier, D. J., Oxford, G. S., and Gereau, R. W. (2003). Protein kinase C phosphorylation sensitizes but does not activate the capsaicin receptor transient receptor potential vanilloid 1 (TRPV1). *Proc. Natl. Acad. Sci. USA* 100, 12480–12485.

55. Numazaki, M., Tominaga, T., Toyooka, H., and Tominaga, M. (2002). Direct phosphorylation of capsaicin receptor VR1 by protein kinase Cepsilon and identification of two target serine residues. *J. Biol. Chem.* 277, 13375–13378.

56. Distler, C., Rathee, P. K., Lips, K. S., Obreja, O., Neuhuber, W., and Kress, M. (2003). Fast Ca^{2+}-induced potentiation of heat-activated ionic currents requires cAMP/PKA signaling and functional AKAP anchoring. *J. Neurophysiol.* 89, 2499–2505.

57. Gu, Q., Kwong, K., and Lee, L. Y. (2003). Ca^{2+} transient evoked by chemical stimulation is enhanced by PGE2 in vagal sensory neurons: Role of cAMP/PKA signaling pathway. *J. Neurophysiol.* 89, 1985–1993.

58. Lopshire, J. C., and Nicol, G. D. (1998). The cAMP transduction cascade mediates the prostaglandin E2 enhancement of the capsaicin-elicited current in rat sensory neurons: Whole-cell and single-channel studies. *J. Neurosci.* 18, 6081–6092.

59. Pitchford, S., and Levine, J. D. (1991). Prostaglandins sensitize nociceptors in cell culture. *Neurosci. Lett.* 132, 105–108.

60. Smith, J. A., Davis, C. L., and Burgess, G. M. (2000). Prostaglandin E2-induced sensitization of bradykinin-evoked responses in rat dorsal root ganglion neurons is mediated by cAMP-dependent protein kinase A. *Eur. J. Neurosci.* 12, 3250–3258.

61. Bhave, G., Zhu, W., Wang, H., Brasier, D. J., Oxford, G. S., and Gereau, R. W. (2002). cAMP-dependent protein kinase regulates desensitization of the capsaicin receptor (VR1) by direct phosphorylation. *Neuron* 35, 721–731.

62. De Petrocellis, L., Harrison, S., Bisogno, T., Tognetto, M., Brandi, I., Smith, G. D., Creminon, C., Davis, J. B., Geppetti, P., and Di Marzo, V. (2001). The vanilloid receptor (VR1)-mediated effects of anandamide are potently enhanced by the cAMP-dependent protein kinase. *J. Neurochem.* 77, 1660–1663.

63. Hu, H. J., Bhave, G., and Gereau, R. W. (2002). Prostaglandin and protein kinase A-dependent modulation of vanilloid receptor function by metabotropic glutamate receptor 5: Potential mechanism for thermal hyperalgesia. *J. Neurosci.* 22, 7444–7452.

64. Rathee, P. K., Distler, C., Obreja, O., Neuhuber, W., Wang, G. K., Wang, S. Y., Nau, C., and Kress, M. (2002). PKA/AKAP/VR-1 module: A common link of Gs-mediated signaling to thermal hyperalgesia. *J. Neurosci.* 22, 4740–4745.

65. Sugiuar, T., Bielefeldt, K., and Gebhart, G. F. (2004). TRPV1 function in mouse colon sensory neurons is enhanced by metabotropic 5-hydroxytryptamine receptor activation. *J. Neurosci.* 24, 9521–9530.

66. Prescott, E. D., and Julius, D. (2003). A modular PIP2 binding site as a determinant of capsaicin receptor sensitivity. *Science* 300, 1284–1288.

67. Chuang, H. H., Prescott, E. D., Kong, H., Shields, S., Jordt, S. E., Basbaum, A. I., Chao, M. V., and Julius, D. (2001). Bradykinin and nerve growth factor release the capsaicin receptor from PtdIns(4,5)P2-mediated inhibition. *Nature* 411, 957–962.

68. Jung, J., Shin, J. S., Lee, S. Y., Hwang, S. W., Koo, J., Cho, H., and Oh, U. (2004). Phosphorylation of vanilloid receptor 1 by Ca^{2+}/calmodulin-dependent kinase II regulates its vanilloid binding. *J. Biol. Chem.* 279, 7048–7054.

69. Zhuang, Z. Y., Xu, H., Clapham, D. E., and Ji, R. R. (2004). Phosphatidylinositol 3-kinase activates ERK in primary sensory neurons and mediates inflammatory heat hyperalgesia through TRPV1 sensitization. *J. Neurosci.* 24, 8300–8309.

70. Piper, A. S., Yeats, J. C., Bevan, S., and Docherty, R. J. (1999). A study of the voltage dependence of capsaicin-activated membrane currents in rat sensory neurones before and after acute desensitization. *J. Physiol.* 518(Pt. 3), 721–733.

71. Liu, L., and Simon, S. A. (1996). Capsaicin-induced currents with distinct desensitization and Ca^{2+} dependence in rat trigeminal ganglion cells. *J. Neurophysiol.* 75, 1503–1514.

72. Koplas, P. A., Rosenberg, R. L., and Oxford, G. S. (1997). The role of calcium in the desensitization of capsaicin responses in rat dorsal root ganglion neurons. *J. Neurosci.* 17, 3525–3537.

73. Docherty, R. J., Yeats, J. C., Bevan, S., and Boddeke, H. W. (1996). Inhibition of calcineurin inhibits the desensitization of capsaicin-evoked currents in cultured dorsal root ganglion neurones from adult rats. *Pflugers Arch.* 431, 828–837.

74. Bernstein, J. E. (1987). Capsaicin in the treatment of dermatologic disease. *Cutis* 39, 352–353.

75. Maggi, C. A. (1991). Capsaicin and primary afferent neurons: From basic science to human therapy? *J. Auton. Nerv. Syst.* 33, 1–14.

76. Numazaki, M., Tominaga, T., Takeuchi, K., Murayama, N., Toyooka, H., and Tominaga, M. (2003). Structural determinant of TRPV1 desensitization interacts with calmodulin. *Proc. Natl. Acad. Sci. USA* 100, 8002–8006.

77. Rosenbaum, T., Gordon-Shaag, A., Munari, M., and Gordon, S. E. (2004). Ca^{2+}/calmodulin modulates TRPV1 activation by capsaicin. *J. Gen. Physiol.* 123, 53–62.

78. Molday, R. S. (1996). Calmodulin regulation of cyclic-nucleotide-gated channels. *Curr. Opin. Neurobiol.* 6, 445–452.

79. Peterson, B. Z., DeMaria, C. D., Adelman, J. P., and Yue, D. T. (1999). Calmodulin is the Ca^{2+} sensor for Ca^{2+}-dependent inactivation of L-type calcium channels. *Neuron* 22, 549–558.

80. Zuhlke, R. D., Pitt, G. S., Deisseroth, K., Tsien, R. W., and Reuter, H. (1999). Calmodulin supports both inactivation and facilitation of L-type calcium channels. *Nature* 399, 159–162.

81. Lee, A., Wong, S. T., Gallagher, D., Li, B., Storm, D. R., Scheuer, T., and Catterall, W. A. (1999). Ca^{2+}/calmodulin binds to and modulates P/Q-type calcium channels. *Nature* 399, 155–159.

82. Ehlers, M. D., Zhang, S., Bernhadt, J. P., and Huganir, R. L. (1996). Inactivation of NMDA receptors by direct interaction of calmodulin with the NR1 subunit. *Cell* 84, 745–755.

83. Zhang, S., Ehlers, M. D., Bernhardt, J. P., Su, C. T., and Huganir, R. L. (1998). Calmodulin mediates calcium-dependent inactivation of *N*-methyl-D-aspartate receptors. *Neuron* 21, 443–453.

84. Chevesich, J., Kreuz, A. J., and Montell, C. (1997). Requirement for the PDZ domain protein, INAD, for localization of the TRP store-operated channel to a signaling complex. *Neuron* 18, 95–105.

85. Scott, K., Sun, Y., Beckingham, K., and Zuker, C. S. (1997). Calmodulin regulation of *Drosophila* light-activated channels and receptor function mediates termination of the light response in vivo. *Cell* 91, 375–383.

86. Davis, J. B., Gray, J., Gunthorpe, M. J., Hatcher, J. P., Davey, P. T., Overend, P., Harries, M. H., Latcham, J., Clapham, C., Atkinson, K., Hughes, S. A., Rance, K., Grau, E., Harper, A. J., Pugh, P. L., Rogers, D. C., Bingham, S., Randall, A., and

Sheardown, S. A. (2000). Vanilloid receptor-1 is essential for inflammatory thermal hyperalgesia. *Nature* 405, 183–187.

87. Hudson, L. J., Bevan, S., Wotherspoon, G., Gentry, C., Fox, A., and Winter, J. (2001). VR1 protein expression increases in undamaged DRG neurons after partial nerve injury. *Eur. J. Neurosci.* 13, 2105–2114.

88. Fukuoka, T., Tokunaga, A., Tachibana, T., Dai, Y., Yamanaka, H., and Noguchi, K. (2002). VR1, but not P2X(3), increases in the spared L4 DRG in rats with L5 spinal nerve ligation. *Pain* 99, 111–120.

89. Caterina, M. J., Rosen, T. A., Tominaga, M., Brake, A. J., and Julius, D. (1999). A capsaicin-receptor homologue with a high threshold for noxious heat. *Nature* 398, 436–441.

90. Ahluwalia, J., Rang, H., and Nagy, I. (2002). The putative role of vanilloid receptor-like protein-1 in mediating high threshold noxious heat-sensitivity in rat cultured primary sensory neurons. *Eur. J. Neurosci.* 16, 1483–1489.

91. Lewinter, R. D., Skinner, K., Julius, D., and Basbaum, A. I. (2004). Immunoreactive TRPV-2 (VRL-1), a capsaicin receptor homolog, in the spinal cord of the rat. *J. Comp. Neurol.* 470, 400–408.

92. Ma, Q. P. (2001). Vanilloid receptor homologue, VRL1, is expressed by both A- and C-fiber sensory neurons. *Neuroreport* 12, 3693–3695.

93. Treede, R. D., Meyer, R. A., Raja, S. N., and Campbell, J. N. (1995). Evidence for two different heat transduction mechanisms in nociceptive primary afferents innervating monkey skin. *J. Physiol.* 483(Pt. 3), 747–758.

94. Woodbury, C. J., Zwick, M., Wang, S., Lawson, J. J., Caterina, M. J., Koltzenburg, M., Albers, K. M., Koerber, H. R., and Davis, B. M. (2004). Nociceptors lacking TRPV1 and TRPV2 have normal heat responses. *J. Neurosci.* 24, 6410–6415.

95. Watanabe, H., Vriens, J., Suh, S. H., Benham, C. D., Droogmans, G., and Nilius, B. (2002). Heat-evoked activation of TRPV4 channels in a HEK293 cell expression system and in native mouse aorta endothelial cells. *J. Biol. Chem.* 277, 47044–47051.

96. Xu, H., Ramsey, I. S., Kotecha, S. A., Moran, M. M., Chong, J. A., Lawson, D., Ge, P., Lilly, J., Silos-Santiago, I., Xie, Y., DiStefano, P. S., Curtis, R., and Clapham, D. E. (2002). TRPV3 is a calcium-permeable temperature-sensitive cation channel. *Nature* 418, 181–186.

97. Smith, G. D., Gunthorpe, M. J., Kelsell, R. E., Hayes, P. D., Reilly, P., Facer, P., Wright, J. E., Jerman, J. C., Walhin, J. P., Ooi, L., Egerton, J., Charles, K. J., Smart, D., Randall, A. D., Anand, P., and Davis, J. B. (2002). TRPV3 is a temperature-sensitive vanilloid receptor-like protein. *Nature* 418, 186–190.

98. Peier, A. M., Reeve, A. J., Andersson, D. A., Moqrich, A., Earley, T. J., Hergarden, A. C., Story, G. M., Colley, S., Hogenesch, J. B., McIntyre, P., Bevan, S., and Patapoutian, A. (2002). A heat-sensitive TRP channel expressed in keratinocytes. *Science* 296, 2046–2049.

99. Guler, A. D., Lee, H., Iida, T., Shimizu, I., Tominaga, M., and Caterina, M. (2002). Heat-evoked activation of the ion channel, TRPV4. *J. Neurosci.* 22, 6408–6414.

100. Liedtke, W., Choe, Y., Marti-Renom, M. A., Bell, A. M., Denis, C. S., Sali, A., Hudspeth, A. J., Friedman, J. M., and Heller, S. (2000). Vanilloid receptor-related osmotically activated channel (VR-OAC), a candidate vertebrate osmoreceptor. *Cell* 103, 525–535.

101. Strotmann, R., Harteneck, C., Nunnenmacher, K., Schultz, G., and Plant, T. D. (2000). OTRPC4, a nonselective cation channel that confers sensitivity to extracellular osmolarity. *Nat. Cell. Biol.* 2, 695–702.

102. Suzuki, M., Mizuno, A., Kodaira, K., and Imai, M. (2003). Impaired pressure sensation in mice lacking TRPV4. *J. Biol. Chem.* 278, 22664–22668.
103. Alessandri-Haber, N., Dina, O. A., Yeh, J. J., Parada, C. A., Reichling, D. B., and Levine, J. D. (2004). Transient receptor potential vanilloid 4 is essential in chemotherapy-induced neuropathic pain in the rat. *J. Neurosci.* 24, 4444–4452.
104. Alessandri-Haber, N., Yeh, J. J., Boyd, A. E., Parada, C. A., Chen, X., Reichling, D. B., and Levine, J. D. (2003). Hypotonicity induces TRPV4-mediated nociception in rat. *Neuron* 39, 497–511.

22

OPIOID RECEPTORS

GAVRIL W. PASTERNAK

Memorial Sloan-Kettering Cancer Center, Laboratory of Molecular Neuropharmacology, New York, New York

22.1	Introduction	745
22.2	Endogenous Opioids	746
	22.2.1 Enkephalins	746
	22.2.2 Dynorphins	747
	22.2.3 β-Endorphin	747
	22.2.4 Orphanin FQ/Nociception	748
22.3	Opioid Receptors	748
	22.3.1 μ Receptors	748
	22.3.2 δ Receptors	751
	22.3.3 κ Receptors	751
22.4	Opioid Receptor Dimerization	752
22.5	Orphanin FQ/Nociceptin and its Receptor	752
22.6	Conclusions	752
	References	753

22.1 INTRODUCTION

The use of opium, a product of the poppy plant, goes back thousands of years. The major analgesic components of opium are morphine and codeine, which are present in relatively high concentrations. Thebaine is another important compound present in opium. Although it is not active, it is widely used to synthesize a number of clinically important opioid analgesics. Following the isolation and purification of morphine and codeine, medicinal chemists synthesized thousands of analogs in an effort to avoid the side effects, which include sedation, respiratory depression, constipation, and abuse potential. Although they were not able to dissociate these actions, they did establish rigid structure–activity relationships for these drugs which, in turn, led to the proposal of distinct binding sites, or receptors, years before they were demonstrated experimentally in 1973 [1–3]. These binding sites were restricted

---

Handbook of Contemporary Neuropharmacology, Edited by David R. Sibley, Israel Hanin, Michael Kuhar, and Phil Skolnick. Copyright © 2007 John Wiley & Sons, Inc.

to nervous tissue and were highly selective for morphine and morphine-like agents. Since then, we have extended our understanding of these receptors and their endogenous ligands and have identified three classes of opioid receptors [4].

22.2 ENDOGENOUS OPIOIDS

The demonstration of opioid receptors quickly led a number of investigators to look for their endogenous ligands, eventually leading to the isolation and identification of a series of opioid peptides (Table 22.1) [5–10]. They fall into three families based upon their precursor peptides and the selectivity for the members of the opioid receptor classes. Each opioid peptide family is generated from a distinct precursor peptide encoded by three different genes. Yet, all the active opioid peptides contain the sequence Tyr–Gly–Gly–Phe–Leu or Tyr–Gly–Gly–Phe–Met as their first five amino acids. The only exception are the endomorphins (Table 22.1). These peptides, which have been isolated from brain [11], are highly μ selective. However, it is not clear whether they are synthesized de novo or generated from a precursor.

22.2.1 Enkephalins

The enkephalins were the first opioid peptides identified, and they played a major role in establishing the explosion within the field of neuropeptides. The enkephalins consist of a pair of pentapeptides that share the same first four amino acids, differing at the fifth with either a methionine (Met^5-enkephalin) or a leucine (Leu^5-enkephalin). They have distinct regional distributions within the brain and are the endogenous ligands for the δ receptors (see below).

Studies of the enkephalins were initially hindered by their lability, due in large part by the actions of peptidases. The demonstration that they could be stabilized by substituting a D-amino acid at position 2 led to the generation of a host of stabilized

TABLE 22.1 Opioid and Related Peptides[a]

[Leu^5]enkephalin	**Tyr–Gly–Gly–Phe–Leu**
[Met^5]enkephalin	**Tyr–Gly–Gly–Phe–Met**
Dynorphin A	**Tyr–Gly–Gly–Phe–Leu**–Arg–Arg–Ile–Arg–Pro–Lys–Leu–Lys–Trp–Asp–Asn–Gln
Dynorphin B	**Tyr–Gly–Gly–Phe–Leu**–Arg–Arg–Gln–Phe–Lys–Val–Val–Thr
α–Neoendorphin	**Tyr–Gly–Gly–Phe–Leu**–Arg–Lys–Tyr–Pro–Lys
β–Neoendorphin	**Tyr–Gly–Gly–Phe–Leu**–Arg–Lys–Tyr–Pro
β–Endorphin	**Tyr–Gly–Gly–Phe–Met**–Thr–Ser–Glu–Lys–Ser–Gln–Thr–Pro–Leu–Val–Thr–Leu–Phe–Lys–Asn–Ala–Ile–Ile–Lys–Asn–Ala–Tyr–Lys–Lys–Gly–Glu
Endomorphin-1	Tyr–Pro–Trp–Phe–NH_2
Endomorphin-2	Tyr–Pro–Phe–Phe–NH_2
Orphanin FQ/ nociceptin	**Phe–Gly–Gly–Phe**–Thr–Gly–Ala–Arg–Lys–Ser–Ala–Arg–Lys–Leu–Ala–Asp–Glu

[a]Common sequences are highlighted.

ENDOGENOUS OPIOIDS   747

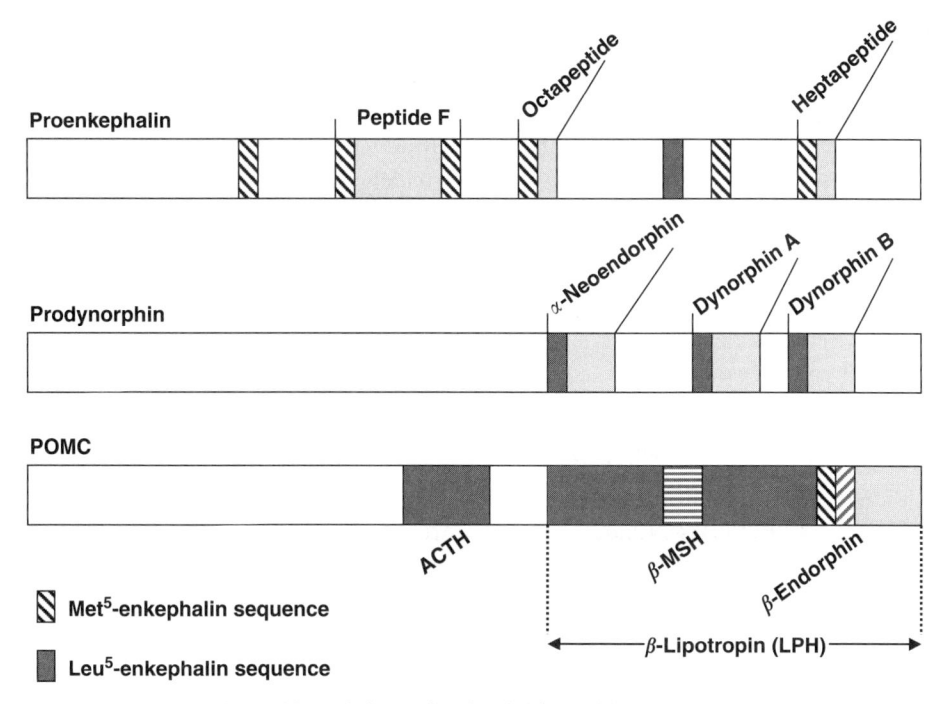

Figure 22.1 Schematic of opioid peptide precursors.

derivatives. Using these compounds, investigators have established that the enkephalins can produce analgesia through receptor mechanisms distinct from those of morphine.

The enkephalins are generated from a larger precursor that contains a number of copies of the enkephalins (Fig. 22.1). There are six copies of Met^5-enkephalin and one copy of Leu^5-enkephalin. However, several of the Met^5-enkephalin may actually be contained in larger peptides (peptide F, the octapeptide, and the heptapeptide). It is not known if these extended peptides are active or simply are broken down to Met^5 enkephalin. Thus, their significance remains unknown.

22.2.2 Dynorphins

There are three major peptides within this family: α-neoendorphin, dynorphin A, and dynorphin B. Each contains the sequence of Leu^5-enkephalin as the first five amino acids. Dynorphin A is the endogenous ligand for κ receptors, specifically κ$_1$. Although dynorphin B and α-neoendorphin also label κ receptors, there has been the suggestion that they may have a slightly different binding selectivity that may be due to the existence of κ receptor subtypes [12]. All three peptides also elicit analgesia through unique receptor mechanisms.

22.2.3 β-Endorphin

β-Endorphin has 31 amino acids, making it the largest of the opioid peptides. Yet, its N-terminus still contains the Met enkephalin sequence. As with dynorphin, there originally were questions as to whether it was pharmacologically relevant or simply the precursor of Met^5-enkephalin. That question was answered with the identification of the enkephalin precursor as well as that for β-endorphin, pro-opiomelanocortin (POMC), which also generates the important peptides adrenocorticotropic hormone (ACTH) and melanocyte-stimulating hormones α-MSH and β-MSH. Unlike the other opioid peptides that are widely distributed within the central nervous system, POMC is synthesized within the brain only in the arcuate nucleus, further distinguishing it from the enkephalins. However, the major location of POMC and its peptides is within the pituitary, where β-endorphin has been shown to be coreleased with ACTH, an important stress hormone responsible for the release of cortisol. This association has suggested the possibility that β-endorphin may be involved with stress analgesia.

22.2.4 Orphanin FQ/Nociception

Although not formally a member of the opioid peptide family, orphanin FQ/nociception (OFQ/N) is strikingly similar in structure to dynorphin A. Like dynorphin A, OFQ/N contains 17 amino acids, but it contains phenylalanine at position 1 instead of tyrosine. OFQ/N labels the opioid receptor-like 1 (ORL1) receptor with very high affinity but does not compete opioid receptor binding. However, if ORL1 receptors are coexpressed with an opioid receptor, OFQ/N acquires the ability to compete opioid binding, presumably due to dimerization of the two receptor classes. Thus, it appears to be closely related to opioids, if not formally one.

22.3 OPIOID RECEPTORS

Opioid receptors were initially proposed based upon the structure–activity relationships of literally hundreds of morphine derivatives. Indeed, the concept of opiate receptors was well entrenched prior to their actual identification in binding assays in 1973 [1–4]. Three major families of opioid receptors were proposed from pharmacological studies and then confirmed in binding assays and then through cloning. Studies in the dog let Martin to propose μ (morphine-preferring) and κ (ketocyclazocine-preferring) receptors, which display high affinity for the dynorphins [13]. This was followed by the identification of δ receptors selective for the enkephalins [5, 14].

22.3.1 μ Receptors

Most of the analgesics that we use to treat pain are morphine-like and act, at least in part, through μ receptors. The μ receptors have a variety of actions. Of these, analgesia is the most commonly desired. Opioid analgesia is particularly intriguing since it does not interfere with primary sensations. Patients retain the ability to feel light touch, temperature, sharp/dull, and vibration, unlike therapy with local anesthetics. Instead, the opiates diminish the subjective "hurt" associated with pain, making these agents quite unique and valuable.

Continued use of morphine-like drugs leads to tolerance, which is defined as a diminished response with a continued dose of a drug or the need to increase the drug dose over time to maintain a response. With the opioids, this is easily seen for all opioid actions, including analgesia, although the rate to which tolerance develops for each one action may vary. Dependence is also associated with μ-opioid use. Dependence is seen through the expression of withdrawal upon the abrupt discontinuation of the opioid or the administration of an opioid antagonist to a subject who has been maintained on an opioid for an extended period of time. The length of time and the dose of the drug determine the severity of the withdrawal syndrome, which in turn is an indication of the degree of dependence. It is important to distinguish between dependence and addiction. Whereas dependence is a physiological response seen in every subject receiving the drugs, addiction is a behavioral drug-seeking response which is actually quite rare when these drugs are used for legitimate medical purposes.

The μ opioids induce a variety of other actions, including sedation, respiratory depression, and inhibition of gastrointestinal transit. Although they have been used to treat diarrhea, this action is more commonly a problematic side-effect manifested as constipation, particularly in pain patients. Sedation is another sideeffect that can be limiting in the use of these agents. Indeed, morphine was named after the Morpheus, who was the god of sleep.

The μ-opiate receptor was first demonstrated biochemically in 1973 with the demonstration of highly selective opioid binding to membranes from the brain [1–3]. Since then, the receptor has been cloned [15–18] and has been identified as a member of the G-protein-coupled receptor family [19]. Like other G-protein-coupled receptors, μ-opioid receptors have seven transmembrane domains with an extracellular N-terminus and an intracellular C-terminus (Fig 22.2a). Following the binding of an opioid to the receptor, the receptor activates a G-protein which then induces a signaling cascade. Opioid receptors are typically inhibitory and act predominantly through G_i and G_o classes of G-proteins.

The concept of multiple μ-opiate receptors goes back 25 years [20] and is particularly important in understanding the clinical actions of these drugs [21, 22]. From the clinical perspective, multiple μ receptors help explain opioid rotation and the variability in responses, observations difficult to reconcile with a single μ-opioid receptor. In opioid rotation, patients highly tolerant to one μ opiate can be switched to a different μ opiate with a markedly enhanced analgesic response to the second drug [23]. This is due to incomplete cross tolerance, consistent with slight differences in the receptor mechanism actions of the two agents. In terms of the sensitivity, some patients respond far better to one μ opioid than another. Both observations can be replicated in animal models. In CXBK mice, morphine is a very weak analgesic with a potency 5- to 10-fold less sensitive than the traditional CD-1 animal. On the other hand, other μ opioids, such as methadone, fentanyl, and heroin, retain full analgesic activity in the CXBK animal, implying that their actions are distinct from those of morphine [4, 22].

The suggestion of multiple μ-opioid receptors has now been confirmed at the molecular level through the identification of a number of splice variants of the μ-opioid receptor MOR-1 in mice, rats, and humans [24–30] (Fig. 22.2b). MOR-1, the μ-opiate receptor that was cloned in 1993, has four exons. Exons 1, 2, and 3 encode the seven transmembrane domains of the receptor while exon 4 encodes the last 12 amino acids in the C-terminus. The major series of splice variants in all three species involve variants that are alternatively spliced downstream of exon 3, with a variety of different exons in place of exon 4. The differences among these variants is restricted to the tip of the C-terminus (Fig. 22.2c). Although some variants share

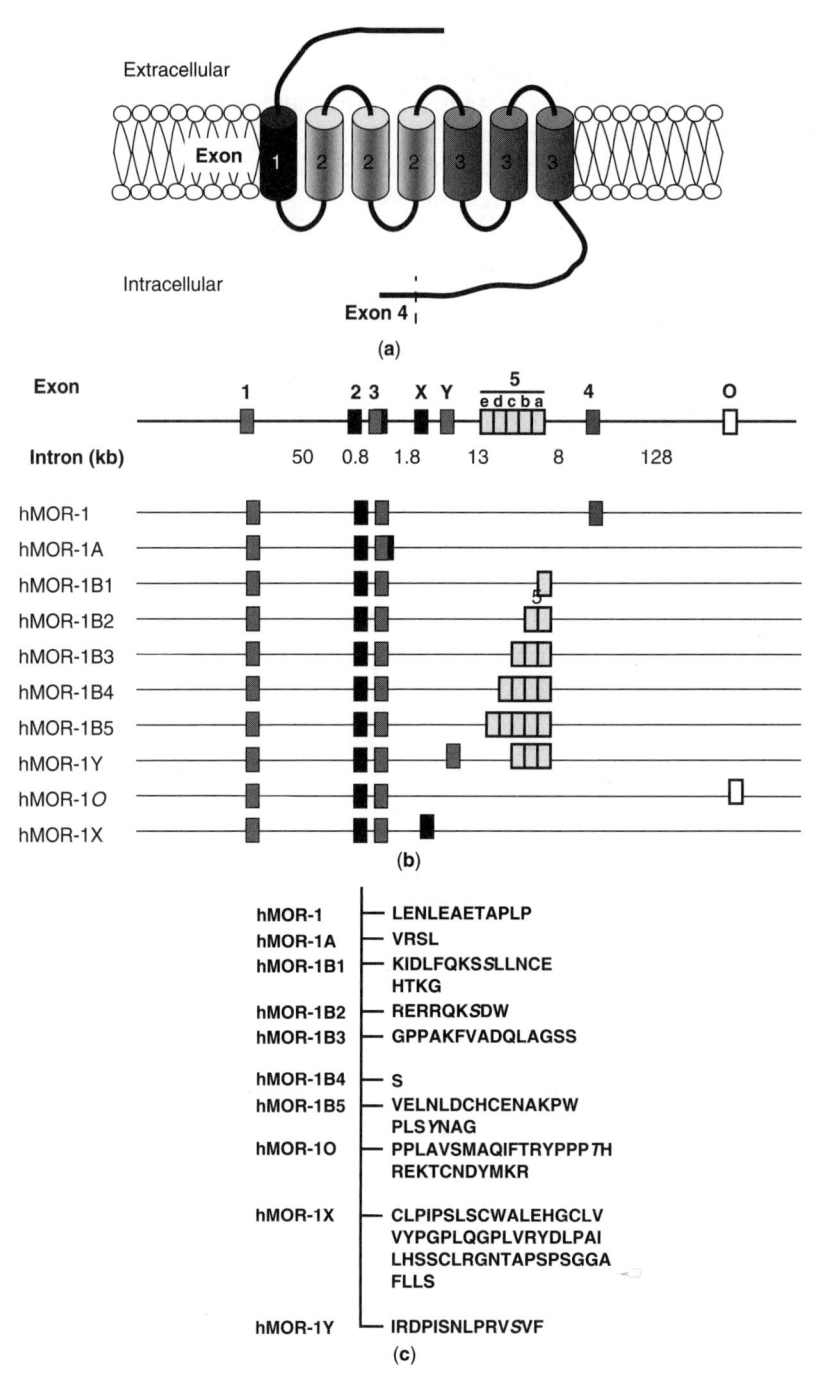

Figure 22.2 Schematic of MOR-1 (a) MOR-1 within membrane. The exons responsible for coding the different regions are indicated. (b) Alternative splicing of MOR-1 in humans. Note that only full-length variants are shown, which involve splicing at the 3′ end. There is another series of 5′spliced variants. (c) Amino acid sequences of alternatively spliced C-terminus of human MOR-1 variants downstream from exon 3.

these spliced exons, all the amino acid sequences downstream of exon 3 are unique and many are identical or highly homologous among species. The binding pockets responsible for the docking of the opioid ligands within the receptor are defined by the seven transmembrane domains. Thus, all these C-terminus splice variants have identical binding pockets, explaining their similar affinities for μ opioids and their high selectivity for μ drugs. However, these changes in the C-terminus do influence the transduction systems and impact on both the efficacy and potency of drugs acting through them [24–26, 29, 31]. In mice, these C-terminus variants also have different distributions regionally and even within cells [32–35]. Furthermore, one variant, MOR-1C, is associated with calcitonin gene–related peptide (CGRP) while MOR-1 is not [32].

In mice, and possibly humans and rats, there is a second series of splice variants at the N-terminus that generate truncated proteins that lack all seven transmembrane domains seen in MOR-1 [28]. The potential pharmacological significance of these variants is not clear, but they have been demonstrated in the brain at both the messenger RNA (mRNA) and protein levels and there are indications that they may be pharmacologically irrelevant.

22.3.2 δ Receptors

The δ receptors were first proposed from studies examining the pharmacology of the enkephalins [14], which are their endogenous ligand. Since then a wide range of synthetic peptides and nonpeptides that are selective for δ receptors have been developed and widely used to characterize the actions of these receptors in animal models. However, there are not any clinically available δ ligands at present and our understanding of their actions in humans is not yet well understood.

The δ receptors are members of the G-protein-coupled receptor family and show marked homology to the μ receptor, particularly in the transmembrane domains. However, the δ receptors are unique in terms of their binding selectivity and are readily distinguished from μ receptors. They are expressed in different regions of the brain and are presumably involved in a variety of distinct physiological responses.

The δ-opioid receptor DOR-1 also has seven transmembrane domains encoded by three exons [36, 37]. Unlike MOR-1, the C-terminus of DOR-1 ends within the third coding exon and there is no C-terminus splicing. Several splice variants of DOR-1 have been reported, but they do not appear to be pharmacologically relevant [38, 39].

22.3.3 κ Receptors

The κ receptors were first proposed from the benzomorphan ketocyclazocine, but we now know that their endogenous ligand is dynorphin A. The κ ligands have been examined clinically and several are available, including pentazocine, nalorphine, and nalbuphine. These early κ drugs were mixed κ agonists–μ antagonists. Studies with more selective κ drugs have confirmed their analgesic activity, but the drugs proved problematic due to their psychotomimetic effects, actions that were also seen with the mixed agonist–antagonist drugs. The highly selective κ drugs that were in clinical trials have been withdrawn.

The κ receptors are also members of the G-protein-coupled receptor family. They were cloned soon after the δ receptors [40–42]. The cloned κ-opioid receptor KOR-1 has three coding exons that encode a seven-transmembrane receptor and the transmembrane domains have high homology with the other members of the opioid receptor family. However, its binding selectivity and distribution within the brain are distinct.

22.4 OPIOID RECEPTOR DIMERIZATION

G-protein-coupled receptors have an additional layer of complexity due to their tendency to associate with themselves (homodimers) or other G-protein-coupled receptors (heterodimers) [43, 44]. Similar observations have been made with opioid receptors [45–48]. In some cases, heterodimers take on pharmacological characteristics unlike those of either receptor expressed alone [46–48]. Thus, this ability to interact with additional receptors to generate pharmacologically unique dimers extends the number of potentially important opioid receptors manyfold. To make matters even more difficult, opioid receptors also can associate with receptors of other classes, as shown between opioid and ß-adrenergic and α-adrenergic receptors [49, 50]. Thus, the presence of three opioid receptors can lead to a host of novel receptor classes due to interactions with other receptors.

22.5 ORPHANIN FQ/NOCICEPTIN AND ITS RECEPTOR

There is a fourth receptor with high homology to the traditional opioid receptors, termed ORL-1 [51–56], which is the receptor for a novel peptide termed nociceptin or orphanin FQ [57, 58]. This 17-amino-acid peptide is distinct from the opioid peptides in that its first amino acid is phenylalanine rather than tyrosine. It displays no appreciable affinity for the traditional opiate receptors. However, the high homology of the ORL-1 receptor with the opioid receptors suggests a common ancestry. Interestingly, OFQ/N is important in the modulation of pain. At low concentrations. OFQ/N is hyperalgesic and enhances pain perception, whereas higher doses are analgesic. The analgesic actions of OFQ/N are reversed by opioid antagonists, which is somewhat unexpected since OFQ/N itself does not bind to opioid receptors. However, when coexpressed, MOR-1 and ORL-1 receptors dimerize and display a unique pharmacological profile in which opioids and OFQ/N can displace each other with a high potency not seen when each receptor is displayed alone [48].

22.6 CONCLUSIONS

The opiate peptides and opiate receptors comprise a highly complex system within the central nervous system (CNS). Although intimately involved with analgesia and pain modulation, they have a host of other functions. Three classes of opioid receptors were proposed from classical pharmacological studies and each family has been cloned. Early work proposing multiple μ-opioid receptors also have been confirmed with the isolation and identification of a host of splice variants of the μ-opioid receptor MOR-1. The complexity of the opioid system is further illustrated by the tendency of opioid receptors to dimerize and associate with other opioid receptors as well as unrelated classes of G-protein-coupled receptors.

REFERENCES

1. Pert, C. B., and Snyder, S. H. (1973). Opiate receptor: Demonstration in nervous tissue. *Science* 179, 1011–1014.
2. Simon, E. J., Hiller, J. M., and Edelman, I. (1973). Stereospecific binding of the potent narcotic analgesic [^{3}H]etorphine to rat-brain homogenate. *Proc. Natl. Acad. Sci. USA* 70, 1947–1949.
3. Terenius, L. (1973). Stereospecific interaction between narcotic analgesics and a synaptic plasma membrane fraction of rat cerebral cortex. *Acta Pharmacol. Toxicol.* 32, 317–320.
4. Snyder, S. H., and Pasternak, G. W. (2003). Historical review: Opioid receptors. *Trends Pharmacol. Sci.* 24, 198–205.
5. Hughes, J., Smith, T. W., Kosterlitz, H. W., Fothergill, L. A., Morgan, B. A., and Morris, H. R. (1975). Identification of two related pentapeptides from the brain with potent opiate agonist activity. *Nature* 258, 577–579.
6. Snyder, S. H. and Matthysse, S. (1975). *Opiate Receptor Mechanisms, Vol. 13: Opiate Receptor Mechanisms*. MIT Press, Boston.
7. Terenius, L., and Wahlstrom, A. (1975). Search for an endogenous ligand for the opiate receptor. *Acta Physiol. Scand.* 94, 74–81.
8. Pasternak, G. W., Goodman, R., and Snyder, S. H. (1975). An endogenous morphine like factor in mammalian brain. *Life Sci.* 16, 1765–1769.
9. Evans, C. J., Hammond, D. L., and Frederickson, R. C. A. (1988). The opioid peptides In *The Opiate Receptors*. G. W. Pasternak, Ed. Humana, Clifton, NJ, pp. 23–74.
10. Reisine, T., and Pasternak, G. W. (1996). Opioid analgesics and antagonists In *Goodman & Gilman's: The Pharmacological Basis of Therapeutics*. J. G. Hardman, and L. E. Limbird, Eds. McGraw-Hill, New York, pp. 521–556.
11. Zadina, J. E., Hackler, L., Ge, L. J., and Kastin, A. J. (1997). A potent and selective endogenous agonist for the μ-opiate receptor. *Nature* 386, 499–502.
12. Clark, J. A., Liu, L., Price, M., Hersh, B., Edelson, M., and Pasternak, G. W. (1989). Kappa opiate receptor multiplicity: Evidence for two U50,488-sensitive kappa$_1$ subtypes and a novel kappa$_3$ subtype. *J. Pharmacol. Exp. Ther.* 251, 461–468.
13. Martin, W. R., Eades, C. G., Thompson, J. A., Huppler, R. E., and Gilbert, P. E. (1976). The effects of morphine and nalorphine-like drugs in the nondependent and morphine-dependent chronic spinal dog. *J. Pharmacol. Exp. Ther.* 197, 517–1977.
14. Lord , J. A. H., Waterfield , A. A., Hughes , J., and Kosterlitz , H. W. (1977). Endogenous opioid peptides. Multiple agonists and receptors. *Nature* 267, 495–499.
15. Chen, Y., Mestek, A., Liu, J., Hurley, J. A., and Yu, L. (1993). Molecular cloning and functional expression of a μ-opioid receptor from rat brain. *Mol. Pharmacol.* 44, 8–12.
16. Eppler, C. M., Hulmes, J. D., Wang, J.-B., Johnson, B., Corbett, M., Luthin, D. R., Uhl, G. R., and Linden, J. (1993). Purification and partial amino acid sequence of a μ opioid receptor from rat brain. *J. Biol. Chem.* 268, 26447–26451.
17. Thompson, R. C., Mansour, A., Akil, H., and Watson, S. J. (1993). Cloning and pharmacological characterization of a rat μ opioid receptor. *Neuron* 11, 903–913.
18. Wang, J. B., Imai, Y., Eppler, C. M., Gregor, P., Spivak, C. E., and Uhl, G. R. (1993). μ Opiate receptor: cDNA cloning and expression. *Proc. Natl. Acad. Sci. USA* 90, 10230–10234.

19. Childers, S. R., and Snyder, S. H. (1978). Guanine nucleotides differentiate agonist and antagonist interactions with opiate receptors. *Life Sci.* 23, 759–762.
20. Wolozin, B. L., and Pasternak, G. W. (1981). Classification of multiple morphine and enkephalin binding sites in the central nervous system. *Proc. Natl. Acad. Sci. USA* 78, 6181–6185.
21. Pasternak, G. W. (2005). Molecular biology of opioid analgesia. *J. Pain Symptom Manag.* 29, S2–S9.
22. Pasternak, G. W. (2004). Multiple opiate receptors: Deja vu all over again. *Neuropharmacology* 47(Suppl. 1), 312–323.
23. Cherny, N., Ripamonti, C., Pereira, J., Davis, C., Fallon, M., McQuay, H., Mercadante, S., Pasternak, G., and Ventafridda, V. (2001). Strategies to manage the adverse effects of oral morphine: An evidence-based report. *J. Clin. Oncol.* 19, 2542–2554.
24. Pan, L., Xu, J., Yu, R., Xu, M., Pan, Y. X., and Pasternak, G. W. (2005). Identification and characterization of six new alternatively spliced variants of the human mu opioid receptor gene, *Oprm*. *Neuroscience* 133, 209–220.
25. Pan, Y. X., Xu, J., Bolan, E., Moskowitz, H. S., Xu, M., and Pasternak, G. W. (2005). Identification of four novel exon 5 splice variants of the mouse mu-opioid receptor gene: Functional consequences of C-terminal splicing. *Mol. Pharmacol.* 68, 866–875.
26. Pasternak, D. A., Pan, L., Xu, J., Yu, R., Xu, M., Pasternak, G. W., and Pan, Y.-X. (2004). Identification of three new alternatively spliced variants of the rat mu opioid receptor gene: Dissociation of affinity and efficacy. *J. Neurochem.* 91, 881–890.
27. Pan, Y. X., Xu, J., Mahurter, L., Xu, M. M., Gilbert, A.-K., and Pasternak, G. W. (2003). Identification and characterization of two new human mu opioid receptor splice variants, hMOR-1O and hMOR-1X. *Biochem. Biophys. Res. Commun.* 301, 1057–1061.
28. Pan, Y.-X., Xu, J., Mahurter, L., Bolan, E. A., Xu, M. M., and Pasternak, G. W. (2001). Generation of the mu opioid receptor (MOR-1) protein by three new splice variants of the *Oprm* gene. *Proc. Natl. Acad. Sci. USA* 98, 14084–14089.
29. Bare, L. A., Mansson, E., and Yang, D. (1994). Expression of two variants of the human mu opioid receptor mRNA in SK-N-SH cells and human brain. *FEBS Lett.* 354, 213–216.
30. Zimprich, A., Simon, T., and Hollt, V. (1995). Cloning and expression of an isoform of the rat µ opioid receptor (rMOR 1 B) which differs in agonist induced desensitization from rMOR1. *FEBS Lett.* 359, 142–146.
31. Bolan, E. A., Pasternak, G. W., and Pan, Y.-X. (2004). Functional analysis of MOR-1 splice variants of the µ opioid receptor gene. *Oprm. Synapse* 51, 11–18.
32. Abbadie, C., Pasternak, G. W., and Aicher, S. A. (2001). Presynaptic localization of the carboxy-terminus epitopes of the mu opioid receptor splice variants MOR-1C and MOR-1D in the superficial laminae of the rat spinal cord. *Neuroscience* 106, 833–842.
33. Abbadie, C., Pan, Y.-X., and Pasternak, G. W. (2000). Differential distribution in rat brain of mu opioid receptor carboxy terminal splice variants MOR-1C and MOR-1-like immunoreactivity: Evidence for region-specific processing. *J. Comp. Neurol.* 419, 244–256.
34. Abbadie, C., Pan, Y.-X., Drake, C. T., and Pasternak, G. W. (2000). Comparative immunhistochemical distributions of carboxy terminus epitopes from the mu opioid receptor splice variants MOR-1D, MOR-1 and MOR-1C in the mouse and rat central nervous systems. *Neuroscience* 100, 141–153.
35. Abbadie, C., Gultekin, S. H., and Pasternak, G. W. (2000). Immunohistochemical localization of the carboxy terminus of the novel mu opioid receptor splice variant MOR-1C within the human spinal cord. *Neuroreport* 11, 1953–1957.

36. Evans, C. J., Keith, D. E., Jr., Morrison, H., Magendzo, K., and Edwards, R. H. (1992). Cloning of a delta opioid receptor by functional expression. *Science* 258, 1952–1955.

37. Kieffer, B. L., Befort, K., Gaveriaux-Ruff, C., and Hirth, C. G. (1992). The δ-opioid receptor: Isolation of a cDNA by expression cloning and pharmacological characterization. *Proc. Natl. Acad. Sci. USA* 89, 12048–12052.

38. Mayer, P., Tischmeyer, H., Jayasinghe, M., Bonnekoh, B., Gollnick, H., Teschemacher, H., and Höllt, V. (2000). A δ opioid receptor lacking the third cytoplasmic loop is generated by atypical mRNA processing in human malignomas. *FEBS Lett.* 480, 156–160.

39. Gavériaux-Ruff, C., Peluso, J., Befort, K., Simonin, F., Zilliox, C., and Kieffer, B. L. (1997). Detection of opioid receptor mRNA by RT-PCR reveals alternative splicing for the δ- and kappa-opioid receptors. *Mol. Brain Res* 48, 298–304.

40. Chen, Y., Mestek, A., Liu, J., and Yu, L. (1993). Molecular cloning of a rat kappa opioid receptor reveals sequence similarities to the μ and δ opioid receptors. *Biochem. J.* 295, 625–628.

41. Li, S., Zhu, J., Chen, C., Chen, Y.-W., Deriel, J. K., Ashby, B., and Liu-Chen, L.-Y. (1993). Molecular cloning and expression of a rat kappa opioid receptor. *Biochem. J.* 295, 629–633.

42. Meng, F., Xie, G.-X., Thompson, R. C., Mansour, A., Goldstein, A., Watson, S. J., and Akil, H. (1993). Cloning and pharmacological characterization of a rat kappa opioid receptor. *Proc. Natl. Acad. Sci. USA* 90, 9954–9958.

43. Pierce, K. L., Premont, R. T., and Lefkowitz, R. J. (2002). Seven-transmembrane receptors. *Nat. Rev. Mol. Cell Biol.* 3, 639–650.

44. Bouvier, M. (2001). Oligomerization of G-protein-coupled transmitter receptors. *Nat. Rev. Neurosci.* 2, 274–286.

45. Cvejic, S., and Devi, L.A. (1997). Dimerization of the delta opioid receptor: Implication for a role in receptor internalization. *J. Biol. Chem.* 272, 26959–26964.

46. Jordan, B. A., and Devi, L. A. (1999). G-protein-coupled receptor heterodimerization modulates receptor function. *Nature* 399, 697–700.

47. George, S. R., Fan, T., Xie, Z., Tse, R., Tam, V., Varghese, G., and O'Dowd, B. F. (2000). Oligomerization of mu- and delta-opioid receptors. Generation of novel functional properties. *J. Biol. Chem.* 275, 26128–26135.

48. Pan, Y.-X., Bolan, E., and Pasternak, G. W. (2002). Dimerization of morphine and orphanin FQ/nociceptin receptors: Generation of a novel opioid receptor subtype. *Biochem. Biophys. Res. Commun.* 297, 659–663.

49. Jordan, B. A., Trapaidze, N., Gomes, I., Nivarthi, R., and Devi, L. A. (2001). Oligomerization of opioid receptors with β_2-adrenergic receptors: A role in trafficking and mitogen-activated protein kinase activation. *Proc. Natl. Acad. Sci. USA* 98, 343–348.

50. Jordan, B. A., Gomes, I., Rios, C., Filipovska, J., and Devi, L. A. (2003). Functional interactions between μ opioid and alpha 2A-adrenergic receptors. *Mol. Pharmacol.* 64, 1317–1324.

51. Bunzow, J. R., Saez, C., Mortrud, M., Bouvier, C., Williams, J. T., Low, M., and Grandy, D. K. (1994). Molecular cloning and tissue distribution of a putative member of the rat opioid receptor gene family that is not a μ, δ or kappa opioid receptor type. *FEBS Lett.* 347, 284–288.

52. Chen, Y., Fan, Y., Liu, J., Mestek, A., Tian, M., Kozak, C. A., and Yu, L. (1994). Molecular cloning, tissue distribution and chromosomal localization of a novel member of the opioid receptor gene family. *FEBS Lett.* 347, 279–283.
53. Keith, D., Jr., Maung, T., Anton, B., and Evans, C. (1994). Isolation of cDNA clones homologous to opioid receptors. *Regul. Pept.* 54, 143–144.
54. Mollereau, C., Parmentier, M., Mailleux, P., Butour, J. L., Moisand, C., Chalon, P., Caput, D., Vassart, G., and Meunier, J. C. (1994). ORL-1, a novel member of the opioid family: Cloning, functional expression and localization. *FEBS Lett.* 341, 33–38.
55. Pan, Y.-X., Cheng, J., Xu, J., and Pasternak, G. W. (1994). Cloning, expression and classification of a kappa$_3$-related opioid receptor using antisense oligodeoxynucleotides. *Regul. Pept.* 54, 217–218.
56. Lachowicz, J. E., Shen, Y., Monsma, F. J., Jr., and Sibley, D. R. (1995). Molecular cloning of a novel G protein-coupled receptor related to the opiate receptor family. *J. Neurochem.* 64, 34–40.
57. Meunier, J. C., Mollereau, C., Toll, L., Suaudeau, C., Moisand, C., Alvinerie, P., Butour, J. L., Guillemot, J. C., Ferrara, P., Monsarrat, B., Mazargull, H., Vassart, G., Parmentier, M., and Costentin, J. (1995). Isolation and structure of the endogenous agonist of the opioid receptor like ORL$_1$ receptor. *Nature* 377, 532–535.
58. Reinscheid, R. K., Nothacker, H. P., Bourson, A., Ardati, A., Henningsen, R. A., Bunzow, J. R., Grandy, D. K., Langen, H., Monsma, F. J., and Civelli, O. (1995). Orphanin FQ: A neuropeptide that activates an opioidlike G protein-coupled receptor. *Science* 270, 792–794.

23

ADVENT OF A NEW GENERATION OF ANTIMIGRAINE MEDICATIONS

ANA RECOBER AND ANDREW F. RUSSO
University of Iowa, Iowa City, Iowa

23.1	Overview		758
23.2	What Is Migraine?		758
	23.2.1	Historical Perspective	758
	23.2.2	Definition of Migraine	758
23.3	Role of CGRP in Migraine		759
	23.3.1	Neurovascular Model	759
	23.3.2	CGRP Synthesis and Actions	760
	23.3.3	Multiple Sites of CGRP Action in Trigeminovasculature	761
	23.3.4	Injection of CGRP Induces Migrainelike Headaches	763
	23.3.5	Therapeutic Efficacy of CGRP Receptor Antagonist	763
23.4	Pharmacological Management of Migraine		764
	23.4.1	Acute Therapy	764
		23.4.1.1 Triptans	764
		23.4.1.2 Nonsteroidal Anti-Inflammatory Drugs and Nonopiate Analgesics	765
		23.4.1.3 Opioids	765
		23.4.1.4 Ergots	765
		23.4.1.5 Valproate	765
		23.4.1.6 Antiemetics	765
	23.4.2	Preventive Therapy	766
		23.4.2.1 Anticonvulsants	766
		23.4.2.2 β-Blockers	767
		23.4.2.3 Antidepressants	767
		23.4.2.4 Calcium Channel Blockers	767
		23.4.2.5 Nonsteroidal Anti-Inflammatory Drugs	768
		23.4.2.6 Botulinum Toxin	768
		23.4.2.7 Other	768
23.5	Future Directions		768
	23.5.1	Potential for Targeted Repression of CGRP Synthesis	768
	23.5.2	Potential for CGRP Antagonists and Migraine Drugs for Other Forms of Pain	768
References			769

Handbook of Contemporary Neuropharmacology, Edited by David R. Sibley, Israel Hanin, Michael Kuhar, and Phil Skolnick. Copyright © 2007 John Wiley & Sons, Inc.

23.1 OVERVIEW

This chapter will address recent developments in the treatment of migraine. The recent promising clinical trials using a new antimigraine medication, BIBN4096BS (see Fig. 23.3 below), heralds the advent of a new generation of therapeutics. BIBN4096BS targets the receptor for the neuropeptide calcitonin gene–related peptide (CGRP), which appears to play a causal role in migraine pain. We will discuss the rationale and therapeutic implications of modulating CGRP, including its potential for acting at multiple sites in the trigeminovasculature. We will then discuss the currently used acute and preventative pharmacological treatments. Of particular interest is the increasing evidence that antiepileptic drugs may be an effective prophylactic treatment for migraine. Future strategies to selectively downregulate CGRP synthesis and the potential use of migraine drugs for other forms of trigeminal-mediated pain, such as temporomandibular disorder and trigeminal neuralgia, will be explored.

23.2 WHAT IS MIGRAINE?

Migraine is a debilitating chronic episodic disorder characterized by attacks of debilitating headaches and other associated sysmptoms. Migraine affects 12% of the general population atleast once a year [1, 2]. It is estimated that the lifetime prevalence may be as high as 18% [3]. It is one of the most underdiagnosed and undertreated neurological diseases [4]. In this section, we will provide a brief review of the history and the now-accepted clinical diagnostic criteria of migraine.

23.2.1 Historical Perspective

People have been suffering from migraine for millenia. The first evidence of migraine is suggested by neolithic skulls from 7000 BCE that show signs of trephination, an ancient procedure that has been used to treat migraine as late as the mid-seventeenth century [5]. Descriptions of migrainelike pain have been found in Babylonian tablets dating back to 3000–4000 BC and Egyptian papyri from 1550 BC [6]. We owe to Hippocrates (c. 400 BCE) the recognition of the syndrome now known as migraine. The term *migraine* originates from the Greek word *hemicrania*, provided by Galen in the second century AD. Despite this long history, it has really only been since the 1990s that significant therapeutic inroads have been made in our understanding and treatment of migraine.

23.2.2 Definition of Migraine

The International Headache Society (IHS) developed in 1988 and reviewed in 2004 a classification system for headaches [7, 8]. But until recently these criteria have been used loosely to define migraine for research purposes. Migraines are divided in two major groups, migraines without aura and migraines with aura. Migraines without aura are defined as headaches lasting 4–72 h (untreated or unsuccessfully treated) with at least two of the following: (1) pulsating quality, (2) unilateral location, (3) moderate or severe intensity, and (4) aggravation by routine physical activity. It has been suggested by some physicians that these criteria can be remembered by the first initial as a "puma" chewing on your brain. In addition to these core criteria, migraine also must fulfill at least one of the following two criteria: (1) nausea and/or vomiting and (2) photophobia and phonophobia. An important point for considering the mechanism behind the pain is that the untreated headache can last for days.

An aura consists in focal neurological phenomena that precede or accompany the headache. The aura can be visual, sensory, or motor and may involve language or brain stem disturbances. Migraines with aura are less common and occur in about 15% of migraineurs [3], although an estimated 30% of migraineurs experience auras at some time [9].

Migraine is a chronic condition, with episodic attacks of variable frequency, that disrupts normal daily activities and has severe economic repercussions [10–12]. Many patients rely on nonprescription medications such as aspirin, acetaminophen, and ibuprofen. However, they often are not effective when pain is moderate to severe and are commonly overused [13, 14]. This can lead to chronic headaches, or "rebound headache." Migraines are more frequent during the most productive years of a person's life. Based on a survey by the World Health Organization, severe migraine was rated as one of the most disabling chronic disorders [15].

There is a marked sex bias among migraineurs [1]. Migraine occurs in 18% of women, in contrast to a 6% frequency in men. In children prior to puberty, the frequency of migraine is about 6% for both boys and girls. After menopause, many, but not all, women report a decrease in migraines. One of the most common triggers of migraines is the timing during estrus cycle. While a molecular explanation for this link has not been forthcoming, several mechanisms have been proposed [16].

23.3 ROLE OF CGRP IN MIGRAINE

A causal role for CGRP during the painful phase of migraine has been a topic of speculation for the past 15 years. In this section, we will describe how CGRP fits into the currently prevailing model for migraine. We will briefly describe the synthesis and known activities of CGRP that support the hypothesis that CGRP contributes to the painful phase of migraine. We will then describe the conclusive evidence from two clinical studies showing that administration of CGRP causes a headache and that a CGRP receptor antagonist can block migraines.

23.3.1 Neurovascular Model

Migraine is now generally accepted to be a neurovascular disorder involving the meningeal and cerebral blood vessels of the cranial vasculature [17–19]. By neurovascular disorder, it is meant that dilation of blood vessels and pain are triggered by neural rather than vascular signals [20, 21]. The identity of those neural signals remains undefined. However, activation of serotonergic and noradrenergic brain stem nuclei has been detected by positron emission tomography during migraine [22, 23]. This suggests the possibility of dysfunction of the aminergic neurons of the brain stem that modulate the craniovasculature. Indeed, given the heterogeneity of migraine, it seems possible that there will be multiple mechanisms by which the pain may be triggered.

Whatever the initial trigger, it is clear that a key player in the pain pathway is the trigeminal ganglion. Nerves from the trigeminal ganglion control cerebral blood flow and provide the pain-sensitive sensory innervation of the cerebrovasculature [24–26]. The trigeminal ganglion is also the major source of CGRP innervation of craniofacial structures and the cerebrovasculature [24, 27]. The ganglion is a heterogeneous collection of neurons with CGRP in $\sim$25% of the neurons, primarily in unmyelinated nociceptive fibers [28]. The importance of trigeminovascular CGRP is highlighted by a report that human cerebral arteries are 10 times more sensitive than coronary arteries to CGRP [29].

While the role of the trigeminal nerves in migraine is increasingly evident, the link between the initiation of migraine and the invocation of the trigeminovascular system is not known. The prevailing current theory is that migraine is initiated by a dysfunction of brain stem neurons that modulate craniovascular sensory input [17]. According to this model, this dysfunction leads to changes in meningeal blood vessel dilation and a reflexlike response of perivascular trigeminal nerves [17, 19]. A complementary model has been proposed in which a wave of cortical spreading depression leads to activation of parasympathetic and trigeminal afferents, which then causes vessel dilation and nociception [30]. Cortical spreading depression is associated with the aura that precedes some migraines [31–33]. This model does not account for migraine without aura, but the authors speculate that the aura may be subclinical. Either way, it is intriguing that a genetically engineered mouse that contains a calcium channel mutation found in familial hemiplegic migraine patients, who tend to have auras, is more susceptible to cortical spreading depression [34]. Mutations in the P/Q calcium channel and Na^+, K^+– adenosine triphosphatase (ATPase) have been identified in these patients [35, 36]. Whether this mouse model has elevated trigeminal activity or CGRP release remains to be seen.

The neurovascular model is consistent with clinical evidence that CGRP levels are elevated in the jugular outflow of migraineurs and decreased upon treatment with triptan antimigraine drugs, coincident with pain relief [4, 17, 37]. Activation of trigeminovascular afferents in the meninges and at the major vessels leads to release of CGRP substance P and neurokinin A. These peptides are known to cause neurogenic inflammation. Neurogenic inflammation is the "sterile" inflammatory response involving vasodilation, plasma extravasation (vessel leakage), and mast cell degranulation [38]. Neurogenic inflammation has been demonstrated upon trigeminal activation in animals, but it has not been established in migraine patients [17]. Release of CGRP and other neuropeptides at the efferent terminals in the brain stem contributes to nociception. This involves central sensitization to lower pain response thresholds and allodynia, which causes previously innocuous stimuli, such as combing of hair, to be painful [39–41]. Thus, peripheral CGRP release is believed to cause vasodilation and neurogenic inflammation and release in the brain stem helps relay nociceptive signals to the central nervous system (CNS) in migraine [42, 43].

23.3.2 CGRP Synthesis and Actions

CGRP was discovered over 20 years ago as an alternative RNA splicing product from the calcitonin gene (Fig. 23.1) [44]. CGRP is prominent in nerve fibers surrounding peripheral and cerebral blood vessels and it is the most potent peptide

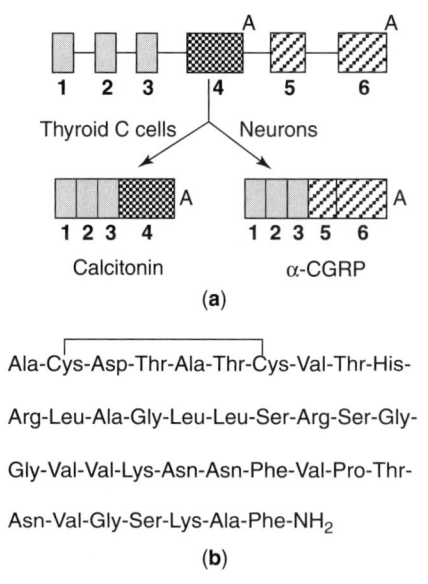

Figure 23.1 Schematic of calcitonin/α-CGRP gene. (a) Alternative processing of primary transcript in thyroid C cells yields primarily calcitonin messenger RNA (mRNA), while CGRP mRNA is the primary product in neurons. The alternative polyadenylation sites following exons 4 and 6 are indicated. (b) Primary sequence of human α-CGRP peptide. The disulfide bond is indicated.

dilator known [24, 45–47]. This vasodilatory activity has been confirmed in two of three lines of CGRP knockout mice [48, 49]. Coincident with vasodilation, CGRP plays an important role in neurogenic inflammation and nociception. CGRP triggers mast cell release of proinflammatory cytokines and inflammatory agents [47]. In a study using homozygous CGRP null mutant mice, CGRP was required for somatic and visceral pain signals associated with neurogenic inflammation [50]. In addition to its actions at the afferent terminals, CGRP modulates nociceptive input via central pathways. Notably, injection of CGRP into the trigeminal nucleus of the brain stem elicits a cardiovascular response that is similar to painful stimuli [51, 52].

Consistent with these biological activities, abnormal levels of CGRP have been implicated in hypertension, migraine, subarachnoid hemorrhage, and myocardial infarction [53]. As described below, the ability of CGRP to induce headache [54] and a CGRP receptor antagonist to alleviate migraine [55] firmly establish the importance of elevated CGRP in migraine pain [42, 43, 56]. While the objective of clinical efforts has been to reduce CGRP actions, elevated CGRP can also be beneficial. For example, following myocardial infarction it is believed that elevated CGRP release plays a protective role during ischemia [57–59].

23.3.3 Multiple Sites of CGRP Action in Trigeminovasculature

There are three potential sites of action for CGRP (Fig. 23.2). The best characterized site of CGRP action is on the vasculature. Human cerebral vessels have functional CGRP receptors and the vascular smooth muscle cells express the calcitonin

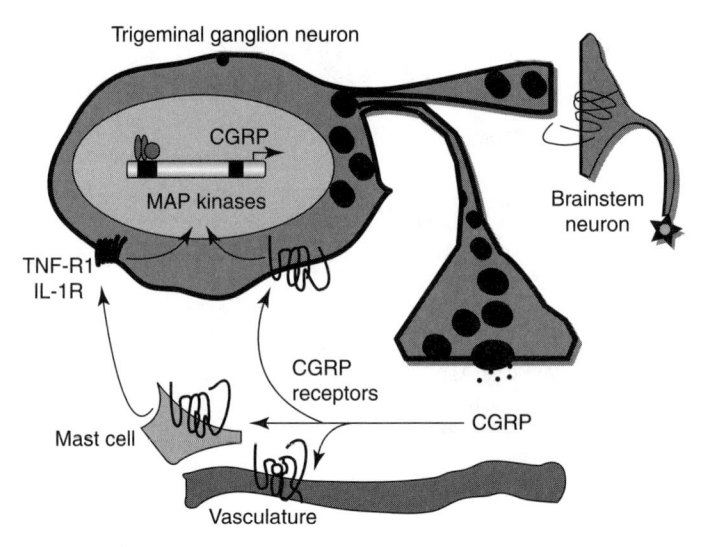

Figure 23.2 Model depicting likely sites of action of CGRP and CGRP antagonist drugs in trigeminovasculature. A pseudounipolar trigeminal ganglion neuron innervating meningeal vessels and projecting to the brain stem is depicted. (1) CGRP receptors are present on the smooth muscle and endothelium of the vasculature. (2) Receptors are present on dural mast cells that can release cytokines and inflammatory agents. (3) There are CGRP receptors on the ganglion neurons and on secondary neurons in the brain stem. The CGRP receptor is shown as a seven-pass transmembrane protein with the associated single-pass RAMP1 protein. Signals from cytokine receptors and the CGRP receptors are predicted to activate mitogen-activated protein (MAP) kinase cascades that stimulate CGRP enhancer activity. The known enhancer elements are indicated.

receptor-like receptor (CLR) and receptor activity modifying protein 1 (RAMP1) proteins that comprise the CGRP receptor [60, 61]. Inhibition of vascular CGRP receptors by the CGRP antagonist BIBN4096BS was shown to inhibit CGRP-induced dilation of the human middle cerebral and middle meningeal arteries [62]. In addition to actions on major vessels, CGRP and presumably the antagonist can also act on receptors located on pial arterioles. Dilation of these meningeal vessels and the associated neurogenic inflammation are believed to be important events in migraine.

The second potential site of CGRP action is on receptors on dural mast cells. CGRP is known to induce mast cell degranulation. Mast cells release histamine and other inflammatory agents and proinflammatory cytokines. In this capacity, the CGRP antagonist should block both meningeal vessel dilation and neurogenic inflammation.

The third potential site is on neurons. There are CGRP receptors on the primary sensory trigeminal ganglion neurons [61] and the second-order sensory neurons within trigeminal nuclei in the caudal brain stem and upper cervical spinal cord [39, 63]. CGRP binding to the ganglion neurons might potentially create a positive-feedback loop with increased CGRP synthesis and secretion. This hypothesis is currently being tested. Inhibition of these CGRP actions by the BIBN4096BS drug would likely reduce the persistent activation of the ganglion neurons. CGRP action on brain stem neurons is known to be involved in relaying nociceptive signals to the thalamus. BIBN4096BS would likely reduce this nociceptive signaling and the sensitization of second-order neurons that is believed to contribute to migraine pain. Inhibition of the trigeminovascular system at either or both of these sites would also be expected to diminish the allodynic effects and effects from autonomic parasympathetic ganglia that are associated with migraine [40].

23.3.4 Injection of CGRP Induces Migrainelike Headaches

The possible causative role of CGRP in migraine has been studied in a double-blind crossover study. Twelve subjects, all of them migraneurs, were administered human CGRP or placebo intravenously on two different days. Two patients developed hypotension and one had an infection, and these three subjects were excluded. Eight of nine patients had immediate headache, within 40 min of the infusion of CGRP versus only one of nine treated with placebo. This immediate headache did not fulfill criteria for migraine. All nine patients had a delayed headache, from 1 to 12 h after the beginning of the infusion of CGRP versus only one receiving placebo. In three of the nine patients treated with CGRP, the delayed headache fulfilled the criteria for migraine [54].

23.3.5 Therapeutic Efficacy of CGRP Receptor Antagonist

The final proof that CGRP plays a causal role in migraine pain is the recently reported efficacy of a novel nonpeptide CGRP receptor antagonist, BIBN4096BS (Fig. 23.3) [55]. Doods and colleagues [64] identified BIBN4096BS as a potent and highly specific antagonist to human CGRP receptors (Boehringer Ingelheim) [29, 62, 64]. BIBN4096BS binds to the human CGRP receptor with over 100-fold higher affinity than the CGRP receptor in other species [29, 64]. BIBN4096BS binds the CLR/RAMP1 protein complex, and the species selectivity appears to be due to BIBN4096BS interactions with RAMP1 [65, 66].

The antagonist BIBN4096BS was shown to be effective in the acute treatment of migraine headache in an international, multicenter, randomized, double-blind European clinical trial [55]. A total of 126 migraineurs were randomized to receive BIBN4096BS or placebo. The patients treated with BIBN4096BS had both decreased headache and improvements in the associated symptoms of nausea, photophobia, phonophobia, and inability to function. The main side effect to the drug was mild

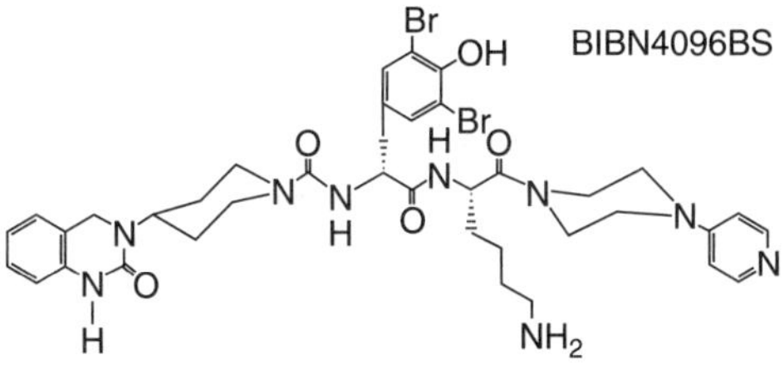

Figure 23.3 Structure of nonpeptide CGRP antagonist BIBN4096BS. BIBN4096BS, developed by Boehringer Ingelheim [64], is schematically represented (1-piperidinecarboxamide, N-[2-[[5-amino-1-[[4-(4-pyridinyl)-1 piperazinyl]carbonyl] pentyl] amino]-1-[(3,5-dibromo-4-hydroxyphenyl) methyl]-2-oxoethyl]-4-(1,4-dihydro-2-oxo-3(2H)-quinazolinyl)-, [R-(R*,S*)]-).

paresthesias that occurred in 7% of the subjects; the other side effects, nausea, headache, dry mouth, and abnormal vision, were very infrequent, 2% each. BIBN4096BS was also effective at treating CGRP-induced headache [67]. Importantly, the drug does not appear to have any adverse cardiovascular effects [68].

The significance of this proof-of-principle result is twofold. First, it presages the development of other CGRP receptor antagonists and agents that interfere with CGRP synthesis or action. Second, the CGRP antagonist is not likely to have the cardiovascular side effects of the currently used triptans.

23.4 PHARMACOLOGICAL MANAGEMENT OF MIGRAINE

The Quality Standards Subcommittee of the American Academy of Neurology developed a practice parameter for physicians in 2000, summarizing the results from evidence-based reviews on the pharmacological, including acute and preventive, as well as nonpharmacological treatments and diagnostic evaluation for migraine patients [69]. This is a very useful resource, but a review of all the drugs would be too extensive for this chapter. We will focus in the following sections on some of the most commonly used drugs included in these guidelines.

23.4.1 Acute Therapy

When a migraine attack occurs, abortive medications are used to arrest the attack or at least decrease the severity and duration of the pain and associated symptoms. An ideal abortive drug should have a rapid onset and long-lasting effect, should be easily administered, preferably orally, and should lack side effects and interactions with other medications. One must also keep in mind the cost of abortive drugs, which ranges from $0.01/unit (generic aspirin) to approximately $15/unit (triptans) and can be as high as $64/unit [dihydroergotamine-45 intra muscular (DHE-45 IM)] [70].

23.4.1.1 Triptans. Perhaps the most significant advance in migraine therapy was the antimigraine drug sumatriptan in the early 1990s. Sumatriptan and the soon-to-follow related triptan drugs provide pain relief for about 60% of migraineurs within 2 h [71]. However, only about 30% of the patients were fully pain free at 2 h and only 20% were still pain free after 24 h. Thus, there is room for improved therapies.

Sumatriptan provided important clues to the underlying mechanisms of migraine pathology [17, 20, 72]. The triptans recognize the 5-hydroxytryptamine (5-HT)$_1$B, 5-HT$_1$D and 5-HT$_1$F serotonin receptors [38, 73]. At the time of the development of sumatriptan, the 5-HT$_1$ receptors were only known to be on blood vessels. Since then functional 5-HT$_1$B, D, F receptors have been found on perivascular trigeminal nerve terminals and the trigeminal nucleus caudalis in the brain stem [39, 74–76]. Consistent with the multiple locations of the 5-HT$_1$ receptors, triptans can inhibit vasodilation of intracranial vessels and inhibit CGRP release to block neurogenic inflammation and central transmission of nociceptive stimuli from trigeminal nerves [38]. The ability of triptan drugs to lower CGRP levels coincident with pain relief is consistent with the causal role of CGRP in migraine discussed in the previous section.

Triptans are also able to repress transcription of the CGRP gene in cultured trigeminal ganglion neurons [56, 77]. Transcriptional repression was seen after 2–4 h, which is close to the estimated half-life of sumatriptan and within the 12 h required for clearance from the body, especially with the newer triptans [17, 78]. While it is risky to extrapolate from cells to people, we speculate that transcriptional repression might lower CGRP levels over the long term. This may be relevant in triptan overuse syndromes, possibly during the withdrawal headache [79, 80].

Unfortunately, the triptans are not miracle drugs. As mentioned above, about one-third of patients do not respond to triptans. In addition, there is a high recurrence rate of the headache [81]. Most importantly, there are potentially lethal side effects. The triptans can cause severe vasoconstriction of coronary arteries [82]. Because of this, triptans are contraindicated in patients with established cardiovascular disease, and they should be used cautiously in patients with cardiovascular risk factors. It is also very important to be aware of the fact that frequent use of triptans is associated with chronic headaches, which proves to be a very disabling condition with poor response to therapy [80]. There are currently seven different triptans in the market. Listed in alphabetic order these are Almotriptan, Eletriptan, Frovatriptan, Naratriptan, Rizatriptan, Sumatriptan, and Zolmitriptan. Their relative efficacies have recently been compared in a meta-analysis of 53 trials [71].

23.4.1.2 Nonsteroidal Anti-Inflammatory Drugs and Nonopiate Analgesics. The most commonly used abortive drugs are likely to be over-the-counter analgesics, nonsteroidal anti-inflamatory drugs, and combination of analgesics with caffeine. These have proven to be effective but are not free of side effects, especially gastrointestinal symptoms. Another important aspect to consider is the risk of chronic daily headaches associated with frequent use of analgesics [83–86].

23.4.1.3 Opioids. Opioids have variable efficacy and are usually reserved as rescue medications or for specific situations like pregnancy, coronary artery disease, or other comorbidities that preclude the use of other drugs.

23.4.1.4 Ergots. Ergotamine and dihydroergotamine have serotonin agonist activity and are vasoconstrictors. Dihyrdroergotamine nasal spray has shown to be effective and well tolerated; other preparations are intramuscular, intravenous, oral tablet, sublingual, and suppository [87, 88].

23.4.1.5 Valproate. Intravenous valproate is also used as abortive treatment in migraines, but its effectiveness needs to be confirmed in randomized, double-blinded, placebo-controlled studies. The doses used in clinical practice are generally well tolerated [89, 90].

23.4.1.6 Antiemetics. Several antiemetic drugs are frequently used in acute migraine either to treat the associated nausea or for their effectiveness on the overall attack. The most common side effect seen with these drugs is sedation. Chlorpromazine, metoclopramide, and prochlorperazine, preferably in intravenous formulation, can be used, although there are some contradictory data [69, 94]. Antiemetics can also increase the effectiveness of other oral abortive drugs by improving delayed gastric emptying associated with acute attacks of migraine [95].

23.4.2 Preventive Therapy

Preventive medications are drugs taken on a daily basis to decrease the frequency, severity, and duration of attacks as well as to improve their responsiveness to abortive treatment and reduce disability. Many migraineurs require a prophylactic approach due to frequent or very debilitating attacks, lack of response to abortive treatment, or inability to use acute drugs due to comorbidities or interaction with other medications. Several groups of medications are used for preventive treatment of migraines: anticonvulsants, antidepressants, β-adrenergic blockers, Ca^{2+} channel blockers, botulinum toxin, and others.

23.4.2.1 Anticonvulsants. Migraines commonly coexist with other chronic neurological and psychiatric conditions. Some of these disorders, such as epilepsy, are also characterized by episodic attacks like migraines. Individuals with epilepsy have a twofold higher risk of suffering from migraine than those without epilepsy. Migraineurs have a higher risk of epilepsy than nonmigraineurs [96].

Several anticonvulsants drugs are also used for migraine prophylaxis. Only two are approved by the Food and Drug Administration (FDA) for such indication. Antiepileptic drugs are used for trigeminal neuralgia and are increasingly being used in migraine therapy [97–100]. While their mechanisms vary, many act via the γ-aminobutyric acid (GABA) system. For example, valproate elevates GABA levels [100]. Indeed, some trigeminal ganglion neurons contain GABA and many have $GABA_A$ receptors [100]. We have found that both $GABA_A$ and $GABA_B$ receptors are present on cultured trigeminal ganglion neurons (unpublished observations). Whether any of these drugs act directly on the trigeminal nerves is speculative. It is generally believed that GABAergic antiepileptics act by inhibiting neural activity in the CNS. The study of these antiepileptic drugs is especially interesting because a better understanding of their mechanisms of action could throw some light on the pathophysiological mechanisms underlying migraine.

Valproate was the first antiepileptic drug approved by the FDA for migraine prophylaxis [101, 102]. The most common side effects of valproate are gastrointestinal, although asthenia, weight gain, alopecia, and tremor are also relatively frequent. Rarely, more severe idiosyncratic adverse reactions like hepatitis, pancreatitis, or hematological disorders can occur. Valproate is potentially teratogenic. An extended-release preparation allows taking valproate only once a day. The starting dose for valproate and all the anticonvulsants is followed by slow tritration to an increased dosage.

Topiramate has shown efficacy in migraine prevention and has been the second and most recent antiepileptic drug approved by the FDA for this purpose [103–106]. Although the exact mechanism of action of topiramate is not fully understood, it is probably related to modulation of GABA and glutamate-mediated neurotransmission as well as its direct activity on α-amino-3-hydroxy-5-methylisoxazole-4-propionic acid (AMPA)/kainate glutamate receptors [97, 98]. The most common side effects are paresthesias, cognitive symptoms and sedation, nausea, anorexia, and weight loss.

Gabapentin is used for several neuropathic conditions as well as for migraine prophylaxis, although more studies are needed to support its use in migraine [69, 107]. Similar to other antiepileptics, Gabapentin is likely to have multiple mechanisms of action, but these are not completely understood [97]. The most common side effects are somnolence and dizziness, which may be minimized by slow titration.

23.4.2.2 **β-Blockers.** The nonselective β blockers propranolol, timolol, and nadolol as well as the selective β_1 blockers atenolol and metoprolol are used in prevention of migraine. Their mechanism of action, although remaining unknown, is thought to be central, at least in part due to β_1 adrenoreceptor antagonism in the ventroposteromedial thalamus [108, 109].

The use of propranolol or timolol appears to be more effective than the other β blockers [110, 111]. Fatigue, depression, nausea, dizziness, and insomnia are the most frequent side effects, although they are usually well tolerated. Nonselective β blockers should not be used in patients with asthma or diabetes. A long-acting formulation of propranolol facilitates compliance by allowing once-a-day administration [112].

23.4.2.3 *Antidepressants.* While the mechanism of antidepressant drugs is not well understood, it is not thought to be due to its effect on underlying depression [113], although more studies are needed to confirm this [114]. Antidepressants produce a decrease in β-adrenergic receptor density and norepinephrine-stimulated cyclic adenosine monophosphate (cAMP) response [87].

Several tricyclic antidepressants (TCAs) are used for migraine prophylaxis: amitriptyline, nortriptyline, protriptyline, doxepin, and imipramine. TCAs upregulate the $GABA_B$ receptor, downregulate the histamine receptor, and enhance the neuronal sensitivity to substance P. Some TCAs are $5-HT_2$ receptor antagonists. Absorption, distribution, and excretion of TCAs are very variable; thus the dose must be individualized. These drugs frequently cause side effects due to their antimuscarinic, antihistaminic, and α-adrenergic activity. They should be used with caution in elderly patients and avoided in patients with arrhythmias due to potential cardiac toxicity. Amitriptyline is the best studied TCA and its use is recommended based on multiple consistent randomized clinical trials [69]. Nortriptyline is a metabolite of amitriptyline and is less sedating.

A second group of antidepressants used in migraine prophylaxis are the selective serotonin reuptake inhibitors (SSRIs): fluoxetine, fluvoxamine, paroxetine, sertraline, and citalopram. All of them have been used with variable results in prevention of migraine. These drugs have less antimuscarinic, antihistaminic, and cardiovascular side effects than TCAs, but the quality of evidence to support their recommendation is not as high as for TCAs [69].

Monoamine oxidase inhibitors (MAOIs) are a third group of antidepressants used in prevention of migraines. Phenelzyne, a nonspecific inhibitor of MAO_A and MAO_B, is considered effective in migraine prophylaxis by experts, but the scientific data available are insufficient. Common side effects of MAOIs are insomnia, orthostatic hypotension, constipation, weight gain, and peripheral edema. Patients on MAOIs must follow a tyramine-restricted diet and avoid certain medications to prevent hypertensive crisis.

23.4.2.4 Calcium Channel Blockers. The strength of evidence to support the use of verapamil and nimodipine for prevention of migraines is not very strong, but these are relatively commonly used drugs. Similarly to what occurs with other prophylactic medications, the physiological mechanisms of action of calcium channel antagonists are unclear. Verapamil is usually well tolerated. Constipation is one of the most common side effects. A sustained-release preparation facilitates compliance.

23.4.2.5 Nonsteroidal Anti-Inflammatory Drugs. Aspirin, ketoprofen, and naproxen can be used in prevention of migraine, although they are not as effective as some of the drugs previously mentioned and they might have significant gastrointestinal and renal side effects [108].

23.4.2.6 Botulinum Toxin. Pericranial injections of botulinum toxin type A (Botox) have recently been introduced as an alternative preventive option for migraine prophylaxis. The evidence available is somewhat inconsistent and further well-designed clinical trials are needed [91, 115].

23.4.2.7 Other. Feverfew is a medicinal herb with undetermined clinical effectiveness. Magnesium supplementation has been studied with contradictory results. The most common side effects were diarrhea and gastric irritation [116]. Riboflavin (vitamin B_2) at high doses is well tolerated and can be used for migraine prevention [117].

23.5 FUTURE DIRECTIONS

23.5.1 Potential for Targeted Repression of CGRP Synthesis

An understanding of the mechanisms by which trigeminal CGRP levels are regulated will allow the development of strategies to specifically lower CGRP levels for the treatment of craniofacial pain disorders such as migraine. We have proposed that MAP kinases are important regulators of CGRP synthesis (Fig. 23.2). $5-HT_1$ receptor agonists can repress CGRP secretion [118] and MAP kinase activation of the 18-bp CGRP enhancer [77, 119]. Based on a recent study, neuronal extracellular regulated kinase (ERK) MAP kinase inhibitors may be a promising strategy for attenuating allodynia in neuropathic pain [120]. A corollary approach will be to stimulate MAP kinase phosphatases. We have found that overexpression of MAP kinase phosphatase-1 lowers CGRP promoter activity [119]. These observations support the significance of future attempts to inhibit MAP kinase activation of CGRP synthesis. A novel approach to repress expression of CGRP synthesis is through posttranscriptional gene silencing. RNA interference (RNAi), a recently described biological process involved in posttranscriptional control of gene expression, could be manipulated to degrade CGRP mRNA, thus preventing its translation into the peptide. Although still far from application in humans, the therapeutic use of RNAi in neurological diseases is currently being explored, and several successes have been described in different animal models of human disease [121].

23.5.2 Potential for CGRP Antagonists and Migraine Drugs for Other Forms of Pain

The role of trigeminal CGRP is of particular significance due to the prevalence of painful craniofacial disorders. For migraine alone, it is estimated that 18 million Americans, including almost one in every five women, suffer an estimated 4 million attacks every week [18, 19]. The chronic pain often precipitates other serious conditions such as depression [122, 123], and there is an enormous financial burden in the billions per year. A large number of people also suffer from other craniofacial pains, with estimates ranging from 5 to 12% of the population [124].

The events in other craniofacial pains, such as the neuropathic pain of trigeminal neuralgia, are even less understood than in migraine [125–127]. Elevated CGRP is associated with temporomandibular joint (TMJ) disorders [128–131] and eye conditions following laser or ocular surgery trauma [132]. Outside the craniofacial structures, elevated CGRP is also associated with other disorders, such as some forms of hypertension [133] and sepsis [134].

Due to the high incidence and generally poor efficacy of current treatments for trigeminal and other chronic-pain disorders, there is a need for improved therapeutic and preventative measures. Some of the drugs used to prevent migraines are also effective in the management of other forms of pain. Specifically, diabetic neuropathy and postherpetic neuralgia have been extensively studied, and TCAs and gabapentin, among others, are frequently used for symptomatic relief in these conditions [135, 136]. In contrast, carbamazepime, which is effective in the treatment of neuropathic pain [137] and is a first-line drug in the management of trigeminal neuralgia [87], has not shown efficacy in the treatment of migraines [138]. It is tempting to speculate that CGRP receptor antagonists might be beneficial in treating other conditions that involve elevated CGRP. Whether CGRP receptor antagonists will be effective in treating these conditions will be of intense basic and clinical interest in the upcoming years.

REFERENCES

1. Stewart, W. F., Lipton, R. B., Celentano, D. D., and Reed, M. L. (1991). Prevalence of migraine headache in the United States. Relation to age, income, race, and other sociodemographic factors. *JAMA* 267(1), 64–69.
2. Lipton, R. B., Stewart, W. F., Diamond, S., Diamond, M. L., and Reed, M. (2001). Prevalence and burden of migraine in the United States: Data from the American Migraine Study II. *Headache* 41(7), 646–657.
3. Rasmussen, B. K., and Olesen, J. (1992). Migraine with aura and migraine without aura: An epidemiological study. *Cephalalgia* 12, 221–228.
4. Ferrari, M. D. (1998). Migraine. *Lancet* 351, 1043–1051.
5. Rapoport, A., and Edmeads, J. (2000). Migraine: The evolution of our knowledge. *Arch. Neurol.* 57, 1221–1223.
6. Rose, F. C. (1995). The history of migraine from Mesopotamian to Medieval times. *Cephalalgia* 15(Suppl. 15), 1–3.
7. Headache Classification Committee of the International Headache Society (1988). Classification and diagnostic criteria for headache disorders, cranial neuralgias and facial pain. *Cephalagia* 8(Suppl. 7), 1–96.
8. Headache Classification Subcommittee of the International Headache Society (IHS) (2004). The International Classification of Headache Disorders (2nd edition). *Cephalalgia* 24(Suppl. 1), 9–160.
9. Launer, L. J., Terwindt, G. M., and Ferrari, M. D. (1999). The prevalence and characteristics of migraine in a population-based cohort: The GEM study. *Neurology* 53(3), 537–542.

10. Hu, X. H., Markson, L. E., Lipton, R. B., Stewart, W. F., and Berger, M. L. (1999). Burden of migraine in the United States: Disability and economic costs. *Arch. Intern. Med.* 159(8), 813–818.
11. Stang, P., Cady, R., Batenhorst, A., and Hoffman, L. (2001). Workplace productivity: A review of the impact of migraine and its treatment. *Pharmacoeconomics* 19(3), 231–244.
12. Ferrari, M. D. (1998). The economic burden of migraine to society. *Pharmacoeconomics* 13(6), 667–676.
13. Wenzel, R. G., Sarvis, C. A., and Krause, M. L. (2003). Over-the-counter drugs for acute migraine attacks: Literature review and recommendations. *Pharmacotherapy* 23(4), 494–505.
14. Gallagher, R. M., and Cutrer, F. M. (2002). Migraine: Diagnosis, management, and new treatment options. *Am. J. Manag. Care* 8(3, Suppl.), S58–S73.
15. Menken, M., Munsat, T. L., and Toole, J. F. (2000). The global burden of disease study: Implications for neurology. *Arch. Neurol.* 57(3), 418–420.
16. Recober, A., and Geweke, L. O. (2005). Menstrual migraine. *Curr. Neurol. Neurosci. Rep.* 5(2), 93–98.
17. Goadsby, P. J., Lipton, R. B., and Ferrari, M. D. (2002). Migraine-current understanding and treatment. *New Engl. J. Med.* 346, 257–270.
18. Parsons, A. A., and Strijbos, P. J. (2003). The neuronal versus vascular hypothesis of migraine and cortical spreading depression. *Curr. Opin. Pharmacol.* 3, 73–77.
19. Pietrobon, D., and Striessnig, J. (2003). Neurobiology of migraine. *Nat. Rev. Neurosci.* 4(5), 386–398.
20. Moskowitz, M. A. (1993). Neurogenic inflammation in the pathophysiology and treatment of migraine. *Neurology* 43(6, Suppl. 3), S16–20.
21. May, A., and Goadsby, P. J. (1999). The trigeminovascular system in humans: Pathophysiologic implications for primary headache syndromes of the neural influences on the cerebral circulation. *J. Cereb. Blood Flow Metab.* 19(2), 115–127.
22. Weiller, C., May, A., Limmroth, V., Juptner, M., Kaube, H., Schayck, R. V., Coenen, H. H., and Diener, H. C. (1995). Brain stem activation in spontaneous human migraine attacks. *Nat. Med.* 1(7), 658–660.
23. Bahra, A., Matharu, M. S., Buchel, C., Frackowiak, R. S., and Goadsby, P. J. (2001). Brainstem activation specific to migraine headache. *Lancet* 357(9261), 1016–1017.
24. McCulloch, J., Uddman, R., Kingman, T. A., and Edvinsson, L. (1986). Calcitonin gene-related peptide: Functional role in cerebrovascular regulation. *Proc. Natl. Acad. Sci. USA* 83, 5731–5735.
25. Linnik, M. D., Sakas, D. E., Uhl, G. R., and Moskowitz, M. A. (1989). Subarachnoid blood and headache: Altered trigeminal tachykinin gene expression. *Ann. Neurol.* 25(2), 179–184.
26. Weber, J. R., Angstwurm, K., Bove, G. M., Burger, W., Einhaulpl, K. M., Dirnagl, U., and Moskowitz, M. A. (1996). The trigeminal nerve and augmentation of regional cerebral blood flow during experimental bacterial meningitis. *J. Cereb. Blood Flow Metab.* 16(6), 1319–1324.
27. O'Conner, T. P., and Van der Kooy, D. (1986). Pattern of intracranial and extracranial projections of trigeminal ganglion cells. *J. Neurosci.* 6, 2200–2207.
28. O'Conner, T. P., and Van der Kooy, D. (1988). Enrichment of a vasoactive neuropeptide (calcitonin gene related peptide) in the trigeminal sensory projection to the intracranial arteries. *J. Neurosci.* 8, 2468–2476.

29. Edvinsson, L., Alm, R., Shaw, D., Rutledge, R. Z., Koblan, K. S., Longmore, J., and Kane, S. A. (2002). Efffect of the CGRP receptor antagonist BIBN4096BS in human cerebral, coronary, and omental arteries and in SK-N-MC cells. *Eur. J. Pharmacol.* 434, 49–53.
30. Bolay, H., Reuter, U., Dunn, A. K., Huang, Z., Boas, D. A., and Moskowitz, M. A. (2002). Intrinsic brain activity triggers trigeminal meningeal afferents in a migraine model. *Nat. Med.* 8, 136–142.
31. Olesen, J., Larsen, B., and Lauritzen, M. (1981). Focal hyperemia followed by spreading oligemia and impaired activation of rCBF in classic migraine. *Ann. Neurol.* 9(4), 344–352.
32. Lauritzen, M. (1994). Pathophysiology of the migraine aura. The spreading depression theory. *Brain* 117(Pt. 1), 199–210.
33. Hadjikhani, N., Sanchez Del Rio, M., Wu, O., Schwartz, D., Bakker, D., Fischl, B., Kwong, K. K., Cutrer, F. M., Rosen, B. R., Tootell, R. B., Sorensen, A. G., and Moskowitz, M. A. (2001). Mechanisms of migraine aura revealed by functional MRI in human visual cortex. *Proc. Natl. Acad. Sci. USA* 98(8), 4687–4692.
34. van den Maagdenberg, A. M., Pietrobon, D., Pizzorusso, T., Kaja, S., Broos, L. A., Cesetti, T., van de Ven, R. C., Tottene, A., van der Kaa, J., Plomp, J. J., Frants, R. R., and Ferrari, M. D. (2004). A Cacna1a knockin migraine mouse model with increased susceptibility to cortical spreading depression. *Neuron* 41, 701–710.
35. Miller, R. J. (1997). Calcium channels prove to be a real headache. *Trends Neurosci.* 20, 189–192.
36. Estevez, M., Estevez, A. O., Cowie, R. H., and Gardner, K. L. (2004). The voltage-gated calcium channel UNC-2 is involved in stress-mediated regulation of tryptophan hydroxylase. *J. Neurochem.* 88, 102–113.
37. Buzzi, M. G., Bonamini, M., and Moskowitz, M. A. (1995). Neurogenic model of migraine. *Cephalalgia* 15, 277–280.
38. Williamson, D. J., and Hargreaves, R. J. (2001). Neurogenic inflammation in the context of migraine. *Microsc. Res. Tech.* 53(3), 167–168.
39. Levy, D., Jakubowski, M., and Burstein, R. (2004). Disruption of communication between peripheral and central trigeminovascular neurons mediates the antimigraine action of 5-HT1B/1D receptor agonists. *Proc. Natl. Acad. Sci. USA* 101(12), 4274–4279.
40. Malick, A., and Burstein, R. (2000). Peripheral and central sensitization during migraine. *Funct. Neurol.* 15(Suppl. 3), 28–35.
41. Yarnitsky, D., Goor-Aryeh, I., Bajwa, Z. H., Ransil, B. I., Cutrer, F. M., Sottile, A., and Burstein, R. (2003). 2003 Wolff Award: Possible parasympathetic contributions to peripheral and central sensitization during migraine. *Headache* 43(7), 704–714.
42. Arulmani, U., Maassenvandenbrink, A., Villalon, C. M., and Saxena, P. R. (2004). Calcitonin gene-related peptide and its role in migraine pathophysiology. *Eur. J. Pharmacol.* 500, 315–330.
43. Edvinsson, L. (2004). Blockade of CGRP receptors in the intracranial vasculature: A new target in the treatment of headache. *Cephalalgia* 24, 611–622.
44. Rosenfeld, M. G., Mermod, J.-J., Amara, S. G., Swanson, L. W., Sawchenko, P. E., Rivier, J., Vale, W. W., and Evans, R. M. (1983). Production of a novel neuropeptide encoded by the calcitonin gene via tissue-specific RNA processing. *Nature* 304, 129–135.
45. Brain, S. D., Williams, T. J., Tippins, J. R., Morris, H. R., and MacIntyre, I. (1985). Calcitonin gene-related peptide is a potent vasodilator. *Nature* 313, 54–56.

46. Brain, S. D., and Grant, A. D. (2004). Vascular actions of calcitonin gene-related peptide and adrenomedullin. *Physiol. Rev.* 84, 903–934.

47. Preibisz, J. J. (1993). Calcitonin gene-related peptide and regulation of human cardiovascular homeostasis. *Am. J. Hypertens.* 6, 434–450.

48. Gangula, P. R., Zhao, H., Supowit, S. C., Wimalawansa, S. J., Dipette, D. J., Westlund, K. N., Gagel, R. F., and Yallampalli, C. (2000). Increased blood pressure in α-calcitonin gene related peptide/calcitonin gene knockout mice. *Hypertension* 35, 470–475.

49. Oh-hashi, Y., Shindo, T., Kurihara, Y., Imai, T., Wang, Y., Morita, H., Imai, Y., Kayaba, Y., Nishimatsu, H., Suematsu, Y., Hirata, Y., Yazaki, Y., Nagai, R., Kuwaki, T., and Kurihara, H. (2001). Elevated sympathetic nervous activity in mice deficient in αCGRP. *Circ. Res.* 89, 983–990.

50. Salmon, A. M., Damaj, M. I., Marubio, L. M., Epping-Jordan, M. P., Merlo-Pich, E., and Changeux, J. P. (2001). Altered neuroadaptation in opiate dependence and neurogenic inflammatory nociception in a-CGRP-deficient mice. *Nat. Neurosci.* 4(4), 357–358.

51. Bereiter, D. A., and Benetti, A. P. (1991). Microinjections of calcitonin gene-related peptide within the trigeminal subnucleus caudalis of the cat affects adrenal and autonomic function. *Brain Res.* 558, 53–62.

52. Allen, G. V., Barbick, B., and Esser, M. J. (1996). Trigeminal-parabrachial connections: Possible pathway for nociception-induced cardiovascular reflex responses. *Brain Res.* 715, 125–135.

53. VanRossum, D., Hanisch, U. -K., and Quirion, R. (1997). Neuroanatomical localization, pharmacological characterization and functions of CGRP, related peptides and their receptors. *Neurosci. Biobehav. Rev.* 21, 649–678.

54. Lassen, L. H., Haderslev, P. A., Jacobsen, V. B., Iversen, H. K., Sperling, B., and Olesen, J. (2002). CGRP may play a causative role in migraine. *Cephalalgia* 22, 54–61.

55. Olesen, J., Diener, H. C., Husstedt, I. W., Goadsby, P. J., Hall, D., Meier, U., Pollentier, S., and Lesko, L. M. (2004). BIBN 4096 BS Clinical Proof of Concept Study Group. Calcitonin gene-related peptide receptor antagonist BIBN 4096 BS for the acute treatment of migraine. *N. Engl. J. Med.* 350, 1104–1110.

56. Durham, P. L. (2004). CGRP-receptor antagonists—A fresh approach to migraine therapy? *N. Engl. J. Med.* 350, 1073–1075.

57. Mair, J., Lechleitner, P., Laengle, T., Wiedermann, C., Diensti, F., and Saria, A. (1990). Plasma CGRP in acute myocardial infarction. *Lancet* 335, 168.

58. Lechleitner, P., Genser, N., Mair, J., Dienstl, A., Haring, C., Wiedermann, C. J., Puschendorf, B., Saria, A., and Dienstl, F. (1992). Calcitonin gene-related peptide in patients with and without early reperfusion after acute myocardial infarction. *Am. Heart J.* 124, 1433–1439.

59. Franco-Cereceda, A., and Liska, J. (2000). Potential of calcitonin gene-related peptide in coronary heart disease. *Pharmacology* 60, 1–8.

60. Oliver, K. R., Wainwright, A., Edvinsson, L., Pickard, J. D., and Hill, R. G. (2002). Immunohistochemical localization of calcitonin receptor-like receptor and receptor activity-modifying proteins in the human cerebral vasculature. *J. Cereb. Blood Flow Metab.* 22(5), 620–629.

61. Moreno, M. J., Cohen, Z., Stanimirovic, D. B., and Hamel, E. (1999). Functional calcitonin gene-related peptide type 1 and adrenomedullin receptors in human trigeminal ganglia, brain vessels, and cerebromicrovascular or astroglial cells in culture. *J. Cereb. Blood Flow Metab.* 19(11), 1270–1278.

62. Moreno, M. J., Abounader, R., Hebert, E., Doods, H., and Hamel, E. (2002). Efficacy of the non-peptide CGRP receptor antagonist BIBN4096BS in blocking CGRP-induced dilations in human and bovine cerebral arteries: Potential implications in acute migraine treatment. *Neuropharmacology* 42(4), 568–576.

63. Storer, R. J., Akerman, S., and Goadsby, P. J. (2004). Calcitonin gene-related peptide (CGRP) modulates nociceptive trigeminovascular transmission in the cat. *Br. J. Pharmacol.* 142(7), 1171–1181.

64. Doods, H., Hallermayer, G., Wu, D., Entzeroth, M., Rudolf, K., Engel, W., and Eberlein, W. (2000). Pharmacological profile of BIBN4096BS, the first selective small molecule CGRP antagonist. *Br. J. Pharmacol.* 129(3), 420–423.

65. Mallee, J. J., Salvatore, C. A., LeBourdelles, B., Oliver, K. R., Longmore, J., Koblan, K. S., and Kane, S. A. (2002). Receptor activity-modifying protein 1 determines the species selectivity of non-peptide CGRP receptor antagonists. *J. Biol. Chem.* 277(16), 14294–14298.

66. Hershey, J. C., Corcoran, H. A., Baskin, E. P., Salvatore, C. A., Mosser, S., Williams, T. M., Koblan, K. S., Hargreaves, R. J., and Kane, S. A. (2005). Investigation of the species selectivity of a nonpeptide CGRP receptor antagonist using a novel pharmacodynamic assay. *Regul. Pept.* 127(1–3), 71–77.

67. Petersen, K. A., Lassen, L. H., Birk, S., Lesko, L., and Olesen, J. (2005). BIBN4096BS antagonizes human alpha-calcitonin gene related peptide-induced headache and extracerebral artery dilatation. *Clin. Pharmacol. Ther.* 77(3), 202–213.

68. Petersen, K. A., Birk, S., Lassen, L. H., Kruuse, C., Jonassen, O., Lesko, L., and Olesen, J. (2005). The CGRP-antagonist, BIBN4096BS does not affect cerebral or systemic haemodynamics in healthy volunteers. *Cephalalgia* 25(2), 139–147.

69. Silberstein, S. D. (2000). Practice parameter: Evidence-based guidelines for migraine headache (an evidence-based review): Report of the Quality Standars Subcommittee of the American Academy of Neurology. *Neurology* 55, 754–762.

70. Adelman, J. U., Adelman, L. C., Freeman, M. C., Von Seggern, R. L., and Drake, J. (2004). Cost considerations of acute migraine treatment. *Headache* 44, 271–285.

71. Ferrari, M. D., Goadsby, P. J., Roon, K. I., and Lipton, R. B. (2002). Triptans (serotonin, 5-HT1B/1D agonists) in migraine: Detailed results and methods of a meta-analysis of 53 trials. *Cephalalgia* 22(8), 633–658.

72. Mathew, N. T. (2001). Pathophysiology, epidemiology, and impact of migraine. *Clin. Cornerstone* 4(3), 1–17.

73. Hamel, E. (1999). The biology of serotonin receptors: Focus on migraine pathophysiology and treatment. *Can. J. Neurol. Sci.* 26(Suppl. 3), S2–6.

74. Longmore, J., Shaw, D., Smith, D., Hopkins, R., McAllister, G., Pickard, J. D., Sirinathsinghji, D. J., Butler, A. J., and Hill, R. G. (1997). Differential distribution of 5HT1D- and 5HT1B-immunoreactivity within the human trigeminocerebrovascular system: Implications for the discovery of new antimigraine drugs. *Cephalalgia* 17(8), 833–842.

75. Potrebic, S., Ahn, A. H., Skinner, K., Fields, H. L., and Basbaum, A. I. (2003). Peptidergic nociceptors of both trigeminal and dorsal root ganglia express serotonin1D receptors: Implications for the selective antimigraine action of triptans. *J. Neurosci.* 23(34), 10988–10997.

76. Goadsby, P. J. (2000). The pharmacology of headache. *Prog. Neurobiol.* 62(5), 509–525.

77. Durham, P. L., and Russo, A. F. (2003). Stimulation of the calcitonin gene-related peptide enhancer by mitogen-activated protein kinases and repression by an antimigraine drug in trigeminal ganglia neurons. *J. Neurosci.* 23, 807–815.
78. Fowler, P. A., Lacey, L. F., Thomas, M., Keene, O. N., Tanner, R. J., and Baber, N. S. (1991). The clinical pharmacology, pharmacokinetics and metabolism of sumatriptan. *Eur. Neurol.* 31, 291–294.
79. Limmroth, V., Kazarawa, Z., Fritsche, G., and Diener, H. C. (1999). Headache after frequent use of new serotonin agonists zolmitriptan and naratriptan. *Lancet* 353(9158), 378.
80. Limmroth, V., Katsarava, Z., Fritsche, G., Przywara, S., and Diener, H. C. (2002). Features of medication overuse headache following overuse of different acute headache drugs. *Neurology* 59(7), 1011–1014.
81. Geraud, G., Keywood, C., and Senard, J. M. (2003). Migraine headache recurrence: Relationship to clinical, pharmacological, and pharmacokinetic properties of triptans. *Headache* 43(4), 376–388.
82. Visser, W. H., Jaspers, N. M., de Vriend, R. H., and Ferrari, M. D. (1996). Chest symptoms after sumatriptan: A two-year clinical practice review in 735 consecutive migraine patients. *Cephalalgia* 16(8), 554–559.
83. Codispoti, J. R., Prior, M. J., Fu, M., Harte, C. M., and Nelson, E. B. (2001). Efficacy of nonprescription doses of ibuprofen for treating migraine headache. A randomized controlled trial. *Headache* 41(7), 665–679.
84. Peroutka, S. J., Lyon, J. A., Swarbrick, J., Lipton, R. B., Kolodner, K., and Goldstein, J. (2004). Efficacy of diclofenac sodium softgel 100 mg with or without caffeine 100 mg in migraine without aura: A randomized, double-blind, crossover study. *Headache* 44(2), 136–141.
85. Lipton, R. B., Stewart, W. F., Ryan, R. E. Jr., Saper, J., Silberstein, S., and Sheftell, F. (1998). Efficacy and safety of acetaminophen, aspirin, and caffeine in alleviating migraine headache pain: Three double-blind, randomized, placebo-controlled trials. *Arch. Neurol.* 55(2), 210–217.
86. The EMSASI Study Group (2004). Placebo-controlled comparison of effervescent acetylsalicylic acid, sumatriptan and ibuprofen in the treatment of migraine attacks. *Cephalalgia* 24, 947–954.
87. Silberstein, S. D., Lipton, R. B., and Dalessio, D. J. (2001). In *Wolff's Headache and Other Head Pain*, 7th ed., Oxford University Press, Oxford.
88. Treves, T. A., Kuritzky, A., Hering, R., and Korczyn, A. D. (1998). Dihydroergotamine nasal spray in the treatment of acute migraine. *Headache* 38(8), 614–617.
89. Stillman, M. J., Zajac, D., and Rybicki, L. A. (2004). Treatment of primary headache disorders with intravenous valproate: Initial outpatient experience. *Headache* 44, 65–69.
90. Tanen, D. A., Miller, S., French, T., and Riffenburgh, R. H. (2003). Intravenous sodium valproate versus prochlorperazine for the emergency department treatment of acute migraine headaches: A prospective, randomized, double-blind trial. *Ann. Emerg. Med.* 41(6), 847–853.
91. Silberstein, S., Mathew, N., Saper, J., and Jenkins, S. (2000). Botulinum toxin type A as a migraine preventive treatment. For the BOTOX Migraine Clinical Research Group. *Headache* 40(6), 445–450.
92. Friedman, B. W., Corbo, J., Lipton, R. B., Bijur, P. E., Esses, D., Solorzano, C., and Gallagher, E. J. (2005). A trial of metoclopramide vs sumatriptan for the emergency department treatment of migraines. *Neurology* 64(3), 463–468.

93. Jones, J., Pack, S., and Chun, E. (1996). Intramuscular prochlorperazine versus metoclopramide as single-agent therapy for the treatment of acute migraine headache. *Am. J. Emerg. Med.* 14(3), 262–264.

94. Coppola, M., Yealy, D. M., and Leibold, R. A. (1995). Randomized, placebo-controlled evaluation of prochlorperazine versus metoclopramide for emergency department treatment of migraine headache. *Ann. Emerg. Med.* 26(5), 541–546.

95. Boyle, R., Behan, P. O., and Sutton, J. A. (1990). A correlation between severity of migraine and delayed gastric emptying measured by an epigastric impedance method. *Br. J. Clin. Pharmacol.* 30(3), 405–409.

96. Silberstein, S. D. (2001). Shared mechanisms and comorbidities in neurologic and psychiatric disorders. *Headache* 41(Suppl. 1), S11–17.

97. Cutrer, F. M. (2004). Antiepileptic drugs: How they work in headache. *Headache* 41(Suppl. 1), S3–10.

98. Rogawski, M. A., and Loscher, W. (2004). The neurobiology of antiepileptic drugs for the treatment of nonepileptic conditions. *Nat. Med.* 10, 685–692.

99. Roudenok, V., Gutjar, L., Antipova, V., and Rogov, Y. (2001). Expression of vasoactive intestinal polypeptide and calcitonin gene-related peptide in human stellate ganglia after acute myocardial infarction. *Ann. Anat.* 183, 341–344.

100. Lee, W. S., Limmroth, V., Ayata, C., Cutrer, F. M., Waeber, C., Yu, X., and Moskowitz, M. A. (1995). Peripheral GABAA receptor-mediated effects of sodium valproate on dural plasma protein extravasation to substance P and trigeminal stimulation. *Br. J. Pharmacol.* 116, 1661–1667.

101. Hering, R., and Kuritzky, A. (1992). Sodium valproate in the prophylactic tratment of migraine: A double-blind study versus placebo. *Cephalalgia* 12, 81–84.

102. Mathew, N. T., Saper, J. R., Silberstein, S. D., Rankin, L., Markley, H. G., Solomon, S., Rapoport, A. M., Silber, C. J., and Deaton, R. L. (1995). Migraine prophylaxis with divalproex. *Arch. Neurol.* 52(3), 281–286.

103. Brandes, J. L., Saper, J. R., Diamond, M., Couch, J. R., Lewis, D. W., Schmitt, J., Neto, W., Schwabe, S., and Jacobs, D. (2004). MIGR-002 Study Group. Topiramate for migraine prevention: A randomized controlled trial. *JAMA* 291, 965–973.

104. Diener, H. C., Tfelt-Hansen, P., Dahlof, C., Lainez, M. J., Sandrini, G., Wang, S. J., Neto, W., Vijapurkar, U., Doyle, A., Jacobs, D., and MIGR-003 Study Group. (2004). Topiramate in migraine prophylaxis: Results from a placebo-controlled trial with propranolol as an active control. *J. Neurol.* 251, 943–950.

105. Silberstein, S. D., Neto, W., Schmitt, J., and Jacobs, D., MIGR-001 Study Group. (2004). Topiramate in migraine prevention: Results of a large controlled trial. *Arch. Neurol.* 61(4), 490–495.

106. Silvestrini, M., Bartolini, M., Coccia, M., Baruffaldi, R., Taffi, R., and Provinciali, L. (2003). Topiramate in the treatment of chronic migraine. *Cephalagia* 23, 820–824.

107. Mathew, N. T., Rapoport, A., Saper, J., Magnus, L., Klapper, J., Ramadan, N., Stacey, B., and Tepper, S. (2001). Efficacy of gabapentin in migraine prophylaxis. *Headache* 41, 119–128.

108. Silberstein, S. D., and Goadsby, P. J. (2002). Migraine: Preventive treatment. *Cephalagia* 22, 491–512.

109. Shields, K. G., and Goadsby, P. J. (2005). Propranolol modulates trigeminovascular responses in thalamic ventroposteromedial nucleus: A role in migraine? *Brain* 128, 86–97.

110. Tfelt-Hansen, P., Standnes, B., Kangasneimi, P., Hakkarainen, H., and Olesen, J. (1984). Timolol vs propranolol vs placebo in common migraine prophylaxis: A double-blind multicenter trial. *Acta. Neurol. Scand.* 69(1), 1–8.

111. Stellar, S., Ahrens, S. P., Meibohm, A. R., and Reines, S. A. (1984). Migraine prevention with timolol: A double-blind crossover study. *JAMA* 252(18), 2576–2580.

112. Carroll, J. D., Reidy, M., Savundra, P. A., Cleave, N., and McAinsh, J. (1990). Long-acting propranolol in the prophylaxis of migraine: A comparative study of two doses. *Cephalalgia* 10, 101–105.

113. Couch, J. R., Ziegler, D., and Hassanein, R. (1976). Amitriptyline in the prophylaxis of migraine: Effectiveness and relationship of antimigraine and antidepressant effects. *Neurology* (26), 121–127.

114. Tomkins, G. E., Jackson, J. L., O'Malley, P. G., Balden, E., and Santoro, J. E. (2001). Treatment of chronic headaches with antidepressants: A meta-analysis. *Am. J. Med.* 111(1), 54–63.

115. Evers, S., Vollmer-Haase, J., Schwaag, S., Rahmann, A., Husstedt, I. W., and Frese, A. (2004). Botulinum toxin A in the prophylactic treatment of migraine—A randomized, double-blind, placebo-controlled study. *Cephalalgia* 24(10), 838–843.

116. Peikert, A., Wilimzig, C., and Kohne-Volland, R. (1996). Prophylaxis of migraine with oral magnesium: Results from a prospective, multicenter, placebo-controlled and double-blind randomized study. *Cephalalgia* 16, 257–263.

117. Schoenen, J., Jacquy, J., and Lenaerts, M. (1998). Effectiveness of high-dose riboflavin in migraine prophylaxis. A randomized controlled trial. *Neurology.* 50, 466–470.

118. Durham, P. L., and Russo, A. F. (1999). Regulation of calcitonin gene-related peptide secretion by a serotonergic antimigraine drug. *J. Neurosci.* 19, 3423–3429.

119. Durham, P. L., and Russo, A. F. (2000). Differential regulation of mitogen-activated protein kinase-responsive genes by the duration of a calcium signal. *Mol. Endocrinol.* 14, 1570–1582.

120. Ciruela, A., Dixon, A. K., Bramwell, S., Gonzalez, M. I., Pinnock, R. D., and Lee, K. (2003). Identification of MEK1 as a novel target for the treatment of neuropathic pain. *Br. J. Pharmacol.* 138, 751–756.

121. Davidson, B. L., and Paulson, H. L. (2004). Molecular medicine for the brain: Silencing of disease genes with RNA interference. *Lancet Neurol.* 3, 145–149.

122. Juang, K. D., Wang, S. J., Fuh, J. L., Lu, S. R., and Su, T. P. (2000). Comorbidity of depressive and anxiety disorders in chronic daily headache and its subtypes. *Headache* 40, 818–823.

123. Merikangas, K. R., Angst, J., and Isler, H. (1990). Migraine and psychopathology: Results of the Zurich cohort study of young adults. *Arch. Gen. Psychiatry* 47, 849–853.

124. Lipton, J. A., Ship, J. A., and Larach-Robinson, D. (1993). Estimated prevalence and distribution of reported orofacial pain in the United States. *J. Am. Dent. Assoc.* 124, 115–121.

125. Elias, W. J., and Burchiel, K. J. (2002). Trigeminal neuralgia and other neuropathic pain syndromes of the head and face. *Curr. Pain Headache Rep.* 6, 115–124.

126. Tal, M. (1999). A Role for inflammation in chronic pain. *Curr. Rev. Pain* 3, 440–446.

127. Zimmermann, M. (2001). Pathobiology of neuropathic pain. *Eur. J. Pharmacol.* 429, 23–37.

128. Kopp, S. (2001). Neuroendocrine, immune, and local responses related to temporomandibular disorders. *J. Orofac. Pain* 15, 9–28.

129. Lundeberg, T., Alstergren, P., Appelgren, A., Appelgren, B., Carleson, J., Kopp, S., and Theodorsson, E. (1996). A model for experimentally induced termporomandibular joint arthritis in rats: effects of carrageenan on neuropeptide-like immunoreactivity. *Neuropeptides* 30, 37–41.

130. Spears, R., Hutchins, B., and Hinton, R. J. (1998). Capsaicin application to the temporomandibular joint alters calcitonin gene-related peptide levels in the trigeminal ganglion of the rat. *J. Orofac. Pain* 12, 108–115.

131. Sessle, B. J. (2001). New insights into peripheral chemical mediators of temporomandibular pain and inflammation. *J. Orofac. Pain.* 15(1), 5.

132. Belmonte, C., Acosta, M. C., and Gallar, J. (2004). Neural basis of sensation in intact and injured corneas. *Exp. Eye Res.* 78(3), 513–525.

133. Goto, K., Miyauchi, T., Homma, S., and Ohshima, N. (1992). Calcitonin gene-related peptide in the regulation of cardiac function. *Ann. NY Acad. Sci.* 657, 194–203.

134. Joyce, C. D., Fiscus, R. R., Wang, X., Dries, D. J., Morris, R. C., and Prinz, R. A. (1990). Calcitonin gene-related peptide levels are elevated in patients with sepsis. *Surgery* 108(6), 1097–1101.

135. Kumar, D., Alvaro, M. S., Julka, I. S., and Marshall, H. J. (1998). Diabetic peripheral neuropathy. Effectiveness of electrotherapy and amitriptyline for symptomatic relief. *Diabetes Care* 21(8), 1322–1325.

136. Backonja, M., Beydoun, A., Edwards, K. R., Schwartz, S. L., Fonseca, V., Hes, M., LaMoreaux, L., and Garofalo, E. (1998). Gabapentin for the symptomatic treatment of painful neuropathy in patients with diabetes mellitus: A randomized controlled trial. *JAMA* 280(21), 1831–1836.

137. Harke, H., Gretenkort, P., Ladleif, H. U., Rahman, S., and Harke, O. (2001). The response of neuropathic pain and pain in complex regional pain syndrome I to carbamazepine and sustained-release morphine in patients pretreated with spinal cord stimulation: A double-blinded randomized study. *Anesth. Analg.* 92(2), 488–495.

138. McQuay, H., Carroll, D., Jadad, A. R., Wiffen, P., and Moore, A. (1995). Anticonvulsant drugs for management of pain: A systematic review. *BMJ* 311(7012), 1047–1052.

INDEX

Absorption pharmacokinetics
  nicotine dependence and withdrawal, 543–544
ABT431 compound
  schizophrenia dopamine hypothesis, 373
N-Acetyl aspartate (NAA)
  glutamate theory of schizophrenia pathological evidence, 292
  schizophrenia analysis, 256–257
  schizophrenia dopamine hypothesis, 289
N-Acetylcysteine (NAC)
  psychostimulant abuse and cystine/glutamate transporter restoration, 576
Acoustic startle
  mouse anxiety models
    neurosteroid effects, 147
Acquired immunodeficiency syndrome (AIDS)
  opiate addiction comorbidity with, 691–694
Acute delivery systems
  nicotine dependence and withdrawal therapy, 547–548
Addictive disorders. *See also* Heroin addiction; specific disorders, e.g. Alcohol abuse
  diagnostic criteria, 456–457
  endocannabinoids, 675–676
  γ-hydroxybutyric acid (GHB) and, 635–636

hallucinogens and, 639–640
nicotine dependence and withdrawal pharmacology, 536–545
  absorption pharmacokinetics, 543–544
  bupropion, 549–550
  cannabinoid antagonists, 550
  distribution pharmacokinetics, 544
  metabolism and elimination pharmacokinetics, 544–545
  nicotine reinforcement neurosubstrates, 537–540
  nicotinic acetylcholine receptors, 537
    functional adaptations, 540–541
  nicotinic antagonists, 548–549
  nicotinic partial agonists, 548
  nonnicotinic agents, 549–551
  opioid antagonists, 550–551
  overview, 545–546
  pharmacokinetics, 543–545
  public health policy and, 551–552
  replacement medications, 546–548
  tricyclic antidepressants, 550
  withdrawal neurosubstrates, 541–543
opiate addiction
  buprenorphine studies, 696–698
  drug discovery survey, 699–700
  epidemiology, 691–694
  future research issues, 698–699
  treatment statistics, 694–696

pharmacotherapy
   history of, 451–457
   reward modulation/countermodulation and, 458–459
   risk factors for addiction development, 457–458
  psychostimulant abuse
   addiction therapy development, 585–586
   chronic exposure-related neurobiology, 579–589
    neurotransmitter/neuroendocrine systems, 580–584
    signal transduction mechanisms and gene expression, 584–585
   future research issues, 588–589
   neuropharmacology, 569–579
    γ-aminobutyric acid, 576–577
    glutamate, 575–576
    hyopthalamic-pituitary-adrenal axis, 577–578
    monoamines, 570–575
    neuropeptides, 578–579
   overview, 567–569
  risk factors for, 455, 457–458
  selective serotonin reuptake inhibitors
   anxiety disorder therapy, 67–69
Adenosine receptors
  anxiety neurobiology and deficits in, 29–30
Aδ fibers
  pain pathways, 711–712
Adolescent patients
  psychostimulant abuse
   chronic exposure and sensitization effects, 581–585
Adrenergic receptors
  antipsychotic drugs mechanisms, 426–427
  psychostimulant abuse, 575
Adrenocorticotropin hormone (ACTH)
  anxiety neurobiology and, 17
  nicotine dependence and withdrawal, 539–540
  psychostimulant abuse, 577–578
   chronic exposure and sensitization effects, 580–585
Adult environmental effects
  anxiety neurobiology, 35
Affective flattening
  in schizophrenia, 255–256
Agonist agents
  psychostimulant abuse therapy, 586–587

AKT1 gene
  dystrobrevin binding protein 1 (DTNBP1) schizophrenia susceptibility, 348–349
Alcohol
  γ-hydroxybutyric acid (GHB) and, 634
  neurosteroid effects and, 157–158
Alcohol abuse
  animal models
   neuroanatomical substrates, 466–467
    behavioral paradigms, 467–470
    central nervous system circuitry, 470–471
   novel substrates, 471
  dopamine neuronal systems and substrates, 471–486
   bed nucleus of stria terminalis, 473–475
   dopaminergic regulation, early research, 472–473
   extracellular dopamine, 485–486
   future research issues, 517–518
   GABAergic interactions with, 486
   lateral hypothalamus, 481–485
   D_2 dopaminergic regulation, hypothesized mechanisms, 481–485
   ventral pallidum, 476–480
    dopaminargic regulation hypothesized mechanisms, 478–480
  GABA$_A$ benzodiazepine receptor complex, molecular biology, 487–501
   alcohol/modulator commonalities, 487–488
   CA1/CA3 hippocampus, 511–516
   efficacy of βCCT/3PBD modulation, GABA$_{A1,2,3,5}$ receptors, 499–501
   future research issues, 517–518
   GABA-DA interaction hypothesis, 496–498
   ligand selectivity with GABA$_{A1}$ subunits, 498–499
   microinjection studies, 505–506
   naltrexone antagonist, 507–511
   novel CNS GABAergic substrates, 498
   oral administration, βCCT/3PBD anxiety reduction, 510–511
   vs. naltrexone, 507–511
   probe applications, 488–493
   site-specific microinjection, 493–496
   subunit selectivity vs. intrinsic efficacy, 516–517

systemic administration, 492–493, 503–504
ventral pallidum, 501–502
overview, 466
Alcohol-preferring rats (P rat line)
alcohol abuse studies
appropriate behavioral paradigms, 467–470
neuroanatomical controls, 469–470
reinforcer-specific controls, 469
central nervous system circuitry in, 470–471
characteristics of, 467
novel neuranatomical substrates, 471
AlloTHDOC
plasma levels, 137–140
Alogia
in schizophrenia, 255–256
α-Amino-3-hydroxy-5-methyl-isoxazole-4-propionic acid (AMPA)
benzodiazepine tolerance, 101
glutamate theory of schizophrenia
history of, 290–291
pathological evidence, 291–292
pharmacological evidence, 294–295
schizophrenia pharmacotherapy
drug development for, 392
Amino acid neurotransmission
anxiety disorder therapy, 72–75
anticonvulsants, 74–75
benzodiazepines, 73–74
Amino acid residues
benzodiazepines
$GABA_A$ receptors, 106–108
D-Amino acid oxidase activator (DAO A)
schizophrenia candidate gene, 327
D-Amino acid oxidase (DAO)
schizophrenia candidate gene, 327
Amisulpiride
schizophrenia therapy
D_2/D_3 and D_4 receptor antagonism and regional specificity, 380
"AMPAkines"
glutamate theory of schizophrenia, 295
Amphetamine
chronic exposure and sensitization effects, 580–585
3,4-methylenedioxymethamphetamine
reinforcement of, 615–616
monoamine neuropharmacology, 571–575
neuropeptide pharmacology and, 579

d-Amphetamine
alcohol abuse studies
dopaminergic receptor systems and substrates, 472–473
Amygdala. See also Extended amygala (EA)
anxiety disorders and, 13–15
Anandamide
appetite regulation and, 671–672
endocannabinoid ligands, 663–664
pain management and, 667–668
pharmacology, 665–675
Anesthesia
neuroactive steroid effects and, 158–159
Animal models. See also Mouse studies
alcohol-motivated behaviors
neuroanatomical substrates, 466–467
behavioral paradigms, 467–470
central nervous system circuitry, 470–471
novel substrates, 471
anxiety neurobiology
anxiety-like behavior in, 10–12
brain imaging studies, 14–15
early-life environmental effects, 33–34
rodent models, 6–9
3,4-methylenedioxymethamphetamine
neurotoxicity, 620–621
behavioral effects, 630–631
neurosteroid effects, 142–152
acoustic/fear-potentiated startle, 147
defensive burying behavior, 149–150
elevated-plus maze, 143–145
Geller/Seifter and Vogel conflict tests, 145–146
light-dark box, 146–147
mild mental stress models and social isolation, 151–152
mirrored chamber, 147–148
modified forced-swim test, 150–151
open-field activity, 148–149
separation-induced ultrasonic vocalizations, 150
obsessive-compulsive disorders (OCD), 224
psychostimulant abuse
chronic exposure and sensitization effects, 581–585
schizophrenia, 263–265
transient receptor potential V1 (TRPV1) receptors, 736
Anticonvulsants
anxiety disorder therapy, 74–75

migraine management, 766–767
Δ^9-tetrahydrocannabinol as, 672–673
Antidepressants
  anxiety disorder therapy, 64–70
    beta blockers, 71
    mirtazapine, 70
    monoamine oxidase inhibitors, 70
    selective serotonin reuptake inhibitors, 66–69
    serotonin and noradrenaline reuptake inhibitors, 69
    serotonin receptor agonists, 70–71
    tricyclic antidpressants, 69–70
  migraine management, 767
  nicotine dependence and withdrawal therapy
    bupropion, 549–550
  tricyclic
    nicotine dependence and withdrawal therapy, 550
Antiemetics
  migraine management, 765
Antihistamines
  anxiety disorder therapy, 75
Antinociception
  cannabinoid analgesics and, 668
Antipsychotics
  anxiety disorder therapy, 71–72
  atypical agents, mechanisms of action
    adrenergic mechanisms, 426–427
    atypical antipsychotics
      5-HT_{2A} receptor, 418–421
    cholinergic mechanisms, 429–430
    clozapine regimens
      dopamine D_2 receptor blockade, 412–415
    glutamatergic mechanisms, 427–429
    neurogenesis, 430
    neurokinin 3 receptors, 430
    partial dopamine agonists, 416–417
    serotonin receptor 5-HT_{1A}-5-HT_{2A} interactions, 424–425
    serotonin receptor 5-HT_{2A}-5-HT_{2C} interactions, 422–424
    serotonin receptor 5-HT_6, 425–426
    serotonin receptors, 417–418
    serotonin release, 426
    sertonin receptor 5-HT_{2A} blockade
      cortical dopamine efflux and cognitive function, 421–422
      extrapyramidal function, 422

  substituted benzamides
    D_1, D_3, and D_4 receptors, 415–416
    table of drugs, 413
    typical vs. atypical drugs, 411–412
  metabolic syndrome with, 254
  obsessive-compulsive disorders
    neuropharmacology, 229–234
    symptom induction from, 234
  schizophrenia therapy
    first-generation (conventional) agents, 383
    glutamate theory of schizophrenia, 294–295
    history of, 370–371
    hypothesized mechanisms of action, 376–382
      D_1 receptors, 380–381
      D_2/D_3 and D_4 antagonism and regional specificity, 380
      D_2 occupancy thresholds and rapid dissociation, 378–380
      D_2 receptor occupancy, 376–378
      dopamine release, 381
      NMDA receptor function, 381
      synthesis reactions, 381–382
    negative affect remediation, 255–256
    psychosis management, 254
    safety and tolerability, 387–388
    second-generation (atypical) agents, 383–387
Anxiety and anxiety disorders
  alcohol abuse and
    βCCT/3PBC anxiety reduction efficacy, 510–511
  clinical management, 60–61
  corticotropin-releasing factor receptor antagonists
    therapeutic potential of, 196–198
  depression and
    pharmacotherapy, 80
  diagnostic criteria, 9–12, 61–62
  3,4-methylenedioxymethamphetamine effects, 630–631
  neuroactive steroids
    alcohol effects, 157–159
    animal models, 142–152
    behavioral effects, 142
    brain and peripheral sources, 135–137
    chemistry and pharmacology, 135–142
    enantiomeric selectivity, 141–142
    $GABA_A$ receptors and ligand-gated ion channels, 137–141

HPA axis function, 154–156
overview, 134–135
stress-induced behaviors, 154–155
neurobiology of
basic principles, 4
early-life environmental effects, 33–37
fear/anxiety circuits, 13–15
genetic susceptibility, 18–19
intracellular regulators, 30–33
knockout mice
neuronal messenger alterations, 24–26
neurotransmitter receptor deficits and CRH proteins, 26–30
mouse genetics studies, 19–24
neurotransmitter systems and neuronal messengers, 15–18
psychological traits
continuous expression of normal personality, 9–10
genetic basis of, 4–6
mouse behavior extrapolation studies, 6–9
pharmacotherapy
anxiolytic drugs, 62–75
amino acid neurotransmission, 72–75
anticonvulsants, 74–75
antidepressants, 64–70
antihistamines, 75
antipsychotics, 71–72
benzodiazepines, 73–74
beta-blockers, 71
lithium, 75
monoamine neurotransmission, 63–72
serotonin receptor agonists, 70–71
depressive disorders, 80
future research issues, 81
generalized anxiety disorder, 77
obsessive-compulsive disorder, 77–78
overview, 60
panic disorder/agoraphobia, 78
phobias, 78, 80
posttraumatic stress disorder, 79
social anxiety disorder, 79–80
treatments chart, 76
"Anxiety-related pathways"
anxiety neurobiology and, 36
Anxiolytic drugs
anxiety disorder pharmacotherapy, 62–75
amino acid neurotransmission, 72–75
anticonvulsants, 74–75
antidepressants, 64–70
antihistamines, 75
antipsychotics, 71–72
benzodiazepines, 73–74
beta-blockers, 71
lithium, 75
mirtazapine, 70
monoamine neurotransmission, 63–72
monoamine oxidase inhibitors, 70
selective serotonin reuptake inhibitors, 66–69
serotonin and noradrenaline reuptake inhibitors, 69
serotonin receptor agonists, 70–71
tricyclic antidepressants, 69–70
corticotropin-releasing factor receptor antagonists
future research issues, 198–199
nonpeptide ligands, 195–196
overview, 177–179
peptide ligand pharmacology, 185–195
ligand binding mechanisms, 190–195
receptor/ligand family structure, 179–185
ligand properties, 180–181
receptor subtypes and distribution, 181–185
therapeutic potential, 196–198
Appetite regulation
cannabinoid receptors and, 670–672
Arachidonic acid derivatives
endocannabinoid ligands, 663–664
transient receptor potential V1 (TRPV1) receptor expression, 732–733
N-Arachidonoyldopamine
endocannabinoid ligands, 663–664
Arachidonoylethanolamide
cannabinoid receptors and, 661–662
O-Arachidonoylethanolamine
endocannabinoid ligands, 663–664
Arousal
autonomic arousal
anxiety neurobiology, 4
animal anxiety-like behavior, 10–12
Asenapine
schizophrenia therapy, 389
Assembly mechanisms
$GABA_A$ receptors
benzodiazepines, 108–110
Astressin
corticotropin-releasing factor receptor antagonists
ligand binding mechanisms, 191–195

Attention-deficit hyperactivity disorder (ADHD)
  obsessive-compulsive disorder comorbidity, 216
  psychostimulant therapy, 568–569, 587
    chronic exposure and sensitization effects, 581–585
Attention deficits
  schizophrenia
    animal models, 263–264
Augmentation strategies
  obsessive-compulsive disorders neuropharmacology, 225, 229–234
Autonomic arousal
  anxiety neurobiology, 4
  animal anxiety-like behavior, 10–12
Autoreceptors
  partial dopamine agonists, 416–417
Avoidance behaviors
  anxiety neurobiology, 4
  animal anxiety-like behavior, 10–12
Avolition
  in schizophrenia, 255–256

Baclofen
  psychostimulant abuse therapy, 588
Basal ganglia-thalamic-frontal loops
  obsessive-compulsive disorders neuropharmacology, 221–222
BC1 RNA
  anxiety neurobiology and, 32
Bed nucleus of stria terminalis (BST)
  alcohol abuse studies
    dopaminergic receptor systems and substrates, 473–475
Behavioral inhibition/activity
  alcohol abuse
    animal models
      neuroanatomical substrates, 466–467
      behavioral paradigms, 467–470
      central nervous system circuitry, 470–471
      novel substrates, 471
    dopamine neuronal systems and substrates, 471–486
      bed nucleus of stria terminalis, 473–475
      dopaminergic regulation, early research, 472–473
      extracellular dopamine, 485–486
      future research issues, 517–518
      GABAergic interactions with, 486

  lateral hypothalamus, 481–485
  ventral pallidum, 476–480
  GABA$_A$ benzodiazepine receptor complex, molecular biology, 487–501
    alcohol/modulator commonalities, 487–488
    CA1/CA3 hippocampus, 511–516
    efficacy of βCCT/3PBD modulation, GABA$_{A1,2,3,5}$ receptors, 499–501
    future research issues, 517–518
    GABA-DA interaction hypothesis, 496–498
    ligand selectivity with GABA$_{A1}$ subunits, 498–499
    microinjection studies, 505–506
    naltrexone antagonist, 507–511
    novel CNS GABAergic substrates, 498
    probe applications, 488–493
    site-specific microinjection, 493–496
    subunit selectivity vs. intrinsic efficacy, 516–517
    systemic administration, 492–493, 503–504
    ventral pallidum, 501–502
  overview, 466
anxiety neurobiology, 4
  animal anxiety-like behavior, 10–12
3,4-methylenedioxymethamphetamine effects, 616–619
  neurotoxic lesions and, 629–631
neurosteroids, 142
psychostimulant abuse
  chronic exposure and sensitization effects, 580–585
Benzamides
  D_1, D_3, and D_4 receptors, 415–416
Benzodiazepines (BZs). See also GABA$_A$ benzodiazepine receptor complex
anxiety disorder therapy, 73–74
flunitrazepam, 637
future research, 116–117
GABA$_A$ benzodiazepine receptor complex
  alcohol abuse studies, 487–501
    alcohol/modulator commonalities, 487–488
    CA1/CA3 hippocampus, 511–516
    efficacy of βCCT/3PBD modulation, GABA$_{A1,2,3,5}$ receptors, 499–501
    future research issues, 517–518

GABA-DA interaction hypothesis, 496–498
ligand selectivity with GABA$_{A1}$ subunits, 498–499
microinjection studies, 505–506
naltrexone antagonist, 507–511
novel CNS GABAergic substrates, 498
oral administration, βCCT/3PBD anxiety reduction, 510–511
vs. naltrexone, 507–511
probe applications, 488–493
site-specific microinjection, 493–496
subunit selectivity vs. intrinsic efficacy, 516–517
systemic administration, 492–493, 503–504
ventral pallidum, 501–502
GABA$_A$ receptors
assembly, clustering, and surface expression, 108–110
binding pocket, 105–108
brain function diversity, 110–112
functional diversity, knockout/knockin models, 112–114
single-cell response modulation, 99–100
structure and function, 93–96
subunit/subtype diversity, 103–104
3,4-methylenedioxymethamphetamine effects on, 628
receptor ligand pharmacology, 97–102
endogenous site, 98–99
metabolism functions, 101–102
single-cell GABA response modulation, 99–100
therapeutic action, 97–98
tolerance and dependence characteristics, 100–101
structure-activity relationships, 114–116
structure and function, 93–96
Beta-blockers
anxiety disorder therapy, 71
migraine management, 767
BIBN4096BS compound
calcitonin gene-related peptide sites and migraine therapy targeting, 762–764
Bicuculline
alcohol abuse studies
GABA$_A$ benzodiazepine receptor complex, 487–488
site-specific microinjection techniques, 494–496
Bifeprunox
schizophrenia therapy, 389
Binding pocket structures
benzodiazepines
GABA$_A$ receptors, 105–108
Biochemical markers
in schizophrenia, 260–262
Biochemistry
3,4-methylenedioxymethamphetamine effects, 616–619
Biogenesis of lysosome-related organelles complex-1 (BLOC1)
dystrobrevin binding protein 1 (DTNBP1) molecular interactions, 353
Biological mechanisms
of schizophrenia, 256–263
Blood alcohol concentration (BAC) levels
alcohol abuse studies in alcohol-preferring rats, 468–470
Body temperature
3,4-methylenedioxymethamphetamine effects on, 617–618
neurotoxicity and, 624–625
Botulinum toxin (Botox)
migraine management, 768
Brain
anxiety disorder-related regions of, 13–15
benzodiazepine distribution, 110–112
3,4-methylenedioxymethamphetamine neurotoxicity
biochemical and functional changes, 631–632
neuroactive steroid sources, 135–137
neuroanatomical control regions
alcohol abuse studies in alcohol-preferring rats, 469–470
circuitry systems, 470–471
psychostimulant abuse, 574–575
Brain-derived neurotrophic factor (BDNF)
anxiety neurobiology, 4
genetic susceptibility studies, 18–19
knockout mice studies, 25–26
receptor deficits and, 29–30
schizophrenia therapy
serotonin receptor 5-HT$_{2A}$ receptor and, 421–422
Brain imaging studies
obsessive-compulsive disorders, 217–222
animal models, 224

neuropharmacological implications, 220–222
schizophrenia, 256–260
Buprenorphine
  opiate addiction therapy
    comparative efficacy studies, 697–698
    implementation issues and pilot studies, 698
    regulatory approval studies, 696–697
Bupropion
  nicotine dependence and withdrawal therapy, 549–550
Buspirone
  anxiety disorder therapy, 70–71
  opiate addiction therapy, 699
Butyrophenones
  schizophrenia therapy
    clinical profile, 383

CA1/CA3 hippocampal fields
  alcohol abuse studies
    $GABA_{A5}$ receptor probes, 511–516
Calcitonin gene-related peptide (CGRP)
  migraine therapy, 759–763
    injection techniques, 763
    neurovascular model, 759–760
    receptor antagonist therapeutic efficacy, 763–764
    synthesis and actions, 760–761
    targeted repression therapy, 768
    trigeminovasculature sites, 761–763
  pain management applications, 768–769
Calcitonin receptor-like receptor (CLR)
  calcitonin gene-related peptide sites and migraine therapy targeting, 762
Calcium/calmodulin-dependent protein kinase II (CaMK II)
  anxiety neurobiology and, 30–33
  benzodiazepine tolerance, 101
Calcium channel blockers
  migraine management, 767–768
  vanilloid receptors and, 728–729
Calmodulin kinase II
  transient receptor potential V1 (TRPV1) receptor sensitization, 735
cAMP response element binding (CREB) protein
  psychostimulant abuse
    chronic exposure and sensitization effects, 585
Cannabinoid hypothesis of schizophrenia pharmacotherapy, 394

Cannabinoid receptors. *See also* Marijuana
  analgesic properties, 666–668
  cannabinoid$_1$ (CB-1) receptor
    addictive disorders
      modulator therapy and, 458–459
    antagonist/agonist medication development, 700
    anxiety neurobiology and deficits in, 29–30
    appetite regulation, 670–672
    cognition and, 669–670
    convulsant effects, 672–673
    emesis modulation, 673–675
    identification of, 661–662
    nicotine dependence and withdrawal therapy
      antagonist agents, 550
    pain management and, 667–668
    prenatal development and, 664–665
    signaling mechanisms, 662–663
  cannabinoid$_2$ (CB-2) receptor
    emesis modulation, 674–675
    pain management and, 668–669
    signaling mechanisms, 662–663
  cognition and, 669–670
  convulsant effects, 672–673
  emesis modulation, 673–675
  future research on, 676
  reward, tolerance, and dependence, 675–676
  in schizophrenia
    animal model, 265
  signaling mechanisms, 662–663
CAPON gene
  schizophrenia molecular genetics, 328
Capsaicin
  cloning of, 727–729
  transient receptor potential V1 (TRPV1) receptor expression, 730–732
Carbamazepine
  anxiety disorder therapy, 75
β-Carboline3-carboxylate-*t*-butyl ester
  alcohol abuse studies
    anxiety reduction with, 510–511
    $GABA_{A1,2,3,5}$ receptor subunit modulation, 499–501
    $GABA_{A1}$ receptor subunit selectivity, 498–499
    microinjection techniques, 505–507
    oral administration, 507–511
    systemic administration, 503–504

β-Carboline antagonist ZK 93426
  alcohol abuse studies
    $GABA_{A5}$ receptor specificity, 514–516
    $GABA_A$ benzodiazepine receptor
      complex, 490–493
    GABAergic modification of dopamine
      agonists, 497
Cardiovascular system
  γ-hydroxybutyric acid (GHB) effects, 634
Caspase-1
  3,4-methylenedioxymethamphetamine
    effects on, 628
Catechol-O-methyl transferase (COMT)
  anxiety neurobiology and
    knockout mice studies, 24–26
  obsessive-compulsive disorders
    metabolism studies, 223
  schizophrenia
    dopamine hypothesis, 373
      genetic evidence, 286–287
      genetics studies, 286–287
      imaging studies, 285–286
    molecular genetics
      chromosomal abnormalities, 328–329
      susceptibility gene identification,
        347–348
    tolcapone targeting of, 389
Cell-cell interactions
  anxiety neurobiology
    neuronal deficits and, 30
Cell membrane-associated proteins
  anxiety neurobiology and
    mouse studies, 19, 21
Central nervous system (CNS)
  alcohol abuse studies in alcohol-preferring
    rats
      circuitry systems, role of, 470–471
      control substrates, 469–470
    γ-hydroxybutyric acid (GHB) effects,
      634
  pain pathways, 712–714
  schizophrenia and, 260–262
Cerebrospinal fluid (CSF)
  corticotropin-releasing factor receptor
    antagonists
      effects on, 177–179
  schizophrenia dopamine hypothesis and,
    288–289
C fibers
  pain pathways, 711–712
  transient receptor potential V1 (TRPV1)
    receptor expression, 729

Chemotherapy
  emesis with
    cannabinoid modulation of, 674–675
Cholecystokinin
  anxiety neurobiology and, 17
  pain management and, 716–717
Cholinergic neurotransmitters
  atypical antipsychotic mechanisms,
    429–430
  schizophrenia neurochemistry and,
    261–262
  schizophrenia pharmacotherapy, 393–394
Chromosomal abnormalities
  schizophrenia molecular genetics, 328–331
    catechol-O-methyltransferase, 328–329
    DISC1 gene, 330–331
    PRODH candidate gene, 329–330
    ZDHHC8 candidate gene, 330
Chromosome mapping
  anxiety neurobiology
    mouse studies, 19, 23
  schizophrenia
    susceptibility gene identification,
      346–351
CL218,872
  alcohol abuse studies
    $GABA_{A1}$ receptor subunit selectivity,
      499
Clomipramine
  obsessive-compulsive disorder therapy,
    69–70
Clonazepam
  obsessive-compulsive disorder therapy,
    234
Clonidine
  schizophrenia pharmacotherapy, 393
Clozapine
  dopamine D_2 receptor blockade, 412–415
  mechanisms of action
    cholinergic mechanisms, 429–430
    serotonin receptor 5-HT_{2A}, 418–421,
      420–421
    serotonin receptor 5-HT_6 and, 425–426
    serotonin receptor 5-HT/D_2 hypothesis,
      417–418
  schizophrenia therapy
    brain-derived neurotrophic factor and,
      421–422
    cholinergic receptor targeting, 393–394
    clinical profile, 387
    dopamine D_2 receptor blockade,
      412–415

history of, 370
safety and tolerability, 388–389
schizophrenia-related psychosis, 254
Clusters
GABA$_A$ receptors
benzodiazepines, 108–110
Cocaine
abuse
3,4-methylenedioxymethamphetamine
reinforcement of, 615–616
monoamine neuropharmacology,
570–575
therapy developments for, 585–588
chronic exposure and sensitization effects,
580–585
neuropeptide pharmacology and, 578–579
Cocaine- and amphetamine-regulated
transcript (CART) peptides
psychostimulant abuse
chronic exposure and sensitization
effects, 585
Cognitive behavior therapy (CBT)
obsessive-compulsive disorders, 219–220
Cognitive function
cannabinoid receptors and, 669–670
3,4-methylenedioxymethamphetamine
and, 630–631
nicotine dependence and withdrawal
withdrawal neurosubstrates, 541–543
schizophrenia, 254–255
animal model, 263–264
glutamatergic receptors, 428–429
neural network analysis, 259
serotonin receptor 5-HT$_{2A}$ receptor
enhancement, 421–422
Comorbid conditions
addictive disorders vulnerability with,
457–458
obsessive-compulsive disorders, 216
opiate addiction, 691–694
Compensatory mechanisms
dopamine hypothesis of schizophrenia,
284–285
Computed tomography (CT)
obsessive-compulsive disorders
brain imaging studies, 217–218
schizophrenia analysis, 256
Conditioned conflict tests
anxiety neurobiology
emotionalty studies in mice, 8–9
Conditioned fear paradigms
emotionality studies in mice, 8–9

Continuous performance test (CPT)
schizophrenia
animal models, 263–264
Cortical dopamine
schizophrenia dopamine hypothesis and,
287–288
serotonin receptor 5-HT$_{2A}$ receptor
enhancement, 421–422
Corticosterone
psychostimulant abuse, 577–578
Corticostriatal-thalamic-cortical loops
integrated glutamate/dopamine
hypotheses of schizophrenia
neurochemistry and, 374–376
Corticotropin-releasing factor (CRF)
alcholol abuse studies
in alcohol-preferring rats, 471
neurosteroid effects
acoustic/fear-potentiated startle, 147
nicotine dependence and withdrawal,
539–540
withdrawal substrate specificity, 543
opiate dependence therapy and, 699
psychostimulant abuse, 577–578
chronic exposure and sensitization
effects, 580–585
Corticotropin-releasing factor receptor
antagonists
anxiolytic applications
future research issues, 198–199
nonpeptide ligands, 195–196
overview, 177–179
peptide ligand pharmacology, 185–195
ligand binding mechanisms, 190–195
receptor/ligand family structure,
179–185
ligand properties, 180–181
receptor subtypes and distribution,
181–185
therapeutic potential, 196–198
Corticotropin-releasing hormone (CRH)
anxiety neurobiology and, 17
knockout mice studies, 25–26
receptor deficits, 28–30
Cortisol
nicotine dependence and withdrawal,
539–540
withdrawal substrate specificity, 543
Cotinine
nicotine dependence and withdrawal
metabolism and elimination
pharmacokinetics, 544–545

Countermodulation therapy
  addictive disorders, 458–459
CP-154,526 antagonist
  opiate dependence therapy and, 699
CRF_1 receptor
  corticotropin-releasing factor receptor
      antagonists, 181–185
    anxiety/depression therapeutic potential
        and, 196–198
    ligand binding mechanisms, 190–195
    nonpeptide ligands, 195–196
    peptide ligand pharmacology, 185–195
$CRF_{2(a)}$ receptor
  corticotropin-releasing factor receptor
      antagonists, 182–185
$CRF_{2(b)}$ receptor
  corticotropin-releasing factor receptor
      antagonists, 182–185
CRF_2 receptor
  corticotropin-releasing factor receptor
      antagonists, 182–185
    ligand binding mechanisms, 190–195
    peptide ligand pharmacology, 185–195
CX516 compound
  schizophrenia pharmacotherapy, 392
Cyclic adenosine monophosphate (cAMP)
  corticotropin-releasing factor receptor
      antagonists
    CRF receptor stimulation, 186–195
  psychostimulant abuse
    chronic exposure and sensitization
        effects, 584–585
Cyclic adenosine monophosphate
      (cAMP)-responsive nuclear
      factors
  anxiety neurobiology and, 32
CYP1A2 enzyme
  3,4-methylenedioxymethamphetamine
      neurotoxicity and, 622
CYP2A6 enzyme
  nicotine dependence and withdrawal
    metabolism and elimination
        pharmacokinetics, 545
Cystine/glutamate transporters
  psychostimulant abuse and, 576
Cytochrome P450 enzymes
  benzodiazepine receptor ligand
      metabolism, 102
  selective serotonin reuptake inhibitors,
      68–69
Cytogenetic abnormalities
  schizophrenia

    susceptibility gene identification,
        346–351
Cytokines
  anxiety neurobiology, 16–18
  knockout mice studies, 26
  3,4-methylenedioxymethamphetamine
      effects on, 627–628

D_1 receptor
  alcohol abuse studies
    bed nucleus of stria terminalis system,
        475
    lateral hypothalamus, dopaminergic
        regulation by, 481–485
    ventral pallidum pathways, 477–480
  psychostimulant abuse
    monoamine neuropharmacology,
        571–575
  schizophrenia dopamine hypothesis
    cortical vs. striatal dopamine, 288
    history, 284–285
    imaging evidence, 286–287
  schizophrenia pharmacotherapy
    antipsychotic agents, 380–381
  schizophrenia therapy
    agonist and antagonists, 390
    substituted benzamides, 415–416
D_2/D_3 receptors
  clozapine D_2 receptor blockade, 414–415
  partial dopamine agonists, 416–417
  psychostimulant abuse therapy,
      586–587
  selective antagonism
    schizophrenia therapy, 380
    substituted benzamides, 416
D_2 receptor
  alcohol abuse studies
    lateral hypothalamus, dopaminergic
        regulation by, 481–485
    ventral pallidum pathways, 477–480
  clozapine blockade, 412–415
  psychostimulant abuse
    chronic exposure and sensitization
        effects, 582–585
    monoamine neuropharmacology,
        571–575
  schizophrenia dopamine hypothesis
    cortical vs. striatal dopamine, 288
    history, 284–285, 371–373
    imaging evidence, 285–286
    pathological evidence, 285
    pharmacological evidence, 287

schizophrenia pharmacotherapy
   antipsychotic occupancy and effect, 376–378
   High 5-HT$_{2A}$ vs., 378
   occupancy thresholds and rapid dissociation, 378–380
   subtherapeutic occupancy time, 382
D$_3$ receptor
   schizophrenia dopamine hypothesis
      genetic evidence, 286–287
      pathological evidence, 285
      pharmacological evidence, 287
   schizophrenia therapy
      antagonist development, 390
      substituted benzamides, 415–416
D$_4$ receptor
   schizophrenia dopamine hypothesis
      pathological evidence, 285
      pharmacological evidence, 287
   schizophrenia therapy
      antagonism and regional specificity, 380
      antagonist development, 390
      substituted benzamides, 415–416
Deep brain stimulation (DBS)
   obsessive-compulsive disorders, 236–237
Defensive burying behavior
   animal anxiety models
      neurosteroid effects, 149–150
Dehydroepiandrosterone
   schizophrenia therapy, 394
Dehydroepiandrosterone sulfate (DHEAS)
   in brain, 137
   schizophrenia therapy, 394
Delta opioid receptors
   structure and function, 751
Dependency risk
   endocannabinoids, 675–676
Depolarization inactivation
   schizophrenia therapy
      D$_2$ receptor occupancy and effect, 376–378
Depression
   anxiety symptoms with pharmacotherapy, 80
   corticotropin-releasing factor receptor antagonists
      therapeutic potential of, 196–198
   neuroactive steroid interactions, 156–157
   stress-induced behavior
      neuroactive steroids, 156–157

Desensitization
   transient receptor potential V1 (TRPV1) receptors, 735–736
Designer drugs. *See also* specific drugs, e.g. 3,4-Methylenedioxy-methamphetamine (MDMA)
   overview, 614
Developmental genes
   obsessive-compulsive disorders, 223–224
Diagnostic criteria
   anxiety disorders, 9–12, 61–62
Diazepam binding inhibitor (DBI)
   benzodiazepine ligands, 98–99
3,4-Dihydroxyamphetamine (HHA)
   3,4-methylenedioxymethamphetamine neurotoxicity and, 622
3,4-Dihyroxy-L-phenylalanine (DOPA)
   schizophrenia dopamine hypothesis, 372–373
Dimerization
   opioid receptors, 752
DISC1 gene
   schizophrenia molecular genetics, 330–331
      molecular interactions, 351–352
      susceptibility identification, 349–350
Discontinuation syndrome
   selective serotonin reuptake inhibitors, 67–69
Distribution kinetics
   nicotine dependence and withdrawal, 544
DOI
   hallucinogens and, 639
   schizophrenia therapy
      serotonin receptor 5-HT$_{2A}$, 420–421
Donepezil
   schizophrenia pharmacotherapy, 393–394
Dopadecarboxylase
   schizophrenia dopamine hypothesis, 372–373
Dopamine agonist
   alcohol abuse studies
      GABAergic modification, 496–498
   partial agonists, 416–417
   psychostimulant abuse therapy, 586–587
   in schizophrenia
      animal models, 264
Dopamine hypothesis of schizophrenia
   cortical vs. striatal dopamine, 287–289
   genetic evidence, 286–287
   glutamate theory consolidated with, 295–296
   history, 284–285

imaging evidence, 285–286
neurochemistry and, 371–373
pathological evidence, 285
pharmacological evidence, 287
postmortem studies, 344
Dopamine neurotransmitters
  addictive disorders
    reward therapy and, 458–459
  anxiety disorder therapy
    antipsychotics, 71–72
  anxiety neurobiology, 15–17
    receptor deficits, 29–30
  3,4-methylenedioxymethamphetamine (MDMA)
    receptor/transporter effects, 617
    reinforcing properties, 614–616
  nicotine dependence and withdrawal
    withdrawal substrates, 542–543
  obsessive-compulsive disorders, 223
  psychostimulant abuse, 569–575
    neuropeptide pharmacology, 579
    neuropharmacology, 570–575
  schizophrenia and, 260–262
    COMT catabolism and, 328
    drug targeting innovations, 389
Dopaminergic receptors
  alcholol abuse studies
    neuronal systems and substrates, 471–486
      bed nucleus of stria terminalis, 473–475
      dopaminergic regulation, early research, 472–473
      extracellular dopamine, 485–486
      future research issues, 517–518
      GABAergic interactions with, 486
      lateral hypothalamus, 481–485
        D_2 dopaminergic regulation, hypothesized mechanisms, 481–485
      ventral pallidum, 476–480
        hypothesized mechanisms, 478–480
  alcohol abuse studies
    in alcohol-preferring rats, 471
  anxiety neurobiology and receptor deficits, 29–30
  nicotine dependence and withdrawal
    nicotine reinforcement substrates, 538–540
  psychostimulant abuse
    chronic exposure and sensitization effects, 582–585
    glutamatergic interactions, 575–576
    monoamine neuropharmacology, 571–575
  schizophrenia molecular genetics
    functional candidate genes, 331–332
Dopamine transporter
  catechol-*O*-methyl transferase
    as schizophrenia susceptibility gene, 347–348
  inhibitors
    psychostimulant therapy targeting, 587–588
  obsessive-compulsive disorders
    abnormalities, 219–220
  psychostimulant abuse
    monoamine neuropharmacology, 573–575
  schizophrenia
    dopamine hypothesis and, 285
Dorsolateral prefrontal cortex (DLPFC)
  schizophrenia dopamine hypothesis, 373
DRD2/DRD3 receptors
  schizophrenia molecular genetics, 331–332
    catechol-*O*-methyl transferase susceptibility gene, 347–348
Drug abuse
  dopaminergic receptor systems and substrates
    bed nucleus of stria terminalis system, 474–475
  rewarding/reinforcing effects in, 459
  stress-induced response
    neuroactive steroid effects and, 159–160
Dyadic encounters
  schizophrenia
    animal models, 264
Dynorphins
  structure and classification, 747
Dysbindin
  dystrobrevin binding protein 1 (DTNBP1)
    molecular interactions, 353
    schizophrenia candidate gene, 326, 348–349
Dystrobrevin binding protein 1 (DTNBP1)
  schizophrenia candidate gene, 325–326
    chomosome mapping, 346
    chromosome identification of, 348–349
    functional implications, 332–333
    molecular interactions, 352–353
Dystrophini-associated glycoprotein complex (DCG)

dystrobrevin binding protein 1
  identification
    schizophrenia candidate gene, 348–349
Electroencephalography (EEG)
  schizophrenia analysis, 256
Elevated-plus maze (EPM)
  animal anxiety-like behavior and, 12
    neurosteroid effects, 143–145
  emotionality studies in mice, 7–9
Elevated-zero maze (EZM)
  emotionality studies in mice, 8–9
Elimination mechanisms
  nicotine dependence and withdrawal, 544–545
Emesis
  antiemetics
    migraine management, 765
    cannabinoid receptors modulation of, 673–675
Emotionality studies
  anxiety neurobiology
    rodent models, 6–9
Enantiomeric selectivity
  neuroactive steroids, 141–142
Endocannabinoid system, 662–665
  cannabinoid receptors and signaling, 662–663
  physiology and pharmacology, 665–675
  prenatal developmental effects, 664–665
  reward, tolerance and dependence mechanisms, 675–676
  synthesis and metabolism, 663–664
Endogenous opioids
  classification, 746–748
Endogenous sites
  benzodiazepine ligands, 98–99
β-Endorphins
  structure and classification, 747–748
Enkephalin neurons
  nicotine dependence and withdrawal, 540
Enkephalins
  structure and function, 746–747
Enthoprotin
  schizophrenia molecular genetics, 328
Environmental factors
  addictive disorders vulnerability, 457–458
  anxiety neurobiology
    early-life experience, 33–34
Epilepsy
  endocannabinoids and, 672–673

ErbB3 gene
  NRG1 molecular interaction, 353–355
  regulator of G-protein signaling 4
    schizophrenia candidate gene, 328
Ergots
  migraine management, 765
Ethanol
  neuroactive steroid effects and, 158–159
Eticlopride
  alcohol abuse studies
    lateral hypothalamus, effects on, 481–485
    ventral pallidum receptor blockade, 478
Excitatory amino acid transporters (EAATs)
  glutamate theory of schizophrenia
    pathological evidence, 292
  schizophrenia genetics
    GRM3 gene, 349
Extended amygala (EA)
  alcohol abuse studies
    dopaminergic receptor systems and substrates, 473–474
    $GABA_A$ benzodiazepine receptor complex manipulation
      site-specific microinjection studies, 493–496
Extracellular dopamine
  alcohol abuse studies
    dopaminergic regulation mechanisms, 485–486
Extrapyramidal symptoms (EPS)
  atypical antipsychotic drugs, 411–412
    clozapine D_2 receptor blockade, 412–415
  schizophrenia therapy
    antipsychotics and, 370–371
    D_2 receptor occupancy and effect, 376–378
    D_2 receptor occupancy thresholds and rapid dissociation, 379–380
    first-generation antipsychotics, 383
    second-generation antipsychotics, 383–388
    serotonin receptor $5\text{-}HT_{2A}$ blockade, 422
Extroversion vs. introversion (E trait)
  anxiety neurobiology, 5–6

Face validity
  animal anxiety-like behavior and, 12
Fatty acid amide hydrolase (FAAH)
  convulsant effects of, 672–673
  emesis modulation, 674–675

endocannabinoid ligands, 664
endocannabinoid physiology and, 666
Fear/anxiety circuits
  anxiety neurobiology, 13–15
Fear-potentiated startle
  mouse anxiety models
    neurosteroid effects, 147
Feverfew
  migraine management, 768
FEZ1 protein
  DISC1 schizophrenia candidate gene
    molecular interactions, 351–352
First-generation antipsychotics (FGAs)
  schizophrenia therapy
    clinical profiles, 383
    D_2 receptor occupancy and effect, 376–378
    history of, 370–371
    NMDA receptor antagonists, 381
    second-generation antipsychotic comparisons, 384–387
Fixed-ratio (FR) schedule
  alcohol abuse studies in alcohol-preferring rats, 469
Flumazenil
  alcohol abuse studies
    $GABA_{A5}$ receptor specificity, 512–516
    $GABA_A$ benzodiazepine receptor complex, 490–493
  endogenous ligand sites, 98–99
Flunitrazepam
  overview, 637
Fluorodeoxyglucose (FDG) studies
  schizophrenia analysis, 257
Fluoxetine
  3,4-methylenedioxymethamphetamine effects on, 616, 627
  nicotine dependence and withdrawal
    withdrawal substrate specificity, 542–543
Fluphenazine
  adrenergic receptor mechanisms, 427
Free-radical formation
  3,4-methylenedioxymethamphetamine neurotoxicity, 624
Frontal cortex abnormalities
  glutamate theory of schizophrenia
    pathological evidence, 292
Functional candidate genes
  schizophrenia molecular genetics, 331–332
Functional imaging studies
  obsessive-compulsive disorders, 219–220
  schizophrenia analysis, 257–260

Fyn tyrosine kinase
  anxiety neurobiology and, 31

$GABA_A$-benzodiazepine receptor complex
  alcohol abuse studies, 487–501
    alcohol/modulator commonalities, 487–488
    CA1/CA3 hippocampus, 511–516
    efficacy of βCCT/3PBD modulation, $GABA_{A1,2,3,5}$ receptors, 499–501
    future research issues, 517–518
    GABA-DA interaction hypothesis, 496–498
    ligand selectivity with $GABA_{A1}$ subunits, 498–499
    microinjection studies, 505–506
    naltrexone antagonist, 507–511
    novel CNS GABAergic substrates, 498
    oral administration, βCCT/3PBD
      anxiety reduction, 510–511
      vs. naltrexone, 507–511
    probe applications, 488–493
    site-specific microinjection, 493–496
    subunit selectivity vs. intrinsic efficacy, 516–517
    systemic administration, 492–493, 503–504
    ventral pallidum, 501–502
GABAergic neurons
  alcohol abuse studies
    in alcohol-preferring rats, 471
    bed nucleus of stria terminalis system, 474
    dopamine agonist modification, 496–498
    $GABA_{A5}$ receptor specificity, 512–516
    novel substrates, 498
    ventral pallidum dopaminergic regulation and, 479–480
  cannabinoid$_1$ (CB-1) receptors and, 672–673
  integrated glutamate/dopamine hypotheses of schizophrenia, 375–376
  psychostimulant abuse, 574–575
    chronic exposure and sensitization effects, 583–585
    γ-aminobutyric acid (GABA) receptors and, 576–577
    novel therapeutic developments, 588

Gabapentin
  anxiety disorder therapy
    amino acid neurotransmission, 75
  migraine management, 766–767
GA-BARAP
  GABA$_A$ receptors
    benzodiazepines, 109–110
"GABA shift" assay
  alcohol abuse studies
    GABA$_A$ benzodiazepine receptor
      complex
        subunit selectivity vs. intrinsic
          efficacy, 517
Galantamine
  schizophrenia pharmacotherapy,
    393–394
γ-aminobutyric acid (GABA) receptors
  addictive disorders
    modulator therapy and, 458–459
  anxiety disorder therapy
    amino acid neurotransmission, 72–75
  anxiety neurobiology and, 15–17
  knockout mice deficit studies, 26–30
  cannabinoid receptors and
    neurotoxicity effects, 673
  GABA$_A$ receptors
    alcohol abuse studies
      novel substrates, 498
      ventral pallidum dopaminergic
        regulation and, 479–480
    benzodiazepines
      assembly, clustering, and surface
        expression, 108–110
      binding pocket, 105–108
      brain function diversity, 110–112
      functional diversity, knockout/
        knockin models, 112–114
      single-cell response modulation,
        99–100
      subunit/subtype diversity, 103–104
    GABA$_{A1}$ subunit
      alcohol abuse studies, 498–501
        microinjection techniques, 505–507
        ventral pallidum selectivity,
          501–503
    GABA$_{A5}$ subunit
      as alcohol substrate probes, 511–516
      neuroactive steroids, 137–141
  GABA$_B$ receptors
    alcohol abuse studies
      ventral pallidum dopaminergic
        regulation and, 479–480

γ-hydroxybutyric acid (GHB)
  mechanisms and, 634–635
  migraine management with
    anticonvulsants, 766–767
  neuroactive steroids
    enantiomeric selectivity, 141–142
  nicotine dependence and withdrawal
    nicotine reinforcement substrates,
      538–540
  NRG1 molecular interaction, 354–355
  psychostimulant abuse and, 576–577
  schizophrenia neurochemistry and,
    261–262
γ-hydroxybutyric acid (GHB)
  addiction risk, 635–636
  mechanism of action, 634–635
  overview, 632–633
  pharmacological effects, 633–634
"Gate control" theory
  classification of, 713–714
Geller-Seifter test
  mouse models of anxiety, 8–9
  neurosteroid effects, 145–146
Gene expression
  psychostimulant abuse
    chronic exposure and sensitization
      effects, 584–585
Gene linkage studies
  schizophrenia, 323–324
    future research issues, 355–356
    susceptibility gene identification,
      344–351
Generalized anxiety disorder (GAD)
  buspirone therapy, 71
  pharmacotherapy, 77
  serotonin/noradrenaline reuptake
    inhibitors, 69
  tricyclic antidepressants, 69–70
Genetic studies. See also Gene linkage
    studies; Molecular genetics
  addictive disorders vulnerability, 457–458
  anxiety neurobiology, 4–6
    environmental effects and, 34–35
    susceptibility studies, 18–19
  glutamate theory of schizophrenia,
    293–294
  obsessive-compulsive disorders, 222–224
    developmental genes, 223–224
    dopamine, 223
    glutamate, 223
    neurotransmitter metabolism, 223
    serotonin, 222–224

schizophrenia, 262–263
  animal models, 264
  dopamine hypothesis, 286–287
  epidemiology, pathophysiology, and
    neurobiology, 323
Gepirone
  anxiety disorder therapy, 71
Glia-derived protein
  $GABA_A$ receptors
    benzodiazepines, 108–110
Glucocorticoid receptor (GR)
  stress-induced behaviors
    neuroactive steroids, 153–154
Glucocorticoid receptor (GR) transcription
    factor
  anxiety neurobiology and, 31
Glucocorticoids
  anxiety neurobiology and, 17
Glucortical hormones
  psychostimulant abuse, 577–578
Glucose utilization
  schizophrenia psychosis
    neural network analysis, 257–258
Glutamate neurotransmitters
  anxiety disorder therapy
    amino acid neurotransmission, 72–75
  nicotine dependence and withdrawal
    withdrawal substrates, 542–543
  obsessive-compulsive disorders, 223
  pain management and, 717
  psychostimulant abuse and, 575–576
  schizophrenia neurochemistry and,
    261–262
    targeted drug development for,
      391–392
Glutamate reuptake inhibitors
  schizophrenia pharmacotherapy,
    391–392
Glutamatergic system
  addictive disorders
    modulator therapy and, 458–459
  atypical antipsychotics, 427–428
  nicotine dependence and withdrawal
    nicotine reinforcement substrates,
      538–540
  psychostimulant abuse, 569–576
    chronic exposure and sensitization
      effects, 583–585
    novel therapeutic developments, 588
  in schizophrenia, 264
    molecular genetics
      functional candidate genes, 331–332

pharmacotherapy
  glutamate reuptake inhibitors,
    391–392
Glutamate theory of schizophrenia
  dopamine hypothesis and, 295–296
  genetic evidence for, 293–294
  history, 289–291
  imaging evidence for, 292–293
  neurochemistry of, 373–374
  pathological evidence for, 291–292
  pharmacological evidence for, 294–295
Glutamic acid decarboxylase (GAD)
  anxiety neurobiology and
    knockout mice studies, 24–26
  schizophrenia susceptibility genetics,
    350–351
Glutathione conjugates
  3,4-methylenedioxymethamphetamine
    neurotoxicity and, 622
Glycine
  schizophrenia pharmacotherapy
    NMDA targeting with, 391–392
Glycine transporter 1 (GlyT1)
  glutamate theory of schizophrenia
    pharmacological evidence, 294–295
Glycine transporter inhibitors
  schizophrenia pharmacotherapy
    NMDA targeting with, 391–392
G-protein coupled receptors (GPCRs)
  corticotropin-releasing factor receptor
    antagonists
    ligand binding mechanisms, 192–195
  delta opioid receptors, 751
  kappa opioid receptors, 751–752
  mu opioid receptors and, 748–751
  regulator of G-protein signaling 4
    schizophrenia candidate gene, 328
G-protein-gated inwardly rectifying K^+
    (GIRK) channels
  anxiety neurobiology and
    receptor deficits and, 29–30
G proteins
  cannabinoid receptors and, 662–663
  psychostimulant abuse
    chronic exposure and sensitization
      effects, 584–585
GRM3 gene
  schizophrenia molecular genetics, 331–332
  susceptibility identification, 349
Group A β-hemolytic streptococcus
    (GABHS) infection
  obsessive-compulsive disorders and, 235

Guanfacine
   schizophrenia pharmacotherapy, 393

Hallucinogens
   LSD, 637–640
      addiction, 639–640
      mechanism of action, 638–639
      pharmacology, 638
Haloperidol
   serotonin receptor 5-HT$_6$ and, 425–426
Hamilton depression and anxiety scales
   corticotropin-releasing factor receptor antagonists
      anxiety/depression therapeutic potential, 197–198
Heat exposure
   transient receptor potential V1 (TRPV1) receptor expression, 730–732
Hepatitis C
   opiate addiction comorbidity with, 691–694
Heroin addiction
   incidence and prevalence, 692–694
   neuropeptide pharmacology and, 578–579
   pharmacotherapy
      history of, 451–457
      treatment statistics, 694–696
High 5-HT$_{2A}$
   schizophrenia therapy
      D$_2$ affinity *vs.*, 378
High alcohol drinking (HAD) rats
   alcohol abuse studies
      characteristics of, 467
Hippocampus
   alcohol abuse studies
      CA1/CA3 fields
         GABA$_{A5}$ receptor probes, 511–516
   anxiety disorders and, 13–15
   3,4-methylenedioxymethamphetamine effects on
      long-term neurochemical effects, 619–620
Homeobox genes
   obsessive-compulsive disorders, 223–224
HTR2A receptor
   schizophrenia molecular genetics, 331–332
Human immunodeficiency virus
   opiate addiction and exposure to, 691–694
Hydroxyl radicals
   3,4-methylenedioxymethamphetamine neurotoxicity and, 627

Hydroxyzine
   anxiety disorder therapy, 75
Hyperdopaminergic state
   schizophrenia dopamine hypothesis and evidence for, 287
Hyperthermia
   3,4-methylenedioxymethamphetamine neurotoxicity and, 624–625
Hypodopaminergia
   schizophrenia dopamine hypothesis, 288–289
Hypothalamic-pituitary-adrenal (HPA) axis
   anxiety neurobiology and, 17
   corticotropin-releasing factor receptor antagonists, 177–179
   nicotine dependence and withdrawal
      nicotine reinforcement substrates, 539–540
      withdrawal substrate specificity, 543
   psychostimulant abuse, 577–578
      chronic exposure and sensitization effects, 580–585
   stress-induced behaviors
      neuroactive steroids, 153–159

Idazozan
   adrenergic receptor mechanisms, 427
Iloperidone
   schizophrenia therapy, 389
Imaging studies
   brain regions
      anxiety disorders and, 13–15
      glutamate theory of schizophrenia, 292–293
   schizophrenia
      dopamine hypothesis, 285–286
Imidazobenzodiazepines
   alcohol abuse studies
      GABA$_{A5}$ receptor specificity, 512–516
Immediate early genes
   psychostimulant abuse
      chronic exposure and sensitization effects, 585
Immune response
   3,4-methylenedioxymethamphetamine effects on, 618
Immunoglobulin therapy
   obsessive-compulsive disorders, 235
Immunomodulatory therapy
   obsessive-compulsive disorders, 235
Indole agents
   serotonin receptor 5-HT$_{2A}$, 418–421

Indolealkylamines, 637–640
  addiction, 639–640
  mechanism of action, 638–639
  pharmacology, 638
Infection
  obsessive-compulsive disorders and, 235
Inflammation
  transient receptor potential V1 (TRPV1) receptor expression, 729
Integrated glutamate/dopamine hypotheses of schizophrenia
  basic principles, 295–297
  pharmacotherapy and, 374–376
Interleukin-1β converting enzyme (ICE)
  3,4-methylenedioxymethamphetamine effects on, 628
Interleukin-1β release
  3,4-methylenedioxymethamphetamine effects on, 628
Intracellular signaling molecules
  anxiety neurobiology and
    mouse studies, 19, 22
    phenotype analysis, 30–33
  psychostimulant abuse
    chronic exposure and sensitization effects, 584–585
  schizophrenia therapy, 394–395
Intrinsic efficacy
  alcohol abuse studies
    GABA$_A$ benzodiazepine receptor complex
      subunit selectivity vs., 516–517
Ionotropic glutamate receptors
  atypical antipsychotics, 427–429

J-domain fragments
  corticotropin-releasing factor receptor antagonists
    ligand binding mechanisms, 192–195

Kainate receptors
  glutamate theory of schizophrenia
    mRNA binding, 291–292
  schizophrenia pharmacotherapy
    drug development for, 392
Kappa opioid receptors
  psychostimulant abuse and, 578–579
  structure and function, 751–752
Ketamine
  glutamate theory of schizophrenia
    history of, 289–290
  overview, 636
  pharmacological effects, 636–637
Ketoconazole
  psychostimulant abuse, 577–578
Knockin mice
  benzodiazepine functional diversity, 112–114
Knockout mice
  anxiety neurobiology
    neuronal messenger alterations, 24–26
    neurotransmitter receptor/CMAP deficits, 26–30
  benzodiazepine functional diversity studies, 112–114
  calcitonin gene-related peptide studies, 760–761
  transient receptor potential V1 (TRPV1) receptor models, 736

LAAM (λ-α-Acetyl methadol)
  addiction pharmacotherapy and, 454–457
  treatment statistics, 695–696
Lamotrigine
  anxiety disorder therapy, 75
  schizophrenia pharmacotherapy
    NMDA targeted drug development, 392–393
Lateral hypothalamus (LH)
  alcohol abuse studies
    dopamine neuronal systems and substrates, 481–485
    D$_2$ dopaminergic regulation, hypothesized mechanisms, 481–485
Leptin
  cannabinoid receptors and, 671–672
Lesion models
  in schizophrenia, 265
Ligand-gated ion channels
  neuroactive steroids, 137–141
Light-dark box
  mouse models of anxiety
    neurosteroid effects, 146–147
LIS1 gene
  DISC1 schizophrenia candidate gene molecular interactions, 351–352
Lithium
  anxiety disorder therapy, 75
Locomotor sensitization
  psychostimulant abuse
    chronic exposure and sensitization effects, 581–585

Lofexidine
    opiate addiction and, 699
Long-term therapy
    selective serotonin reuptake inhibitors, 68–69
LY206130
    nicotine dependence and withdrawal
        withdrawal substrate specificity, 542–543
LY274600
    nicotine dependence and withdrawal
        withdrawal substrate specificity, 542–543
LY354740 Glu analog
    nicotine dependence and withdrawal
        withdrawal substrate specificity, 542–543
Lysergic acid diethylamide (LSD), 637–640
    addiction, 639–640
    mechanism of action, 638–639
    pharmacology, 638

M100907 compound
    schizophrenia therapy
        serotonin receptor 5-HT$_{2A}$, 419–421
Magnetic resonance imaging (MRI)
    obsessive-compulsive disorders
        brain imaging studies, 217–218, 220
    schizophrenia analysis, 256
Magnetic resonance spectroscopy (MRS)
    glutamate theory of schizophrenia, 293
    schizophrenia analysis, 256–257
MAPK/ERK signaling
    anxiety neurobiology and, 36–37
Marijuana
    endocannabinoid system, 662–665
        cannabinoid receptors and signaling, 662–663
        prenatal developmental effects, 664–665
        reward, tolerance and dependence mechanisms, 675–676
        synthesis and metabolism, 663–664
    future research on, 676
    pharmacology
        appetite regulation, 670–672
        cognitive function, 669–670
        emesis, 673–674
        endocannabinoid system physiology, 665–666
        neurotoxicity, 672–673
        overview, 659–662
        pain management, 666–669

Mast cells
    calcitonin gene-related peptide sites and migraine therapy targeting, 762
MATRICS program
    schizophrenia-related cognitive dysfunction, 254–255
Mazindol
    psychostimulant abuse therapy, 587
mCCP serotonin receptor agonist
    obsessive-compulsive disorders, 234
Mecamylamine
    nicotine dependence and withdrawal therapy, 549
Medial prefrontal cortex (MPFC)
    anxiety neurobiology
        brain imaging studies, 15
Melanocyte-inhibiting factor (MIF) peptides
    pain management and
Memantine
    schizophrenia pharmacotherapy, 392
Memory deficits
    cannabinoid receptors and, 669–670
    3,4-methylenedioxymethamphetamine and, 630–631
    schizophrenia
        animal models, 263
    schizophrenia and, 254–255
Mesoaccumbens system
    alcohol abuse studies
        dopaminergic receptor systems and substrates, 472–473
        GABA$_A$ benzodiazepine receptor complex
            site-specific microinjection techniques, 494–496
Mesolimbic pathway
    alcohol abuse studies
        dopaminergic receptor systems and substrates, 472–473
    psychostimulant abuse
        dopamine system, 574–575
Mesopallidal system
    alcohol abuse studies, 476–480
Metabolic syndrome
    antipsychotics and, 254
Metabolism kinetics
    endocannabinoid system, 663–664
    3,4-methylenedioxymethamphetamine neurotoxicity and, 621–622
    nicotine dependence and withdrawal, 544–545

Metabolites
  3,4-methylenedioxymethamphetamine
    neurotoxicity and mechanisms of,
    621–622
Metabotropic glutamate receptors
  atypical antipsychotics, 427–429
  glutamate theory of schizophrenia,
    293–294
    history of, 290–291
    pathological evidence, 292
  psychostimulant abuse, 576
  schizophrenia pharmacotherapy
    group II receptor targeting, 391–392
Methadone
  heroin addiction pharmacotherapy
    history of, 453–457
  in "office-based practice," 700
  opiate addiction therapy
    buprenorphine comparisons with,
    697–698
  psychostimulant abuse therapy, 585–586
  treatment statistics, 694–696
Methamphetamine. *See also* 3,4-Methylene-
    dioxymethamphetamine (MDMA)
  3,4-methylenedioxymethamphetamine
    and
    behavioral effects, 630–631
    monoamine neuropharmacology, 571–575
α-Methylparatyrosine (AMPT)
  schizophrenia dopamine hypothesis,
    372–373
  schizophrenia therapy
    D_2 receptor occupancy and effect,
    376–378
Methylation techniques
  3,4-methylenedioxymethamphetamine
    neurotoxicity and, 622
3,4-Methylenedioxyamphetamine (MDA)
  3,4-methylenedioxymethamphetamine
    neurotoxicity and, 621–622
3,4-Methylenedioxymethamphetamine
    (MDMA)
  behavioral effects, 618–619
  body temperature effects, 617–618
  brain biochemistry and function, 631–632
  monoamine release, 616
  neuroendocrine and immune responses,
    618
  neurotoxicity, 619–628
    animal models, 620–621
    cytokines and microglia, 627–628
    hyperthermia, 624–625

long-term neurochemical change,
    619–620
  metabolite mechanisms, 621–622
  monoaminergic transporter, 625–627
  oxidative stress, 623–624
neurotoxic lesions
  behavioral effects, 629–631
  thermoregulation effects, 629
neurotransmitter receptors and
    transporters, 617
overview, 614
reinforcing properties, 614–616
tryptophan hydroxylase, 616–617
Methylphenidate
  chronic exposure and sensitization effects,
    580–585
  monoamine neuropharmacology, 571–575
  psychostimulant abuse therapy, 587
Microglia
  3,4-methylenedioxymethamphetamine
    effects on, 627–628
Microinjection studies
  alcohol abuse
    $GABA_A$ benzodiazepine receptor
      complex modulation, 505–507
Migraine headaches
  history and definition, 758–759
  therapy
    calcitonin gene-related peptide and,
      759–763
      injection techniques, 763
      neurovascular model, 759–760
      receptor antagonist therapeutic
        efficacy, 763–764
      synthesis and actions, 760–761
      trigeminovasculature sites, 761–763
    future trends in, 768–769
    history of, 758–759
    migraine diagnostic criteria, 758–759
    overview, 758
    pharmacology, 764–768
      acute therapy, 764–765
      preventive therapy, 766–768
Mild mental stress models
  neurosteroid effects, 151–152
Mineralocorticoid receptors
  psychostimulant abuse, 577–578
Mirrored chamber
  mouse anxiety models
    neurosteroid effects, 147–148
Mirtazapine
  anxiety disorder therapy, 70

Missense mutations
  PRODH gene
    schizophrenia molecular genetics, 329–330
Mitogen-activated protein kinase
  transient receptor potential V1 (TRPV1) receptor expression, 729
Mitotic inhibitor methylazoxymethanol (MAM)
  in schizophrenia, 265
Moclobemide
  anxiety disorder therapy, 70
Modafinil
  psychostimulant abuse therapy, 588
  schizophrenia therapy, 389
Modified forced-swim test
  animal anxiety models
    neurosteroid effects, 150–151
Modulation therapy
  addictive disorders, 458–459
Molecular genetics
  corticotropin-releasing factor receptor antagonists
    ligand binding mechanisms, 191–195
  $GABA_A$ benzodiazepine receptor complex
    alcohol abuse studies, 487–501
      alcohol/modulator commonalities, 487–488
      CA1/CA3 hippocampus, 511–516
      efficacy of $\beta CCT/3PBD$ modulation, $GABA_{A1,2,3,5}$ receptors, 499–501
      future research issues, 517–518
      GABA-DA interaction hypothesis, 496–498
      ligand selectivity with $GABA_{A1}$ subunits, 498–499
      microinjection studies, 505–506
      naltrexone antagonist, 507–511
      novel CNS GABAergic substrates, 498
      oral administration, $\beta CCT/3PBD$ anxiety reduction, 510–511
      vs. naltrexone, 507–511
      probe applications, 488–493
      site-specific microinjection, 493–496
      subunit selectivity vs. intrinsic efficacy, 516–517
      systemic administration, 492–493, 503–504
      ventral pallidum, 501–502
  schizophrenia, 323–325
    candidate genes, 325–328
    chromosomal abnormalities, 328–331
    functional candidate genes, 331–332
    future research issues, 333
    gene linkage studies, 323–324
    neurochemistry and, 261–262
    positional candidate genes, 325
    susceptibility genes, 351–355
      DISC1 gene, 351–352
      DTNBP1 gene, 352–353
      function, 332–333
      NRG1 gene, 353–355
Molecular path model
  benzodiazepine activity, 115
Molecular targeting
  schizophrenia-related cognitive dysfunction therapy, 254–255
Monoamine neurotransmitters
  anxiety disorder anxiolytics, 63–72
    antidepressants, 64–70
    antipsychotics, 71–72
    beta blockers, 71
  cannabinoid analgesics and, 668–669
  dopamine hypothesis of schizophrenia, 371–373
  3,4-methylenedioxymethamphetamine effects, 616
  psychostimulant abuse and, 569–575
Monoamine oxidase inhibitors (MAOIs)
  anxiety disorder therapy, 70
  obsessive-compulsive disorders metabolism studies, 223
  schizophrenia therapy, 394
Monoaminergic transporter
  3,4-methylenedioxymethamphetamine neurotoxicity and, 625–627
Monotherapies
  obsessive-compulsive disorders controlled trials, 225
MOR-1 opioid receptor
  pain management and, 716–717
  structure and function, 748–751
Morphine compounds
  mu opioid receptors and, 748–751
  obsessive-compulsive disorder therapy, 234
  peripheral-central interactions, 719–721
  spinal-supraspinal interactions, 718–720
Mouse studies
  anxiety neurobiology
    anxiety-like behavior, genetically altered mice, 19–24

neuroticism (N trait), 6–9
  oligogenic anxiety-like conditions, 32–33
  QTL studies, 19
  benzodiazepine functional diversity, 112–114
MPEP antagonist
  psychostimulant abuse and, 576
Multipoint linkage analysis
  anxiety neurobiology, 4
Mu opoid receptors
  obsessive-compulsive disorders, 234
  psychostimulant abuse and, 578–579
  structure and function, 748–751
Muscarinic receptor agonists
  atypical antipsychotics and cholinergic agents, 429–430
  schizophrenia therapy, 393–394
Muscimol
  alcohol abuse studies
    GABA$_A$ benzodiazepine receptor complex manipulation, 494–496

Naloxone
  nicotine dependence and withdrawal, 540
  opiate addiction therapy
    regulatory studies, 696–697
Naltrexone
  alcohol abuse studies
    oral administration of βCCT/3PBC vs., 507–511
  nicotine dependence and withdrawal, 540
    pharmacotherapy, 550–551
  opiate addiction therapy, 698–699
  psychostimulant abuse therapy, 585–586
NAN-190 antagonists
  nicotine dependence and withdrawal
    withdrawal substrate specificity, 542–543
N-back task analysis
  schizophrenia cognitive dysfunction and, 259
NDMC metabolite
  cholinergic mechanisms and, 429–430
N-domain fragments
  corticotropin-releasing factor receptor antagonists
    ligand binding mechanisms, 192–195
Negative affect
  in schizophrenia, 255–256
    neural network studies, 258–259

NEO-five factor inventory (NEO-FFI)
  anxiety neurobiology
    genetic susceptibility studies, 18–19
NEO personality inventory
  anxiety neurobiology, 5–6
  human personality traits, 9–12
Neospinothalamic pain pathways
  classification of, 711–714
Nerve-growth factor (NGF)
  transient receptor potential V1 (TRPV1) receptor expression, 729
Neural networks
  glutamate theory of schizophrenia
    history of, 290–291
  schizophrenia
    cognitive dysfunction and, 259
    future research issues, 266
    negative affect and, 255–256, 258–259
    psychosis and, 257–258
Neuregulin I (NRG1)
  schizophrenia candidate gene, 326–327
  ErbB3 receptor, 328
  functional implications, 332–333
  molecular interactions, 352–353
  susceptibility identification, 350
Neuroactive steroids
  anxiety disorders
    alcohol effects, 157–159
    animal models, 142–152
    behavioral effects, 142
    brain and peripheral sources, 135–137
    chemistry and pharmacology, 135–142
    enantiomeric selectivity, 141–142
    GABA$_A$ receptors and ligand-gated ion channels, 137–141
    HPA axis function, 154–156
    overview, 134–135
  stress-induced behaviors
    drug abuse relapse, 159–160
    HPA axis, 153–154
    overview, 152–153
Neuroanatomical controls
  alcohol abuse studies in alcohol-preferring rats, 469–470
Neurobiology
  obsessive-compulsive disorders, 216–224
    brain imaging studies, 217–222
    functional imaging studies, 219–220
    magnetic resonance spectroscopy, 220

Neurochemistry
  3,4-Methylenedioxymethamphetamine
      (MDMA) neurotoxicity
    long-term changes in, 619–620
  schizophrenia, 260–262
    hypotheses, 371–376
      dopamine hypothesis, 371–373
      glutamate receptor hypothesis,
          373–374
      integrated dopamine/glutamate
          hypotheses, 374–376
Neurodevelopmental animal model
    schizophrenia, 265
Neuroendocrine systems
  3,4-methylcnedioxymethamphetamine
      effects on, 618
  psychostimulant abuse
    chronic exposure and sensitization
        effects, 580–585
Neurogenesis
  atypical antipsychotics and, 430
  schizophrenia
    disruption of, 265
Neurogenic inflammation
  vanilloid receptors and, 728–729
Neuroimaging studies
  3,4-methylenedioxymethamphetamine
      neurotoxicity
    brain biochemical and functional
        changes, 631–632
  obsessive-compulsive disorders,
      219–220
  psychostimulant abuse
    chronic exposure and sensitization
        effects, 582–585
    monoamine neuropharmacology,
        573–575
Neurokinin 3 receptors
  antipsychotic mechanisms with, 430
Neurokinin antagonists
  schizophrenia therapy, 391
Neuronal cell adhesion molecules (NCAM)
  anxiety neurobiology, 30
Neuronal pathways
  anxiety neurobiology and, 15–18
    knockout mice studies, 24–26
    mouse studies, 19–20
  pain management
    anatomical drug interactions,
        718–720
    descending modulatory pathways,
        712–714

neospinothalamic/paleospinothalamic
    pathways, 711–712
  overview, 709–710
Neuronal systems and substrates
  calcitonin gene-related peptide sites and
      migraine therapy targeting, 762
  dopaminergic receptors
    alcholol abuse studies, 471–486
      bed nucleus of stria terminalis,
          473–475
      dopaminergic regulation, early
          research, 472–473
      extracellular dopamine, 485–486
      future research issues, 517–518
      GABAergic interactions with, 486
      lateral hypothalamus, 481–485
        D_2 dopaminergic regulation,
            hypothesized mechanisms,
            481–485
      ventral pallidum, 476–480
        dopaminargic regulation
            hypothesized mechanisms,
            478–480
  nicotine dependence and withdrawal
    nicotine reinforcement substrates,
        537–540
    withdrawal neurosubstrates, 541–543
Neuropeptide FF
  pain management and, 716–717
Neuropeptides
  anxiety neurobiology, 16–17
  psychostimulant abuse and, 578–579
Neuropeptide Y (NPY)
  alcholol abuse studies
    in alcohol-preferring rats, 471
  anxiety neurobiology and, 17
    knockout mice studies, 25–26
Neuropharmacology
  obsessive-compulsive disorders, 225–235
    antipsychotic agents, 229–234
    augmenting agents, 225, 229–234
    brain imaging studies, 220–222
    current trials, 234
    monotherapy trials, 225
    serotonin uptake inhibitor efficacy,
        226–228
  schizophrenia dopamine hypothesis, 287
Neuroprotective agents
  3,4-methylenedioxymethamphetamine
      neurotoxicity and, 625
Neuroreceptor imaging
  schizophrenia, 259–260

Neurosteroids
    schizophrenia therapy, 394
Neurosurgery
    obsessive-compulsive disorders, 235–237
Neurotensin agonist/antagonist
    psychostimulant abuse and, 579
    schizophrenia therapy, 390
Neuroticism (N trait)
    anxiety neurobiology, 5–6
    mouse behavior, 6–9
Neurotoxicity
    cannabinoid receptors and, 672–673
    3,4-Methylenedioxymethamphetamine
        (MDMA), 619–628
        animal models, 620–621
        cytokines and microglia, 627–628
        hyperthermia, 624–625
        long-term neurochemical change,
            619–620
        metabolite mechanisms, 621–622
        monoaminergic transporter, 625–627
        oxidative stress, 623–624
Neurotransmitters. *See also* specific
        Neurotransmitters
    addictive disorders
        modulator therapy and, 458–459
    anxiety neurobiology
        knockout mice studies, 24–26
    anxiety neurobiology and, 15–18
    endocannabinoid system, 663
    3,4-methylenedioxymethamphetamine
        effects on
        receptor/transporter effects, 617
    obsessive-compulsive disorders
        metabolism studies, 223
    pain neuropharmacology, 714–717
        drug action localization, 718
    psychostimulant abuse
        chronic exposure and sensitization
            effects, 580–581, 583–585
Neurovascular model
    migraine therapy, calcitonin gene-related
        peptide, 759–760
NF-κB transcription factor family
    anxiety neurobiology and, 31
Nicotine
    basic properties, 535–536
    patches
        obsessive-compulsive disorder therapy,
            234
    pharmacology, 536–545
        absorption pharmacokinetics, 543–544

dependence and withdrawal therapy
    bupropion, 549–550
    cannabinoid antagonists, 550
    nicotinic antagonists, 548–549
    nicotinic partial agonists, 548
    nonnicotinic agents, 549–551
    opioid antagonists, 550–551
    overview, 545–546
    public health policy and, 551–552
    replacement medications, 546–548
    tricyclic antidepressants, 550
distribution pharmacokinetics, 544
metabolism and elimination
    pharmacokinetics, 544–545
nicotine reinforcement neurosubstrates,
    537–540
nicotinic acetylcholine receptors,
    537
    functional adaptations, 540–541
    withdrawal neurosubstrates, 541–543
Nicotine gum
    nicotine dependence and withdrawal
        therapy, 547–548
Nicotine-N-oxide
    nicotine dependence and withdrawal
    metabolism and elimination
        pharmacokinetics, 544–545
Nicotinic acetylcholine receptors (nAChRs)
    nicotine dependence and withdrawal
        classification and function, 537
        functional adaptations mechanisms,
            540–541
        nicotine reinforcement substrates,
            538–540
        nicotinic partial agonist therapy,
            548
        nicotinic partial antagonist therapy,
            548–549
        overview, 536–537
        withdrawal substrates, 542–543
    NRG1 molecular interaction, 354–355
    schizophrenia pharmacotherapy
        cholinergic agents, 393–394
Nicotinic agonists
    anxiety neurobiology and
        receptor deficits and, 29–30
Nicotinic antagonists
    nicotine dependence and withdrawal
        therapy, 548
Nicotinic partial agonists
    nicotine dependence and withdrawal
        therapy, 548

Nitric oxide synthase (NOS) inhibitor
   3,4-methylenedioxymethamphetamine
     neurotoxicity, 623–624
Nitrogen ohne radikal (NOR) metabolites
   benzodiazepine receptor ligand
     metabolism, 102
NMDA (*N*-methyl-D-aspartic acid)
   receptors
   addictive disorder pharmacotherapy
     methadone interactions, 456–457
   consolidated glutamate/dopamine
     hypotheses, 295–296
   glutamate theory of schizophrenia
     history of, 289–290
     imaging studies, 293
     neurochemistry of, 373–374
     pathological evidence, 291–292
     pharmacological evidence, 294–295
   ketamine effects on, 636–637
   obsessive-compulsive disorders
     glutamate genetic studies, 223
   pain management and, 717
   schizophrenia pharmacotherapy
     first- and second-generation
       antipsychotics, 381
     targeted drug development for, 391–392
   schizophrenia psychosis, 257–258
Nociception
   defined, 710
   drug action localization, 718
   pain pathways and, 711–712
   transient receptor potential V2 (TRPV2),
     736–737
Nonopiate analgesics
   migraine management, 765
Nonpeptide ligands
   corticotropin-releasing factor receptor
     antagonists, 195–196
Nonpharmacological therapy
   obsessive-compulsive disorders and,
     235–237
Nonsteroidal anti-inflammatory drugs
   migraine management, 765, 768
Noradrenergic systems
   psychostimulant abuse
     chronic exposure and sensitization
       effects, 584
   schizophrenia pharmacotherapy, 393
Norepinephrine (NE)
   alcohol abuse studies
     dopaminergic receptor systems and
       substrates, 472–473
   anxiety neurobiology, 15–17
   3,4-methylenedioxymethamphetamine
     effects on, 616
   receptor/transporter effects, 617
   psychostimulant abuse
     chronic exposure and sensitization
       effects, 584
     neuropharmacology, 570–575
   schizophrenia pharmacotherapy
     noradrenergic agent development, 393
Norepinephrine transporter (NET)
   anxiety neurobiology and
     knockout mice studies, 24–26
Nucleus accumbens (NAcc)
   alcohol abuse studies
     in alcohol-preferring rats, 470–471
     dopaminergic receptor systems and
       substrates, 471–472
     $GABA_A$ benzodiazepine receptor
       complex manipulation
       site-specific microinjection studies,
         493–496
   3,4-methylenedioxymethamphetamine
     (MDMA)
     reinforcing properties, 614–616
NUDEL gene
   DISC1 schizophrenia candidate gene
     molecular interactions, 351–352
Nur transcription factors
   schizophrenia therapy
     dopamine neurotransmission and,
       422

Obsessive-compulsive disorders (OCD)
   animal models, 224
   brain regions related to, 13–15
   clinical psychopharmacology, 225–235
     antipsychotic agents, 229–234
     augmenting agents, 225, 229–234
     current trials, 234
     monotherapy trials, 225
     serotonin uptake inhibitor efficacy,
       226–228
   deep brain stimulation, 236–237
   defined, 216
   diagnostic criteria, 10–12, 216
   genetic studies, 222–224
     developmental genes, 223–224
     dopamine, 223
     glutamate, 223
     neurotransmitter metabolism, 223
     serotonin, 222–224

immunomodulatory treatments, 235
neurobiology, 216–224
  brain imaging studies, 217–222
  functional imaging studies, 219–220
  magnetic resonance spectroscopy, 220
neuropharmacology
  brain imaging studies, 220–222
neurosurgery, 235–237
nonpharmacological experimental treatments, 235–237
pharmacotherapy, 77–78
serotonin/noradrenaline reuptake inhibitors, 69
summary of therapeutic advances, 237
symptom induction, 234
transcranial magnetic stimulation, 236
tricyclic antidepressants, 69–70
Ocapridone
  schizophrenia therapy, 389
8-OH-DPAT
  nicotine dependence and withdrawal
    withdrawal substrate specificity, 542–543
  serotonin receptors 5-HT$_{2A}$-5-HT$_{2C}$ interactions, 422–424
Olanzapine
  D$_2$ receptor blockade, 414–415
  neurogenesis and, 430
  schizophrenia therapy
    brain-derived neurotrophic factor and, 421–422
    clinical profile, 383–387
    D$_2$ receptor occupancy and effect, 376–378
    safety and tolerability, 388–389
    serotonin receptor 5-HT$_{2A}$, 420–421
Oligogenic anxiety-like conditions
  anxiety neurobiology
    mouse studies, 32–33
Open-field activity
  mouse anxiety models
    neurosteroid effects, 148–149
Opiates
  addiction and
    buprenorphine studies, 696–698
    drug discovery survey, 699–700
    epidemiology, 691–694
    future research issues, 698–699
    treatment statistics, 694–696
  pain management
    anatomical interactions, 718–720

Opioid agonists/antagonists
  migraine management, 765
  nicotine dependence and withdrawal therapy, 550–551
Opioid receptor system
  addictive disorders
    reward therapy and, 458–459
  alcohol abuse studies
    oral administration of βCCT/3PBC vs. agonists, 507–511
  delta receptors, 751
  dimerization, 752
  endogenous opioids, 746–748
  future research on, 752
  kappa receptors, 751–752
  mu receptors, 748–751
  nicotine dependence and withdrawal, 540
    withdrawal substrate specificity, 543
  orphanin FQ/nociceptin and receptor, 752
  overview, 745–746
  pain management and, 716–717
    targeting mechanisms, 718
  psychostimulant abuse and, 578–579
    chronic exposure and sensitization effects, 584
  short-acting
    addiction pharmacotherapy and, 453–457
Orbitofrontal-dorsomedial thalamic loop
  obsessive-compulsive disorders
    neuropharmacology, 221–222
Orphanin FQ/nociceptin (OFQ/N) receptor
  anxiety neurobiology and
    knockout mice studies, 25–26
  structure and function, 748, 752
Oxidative stress
  3,4-methylenedioxymethamphetamine neurotoxicity and, 623–624
Oxycodone
  abuse of
    incidence and prevalence, 692–694

Pain perception and management
  calcitonin gene-related peptide for, 768–769
  marijuana and, 666–668
  neuronal pathways
    descending modulatory pathways, 712–714
    neospinothalamic/paleospinothalamic pathways, 711–712
    overview, 709–710

neuropharmacology, 714–717
  anatomically-based interactions, 718–721
  drug targeting mechanisms, 718
transient receptor potential V1 (TRPV1) receptors
  antagonists, 733
  capsaicin, protons, and heat, 730–732
  chemical activators, 732–733
  cloning of, 728–729
  desensitization, 735–736
  expression, 729
  knockout mouse models, 736
  nociception channels, 736–737
  sensitization, 733–735
Paleospinothalamic pain pathways
  classification of, 711–712
Paliperodone
  schizophrenia therapy, 389
Panic disorders
  anticonvulsant therapy, 74–75
  anxiety disorder therapy, 78
  brain regions related to, 13–15
  diagnostic criteria, 10–12
  neuroactive steroids, 155
Peptide ligands
  corticotropin-releasing factor receptor antagonists
    basic properties, 180–181
    CRF_1/CRF_2 binding mechanisms, 190–195
    CRF_1/CRF_2 pharmacology, 185–195
    CRF_1/CRF_2 receptor pharmacology, 185–195
    structure and function, 179–185
    subtypes and distribution, 181–185
Periaqueductal gray (PAG) stimulation
  cannabinoid analgesics and, 667–668
Peripheral benzodiazepine receptors (PBRs)
  stress-induced behavior
    neuroactive steroids, 155–156
Personality traits
  continuous expression
    anxiety neurobiology, 9–12
Pharmacophore models
  benzodiazepine activity, 116
Pharmacotherapy
  addictive disorders
    history of, 451–457
    reward modulation/countermodulation and, 458–459

risk factors for addiction development, 457–458
anxiety disorders
  anxiolytic drugs, 62–75
    amino acid neurotransmission, 72–75
    anticonvulsants, 74–75
    antidepressants, 64–70
    antihistamines, 75
    antipsychotics, 71–72
    benzodiazepines, 73–74
    beta-blockers, 71
    lithium, 75
    monoamine neurotransmission, 63–72
    serotonin receptor agonists, 70–71
  depressive disorders, 80
  future research issues, 81
  generalized anxiety disorder, 77
  obsessive-compulsive disorder, 77–78
  overview, 60
  panic disorder/agoraphobia, 78
  phobias, 78, 80
  posttraumatic stress disorder, 79
  social anxiety disorder, 79–80
  treatments chart, 76
obsessive-compulsive disorders
  overview, 216
schizophrenia
  antipsychotic drug profiles
    first-generation (conventional) agents, 383
    safety and tolerability, 387–388
    second-generation (atypical) agents, 383–387
  antipsychotic mechanisms of action, 376–382
    D_1 receptors, 380–381
    D_2/D_3 and D_4 antagonism and regional specificity, 380
    D_2 occupancy thresholds and rapid dissociation, 378–380
    D_2 receptor occupancy, 376–378
    dopamine release, 381
    NMDA receptor function, 381
    synthesis reactions, 381–382
  current developments and future directions, 388–394
    cannabinoid hypothesis, 394
    cholinergic agents, 393–394
    D_1 agonists and antagonists, 390
    D_3 antagonists, 390
    D_4 antagonists, 390

dopamine system targeting, 389
glutamate system targeting, 391–393
neurokinin antagonists, 391
neurosteroids, 394
neurotensin agonist/antagonist, 390
noradrenergic agents, 393
future research issues, 394–395
high 5-HT$_{2A}$ vs. D$_2$ affinity, 378
neurochemical hypotheses, 371–376
overview, 370–371
Phencyclidine. *See also* Ketamine
glutamate theory of schizophrenia
history of, 289–290
neurochemistry of, 374
ketamine derivative, 636–637
schizophrenia neurochemistry and, 260–262
Phenothiazines
schizophrenia therapy
clinical profiles, 383
Phenotype analysis
obsessive-compulsive disorders, 237
schizophrenia, 262–263
genetic epidemiology, 322–323
Phenylalkylamines, 637–640
addiction, 639–640
mechanism of action, 638–639
pharmacology, 638
α-Phenyl-*N-tert*-butyl nitrone (PBN)
3,4-methylenedioxymethamphetamine neurotoxicity
oxidative stress, 623–624
Phobias
brain regions related to, 13–15
pharmacotherapy, 79–80
Phosphoinositol 3-kinase-AKT signaling pathway
dystrobrevin binding protein 1 (DTNBP1)
molecular interactions, 353
Phosphoinositol-4,5-bisphosphate (PIP$_2$)
transient receptor potential V1 (TRPV1)
receptor sensitization, 734–735
Phospholipase C
transient receptor potential V1 (TRPV1)
receptor sensitization, 734–735
Phosphorus MRS
schizophrenia analysis, 257
Picrotoxin
alcohol abuse studies
GABA$_A$ benzodiazepine receptor complex, 487–488

GABAergic modification of dopamine agonists, 496–497
p-MPPI receptor antagonist
nicotine dependence and withdrawal
withdrawal substrate specificity, 542–543
Positional candidate genes
schizophrenia genetics, 325
Positional cloning
schizophrenia genetics, 324
Positron emission tomography (PET)
obsessive-compulsive disorders, 219–220
schizophrenia
dopamine hypothesis, 286
schizophrenia analysis, 257
Postmortem studies
schizophrenia, 260–262
dopamine hypothesis and, 285
future research issues, 355–356
overview, 343–344
susceptibility gene identification, 344–351
susceptibility gene interactions, 351–355
Postpartum depression
neuroactive steroids, 156–157
Posttraumatic stress disorder (PTSD)
anticonvulsant therapy, 74–75
brain regions related to, 13–15
diagnostic criteria, 10–12
mirtazapine therapy, 70
neuroactive steroids, 154–155
pharmacotherapy, 79
PPP3CC gene
schizophrenia molecular genetics, 328
P rat line. *See* Alcohol-preferring rats
Predictive validity
animal anxiety-like behavior and, 12
"Preemptive analgesia"
pain management and, 717
Prefrontal cortex (PFC)
integrated glutamate/dopamine hypotheses of schizophrenia, 374–376
Pregnancy
marijuana effects in, 664–665
3,4-methylenedioxymethamphetamine and, 630–631
Pregnenolone sulfate (PREGS)
in brain, 137
Prenatal development
marijuana effects on, 664–665

Prescription drugs. *See also* Opiates
abuse of
incidence and prevalence, 692–694
Preventive therapy
migraine management, 766–768
PRODH gene
schizophrenia molecular genetics, 329–330
Prodromal period
schizophrenia therapy
second-generation antipsychotics, 386–387
Progesterone levels
depression
neuroactive steroids, 156–157
Pro-opiomelanocortin peptide group
nicotine dependence and withdrawal, 540
3-Propoxy-β-carboline hydrochloride (3BPC)
alcohol abuse studies
anxiety reduction with, 510–511
$GABA_{A1,2,3,5}$ receptor subunit modulation, 499–501
$GABA_{A1}$ receptor subunit selectivity, 498–499
microinjection techniques, 505–507
oral administration, 507–511
systemic administration, 503–504
Protein kinase A
transient receptor potential V1 (TRPV1) receptor sensitization, 733–735
Protein kinase C
transient receptor potential V1 (TRPV1) receptor sensitization, 733–735
Protein kinase C_γ
anxiety neurobiology and, 31
Protons
transient receptor potential V1 (TRPV1) receptor expression, 730–732
Psilocybin
schizophrenia therapy
serotonin receptor 5-HT_{2A}, 420–421
Psychoeducation
anxiety management with, 60–61
Psychological traits
anxiety neurobiology
continuous expression of normal personality, 9–10
genetic basis of, 4–6
mouse behavior extrapolation studies, 6–9
Psychosis
in schizophrenia, 253–254

animal models, 264–265
neural network studies, 257–258
second-generation antipsychotics and, 386–387
Psychostimulants
abuse-related neuropharmacology, 569–579
γ-aminobutyric acid, 576–577
glutamate, 575–576
hyopthalamic-pituitary-adrenal axis, 577–578
monoamines, 570–575
neuropeptides, 578–579
addiction therapy development, 585–586
chronic exposure-related neurobiology, 579–589
neurotransmitter/neuroendocrine systems, 580–584
signal transduction mechanisms and gene expression, 584–585
future research issues, 588–589
therapeutic applications of, 567–569
Public health policy
nicotine dependency and withdrawal therapy, 551–552
Pyrazolopyrimidine
corticotropin-releasing factor receptor antagonists
anxiety/depression therapeutic potential, 197–198
Pyrazoloquinoline
alcohol abuse studies
$GABA_A$ benzodiazepine receptor complex, 490–493

Quantitative behavioral genetics
anxiety neurobiology, 6
Quantitative trait locus (QTL) analysis
anxiety neurobiology, 4
emotionality studies in mice, 8–9
mice studies, 19
oligogenic anxiety-like conditions, 32–33
Quetiapine
schizophrenia therapy
clinical profile, 383–387
safety and tolerability, 389
Quinelorane
alcohol abuse studies
dopaminergic receptor systems and substrates, 472–473

Quinpirole
  alcohol abuse studies
    dopaminergic receptor systems and substrates, 472–473

Raclopride
  alcohol abuse studies
    dopaminergic receptor systems and substrates, 472–473
    chronic exposure and sensitization effects, 582–585
^{11}C-Raclopride
  striatal D_2 receptor blockade, 414–415
Radiolabeled peptides
  corticotropin-releasing factor receptor antagonists
    peptide ligand pharmacology, 187–195
Rapid dissociation
  schizophrenia pharmacotherapy
    D_2 receptor occupancy thresholds, 379–380
Receptor activity modifying protein 1 (RAMP1)
  calcitonin gene-related peptide sites and migraine therapy targeting, 762
Receptor density assessment
  schizophrenia
    dopamine hypothesis and, 285
  schizophrenia neuroreceptor imaging, 259–260
Receptor ligand pharmacology
  benzodiazepines, 97–102
    endogenous site, 98–99
    metabolism functions, 101–102
    single-cell GABA response modulation, 99–100
    therapeutic action, 97–98
    tolerance and dependence characteristics, 100–101
Regional cerebral blood flow (rCBF)
  schizophrenia, 257–259
Regional specificity
  schizophrenia therapy
    D_2/D_3 and D_4 receptor antagonism and, 380
"Region-specific" neuroanatomical controls
  alcohol abuse studies in alcohol-preferring rats, 469–470
Regulator of G-protein signaling 4 (RGS4)
  schizophrenia candidate gene, 328
  susceptibility identification, 351

Reinforcing mechanisms
  alcohol abuse studies in alcohol-preferring rats, 469
  3,4-methylenedioxymethamphetamine (MDMA), 614–616
Resinferatoxin (RTX)
  cloning of, 727–729
  transient receptor potential V1 (TRPV1) receptor expression, 733
Respiratory system
  γ-hydroxybutyric acid (GHB) effects, 634
Reuptake inhibitors
  psychostimulant abuse
    monoamine neuropharmacology, 571–575
Reversible inhibitor of monoamine oxidase A (RIMA)
  anxiety disorder therapy, 70
Reward effects
  addictive disorders, 458–459
  endocannabinoids and, 675–676
  3,4-methylenedioxymethamphetamine (MDMA), 614–616
  psychostimulant abuse
    chronic exposure and sensitization effects, 581–585
Rhodopsin
  corticotropin-releasing factor receptor antagonists
    ligand binding mechanisms, 191–195
Riluzole
  obsessive-compulsive disorder therapy, 234
Rimonabant
  appetite regulation, 670–672
  cannabinoid receptors and, 661–662
  cognition and, 669–670
  endocannabinoid physiology and, 665–675
  nicotine dependence and withdrawal therapy, 550
  opiate dependence therapy and, 699
  pain management and, 667–668
  reward, tolerance, and dependence, 675–676
Risperidone
  neurogenesis and, 430
  schizophrenia therapy
    clinical profile, 383–387
    safety and tolerability, 389
    serotonin receptor 5-HT$_{2A}$, 418–421

Ritanserin
    3,4-methylenedioxymethamphetamine
        effects on, 616
RO19-4603 inverse agonist
    alcohol abuse studies
        GABA$_A$ benzodiazepine receptor
            complex, 488–493
            site-specific microinjection
                techniques, 494–496
            systemic administration studies,
                492–493
Rohypnol. See Flunitrazepam
ROI15-4513 inverse agonist
    alcohol abuse studies
        GABA$_A$ benzodiazepine receptor
            complex
                alcohol-modulator commonalities,
                    487–488
RU34000 imidazopyrimidine inverse agonist
    alcohol abuse studies
        GABA$_A$ benzodiazepine receptor
            complex, 490–493
            site-specific microinjection
                techniques, 496
RY 023 inverse agonist
    alcohol abuse studies
        GABA$_{A5}$ receptor specificity,
            512–516

Safety
    schizophrenia therapy
        second-generation antipsychotics,
            387–388
Samson test procedure
    alcohol abuse studies in alcohol-preferring
        rats, 468–470
SB-271046
    serotonin receptor 5-HT$_6$ and,
        425–426
SB-399885
    serotonin receptor 5-HT$_6$ and, 426
SCH 23390 compound
    alcohol abuse studies
        bed nucleus of stria terminalis system,
            475
        lateral hypothalamus, effects on,
            481–485
        ventral pallidum receptor blockade,
            477–480
Schizophrenia
    animal models, 263–265
    biological mechanisms, 256–263
    brain imaging studies, 256–260
    characteristics of, 252
    clinical phenomenology and treatment,
        252–256
    cognitive dysfunction, 254–255
    dopamine hypothesis
        cortical vs. striatal dopamine, 287–289
        genetic evidence, 286–287
        history, 284–285
        imaging evidence, 285–286
        pathological evidence, 285
        pharmacological evidence, 287
        pharmacotherapy, 371–373
    evolution of theories on, 283–284
    future research issues, 265–266
    genetic epidemiology, 321–323
        phenotype definition, 322–323
    genetics and phenotypes, 262–263
    glutamate theory of
        genetic evidence for, 293–294
        history, 289–291
        imaging evidence for, 292–293
        pathological evidence for, 291–292
        pharmacological evidence for,
            294–295
        pharmacotherapy, 373–374
    integrated glutamate/dopamine
        hypotheses, 295–297
        pharmacotherapy, 374–376
    molecular genetics, 323–325
        candidate genes, 325–328
        chromosomal abnormalities, 328–331
        functional candidate genes, 331–332
        future research issues, 333
        susceptibility gene function, 332–333
    negative affect, 255–256
    neural network studies and, 255–259
    neurochemistry, 260–262
    neurogenesis in, 430
    neuroreceptor imaging, 259–260
    pharmacotherapy
        antipsychotic drug profiles
            first-generation (conventional)
                agents, 383
            safety and tolerability, 387–388
            second-generation (atypical) agents,
                383–387
        antipsychotic mechanisms of action,
            376–382
            D$_1$ receptors, 380–381
            D$_2$/D$_3$ and D$_4$ antagonism and
                regional specificity, 380

D_2 occupancy thresholds and rapid
  dissociation, 378–380
D_2 receptor occupancy, 376–378
dopamine release, 381
NMDA receptor function, 381
synthesis reactions, 381–382
current developments and future
  directions, 388–394
  cannabinoid hypothesis, 394
  cholinergic agents, 393–394
  D_1 agonists and antagonists, 390
  D_3 antagonists, 390
  D_4 antagonists, 390
  dopamine system targeting, 389
  glutamate system targeting, 391–393
  neurokinin antagonists, 391
  neurosteroids, 394
  neurotensin agonist/antagonist, 390
  noradrenergic agents, 393
future research issues, 394–395
high 5-HT_{2A} vs. D_2 affinity, 378
neurochemical hypotheses, 371–376
overview, 370–371
postmortem studies, 260–262
dopamine hypothesis and, 285
future research issues, 355–356
overview, 343–344
susceptibility gene identification,
  344–351
susceptibility gene interactions, 351–355
prevalence, 252–253
psychosis and, 253–254
symptom classification, 253
Second-generation antipsychotics (SGAs)
schizophrenia therapy
  clinical profile, 383–387
  D_2/D_3 and D_4 receptor antagonism and
    regional specificity, 380
  D_2 receptor occupancy thresholds and
    rapid dissociation, 378–380
  history of, 370–371
  NMDA receptor antagonists, 381
  safety and tolerability, 387–388
Selective serotonin reuptake inhibitors
  (SSRIs)
anxiety disorder therapy, 66–69
obsessive-compulsive disorders
  controlled trials, 225
panic disorder therapy, 78
posttraumatic stress disorder therapy,
  79
social anxiety disorder therapy, 79–80

Selegiline
  schizophrenia therapy, 394
Sensitivity
  psychostimulant abuse and reduction of
    neurobiology of, 579–585
  transient receptor potential V1 (TRPV1)
    receptor expression, 733–735
Sensory neurons
  pain pathways, 711–712
Separation-induced ultrasonic vocalizations
  animal anxiety models
    neurosteroid effects, 150
Sequence homology
  corticotropin-releasing factor receptor
    antagonists
    ligand binding mechanisms, 191–195
Serotonin (5-HT)
  antipsychotic drugs and release of, 426
  anxiety disorder anxiolytics
    monoamine neurotransmission, 63–72
  anxiety neurobiology, 4
    genetic susceptibility studies, 18–19
    neurotransmission mechanisms, 15–17
  3,4-methylenedioxymethamphetamine
    effects on, 616
    long-term neurochemical effects, 619–620
    oxidative stress, 623–624
    receptor/transporter effects, 617
  nicotine dependence and withdrawal
    withdrawal substrates, 542–543
  obsessive-compulsive disorders
    genetic studies, 222–224
  psychostimulant abuse
    neuropharmacology, 570–575
Serotonin and noradrenaline reuptake
  inhibitors (SNRI)
  anxiety disorder therapy, 69
Serotonin hypothesis
  obsessive-compulsive disorders
    neuropharmacology, 221–222
Serotonin receptor 5-HT/D_2 hypothesis
  atypical antipsychotics, 417–418
  serotonin receptor 5-HT_{2A}, 419–421
Serotonin receptors
  atypical antipsychotics
    adrenergic mechanisms, 426–427
    serotonin receptor 5-HT_{1A}-5-HT_{2A}
      interactions, 421–425
    serotonin receptor 5-HT_{2A}, 418–421
      cortical dopamine efflux and
        cognitive function, 421–422
      extrapyramidal function, 422

serotonin receptor 5-HT$_{2A}$-5-HT$_{2C}$
  receptor interactions, 422–424
serotonin receptor 5-HT/D$_2$ hypothesis,
  417–418
schizophrenia neurochemistry and,
  261–262
schizophrenia pharmacotherapy
  serotonin receptor 5-HT$_{2A}$
    D$_2$ antagonism and, 381
  serotonin 5-HT$_{1A}$
    nicotine dependence and withdrawal,
      542–543
  serotonin 5-HT$_{2C}$ receptors
    psychostimulant abuse, 574–575
  serotonin receptor 5-HT$_{1A}$
    anxiety disorder therapy, 70–71
    anxiety neurobiology and
      knockout mice deficit studies, 27–30
  serotonin receptor 5-HT$_{1B}$
    anxiety neurobiology and
      knockout mice deficit studies, 28–30
  serotonin receptor 5-HT$_{2A}$
    cortical dopamine efflux and cognitive
      function, 421–422
    extrapyramidal function, 422
    LSD downregulation of, 638–640
    schizophrenia pharmacotherapy
      D$_2$ antagonism and, 381
  serotonin receptor 5-HT$_6$ interactions
    atypical antipsychotics, 425–426
  triptan therapy for migraines, 764–765
Serotonin reuptake inhibitors (SRIs)
  obsessive-compulsive disorders
    brain neuropharmacology, 221–222
    neuropharmacology, 226–228
Serotonin transporter (5-HTT)
  anxiety neurobiology
    environmental effects and, 34–35
  anxiety neurobiology and
    knockout mice studies, 24–26
  3,4-methylenedioxymethamphetamine
    neurotoxicity and, 625–627
  obsessive-compulsive disorders
    abnormalities, 219–220
    genetic studies, 222–224
Serotonin transporter (SERT) antagonists
  obsessive-compulsive disorders, 223
Sertindole
  schizophrenia therapy
    clinical profile, 383–387
Signal transduction mechanisms
  psychostimulant abuse

chronic exposure and sensitization
  effects, 584–585
Single-nucleotide polymorphisms (SNPs)
  addictive disorders vulnerability, 457–458
  catechol-O-methyl transferase
    as schizophrenia susceptibility gene,
      347–348
  schizophrenia genetics
    DISC1 molecular interactions, 352
    GRM3 gene, 349
    positional candidate genes, 325
Single-photon-emission computerized
  tomography (SPECT)
  schizophrenia analysis, 257
Site-specific microinjection studies
  alcohol abuse
    GABA$_A$ benzodiazepine receptor
      complex manipulation, 493–496
Smoking. *See* Nicotine
Social anxiety disorder
  pharmacotherapy, 79–80
Social interaction paradigm
  3,4-methylenedioxymethamphetamine
    effects on, 630–631
Social isolation
  animal anxiety model
    neurosteroid effects, 151–152
  schizophrenia
    animal models, 264
Soluble N-ethylmaleimide-sensitive factor
  attachment protein receptors
  (SNAREs)
    dystrobrevin binding protein 1 (DTNBP1)
      molecular interactions, 353
"Speedball" psychostimulant combination
  neuropeptide pharmacology and, 578–579
Splice variants
  corticotropin-releasing factor receptor
    antagonists
    receptor subunits, 182–185
SR48692
  psychostimulant abuse
    neuropeptide pharmacology and, 579
SR144528 antagonist
  cannabinoid receptors and, 661–662
Stimulant medications
  psychostimulant therapy, 587–588
Stress
  addictive disorders and response to, 459
  cannabinoid analgesics and, 667–668
  neuroactive steroid interactions
    drug abuse relapse, 159–160

HPA axis, 153–154
  overview, 152–153
  psychostimulant abuse
    chronic exposure and sensitization effects, 580–585
    neuropharmacology and, 577–578
Striatal dopamine receptors
  atypical antipsychotic drugs
    clozapine D_2 receptor blockade, 414–415
  schizophrenia dopamine hypothesis and, 287–288
Structural studies
  obsessive-compulsive disorders, 217–218
Structure-activity relationships (SARs)
  benzodiazepines, 114–116
Substance P
  anxiety neurobiology and, 17
Substantia nigra
  clozapine D_2 receptor blockade, 414–415
Sucrose-fading technique
  alcohol abuse studies in alcohol-preferring rats, 467–470
Sulfate fraction
  neuroactive steroids
    in brain, 137
Sulpiride
  alcohol abuse studies
    dopaminergic receptor systems and substrates, 472–473
    ventral pallidum receptor blockade, 477–480
Sumatriptan
  migraine management with, 764–765
  obsessive-compulsive disorders, 234
Susceptibility genes
  schizophrenia
    future research issues, 355–356
    gene linkage studies, 324
    molecular genetics
      functional implications, 332–333
    molecular interactions, 351–355
    postmortem studies
      overview, 343–344
      susceptibility gene identification, 344–351
      susceptibility gene interactions, 351–355
Sweetened cocktail solution procedure
  alcohol abuse studies in alcohol-preferring rats, 468–470

Synapsin I proteins
  dystrobrevin binding protein 1 (DTNBP1) molecular interactions, 353
Synaptosomal-associated protein 25 (SNAP25)
  dystrobrevin binding protein 1 (DTNBP1) molecular interactions, 353
Synthesis
  antipsychotics
    schizophrenia pharmacotherapy, 381–382
  endocannabinoid system, 663–664
Systemic administration studies
  alcohol abuse studies
    $GABA_A$ benzodiazepine receptor complex, 492–493
Systems biology theory
  schizophrenia and, 255–256
"Systems neuroscience"
  schizophrenia dopamine hypothesis and, 288

T-butyl agents
  alcohol abuse studies
    $GABA_A$ benzodiazepine receptor complex
      site-specific microinjection techniques, 494–496
Δ^9-Tetrahydrocannabinol
  analgesic properties, 666–669
  appetite regulation, 670–672
  cannabinoid receptor binding, 663
  cognition and, 669–670
  emesis modulation, 674–675
  endocannabinoid physiology and, 665–675
  isolation off, 660–661
  neurotoxicity effects, 672–673
  prenatal development and, 664–665
  reward, tolerance, and dependence, 675–676
Thermoregulation
  3,4-methylenedioxymethamphetamine effects on, 629
Thioxanthine
  schizophrenia therapy
    clinical profile, 383
THIP agonist
  alcohol abuse studies
    $GABA_A$ benzodiazepine receptor complex, 488–493

Tiagabine
   psychostimulant abuse therapy, 588
Tissue injury
   transient receptor potential V1 (TRPV1)
      receptor expression, 729–732
Tolcapone
   schizophrenia therapy, 389
Tolerability
   schizophrenia therapy
      second-generation antipsychotics, 387–388
Tolerance mechanisms
   benzodiazepines, 100
   endocannabinoids, 675–676
   psychostimulant abuse
      neurobiology of, 579–585
Topiramate
   migraine management, 766
   psychostimulant abuse therapy, 688
Topological analysis
   corticotropin-releasing factor receptor antagonists
      receptor subunits, 183–185
Tourette's disorder
   obsessive-compulsive disorder comorbidity, 216
Tramadol
   obsessive-compulsive disorder therapy, 234
Transcranial magnetic stimulation (TMS)
   obsessive-compulsive disorders, 236
Transcriptional regulators
   anxiety neurobiology and
      mouse studies, 19, 22
Transdermal nicotine patch
   mecamylamine in conjunction with, 549
   nicotine dependence and withdrawal therapy, 546–547
   obsessive-compulsive disorder therapy, 234
Transient receptor potential V1 (TRPV1) receptors
   analgesic properties, 668–669
   antagonists, 733
   capsaicin, protons, and heat, 730–732
   chemical activators, 732–733
   cloning of, 728–729
   desensitization, 735–736
   endocannabinoid ligands, 664
   expression, 729
   knockout mouse models, 736
   nociception channels, 736–737
   sensitization, 733–735

Transient receptor potential V2 (TRPV2)
   nociception and, 736–737
Transient receptor potential V3 (TRPV3)
   nociception and, 737
Transient receptor potential V4 (TRPV4)
   nociception and, 737
TRAR4 gene
   schizophrenia molecular genetics, 328
Treatment Episode Data Set (TEDS)
   opiate treatment statistics, 694–696
Tricyclic antidepressants (TCAs)
   anxiety disorder therapy, 69–70
   nicotine dependence and withdrawal therapy, 550
   panic disorder therapy, 78
   psychostimulant abuse therapy, 586–587
Trigeminal ganglion
   migraine therapy targeting of, 760
Trigeminovasculature system
   calcitonin gene-related peptide sites and migraine therapy targeting, 761–762
Triptans
   migraine management with, 764–765
Tryptophan hydroxylase
   3,4-methylenedioxymethamphetamine effects on, 616–617
Two-bottle water choice procedure
   alcohol abuse studies in alcohol-preferring rats, 468–470
Tyrosine-hydroxylase
   schizophrenia dopamine hypothesis and, 288–289
Tyrosine kinase B (trkB)
   anxiety neurobiology
      receptor deficits and, 29–30

Urocortins
   corticotropin-releasing factor receptor antagonists
      ligand structure, 180–181

Val66Met substitution polymorphism
   anxiety neurobiology
      genetic susceptibility studies, 18–19
   schizophrenia
      serotonin receptor 5-HT$_{2A}$ receptor and, 421–422
Valproate
   anxiety disorder therapy, 75
   migraine management, 765–766

Vanilloid receptors
  cloning, 727–729
  transient receptor potential V1 expression, 729
    antagonists, 733
    capsaicin, protons, and heat, 730–732
    chemical activators, 732–733
    desensitization, 735–736
    knockout mouse models, 736
    nociception channels, 736–737
    sensitization, 731–735
Varenicline
  nicotine dependence and withdrawal therapy, 548
Variable numbers of tandem repeats (VNTR)
  obsessive-compulsive disorders
    dopamine genetics, 223
Velocardiofacial syndrome gene
  schizophrenia
    chomosome mapping, 346
    COMT catabolism and, 329
Venlafaxine
  anxiety disorder therapy, 69
  obsessive-compulsive disorder therapy, 234
Ventral hippocampal lesions
  in schizophrenia
    animal models, 265
Ventral pallidum
  alcohol abuse studies, 476–480
    dopaminergic regulation hypotheses, 478–480
    $GABA_{A1}$ subunit probe selectivity, 501–503
    GABAergic modification of dopamine agonists, 497–498
Ventral tegmental area (VTA)
  alcohol abuse studies
    dopaminergic receptor systems and substrates, 472–473
  alcohol abuse studies in alcohol-preferring rats
    control substrates in, 470
  atypical antipsychotic drug mechanisms in clozapine D_2 receptors, 414–415
  cannabinoid receptors in, 675–676
  integrated glutamate/dopamine hypotheses of schizophrenia, 375–376
  nicotine dependence and withdrawal

    nicotine reinforcement substrates, 538–540
    withdrawal substrates, 542–543
  psychostimulant abuse
    monoamine neuropharmacology, 571–575
    neuropeptide pharmacology, 578–579
Vesicular glutamate transporter
  glutamate theory of schizophrenia
    pathological evidence, 292
Vesicular monoamine transporter (VMAT) protein
  dopamine hypothesis of schizophrenia, 284–285
Visual system
  γ-hydroxybutyric acid (GHB) effects, 634
Vitamin D receptor (VDR)
  anxiety neurobiology and, 32
Vogel conflict test
  mouse models of anxiety
    neurosteroid effects, 145–146
Vogel punished drinking test
  emotionality studies in mice, 8–9

WAY-100635 compound
  $5-HT_{2A}$-$5-HT_{2C}$ receptor interactions, 422–424
  nicotine dependence and withdrawal
    withdrawal substrate specificity, 542–543
WIN 55,212-2
  analgesic properties, 666–668
  convulsant effects of, 673
  pain management and, 667–668
Wisconsin card sort task (WCST)
  schizophrenia dopamine hypothesis
    genetic evidence, 286–287
Withdrawal syndrome
  benzodiazepines, 74
  nicotine dependence and withdrawal
    withdrawal neurosubstrates, 541–543
  opiate addiction and, 699

ZDHHC8 candidate gene
  schizophrenia molecular genetics, 330
Ziprasidone
  schizophrenia therapy
    safety and tolerability, 389
Zolpidem
  alcohol abuse studies
    $GABA_{A1}$ receptor subunit selectivity, 499

CUMULATIVE INDEX

Numbers in *italic* indicate the volume in which the entry appears.

AB1-42, Alzheimer's disease, invertebrate models, *3:*579–582
Abecarnil, GABA$_A$ subunit pharmacology, allosteric ligand modulation, *1:*503–506
Absorption pharmacokinetics, nicotine dependence and withdrawal, *2:*543–544
ABT-418 nicotinic agonist, dementia disorders and, *3:*467–468
ABT431 compound, schizophrenia dopamine hypothesis, *2:*373
ACEA 1021/1031 agents, stroke management, *3:*358
Acetylcholine (ACh):
  action potential research on, *1:*26–27
  early research on, *1:*17
  Feldberg's research on, *1:*20–21
  H$_3$ receptor release, *1:*316
  Loewi's experiments in, *1:*18–19
  muscarinic receptors:
    activation mechanisms, *1:*155
    dimerization, *1:*166–167
    distribution, *1:*149
    G-protein coupling properties, *1:*155–156
      RGS proteins, *1:*158
    ion channels, *1:*160–162
    ligand binding mechanisms, *1:*152–154
      agonists, *1:*152
      allosteric ligands, *1:*153–154
      antagonists, *1:*152–153
    clinical applications, *1:*154
    MAPK pathways modulation, *1:*159
    phenotypic mouse analysis, *1:*167–177
      agonist-induced tremor and hypothermia, *1:*170–171
      amylase secretion, exocrine pancreas, *1:*175
      analgesia, *1:*170
      autoreceptors, *1:*171
      cardiovascular system, *1:*175–176
      cytolytic T cells, *1:*177
      drug abuse effects, *1:*173
      epileptic seizures, *1:*169
      food intake stimulation, *1:*171
      gastric acid secretion, *1:*175
      inhibitory hippocampal synapse suppression, *1:*172
      learning and memory functions, *1:*168–169
      locomotor activity, *1:*169–170
      nucleus accumbens, dopamine effects, *1:*172–173
      pancreatic islet insulin and glucagon secretion, *1:*174–175
      peripheral autoreceptors and heteroreceptors, *1:*176
      prepulse inhibition and haloperidol-induced catalepsy, *1:*172
      salivary secretion, *1:*174

Handbook of Contemporary Neuropharmacology, Edited by David R. Sibley, Israel Hanin, Michael Kuhar, and Phil Skolnick. Copyright © 2007 John Wiley & Sons, Inc.

skin functions, *1:*177
smooth muscle functions, *1:*173–174
striatal dopamine release modulation, *1:*171–172
regulatory mechanisms, *1:*162–166
downregulation, *1:*163–164
internatlizations, *1:*162–163
phosphorylation, *1:*164–166
resensitization, *1:*166
uncoupling, *1:*162
research background, *1:*148–149
signaling pathways, *1:*158–159
structural features, *1:*149–151
neuropeptide electrophysiology and, *1:*676–677
neurotransmitter transporters:
choline, *1:*714–715
vesicular transporters, *1:*716–717
Torpedo electric organ, *1:*109–110
transmitter inactivation, *1:*51–52
Acetylcholine binding protein (AChBP), $GABA_A$ receptor activation, agonist binding site architecture, *1:*495
Acetylcholinesterase:
early research on, *1:*23
inhibitors, dementia disorders and, *3:*463–465
nicotinic acetylcholine receptor and, *1:*28
N-Acetyl aspartate (NAA):
glutamate theory of schizophrenia, pathological evidence, *2:*292
schizophrenia analysis, *2:*256–257
schizophrenia dopamine hypothesis, *2:*289
N-Acetylcysteine (NAC), psychostimulant abuse and, cystine/glutamate transporter restoration, *2:*576
Acoustic startle, mouse anxiety models, neurosteroid effects, *2:*147
1S,3R-ACPD, mGlu group I selective orthosteric agonists, *1:*423
Acquired immunodeficiency syndrome (AIDS):
alcohol abuse and, *3:*716
cholinergic system, *3:*711–712
clinical features, *3:*694–695
dementia and, *3:*711–712
drug abuse and, *3:*712–716
methamphetamine/cocaine, *3:*713–715
opioid drugs, *3:*715–716
excitatory amino acid neurotransmitters, *3:*711

future neuropharmacology issues, *3:*718
lipid metabolism alterations, *3:*707
neurodegenerative diseases and, *3:*716–718
neuropathology, *3:*695–704
cell death cascades, *3:*704–707
apoptosis, *3:*704–705
excitotoxicity, *3:*705–706
neural progenitor cells, *3:*706–707
oxidative stress, *3:*706
chemokines in, *3:*697–698
neurodegenerative mechanisms, *3:*699
neuropharmacology, features of, *3:*694–695
neurotoxic proteins, *3:*699–704
glycoproteins gp120 and gp41, *3:*699, *3:*701
Nef protein, *3:*703
neurobiology of, *3:*700
Rev protein, *3:*704
Tat protein, *3:*701–703
Vpr protein, *3:*703
Vpu protein, *3:*704
nigrostriatal system, *3:*707–711
dopamine mediators, *3:*709–711
opiate addiction comorbidity with, *2:*691–694
pathogenesis, *3:*695
Action potentials:
early research on, *1:*25–27
voltage-gated potassium channels, K_V subunits, structure and function, *1:*628–630
Activin, vascular endothelial growth factor and, *1:*809
Acute delivery systems, nicotine dependence and withdrawal therapy, *2:*547–548
Acute motor axonal neuropathy (AMAN), pathology, *3:*614
Acylated peptide hormones, ghrelin receptor ligands, *3:*766–768
Adaptor proteins, tyrosine kinase receptor signaling, *3:*243–245
Addiction. *See* Substance abuse
Addictive disorders. *See also* Heroin addiction; specific disorders, e.g. Alcohol abuse
diagnostic criteria, *2:*456–457
endocannabinoids, *2:*675–676
γ-hydroxybutyric acid (GHB) and, *2:*635–636
hallucinogens and, *2:*639–640

hypocretin/orexin system, *3:*135
nicotine dependence and withdrawal,
  pharmacology, *2:*536–545
  absorption pharmacokinetics,
    *2:*543–544
  bupropion, *2:*549–550
  cannabinoid antagonists, *2:*550
  distribution pharmacokinetics, *2:*544
  metabolism and elimination
    pharmacokinetics, *2:*544–545
  nicotine reinforcement neurosubstrates,
    *2:*537–540
  nicotinic acetylcholine receptors,
    *2:*537
    functional adaptations, *2:*540–541
  nicotinic antagonists, *2:*548–549
  nicotinic partial agonists, *2:*548
  nonnicotinic agents, *2:*549–551
  opioid antagonists, *2:*550–551
  overview, *2:*545–546
  pharmacokinetics, *2:*543–545
  public health policy and, *2:*551–552
  replacement medications, *2:*546–548
  tricyclic antidepressants, *2:*550
  withdrawal neurosubstrates, *2:*541–543
opiate addiction:
  buprenorphine studies, *2:*696–698
  drug discovery survey, *2:*699–700
  epidemiology, *2:*691–694
  future research issues, *2:*698–699
  treatment statistics, *2:*694–696
pharmacotherapy:
  history of, *2:*451–457
  reward modulation/countermodulation
    and, *2:*458–459
  risk factors for addiction development,
    *2:*457–458
psychostimulant abuse:
  addiction therapy development,
    *2:*585–586
  chronic exposure-related neurobiology,
    *2:*579–589
    neurotransmitter/neuroendocrine
      systems, *2:*580–584
    signal transduction mechanisms and
      gene expression, *2:*584–585
  future research issues, *2:*588–589
  neuropharmacology, *2:*569–579
    γ-aminobutyric acid, *2:*576–577
    glutamate, *2:*575–576
    hyopthalamic-pituitary-adrenal axis,
      *2:*577–578

monoamines, *2:*570–575
neuropeptides, *2:*578–579
overview, *2:*567–569
risk factors for, *2:*455, *2:*457–458
selective serotonin reuptake inhibitors,
  anxiety disorder therapy, *2:*67–69
Adenosine A_{2A} receptors:
  neuroinflammation, purinergic receptor
    modulation and, *3:*643–644
  Parkinson's disease treatment, *3:*505–506
Adenosine deaminase (ADA) deficiency,
  neuroinflammation and, *3:*643–644
Adenosine diphosphate (ADP) ribosylation
  factor (ARF) family, $GABA_B$
  receptor trafficking and
  heteromization, *1:*577–578
Adenosine receptors, anxiety neurobiology
  and, deficits in, *2:*29–30
Adenosine triphosphate (ATP):
  adipose tissue cell types and depots,
    *3:*786–789
  ischemic brain injury, *3:*351–353
  plasma membrane glutamate transporters,
    *1:*709–711
  second messengers and, *1:*31–32
  synapse research and, 23
Adenylate cyclase:
  $GABA_B$ receptors, effector systems,
    *1:*582–583
  H_3 receptor, *1:*314–315
  lithium mechanism in bipolar disorder
    patients, *1:*868–869
Adenylyl cyclase:
  adipose tissue signaling and, *3:*802–803
  α_2 adrenergic receptor regulation, signal
    transduction pathways, *1:*206
  cyclic nucleotide second messenger
    signaling, *1:*72–77
  heterotrimeric G proteins, *1:*62–63
  muscarinic acetylcholine receptors,
    G-protein-coupling properties,
    *1:*156
Aδ fibers, pain pathways, *2:*711–712
Adhesion molecules, inflammation
  mechanisms, *3:*624–625
Adipocytes:
  ghrelin modulation, *3:*775
  leptin secretion and, *3:*735–736
  proliferation, sympathetic nervous system
    innervation and, *3:*797–799
  white *vs.* brown molecular features,
    *3:*787–789

Adipose tissue. *See also* Brown adipose tissue; White adipose tissue
  catecholamine signaling mechanisms, 3:801–803
  cell types and depots, 3:786–789
  future research issues, 3:804
  glyceroneogenesis, 3:799–801
  sympathetic nervous system innervation, 3:789–797
    adipocyte prolierative capacity, 3:797–799
    anterograde tract-testing, SNS to WAT, 3:792–797
    retrograde tracing neuroanatomical studies, 3:790–792
  white *vs.* brown adipocytes, 3:787–789
Adolescent patients, psychostimulant abuse, 2:581–585
Adrenaline, early research on, 1:15–16
Adrenergic agonists:
  attention-deficit hyperactivity disorder therapy, 3:299–300
  autism spectrum disorders, 3:330
  Tourette's syndrome therapy, 3:276–277
Adrenergic neurotransmitters, cataplexy therapy, animal models, 3:109–110
Adrenergic receptors. *See also* α and β-adrenergic receptors
  antipsychotic drugs mechanisms, 2:426–427
  historical perspective, 1:194–195
  psychostimulant abuse, 2:575
α-adrenergic receptors:
  α_1-adrenergic receptor:
    general characteristics, 1:201–203
    physiological roles, 1:203–204
    signal transduction pathways, 1:203
  α_2-adrenergic receptor:
    general characteristics, 1:204–206
    physiological roles, 1:207–209
    signal transduction pathways, 1:206
  historical perspective, 1:196
  subdivision of, 1:196
β-adrenergic receptors:
  general characteristics and regulation, 1:209–210
  physiological roles, 1:211–213
  signal transduction pathways, 1:210–211
  subdivision of, 1:195–196
Adrenergic transmitters, early research on, 1:29–30

Adrenocorticotropic hormone (ACTH):
  anxiety neurobiology and, 2:17
  neuropeptides and, 1:670–671
    behavioral techniques, 1:677–678
    opioid family gene duplication, 1:680–682
  nicotine dependence and withdrawal, 2:539–540
  psychostimulant abuse, 2:577–578
    chronic exposure and sensitization effects, 2:580–585
  for secondary generalized epilepsy, 3:424
Adrenoreceptors, white adipose tissue innervation, 3:789–797
Adult environmental effects, anxiety neurobiology, 2:35
Adult respiratory distress syndrome (ARDS), adenosine pathway and purinergic receptor modulation, 3:644
Advanced sleep phase syndrome (ASPS), circadian rhythms, melatonin receptor modulation, 3:58
AF102B agonist, dementia disorders and, 3:466
Affective disorders:
  autism spectrum disorder and, 3:333
  circadian rhythms and, 3:15–17
Affective flattening, in schizophrenia, 2:255–256
Afferent neurons:
  histaminergic neurons, 1:303–305
  hypocretins at, 3:130
Affinity mechanisms, GABA$_A$ receptors, desensitization and deactivation, 1:498–499
Aftereffects, circadian rhythms, 3:6
Afterhyperpolarization (AHP), small-conductance calcium-activated potassium channels, 1:631–632
Agatoxins, voltage-gated calcium ion channels, Ca$_v$2 family, 1:649
Age of onset modifiers, idiopathic Parkinson's disease, 3:542
Aggression, autism spectrum disorders, 3:334
Agomelatine, melatonin receptor targeting, 3:57–58
  depression therapy, 3:59–61
Agonist chelation hypothesis, GABA$_A$ receptor activation, 1:493–494
  binding site architecture, 1:494–495

Agonists:
    α_1 adrenergic receptors, *1:*202–203
    $GABA_A$ receptor activation, *1:*492–495
        allosteric ligand modulation,
            *1:*500–506
        glutamate transporter regulation, *1:*728
        muscarinic acetylcholine receptor, ligand
            binding, *1:*152
        neuropeptide receptors, *1:*675
        serotonin receptor families, *1:*263–267
        upregulation, nicotinic acetylcholine
            receptor, *1:*127–130
Agouti-related peptide (AgRP):
    antiobesity therapy, axokine, *3:*823–824
    hypocretin/orexin system and, *3:*132–134
A kinase anchoring proteins (AKAPs),
    $GABA_A$ phosphorylation, *1:*482
AKT1 gene, dystrobrevin binding protein 1
    (DTNBP1), schizophrenia
    susceptibility, *2:*348–349
Alcohol:
    $GABA_A$ receptor modulation, *1:*511–516,
        *1:*516
    γ-hydroxybutyric acid (GHB) and,
        *2:*634
    histaminergic neuron activity, *1:*321–322
    neuroactive steroid effects and, *2:*158–159
    neurosteroid effects and, *2:*157–158
Alcohol abuse:
    animal models, neuroanatomical
        substrates, *2:*466–467
        behavioral paradigms, *2:*467–470
        central nervous system circuitry,
            *2:*470–471
        novel substrates, *2:*471
    dopamine neuronal systems and
        substrates, *2:*471–486
        bed nucleus of stria terminalis,
            *2:*473–475
        dopaminergic regulation, early
            research, *2:*472–473
        extracellular dopamine, *2:*485–486
        future research issues, *2:*517–518
        GABAergic interactions with, *2:*486
        lateral hypothalamus, *2:*481–485
            D_2 dopaminergic regulation,
                hypothesized mechanisms,
                *2:*481–485
        ventral pallidum, *2:*476–480
            dopaminargic regulation
                hypothesized mechanisms,
                *2:*478–480

    $GABA_A$ benzodiazepine receptor
        complex, molecular biology,
        *2:*487–501
        alcohol/modulator commonalities,
            *2:*487–488
        CA1/CA3 hippocampus, *2:*511–516
        efficacy of βCCT/3PBD modulation,
            $GABA_{A1,2,3,5}$ receptors, *2:*499–501
        future research issues, *2:*517–518
        GABA-DA interaction hypothesis,
            *2:*496–498
        ligand selectivity with $GABA_{A1}$
            subunits, *2:*498–499
        microinjection studies, *2:*505–506
        naltrexone antagonist, *2:*507–511
        novel CNS GABAergic substrates,
            *2:*498
        oral administration, βCCT/3PBD:
            anxiety reduction, *2:*510–511
            vs. naltrexone, *2:*507–511
        probe applications, *2:*488–493
        site-specific microinjection, *2:*493–496
        subunit selectivity *vs.* intrinsic efficacy,
            *2:*516–517
        systemic administration, *2:*492–493,
            *2:*503–504
        ventral pallidum, *2:*501–502
    HIV neuropharmacology and, *3:*716
    idiopathic Parkinson's disease and, *3:*544
    overview, *2:*466
Alcohol-preferring rats (P rat line), alcohol
    abuse studies:
    appropriate behavioral paradigms,
        *2:*467–470
        neuroanatomical controls, *2:*469–470
        reinforcer-specific controls, *2:*469
    central nervous system circuitry in,
        *2:*470–471
    characteristics of, *2:*467
    novel neuranatomical substrates, *2:*471
Aldo-keto reductase family, voltage-gated
    potassium channels, *1:*627–628
ALE-0540, nerve growth factor inhibitor,
    *3:*232
Alemtuzumab, multiple sclerosis therapy,
    *3:*677–679, *3:*686
Allopregnanolone, $GABA_A$ receptor
    modulation, *1:*515
Allosteric potentiators and antagonists:
    $GABA_A$ receptors:
        benzodiazepine recognition site,
            *1:*499–506

benzodiazepine structural determinants, 1:507–509
transmembrane domains, 1:516–518
unidentified sites, 1:519–520
$GABA_B$ receptors, 1:590–592
subunits, 1:580
ionotropic glutamate receptors, 1:385–397
AMPA antagonists, 1:395–396
AMPA potentiators, 1:390–395
kainate receptor antagonists, 1:397
kainate receptor potentiators, 1:396
NMDA receptor antagonists, 1:386–390
NMDA receptor potentiators, 1:385–386
metabotropic glutamate receptors:
mGlu1 antagonists, 1:436–437
mGlu1 potentiators, 1:435–436
mGlu2/3 antagonists, 1:439–440
mGlu2 potentiators, 1:437–439
mGlu4 potentiators, 1:440–441
mGlu5 antagonists, 1:443–445
mGlu5 potentiators, 1:441–443
mGlu7 antagonists, 1:445
muscarinic acetylcholine receptor, 1:153–154
AlloTHDOC, plasma levels, 2:137–140
Alogia, in schizophrenia, 2:255–256
α_1 interaction domain (AID), voltage-gated calcium channels, 1:644
Alzheimer's disease (AD):
acetylcholinesterase inhibitors and, 3:463–465
diagnostic criteria, 3:462
dopaminergic drugs, 1:237
$GABA_A$ α_5 subunit pharmacology, 1:489
glutamate receptor ligands, 3:469–471
histaminergic neuron activity, 1:327–328
invertebrate models, 3:579–582
KCNQ channels and, 1:633
muscarinic receptor drugs and, 3:465–469
neuropathies and, 3:227–228
nicotinic agonists, 3:469
nitric oxide and, 1:754
plasma membrane glutamate transporter, 1:719
therapeutic targets, 3:471–473
Amantidine:
autism spectrum disorders, 3:332
Parkinson's disease treatment, 3:496–497

Amino acid neurotransmitters:
anxiety disorder therapy, 2:72–75
anticonvulsants, 2:74–75
benzodiazepines, 2:73–74
early research on, 1:32
intercellular signaling and, 1:42–44
D-Amino acid oxidase (DAO), schizophrenia candidate gene, 2:327
D-Amino acid oxidase activator (DAO A), schizophrenia candidate gene, 2:327
Amino acid residues:
benzodiazepines, $GABA_A$ receptors, 2:106–108
$GABA_A$ receptors:
activation, agonist binding site architecture, 1:494–495
assembly, 1:478
modulation, allosteric structural determinants, 1:508–509
1-Amino-cyclopentane-1,3-dicarboxylic acid (ACPD), mGlu group I selective orthosteric agonists, 1:423
Aminocyclopropylcarboxylic acid (ACC), NMDA allosteric potentiators, 1:386
α-Amino-3-hydroxy-5-methyl-isoxazole-4-propionic acid (AMPA) receptors:
allosteric antagonists, 1:395–396
allosteric potentiators, 1:390–395
antiepileptic drugs and, topiramate, 3:416–417
benzodiazepine tolerance, 2:101
dementia disorders and, 3:470
glutamate theory of schizophrenia:
history of, 2:290–291
pathological evidence, 2:291–292
pharmacological evidence, 2:294–295
kainate receptor orthosteric agonists, 1:381
mGlu group I selective orthosteric agonists, quisqualate, 1:423
neurogenesis and, 3:208
neurotrophic factor synthesis and, 3:232
orthosteric agonists, 1:376–377
orthosteric antagonists, 1:377–378
schizophrenia pharmacotherapy, drug development for, 2:392
stroke and:
ischemic brain injury, 3:351–353

receptor antagonists, 3:361–363
structure and function, 1:370–371
(R,S)-1-Aminoindan-1,5-dicarboxylic acid (AIDA), mGlu I selective orthosteric antagonists, 1:425
2R,4R-4-Aminopyrrolidine-2,4-dicarboxylate (2R,4R-APDC), mGlu II selective orthosteric agonists, 1:429
Amisulpiride:
 schizophrenia therapy, D_2/D_3 and D_4 receptor antagonism and regional specificity, 2:380
 Tourette's syndrome therapy, 3:276
AMPA. See α-Amino-3-hydroxy-5-methyl-isoxazole-4-propionic acid (AMPA) receptors
AMP-activated kinase (AMPK), ghrelin effects and, 3:773
"AMPAkines," glutamate theory of schizophrenia, 2:295
Amphetamines:
 attention-deficit hyperactivity disorder therapy, 3:296–298
 chronic exposure and sensitization effects, 2:580–585
 derivatives, serotonin synthesis, 1:261
 3,4-methylenedioxymethamphetamine reinforcement of, 2:615–616
 monoamine neuropharmacology, 2:571–575
 narcolepsy therapy:
  adverse effects, 3:98
  cerebrospinal fluid hypocretin-1 assessment, 3:84
  drug interactions, 3:98, 3:100
  excessive daytime sleepiness and, 3:90–100
  histocompatibility human leukocyte antigen testing, 3:84
  molecular targeting, 3:93–94
  polysomnography, 3:83
 neuropeptide pharmacology and, 2:579
 stroke therapy and, 3:377
 traumatic brain injury and, 3:453–454
d-Amphetamine, alcohol abuse studies, dopaminergic receptor systems and substrates, 2:472–473
Amygdala. See also Extended amygala (EA)
 anxiety disorders and, 2:13–15

Amylase secretion, exocrine pancreas, muscarinic acetylcholine receptor deficiency, 1:175
β-Amyloid peptide:
 in HIV patients, 3:717–718
 neurodegenerative disease, immunization modulation of, 3:644–645
Amyloid precursor protein (APP):
 Alzheimer's disease, invertebrate models, 3:579–582
 in HIV patients, 3:717–718
Amyotrophic lateral sclerosis (ALS):
 neurotrophic factor therapy and, 3:225–227
 nitric oxide and, 1:754
 plasma membrane glutamate transporter, 1:718–719
Analgesia:
 α_2 adrenergic receptor physiology, 1:207–208
 muscarinic acetylcholine receptor deficiency, 1:170
Anandamide:
 appetite regulation and, 2:671–672
 endocannabinoid ligands, 2:663–664
 pain management and, 2:667–668
 pharmacology, 2:665–675
Anesthesias:
 $GABA_A$ receptor:
  β subunit pharmacology, 1:490–491
  modulation, 1:511–516
 hypocretin/orexin system, 3:136
 neuroactive steroid effects and, 2:158–159
 voltage-gated sodium ion channels and, 1:643
Angina therapy, voltage-gated calcium channels, Ca_v1 family, 1:648
Angiogenesis, prokineticins and, 3:169–170
Angiotensin-converting enzyme (ACE), neuropeptide inactivation, 1:687–688
Animal models. See also Invertebrate models; Mouse studies
 alcohol-motivated behaviors, neuroanatomical substrates, 2:466–467
 behavioral paradigms, 2:467–470
 central nervous system circuitry, 2:470–471
 novel substrates, 2:471
 antidepressants and hippocampal neurogenesis, 1:833

antiepileptic drugs, topiramate, 3:416–417
anxiety neurobiology:
   anxiety-like behavior in, 2:10–12
   brain imaging studies, 2:14–15
   early-life environmental effects, 2:33–34
   rodent models, 2:6–9
circadian rhythms:
   mammalian models, 3:10–13
   nonmammalian models, 3:6–9
curare research on, 1:5–7
human autoimmune neuropathies, 3:615
invertebrate models, neurodegenerative disease:
   Alzheimer's disease, 3:579–582
   Caenorhabditis elegans system, 3:568–569
   Drosophila melanogaster, 3:569
   early research, 3:567–568
   future applications, 3:582–583
   genetic and molecular pathways, 3:568
   Huntington's disease trinucleotide repeats, 3:577–579
   Parkinson's disease, dopamine neuron cell death, 3:569–577
3,4-methylenedioxymethamphetamine neurotoxicity, 2:620–621
   behavioral effects, 2:630–631
myelin disorders, experimental allergic encephalomyelitis, 3:611–612
narcolepsy:
   hypocretin-1 deficiency, 3:86
   modafinil therapy, 3:102–103
neurosteroid effects, 2:142–152
   acoustics/fear-potentiated startle, 2:147
   defensive burying behavior, 2:149–150
   elevated-plus maze, 2:143–145
   Geller/Seifter and Vogel conflict tests, 2:145–146
   light-dark box, 2:146–147
   mild mental stress models and social isolation, 2:151–152
   mirrored chamber, 2:147–148
   modified forced-swim test, 2:150–151
   open-field activity, 2:148–149
   separation-induced ultrasonic vocalizations, 2:150
obsessive-compulsive disorders (OCD), 2:224
pharmacology research and, 1:11
psychostimulant abuse, chronic exposure and sensitization effects, 2:581–585
schizophrenia, 2:263–265

stroke and:
   global and focal ischemia, 3:353–354
   NMDA receptor antagonists, 3:355–356
transient receptor potential V1 (TRPV1) receptors, 2:736
Aniracetam, AMPA receptor allosteric potentiators, 1:390–391
Anterograde tract-tracing, sympathetic nervous system innervation, white adipose tissue, 3:792–797
Antiadhesion molecules, stroke management, 3:369–370
Antianxiety drugs. *See also* Anxiolytic drugs
   $GABA_A$ subunit pharmacology:
      allosteric ligand modulation, 1:503–506
      α subunits, 1:483–490, 1:509–511
         $α_1$ subunit, 1:484, 1:488
         $α_2$ subunit, 1:488
         $α_3$ subunit, 1:488
         $α_4$ subunit, 1:488–489
         $α_5$ subunit, 1:489
         $α_6$ subunit, 1:489–490
      electrophysiology, 1:486–487
      modulator selectivity, 1:484
      terminology, 1:483
   $GABA_B$ receptor targeting, 1:594–595
   mGlu 2 selective orthosteric antagonists, 1:430–431
   mGlu2 receptor:
      allosteric potentiators, 1:439
      selective orthosteric agonists, 1:427–429
   mGlu5 allosteric antagonists, 1:443–444
   serotonin receptor 5-HT_{2C} and, 1:272–273
   serotonin receptors, 1:263–266
Antiapoptotic signaling, p75 neurotrophin receptor, 3:246–247
Antiarrhythmics:
   KCNH potassium channels, 1:634
   voltage-gated calcium channels, Ca_v1 family, 1:648
   voltage-gated sodium ion channels and, 1:642
Anticholinergic agents, Parkinson's disease treatment, 3:496, 3:502
Anticonvulsant drugs. *See also* Antiepileptic drugs (AEDS)
   AMPA receptor allosteric antagonists, 1:396
   anxiety disorder therapy, 2:74–75
   autism spectrum disorder therapy, 3:332–333

in bipolar disorder patients, 1:869–870
GABA$_A$ receptor:
    GABA$_A$ α$_1$ subunit pharmacology,
        1:484–485, 1:488
    modulation, 1:511–516
GABA$_B$ receptor modulation, 1:595
histamine neuron physiology, 1:326
mGlu 1 selective orthosteric antagonists,
    1:425–426
mGlu 2 selective orthosteric agonists,
    1:428–429
migraine management, 2:766–767
Antidepressants. See also specific
        antidepressants, e.g. Tricyclic
        antidepressants
    β-adrenergic receptor activation, 1:210
    anxiety disorder therapy, 2:64–70
        beta blockers, 2:71
        mirtazapine, 2:70
        monoamine oxidase inhibitors, 2:70
        selective serotonin reuptake inhibitors,
            2:66–69
        serotonin and noradrenaline reuptake
            inhibitors, 2:69
        serotonin receptor agonists, 2:70–71
        tricyclic antidpressants, 2:69–70
    cataplexy therapy, 3:114–115
        historical overview, 3:106–107
        second- and third-generation, 3:108
        tricyclic antidepressants, 3:107–109
    circadian rhythms and, 3:18–20
    GABA$_B$ receptor targeting, 1:594–595
    hippocampal neurogenesis and:
        adult neurogenesis stages, 1:827–828
        behavioral and animal models, 1:833
        depression physiology and, 1:823–824,
            1:826–827
        future research on, 1:833
        monoamines and, 1:822–823
        research background, 1:821–822
        serotonin/norepinephrine regulation,
            1:831–833
        stress and monamine hypotheses,
            1:825–826
        stress hormone neurogenesis regulation,
            1:829–830
    histaminergic neuron activity, 1:329
    melatonin receptors, therapeutic targeting
        of, 3:58–61
    mGlu II selective orthosteric antagonists,
        1:431
    migraine management, 2:767

neurogenesis and, 3:209–210
neurotrophic factor expression and,
    1:804–806
    BDNF expression, 1:804–805
    models for, 1:805–806
    neurogenesis in adults and, 1:806–808
nicotine dependence and withdrawal
    therapy, bupropion, 2:549–550
serotonin receptors, 1:263–266
    serotonin receptor 5-HT$_{2C}$ and,
        1:272–273
sleep effects of, 3:17–18
Antidiabetic agents, β-adrenergic receptor
    physiology, 1:212–213
Antidiuretic hormone (ADH). See
    Vasopressin
Antiemetics. See also Nausea and vomiting
    migraine management, 2:765
Antiepileptic drugs (AEDs). See also
        Anticonvulsant drugs
    epilepsy management, 3:404–405
        calcium channels, 3:413–414
        clinical efficacy, 3:417–418
        clinical prediction markers, 3:420
        combination therapy, 3:423–424
        development and testing, 3:418–420
        felbamate interactions, 3:414–415
        GABA$_A$ receptor and, 3:411–412
        generalized absence epilepsy, 3:421
        localization-related epilepsy, 3:421–423
        mechanisms of action, 3:408–410
        metabotropic glutamate receptors,
            3:413
        mixed actions, 3:414–418, 3:422
        secondary generalized epilepsies, 3:424
        selection criteria, 3:421–424
        sodium channel modulation, 3:411
        special population requirements,
            3:424–425
        synaptic vesicle protein, 3:414
        topiramate interactions, 3:415–418
        toxicity detection, limitations of,
            3:420–421
    molecular targeting, 3:409–410
    pharmacokinetic characteristics, drug
        interactions and serum levels, 3:422
    Δ^9-tetrahydrocannabinol as, 2:672–673
Antigen-presenting cells (APC),
        neuroinflammation, 3:626
    astrocytes and, 3:627
Antigen-specific T cells, inflammation
        mechanisms, 3:625

Antiglutamate agents, Parkinson's disease treatment, 3:496–497
Antihistamines:
  anxiety disorder therapy, 2:75
  arousal mechanisms, 1:323–324
  KCNH potassium channels, 1:634
  sedative/hypnotics and, 3:188
Anti-inflammatory agents:
  stroke management, 3:367–371
  traumatic brain injury and, 3:447–449
Antinociception, cannabinoid analgesics and, 2:668
Anti-NoGo agents, stroke therapy, 3:377–378
Antiobesity agents:
  β-adrenergic receptor physiology, 1:212–213
  current development of, 3:821–831
    axokine, 3:822–824
    CCK_A receptor agonists, 3:830–831
    future research issues, 3:831–833
    MC4 receptor agonists, 3:828–829
    MCH receptor-1 antagonists, 3:829–830
    orlistat, 3:820–821
    PYY3-36 peptide agonists, 3:831
    rimonabant, 3:824–828
    serotonin receptor 5-HT_{2C} agonists, 3:828
  FDA-approved drugs, 3:819
  future research issues, 3:832–833
  historic perspective on, 3:817–818
  orlistat, 3:820–821
  sibutramine, 3:818–820
Antioxidants:
  neuroinflammation and, 3:636–637
  Parkinson's disease therapy, 3:504–505
  stroke management, 3:371–372
Antiproliferative/proliferative mechanisms, ghrelin modulation, 3:776
Antipsychotics:
  α_2-adrenergic receptor physiology, 1:209
  anxiety disorder therapy, 2:71–72
  attention-deficit hyperactivity disorder therapy, 3:301
  atypical agents, mechanisms of action:
    adrenergic mechanisms, 2:426–427
    atypical antipsychotics, 5-HT_{2A} receptor, 2:418–421
    cholinergic mechanisms, 2:429–430
    clozapine regimens, dopamine D_2 receptor blockade, 2:412–415

  glutamatergic mechanisms, 2:427–429
  neurogenesis, 2:430
  neurokinin 3 receptors, 2:430
  partial dopamine agonists, 2:416–417
  serotonin receptors, 2:417–418
    serotonin receptor 5-HT_{1A}-5-HT_{2A} interactions, 2:424–425
    serotonin receptor 5-HT_{2A}-5-HT_{2C} interactions, 2:422–424
    serotonin receptor 5-HT_{2A} blockade:
      cortical dopamine efflux and cognitive function, 2:421–422
      extrapyramidal function, 2:422
    serotonin receptor 5-HT_6, 2:425–426
  serotonin release, 2:426
  substituted benzamides, D_1, D_3, and D_4 receptors, 2:415–416
  table of drugs, 2:413
  typical vs. atypical drugs, 2:411–412
autism spectrum disorders:
  atypical agents, 3:326–330
  typical agents, 3:325–326
in bipolar disorder patients, 1:869–870
histaminergic neuron activity, 1:327
metabolic syndrome with, 2:254
mGlu2 receptors:
  allosteric potentiators, 1:439
  selective orthosteric agonists, 1:427–429
obsessive-compulsive disorders:
  neuropharmacology, 2:229–234
  symptom induction from, 2:234
schizophrenia therapy:
  first-generation (conventional) agents, 2:383
  glutamate theory of schizophrenia, 2:294–295
  history of, 2:370–371
  hypothesized mechanisms of action, 2:376–382
    D_1 receptors, 2:380–381
    D_2/D_3 and D_4 antagonism and regional specificity, 2:380
    D_2 receptors:
      occupancy, 2:376–378
      occupancy thresholds and rapid dissociation, 2:378–380
    dopamine release, 2:381
    NMDA receptor function, 2:381
    synthesis reactions, 2:381–382
  negative affect remediation, 2:255–256
  psychosis management, 2:254
  safety and tolerability, 2:387–388

second-generation (atypical) agents, 2:383–387
serotonin receptors:
serotonin receptor 5-HT$_6$ family, 1:275
Anxiety and anxiety disorders:
alcohol abuse and, βCCT/3PBC anxiety reduction efficacy, 2:510–511
clinical management, 2:60–61
corticotropin-releasing factor receptor antagonists, therapeutic potential of, 2:196–198
depression and, pharmacotherapy, 2:80
diagnostic criteria, 2:9–12, 2:61–62
histaminergic neuron activity, 1:329
3,4-methylenedioxymethamphetamine effects, 2:630–631
neuroactive steroids:
alcohol effects, 2:157–159
animal models, 2:142–152
behavioral effects, 2:142
brain and peripheral sources, 2:135–137
chemistry and pharmacology, 2:135–142
enantiomeric selectivity, 2:141–142
GABA$_A$ receptors and ligand-gated ion channels, 2:137–141
HPA axis function, 2:154–156
overview, 2:134–135
stress-induced behaviors, 2:154–155
neurobiology of:
basic principles, 2:4
early-life environmental effects, 2:33–37
fear/anxiety circuits, 2:13–15
genetic susceptibility, 2:18–19
intracellular regulators, 2:30–33
knockout mice:
neuronal messenger alterations, 2:24–26
neurotransmitter receptor deficits and CRH proteins, 2:26–30
mouse genetics studies, 2:19–24
neurotransmitter systems and neuronal messengers, 2:15–18
psychological traits:
continuous expression of normal personality, 2:9–10
genetic basis of, 2:4–6
mouse behavior extrapolation studies, 2:6–9
Parkinson's disease treatment and, 3:500–501

pharmacotherapy:
anxiolytic drugs, 2:62–75
amino acid neurotransmission, 2:72–75
anticonvulsants, 2:74–75
antidepressants, 2:64–70
antihistamines, 2:75
antipsychotics, 2:71–72
benzodiazepines, 2:73–74
beta-blockers, 2:71
lithium, 2:75
monoamine neurotransmission, 2:63–72
serotonin receptor agonists, 2:70–71
depressive disorders, 2:80
future research issues, 2:81
generalized anxiety disorder, 2:77
obsessive-compulsive disorder, 2:77–78
overview, 2:60
panic disorder/agoraphobia, 2:78
phobias, 2:78, 2:80
posttraumatic stress disorder, 2:79
social anxiety disorder, 2:79–80
treatments chart, 2:76
serotonin receptors:
serotonin receptor 5-HT$_{2B}$, 1:271
serotonin transporters and, 1:720
"Anxiety-related pathways," anxiety neurobiology and, 2:36
Anxiolytic drugs:
anxiety disorder pharmacotherapy, 2:62–75
amino acid neurotransmission, 2:72–75
anticonvulsants, 2:74–75
antidepressants, 2:64–70
antihistamines, 2:75
antipsychotics, 2:71–72
benzodiazepines, 2:73–74
beta-blockers, 2:71
lithium, 2:75
mirtazapine, 2:70
monoamine neurotransmission, 2:63–72
monoamine oxidase inhibitors, 2:70
selective serotonin reuptake inhibitors, 2:66–69
serotonin and noradrenaline reuptake inhibitors, 2:69
serotonin receptor agonists, 2:70–71
tricyclic antidepressants, 2:69–70
corticotropin-releasing factor receptor antagonists:
future research issues, 2:198–199

nonpeptide ligands, 2:195–196
overview, 2:177–179
peptide ligand pharmacology,
  2:185–195
  ligand binding mechanisms,
    2:190–195
  receptor/ligand family structure,
    2:179–185
    ligand properties, 2:180–181
    receptor subtypes and distribution,
      2:181–185
  therapeutic potential, 2:196–198
AP-1 complex, amino acid
  neurotransmitters, 1:44
Apamin, small-conductance
  calcium-activated potassium
  channels, 1:632
Aplysia californica, circadian rhythmicity, 3:9
Apomorphine, Parkinson's disease
  treatment, 3:493–494, 3:505
Apoptosis mechanisms:
  HIV neuropathology, 3:704–705
  neuroinflammation and, modulation of,
    3:637–638
  stroke management, 3:372–373
Appetite regulation:
  cannabinoid receptors and, 2:670–672
  ghrelin effects, 3:772–773
  histaminergic neuron activity, 1:325–326
  hypocretin/orexin system, 3:132–134
  leptin signaling and, 3:740–743
  muscarinic acetylcholine receptor
    deficiency, 1:171
  prokineticins and, 3:168–169
  serotonin receptor 5-HT$_{2C}$, 1:272–273
Arachidonic acid derivatives:
  endocannabinoid ligands, 2:663–664
  transient receptor potential V1 (TRPV1)
    receptor expression, 2:732–733
Arachidonic acid pathways,
  neuroinflammation and, 3:630
  pharmocological activation of, 3:634–635
N-Arachidonoyldopamine,
  endocannabinoid ligands,
  2:663–664
Arachidonoylethanolamide, cannabinoid
  receptors and, 2:661–662
O-Arachidonoylethanolamine,
  endocannabinoid ligands,
  2:663–664
Arginine vasopressin, neuropeptide
  receptors, 1:689

Aripiprazole, autism spectrum disorders,
  3:327–328
Aromatic amino acid decarboxylase
  (AAAD):
  dopamine synthesis, 1:223–224
  Parkinson's disease, neurochemistry,
    3:481–483
  serotonin synthesis, 1:260–261
Arousal:
  autonomic arousal, anxiety neurobiology,
    2:4
  animal anxiety-like behavior, 2:10–12
  histamine neuron physiology, 1:322–324
  hypocretin/orexin system, 3:139–144
    cholinergic systems, 3:143–144
    dopaminergic systems, 3:143
    feeding and motivation integration,
      3:144
    histaminergic systems, 3:142–143
    lateral hypothalamic neurons,
      3:140–141
    noradrenergic systems, 3:141–142
    serotonergic systems, 3:142
  sleep and, circadian rhythms:
    chronopharmacology, 3:15–23
    functional importance, 3:4
    future research issues, 3:23–24
    mammallian structural models,
      3:10–13
    nonmammalian structural models,
      3:6–10
    properties, 3:4–6
    superchiasmatic nucleus period and
      phase, 3:13–15
Arrhythmias:
  KCNH potassium channels, 1:634
  voltage-gated calcium channels, Ca$_v$1
    family, 1:648
  voltage-gated sodium ion channels and,
    1:642
Artemin (ARTN), discovery of, 3:221–223
2-Arylureidobenzoic acids, kainate receptor
  allosteric antagonists, 1:397
Aschoff's rules, circadian rhythms,
  3:5–6
Asenapine, schizophrenia therapy, 2:389
Assembly mechanisms, GABA$_A$ receptor,
  1:477–478
  benzodiazepines, 2:108–110
Astressin, corticotropin-releasing factor
  receptor antagonists, ligand
  binding mechanisms, 2:191–195

Astrocytes:
  HIV neuropathogenesis and, *3:*697
  neuroinflammation and, *3:*627
    cytokine/chemokine expression, *3:*632
Ataxin-3, Huntingdon's disease, invertebrate model, *3:*578–579
Atomoxetine, attention-deficit hyperactivity disorder therapy, *3:*299
Atorvastatin, multiple sclerosis therapy, *3:*667
ATPA, kainate receptor orthosteric agonists, *1:*381
Atropine, early research on, *1:*10
Attention-deficit hyperactivity disorder (ADHD):
  clinical management issues, *3:*301–302
  diagnostic criteria, *3:*291–292
  dopaminergic drugs, *1:*237–238
  dopamine transporters and, *1:*721
  evaluation, *3:*292–293
  GABA$_B$ receptor targeting, *1:*592–593
  histaminergic neuron activity, *1:*329
  obsessive-compulsive disorder comorbidity, *2:*216
  pharmacotherapy, *3:*293–301
    adverse effects, *3:*298
    amphetamines, *3:*296–298
    antipsychotics, *3:*301
    atomoxetine, *3:*299
    bupropion, *3:*300–301
    clonidine/guanfacine, *3:*299–300
    dexmethylphenidate, *3:*296
    methylphenidate hydrochloride, *3:*294–296
    modafinil, *3:*301
    nonstimulants, *3:*299–301
    stimulants, *3:*293–298
    tricyclic antidepressants, *3:*299
    venlafaxine, *3:*301
  psychostimulant therapy, *2:*568–569, *2:*587
    chronic exposure and sensitization effects, *2:*581–585
  Tourette's syndrome comorbidity, *3:*266–268, *3:*276–277
  treatment rationale, *3:*292
Attention deficits, schizophrenia, animal models, *2:*263–264
Auditory function, KCNQ channel action on, *1:*632–633

Augmentation strategies, obsessive-compulsive disorders, neuropharmacology, *2:*225, *2:*229–234
Autism spectrum disorders:
  aggression/self-injury, *3:*334
  anxiety and depression, *3:*334
  dopaminergic drugs, *1:*237
  interfering repetitive behaviors, *3:*334
  motor hyperactivity and inattention, *3:*333–334
  overview, *3:*320–321
  pharmacology, *3:*321–333
    adrenergic agonists, *3:*330
    amantidine, *3:*332
    antiepileptic drugs, *3:*332–333
    antipsychotics, *3:*325–328
    atypical antipsychotics, *3:*326
    clomipramine, *3:*322
    clonidine, *3:*330
    clozapine, *3:*326
    d-cycloserine, *3:*332
    dopaminergic medications, *3:*325–330
    fluoxetine, *3:*323–324
    fluvoxamine, *3:*322–323
    glutamatergic medications, *3:*331–332
    guanfacine, *3:*330–331
    haloperidol, *3:*325
    lamotrigine, *3:*332
    methylphenidate, *3:*329–330
    mirtazapine, *3:*331
    olanzapine, quetiapine, ziprasidone, and aripiprazole, *3:*327–328
    pimozide, *3:*325–326
    risperidone, *3:*326–327
    serotonergic medications, *3:*321–325
    sertraline, citalopram, escitalopram, and paroxetine, *3:*324–325
    stimulants, *3:*328–330
    venlafaxine, *3:*331
  serotonin transporters and, *1:*720
  syndromes within, *3:*333–335
Autoimmune disease:
  demyelinating disorders of PNS, *3:*613–615
  human autoimmune neuropathies, *3:*613–614
  nitric oxide physiology, *1:*745
  Tourette's syndrome and, *3:*268–269
Autonomic arousal, anxiety neurobiology, *2:*4
  animal anxiety-like behavior, *2:*10–12

Autonomic nervous system:
  early research on, 1:13
  hypocretin/orexin system, 3:134–135
Autoradiography, neuropeptide identification, 1:673–674
Autoreceptors:
  chemical transmission, 1:50–51
  H_3 receptor, 1:314–315
  muscarinic acetylcholine receptor deficiency, 1:171
    peripheral agents, 1:176
  partial dopamine agonists, 2:416–417
  serotonin receptor families, 1:263–267
Autosomal-dominant (AD) Parkinsonism, genetic mutations in, 3:527
Autosomal-recessive (AR) Parkinsonism:
  genetic mutations in, 3:527
  juvenile parkinsonism, *parkin* gene mutations and, 3:530–532
Avoidance behaviors, anxiety neurobiology, 2:4
  animal anxiety-like behavior, 2:10–12
Avolition, in schizophrenia, 2:255–256
Avonex, multiple sclerosis therapy, 3:684–685
Axokine, antiobesity therapy, 3:822–824

B7 molecule, inflammation and, 3:631
Backpropagation action potentials, voltage-gated potassium channels, K_V subunits, structure and function, 1:629–630
Baclofen:
  $GABA_B$ receptors, 1:469
    anxiety and depression therapy, 1:594–595
    targeting, 1:592–593
  psychostimulant abuse therapy, 2:588
  Tourette's syndrome, 3:277
Barbiturates:
  as epilepsy therapy, 3:423
  $GABA_A$ receptor binding site, 3:181
  structure and function, 3:184–187
Barium:
  second messengers and, 1:31–32
  voltage-gated potassium channels, K_V subunits, structure and function, 1:630
Basal ganglia:
  Parkinson's disease, neurochemistry, 3:482–483
  Tourette's syndrome, 3:269–270

Basal ganglia-thalamic-frontal loops, obsessive-compulsive disorders, neuropharmacology, 2:221–222
BAY367620, mGlu1 allosteric antagonists, 1:437
BC1 RNA, anxiety neurobiology and, 2:32
Bcl-2 family proteins, stroke management, 3:373
Bed nucleus of stria terminalis (BST), alcohol abuse studies, dopaminergic receptor systems and substrates, 2:473–475
Behavioral inhibition/activity:
  alcohol abuse:
    animal models, neuroanatomical substrates, 2:466–467
    behavioral paradigms, 2:467–470
    central nervous system circuitry, 2:470–471
    novel substrates, 2:471
  dopamine neuronal systems and substrates, 2:471–486
    bed nucleus of stria terminalis, 2:473–475
    dopaminergic regulation, early research, 2:472–473
    extracellular dopamine, 2:485–486
    future research issues, 2:517–518
    GABAergic interactions with, 2:486
    lateral hypothalamus, 2:481–485
    ventral pallidum, 2:476–480
  $GABA_A$ benzodiazepine receptor complex, molecular biology, 2:487–501
    alcohol/modulator commonalities, 2:487–488
    CA1/CA3 hippocampus, 2:511–516
    efficacy of $\beta CCT/3PBD$ modulation, $GABA_{A1,2,3,5}$ receptors, 2:499–501
    future research issues, 2:517–518
    GABA-DA interaction hypothesis, 2:496–498
    ligand selectivity with $GABA_{A1}$ subunits, 2:498–499
    microinjection studies, 2:505–506
    naltrexone antagonist, 2:507–511
    novel CNS GABAergic substrates, 2:498
    probe applications, 2:488–493
    site-specific microinjection, 2:493–496

subunit selectivity *vs.* intrinsic
efficacy, 2:516–517
systemic administration, 2:492–493,
2:503–504
ventral pallidum, 2:501–502
overview, 2:466
antidepressants and hippocampal
neurogenesis, 1:833
anxiety neurobiology, 2:4
animal anxiety-like behavior, 2:10–12
autism spectrum disorders, 3:334
hypocretin/orexin system, 3:144
melatonin modulation of circadian
rhythms, 3:54–57
3,4-methylenedioxymethamphetamine
effects, 2:616–619
neurotoxic lesions and, 2:629–631
neuropeptide electrophysiology and,
1:677–678
neurosteroids, 2:142
neurotrophic factors and, 1:808–809
psychostimulant abuse, chronic exposure
and sensitization effects,
2:580–585
Tourette's syndrome therapy, 3:277–278
Benign neonatal familial convulsion
(BNFC), KCNQ channels and,
1:633
Benserazide, Parkinson's disease treatment,
3:484–487
Benzamides:
AMPA receptor allosteric potentiators,
1:390
D_1, D_3, and D_4 receptors, 2:415–416
NMDA receptor allosteric antagonists,
1:390
Benzedrine, attention-deficit hyperactivity
disorder therapy, 3:296–298
Benzhexol, Parkinson's disease treatment,
3:496
Benzimidazoles, NMDA receptor allosteric
antagonists, 1:390
2,3-Benzodiazepine, AMPA receptor
allosteric antagonists, 1:395
Benzodiazepines (BZs). *See also* $GABA_A$
benzodiazepine receptor complex
anxiety disorder therapy, 2:73–74
circadian rhythms and, 3:20–21
epilepsy efficacy, 3:417–418
as epilepsy therapy, 3:423
flunitrazepam, 2:637
future research, 2:116–117

$GABA_A$-benzodiazepine receptor
complex, alcohol abuse studies,
2:487–501
alcohol/modulator commonalities,
2:487–488
CA1/CA3 hippocampus, 2:511–516
efficacy of $\beta CCT/3PBD$ modulation,
$GABA_{A1,2,3,5}$ receptors,
2:499–501
future research issues, 2:517–518
GABA-DA interaction hypothesis,
2:496–498
ligand selectivity with $GABA_{A1}$
subunits, 2:498–499
microinjection studies, 2:505–506
naltrexone antagonist, 2:507–511
novel CNS GABAergic substrates,
2:498
oral administration, $\beta CCT/3PBD$:
anxiety reduction, 2:510–511
vs. naltrexone, 2:507–511
probe applications, 2:488–493
site-specific microinjection, 2:493–496
subunit selectivity *vs.* intrinsic efficacy,
2:516–517
systemic administration, 2:492–493,
2:503–504
ventral pallidum, 2:501–502
$GABA_A$ receptors:
allosteric binding, 1:499–506
allosteric structural determinants,
1:507–509
assembly, clustering, and surface
expression, 2:108–110
binding pocket, 2:105–108
binding sites, 1:506–507, 3:180–181
brain function diversity, 2:110–112
functional diversity, knockout/knockin
models, 2:112–114
single-cell response modulation,
2:99–100
structure and function, 2:93–96
subunit pharmacology:
α subunits, 1:483–490, 1:509–511
α_1 subunit, 1:484, 1:488
α_2 subunit, 1:488
α_3 subunit, 1:488
α_4 subunit, 1:488–489
α_5 subunit, 1:489
α_6 subunit, 1:489–490
electrophysiology, 1:486–487
modulator selectivity, 1:484

γ subunit isoforms, *1:*509–511
   terminology, *1:*483
   subunit/subtype diversity, *2:*103–104
   3,4-methylenedioxymethamphetamine
      effects on, *2:*628
   receptor ligand pharmacology, *2:*97–102
      endogenous site, *2:*98–99
      metabolism functions, *2:*101–102
      single-cell GABA response modulation, *2:*99–100
      therapeutic action, *2:*97–98
      tolerance and dependence characteristics, *2:*100–101
   sedative/hypnotic functions, *3:*187–188
   stroke management, *3:*362
   structure-activity relationships, *2:*114–116
   structure and function, *2:*93–96
Benzothiadiazides, AMPA receptor allosteric potentiators, *1:*390–392
Benztropine, Parkinson's disease treatment, *3:*496
Beta-blockers:
   anxiety disorder therapy, *2:*71
   migraine management, *2:*767
Betaseron, multiple sclerosis therapy, *3:*674–675
Biarypropylsulfonamides, AMPA receptor allosteric potentiators, *1:*393
BIBN4096BS compound, calcitonin gene-related peptide sites and migraine therapy targeting, *2:*762–764
Bicuculline:
   alcohol abuse studies, GABA$_A$ benzodiazepine receptor complex, *2:*487–488
      site-specific microinjection techniques, *2:*494–496
   GABA$_A$ receptor inhibition, *1:*468–469
Bifeprunox, schizophrenia therapy, *2:*389
Binding affinities, GABA$_A$ subunit selectivity, *1:*484–485
Binding pocket structures, benzodiazepines, GABA$_A$ receptors, *2:*105–108
Bioassays, neuropeptide identification, *1:*671
Biochemical markers, in schizophrenia, *2:*260–262
Biochemistry, 3,4-methylenedioxy-methamphetamine effects, *2:*616–619

Biogenesis of lysosome-related organelles complex-1 (BLOC1), dystrobrevin binding protein 1 (DTNBP1), molecular interactions, *2:*353
Biological antagonists, neurotrophic factors as, *3:*231
Biological mechanisms, of schizophrenia, *2:*256–263
Biosynthesis:
   classical neurotransmitters, *1:*42–43
   histamine metabolism, *1:*305–306
   neuropeptides, *1:*685–687
      preprohormones, *1:*686
      prohormones, *1:*686
      tissue specificity, *1:*687
Biotin-switch method, nitrosothiol detection, *1:*748
Bipolar disorder:
   dopaminergic drugs, *1:*237
   neurobiology of:
      genetics, *1:*860–861
      peripheral neurochemistry, *1:*863–864
      postmortem findings, *1:*861–863
      research background, *1:*859
      in vivo imaging, *1:*863
   pharmacology:
      anticonvulsant antibipolar compounds, *1:*869–870
      lithium mechanism of action, *1:*864–869
Blood alcohol concentration (BAC) levels, alcohol abuse studies in alcohol-preferring rats, *2:*468–470
Blood-brain barrier (BBB):
   HIV neuropathogenesis and, *3:*696–697
   inflammation and, *3:*624–625
      pharmacological activation, *3:*633
   neuropeptides in, *1:*692–693
Blood-derived inflammatory cells, neuroinflammation, *3:*628
Blood pressure, norepinephrine/epinephrine physiology and, *1:*197–198
Blood vessels, muscarinic acetylcholine receptor deficiency, *1:*176
BMAL1 protein:
   circadian rhythms, animal models, *3:*12
   melatonin receptors and, *3:*50–51
Body composition, ghrelin modulation, *3:*775
Body temperature, 3,4-methylenedioxy-methamphetamine effects on, *2:*617–618
   neurotoxicity and, *2:*624–625

Bone morphogenetic proteins (BMP), stroke and, 3:375–377
Bone resorption and formation, ghrelin modulation, 3:776
Botulinium toxin (Botox), migraine management, 2:768
Bovine rhodopsin, muscarinic acetylcholine receptor structure, 1:149–151
Bphs gene, H_1 receptor in, 1:307–309
Brain:
   anxiety disorder-related regions of, 2:13–15
   benzodiazepine distribution, 2:110–112
   development:
      in bipolar disorder patients, 1:860–861
      $GABA_A$ receptor subunit distribution and, 1:471–473
      GABA transporters and, 1:467–468
      hippocampal neurogenesis and depression and, 1:826–827
      voltage-gated sodium ion channels, 1:640–641
   imaging studies:
      brain regions, anxiety disorders and, 2:13–15
      depressed patients, 1:802
      glutamate theory of schizophrenia, 2:292–293
      obsessive-compulsive disorders, 2:217–222
         animal models, 2:224
         neuropharmacological implications, 2:220–222
      schizophrenia, 2:256–260
      schizophrenia, dopamine hypothesis, 2:285–286
   immunoreceptors, inflammation and, 3:631–632
   injury:
      neurotrophic factors and, 3:229–230
      stroke and:
         classification, 3:350
         mechanisms of, 3:351–353
         poststroke repair approaches, 3:375–379
         repair approaches, 3:377–379
      traumatic:
         characteristics and classification, 3:443–446
         future research issues, 3:454
         neural regeneration, 3:452–453
         neuroplasticity, 3:453–454
         neuroprotective agents, 3:446–451
            anti-inflammatory agents, 3:447–449
            free-radical scavengers, 3:447
            neuroactive steroids/neurosteroids, 3:450–451
            neurotransmitter agonists/antagonists, 3:449–450
3,4-methylenedioxymethamphetamine neurotoxicity, biochemical and functional changes, 2:631–632
neuroactive steroid sources, 2:135–137
neuroanatomical control regions:
   alcohol abuse studies in alcohol-preferring rats, 2:469–470
   circuitry systems, 2:470–471
   psychostimulant abuse, 2:574–575
neurotransmitters, histamine:
   biosynthesis, 1:305–306
   early history, 1:300–301
   inactivation, 1:306–307
   metabolism, 1:305–307
   molecular pharmacology, receptor subtypes, 1:307–317
      H_1 receptor, 1:307–312
      H_2 receptor, 1:312–314
      H_3 receptor, 1:314–316
      H_4 receptor, 1:316
      NMDA receptor interaction, 1:316–317
   neuron activity and control, 1:317–322
      electrophysiology, 1:317
      pharmacological changes, 1:321–322
      in vitro modulation, 1:317–319
      in vivo changes, 1:319–321
   neuronal organization, 1:301–305
      afferents, 1:303–305
      histaminergic pathways, 1:303
      perikarya, 1:301–303
   neuron physiology, 1:322–326
      arousal, 1:322–324
      cognitive functions, 1:324
      nociception, 1:326
      pituitary hormone secretion, 1:324–325
      satiation, 1:325–326
      seizuers, 1:326
   neuropsychiatric disease, 1:327–329
      Alzheimer's disease, 1:327–328
      anxiety/ADHD, 1:329
      Parkinson's disease, 1:328

schizophrenia and antipsychotic
actions, *1:*327
sedative/hypnotic action sites in,
*3:*181–184
Brain-derived neurotrophic factor (BDNF):
AMPA receptor allosteric potentiators,
*1:*394–395
amyotrophic lateral sclerosis and,
*3:*226–227
antidepressant treatments and expression
of, *1:*804–805
5-HT neuronal growth and, *1:*807–808
adult neurogenesis and, *1:*806–808
stress-monoamine convergence in
depression, *1:*825–826
anxiety neurobiology, *2:*4
genetic susceptibility studies, *2:*18–19
knockout mice studies, *2:*25–26
receptor deficits and, *2:*29–30
cognitive function and, *3:*228
in depressed patients, *1:*800–801
depression and, *3:*229–230
depression models and, *1:*808
discovery of, *3:*221–223
$GABA_A$ phosphorylation, *1:*482
genetic studies in mood disorders, *1:*803
HIV neuropathology, Tax protein and,
*3:*705
indirect modulators of, *3:*232
intracellular signaling, *1:*791–792
lithium mechanism in bipolar disorder
and, *1:*868–869
neurogenesis and, *3:*206, *3:*224
neuroinflammatory mechanisms, *3:*641
neuronal maturation regulation, *3:*224
neurotrophins and, *3:*238
obesity and weight control, *3:*229–230
p75 neurotrophin receptor signaling,
*3:*246–247
pain perception and management, *3:*229
Parkinson's disease and, *3:*228–229
schizophrenia therapy, serotonin receptor
5-HT_{2A} receptor and, *2:*421–422
stress influence on, *1:*794
adrenal glucocorticoids, *1:*796–797
alterations in, *1:*794–795
cytokine alterations, *1:*797
neurogenesis and, *1:*799–800
regulation mechanisms, *1:*795–796
serotonin receptors, *1:*797
structure of, *3:*240
synaptic function and, *3:*239

Breast cancer resistance protein (BCRP),
drug-resistant epilepsy, *3:*425–426
Bretazenil, $GABA_A$ subunit pharmacology,
allosteric ligand modulation,
*1:*504–506
Bromocriptine, Parkinson's disease
treatment, *3:*488, *3:*490
Brown adipose tissue (BAT):
classification, *3:*786–789
glyceroneogenesis control, lipolysis and
thermogenesis, *3:*799–801
leptin and energy expenditure, *3:*744
molecular features, *3:*787–789
Brugada syndrome, voltage-gated sodium
ion channels and, *1:*642
α-Bungarotoxin, nicotinic acetylcholine
receptor and, *1:*28
Buprenorphine, opiate addiction therapy:
comparative efficacy studies, *2:*697–698
implementation issues and pilot studies,
*2:*698
regulatory approval studies, *2:*696–697
Bupropion:
attention-deficit hyperactivity disorder
therapy, *3:*300–301
narcolepsy therapy, *3:*103–104
nicotine dependence and withdrawal
therapy, *2:*549–550
Buspirone:
anxiety disorder therapy, *2:*70–71
opiate addiction therapy, *2:*699
γ-Butyrolactones, $GABA_A$ receptor
modulation, *1:*519–520
Butyrophenones, schizophrenia therapy,
clinical profile, *2:*383

CA1/CA3 hippocampal fields, alcohol abuse
studies, $GABA_{A5}$ receptor probes,
*2:*511–516
CA1 pyramidal neurons, $GABA_A$ receptor
distribution on, *1:*474–475
CA3 pyramidal neurons, stress and, *1:*800
CAAT-enhancing binding proteins (C/EBP),
leptin secretion and expression of,
*3:*735–736
Cabergolline, Parkinson's disease treatment,
*3:*491
Caenorhabditis elegans, neurodegenerative
disease model:
Alzheimer's disease, *3:*580–582
genetic and molecular pathways,
*3:*568–569

Huntingdon's disease trinucleotide
  repeats, 3:577–579
Parkinson's disease cell death, 3:570–577
Caffeine:
  idiopathic Parkinson's disease and, 3:544
  narcolepsy therapy, 3:104–105
  Parkinson's disease and, 3:505
Calcitonin gene-related peptide (CGRP):
  migraine therapy, 2:759–763
    injection techniques, 2:763
    neurovascular model, 2:759–760
    receptor antagonist therapeutic efficacy,
      2:763–764
    synthesis and actions, 2:760–761
    targeted repression therapy, 2:768
    trigeminovasculature sites, 2:761–763
  pain management applications, 2:768–769
Calcitonin receptor-like receptor (CLR),
    calcitonin gene-related peptide sites
    and migraine therapy targeting,
    2:762
Calcium-activated potassium channels,
    structure and function, 1:630–632
Calcium-calmodulin-dependent protein
    kinase II (CaMK II):
  amino acid neurotransmitters, 1:43–44
  anxiety neurobiology and, 2:30–33
  benzodiazepine tolerance, 2:101
  GABA transporters, 1:467–468
  transient receptor potential V1 (TRPV1)
    receptor sensitization, 2:735
Calcium channel blockers:
  migraine management, 2:767–768
  vanilloid receptors and, 2:728–729
Calcium channels:
  amino acid neurotransmitters, 1:43–44
  in bipolar disorder patients, 1:862
  calmodulin mediator, 1:85–87
  cyclic nucleotide second messenger
    signaling, adenylyl cyclase, 1:72–77
  $GABA_B$ receptors, effector systems,
    1:581–582
  H_1 receptor signaling, 1:309
  histaminergic neuron activity, 1:317–319
  hypocretin/orexin system, 3:132
  muscarinic acetylcholine receptor
    modulation, 1:161
  neuroinflammation and, 3:642
  signaling molecules, 1:83–85
  stroke and:
    ischemic brain injury, 3:351–353
    neuronal channel blockers, 3:366–367

subunits, antiepileptic drug modulation,
    3:413–414
  suprachiasmatic nucleus, 3:13–15
  T-type, antiepileptic drug modulation,
    3:413
  voltage-gated ion channels, 1:643–650
    α subunits, 1:644–645
    αδ subunits, 1:646
    auxiliary subunit modulators, 1:650
    β subunits, 1:645–646
    Ca_v1 family, 1:647–648
    Ca_v2 family, 1:648–649
    Ca_v3 family, 1:649–650
    γ subunits, 1:646
    general blockers, 1:647
    genetics, 1:619–620
    miscellaneous channels, 1:650–651
Calcium metabolism, 1:30–31
Calmodulin:
  calcium channel modulation, 1:85–87
  Ca_v1 family, 1:647–648
  intermediate-conductance
    calcium-activated potassium
    channels, 1:631
CamKII, $GABA_A$ receptor
    phosphorylation, 1:481–482
cAMP response element binding (CREB)
    protein:
  amino acid neurotransmitters, 1:44
  BDNF regulation and, 1:805
  calcium channel modulation, Ca_v1 family,
    1:647–648
  cognitive function and, 3:228
  HIV neuropathology and, apoptosis and,
    3:705
  Huntingdon's disease, invertebrate model,
    3:579
  leptin secretion and expression of,
    3:735–736
  lithium mechanism in bipolar disorder
    and, 1:868–869
  melatonin receptors, supersensitization,
    3:54
  psychostimulant abuse, chronic exposure
    and sensitization effects, 2:585
Cannabinoid hypothesis of schizophrenia,
    pharmacotherapy, 2:394
Cannabinoid receptors. See also
    Endocannabinoids; Marijuana
  analgesic properties, 2:666–668
  antiobesity therapy, 3:825–828
  cannabinoid$_1$ (CB-1) receptor:

addictive disorders, modulator therapy
and, 2:458–459
antagonist/agonist medication
development, 2:700
anxiety neurobiology and, deficits in,
2:29–30
appetite regulation, 2:670–672
cognition and, 2:669–670
convulsant effects, 2:672–673
emesis modulation, 2:673–675
identification of, 2:661–662
nicotine dependence and withdrawal
therapy, antagonist agents, 2:550
pain management and, 2:667–668
prenatal development and, 2:664–665
signaling mechanisms, 2:662–663
cannabinoid$_2$ (CB-2) receptor:
emesis modulation, 2:674–675
pain management and, 2:668–669
signaling mechanisms, 2:662–663
cognition and, 2:669–670
convulsant effects, 2:672–673
emesis modulation, 2:673–675
future research on, 2:676
neuroinflammation and, modulation
mechanisms, 3:641–642
reward, tolerance, and dependence,
2:675–676
in schizophrenia, animal model, 2:265
signaling mechanisms, 2:662–663
CAPON gene, schizophrenia molecular
genetics, 2:328
Capsaicin:
cloning of, 2:727–729
transient receptor potential V1 (TRPV1)
receptor expression, 2:730–732
Carbamazepine:
anxiety disorder therapy, 2:75
development and testing, 3:419
epilepsy efficacy, 3:417–418
focal/localization-related epilepsy therapy,
3:421, 3:423
Carbidopa, Parkinson's disease treatment,
3:484–487
β-Carboline3-carboxylate-*t*-butyl ester,
alcohol abuse studies:
anxiety reduction with, 2:510–511
GABA$_{A1,2,3,5}$ receptor subunit
modulation, 2:499–501
GABA$_{A1}$ receptor subunit selectivity,
2:498–499
microinjection techniques, 2:505–507

oral administration, 2:507–511
systemic administration, 2:503–504
β-Carboline antagonist ZK 93426, alcohol
abuse studies:
GABA$_{A5}$ receptor specificity, 2:514–516
GABA$_A$ benzodiazepine receptor
complex, 2:490–493
GABAergic modification of dopamine
agonists, 2:497
Carbonic anhydrase, topiramate and,
3:416–417
Carbon monoxide, as signaling molecule,
1:756–757
2-(Carboxycyclopropyl)glycines (CCGs),
mGlu II selective orthosteric
agonists, 1:426
S4-Carboxy phenylglycine (*S-4*CPG), mGlu
group I selective orthosteric
antagonists, 1:424–425
Cardiovascular system. *See also*
Arrhythmias
α$_2$-adrenergic receptor physiology,
1:208–209
β-adrenergic receptor physiology,
1:211–212
γ-hydroxybutyric acid (GHB) effects,
2:634
ghrelin effects, 3:774–775
KCNQ channel action on, 1:632–633
muscarinic acetylcholine receptor
deficiency, 1:175–176
voltage-gated calcium channels, 1:647–648
voltage-gated sodium ion channels,
1:640–641
Carrier-mediated mechanisms, blood-brain
barrier neuropeptides and,
1:692–693
Caspase-1, 3,4-methylenedioxy-
methamphetamine effects on, 2:628
Caspase inhibitors:
HIV neurotoxicity, Vpr protein, 3:703
stroke management, 3:372–373
Catalepsy, muscarinic acetylcholine receptor
deficiency, 1:172
Cataplexy:
defined, 3:82
mazindol therapy, 3:103
narcolepsy pathophysiology, 3:85
human leukocyte antigen and, 3:85–86
pharmacological treatment:
antidepressants, 3:114–115
future anticataplectics, 3:113–114

historical overview, 3:106–107
monoamine oxidase inhibitors, 3:111
neurotransmission, animal studies, 3:109–110
receptor subtypes, 3:110–111
second- and third-generation antidepressants, 3:108
sodium oxybate, 3:112
tricyclic antidepressants, 3:107–109
Catecholamines:
early research on, 1:30–31
signaling, in adipose tissues, 3:801–803
Catechol-*O*-methyl transferase (COMT):
anxiety neurobiology and, knockout mice studies, 2:24–26
dopamine synthesis, 1:224
norephinephrine neurochemistry, 1:198–199
obsessive-compulsive disorders, metabolism studies, 2:223
Parkinson's disease, neurochemistry, 3:481–483
schizophrenia:
dopamine hypothesis, 2:373
genetic evidence, 2:286–287
genetics studies, 2:286–287
imaging studies, 2:285–286
molecular genetics, chromosomal abnormalities, 2:328–329
susceptibility gene identification, 2:347–348
tolcapone targeting of, 2:389
Cation channels, muscarinic acetylcholine receptor modulation, 1:161
CCK$_A$ receptor agonist, antiobesity therapy, 3:830–831
CD9 protein, structure and function, 3:608–609
CD40 molecule, inflammation and, 3:631
CD80 molecule, inflammation and, 3:631
CD86 molecule, inflammation and, 3:631
CDPPB, mGlu5 allosteric potentiators, 1:442–443
Cell autonomy, Circadian rhythmicity, 3:8
Cell-cell interactions, anxiety neurobiology, neuronal deficits and, 2:30
Cell death cascades, human immunodeficiency virus neuropathology, 3:704–707
apoptosis, 3:704–705
excitotoxicity, 3:705–706
neural progenitor cells, 3:706–707
oxidative stress, 3:706
Cell membrane-associated proteins, anxiety neurobiology and, mouse studies, 2:19, 2:21
Cell survival, nitrosylation and, 1:752
Cellular migration, neural inflammation and, pharmacological activation, 3:633
Cellular pathways, nitrosylation in:
cell survival, 1:752
extracellular matrix, 1:751–752
gene transcription, 1:750–571
ion channels, 1:748–749
protein-protein interactions, 1:749–750
vesicular transport, 1:751
Central nervous system (CNS):
β-adrenergic receptor physiology, 1:211–212
adrenergic transmitters in, 1:29–30
alcohol abuse studies in alcohol-preferring rats:
circuitry systems, role of, 2:470–471
control substrates, 2:469–470
AMPA receptors, 1:370–371
GABA$_A$ receptor subunit distribution in, 1:471–473
γ-hydroxybutyric acid (GHB) effects, 2:634
HIV neuropathogenesis and, 3:696–697
inflammation mechanisms in, 3:622–625
kainate receptors, 1:372
melatonin receptors:
circadian rhythm modulation, 3:54–57
clock genes and, 3:50–51
desensitization, 3:52–53
historical perspective, 3:38–40
melatonin production, 3:40–41
molecular pharmacology, 3:42–44
molecular structure, 3:41–42
overview, 3:37–38
regulatory mechanisms, 3:51–54
signaling mechanisms, 3:44–46
supersensitization, 3:54
suprachiasmatic nucleus, 3:46–54
circadian inputs and outputs, 3:46–47
receptor localization, signaling, and function, 3:47–50
as therapeutic targets, 3:57–61
circadian rhythms, 3:58
depression, 3:58–61
sleep, 3:57–58
NMDA receptors, 1:369–370

pain pathways, 2:712–714
schizophrenia and, 2:260–262
serotonin receptors, 1:258–259
  serotonin receptor 5-HT$_3$, 1:273
  serotonin receptor 5-HT$_4$, 1:274
  serotonin receptor 5-HT$_\gamma$, 1:275–276
voltage-gated calcium ion channels, Ca$_v$2 family, 1:648–649
voltage-gated sodium ion channels, 1:640–641
CEP-1347 compound, Parkinson's disease and, 3:229
Ceramide production, HIV lipid metabolism and, 3:707
Cerebroside/sulfatide lipids, in myelin, 3:594–596
Cerebrospinal fluid (CSF):
  blood-brain barrier neuropeptides and, 1:692–693
  corticotropin-releasing factor receptor antagonists, effects on, 2:177–179
  hypocretin/orexin system, narcolepsy and, 3:138–139
  narcolepsy evaluation, hypocretin-1 assessment, 3:84
  schizophrenia dopamine hypothesis and, 2:288–289
Cerostat/Aptiganel, stroke management, 3:359
Cerovive, stroke management, 3:371–372
Cesium, voltage-gated potassium channels, K$_V$ subunits, structure and function, 1:630
C fibers:
  pain pathways, 2:711–712
  transient receptor potential V1 (TRPV1) receptor expression, 2:729
Channel blockers. *See also* specific Ion channels, e.g. Calcium channel
  GABA receptor binding sites, 1:518–519
  NMDA receptor allosteric antagonists, 1:387–389
  voltage-gated calcium ion channels, Ca$_v$2 family, 1:649
Channel-gating process, GABA$_A$ receptor activation, 1:492–494
  binding transduction to, 1:495–497
Channelopathies, voltage-gated sodium ion channels, 1:641–642
Channel pore structures, GABA$_A$ receptor activation, 1:497–498

Charcot-Marie-Tooth, neurotrophic factor therapy, 3:227
Charybdotoxin, intermediate-conductance calcium-activated potassium channels, 1:631
Chemical neurotransmitters, categories of, 1:40–41
Chemokines:
  HIV neuropathogenesis and, 3:697–699
  inhibitors, stroke management and, 3:369
  neuroinflammation and, 3:629–632
  receptor-directed pharmacological approaches to, 3:633–634
Chemotherapy:
  emesis with, cannabinoid modulation of, 2:674–675
  multiple sclerosis, mitoxantrone, 3:676–677
Chimeric receptors, GABA$_A$ receptor modulation, allosteric structural determinants, 1:508–509
Chlordiazepoxide (CDPX), GABA$_A$ receptor modulation, 1:499–500
Chloride channels:
  early research on, 1:29
  GABA receptors and, 1:468–469
  muscarinic acetylcholine receptor modulation, 1:161–162
  voltage-gated channels, 1:649–650
(R,S)-2-Chloro-5-hydroxyphenylglycine (CHPG), mGlu group I selective orthosteric agonists, 1:424
Cholecystokinin (CCK):
  antiobesity therapy, 3:830–831
  anxiety neurobiology and, 2:17
  leptin signaling and and feeding regulation, 3:743
  neuropeptides and, 1:670–671
  pain management and, 2:716–717
Cholesterol, in myelin, 3:594–596
Choline acetyltransferase (CHAT):
  HIV-associated dementia and, 3:711–712
  structure and function, 1:714–715
Choline neurotransmitter transporters (CHT), structure and function, 1:714–715
Cholinergic neurotransmitters:
  atypical antipsychotic mechanisms, 2:429–430
  hypocretin/orexin system, arousal mechanisms, 3:143–144
  neurogenesis and, 3:208–209

schizophrenia:
  neurochemistry, 2:261–262
  pharmacotherapy, 2:393–394
Chromosomal abnormalities, schizophrenia molecular genetics, 2:328–331
  catechol-O-methyltransferase, 2:328–329
  DISC1 gene, 2:330–331
  PRODH candidate gene, 2:329–330
  ZDHHC8 candidate gene, 2:330
Chromosome mapping:
  anxiety neurobiology, mouse studies, 2:19, 2:23
  hypocretin/orexin system, 3:127
  schizophrenia, susceptibility gene identification, 2:346–351
Chronic inflammatory demyelinating polyneuropathy (CIDP), myelin pathology, 3:613–614
Chronopharmacology, circadian rhythms, 3:15
Chrysin, $GABA_A$ subunit pharmacology, allosteric ligand modulation, 1:505–506
Ciliary neurotrophic factor (CNTF):
  amyotrophic lateral sclerosis, 3:226–227
  antiobesity therapy, axokine, 3:822–824
  depression and, 3:229–230
  therapeutic applications, 3:226
Ciproxifan, histamine neuron physiology and, 1:324
Circadian rhythms:
  antidepressant effects on, 3:18–20
  chronopharmacology, 3:15–23
  functional importance, 3:4
  future research issues, 3:23–24
  histaminergic neuron activity, 1:319–322
  mammallian structural models, 3:10–13
  melatonin receptor modulation, 3:54–57
    therapeutic targeting, 3:58
  neurotrophins and, 3:239
  nonmammalian structural models, 3:6–10
  prokineticin regulation, 3:167–168
  properties, 3:4–6
  reproductive cycle depression:
    future research issues, 1:852–853
    neuroendocrine compounds:
      cross-reproductive cycle analysis, 1:851–853
      menopause, 1:849–851
        cortisol, 1:850
        melatonin, 1:849–850
        prolactin, 1:850–851

        thyroid-stimulating hormone, 1:850
      menstrual cycle, 1:844–846
        cortisol, 1:845
        melatonin, 1:844–845
        prolactin, 1:846
        thyroid-stimulating hormone, 1:845
      postpartum depression, 1:848–849
        cortisol, 1:848
        estradiol, 1:849
        melatonin, 1:848
        prolactin, 1:848–849
        thyroid-stimulating hormone, 1:848
      pregnancy, 1:846–847
        cortisol, 1:847
        melatonin, 1:846–847
        prolactin, 1:847
        thyroid-stimulating hormone, 1:847
    research background, 1:844
  superchiasmatic nucleus:
    inputs and outputs, 3:46–47
    period and phase, 3:13–15
Cisplatin-induced neuropathy, neurotrophic factors and, 3:227
Citalopram, autism spectrum disorders, 3:324–325
CL218,872 compound:
  alcohol abuse studies, $GABA_{A1}$ receptor subunit selectivity, 2:499
CL-218,872 compound:
  $GABA_A$ receptor activation, benzodiazepine binding sites, 1:510–511
Clathrin-mediated endocytosis, $GABA_A$ receptor trafficking, 1:480–481
Claudin protein family, structure and function, 3:608
"Clinically isolated syndrome" (CIS) of demyelination, betaseron therapy and, 3:675
Clinical markers, antiepileptic drug efficacy, 3:420
Clock genes:
  circadian rhythms, animal models, 3:12
  melatonin receptors and, 3:50–51
    supersensitization function, 3:54
  prokineticin regulation, 3:167–168
Clock neurons, synchronization and modulation, 3:8–9

Clomipramine:
  attention-deficit hyperactivity disorder therapy, 3:299
  autism spectrum disorders, 3:322
  obsessive-compulsive disorder therapy, 2:69–70
Clonazepam:
  GABA$_A$ α_3 subunit pharmacology, 1:488
  obsessive-compulsive disorder therapy, 2:234
  Parkinson-related sleep disturbance, 3:504
Clonidine:
  attention-deficit hyperactivity disorder therapy, 3:299–300
  autism spectrum disorders, 3:330
  circadian rhythms and, 3:19–20
  schizophrenia pharmacotherapy, 2:393
  Tourette's syndrome therapy, 3:274–276
Cloning experiments:
  cyclic nucleotide second messenger signaling, adenylyl cyclase, 1:74–75
  GABA$_B$ receptors, 1:571–572
  glutamate receptors, 1:397–398
  NMDA receptors, 1:369–370
  voltage-gated ion channels, 1:619–620
Clostridium botulinum, synaptic vesicle action and, 1:27
Clotrimazole, intermediate-conductance calcium-activated potassium channels, 1:631
Clozapine:
  autism spectrum disorders, 3:326
  dopamine D$_2$ receptor blockade, 2:412–415
  mechanisms of action:
    cholinergic mechanisms, 2:429–430
    serotonin receptor 5-HT$_{2A}$, 2:418–421, 2:420–421
    serotonin receptor 5-HT$_6$ and, 2:425–426
    serotonin receptor 5-HT/D$_2$ hypothesis, 2:417–418
  schizophrenia therapy:
    brain-derived neurotrophic factor and, 2:421–422
    cholinergic receptor targeting, 2:393–394
    clinical profile, 2:387
    dopamine D$_2$ receptor blockade, 2:412–415
    history of, 2:370

  safety and tolerability, 2:388–389
  schizophrenia-related psychosis, 2:254
  vesicular transporters and, 1:723
Clustering behavior, GABA$_A$ receptors, 1:478–480
Clusters, GABA$_A$ receptors, benzodiazepines, 2:108–110
CNS 1102 antagonist, stroke and, 3:357
Cocaine:
  abuse:
    3,4-methylenedioxymethamphetamine reinforcement of, 2:615–616
    monoamine neuropharmacology, 2:570–575
    therapy developments for, 2:585–588
  chronic exposure and sensitization effects, 2:580–585
  HIV/AIDS and, 3:713–715
  neuropeptide pharmacology and, 2:578–579
Cocaine- and amphetamine-regulated transcript (CART):
  antiobesity therapy, axokine, 3:823–824
  leptin signaling and and feeding regulation, 3:741–743
  psychostimulant abuse, chronic exposure and sensitization effects, 2:585
  stress response and, 1:695
Cockroach, circadian rhythms in, 3:10
Coenzyme Q$_{10}$, Parkinson's disease treatment, 3:504–505
Cognitive behavior therapy (CBT), obsessive-compulsive disorders, 2:219–220
Cognitive function. *See also* Dementia
  cannabinoid receptors and, 2:669–670
  GABA$_A$ subunit pharmacology:
    allosteric ligand modulation, 1:505–506
    GABA$_A$ α_5 subunit, 1:489
  GABA$_B$ receptor targeting, 1:592–593
  histamine neuron physiology, 1:324
  in HIV patients, 3:717–718
  3,4-methylenedioxymethamphetamine and, 2:630–631
  neural system diversity and, 3:461–463
  neuropathies and, 3:227–228
  nicotine dependence and withdrawal, withdrawal neurosubstrates, 2:541–543
  schizophrenia, 2:254–255
    animal model, 2:263–264
    glutamatergic receptors, 2:428–429

neural network analysis, 2:259
   serotonin receptor 5-HT$_{2A}$ receptor enhancement, 2:421–422
   traumatic brain injury and, 3:446
Colorimetry, nitrosothiol detection, 1:748
Comorbid conditions:
   addictive disorders vulnerability with, 2:457–458
   obsessive-compulsive disorders, 2:216
   opiate addiction, 2:691–694
   Tourette's syndrome, 3:266–268
Compensatory mechanisms, dopamine hypothesis of schizophrenia, 2:284–285
Complexins, in bipolar disorder patients, 1:861–862
Computed tomography (CT):
   obsessive-compulsive disorders, brain imaging studies, 2:217–218
   schizophrenia analysis, 2:256
Concanavlin A, kainate receptor allosteric potentiators, 1:396
Conditioned conflict tests, anxiety neurobiology, emotionalty studies in mice, 2:8–9
Conditioned fear paradigms, emotionality studies in mice, 2:8–9
Congenital stationary night blilndness (CSNB2), voltage-gated calcium channels, Ca$_v$1 family, 1:648
Connexins, structure and function, 3:609
Conotoxins:
   nicotinic acetylcholine receptors, 1:124
   stroke management, calcium channel blocker, 3:366–367
   voltage-gated calcium ion channels, Ca$_v$2 family, 1:649
Constipation, Parkinson's disease and, 3:503
Continuous performance test (CPT), schizophrenia, animal models, 2:263–264
COPI components, GABA$_B$ receptor trafficking and heteromization, 1:576–578
Cortical dopamine:
   schizophrenia dopamine hypothesis and, 2:287–288
   serotonin receptor 5-HT$_{2A}$ receptor enhancement, 2:421–422
Cortical neurons:
   HIV neuropathology, apoptosis and, 3:705
   Tourette's syndrome, 3:270

Corticosteroids:
   multiple sclerosis acute relapse, treatment of, 3:672–673
   neurogenesis and, 3:206–207
   traumatic brain injury and, 3:448–449
Corticosterone, psychostimulant abuse, 2:577–578
Corticostriatal-thalamic-cortical loops, integrated glutamate/dopamine hypotheses of schizophrenia, neurochemistry and, 2:374–376
Corticotropin-releasing factor (CRF):
   alcholol abuse studies, in alcohol-preferring rats, 2:471
   hypocretin/orexin system, 3:135
   neurosteroid effects, acoustic/fear-potentiated startle, 2:147
   nicotine dependence and withdrawal, 2:539–540
      withdrawal substrate specificity, 2:543
   opiate dependence therapy and, 2:699
   psychostimulant abuse, 2:577–578
   chronic exposure and sensitization effects, 2:580–585
   receptor antagonists, anxiolytic applications:
      future research issues, 2:198–199
      nonpeptide ligands, 2:195–196
      overview, 2:177–179
      peptide ligand pharmacology, 2:185–195
         ligand binding mechanisms, 2:190–195
      receptor/ligand family structure, 2:179–185
         ligand properties, 2:180–181
         receptor subtypes and distribution, 2:181–185
      therapeutic potential, 2:196–198
Corticotropin-releasing hormone (CRH):
   anxiety neurobiology and, 2:17
   knockout mice studies, 2:25–26
   receptor deficits, 2:28–30
   stress response and, 1:694–695
Cortisol:
   circadian rhythms and release of, 3:19–20
   depression and levels of:
      in menopause, 1:850
      during menstrual cycle, 1:845
      postpartum depression, 1:848
      in pregnancy, 1:846–847

nicotine dependence and withdrawal, 2:539–540
    withdrawal substrate specificity, 2:543
Costimulatory molecules, inflammation and, 3:631
Cotinine, nicotine dependence and withdrawal, metabolism and elimination pharmacokinetics, 2:544–545
Countermodulation therapy, addictive disorders, 2:458–459
CP-154,526 antagonist, opiate dependence therapy and, 2:699
CPCCOEt, mGlu1 allosteric antagonists, 1:436–437
CPPHA, mGlu5 allosteric potentiators, 1:442
CRF_1 receptor, corticotropin-releasing factor receptor antagonists, 2:181–185
    anxiety/depression therapeutic potential and, 2:196–198
    ligand binding mechanisms, 2:190–195
    nonpeptide ligands, 2:195–196
    peptide ligand pharmacology, 2:185–195
CRF_2 receptor, corticotropin-releasing factor receptor antagonists, 2:182–185
    ligand binding mechanisms, 2:190–195
    peptide ligand pharmacology, 2:185–195
$CRF_{2(a)}$ receptor, corticotropin-releasing factor receptor antagonists, 2:182–185
$CRF_{2(b)}$ receptor, corticotropin-releasing factor receptor antagonists, 2:182–185
Cryptochrome genes, melatonin receptors, 3:50–51
Curare:
    action of, 1:4–5
    Bernard's research on, 1:4–7
CX516 compound, schizophrenia pharmacotherapy, 2:392
CX546, AMPA receptor allosteric potentiators, 1:390–391
CX614, AMPA receptor allosteric potentiators, 1:393–395
Cycle regulation, G proteins, 1:64–65
Cyclic adenosine monophosphate (cAMP):
    α_1 adrenergic receptors, 1:203
    in bipolar disorder patients, 1:861–862
    corticotropin-releasing factor receptor antagonists, CRF receptor stimulation, 2:186–195
    cyclic nucleotide second messenger signaling, 1:75, 1:78
    melatonin receptors, supersensitization, 3:54
    neuroinflammation and, modulating agents, 3:635–636
    psychostimulant abuse, chronic exposure and sensitization effects, 2:584–585
    second messengers and, 1:32
Cyclic adenosine monophosphate (cAMP)-responsive nuclear factors, anxiety neurobiology and, 2:32
Cyclic guanosine monophosphate (cGMP):
    cyclic nucleotide second messenger signaling, cellular targets, 1:80–81
    $GABA_A$ phosphorylation, 1:481–482
    neuroinflammation and, modulating agents, 3:635–636
    nitric oxide physiology, 1:745
$2',3'$-Cyclic nucleotide $3'$-phosphodiesterase (CNP), structure and function, 3:603–604
Cyclic nucleotide-gated (CNG) channels, structure and function, 1:649–650
Cyclic nucleotide second messengers, intracellular signaling, 1:72–81
    adenylyl cyclase, 1:72–77
    cAMP targets, 1:75, 1:78
    cGMP targets, 1:80–81
    guanylyl cyclase, 1:78–80
Cyclooxygenase (COX1) inhibitors, neuroinflammation, arachidonic acid/prostaglandin pathways, 3:634–635
Cyclooxygenase (COX2) inhibitors:
    neuroinflammation, arachidonic acid/prostaglandin pathways, 3:634–635
    traumatic brain injury and, 3:448–449
Cyclopropylglutamate (CCG), NMDA orthosteric agonists, 1:373
(R,S)-α-Cyclopropyl-4-phosphono-phenylglycine (CPPG), mGlu III selective orthosteric agonists, 1:435
d-Cycloserine, autism spectrum disorders, 3:332
Cyclothiazide, AMPA receptor allosteric potentiators, 1:390–395

CYP1A2 enzyme, 3,4-methylenedioxy-methamphetamine neurotoxicity and, 2:622
CYP2A6 enzyme, nicotine dependence and withdrawal, metabolism and elimination pharmacokinetics, 2:545
cyPPTS, mGlu2 allosteric potentiators, 1:438–439
Cys loop ligand-gated ion channel superfamily:
 GABA$_A$ receptor activation, 1:493–494
  channel pore complex, 1:497–498
 GABA receptors and, 1:468–469
Cysteine residues, nitric oxide nitrosylation, 1:747
Cysteines, melatonin receptor molecular structure, 3:42
Cystine, nicotinic acetylcholine receptors, 1:120
Cystine/glutamate transporters, psychostimulant abuse and, 2:576
Cystinyl leukotriene, mGlu2 allosteric potentiators, 1:439
Cytochemical assay, neuropeptide identification, 1:673
Cytochrome P450 enzymes:
 benzodiazepine receptor ligand metabolism, 2:102
 selective serotonin reuptake inhibitors, 2:68–69
 Tourette's syndrome therapy, 3:274–276
Cytogenetic abnormalities, schizophrenia, susceptibility gene identification, 2:346–351
Cytokines:
 anxiety neurobiology, 2:16–18
  knockout mice studies, 2:26
 circadian rhythms and, 3:21–23
 3,4-methylenedioxymethamphetamine effects on, 2:627–628
 multiple sclerosis therapy, daclizumab agents, 3:685–686
 neuroinflammation:
  arachidonic acid pathways, 3:630
  astrocytes and, 3:627
  minocycline inhibition and, 3:645–646
  proinflammatory pathway modulation, 3:638–639
  receptor-directed pharmacological approaches to, 3:633–634
  structure and function, 3:628–629

neuropeptide receptors, 1:691
stress response and, neurotrophins and, 1:797
stroke and:
 ischemic brain injury, 3:352–353
 management through inhibition of, 3:368–369
 traumatic brain injury and, 3:447–449
Cytolytic T cells, muscarinic acetylcholine receptor deficiency, 1:177
Cytoplasmic proteins:
 sodium voltage-gated ion channels, 1:636
 voltage-gated potassium channels, 1:627–628
Cytoskeletal proteins, voltage-gated potassium channels, 1:628

D_1 receptor:
 alcohol abuse studies:
  bed nucleus of stria terminalis system, 2:475
  lateral hypothalamus, dopaminergic regulation by, 2:481–485
  ventral pallidum pathways, 2:477–480
 psychostimulant abuse, monoamine neuropharmacology, 2:571–575
 schizophrenia dopamine hypothesis:
  cortical vs. striatal dopamine, 2:288
  history, 2:284–285
  imaging evidence, 2:286–287
 schizophrenia pharmacotherapy, antipsychotic agents, 2:380–381
 schizophrenia therapy, agonist and antagonists, 2:390
 subfamily, 1:225–227
 substituted benzamides, 2:415–416
D-2-amino-5-phosphonopentonoate (D-AP5), NMDA orthosteric antagonists, 1:373–375
D_2/D_3 receptors:
 cataplexy therapy, 3:110–111
  novel anticataplectics, 3:113–114
 clozapine D_2 receptor blockade, 2:414–415
 partial dopamine agonists, 2:416–417
 psychostimulant abuse therapy, 2:586–587
 selective antagonism, schizophrenia therapy, 2:380
 substituted benzamides, 2:416
 Tourette's syndrome therapy, 3:276

D$_2$ receptor:
  alcohol abuse studies:
    lateral hypothalamus, dopaminergic regulation by, 2:481–485
    ventral pallidum pathways, 2:477–480
  clozapine blockade, 2:412–415
  psychostimulant abuse:
    chronic exposure and sensitization effects, 2:582–585
    monoamine neuropharmacology, 2:571–575
  schizophrenia dopamine hypothesis:
    cortical vs. striatal dopamine, 2:288
    history, 2:284–285, 2:371–373
    imaging evidence, 2:285–286
    pathological evidence, 2:285
    pharmacological evidence, 2:287
  schizophrenia pharmacotherapy:
    antipsychotic occupancy and effect, 2:376–378
    High 5-HT$_{2A}$ vs., 2:378
    occupancy thresholds and rapid dissociation, 2:378–380
    subtherapeutic occupancy time, 2:382
  subfamily, 1:227–230
D$_3$ receptor:
  schizophrenia dopamine hypothesis:
    genetic evidence, 2:286–287
    pathological evidence, 2:285
    pharmacological evidence, 2:287
  schizophrenia therapy, antagonist development, 2:390
  substituted benzamides, 2:415–416
  subunit, properties of, 1:229–230
D$_4$ receptor:
  schizophrenia dopamine hypothesis:
    pathological evidence, 2:285
    pharmacological evidence, 2:287
  schizophrenia therapy:
    antagonism and regional specificity, 2:380
    antagonist development, 2:390
    substituted benzamides, 2:415–416
  subunit, properties of, 1:230
Daclizumab, multiple sclerosis therapy, 3:685–686
DAG activation, protein kinase C, 1:85
Dardarin mutation, familial Parkinson's disease and mutation of, LRRK2 gene and, 3:538–539
DARPP-32, protein phosphatases integration, 1:95–96
Daytime sleep studies, narcolepsy evaluation, 3:83
D-CPP-ene NMDA antagonist, stroke management and, 3:356–357, 3:360
Deactivation, GABA$_A$ receptors, 1:498–499
Deafness, KCNQ channels and, 1:632–633
Death domain:
  p75 neurotrophin receptor structure and, 3:241
  stroke management, 3:373
Decahydroisoquinolines:
  AMPA receptor orthosteric antagonists, 1:377–378
  kainate receptor orthosteric antagonists, 1:383–385
  stroke management, 3:362
Decarboxylase inhibitor, Parkinson's disease treatment, levodopa with, 3:484–487
Decarboxylation, dopamine synthesis, 1:54–55
Deep brain stimulation (DBS), obsessive-compulsive disorders, 2:236–237
Deep sleep phase syndrome (DSPS), circadian rhythms, melatonin receptor modulation, 3:58
Defensive burying behavior, animal anxiety models, neurosteroid effects, 2:149–150
Degradation reactions, serotonin, 1:261–262
Dehydroepiandrosterone, schizophrenia therapy, 2:394
Dehydroepiandrosterone sulfate (DHEAS):
  in brain, 2:137
  schizophrenia therapy, 2:394
Delta opioid receptors, structure and function, 2:751
Dementia:
  acetylcholinesterase inhibitors and, 3:463–465
  glutamate receptor ligands, 3:469–471
  HIV-associated dementia (HAD):
    alcohol abuse and, 3:716
    apoptosis mechanisms, 3:704–705
    classification, 3:694–695
    epidemiology and pathogenesis, 3:695–696
    lipid metabolism and, 3:707
    methamphetamine/cocaine abuse and, 3:713–715

neurodegenerative disease and, *3:*716–718
neurotransmitters and, *3:*711–712
nigrostriatal system and, *3:*708–710
Vpu protein and, *3:*704
muscarinic receptor drugs and, *3:*465–469
nicotinic agonists, *3:*469
Parkinson's disease and, *3:*502
therapeutic targets, *3:*471–473
Dendrotoxins, voltage-gated potassium channels, K$_V$ subunits, structure and function, *1:*630
Dependency risk, endocannabinoids, *2:*675–676
Depolarization inactivation, schizophrenia therapy, D$_2$ receptor occupancy and effect, *2:*376–378
Depolarization responses:
GABA receptors, *1:*468–469
voltage-gated calcium channels, *1:*647–648
voltage-gated sodium ion channels, *1:*640
L-Deprenyl, narcolepsy therapy, *3:*104
Deprenyl and Tocopherol Antioxidative Therapy of Parkinsonism (DATATOP), *3:*504–505
Depression:
anxiety symptoms with, pharmacotherapy, *2:*80
autism spectrum disorders, *3:*334
corticotropin-releasing factor receptor antagonists, therapeutic potential of, *2:*196–198
hippocampal neurogenesis and treatment for:
adult neurogenesis stages, *1:*827–828
behavioral and animal models, *1:*833
depression physiology and, *1:*823–824, *1:*826–827
future research on, *1:*833
monoamines and, *1:*822–823
research background, *1:*821–822
serotonin/norepinephrine regulation, *1:*831–833
stress and monamine hypotheses, *1:*825–826
stress hormone neurogenesis regulation, *1:*829–830
melatonin receptors, therapeutic targeting of, *3:*58–61
neuroactive steroid interactions, *2:*156–157
neurotrophic factors and, *3:*229–230

neurotrophic factors in, *1:*800–802
antidepressant therapies:
BDNR expression and, *1:*804–806
neurogenesis and, *1:*806–808
BDNF levels, *1:*800–801
Brain-derived neurotrophic factor and models of, *1:*808
fibroblast growth factor levels, *1:*802
structural and cellular alterations, *1:*802–803
Parkinson's disease treatment and, *3:*500–501
in reproductive cycle, circadian studies of neuroendocrine compounds:
cross-reproductive cycle analysis, *1:*851–853
future research issues, *1:*852–853
menopause, *1:*849–851
cortisol, *1:*850
melatonin, *1:*849–850
prolactin, *1:*850–851
thyroid-stimulating hormone, *1:*850
menstrual cycle, *1:*844–846
cortisol, *1:*845
melatonin, *1:*844–845
prolactin, *1:*846
thyroid-stimulating hormone, *1:*845
postpartum depression, *1:*848–849
cortisol, *1:*848
estradiol, *1:*849
melatonin, *1:*848
prolactin, *1:*848–849
thyroid-stimulating hormone, *1:*848
pregnancy, *1:*846–847
cortisol, *1:*847
melatonin, *1:*846–847
prolactin, *1:*847
thyroid-stimulating hormone, *1:*847
research background, *1:*844
serotonin transporters and, *1:*720
stress-induced behavior, neuroactive steroids, *2:*156–157
Desensitization:
α$_1$ adrenergic receptors, *1:*202–203
β-adrenergic receptor activation, *1:*210
AMPA receptor allosteric potentiators, *1:*393–395
GABA$_A$ receptors, *1:*498–499
GABA$_B$ receptors, *1:*584–585
melatonin receptors, *3:*52–53
neuropeptide receptors, *1:*688–689

of nicotinic acetylcholine receptor, *1:*125–127
transient receptor potential V1 (TRPV1) receptors, *2:*735–736
Designer drugs. *See also* specific drugs, e.g. *2:*3,*2:*4-Methylenedioxy-methamphetamine (MDMA)
overview, *2:*614
Desipramine, attention-deficit hyperactivity disorder therapy, *3:*299
Developmental genes, obsessive-compulsive disorders, *2:*223–224
Dexmethylphenidate, attention-deficit hyperactivity disorder therapy, *3:*296
Diabetes mellitus, β-adrenergic receptor physiology, *1:*212–213
Diagnostic criteria, anxiety disorders, *2:*9–12, *2:*61–62
Diazepam:
GABA$_A$ receptor:
α_1 subunit pharmacology, *1:*484–485, *1:*488
modulation, *1:*499
γ subunit isoforms, *1:*509–511
Diazepam binding inhibitor (DBI), benzodiazepine ligands, *2:*98–99
2′,3′-Dicarboxycyclopropylglycine analog (DCG-IV), mGlu II selective orthosteric agonists, *1:*426–427
Diet, epilepsy management and, *3:*427
Diethylpropion, as anti-obesity agent, *3:*817–818
3,3′-Difluorobenzaldazine, mGlu5 allosteric potentiators, *1:*441–442
Dihydroergocryptine, Parkinson's disease treatment, *3:*491
3,4-Dihydroxyamphetamine (HHA), 3,4-methylenedioxy-methamphetamine neurotoxicity and, *2:*622
3,4-Dihydroxyphenylacetic acid (DOPAC):
human immunodeficiency virus: methamphetamine/cocaine abuse and, *3:*714–715
nigrostriatal system and, *3:*709
Parkinson's disease, neurochemistry, *3:*481–483
3,4-Dihydroxy-L-phenylalanine (DOPA):
early research on, *1:*30–31
norephinephrine/epinephrine neurochemistry, *1:*198–199

schizophrenia dopamine hypothesis, *2:*372–373
3,5-Dihydroxyphenylglycine (3,5-DHPG), mGlu group I selective orthosteric agonists, *1:*423–424
Diisopropyl phosphorofluoridate (DFP), synapse research and, *1:*23
Dimerization:
α_1 adrenergic receptors, *1:*201–203
muscarinic acetylcholine receptors, *1:*166–167
opioid receptors, *2:*752
Dipeptidyl-peptidase IV (DPP IV), neuropeptide inactivation, *1:*687–688
Diphasic dyskinesia, Parkinson's disease treatment and, *3:*499
DISC1 gene, schizophrenia molecular genetics, *2:*330–331
molecular interactions, *2:*351–352
susceptibility identification, *2:*349–350
Discontinuation syndrome, selective serotonin reuptake inhibitors, *2:*67–69
Disease, G proteins and, *1:*66
Distribution kinetics, nicotine dependence and withdrawal, *2:*544
Disturbed nocturnal sleep, treatment of, *3:*112
DJ-1 gene, familial Parkinson's disease and, *3:*535–536
DMPP agonist, nicotinic acetylcholine receptors, *1:*120
DOI:
hallucinogens and, *2:*639
schizophrenia therapy, serotonin receptor 5-HT$_{2A}$, *2:*420–421
Donepezil:
dementia disorders and, *3:*464–465
schizophrenia pharmacotherapy, *2:*393–394
Dopadecarboxylase, schizophrenia dopamine hypothesis, *2:*372–373
Dopamine agonists:
alcohol abuse studies, GABAergic modification, *2:*496–498
human immunodeficiency virus and, nigrostriatal system, *3:*708–710
Parkinson's disease treatment, *3:*488–494
antioxidant effects, *3:*504–505
apomorphine, *3:*493–494
bromocriptine, *3:*488, *3:*490

cabergoline, *3:*491
monoamine oxidase type B inhibitor, *3:*494
pergolide, *3:*490–491
piribedil, *3:*493
pramipexole, *3:*491–492
ropinirole, *3:*492
partial agonists, *2:*416–417
pharmacology of, *3:*489
psychostimulant abuse therapy, *2:*586–587
in schizophrenia, animal models, *2:*264
Dopamine hypothesis of schizophrenia:
cortical *vs.* striatal dopamine, *2:*287–289
genetic evidence, *2:*286–287
glutamate theory consolidated with, *2:*295–296
history, *2:*284–285
imaging evidence, *2:*285–286
neurochemistry and, *2:*371–373
pathological evidence, *2:*285
pharmacological evidence, *2:*287
postmortem studies, *2:*344
Dopamine neurotransmitters:
addictive disorders, reward therapy and, *2:*458–459
anxiety disorder therapy, antipsychotics, *2:*71–72
anxiety neurobiology, *2:*15–17
receptor deficits, *2:*29–30
attention-deficit hyperactivity disorder, *1:*237–238
basic properties, *1:*221–222
bipolar disorders, *1:*237
chemistry and metabolism, *1:*222–224
classification and molecular properties, *1:*225–230
D_1 receptor subfamily, *1:*225–227
D_2 receptor subfamily, *1:*227–230
drug applications, *1:*236–239
H_3 receptor synthesis, *1:*315–316
histaminergic neuron activity, Parkinson's disease, *1:*328
hypocretin/orexin system, arousal mechanisms, *3:*143
mechanisms, *1:*54–55
3,4-methylenedioxymethamphetamine (MDMA):
receptor/transporter effects, *2:*617
reinforcing properties, *2:*614–616
muscarinic acetylcholine receptor deficiency:

efflux nucleus accumbens, *1:*172–173
striatal release, *1:*171–172
narcolepsy therapy:
amphetamine targeting, *3:*92–94
adverse effects, *3:*98
anatomical substrates, *3:*97–98
drug interactions, *3:*98, *3:*100
EEG arousal and, *3:*94–97
modafinil, *3:*102–103
nicotine dependence and withdrawal, withdrawal substrates, *2:*542–543
obsessive-compulsive disorders, *2:*223
Parkinson's disease, *1:*236
Parkinson's disease neurochemistry and, *3:*481–483
invertebrate models of cell death, *3:*569–577
polymorphisms, splice variants and SNPs, *1:*234–236
psychostimulant abuse, *2:*569–575
neuropeptide pharmacology, *2:*579
neuropharmacology, *2:*570–575
schizophrenia, *1:*237, *2:*260–262
COMT catabolism and, *2:*328
drug targeting innovations, *2:*389
signal transduction pathways, *1:*230–232
structure-affinity/structure-activity relationships, *1:*232–234
substance abuse, *1:*238
Tourette's syndrome, *3:*270–273
Dopaminergic receptors:
alcholol abuse studies, neuronal systems and substrates, *2:*471–486
bed nucleus of stria terminalis, *2:*473–475
dopaminergic regulation, early research, *2:*472–473
extracellular dopamine, *2:*485–486
future research issues, *2:*517–518
GABAergic interactions with, *2:*486
lateral hypothalamus, *2:*481–485
D_2 dopaminergic regulation, hypothesized mechanisms, *2:*481–485
ventral pallidum, *2:*476–480
hypothesized mechanisms, *2:*478–480
alcohol abuse studies, in alcohol-preferring rats, *2:*471
anxiety neurobiology and receptor deficits, *2:*29–30
autism spectrum disorders, medications, *3:*325–330

human immunodeficiency virus:
  nigrostriatal system and, 3:710–711
  opioid abuse and, 3:715–716
nicotine dependence and withdrawal, nicotine reinforcement substrates, 2:538–540
psychostimulant abuse:
  chronic exposure and sensitization effects, 2:582–585
  glutamatergic interactions, 2:575–576
  monoamine neuropharmacology, 2:571–575
  schizophrenia molecular genetics, functional candidate genes, 2:331–332
Tourette's syndrome, 3:266–267
Dopamine transporters:
  attention-deficit hyperactivity disorder therapy, 3:297–298
  catechol-O-methyl transferase, as schizophrenia susceptibility gene, 2:347–348
  chronic substrate treatment, 1:726
  clinical relevance, 1:721
  inhibitors, psychostimulant therapy targeting, 2:587–588
  multiple interactions, 1:723–724
  obsessive-compulsive disorders, abnormalities, 2:219–220
  polymorphisms, 1:724–725
  psychostimulant abuse, monoamine neuropharmacology, 2:573–575
  schizophrenia, dopamine hypothesis and, 2:285
  structure and function, 1:712–713
Dopaminomimetic agents, Parkinson's disease, 3:484–496
  apomorphine, 3:493–494
  bromocriptine, 3:488, 3:490
  cabergoline, 3:491
  COMT inhibitors, 3:495
  dihydroergocryptine, 3:491
  dopamine agonists, 3:488–494
  entacapone, 3:496
  levodopa plus peripheral decarboxylase inhibitor, 3:484–487
  levodopa slow-release formulations, 3:487–488
  lisuride, 3:491
  monoamine oxidase type B inhibitor, 3:494
  pergolide, 3:490–491
  piribedil, 3:493
  pramipexole, 3:491–492
  rasagiline, 3:495
  ropinirole, 3:492
  selegiline, 3:494–495
  stalevo, 3:496
  tolcapone, 3:495
Dorsolateral prefrontal cortex (DLPFC), schizophrenia dopamine hypothesis, 2:373
Dose failure, Parkinson's disease treatment and, 3:499
Downregulation:
  muscarinic acetylcholine receptors, 1:163–164
  neuropeptide receptors, 1:688–689
Downstream signaling molecules, ion channel modulation, 1:69–70
Downstream techniques, stroke management, 3:366–373
DRD2/DRD3 receptors, schizophrenia molecular genetics, 2:331–332
  catechol-O-methyl transferase susceptibility gene, 2:347–348
Drosophila models:
  Alzheimer's disease, 3:580–582
  drug effects in, 3:7–8
  Huntingdon's disease trinucleotide repeats, 3:578–579
  neurodegenerative disease:
    genetic and molecular pathways, 3:569
    Parkinson's disease cell death, 3:570–577
  rhythmicity in, 3:7
Drug abuse. See also Addictive disorders; specific drugs, e.g. Psychostimulants
  dopaminergic drugs for, 1:238–239
  dopaminergic receptor systems and substrates, bed nucleus of stria terminalis system, 2:474–475
  Drosophila models, 3:7–8
  GABA$_B$ receptor targeting, 1:593–594
  in HIV/AIDS, 3:712–716
    methamphetamine/cocaine, 3:713–715
    opioid drugs, 3:715–716
  muscarinic acetylcholine receptor deficiency, 1:173
  rewarding/reinforcing effects in, 2:459
  sereotonin receptor 5-HT$_{2C}$ and, 1:272–273
  serotonin transporters and, 1:720

stress-induced response, neuroactive steroid effects and, 2:159–160
Drug discovery, neurotrophic factors and, 3:230–232
Drug interactions:
  α_1 adrenergic receptors, 1:202–203
  dopaminergic receptors, 1:236–239
    attention-deficit hyperactivity disorder, 1:237–238
    bipolar disorders, 1:237
    Parkinson's disease, 1:236
    schizophrenia, 1:237
  muscarinic acetylcholine receptors, 1:154
  narcolepsy therapy, amphetamines, 3:98, 3:100
Drug-resistant epilepsy, 3:425–426
Dyadic encounters, schizophrenia, animal models, 2:264
Dynorphins, structure and classification, 2:747
Dysbindin, dystrobrevin binding protein 1 (DTNBP1):
  molecular interactions, 2:353
  schizophrenia candidate gene, 2:326, 2:348–349
Dysiherbaine, kainate receptor orthosteric agonists, 1:380
Dyskinesia, Parkinson's disease treatment and:
  classification of, 3:499
  levodopa agents, 3:487
Dystrobrevin binding protein 1 (DTNBP1), schizophrenia candidate gene, 2:325–326
  chomosome mapping, 2:346
  chromosome identification of, 2:348–349
  functional implications, 2:332–333
  molecular interactions, 2:352–353
Dystrophin-associated glycoprotein complex (DCG), dystrobrevin binding protein 1 identification, schizophrenia candidate gene, 2:348–349

EAG genes, KCNH potassium channels, 1:633–634
Effector systems, $GABA_B$ receptors, 1:580–583
  adenylate cyclase, 1:582–583
  calcium channels, 1:581–582
  G-protein-dependent/independent $GABA_B$ effects, 1:580–581
  MAPKs, 1:583
  potassium channels, 1:582
Electrical stimulation, epilepsy management, 3:427
Electrocoagulation model, stroke-related global and focal ischemia, 3:353–354
Electroencephalogram (EEG):
  epilepsy investigation, 3:405–407
  narcolepsy therapy, dopaminergic neurotransmission and, 3:94–95
Electroencephalography (EEG), schizophrenia analysis, 2:256
Electrophysiology:
  histaminergic neuron activity, 1:317
  neuropeptides, 1:675–677
    neurohormones, 1:675–676
    neuromodulators, 1:676–677
    neurotransmitters, 1:676
  potassium channels, 1:625
Electrospray ionization mass spectrometry (ESI-MS), nitrosothiol detection, 1:747–748
Elevated-plus maze (EPM):
  animal anxiety-like behavior and, 2:12
  neurosteroid effects, 2:143–145
  emotionalty studies in mice, 2:7–9
Elevated-zero maze (EZM), emotionalty studies in mice, 2:8–9
Elimination mechanisms, nicotine dependence and withdrawal, 2:544–545
Eliprodil, stroke management, 3:357, 3:359
ELK genes, KCNH potassium channels, 1:633–634
Emesis. See Nausea and vomiting
Emotionality studies, anxiety neurobiology, rodent models, 2:6–9
Enantiomeric selectivity, neuroactive steroids, 2:141–142
Endocannabinoids, 2:662–665
  cannabinoid receptors and signaling, 2:662–663
  packaging of, 1:46
  physiology and pharmacology, 2:665–675
  prenatal developmental effects, 2:664–665
  reward, tolerance and dependence mechanisms, 2:675–676
  synthesis and metabolism, 1:45, 2:663–664
Endocrine system, hypocretin/orexin system, 3:134–135

Endocytosis, neuropeptide receptor downregulation, *1:*688–689
Endogenous opioids, classification, *2:*746–748
Endogenous sites, benzodiazepine ligands, *2:*98–99
β-Endorphins, structure and classification, *2:*747–748
Endothelial cells, neuroinflammation, *3:*627
　pharmacological activation, *3:*633
Endothelium-derived relaxing factor (EDRF), nitric oxide and, *1:*743–745
End-plate potentials, early research on, *1:*26–27
Energy expenditure, leptin and, *3:*743–744
Enkephalins:
　nicotine dependence and withdrawal, *2:*540
　structure and function, *2:*746–747
Enthoprotin, schizophrenia molecular genetics, *2:*328
Entrainment stimuli:
　circadian rhythms, *3:*5
　clock neuron synchronization and modulation, *3:*8–9
Environmental factors:
　addictive disorders vulnerability, *2:*457–458
　anxiety neurobiology, early-life experience, *2:*33–34
　idiopathic Parkinson's disease and, *3:*543–545
　Tourette's syndrome, *3:*267–269
Enzymes:
　in myelin, *3:*609–610
　neurotransmitter biosynthesis, *1:*42–43
Ephedrine, as anti-obesity agent, *3:*817–818
Epibatidine, nicotinic acetylcholine receptors, *1:*121
Epilepsy:
　acute seizures and status epilepticus, *3:*427–428
　alternative therapies, *3:*426–427
　antiepileptic drugs, *3:*404–405
　　calcium channels, *3:*413–414
　　clinical efficacy, *3:*418
　　clinical prediction markers, *3:*420
　　combination therapy, *3:*423–424
　　development and testing, *3:*418–420
　　felbamate interactions, *3:*414–415
　　GABA$_A$ receptor and, *3:*411–412
　　generalized absence epilepsy, *3:*421
　　localization-related epilepsy, *3:*421–423
　　mechanisms of action, *3:*408–410
　　metabotropic glutamate receptors, *3:*413
　　mixed actions, *3:*414–418, *3:*422
　　secondary generalized epilepsies, *3:*424
　　selection criteria, *3:*421–424
　　sodium channel modulation, *3:*411
　　special population requirements, *3:*424–425
　　synaptic vesicle protein, *3:*414
　　topiramate interactions, *3:*415–418
　　toxicity detection, limitations of, *3:*420–421
　child-onset absence, classification, *3:*405–406
　classification, *3:*404–405
　clinical investigation, *3:*405–408
　diet and, *3:*427
　drug-resistant, *3:*425–426
　electrical stimulation therapy, *3:*427
　endocannabinoids and, *2:*672–673
　focal/localization-related epilepsy:
　　classification, *3:*405–406
　　prognosis, *3:*408
　　therapy for, *3:*421, *3:*423
　future research issues, *3:*428–429
　GABA$_A$ β subunit pharmacology, *1:*490–491
　GABA$_B$ receptor therapy, *1:*595
　generalized absence form, therapy options, *3:*421
　histamine neuron physiology, *1:*326
　muscarinic acetylcholine receptor deficiency, *1:*169
　NMDA orthosteric antagonists, *1:*375–377
　prognosis of, *3:*407–408
　secondary generalized epilepsy syndrome:
　　classification, *3:*405–406
　　therapy options, *3:*424
　surgical management of, *3:*426
　temporal lobe epilepsy:
　　classification, *3:*405–406
　　surgical treatment, *3:*426
　voltage-gated sodium ion channels and, *1:*642
Epinephrine:
　α-adrenergic receptors, α$_2$-adrenergic receptor, *1:*205–206

β-adrenergic receptor activation, *1:*209–210
basic properties, *1:*193
dopamine synthesis, *1:*223–224
historical perspective, *1:*194–196
neurochemistry, *1:*198–199
physiology, *1:*197–198
white adipose tissue innervation, *3:*789–797
Episodic ataxia type 1 (EA-1), voltage-gated potassium channels, K_V subunits, structure and function, *1:*629–630
EPO receptor (EPOR), stroke therapy and, *3:*377
ErbB3 gene:
NRG1 molecular interaction, *2:*353–355
regulator of G-protein signaling 4 schizophrenia candidate gene, *2:*328
Ergot:
early research on, *1:*15–16
migraine management, *2:*765
Erythropoietin (EPO):
neuroinflammatory mechanisms, *3:*641
stroke therapy and, *3:*377
Escitalopram, autism spectrum disorders, *3:*324–325
Estradiol, postpartum depression and levels of, *1:*849
Estrogen receptors, histaminergic neuron activity, *1:*325
Estrogen response element (ERE), leptin receptor expression and, *3:*738–739
Estrogens:
neuroinflammation and, *3:*645
traumatic brain injury and, *3:*450–451
Ethanol. *See* Alcohol
Ethosuximide:
development and testing, *3:*419
epilepsy efficacy, *3:*417–418
for generalized absence epilepsy, *3:*421
T-type calcium channel modulation, *3:*413
Eticlopride, alcohol abuse studies:
lateral hypothalamus, effects on, *2:*481–485
ventral pallidum receptor blockade, *2:*478
Evolutionary relationships:
neuropeptides, *1:*679–685
gene duplication, *1:*680–685
gene splicing, *1:*685
neurohypophyseal family, *1:*682–684
NPY family, *1:*684
opioid family, *1:*680–682
structural conservation, *1:*679–680
voltage-gated ion channels, *1:*619–620
Excessive daytime sleepiness (EDS):
idiopathic hypersomnia and, *3:*84
mazindol therapy, *3:*103
narcolepsy, *3:*80–82
amphetamines, *3:*90–100
drug interactions with, *3:*98, *3:*100
molecular targeting of, *3:*93–94
side effects, *3:*98
bupropion, *3:*103–105
caffeine, *3:*104–105
dopamine neurotransmitters, substrates, *3:*97–98
dopamine neurotransmitters and EEG arousal, *3:*94–97
future stimulant development, *3:*105–106
mazindol, *3:*103
modafinal, *3:*100–103
nonamphetamine stimulants, *3:*99–105
pharmacological treatment, *3:*90–100
selegiline, *3:*104
Excitatory amino acid transporters (EAATs):
glutamate neurotransmitters, *1:*53–54
glutamate theory of schizophrenia, pathological evidence, *2:*292
plasma membrane glutamate transporter, clinical relevance, *1:*718–719
plasma membrane glutamate transporters, *1:*708–711
schizophrenia genetics, GRM3 gene, *2:*349
stroke management, *3:*365–366
Excitatory mechanisms in stroke:
AMPA receptor antagonists, *3:*361–363
amphetamine and neurotransmitter modulators, *3:*377
antiadhesion molecules, *3:*369–370
anti-nogo (IN-1) inhibitors, *3:*377–378
antioxidants, *3:*371–372
apoptosis and caspase inhibitors, *3:*372–373
basic characteristics and symptoms, *3:*348–349
brain injury with:
classification, *3:*350
mechanisms of, *3:*351–353
repair approaches, *3:*377–379

calcium channel blockers, 3:366–367
chemokine inhibition, 3:369
cytokine inhibition, 3:368–369
decahydroisoguinolines, 3:362
down-stream approaches, 3:367–368
erythropoietin, 3:377
global/focal ischemia, animal models, 3:353–354
glutamate/glutamatergic receptors, 3:354–355, 3:361–366
glutamate release inhibitors, 3:366–367
glutamate transporters, 3:365–366
growth factors, 3:375–377
GYKI 52466/related benzodiazepines, 3:362
inflammatory pathways, 3:368
kainate receptor antagonists, 3:363
metabotropic glutamate receptors, 3:363–365
NBQX/related quinoxalinediones, 3:361–362
neuroprotective techniques, 3:366–373
  development criteria, 3:374
nitric oxide synthase inhibition, 3:370–371
NMDA receptor antagonists, 3:354–359
  clinical trial data, 3:358–359
  competitive/noncompetitive agonists, 3:356–357
  glycine site antagonists, 3:357–358
  MK-801 compound, 3:355–356
  polyamine site antagonists, 3:357
  side effects, 3:359–360
p38 inhibition, 3:369
prevalence and incidence, 3:349–350
sodium channel blockers, 3:367
sonic hedgehog approach, 3:378
stem cell approach, 3:378–379
time window issues, 3:360–361
upstream techniques, 3:366–373
Excitatory neurotransmitters, hypocretin/orexin system, 3:131–132
Excitatory postsynaptic potentials (EPSPs):
  early research on, 1:28–29
  mGlu2 allosteric potentiators, 1:438–439
  neuropeptides and, 1:676–677
Excitatory reponses:
  H_1 receptor, 1:309–311
  H_2 receptor, 1:312–313
Excitotoxicity cell death, human immunodeficiency virus and, 3:705–706

Exocrine pancreas, amylase secretion, muscarinic acetylcholine receptor deficiency, 1:175
Exocytosis, neuropeptide electrophysiology, 1:676
Experimental allergic encephalomyelitis (EAE):
  natalizumab, 3:684–685
  novel therapy for, 3:678–679
  pathogenesis, cytokines and, 3:628–629
  pathophysiology, 3:611–612
  statin therapy, 3:668
Extended amygala (EA), alcohol abuse studies:
  dopaminergic receptor systems and substrates, 2:473–474
  $GABA_A$ benzodiazepine receptor complex manipulation, site-specific microinjection studies, 2:493–496
Extended-release stimulants, attention-deficit hyperactivity disorder therapy, 3:295
Extracellular calcium, $GABA_B$ receptor modulation, 1:584
Extracellular catabolism, dopamine synthesis, 1:55
Extracellular domain (ECD), $GABA_B$ receptors:
  modulation, 1:585–587
  sites, 1:578–579
  subtypes, 1:573–575
Extracellular dopamine, alcohol abuse studies, dopaminergic regulation mechanisms, 2:485–486
Extracellular inactivation, neuropeptides, 1:687–688
Extracellular matrix (ECM), nitrosylation and, 1:751–752
Extracellular signal-related kinases (ERK):
  brain-derived neurotrophic factor in depressed patients and, 1:801
  ERK1/ERK2 protein kinases, tyrosine kinase receptor signal transduction, 3:243
  $GABA_B$ receptors, effector systems, 1:583
  lithium mechanism in bipolar disorder patients, 1:867–869
  muscarinic acetylcholine receptor modulation, 1:159
  phosphorylation, 1:89–90

Extrapyramidal symptoms (EPS):
  atypical antipsychotic drugs, 2:411–412
    clozapine D_2 receptor blockade, 2:412–415
  schizophrenia therapy:
    antipsychotics and, 2:370–371
    D_2 receptor occupancy and effect, 2:376–378
    D_2 receptor occupancy thresholds and rapid dissociation, 2:379–380
    first-generation antipsychotics, 2:383
    second-generation antipsychotics, 2:383–388
    serotonin receptor 5-HT_{2A} blockade, 2:422
  Tourette's syndrome therapy, 3:274–276
Extrasynaptic receptors, $GABA_A$ receptor structure, sedative/hypnotic mechanisms, 3:180
Extroversion vs. introversion (E trait), anxiety neurobiology, 2:5–6

Face validity, animal anxiety-like behavior and, 2:12
"Fail-safe" mechanism, stress response and, 1:695
Famotidine, histaminergic neuron activity, 1:327
Fas-associated death domain (FADD) protein, stroke management, 3:373
Fast inactivation, potassium channels, 1:627
Fatty acid amide hydrolase (FAAH):
  convulsant effects of, 2:672–673
  emesis modulation, 2:674–675
  endocannabinoid ligands, 2:664
  endocannabinoid physiology and, 2:666
Fatty acid binding proteins (FABP), protein 2, 3:603
Fatty acids:
  $GABA_A$ receptor modulation, 1:520
  metabolism, overview of, 3:785–786
Fear/anxiety circuits, anxiety neurobiology, 2:13–15
Fear-potentiated startle, mouse anxiety models, neurosteroid effects, 2:147
Feeding mechanisms. See also Appetite regulation
  ghrelin effects, 3:772–773
  histaminergic neuron activity, 1:320–322
  hypocretin/orexin system, 3:132–134
    arousal integration, 3:144
  leptin signaling and, 3:740–743

  muscarinic acetylcholine receptor deficiency, 1:171
  prokineticin regulation, 3:168–169
Felbamate:
  epilepsy efficacy, 3:417–418
  ionotropic glutamate receptor modulation, 3:413
  for secondary generalized epilepsy, 3:424
  target interactions of, 3:414–415
Feverfew, migraine management, 2:768
FEZ1 protein, DISC1 schizophrenia candidate gene, molecular interactions, 2:351–352
Fibroblast growth factor (FGF):
  antidepressant influences on, 1:805–806
  in depressed patients, 1:802
  intracellular signaling, 1:793
  stroke therapy and, 3:375–377
Filamin, voltage-gated potassium channels, 1:628
First-generation antipsychotics (FGAs), schizophrenia therapy:
  clinical profiles, 2:383
  D_2 receptor occupancy and effect, 2:376–378
  history of, 2:370–371
  NMDA receptor antagonists, 2:381
  second-generation antipsychotic comparisons, 2:384–387
Fixed-ratio (FR) schedule, alcohol abuse studies in alcohol-preferring rats, 2:469
FKBP5 cochaperone, stress-monoamine convergence in depression, 1:825–826
FKBP12 protein, multiple sclerosis therapy, 3:667
Flavonoids, $GABA_A$ subunit pharmacology, allosteric ligand modulation, 1:505–506
Flenfluramine, as anti-obesity agent, 3:818
Flip/flop exons:
  AMPA receptor allosteric potentiators, 1:393
  AMPA receptors, 1:370–371
Fluid extravasation, inflammation and, pharmacological activation, 3:633
Flumazenil:
  alcohol abuse studies:
    $GABA_{A5}$ receptor specificity, 2:512–516
    $GABA_A$ benzodiazepine receptor complex, 2:490–493

endogenous ligand sites, 2:98–99
GABA$_A$ α$_6$ subunit pharmacology,
    1:489–490
Flunitrazepam, overview, 2:637
Fluorodeoxyglucose (FDG) studies,
    schizophrenia analysis, 2:257
Fluorometry, nitrosothiol detection, 1:748
Fluoxetine:
    autism spectrum disorders, 3:323–324
    circadian rhythms and, antidepressant
        effects, 3:19–20
    3,4-methylenedioxymethamphetamine
        effects on, 2:616, 2:627
    neurogenesis and, 3:209–210
    nicotine dependence and withdrawal,
        withdrawal substrate specificity,
        2:542–543
Fluphenazine, adrenergic receptor
    mechanisms, 2:427
Fluvoxamine:
    autism spectrum disorders, 3:322–323
    circadian rhythms and release of, 3:20
Follicle-stimulating hormone, in menopause,
    1:851
4P-PDOT antagonist, melatonin receptor
    molecular pharmacology, 3:43–44
    circadian rhythm modulation, 3:55–57
    desensitization function, 3:53
    in suprachiasmatic nucleus, 3:49–50
Free-radical formation:
    3,4-methylenedioxymethamphetamine
        neurotoxicity, 2:624
    traumatic brain injury and, 3:447
Frontal cortex abnormalities, glutamate
    theory of schizophrenia,
    pathological evidence, 2:292
FTY720 agent, multiple sclerosis therapy,
    3:689
Functional candidate genes, schizophrenia
    molecular genetics, 2:331–332
Functional imaging studies:
    obsessive-compulsive disorders, 2:219–220
    schizophrenia analysis, 2:257–260
Functional recovery, stroke therapy and,
    3:375–379
Fyn tyrosine kinase, anxiety neurobiology
    and, 2:31

GABA$_A$-benzodiazepine receptor complex,
    alcohol abuse studies, 2:487–501
    alcohol/modulator commonalities,
        2:487–488

CA1/CA3 hippocampus, 2:511–516
efficacy of βCCT/3PBD modulation,
    GABA$_{A1,2,3,5}$ receptors, 2:499–501
future research issues, 2:517–518
GABA-DA interaction hypothesis,
    2:496–498
ligand selectivity with GABA$_{A1}$ subunits,
    2:498–499
microinjection studies, 2:505–506
naltrexone antagonist, 2:507–511
novel CNS GABAergic substrates, 2:498
oral administration, βCCT/3PBD:
    anxiety reduction, 2:510–511
    vs. naltrexone, 2:507–511
probe applications, 2:488–493
site-specific microinjection, 2:493–496
subunit selectivity vs. intrinsic efficacy,
    2:516–517
systemic administration, 2:492–493,
    2:503–504
ventral pallidum, 2:501–502
GABAergic neurons:
    alcohol abuse studies:
        in alcohol-preferring rats, 2:471
        bed nucleus of stria terminalis system,
            2:474
        dopamine agonist modification,
            2:496–498
        GABA$_{A5}$ receptor specificity, 2:512–516
        novel substrates, 2:498
        ventral pallidum dopaminergic
            regulation and, 2:479–480
    cannabinoid$_1$ (CB-1) receptors and,
        2:672–673
    H$_2$ receptor, 1:313
    histaminergic neuron activity, 1:319–322
    integrated glutamate/dopamine
        hypotheses of schizophrenia,
        2:375–376
    Parkinson's disease treatment and,
        3:505–506
    psychostimulant abuse, 2:574–575
        chronic exposure and sensitization
            effects, 2:583–585
        γ-aminobutyric acid (GABA) receptors
            and, 2:576–577
        novel therapeutic developments, 2:588
    sedative/hypnotic action sites, 3:184
    Tourette's syndrome and, 3:270–273
Gabapentin:
    anxiety disorder therapy, amino acid
        neurotransmission, 2:75

calcium channel modulation, *3:*413–414
epilepsy efficacy, *3:*417–418
migraine management, *2:*766–767
voltage-gated calcium ion channels,
    auxiliary subunit modulators,
    *1:*650
GABARAP polypeptide, GABA$_A$ receptors:
    benzodiazepines, *2:*109–110
    trafficking, *1:*478–480
"GABA shift" assay, alcohol abuse studies,
    GABA$_A$ benzodiazepine receptor
    complex, subunit selectivity *vs.*
    intrinsic efficacy, *2:*517
GABA transporters (GATs), structure and
    function, *1:*711–712
GAD protein, in bipolar disorder patients,
    *1:*862
Galanin, histaminergic neuron activity,
    *1:*318–319
Galantamine:
    dementia disorders and, *3:*463–465
    schizophrenia pharmacotherapy,
    *2:*393–394
γ-aminobutyric acid (GABA) receptors:
    addictive disorders, modulator therapy
    and, *2:*458–459
    adult neurogenesis and, *1:*829
    agonist binding site architecture,
    *1:*494–495
    anxiety disorder therapy, amino acid
    neurotransmission, *2:*72–75
    anxiety neurobiology and, *2:*15–17
        knockout mice deficit studies,
        *2:*26–30
    binding-to-gating transduction, *1:*495–497
    in bipolar disorder patients, *1:*861–862
    cannabinoid receptors and, neurotoxicity
    effects, *2:*673
    channel blocker binding sites, *1:*518–519
    channel pore ion selectivity, *1:*497–498
    early research on, *1:*32, *1:*466
    GABA$_A$ receptors:
        alcohol abuse studies:
            novel substrates, *2:*498
            ventral pallidum dopaminergic
            regulation and, *2:*479–480
        allosteric modulation:
            benzodiazepine recognition site,
            *1:*499–506
            structural determinants, *1:*507–509
        α$_1$ subunit:
            alcohol abuse studies, *2:*498–501
            microinjection techniques,
            *2:*505–507
            ventral pallidum selectivity,
            *2:*501–503
        α subunit, *1:*483–490, *1:*509–511
            α$_1$ subunit, *1:*484, *1:*488
            α$_2$ subunit, *1:*488
            α$_3$ subunit, *1:*488
            α$_4$ subunit, *1:*488–489
            α$_5$ subunit, *1:*489
            as alcohol substrate probes,
            *2:*511–516
            α$_6$ subunit, *1:*489–490
            electrophysiology, *1:*486–487
            modulator selectivity, *1:*484
            terminology, *1:*483
        antiepileptic drugs and, *3:*411–412
            felbamate, *3:*414–415
            topiramate, *3:*415–416
        assembly, *1:*477–478
        benzodiazepine binding site, *1:*506–507
            subunit isoforms, *1:*509–511
        benzodiazepines:
            assembly, clustering, and surface
            expression, *2:*108–110
            binding pocket, *2:*105–108
            brain function diversity, *2:*110–112
            functional diversity, knockout/
            knockin models, *2:*112–114
            single-cell response modulation,
            *2:*99–100
            subunit/subtype diversity, *2:*103–104
        β subunit pharmacology, *1:*490–491
        δ subunit pharmacology, *1:*491–492
        desensitization and deactivation,
        *1:*498–499
        ε subunit distribution, *1:*472, *1:*492
        γ subunit pharmacology, *1:*491–492,
        *1:*509–511
        hetero-oligomeric structure, *1:*476–477
        homo-oligomeric structure, *1:*476
        modulation mechanisms, *1:*511–516
        neuroactive steroids, *2:*137–141
        pharmacology, *1:*482–483
        phosphorylation, *1:*481–482
        π subunit distribution, *1:*472, *1:*492
        rare subunits, *1:*492
        ρ subunit distribution, *1:*472
        sedatives:
            benzodiazepine binding, *3:*190–192
            pharmacology, *3:*180–181
            structure, *3:*178–180

structure, *1:*475
subcellular distribution, *1:*473–475
θ subunit distribution, *1:*472, *1:*492
trafficking, *1:*478–481
transmembrane domain allosteric sites, subunits, *1:*516–518
unidentified allosteric modulation, *1:*519–520
GABA$_B$ receptors:
alcohol abuse studies, ventral pallidum dopaminergic regulation and, *2:*479–480
deficient mice, *1:*587–588
effector systems, *1:*580–583
endogenous GABA$_B$ ligands, *1:*588–589
endogenous ligands, *1:*588–589
expression cloning, *1:*571–572
γ-hydroxybutyric acid (GHB) mechanisms and, *2:*634–635
G-protein coupling determinants, *1:*579–580
ligand binding sites, *1:*578–579
modulation, *1:*584–586
 extracellular calcium, *1:*584
 interacting proteins, *1:*585–587
 phosphorylation and desensitization, *1:*584–585
modulation mechanisms, *1:*584–586
molecular subtypes, *1:*572–575
novel compounds, *1:*590–592
structure and function, *1:*570–571
trafficking and heteromization, *1:*575–578
histaminergic perikarya, *1:*302–303
ion channel modulation, protein-protein interaction, *1:*70–71
metabotropic receptors:
agonists and competitive antagonists, *1:*589–590
disease and, *1:*592–597
 anxiety and depression, *1:*594–595
 drug addiction, *1:*593–594
 epilepsy, *1:*595
 gene linkage studies, *1:*596–597
 nociception, *1:*595–596
 therapeutic targeting, GABA$_B$ receptors, *1:*592–593
 tumor cell growth and migration, *1:*596
effector systems, *1:*580–583
 adenylate cyclase, *1:*582–583
 calcium channels, *1:*581–582

G-protein-dependent/indepdendent GABA$_B$ effects, *1:*580–581
 MAPKs, *1:*583
 potassium channels, *1:*582
research background, *1:*570–571
structural properties, *1:*571–580
 allosteric interactions, *1:*580
 expression cloning, *1:*571–572
 G-protein coupling determinants, *1:*579–580
 liganding binding sites, *1:*578–579
 molecular subtypes, *1:*572–575
 surface trafficking and heteromerization, *1:*575–578
migraine management with anticonvulsants, *2:*766–767
narcolepsy therapy, modafinil, *3:*101–103
neuroactive steroids, enantiomeric selectivity, *2:*141–142
neuropeptides and, *1:*671
nicotine dependence and withdrawal, nicotine reinforcement substrates, *2:*538–540
NRG1 molecular interaction, *2:*354–355
plasma membrane neurotransmitter transporters:
 clinical relevance, *1:*721–722
 interacting protein regulation, *1:*728
 structure and function, *1:*711–712
psychostimulant abuse and, *2:*576–577
receptor classifications A, B, and C, *1:*468–469
schizophrenia neurochemistry and, *2:*261–262
structural determinants of activation, *1:*492–494
subunit genes, *1:*469–470
 central nervous system distribution, *1:*471–473
suprachiasmatic nucleus and, *3:*13–15
transmitter inactivation, *1:*51–52
transporters, *1:*467–468
traumatic brain injury and, *3:*451
γ-hydroxybutyric acid (GHB):
 addiction risk, *2:*635–636
 cataplexy therapy, *3:*112
 disturbed nocturnal sleep therapy, *3:*112
 mechanism of action, *2:*634–635
 overview, *2:*632–633
 pharmacological effects, *2:*633–634
 sleep paralysis and hypnagogic hallucination therapy, *3:*112

Gamma glutamate analogs, kainate receptor orthosteric agonists, *1:*378–379
γ-glutamyl transpeptidase, nitric oxide nitrosilyation, *1:*747
Ganaxolone, GABA$_A$ receptor modulation, *1:*515–516
Gaseous signaling:
  carbon monoxide, *1:*756–757
  future research, *1:*757
  nitric oxide:
    basic principles, *1:*743–744
    neurodegeneration and, *1:*754
    nitrosothiol detection, *1:*747–748
    nitrosylation mechanism, *1:*745–747
      cell survival, *1:*752
      extracellular matrix, *1:*751–752
      gene transport, *1:*750–751
      ion channels, *1:*748–749
      Parkinson's disease and, *1:*755–756
      protein-protein interactions, *1:*749–750
      S nitrosylation physiology, *1:*752–754
      vesicular transport, *1:*751
    physiological role, *1:*745
  packaging of, *1:*46
  synthesis, *1:*45
Gastic acid secretion, muscarinic acetylcholine receptor deficiency, *1:*175
Gastrointestinal tract:
  disorders, serotonin transporters and, *1:*720
  ghrelin modulation, *3:*776
"Gate control" theory, classification of, *2:*713–714
Gating mechanisms, voltage-gated potassium channels, *1:*626–627
Gavestinel, stroke management, *3:*359
GBA polymorphisms, idiopathic Parkinson's disease and, *3:*543
Gβγ signaling, to ion channels, *1:*67–69
GBR12909, narcolepsy therapy, dopaminergic neurotransmission, *3:*94–95
Geller-Seifter conflict test:
  mGlu5 allosteric antagonists, *1:*444
  mouse models of anxiety, *2:*8–9
  neurosteroid effects, *2:*145–146
Gene duplication, neuropeptides, *1:*680–682
Gene expression:
  neuropeptides, *1:*685
  psychostimulant abuse, chronic exposure and sensitization effects, *2:*584–585

Gene linkage studies, schizophrenia, *2:*323–324
  future research issues, *2:*355–356
  susceptibility gene identification, *2:*344–351
Generalized anxiety disorder (GAD):
  buspirone therapy, *2:*71
  pharmacotherapy, *2:*77
  serotonin/noradrenaline reuptake inhibitors, *2:*69
  tricyclic antidepressants, *2:*69–70
Gene splicing:
  neuropeptides, *1:*685
  plasma membrane transporter regulation, *1:*725
Gene therapy, vesicular transporters and, *1:*723
Genetic absence-epilepsy rats from Strasbourg (GAERS), GABA$_B$ receptors, *1:*595
Genetic studies. *See also* Gene linkage studies; Molecular genetics
  addictive disorders vulnerability, *2:*457–458
  α$_1$ adrenergic receptors, *1:*201–202
  β-adrenergic receptor physiology, *1:*211–213
  anxiety neurobiology, *2:*4–6
    environmental effects and, *2:*34–35
    susceptibility studies, *2:*18–19
  BDNF in mood disorders, *1:*803
  bipolar disorder, *1:*860
  GABA$_A$ receptor subunits, *1:*469–470
  GABA$_B$ receptor targeting, *1:*596–597
  glutamate theory of schizophrenia, *2:*293–294
  neuropeptides, *1:*678–679
    knockout mice, *1:*678
    transgenic animals, *1:*678
  norepinephrine transporter, *1:*200–201
  obsessive-compulsive disorders, *2:*222–224
    developmental genes, *2:*223–224
    dopamine, *2:*223
    glutamate, *2:*223
    neurotransmitter metabolism, *2:*223
    serotonin, *2:*222–224
  Parkinson's disease and, *1:*755–756
  schizophrenia, *2:*262–263
    animal models, *2:*264
    dopamine hypothesis, *2:*286–287

epidemiology, pathophysiology, and neurobiology, 2:323
Tourette's syndrome, 3:266–267
Gene transcription, nitrosylation and, 1:750–751
Genome sequencing, potassium channels, 1:621–623
Genomics:
neuropeptides and, 1:678–679
Tourette's syndrome, 3:267
Gephyrin, GABA$_A$ receptor clusters, 1:478–480
Gepirone, anxiety disorder therapy, 2:71
GHB (Xyrem), GABA$_B$ receptor targeting, 1:592–593
Ghrelin:
acylated peptide hormone, 3:766–768
adipocyte and body composition modulation, 3:774
agonists/antagonists, 3:777
antiproliferative/proliferative effect, 3:776
appetite and metabolic regulation, 3:772–773
bone effects, 3:776
cardiovacsular action, 3:774–775
expression pattern, 3:768–769
gastrointestinal tract function, 3:776
growth hormone secretagogues, 3:769
growth hormone secretion, 3:773–774
immune system modulation, 3:775
pancreas function and insulin resistance, 3:775–776
peripheral function, 3:774–776
receptor:
constitutive activity, 3:770–771
homologous subfamily, 3:771–772
receptor ligands, 3:766–769
research history on, 3:766
sympathetic nervous system, 3:774
thyroid function, 3:775
Giant depolarizing potentials, GABA transporters, 1:467–468
GLAST knockout mice, plasma membrane glutamate transporters, 1:711
Glatiramer acetate, multiple sclerosis therapy, 3:676
Glia-derived protein, GABA$_A$ receptors, benzodiazepines, 2:108–110
Glial cells:
human immunodeficiency virus, excitotoxicity cell death, 3:706

myelin-forming, 3:592–593
neurotrophins and, 3:239
Glial-derived neurotrophic factor (GDNF):
amyotrophic lateral sclerosis and, 3:226–227
discovery of, 3:221–223
future research on, 3:232–233
neuroinflammatory mechanisms, 3:641
neuronal maturation regulation, 3:224
pain perception and management, 3:229
Parkinson's disease and, 3:228–229, 3:505
Glial-derived neurotrophic factor (GDNF), intracellular signaling, 1:793–794
Glial proliferation:
antidepressant influences on, 1:807
stress and, 1:800
Glial transporters, stroke management, 3:365–366
GLT1 knockout mice, plasma membrane glutamate transporters, 1:711
Glucagon-like peptide 1 (GLP1), leptin signaling and and feeding regulation, 3:743
Glucagon-like peptides, neuropeptide inactivation, 1:687–688
Glucagon secretion, muscarinic acetylcholine receptor deficiency, 1:174–175
Glucocorticoid receptor (GR), stress-induced behaviors, neuroactive steroids, 2:153–154
Glucocorticoid receptor (GR) transcription factor, anxiety neurobiology and, 2:31
Glucocorticoids:
anxiety neurobiology and, 2:17
in bipolar disorder patients, 1:861–862
neurogenesis regulation by, 1:830
psychostimulant abuse, 2:577–578
stress response, 1:694–695
influence on BDNF, 1:796–797
Glucose, leptin effect on, 3:746–747
Glucose-related protein 78 (GRP78), in bipolar disorder patients, 1:870
Glucose utilization, schizophrenia psychosis, neural network analysis, 2:257–258
Glutamate neurotransmitters:
anxiety disorder therapy, amino acid neurotransmission, 2:72–75
ionotropic receptors:
allosteric potentiators and antagonists, 1:385–397

AMPA receptors, *1:*370–371
  allosteric antagonists, *1:*395–396
  allosteric potentiators, *1:*390–395
  orthosteric agonists, *1:*376–377,
    *1:*378–381
  orthosteric antagonists, *1:*377–378,
    *1:*381–385
classification and background,
  *1:*365–366
future research issues, *1:*397–398
kainate receptors, *1:*371–372
  allosteric antagonists, *1:*397
  allosteric potentiators, *1:*396
NMDA receptors, *1:*367–370
  allosteric antagonists, *1:*386–390
  allosteric potentiators, *1:*385–386
  orthosteric agonists, *1:*373
  orthosteric antagonists, *1:*373–376
orthosteric pharmacological agents,
  *1:*373–385
subtypes, *1:*366–367
synthesis and storage, *1:*366
metabotropic receptors:
  allosteric potentiators and antagonists:
    mGlu1 antagonists, *1:*436–437
    mGlu1 potentiators, *1:*435–436
    mGlu2/3 antagonists, *1:*439–440
    mGlu2 potentiators, *1:*437–439
    mGlu4 potentiators, *1:*440–441
    mGlu5 antagonists, *1:*443–445
    mGlu5 potentiators, *1:*441–443
    mGlu7 antagonists, *1:*445
  background and classification,
    *1:*421–422
  future research issues, *1:*445–446
  orthosteric agents:
    group III selective agonists,
      *1:*431–433
    group III selective antagonists,
      *1:*433–435
    group II selective agonists, *1:*426–429
    group II selective antagonists,
      *1:*429–431
    group I selective agonists, *1:*423–424
    group I selective antagonists,
      *1:*424–426
neurogenesis and, *3:*207–208
neurotransmitter mechanisms, *1:*53–54
  plasma membrane neurotransmitter
    transporters:
      clinical relevance, *1:*718–719
      interacting proteins, *1:*728
      second messenger regulation,
        *1:*727–728
      structure and function, *1:*708–711
    vesicular transporters:
      clinical relevance, *1:*723
      structure and function, *1:*716
nicotine dependence and withdrawal,
  withdrawal substrates, *2:*542–543
obsessive-compulsive disorders, *2:*223
pain management and, *2:*717
Parkinson's disease treatment, *3:*504–505
psychostimulant abuse and, *2:*575–576
schizophrenia neurochemistry and,
  *2:*261–262
targeted drug development for,
  *2:*391–392
stroke and:
  ischemic brain injury, *3:*351–353
  NMDA receptor antagonists,
    *3:*354–355
  release inhibitors, *3:*366–367
Tourette's syndrome, *3:*272
traumatic brain injury and, *3:*449–450
Glutamate reuptake inhibitors,
  schizophrenia pharmacotherapy,
  *2:*391–392
Glutamatergic receptors:
  addictive disorders, modulator therapy
    and, *2:*458–459
  atypical antipsychotics, *2:*427–428
  autism spectrum disorders, medications,
    *3:*331–332
  dementia disorders and, *3:*469–470
  human immunodeficiency virus and,
    excitotoxicity cell death, *3:*705–706
  nicotine dependence and withdrawal,
    nicotine reinforcement substrates,
    *2:*538–540
  psychostimulant abuse, *2:*569–576
    chronic exposure and sensitization
      effects, *2:*583–585
    novel therapeutic developments, *2:*588
  in schizophrenia, *2:*264
    molecular genetics, functional
      candidate genes, *2:*331–332
    pharmacotherapy, glutamate reuptake
      inhibitors, *2:*391–392
  stroke pathophysiology and, *3:*354, *3:*355,
    *3:*361–366
    AMPA receptor antagonists, *3:*361–363
    glutamate transporters, *3:*365–366
    kainate receptor agonists, *3:*363

metabotropic glutamate receptors, 3:363–365
Glutamate theory of schizophrenia:
  dopamine hypothesis and, 2:295–296
  genetic evidence for, 2:293–294
  history, 2:289–291
  imaging evidence for, 2:292–293
  neurochemistry of, 2:373–374
  pathological evidence for, 2:291–292
  pharmacological evidence for, 2:294–295
Glutamate transporters, stroke management, 3:365–366
Glutamic acid decarboxylase (GAD):
  anxiety neurobiology and, knockout mice studies, 2:24–26
  GABA catalysis, 1:466
  schizophrenia susceptibility genetics, 2:350–351
Glutamine neurotransmitter transporter, structure and function, 1:715
Glutaminergic signaling, in bipolar disorder patients, 1:862–863
γ-D-Glutamylaminomethylsulfonic acid (GAMS)
  kainate receptor orthosteric antagonists, 1:385
Glutathione conjugates, 3,4-methylenedioxy-methamphetamine neurotoxicity and, 2:622
Glyceroneogenesis, lipolysis and thermogenesis, 3:799–801
Glycine:
  binding site agonists, NMDA allosteric potentiators, 1:385–386
  competitive site antagonists, NMDA receptors, 1:386–389
  early research on, 1:32
  neurotransmitter transporters:
    clinical relevance, 1:722–723
    structure and function, 1:712
  schizophrenia pharmacotherapy, NMDA targeting with, 2:391–392
Glycine site antagonists, NMDA receptor, stroke management, 3:357–359
Glycine transporter 1 (GlyT1), glutamate theory of schizophrenia, pharmacological evidence, 2:294–295
Glycine transporter inhibitors, schizophrenia pharmacotherapy, NMDA targeting with, 2:391–392

Glycogen breakdown, second messengers and, 1:31–32
Glycogen synthase kinase-3 (GSK-3), lithium mechanism in bipolar disorder patients, 1:864–869
Glycolipids, human neuropathy targeting, 3:614
Glycoproteins. See also specific glycoproteins, e.g. Gp120
  human immunodeficiency virus, 3:699, 3:701
  human neuropathy targeting, 3:614
  in myelin, 3:604–607
Glycosylation, plasma membrane transporter regulation, 1:725–726
GM6001 inhibitor, neuroinflammation and, 3:633
Golgi-specific DHHC zinc finger protein (GODZ), $GABA_A$ receptor trafficking, 1:480
Gonadotropin-releasing hormone (GnRH), neuropeptides and, 1:676
Gp41 protein, human immunodeficiency virus, 3:699, 3:701
Gp120 protein, human immunodeficiency virus, 3:699, 3:701
  alcohol abuse and, 3:716
  excitotoxicity cell death, 3:705–706
  nigrostriatal system and, 3:709–710
Gp130 cytokine receptor subunit, inflammation mechanisms, 3:640
G protein:
  in bipolar disorder patients, 1:861–862
  cannabinoid receptors and, 2:662–663
  ghrelin receptor activity, 3:770
  muscarinic acetylcholine receptors, selectivity, 1:157–158
  psychostimulant abuse, chronic exposure and sensitization effects, 2:584–585
  signal transducers, 1:60–66
    cycle regulations, 1:64–65
    disease and, 1:67
    heterotrimeric protein structure, 1:60–63
    RGS proteins, 1:65–66
    small proteins, 1:63–64
G-protein-activated inwardly rectifying K^+ (GIRK) channel:
  anxiety neurobiology and, receptor deficits and, 2:29–30
  signaling mechanisms, 1:67–69
  structure and function, 1:635

G-protein coupled receptors (GPCRs). *See also* Adrenergic receptors
  chemical release, 1:48–50
  corticotropin-releasing factor receptor antagonists, ligand binding mechanisms, 2:192–195
  delta opioid receptors, 2:751
  dopamine, 1:225
  dopamine signal transducers, 1:230–232
  GABA$_B$ receptors:
    dependent and independent effects, 1:580–581
    molecular determinants, 1:579–580
  glutamate neurotransmitters, 1:53–54
  hypocretin/orexin system, 3:126–127
    receptors, 3:128
  ion channel modulation, 1:66–71
    downstream signaling molecules, 1:69–70
    G$\beta\gamma$ signaling, 1:67–69
    protein-protein interactions, 1:70–71
  kappa opioid receptors, 2:751–752
  melatonin receptor molecular structure, 3:41–44
  mu opioid receptors and, 2:748–751
  muscarinic acetylcholine receptors:
    basic properties, 1:155–157
    downregulation, 1:163–164
    internalization, 1:162–163
    RGS proteins, 1:158
    uncoupling, 1:162
  muscarinic acetylcholine receptors and, 1:149–151
  neuropeptide receptors, 1:689–690
  regulator of G-protein signaling 4 schizophrenia candidate gene, 2:328
G-protein receptor kinases (GRKs):
  α_2-adrenergic receptor regulation, 1:205–206
  D$_1$ receptor subfamily, 1:225–227
  muscarinic acetylcholine receptor phosphorylation, 1:164–166
  phosphorylation, 1:90–92
  RGS protein function, 1:65–66
Green fluorescent protein (GFP), invertebrate neurodegenerative disease models, Parkinson's disease cell death, 3:570–577
GRM3 gene, schizophrenia molecular genetics, 2:331–332
  susceptibility identification, 2:349

Group A β-hemolytic streptococcus (GABHS) infection, obsessive-compulsive disorders and, 2:235
Growth factors:
  amyotrophic lateral sclerosis and, 3:226–227
  inflammation mechanisms, 3:639–641
  intercellular signaling, 1:44–45, 1:46
  neurogenesis and, 3:210–211
  neurotrophin structure and, 3:240
  stroke therapy and, 3:375–377
Growth hormone-releasing hormone (GHRH), ghrelin effects and, 3:774
Growth hormone secretagogues (GHS):
  classification of, 3:766
  ghrelin receptor evaluation, 3:770
  ghrelin receptor ligands and, 3:769
Growth hormone secretion, ghrelin effects and, 3:773–774
GTPase-activating proteins (GAPs), cycle regulation, 1:64–65
GTS-21 nicotinic agonist, dementia disorders and, 3:468–469
Guanfacine:
  attention-deficit hyperactivity disorder therapy, 3:299–300
  autism spectrum disorders, 3:330–331
  schizophrenia pharmacotherapy, 2:393
Guanine nucleotide exchange factors (GEFs), small G proteins, 1:63–64
Guanosine diphosphate (GDP):
  dopamine signal transducers, 1:231–232
  heterotrimeric G protein binding, 1:60–73
Guanosine triphosphate (GTP), heterotrimeric G protein binding, 1:60–73
Guanylate cyclase (cGMP) receptors:
  neuropeptides, 1:691
  nitric oxide gaseous signaling, nitrosylation, 1:745–747
Guanylyl cyclases (GCs), cyclic nucleotide second messenger signaling, 1:78–80
Guillain-Barré syndrome, myelin pathology, 3:613–614
GYKI 52466 antagonist, stroke management, 3:362

H$_1$ receptor:
  arousal mechanisms, 1:323–324
  molecular pharmacology, 1:307–312

brain tissue responses, *1:*309–311
distribution, *1:*311–312
signaling mechanisms, *1:*309
structure and properties, *1:*307–309
H_2 receptor, molecular pharmacology, *1:*312–314
H_3 receptor:
cognitive functions, *1:*324
histaminergic neuron activity, *1:*321–322
molecular pharmacology, *1:*314–316
H_4 receptor, molecular pharmacology, *1:*316
Habit reversal training, Tourette's syndrome therapy, *3:*277–278
Hallucinations:
hypnagogic hallucinations:
symptoms of, *3:*83
treatment of, *3:*112
hypnopompic hallucinations, symptoms of, *3:*83
Parkinson's disease and, *3:*502–503
Hallucinogens, LSD, *2:*637–640
addiction, *2:*639–640
mechanism of action, *2:*638–639
pharmacology, *2:*638
Haloperidol:
autism spectrum disorders, *3:*325
serotonin receptor 5-HT_6 and, *2:*425–426
Tourette's syndrome and, *3:*273–276
Haloperidol-induced catalepsy, muscarinic acetylcholine receptor deficiency, *1:*172
Hamilton depression and anxiety scales, corticotropin-releasing factor receptor antagonists, anxiety/depression therapeutic potential, *2:*197–198
HCRT gene, hypocretin/orexin system, *3:*127
HCRTR2 gene, hypocretin/orexin system, narcolepsy and, *3:*137–138
Heart function, muscarinic acetylcholine receptor deficiency, *1:*175
Heat exposure, transient receptor potential V1 (TRPV1) receptor expression, *2:*730–732
Hematopoiesis, prokineticins and, *3:*170–171
Hemizygosity:
parkin gene mutations, familial Parkinsonism, *3:*531–532
PINK1 gene mutation and, *3:*533–535

Hepatitis C, opiate addiction comorbidity with, *2:*691–694
HERG gene:
KCNH potassium channels and, *1:*633–634
voltage-gated potassium channels, *1:*623
Heroin addiction:
incidence and prevalence, *2:*692–694
neuropeptide pharmacology and, *2:*578–579
pharmacotherapy, history of, *2:*451–457
treatment statistics, *2:*694–696
3-Heteroaryl-5,6bis(aryl)-1-methyl-2-pyridone, $GABA_A$ α_3 subunit pharmacology, *1:*488
Heteromeric structure:
$GABA_B$ receptors, *1:*575–578
nicotinic acetylcholine receptors, *1:*112–113, *1:*116–125
Hetero-oligomeric receptors, $GABA_A$ receptors, subunit subtype composition, *1:*476–477
Heteroreceptors, muscarinic acetylcholine receptor deficiency, *1:*176
Heterotrimeric G proteins, structure and function, *1:*60–63
Hexamethonium blockers, nicotinic acetylcholine receptors, *1:*121
High 5-HT_{2A}, schizophrenia therapy, D_2 affinity *vs.*, *2:*378
High alcohol drinking (HAD) rats, alcohol abuse studies, characteristics of, *2:*467
High-density lipoprotein (HDL), antiobesity therapy, rimonabant and, *3:*827–828
Highly active antiretroviral therapy (HAART), HIV neuropharmacology and, *3:*694–695
methamphetamine/cocaine abuse and, *3:*714–715
neurodegenerative disease and, *3:*716–718
High-throughput screening, neurodegenerative disease, invertebrate models, *3:*582–583
Hippocampal system:
alcohol abuse studies, CA1/CA3 fields, $GABA_{A5}$ receptor probes, *2:*511–516
anatomy and physiology, *1:*823–824

antidepressants and neurogenesis in:
  adult neurogenesis stages, *1:*827–828
  behavioral and animal models, *1:*833
  depression physiology and, *1:*823–824, *1:*826–827
  future research on, *1:*833
  monoamines and, *1:*822–823
  research background, *1:*821–822
  serotonin/norepinephrine regulation, *1:*831–833
  stress and monamine hypotheses, *1:*825–826
  stress hormone neurogenesis regulation, *1:*829–830
anxiety disorders and, *2:*13–15
hypocretin/orexin system, plasticity of, *3:*136
3,4-methylenedioxymethamphetamine effects on, long-term neurochemical effects, *2:*619–620
neuronal survival mechanisms, *3:*205–206
synapses:
  5-HT$_\gamma$ receptor family, *1:*276
  mGlu5 allosteric potentiators, *1:*441–442
  muscarinic acetylcholine receptor deficiency and suppression of, *1:*172
  neurotrophins and, stress and neurogenesis in, *1:*798–799
  vesicular transporters and, *1:*723
Hispidulin, GABA$_A$ subunit pharmacology, allosteric ligand modulation, *1:*506
Histamine:
  in brain:
    biosynthesis, *1:*305–306
    early history, *1:*300–301
    inactivation, *1:*306–307
    metabolism, *1:*305–307
    molecular pharmacology, receptor subtypes, *1:*307–317
      H$_1$ receptor, *1:*307–312
      H$_2$ receptor, *1:*312–314
      H$_3$ receptor, *1:*314–316
      H$_4$ receptor, *1:*316
      NMDA receptor interaction, *1:*316–317
    neuron activity and control, *1:*317–322
      electrophysiology, *1:*317
      pharmacological changes, *1:*321–322
      in vitro modulation, *1:*317–319
      in vivo changes, *1:*319–321
    neuronal organization, *1:*301–305
      afferents, *1:*303–305
      histaminergic pathways, *1:*303
      perikarya, *1:*301–303
    neuron physiology, *1:*322–326
      arousal, *1:*322–324
      cognitive functions, *1:*324
      nociception, *1:*326
      pituitary hormone secretion, *1:*324–325
      satiation, *1:*325–326
      seizuers, *1:*326
    neuropsychiatric disease, *1:*327–329
      Alzheimer's disease, *1:*327–328
      anxiety/ADHD, *1:*329
      Parkinson's disease, *1:*328
      schizophrenia and antipsychotic actions, *1:*327
    early research on, *1:*16–17
  hypocretin/orexin system, arousal mechanisms, *3:*142–143
  narcolepsy therapy, *3:*105–106
Histamine *N*-methyltransferase (HMT), histamine inactivation, *1:*306–307
Histaminergic pathways, structure and function, *1:*303
Histaminergic perikarya, structure and function, *1:*301–303
Histidine residues, sedative/hypnotic binding, *3:*190–192
L-Histidine decarboxylase (HDC):
  histamine neuron physiology, arousal mechanisms, *1:*322–324
  histaminergic perikarya and, *1:*301–303
Histochemistry, neuropeptide identification, *1:*674
HIV-associated dementia (HAD):
  alcohol abuse and, *3:*716
  apoptosis mechanisms, *3:*704–705
  classification, *3:*694–695
  epidemiology and pathogenesis, *3:*695–696
  lipid metabolism and, *3:*707
  methamphetamine/cocaine abuse and, *3:*713–715
  neurodegenerative disease and, *3:*716–718
  neurotransmitters and, *3:*711–712
  nigrostriatal system and, *3:*708–710
  Vpu protein and, *3:*704
Homeobox genes, obsessive-compulsive disorders, *2:*223–224

Homologous residues, GABA$_A$ receptor activation, channel gating binding, *1:*497
Homologs:
  ghrelin receptors, *3:*771–772
  p75 neurotrophin receptor structure, *3:*241
Homooligomeric receptors:
  GABA$_A$ receptors, *1:*476
  GABA$_C$ receptor inhibition
Homovanillic acid (HVA), Parkinson's disease, neurochemistry, *3:*481–483
Hormones, neuroinflammation and, *3:*645
HTR2A receptor, schizophrenia molecular genetics, *2:*331–332
Human autoimmune neuropathies, *3:*613–614
  animal models, *3:*615
Human immunodeficiency virus (HIV). *See also* HIV-associated dementia (HAD)
  alcohol abuse and, *3:*716
  cholinergic system, *3:*711–712
  clinical features, *3:*694–695
  dementia and, *3:*711–712
  drug abuse and, *3:*712–716
    methamphetamine/cocaine, *3:*713–715
    opioid drugs, *3:*715–716
  excitatory amino acid neurotransmitters, *3:*711
  future neuropharmacology issues, *3:*718
  lipid metabolism alterations, *3:*707
  neurodegenerative diseases and, *3:*716–718
  neuropathology, *3:*695–704
    cell death cascades, *3:*704–707
      apoptosis, *3:*704–705
      excitotoxicity, *3:*705–706
      neural progenitor cells, *3:*706–707
      oxidative stress, *3:*706
    chemokines in, *3:*697–698
    neurodegenerative mechanisms, *3:*699
  neuropharmacology:
    features of, *3:*694–695
    future research issues, *3:*718
  neurotoxic proteins, *3:*699–704
    glycoproteins gp120 and gp41, *3:*699, *3:*701
    Nef protein, *3:*703
    neurobiology of, *3:*700
    Rev protein, *3:*704
    Tat protein, *3:*701–703
    Vpr protein, *3:*703
    Vpu protein, *3:*704
  nigrostriatal system, *3:*707–711
    dopamine mediators, *3:*709–711
  opiate addiction and exposure to, *2:*691–694, *3:*715–716
  pathogenesis, *3:*695
Human leukocyte antigen (HLA):
  narcolepsy evaluation, *3:*84
  narcolepsy pathophysiology, immune system and, *3:*85–86
  neuroinflammation and, *3:*626
Huntington's disease:
  H$_1$ receptor distribution, *1:*313–314
  invertebrate models of trinucleotide repeats, *3:*577–579
7-Hydroxyiminocyclopropan[*b*]chromene-1α-carboxylic acid, mGlu1 allosteric antagonists, *1:*436–437
Hydroxyindole-*O*-methyl transferase (HIOMT), melatonin production, *3:*40–41
Hydroxylation, dopamine synthesis, *1:*54–55
Hydroxyl radicals, 3,4-methylenedioxymethamphetamine neurotoxicity and, *2:*627
3-Hydroxy-3-methylglutaryl coenzyme A (HMG-CoA), multiple sclerosis therapy, *3:*687
5-Hydroxytryptamine (5-HT). *See also* *1:*5-HT$_{1:1}$ *receptor family; Serotonin systems*
Hydroxyzine, anxiety disorder therapy, *2:*75
Hyperdopaminergic state, schizophrenia dopamine hypothesis and evidence for, *2:*287
Hyperkalemic periodic paralysis (HyperPP), voltage-gated sodium ion channels and, *1:*641–642
Hyperpolarization-activated channels (HCN), structure and function, *1:*649–650
Hyperserotonin hypothesis, autism spectrum disorders, *3:*321–322
Hypertension therapy, voltage-gated calcium channels, Ca$_v$1 family, *1:*648
Hyperthermia, 3,4-methylenedioxymethamphetamine neurotoxicity and, *2:*624–625
Hyperzine A, dementia disorders and, *3:*463

Hypnagogic hallucinations:
    symptoms of, 3:83
    treatment of, 3:112
Hypnopompic hallucinations, symptoms of, 3:83
Hypnotics:
    barbiturate-like drugs, 3:187
    barbiturates, 3:184–187
    basic principles, 3:177–178
    benzodiazepines, 3:187–188
    brain sites of action, 3:181–184
    $GABA_A$ receptors:
        pharmacology, 3:180–181
        structure, 3:178–180
    mouse studies, 3:190–192
    new agents, 3:188–190
    non-$GABA_A$ receptor agents, 3:188
    safe development of, 3:184–190
Hypocellularity, adipocyte proliferative capacity, 3:797–799
Hypocretin-1:
    cataplexy therapy, 3:113–114
    narcolepsy evaluation, in cerebrospinal fluid, 3:84
    narcolepsy pathophysiology, deficiency in, animal models, 3:86
    narcolepsy therapy, future research issues, 3:105—106
Hypocretin-2, history of, 3:127
Hypocretin/orexin system:
    afferents, 3:130
    agonists/antagonists, 3:128
    arousal, feeding behavior and motivation integration, 3:144–145
    arousal circuitry, 3:139–144
        cholinergic systems, 3:143–144
        dopaminergic systems, 3:143
        histaminergic systems, 3:142–143
        lateral hypothalamic neurons, 3:140–141
        noradrenergic systems, 3:141–142
        serotonergic systems, 3:142
    autonomic endocrine effects, 3:134–135
    excitatory neurotransmitters, 3:131–132
    feeding and metabolism, 3:132–134
    fiber projections, 3:129–130
    hippocampal plasticity, 3:136
    hypocretin cell bodies, 3:128–131
    hypocretin discovery, 3:126–127
    lateral hypothalamus, 3:125–126
    motivation and addiction, 3:135
    narcolepsy pathophysiology, 3:136–139
    sleep regulation and, 3:86–89
    pain and anesthesia, 3:136
    receptors, 3:128
        distribution of, 3:130–131
        at synapses, 3:130
Hypodopaminergia, schizophrenia dopamine hypothesis, 2:288–289
Hypothalamic pathway, sedative/hypnotic action sites, 3:182–184
Hypothalamic-pituitary-adrenal (HPA) axis:
    anxiety neurobiology and, 2:17
    circadian rhythms and release of, 3:19–20
    corticotropin-releasing factor receptor antagonists, 2:177–179
    hippocampal neurogenesis and depression and, 1:827
    nicotine dependence and withdrawal:
        nicotine reinforcement substrates, 2:539–540
        withdrawal substrate specificity, 2:543
    psychostimulant abuse, 2:577–578
        chronic exposure and sensitization effects, 2:580–585
    stress-induced behaviors, neuroactive steroids, 2:153–159
    stress response and, 1:694–695
Hypothalamic-pituitary pathways, neuropeptides, 1:692
Hypothalamic release-stimulating/ release-inhibiting actions, neuropeptides, 1:691
Hypothalamus:
    circadian rhythms and, 3:23–24
    histamine neuron physiology:
        arousal mechanisms, 1:323–324
        satiation effects, 1:325–326
    leptin signaling and and feeding regulation, 3:741–743
    neuropeptide control, 1:691–692
Hypothermia, muscarinic acetylcholine receptor deficiency, 1:170–171
Hypoxia, S nitrosylation physiology and, 1:753–754

Idazozan, adrenergic receptor mechanisms, 2:427
Idiopathic hypersomnia:
    classification of, 3:84
    modafinil therapy, 3:100–103

Idiopathic Parkinson's disease (IPD):
  genetics and, *3:*542–543
  parkin gene mutations, *3:*531–532
IDRA 21 receptor modulator, dementia disorders and, *3:*470
Ifenprodil:
  NMDA receptor allosteric antagonists, *1:*390
  stroke management, *3:*357
IGF binding proteins (IGFBPs), stroke and, *3:*376–377
Iloperidone, schizophrenia therapy, *2:*389
Imidazenil, GABA$_A$ subunit pharmacology, allosteric ligand modulation, *1:*504–506
Imidazobenzodiazepines, alcohol abuse studies, GABA$_{A5}$ receptor specificity, *2:*512–516
Iminodibenzyl derivatives, early research on, *1:*30
Imipramine, early research on, *1:*30–31
Immediate early genes:
  neuropeptide identification, *1:*673
  psychostimulant abuse, chronic exposure and sensitization effects, *2:*585
Immediate-release stimulants, attention-deficit hyperactivity disorder therapy, *3:*294
Immune response, 3,4-methylenedioxy-methamphetamine effects on, *2:*618
Immune system:
  ghrelin modulation, *3:*775
  narcolepsy pathophysiology and, *3:*85–86
Immunization techniques, neuroinflammation modulation, *3:*644–645
Immunocytochemistry, neuropeptide identification, *1:*673
Immunoglobulin therapy, obsessive-compulsive disorders, *2:*235
Immunomodulatory therapy:
  multiple sclerosis, *3:*674–676
    novel drug development, *3:*687–688
  obsessive-compulsive disorders, *2:*235
Immunoreceptors, inflammation and, *3:*631–632
Immunosuppression, intermediate-conductance calcium-activated potassium channels, *1:*631

Inactivation:
  histamines, *1:*306–307
  neuropeptides, *1:*687–688
    extracellular inactivation, *1:*687–688
  neurotransmitters, *1:*50–52
  of nicotinic acetylcholine receptor, *1:*125–127
  potassium ion channels, *1:*627
Indole agents, serotonin receptor 5-HT$_{2A}$, *2:*418–421
Indolealkylamines, *2:*637–640
  addiction, *2:*639–640
  mechanism of action, *2:*638–639
  pharmacology, *2:*638
Indoleamine 2,3-deoxygenase (IDO), inflammation mechanisms, *3:*625
  tryptophan metabolism and, *3:*644
Infection:
  obsessive-compulsive disorders and, *2:*235
  Tourette's syndrome, *3:*268–269
Inflammation. *See also* Neuroinflammation
  basic principles of, *3:*622–623
  brain immunoreceptors, *3:*631–632
  central nervous system response, *3:*623–624
    blood-brain barrier, *3:*624–625
  costimulatory molecules, *3:*631
  major histocompatibility classes, *3:*631
  neuroinflammation:
    antigen-presenting cells, *3:*626
    arachidonic acid pathways, *3:*630
    astrocytes, *3:*627
    blood-derived inflammatory cells, *3:*628
    chemokines, *3:*629–630
    cytokines, *3:*628–629
    endothelial cells, *3:*627
    growth factors, *3:*639–641
    humoral components, *3:*628–630
    immunization approaches, *3:*644–645
    microglia, *3:*626–627
    neurons, *3:*628
    pharmacological modification, *3:*645–646
    radical formation and oxidative damage, *3:*630
  pharmacology, *3:*632–646
    adenosine pathway purinergic receptor modulation, *3:*643–644
    antioxidants, *3:*636–637
    apoptosis modulation, *3:*637–638
    arachidonic acid/prostaglandin pathways, *3:*634–635

cAMP/cGMP modulation, *3:*635–636
cannabinoid receptor modulation,
  *3:*641–642
central nervous system migration,
  *3:*633
chimokine-directed approaches,
  *3:*633–634
estrogen/hormones, *3:*645
future research issues, *3:*646
indoleamine deoxygenase and
  tryptophan metabolism,
  *3:*644
ion-channel approaches, *3:*642
proinflammatory pathway modulation,
  *3:*638–639
statins, *3:*643
vitamin D derivatives, *3:*642–643
toll-like receptors, *3:*631–632
transient receptor potential V1
  (TRPV1) receptor expression,
  *2:*729
Inflammatory cascade, traumatic brain
  injury and, *3:*447–449
Inflammatory molecules, circadian rhythms
  and, *3:*21
Inflammatory pathways, stroke
  management, *3:*368
Inhibitory postsynaptic potential (IPSP):
  early research on, *1:*29
  neuropeptides and, *1:*676–677
INO1 gene, lithium mechanism in bipolar
  disorder and, *1:*869
Inositol depletion, lithium mechanism in
  bipolar disorder and, *1:*869
In situ hybridization, neuropeptide
  identification, *1:*674
Insulin:
  β-adrenergic receptor physiology,
    *1:*212–213
  GABA$_A$ receptor trafficking, *1:*480
  ghrelin modulation, *3:*775–776
  leptin and, *3:*745–746
  muscarinic acetylcholine receptor
    deficiency, *1:*174–175
  neurotrophic factors and, *1:*763
Insulin-like growth factor-1 (IGF-1):
  amyotrophic lateral sclerosis, *3:*226–227
  depression models and, *1:*809
  ghrelin modulation, *3:*776
  inflammation mechanisms, *3:*640–641
  intracellular signaling, *1:*763
  stroke and, *3:*376–377

Integrated glutamate/dopamine hypotheses
  of schizophrenia:
  basic principles, *2:*295–297
  pharmacotherapy and, *2:*374–376
Integrins, Tat protein binding, HIV
  immunodeficiency and, *3:*702–703
Interacting proteins:
  GABA$_B$ receptor modulation, *1:*585–587
  G-protein-coupled receptors, *1:*70–71
  plasma membrane transporter regulation,
    *1:*728
  voltage-gated potassium channels,
    *1:*627–628
Intercellular adhesion molecule-1 (ICAM-1):
  inflammation mechanisms, *3:*624–625
  statin therapy and, *3:*643
  stroke management, *3:*369–370
Intercellular signaling, synaptic
  transmission:
  basic principles, *1:*40–41
  classical transmitters, *1:*45–46
  dopamine neurotransmitters, *1:*54–56
  endocannabinoids, purines, and gaseous
    transmitters, *1:*46
  glutamate neurotransmitters, *1:*52–54
  peptide transmitters and growth factors,
    *1:*46
  postsynaptic receptors, *1:*48–50
  presynaptic receptors, *1:*50–51
  synaptic release, *1:*46–48
  transmitter inactivation, *1:*51–52
  transmitter packaging, *1:*45–46
  transmitter synthesis, *1:*41–45
    amine transmitters, *1:*42–44
    endocannabinoids, *1:*45
    gaseous transmitters, *1:*45
    neuropeptides, neurotrophins, and
      growth factors, *1:*44–45
  vesicle-dependent release, *1:*46–47
  vesicle-independent release, *1:*47–48
Interference RNA (RNAi):
  Huntingdon's disease trinucleotide
    repeats, invertebrate model,
    *3:*577–579
  Parkinson's disease, invertebrate models,
    *3:*573–577
Interferon β1b, multiple sclerosis therapy,
  *3:*674–675
Interleukin-1β converting enzyme (ICE),
  3,4-methylenedioxy-
  methamphetamine effects on,
  *2:*628

Interleukin-1β (IL-β):
  release, 3,4-methylenedioxy-
    methamphetamine effects on, 2:628
  stress response and, 1:797
Intermediate-conductance calcium-activated
    potassium channels (IK channels),
    structure and function, 1:631
Internalization, muscarinic acetylcholine
    receptors, 1:162–163
Intracellular signaling:
  anxiety neurobiology and:
    mouse studies, 2:19, 2:22
    phenotype analysis, 2:30–33
  GABA$_B$ receptor modulation, 1:585–586
  neuropeptide degradation, 1:687
  neurotrophic factors, 1:791–794
    fibroblast growth factor, 1:793
    insulin/insulin-like growth factor,
      1:793
    nerve growth factor family, 1:791–792
    transforming growth factor-beta,
      1:793–794
    vascular endothelial growth factor,
      1:792–793
  psychostimulant abuse, chronic exposure
    and sensitization effects, 2:584–585
  schizophrenia therapy, 2:394–395
  synaptic transmission:
    basic principles, 1:59–60
    calcium channel calmodulin mediator,
      1:85–87
    calcium channel signaling molecules,
      1:83–85
    cyclic nucleotide second messengers,
      1:72–81
      adenylyl cyclase, 1:72–77
      cAMP targets, 1:75, 1:78
      cGMP cellular targets, 1:80–81
      guanylyl cyclase, 1:78–80
    DAG activation of protein kinase C,
      1:85
    GPCR-G protein ion channel
      modulation, 1:66–71
      downstream signaling molecules,
        1:69–70
      Gβγ signaling, 1:67–69
      protein-protein interactions, 1:70–71
    G protein signal transducers, 1:60–66
      cycle regulations, 1:64–65
      disease and, 1:67
      heterotrimeric protein structure,
        1:60–63

      RGS proteins, 1:65–66
      small proteins, 1:63–64
    IP$_3$ and phosphoinositide signaling
      molecules, 1:81–83
    protein phosphorylation, 1:87–96
      G-protein-coupled receptor kinases,
        1:90–92
      mitogen-activated protein kinase,
        1:89–90
      protein tyrosine kinase, 1:87–89
      protein tyrosines phosphatases,
        1:92–94
      serine/threonine phosphatases,
        1:94–96
Intrinsic efficacy, alcohol abuse studies,
    GABA$_A$ benzodiazepine receptor
    complex, subunit selectivity vs.,
    2:516–517
Introns, H$_3$ receptor, 1:314–315
Inverse agonism, GABA$_A$ receptor
    activation, allosteric ligand
    modulation, 1:500–506
Invertebrate models, neurodegenerative
    disease:
  Alzheimer's disease, 3:579–582
  Caenorhabditis elegans system, 3:568–569
  Drosophila melanogaster, 3:569
  early research, 3:567–568
  future applications, 3:582–583
  genetic and molecular pathways, 3:568
  Huntington's disease trinucleotide repeats,
    3:577–579
  Parkinson's disease, dopamine neuron cell
    death, 3:569–577
In vitro modulation, histaminergic neuron
    activity, 1:317–319
In vivo modulation:
  in bipolar disorder patients, 1:863
  GABA$_B$ deficient mice, 1:587–588
  histaminergic neuron activity, 1:319–322
Inwardly rectifying potassium, structure and
    function, 1:634–635
2-[^{125}I]Iodomelatonin, development of,
    3:39–40
Ion channels:
  circadian rhythms and, 3:9
  early research on, 1:25
  GABA$_A$ receptor activation, channel pore
    complex, 1:497–498
  GABA$_B$ receptor and, 1:469
  G-protein-coupled receptor modulation,
    1:66–71

downstream signaling molecules, 1:69–70
Gβγ signaling, 1:67–69
protein-protein interactions, 1:70–71
muscarinic acetylcholine receptor modulation, 1:160–162
myelin pronodal proteins and, 3:609
neuroinflammation and, 3:642
nitrosylation in, 1:748–759
Ionotropic glutamate receptors:
antiepileptic drugs and, 3:413
atypical antipsychotics, 2:427–429
Ionotropic receptors:
chemical release, 1:48–50
glutamate receptors:
allosteric potentiators and antagonists, 1:385–397
AMPA receptors, 1:370–371
allosteric antagonists, 1:395–396
allosteric potentiators, 1:390–395
orthosteric agonists, 1:376–377, 1:378–381
orthosteric antagonists, 1:377–378, 1:381–385
classification and background, 1:365–366
future research issues, 1:397–398
kainate receptors, 1:371–372
allosteric antagonists, 1:397
allosteric potentiators, 1:396
NMDA receptors, 1:367–370
allosteric antagonists, 1:386–390
allosteric potentiators, 1:385–386
orthosteric agonists, 1:373
orthosteric antagonists, 1:373–376
orthosteric pharmacological agents, 1:373–385
subtypes, 1:366–367
synthesis and storage, 1:366
IP$_3$ signaling molecules, intracellular signaling, 1:81–83
Ischemia. See Stroke therapy
Isoquinolin-pyrimidines, NMDA receptor allosteric antagonists, 1:390
Isoreceptors, neuropeptides, 1:689

Janus kinase (Jak) gene, leptin secretion and, 3:737–739
JC virus, 5-HT$_{2A}$ receptors and, 1:271
J-domain fragments, corticotropin-releasing factor receptor antagonists, ligand binding mechanisms, 2:192–195
Jervall-Lange-Nielsen syndrome, KCNQ channels and, 1:632–633
Jet lag, circadian rhythms, 3:15
Jun-N-terminal kinase (JNK):
p75 neurotrophin receptor signaling, 3:246–247
Parkinson's disease and, 3:228–229
JWS-USC-751X, dementia disorders therapy and, 3:471–473

K36, GABA$_A$ subunit pharmacology, allosteric ligand modulation, 1:505–506
K252a inhibitor, tyrosine kinase receptor blockade, 3:232
Kainate receptors:
allosteric antagonists, 1:397
allosteric potentiators, 1:396
antiepileptic drugs and, topiramate, 3:416–417
glutamate theory of schizophrenia, mRNA binding, 2:291–292
neurogenesis and, 3:208
orthosteric agonists, 1:378–381
orthosteric antagonists, 1:381–385
schizophrenia pharmacotherapy, drug development for, 2:392
stroke and:
antagonists, 3:363
ischemic brain injury, 3:351–353
structure and function, 1:371–372
Kappa opioid receptors:
psychostimulant abuse and, 2:578–579
structure and function, 2:751–752
K$^+$ channel interacting protein (KChIPs), voltage-gated potassium channels, 1:628
KCNE proteins, voltage-gated potassium channels, 1:628
KCNH potassium channels:
clinical conditions and, 1:633–634
structure and function, 1:623
KCNQ channels:
clinical applications, 1:632–633
structure and function, 1:623
KcsA channel, gating mechanism, 1:626–627
Ketamine:
glutamate theory of schizophrenia, history of, 2:289–290
NMDA receptor allosteric antagonists, 1:389–390
NMDA receptors, 1:368–370

overview, 2:636
pharmacological effects, 2:636–637
Ketanserin, narcolepsy therapy, GABA inhibition, 3:101–102
Ketoconazole, psychostimulant abuse, 2:577–578
Knockin mice, benzodiazepine functional diversity, 2:112–114
Knockout mice:
 anxiety neurobiology:
  neuronal messenger alterations, 2:24–26
  neurotransmitter receptor/CMAP deficits, 2:26–30
 benzodiazepine functional diversity studies, 2:112–114
 calcitonin gene-related peptide studies, 2:760–761
 $GABA_A$ subunit pharmacology, α subunits, $α_1$ subunit, 1:484, 1:488
 $GABA_B$ deficient mice, 1:587–588
 neuropeptide gene targeting in, 1:678
 plasma membrane glutamate transporters, 1:711
 transient receptor potential V1 (TRPV1) receptor models, 2:736
Kufor Rakeb disease (KRD), familial Parkinson's disease and, 3:541
Kymarenic acid, kainate receptor orthosteric antagonists, 1:385
Kynuremic acid, NMDA receptor allosteric antagonists, 1:387

L-4-phosphono-2-aminobutyric acid (L-AP4), mGlu III selective orthosteric agonists, 1:433–435
L-655,708, $GABA_A$ $α_5$ subunit pharmacology, 1:489
L-838,417, $GABA_A$ subunit pharmacology, allosteric ligand modulation, 1:505–506
LAAM (λ-α-Acetyl methadol):
 addiction pharmacotherapy and, 2:454–457
 treatment statistics, 2:695–696
Lamotrigine:
 anxiety disorder therapy, 2:75
 autism spectrum disorders, 3:332
 epilepsy efficacy, 3:417–418
 schizophrenia pharmacotherapy, NMDA targeted drug development, 2:392–393
 for secondary generalized epilepsy, 3:424
 stroke management, 3:367
Large-conductance calcium-activated potassium channels (BK channels), structure and function, 1:630–631
Large dense-core vesicles (LDCVs), neuropeptide electrophysiology, 1:675–676
Lateral hypothalamus (LH):
 alcohol abuse studies, dopamine neuronal systems and substrates, 2:481–485
 D_2 dopaminergic regulation, hypothesized mechanisms, 2:481–485
 hypocretin/orexin system, 3:125–126
  cell bodies, 3:128–129
  fiber projections, 3:129–130
  self-stimulation (LHSS), 3:135
Lazaroids, stroke management, 3:371–372
Learning function, muscarinic acetylcholine receptor deficiency, 1:168–169
Learning-related survival mechanisms, neurogenesis, 3:204–206
Lennox-Gastaut syndrome:
 felbamate therapy, 3:414–415, 3:418
 therapy options for, 3:421, 3:424
Leptin:
 cannabinoid receptors and, 2:671–672
 early research, 3:733–734
 energy expenditure and, 3:743–744
 food intake regulation, 3:740–743
 OB gene expression and, 3:734–736
 peripheral nutrient utilization, 3:744–748
 receptor expression, 3:736–739
 signaling inhibition and resistance, 3:739–740
Lesion models, in schizophrenia, 2:265
Leucine binding protein (LBP), $GABA_B$ receptor sites, 1:578–579
Leucine residues, $GABA_A$ receptor activation, channel pore complex, 1:497–498
Leucine-rich repeat kinase 2 (LRRK2) gene, familial Parkinson's disease and mutation of, 3:536–539
Leukotriene D4 (LTDR), mGlu2 allosteric potentiators, 1:439
Levetiracetam:
 drug-resistant epilepsy, 3:425–426
 synaptic vesicle protein SV2A modulation, 3:414

Levoamphetamine, attention-deficit hyperactivity disorder therapy, 3:297–298
Levodopa:
 human immunodeficiency virus, nigrostriatal system and, 3:710
 Parkinson's disease treatment:
  peripheral decarboxylase inhibitor with, 3:484–487
  slow-release formulations, 3:487–488
Lewy bodies:
 familial Parkinsonism and, PARK 1 and PARK4 mutations, 3:527–529
 Parkinson's disease, invertebrate models of cell death, 3:570–577
Lifestyle factors, idiopathic Parkinson's disease and, 3:544
Ligand binding core (LBC), AMPA receptors, 1:370–371
 allosteric potentiators, 1:393–395
 orthosteric agonists, 1:377
Ligand binding domain (LBD):
 dopamine, 1:233–234
 $GABA_A$ receptors:
  agonist binding site architecture, 1:494–495
  allosteric ligand modulation, 1:499–506
  assembly, 1:477–478
 $GABA_B$ receptor sites, 1:578–579
 muscarinic acetylcholine receptors (mAChRs), 1:152–154
  agonists, 1:152
  allosteric ligands, 1:153–154
  antagonists, 1:152–153
  clinical applications, 1:154
 serotonin receptor families, 1:263–267
Ligand-gated ion channels:
 $5-HT_3$ receptor family and, 1:273
 $GABA_A$ receptors, desensitization and deactivation, 1:498–499
 glutamate neurotransmitters, 1:53–54
 neuroactive steroids, 2:137–141
Light-dark box, mouse models of anxiety, neurosteroid effects, 2:146–147
Light-dark cycles, circadian rhythms, 3:5
Lipid metabolism:
 human immunodeficiency virus and, 3:707
 leptin effect on, 3:746–747
Lipolysis:
 adipose tissue signaling and, 3:802–803
 glyceroneogenesis, 3:799–801
 leptin effect on, 3:747–748

Lipostatic hypothesis, 3:733–734
LIS1 gene, DISC1 schizophrenia candidate gene, molecular interactions, 2:351–352
Lisuride, Parkinson's disease treatment, 3:491
Lithium:
 anxiety disorder therapy, 2:75
 in bipolar disorder patients, 1:864–869
 circadian rhythms and, 3:15–17
Lobeline, vesicular transporters and, 1:723
Localization studies:
 H_1 receptor distribution, 1:311–312
 H_2 receptor, 1:313–314
 H_3 receptors, 1:316
Locomotor activity:
 $GABA_A$ α_6 subunit pharmacology, 1:489–490
 mGlu5 allosteric potentiators, 1:442–443
 mGlu II selective orthosteric antagonists, 1:431
 muscarinic acetylcholine receptor deficiency, 1:169–170
 psychostimulant abuse, chronic exposure and sensitization effects, 2:581–585
Lofexidine, opiate addiction and, 2:699
Long-QT syndrome:
 KCNQ channels and, 1:632–633
 voltage-gated sodium ion channels and, 1:642
Long-term potentiation (LTP):
 adult neurogenesis and, 1:829
 brain-derived neurotrophic factor synthesis and, 3:224–225
 glutamate receptors and, 3:470
 hypocretin/orexin system, 3:136
Long-term therapy, selective serotonin reuptake inhibitors, 2:68–69
Lubeluzole, stroke management, 3:367
Luteinizing hormone (LH), hypocretin/orexin system, 3:134–135
Luteinizing hormone releasing hormone (LHRH), histaminergic neuron activity, 1:325
Luzindole:
 melatonin receptor inhibition, 3:39
 in suprachiasmatic nucleus, 3:49–50
 melatonin receptor molecular pharmacology, 3:43–44
LY34195, mGlu II selective orthosteric antagonists, 1:430–431

LY206130, nicotine dependence and withdrawal, withdrawal substrate specificity, 2:542–543
LY274600, nicotine dependence and withdrawal, withdrawal substrate specificity, 2:542–543
LY354740, mGlu II selective orthosteric agonists, 1:426–428
LY354740 Glu analog, nicotine dependence and withdrawal, withdrawal substrate specificity, 2:542–543
LY367385, mGlu I selective orthosteric antagonists, 1:425–426
LY377770 antagonist, stroke and, kainate receptors, 3:363
LY379268/LY389795, mGlu II selective orthosteric agonists, 1:428–429
LY392098, AMPA receptor allosteric potentiators, 1:390–391
LY487379, mGlu2 allosteric potentiators, 1:437–439
LY520303, mGlu II selective orthosteric agonists, 1:426–427
LY4464333, mGlu II selective orthosteric agonists, 1:426–427
Lysergic acid diethylamide (LSD), 2:637–640
  addiction, 2:639–640
  mechanism of action, 2:638–639
  pharmacology, 2:638

M100907 compound, schizophrenia therapy, serotonin receptor 5-HT$_{2A}$, 2:419–421
MAdCAM-1, inflammation mechanisms, 3:624–625
Madopar, Parkinson's disease treatment, 3:484–487
  slow-release formulations, 3:487–488
Magnesium ions:
  NMDA receptor allosteric antagonists, 1:387–389
  second messengers and, 1:31–32
Magnetic resonance imaging (MRI):
  obsessive-compulsive disorders, brain imaging studies, 2:217–218, 2:220
  schizophrenia analysis, 2:256
Magnetic resonance spectroscopy (MRS):
  glutamate theory of schizophrenia, 2:293
  schizophrenia analysis, 2:256–257
Magnetoencephalography (MEG), epilepsy diagnosis, 3:407

Magnocellular system, hypothalamic-pituitary pathways, 1:692
Major depressive disorder (MDD). See Depression
Major histocompatibility complex (MHC), neuroinflammation and, 3:626–627
  class I/II immunoreceptors, 3:631
MAPK/ERK signaling, anxiety neurobiology and, 2:36–37
Marijuana. See also Cannabinoid receptors
  endocannabinoid system, 2:662–665
    cannabinoid receptors and signaling, 2:662–663
    prenatal developmental effects, 2:664–665
    reward, tolerance and dependence mechanisms, 2:675–676
    synthesis and metabolism, 2:663–664
  future research on, 2:676
  pharmacology:
    appetite regulation, 2:670–672
    cognitive function, 2:669–670
    emesis, 2:673–674
    endocannabinoid system physiology, 2:665–666
    neurotoxicity, 2:672–673
    overview, 2:659–662
    pain management, 2:666–669
Marine products, kainate receptor orthosteric agonists, 1:379–381
Mast cells, calcitonin gene-related peptide sites and migraine therapy targeting, 2:762
MATRICS program, schizophrenia-related cognitive dysfunction, 2:254–255
Matrix metalloproteinases (MMPs):
  neuroinflammation and, 3:633
    minocycline inhibition, 3:645–656
  nitrosylation and, 1:751–752
  Tat protein promotion of, 3:703
Mazindol:
  narcolepsy therapy, 3:103
  psychostimulant abuse therapy, 2:587
MC4 receptor agonist, antiobesity therapy, 3:828–829
mCCP serotonin receptor agonist, obsessive-compulsive disorders, 2:234
MCG-1, mGlu II selective orthosteric agonists, 1:426–427

MCH peptide, hypocretin/orexin system, 3:129
MCH receptor-1 antagonists, antiobesity therapy, 3:829–830
McN-A-343 muscarinic agonist, cardiovascular effects, 1:176
Mecamylamine, nicotine dependence and withdrawal therapy, 2:549
Mecamylamine, nicotinic acetylcholine receptors, 1:121
Medial prefrontal cortex (MPFC), anxiety neurobiology, brain imaging studies, 2:15
Melanin-concentrating hormone (MCH), leptin signaling and and feeding regulation, 3:743
Melanocortin:
  neuropeptide receptors, 1:690
  pathways, leptin signaling and feeding regulation, 3:741–743
Melanocyte-inhibiting factor (MIF) peptides, pain management and
Melanocyte-stimulating hormone (MSH), neuropeptides and, 1:677–678
Melatonin:
  central nervous system receptors:
    circadian rhythm modulation, 3:54–57
    clock genes and, 3:50–51
    desensitization, 3:52–53
    historical perspective, 3:38–40
    melatonin production, 3:40–41
    molecular pharmacology, 3:42–44
    molecular structure, 3:41–42
    overview, 3:37–38
    regulatory mechanisms, 3:51–54
    signaling mechanisms, 3:44–46
    supersensitization, 3:54
    suprachiasmatic nucleus, 3:46–54
      circadian inputs and outputs, 3:46–47
      receptor localization, signaling, and function, 3:47–50
    as therapeutic targets, 3:57–61
      circadian rhythms, 3:58
      depression, 3:58–61
      sleep, 3:57–58
  circadian rhythm modulation, 3:54–57
  depression and levels of:
    in menopause, 1:849–850
    during menstrual cycle, 1:844–845
    postpartum depression, 1:848
    in pregnancy, 1:846–847
  desensitization function, 3:52–53
  regulatory mechanisms, 3:51–54
  reproductive-cycle depression and levels of, in menstrual cycle, 1:844–845
  sedative/hypnotics and, 3:188
  supersensitization function, 3:54
  in suprachiasmatic nucleus, localization, signaling, and function, 3:47–50
  therapeutic targeting of, 3:57–61
    circadian rhythms, 3:58
    depression, 3:58–61
    sleep, 3:57–58
  white adipose tissue innervation, 3:794–797
Memantine:
  dementia disorders and, 3:470
  schizophrenia pharmacotherapy, 2:392
Membrane activity, circadian rhythms, 3:12
Membrane-associated guanylate kinase (MAGUK) family, voltage-gated calcium channels, β subunits, 1:645–646
Membrane potentials:
  early research on, 1:25–27
  inward rectification, with potassium channels, 1:634–635
Memory. See also Cognitive function; Dementia
  brain-derived neurotrophic factor synthesis and, 3:224–225
  cannabinoid receptors and, 2:669–670
  3,4-methylenedioxymethamphetamine and, 2:630–631
  muscarinic acetylcholine receptor deficiency, 1:168–169
  schizophrenia, animal models, 2:263
  schizophrenia and, 2:254–255
  traumatic brain injury and, 3:446
Menopause, neuroendocrine abnormalities and depression in, 1:849–851
Menstrual cycle depression, neuroendocrine abnormalities, 1:844–846, 1:851
  cortisol, 1:845
  melatonin, 1:844–845
  prolactin, 1:846
  thyroid-stimulating hormone, 1:845
Mesial temporal sclerosis (MTS), epilepsy and, 3:405
Mesoaccumbens system, alcohol abuse studies:
  dopaminergic receptor systems and substrates, 2:472–473

GABA$_A$ benzodiazepine receptor
  complex, site-specific
  microinjection techniques,
  2:494–496
Mesolimbic pathway:
  alcohol abuse studies, dopaminergic
    receptor systems and substrates,
    2:472–473
  psychostimulant abuse, dopamine system,
    2:574–575
Mesopallidal system, alcohol abuse studies,
  2:476–480
Messenger RNA (mRNA):
  D$_1$ receptor expression, 1:226–227
  D$_2$ receptor expression, 1:229–230
  hypocretin receptor distribution,
    3:130–131
  large-conductance calcium-activated
    potassium channels, structure and
    function, 1:630–631
  mGlu group I selective orthosteric
    agonists, 1:423
Metabolic syndrome, antipsychotics and,
  2:254
Metabolism kinetics:
  endocannabinoid system, 2:663–664
  ghrelin effects, 3:772–773
  hypocretin/orexin system, 3:132–134
  leptin gene, 3:733–734
  3,4-methylenedioxymethamphetamine
    neurotoxicity and, 2:621–622
  nicotine dependence and withdrawal,
    2:544–545
Metabolites, 3,4-methylenedioxy-
  methamphetamine neurotoxicity
  and mechanisms of, 2:621–622
Metabotropic receptors:
  γ-amino butyric acid (GABA) receptors:
    agonists and competitive antagonists,
      1:589–590
    disease and, 1:592–597
      anxiety and depression, 1:594–595
      drug addiction, 1:593–594
      epilepsy, 1:595
      gene linkage studies, 1:596–597
      nociception, 1:595–596
      therapeutic targeting, GABA$_B$
        receptors, 1:592–593
      tumor cell growth and migration,
        1:596
    effector systems, 1:580–583
      adenylate cyclase, 1:582–583
      calcium channels, 1:581–582
      G-protein-dependent/indepdendent
        GABA$_B$ effects, 1:580–581
      MAPKs, 1:583
      potassium channels, 1:582
    endogenous GABA$_B$ ligands,
      1:588–589
    GABA$_B$ receptors:
      deficient mice, 1:587–588
      modulation, 1:584–586
        extracellular calcium, 1:584
        interacting proteins, 1:585–587
        phosphorylation and
          desensitization, 1:584–585
      novel compounds, 1:590–592
      research background, 1:570–571
      structural properties, 1:571–580
        allosteric interactions, 1:580
        expression cloning, 1:571–572
        G-protein coupling determinants,
          1:579–580
        liganding binding sites, 1:578–579
        molecular subtypes, 1:572–575
        surface trafficking and
          heteromerization, 1:575–578
  glutamate receptors:
    allosteric potentiators and antagonists:
      mGlu1 antagonists, 1:436–437
      mGlu1 potentiators, 1:435–436
      mGlu2/3 antagonists, 1:439–440
      mGlu2 potentiators, 1:437–439
      mGlu4 potentiators, 1:440–441
      mGlu5 antagonists, 1:443–445
      mGlu5 potentiators, 1:441–443
      mGlu7 antagonists, 1:445
    atypical antipsychotics, 2:427–429
    background and classification,
      1:421–422
    future research issues, 1:445–446
    glutamate theory of schizophrenia,
      2:293–294
    history of, 2:290–291
    pathological evidence, 2:292
    neurogenesis and, 3:208
    orthosteric agents:
      group 1 selective agonists, 1:423–424
      group 1 selective antagonists,
        1:424–426
      group 2 selective agonists, 1:426–429
      group 2 selective antagonists,
        1:429–431
      group 3 selective agonists, 1:431–433

group 3 selective antagonists,
  1:433–435
psychostimulant abuse, 2:576
schizophrenia pharmacotherapy, group
  II receptor targeting, 2:391–392
stroke management, 3:363–365
Metal ions, voltage-gated calcium channel
  blockers, 1:647
Methadone:
  heroin addiction pharmacotherapy,
    history of, 2:453–457
  in "office-based practice," 2:700
  opiate addiction therapy, buprenorphine
    comparisons with, 2:697–698
  psychostimulant abuse therapy, 2:585–586
  treatment statistics, 2:694–696
Methamphetamine. See also 2:3,2:4-
    Methylenedioxymethamphetamine
    (MDMA)
  histaminergic neuron activity, 1:327
  HIV/AIDS and abuse of, 3:713–715
  3,4-methylenedioxymethamphetamine
    and, behavioral effects, 2:630–631
  monoamine neuropharmacology,
    2:571–575
3-Methoxy-4-hydroxyphenol-glycol
    (MHPG), norephinephrine
    neurochemistry, 1:198–199
3-(2-Methoxy-phenyl)-5-methyl-6-phenyl-
    5H-isoxazolol[4,5-c]pyridin-4-one,
    mGlu7 allosteric antagonists, 1:445
Methylation techniques, 3,4-methylene-
    dioxymethamphetamine
    neurotoxicity and, 2:622
(2S,1′S,2′S)-2-Methyl-2(2′-carboxy-
    cyclopropyl)glycine (MCCG),
    mGlu II selective orthosteric
    antagonists, 1:429–430
S-α-Methyl-4-carboxyphenylglycine
    (S-MCPG), mGlu I selective
    orthosteric antagonists, 1:425
N-Methyl-D-aspartic acid receptors. See
    NMDA (N-methyl-D-aspartic
    acid) receptors
3,4-Methylenedioxyamphetamine (MDA),
    3,4-methylenedioxy-
    methamphetamine neurotoxicity
    and, 2:621–622
3,4-Methylenedioxymethamphetamine
    (MDMA):
  behavioral effects, 2:618–619
  body temperature effects, 2:617–618

brain biochemistry and function,
  2:631–632
monoamine release, 2:616
neuroendocrine and immune responses,
  2:618
neurotoxicity, 2:619–628
  animal models, 2:620–621
  cytokines and microglia, 2:627–628
  hyperthermia, 2:624–625
  long-term neurochemical change,
    2:619–620
  metabolite mechanisms, 2:621–622
  monoaminergic transporter,
    2:625–627
  oxidative stress, 2:623–624
neurotoxic lesions:
  behavioral effects, 2:629–631
  thermoregulation effects, 2:629
neurotransmitter receptors and
  transporters, 2:617
overview, 2:614
reinforcing properties, 2:614–616
tryptophan hydroxylase, 2:616–617
Methyl methanethiosulfonate, nitrosothiol
  detection, 1:748
α-Methylparatyrosine (AMPT):
  schizophrenia dopamine hypothesis,
    2:372–373
  schizophrenia therapy, D_2 receptor
    occupancy and effect, 2:376–378
Methylphenidate:
  attention-deficit hyperactivity disorder,
    3:294–296
  autism spectrum disorders, 3:329–330
  chronic exposure and sensitization effects,
    2:580–585
  monoamine neuropharmacology,
    2:571–575
  narcolepsy therapy, 3:90–93
  psychostimulant abuse therapy, 2:587
1-Methyl-4-phenyl-1,2,3,6-tetra-
    hydropyridine (MPTP):
  parkin gene mutations and, 3:532
  Parkinson's disease, 1:755
  pathogenesis, 3:546
(R,S)-α-Methyl-4-phosphonophenylglyine
    (MPPG), mGlu III selective
    orthosteric agonists, 1:434–435
Methylprednisolone, traumatic brain injury
    and, 3:448–449
MGS0028, mGlu II selective orthosteric
    agonists, 1:429

MGS0039, mGlu II selective orthosteric antagonists, 1:431
Microdomains, dopamine, 1:233–234
Microglia:
  3,4-methylenedioxymethamphetamine effects on, 2:627–628
  neuroinflammation and, 3:626–627
Microinjection studies, alcohol abuse, $GABA_A$ benzodiazepine receptor complex modulation, 2:505–507
Middle cerebral artery occlusion (MCAO), stroke-related global and focal ischemia, 3:353–354
Migraine headaches:
  history and definition, 2:758–759
  therapy:
    calcitonin gene-related peptide and, 2:759–763
      injection techniques, 2:763
      neurovascular model, 2:759–760
      receptor antagonist therapeutic efficacy, 2:763–764
      synthesis and actions, 2:760–761
      trigeminovasculature sites, 2:761–763
    future trends in, 2:768–769
    history of, 2:758–759
    migraine diagnostic criteria, 2:758–759
    overview, 2:758
    pharmacology, 2:764–768
      acute therapy, 2:764–765
      preventive therapy, 2:766–768
Mild cognitive impairment, diagnostic criteria, 3:462
Mild cognitive motor disorder (MCMD), HIV neuropharmacology and, 3:694–696
Mild mental stress models, neurosteroid effects, 2:151–152
Mineralocorticoid receptors, psychostimulant abuse, 2:577–578
Miniature end-plate potentials (MEPPS), early research on, 1:26–27
Minocycline:
  multiple sclerosis therapy, 3:679
  neuroinflammation therapy with, 3:645–646
Mirrored chamber, mouse anxiety models, neurosteroid effects, 2:147–148
Mirtazapine:
  anxiety disorder therapy, 2:70
  autism spectrum disorders, 3:331, 3:334

Missense mutations:
  familial Parkinson's disease and, PINK1 gene mutation and, 3:534–535
  PRODH gene, schizophrenia molecular genetics, 2:329–330
Mitochondrial DNA, idiopathic Parkinson's disease and, 3:543
Mitochondrial dysfunction, Parkinson's disease pathogenesis and, 3:545–547
Mitogen-activated protein kinase (MAPK):
  adipose tissue signaling and, 3:802–803
  α_1 adrenergic receptor signal transduction pathways, 1:203
  $GABA_B$ receptors, effector systems, 1:583
  lithium mechanism in bipolar disorder patients, 1:867–869
  muscarinic acetylcholine receptor modulation, 1:159
  phosphorylation, 1:89–90
  receptor-like PTPs, 1:92–94
  small G proteins, 1:63–64
  transient receptor potential V1 (TRPV1) receptor expression, 2:729
Mitotic inhibitor methylazoxymethanol (MAM), in schizophrenia, 2:265
Mitoxantrone, multiple sclerosis therapy, 3:676–677
MK-801 antagonist:
  human immunodeficiency virus, nigrostriatal system and, 3:709
  stroke and NMDA receptors, 3:355–356, 3:361
Moclobemide, anxiety disorder therapy, 2:70
Modafinil:
  attention-deficit hyperactivity disorder therapy, 3:301
  narcolepsy therapy, 3:100–103
    limits of, 3:114
  Parkinson-related sleep disturbance, 3:504
  psychostimulant abuse therapy, 2:588
  schizophrenia therapy, 2:389
Modified forced-swim test, animal anxiety models, neurosteroid effects, 2:150–151
Modulation therapy, addictive disorders, 2:458–459
Molecular feedback loops, circadian rhythms, animal models, 3:11–12

Molecular genetics:
　corticotropin-releasing factor receptor antagonists, ligand binding mechanisms, 2:191–195
　GABA$_A$ benzodiazepine receptor complex, alcohol abuse studies, 2:487–501
　　alcohol/modulator commonalities, 2:487–488
　　CA1/CA3 hippocampus, 2:511–516
　　efficacy of βCCT/3PBD modulation, GABA$_{A1,2,3,5}$ receptors, 2:499–501
　　future research issues, 2:517–518
　　GABA-DA interaction hypothesis, 2:496–498
　　ligand selectivity with GABA$_{A1}$ subunits, 2:498–499
　　microinjection studies, 2:505–506
　　naltrexone antagonist, 2:507–511
　　novel CNS GABAergic substrates, 2:498
　　oral administration, βCCT/3PBD: anxiety reduction, 2:510–511
　　　vs. naltrexone, 2:507–511
　　probe applications, 2:488–493
　　site-specific microinjection, 2:493–496
　　subunit selectivity vs. intrinsic efficacy, 2:516–517
　　systemic administration, 2:492–493, 2:503–504
　　ventral pallidum, 2:501–502
　rhythmicity, Drosophila models, 3:7
　schizophrenia, 2:323–325
　　candidate genes, 2:325–328
　　chromosomal abnormalities, 2:328–331
　　functional candidate genes, 2:331–332
　　future research issues, 2:333
　　gene linkage studies, 2:323–324
　　neurochemistry and, 2:261–262
　　positional candidate genes, 2:325
　　susceptibility genes, 2:351–355
　　　DISC1 gene, 2:351–352
　　　DTNBP1 gene, 2:352–353
　　　function, 2:332–333
　　　NRG1 gene, 2:353–355
Molecular path model, benzodiazepine activity, 2:115
Molecular targeting:
　narcolepsy therapy, amphetamines, 3:93–94
　schizophrenia-related cognitive dysfunction therapy, 2:254–255

Monoamine neurotransmitters:
　anxiety disorder anxiolytics, 2:63–72
　antidepressants, 2:64–70
　antipsychotics, 2:71–72
　beta blockers, 2:71
　attention-deficit hyperactivity disorder therapy, 3:297–298
　autism spectrum disorders, 3:331
　cannabinoid analgesics and, 2:668–669
　dopamine hypothesis of schizophrenia, 2:371–373
　3,4-methylenedioxymethamphetamine effects, 2:616
　narcolepsy pathophysiology, hypocretin/orexin system, 3:87–89
　psychostimulant abuse and, 2:569–575
Monoamine oxidase B (MAOB), Parkinson's disease and, 1:755
Monoamine oxidase inhibitors (MAOIs):
　anxiety disorder therapy, 2:70
　cataplexy therapy, 3:111, 3:114–115
　circadian rhythms and, antidepressant effects, 3:19–20
　obsessive-compulsive disorders, metabolism studies, 2:223
　Parkinson's disease:
　　neurochemistry of, 3:481–483
　　type B inhibitor (MAO$_B$), 3:494–496
　schizophrenia therapy, 2:394
Monoamine oxidase (MAO):
　α$_2$-adrenergic receptor regulation, 1:205–206
　dopamine inhibition, 1:223–224
　mGlu5 allosteric antagonists, 1:443–444
　norephinephrine neurochemistry, 1:198–199
　serotonin degradation and reuptake, 1:261–262
Monoaminergic transporter, 3,4-methylenedioxymethamphetamine neurotoxicity and, 2:625–627
Monoamines:
　antidepressants and, hippocampal neurogenesis and, 1:822–823
　neurotransmitter inactivation, 1:51–52
　plasma membrane transporters, 1:719–720
　stress and depression convergence in, 1:825–826
　vesicular monoamine neurotransmitter transporters, 1:716–717, 1:723

Monoclonal antibodies, multiple sclerosis
    therapy, 3:677–679
  new drug development, 3:684–687
Monogenetic Parkinsonism:
  causative mutations, 3:527–539
  genetic mutations in, 3:525–541
  non-PARK mutations, 3:540
  PARK1 loci, 3:527–529
  PARK2 (parkin) mutations, 3:529–532
  PARK3 mutations, 3:541
  PARK4 loci, 3:527–529
  PARK5 (UCH-L1) mutation, 3:539–540
  PARK6 (PINK1) mutations, 3:532–535
  PARK7 (DJ-1) mutations, 3:535–536
  PARK8 (LRRK2) mutation, 3:536–539
  PARK9 mutations, 3:541
  PARK10 mutations, 3:541
  PARK11 mutations, 3:541
  Parkinsonism loci, 3:540–541
  PARK loci, 3:526–527
  potential causative mutations, 3:539–541
Monosynaptic H reflex, narcolepsy
    pathophysiology, 3:85
Monotherapies:
  antiepileptic drugs, 3:419–420
  obsessive-compulsive disorders, controlled
    trials, 2:225
Mood disorders. See also specific disorders,
    e.g. Depression
  neurotrophic factors:
    antidepressants:
      BDNR expression and, 1:804–806
      neurogenesis and, 1:806–808
    behavioral effects, 1:808–809
    brain-derived neurotrophic factor
      genetics, 1:803
    depressed patients, 1:800–802
      structural and cellular alterations,
        1:802–803
    intracellular signaling cascades,
      1:791–794
    fibroblast growth factor, 1:793
    insulin/insulin-like growth factor,
      1:793
    nerve growth factor family,
      1:791–792
    transforming growth factor-beta,
      1:793–794
    vascular endothelial growth factor,
      1:792–793
  research background, 1:790
  stress and, 1:794–797

  adrenal glucocorticoids, 1:796–797
  adult neurogenesis and morphology,
    1:797–800
    hippocampus, 1:798
    alterations in, 1:794–795
  brain-derived neurotrophic factor,
    1:794–796
  cytokines, 1:797
  glial proliferation, 1:800
  serotonin receptors, 1:797
  vascular endothelial growth factor,
    1:797
MOR-1 opioid receptor:
  pain management and, 2:716–717
  structure and function, 2:748–751
Morphine compounds:
  mu opioid receptors and, 2:748–751
  obsessive-compulsive disorder therapy,
    2:234
  peripheral-central interactions,
    2:719–721
  spinal-supraspinal interactions, 2:718–720
Morphometric studies, depressed patients,
    neurotrophic factors and,
    1:802–803
Motilin receptor, ghrelin and, 3:771–772
Motivation response, hypocretin/orexin
    system, 3:135
  arousal and feeding behavior integration,
    3:144
Motor fluctuation, Parkinson's disease
    treatment and:
  classification of, 3:496–499
  levodopa agents, 3:487
Motor hyperactivity/inattention, autism
    spectrum disorder, 3:333–334
Motor neuron diseases, plasma membrane
    glutamate transporter,
    1:718–719
Mouse models:
  anxiety neurobiology:
    anxiety-like behavior, genetically
      altered mice, 2:19–24
    neuroticism (N trait), 2:6–9
    oligogenic anxiety-like conditions,
      2:32–33
    QTL studies, 2:19
  benzodiazepine functional diversity,
    2:112–114
  circadian rhythms, 3:4–5
    rhythmicity in, 3:8
  sedative/hypnotics, 3:190–192

MPEP:
  mGlu4 allosteric antagonists, *1:*440–441
  mGlu5 allosteric antagonists, *1:*443–444
MPEP antagonist, psychostimulant abuse and, *2:*576
MTEP, mGlu5 allosteric antagonists, *1:*444
MthK channel, gating mechanism, *1:*626–627
Multidrug resistance, drug-resistant epilepsy, *3:*425–426
Multidrug transporters, drug-resistant epilepsy, *3:*425–426
Multifocal leukoencephalopathy (PML), 5-HT$_{2A}$ receptors and, *1:*271
Multifocal motor neuropathy (MMN), characteristics of, *3:*614–615
Multinucleated giant cells (MNGCs), HIV neuropathogenesis and, *3:*697
Multiple sclerosis (MS):
  acute relapses, treatment of, *3:*672–674
  chemotherapy agents, *3:*676–677
  classification of, *3:*671–672
  immunomodulatory therapies, *3:*674–676
  monoclonal antibody therapy, *3:*677–678
    new drug development, *3:*684–687
  myelin pathology and, *3:*612–613
  new drug development, *3:*678–679
    immunomodulator/suppressants, *3:*687–689
    overview, *3:*683–684
  nitric oxide physiology, *1:*745
  voltage-gated sodium ion channels, *1:*640–641
Multipoint linkage analysis, anxiety neurobiology, *2:*4
Mu opioid receptors:
  obsessive-compulsive disorders, *2:*234
  psychostimulant abuse and, *2:*578–579
  structure and function, *2:*748–751
Muscarinic acetylcholine receptors (mAChRs):
  activation mechanisms, *1:*155
  dimerization, *1:*166–167
  distribution, *1:*149
  G-protein coupling properties, *1:*155–157
    RGS proteins, *1:*158
  G protein selectivity, *1:*157–158
  ion channels, *1:*160–162
  ligand binding mechanisms, *1:*152–154
    agonists, *1:*152
    allosteric ligands, *1:*153–154
    antagonists, *1:*152–153
    clinical applications, *1:*154
  MAPK pathways modulation, *1:*159
  phenotypic mouse analysis, *1:*167–177
    agonist-induced tremor and hypothermia, *1:*170–171
    amylase secretion, exocrine pancreas, *1:*175
    analgesia, *1:*170
    autoreceptors, *1:*171
    cardiovascular system, *1:*175–176
    cytolytic T cells, *1:*177
    drug abuse effects, *1:*173
    epileptic seizures, *1:*169
    food intake stimulation, *1:*171
    gastric acid secretion, *1:*175
    inhibitory hippocampal synapse suppression, *1:*172
    learning and memory functions, *1:*168–169
    locomotor activity, *1:*169–170
    nucleus accumbens, dopamine effects, *1:*172–173
    pancreatic islet insulin and glucagon secretion, *1:*174–175
    peripheral autoreceptors and heteroreceptors, *1:*176
    prepulse inhibition and haloperidol-induced catalepsy, *1:*172
    salivary secretion, *1:*174
    skin functions, *1:*177
    smooth muscle functions, *1:*173–174
    striatal dopamine release modulation, *1:*171–172
  regulatory mechanisms, *1:*162–166
    downregulation, *1:*163–164
    internalizations, *1:*162–163
    phosphorylation, *1:*164–166
    resensitization, *1:*166
    uncoupling, *1:*162
  research background, *1:*148–149
  signaling pathways, *1:*158–159
  structural features, *1:*149–151
Muscarinic receptor agonists:
  atypical antipsychotics and, cholinergic agents, *2:*429–430
  dementia disorders and, *3:*465–466
  schizophrenia therapy, *2:*393–394

Muscimol, alcohol abuse studies, $GABA_A$ benzodiazepine receptor complex manipulation, 2:494–496
Mutagenesis:
　$GABA_A$ receptor activation:
　　benzodiazepine binding sites, 1:506–507, 1:509–511
　　channel gating binding, 1:496–497
　　potassium channels, voltage activation, 1:625–626
Mutations, in G proteins, 1:66
Myelin:
　CD9 protein in, 3:608
　claudin protein family in, 3:608
　CNS proteins, 3:596–599
　composition, 3:592–609
　　lipids, 3:594–596
　connexins in, 3:609
　2′,3′-cyclic nucleotide 3′-phosphodiesterase, 3:603–604
　disorders, 3:611–615
　　autoimmune demyelinating diseases, 3:611–615
　　axon-glia disruptions, 3:611
　　experimental allergic encephalomyelitis, 3:611–612
　　multiple sclerosis, 3:612–613
　enzymes in, 3:609–610
　future research issues, 3:615–616
　glycoproteins in, 3:604–607
　myelin and lymphocyte protein and plasmolipin, 3:608
　myelin basic protein, 3:598–599, 3:602–603
　paranodal proteins, 3:609
　peripheral myelin protein-22, 3:601–602
　PNS proteins, 3:599–603
　protein 2, 3:603
　protein locations in, 3:600
　protein zero in, 3:599–601
　proteolipid protein, 3:596–598
　receptors, 3:610
　structure of, 3:592
　　molecular organization, 3:592, 3:595
　　sheath structures, 3:592, 3:594
　tetraspan proteins in, 3:607–608
Myelin and lymphocyte protein (MAL), structure and function, 3:608
Myelin-associated glycoprotein (MAG):
　multiple sclerosis and, 3:613
　stroke therapy, 3:377–378
　structure and function, 3:604–606

Myelin basic protein (MBP):
　peripheral form, 3:602–603
　structure and function, 3:596–598
Myelin oligodendrocyte glycoprotein (MOG):
　multiple sclerosis and, 3:613
　structure and function, 3:606–607
Myotonias, voltage-gated sodium ion channels and, 1:641–642
Myristoylated alanine rich C-kinase substrate (MARCKS), lithium mechanism in bipolar disorder patients, 1:868–869

Naloxone:
　nicotine dependence and withdrawal, 2:540
　opiate addiction therapy, regulatory studies, 2:696–697
Naltrexone:
　alcohol abuse studies, oral administration of $\beta CCT/3PBC$ vs., 2:507–511
　nicotine dependence and withdrawal, 2:540
　pharmacotherapy, 2:550–551
　opiate addiction therapy, 2:698–699
　psychostimulant abuse therapy, 2:585–586
NAN-190 antagonists, nicotine dependence and withdrawal, withdrawal substrate specificity, 2:542–543
Narcolepsy:
　evaluation, 3:83–84
　　cerebrospinal fluid hypocretin-1 assessment, 3:84
　　histocompatibility human leukocyte antigen testing, 3:84
　　polysomnography, 3:83
　future research issues, 3:114–115
　idiopathic hypersomnia, 3:84
　overview of, 3:80
　pathophysiology, 3:84–89
　　human leukocyte antigen analysis, 3:85–86
　　hypocretin/orexin system, 3:136–138
　　hypocretin/orexin system and sleep regulation, 3:86–89
　　hypocretin transmission, animal models, 3:86
　　symptoms analysis, 3:84–85
　symptoms of, 3:80–83
　　cataplexy, 3:83

excessive daytime sleepiness, 3:82, 3:84, 3:90–92
hypnagogic/hypnopompic hallucinations, 3:83
sleep paralysis, 3:83
treatment of, 3:90–100
  amphetamines, 3:90–100
    drug interactions with, 3:98, 3:100
    molecular targeting of, 3:93–94
    side effects, 3:98
  bupropion, 3:103–105
  caffeine, 3:104–105
  dopamine neurotransmitters, substrates, 3:97–98
  dopamine neurotransmitters and EEG arousal, 3:94–97
  future stimulant development, 3:105–106
  mazindol, 3:103
  modafinal, 3:100–103
  monoamine oxidase inhibitor reduction of, 3:111
  nonamphetamine stimulants, 3:99–105
  selegiline, 3:104
Natalizumab, multiple sclerosis therapy, 3:677–679, 3:684–685
National Institute for Medical Research, establishment of, 1:17–18
Natural products, AMPA receptor orthosteric agonists, 1:376–377
Nausea and vomiting:
  antiemetics, migraine management, 2:765
  cannabinoid receptors modulation of, 2:673–675
  Parkinson's disease treatment and, 3:500
    levodopa agents, 3:486–487
N-back task analysis, schizophrenia cognitive dysfunction and, 2:259
NBI-31772 molecule, stroke therapy, 3:376–377
NBQX antagonist, stroke and, 3:361–362
NDMC metabolite, cholinergic mechanisms and, 2:429–430
N-domain fragments, corticotropin-releasing factor receptor antagonists, ligand binding mechanisms, 2:192–195
Negative affect, in schizophrenia, 2:255–256
  neural network studies, 2:258–259
Negative modulators:
  GABA$_A$ receptors subunit pharmacology, 1:483–491

GABA$_A$ α_1 subunit, 1:488
GABA$_A$ δ subunit, 1:492
GABA$_A$ γ subunit, 1:491
Neodysiherbaine, kainate receptor orthosteric agonists, 1:380
NEO-five factor inventory (NEO-FFI), anxiety neurobiology, genetic susceptibility studies, 2:18–19
NEO personality inventory, anxiety neurobiology, 2:5–6
  human personality traits, 2:9–12
Neospinothalamic pain pathways, classification of, 2:711–714
Nerve growth factor (NGF):
  cognitive function and, 3:228
  discovery, 3:221–222
  inflammation mechanisms, 3:641
  neuronal maturation regulation, 3:224
  neuropathies and, 3:227
  neurotrophins and, 3:237–238
    signaling mechanisms, 3:239
  p75 neurotrophin receptor:
    signaling, 3:246–247
    structure, 3:240–241
  pain perception and management, 3:229
  peripheral nervous system and, 3:225
  receptors and kinases in, 1:791–792
  structure of, 3:240
  transient receptor potential V1 (TRPV1) receptor expression, 2:729
  tyrosine kinase receptor structure and, 3:241–242
Nerve injury, voltage-gated sodium ion channels, 1:640–641
N-ethylmaleimide-sensitive factor (NSF):
  GABA$_A$ receptor trafficking, 1:480
  nitrosylation and, 1:751
Neural networks:
  glutamate theory of schizophrenia, history of, 2:290–291
  schizophrenia:
    cognitive dysfunction and, 2:259
    future research issues, 2:266
    negative affect and, 2:255–256, 2:258–259
    psychosis and, 2:257–258
Neural progenitor cells, human immunodeficiency virus and, 3:706–707
Neural regeneration, traumatic brain injury and, 3:452–453

Neuregulin I (NRG1), schizophrenia
  candidate gene, 2:326–327
  ErbB3 receptor, 2:328
  functional implications, 2:332–333
  molecular interactions, 2:352–353
  susceptibility identification, 2:350
Neurite outgrowth inhibitor (NoGo), stroke
  therapy, 3:377–378
Neuroactive steroids/neurosteroids:
  anxiety disorders:
    alcohol effects, 2:157–159
    animal models, 2:142–152
    behavioral effects, 2:142
    brain and peripheral sources, 2:135–137
    chemistry and pharmacology,
      2:135–142
    enantiomeric selectivity, 2:141–142
    $GABA_A$ receptors and ligand-gated ion
      channels, 2:137–141
    HPA axis function, 2:154–156
    overview, 2:134–135
  $GABA_A$ receptors:
    δ subunit pharmacology, 1:491–492
    modulation, 1:511–516
      transmembrane domains, 1:518
  schizophrenia therapy, 2:394
  stress-induced behaviors:
    drug abuse relapse, 2:159–160
    HPA axis, 2:153–154
    overview, 2:152–153
  traumatic brain injury and, 3:450–451
Neuroanatomy:
  alcohol abuse studies in alcohol-preferring
    rats, 2:469–470
  bipolar disorder, 1:860–861
  Tourette's syndrome, 3:269–270
Neurobiology, obsessive-compulsive
  disorders, 2:216–224
  brain imaging studies, 2:217–222
  functional imaging studies, 2:219–220
  magnetic resonance spectroscopy,
    2:220
Neurochemistry:
  bipolar disorder, 1:861–862
  dementia disorders and, 3:462–463
  3,4-Methylenedioxymethamphetamine
    (MDMA) neurotoxicity, long-term
    changes in, 2:619–620
  Parkinson's disease, 3:481–483
  schizophrenia, 2:260–262
    hypotheses, 2:371–376
      dopamine hypothesis, 2:371–373

glutamate receptor hypothesis,
  2:373–374
integrated dopamine/glutamate
  hypotheses, 2:374–376
Tourette's syndrome, 3:270–273
white adipose tissue innervation,
  3:794–797
Neurodegenerative disease:
  extra/intracellular protein aggregates and,
    3:644–645
  HIV neuropathogenesis and, 3:699,
    3:716–718
  inflammation mechanisms in, 3:622–623
  invertebrate models:
    Alzheimer's disease, 3:579–582
    Caenorhabditis elegans system,
      3:568–569
    Drosophila melanogaster, 3:569
    early research, 3:567–568
    future applications, 3:582–583
    genetic and molecular pathways, 3:568
    Huntington's disease trinucleotide
      repeats, 3:577–579
    Parkinson's disease, dopamine neuron
      cell death, 3:569–577
  nitric oxide and, 1:754
Neurodevelopmental animal model,
  schizophrenia, 2:265
Neuroendocrine compounds:
  circadian studies of reproductive cycle
    depression:
    cross-reproductive cycle analysis,
      1:851–853
    menopause, 1:849–851
      cortisol, 1:850
      melatonin, 1:849–850
      prolactin, 1:850–851
      thyroid-stimulating hormone, 1:850
    menstrual cycle, 1:844–846
      cortisol, 1:845
      melatonin, 1:844–845
      prolactin, 1:846
      thyroid-stimulating hormone, 1:845
    postpartum depression, 1:848–849
      cortisol, 1:848
      estradiol, 1:849
      melatonin, 1:848
      prolactin, 1:848–849
      thyroid-stimulating hormone, 1:848
    pregnancy, 1:846–847
      cortisol, 1:847
      melatonin, 1:846–847

prolactin, *1:*847
thyroid-stimulating hormone, *1:*847
research background, *1:*844
3,4-methylenedioxymethamphetamine effects on, *2:*618
neuropeptide electrophysiology, *1:*675–676
psychostimulant abuse, chronic exposure and sensitization effects, *2:*580–585
Neurogenesis:
adult stages of, *1:*827–829
antidepressant influences on, *1:*806–808
atypical antipsychotics and, *2:*430
neurotrophin regulation of, *3:*224
prokineticins and, *3:*171–172
regulation in adults:
future research issues, *3:*211–212
multiple regulation points, *3:*204
overview, *3:*203–204
proliferation, *3:*206–211
survival, *3:*204–206
schizophrenia, disruption of, *2:*265
serotonin/norepinephrine regulation, *1:*831–833
stress and:
hormone regulation, *1:*829–830
neurotrophins and, *1:*797–800
Neurogenic inflammation, vanilloid receptors and, *2:*728–729
Neurohypophyseal gene family, neuropeptides and, *1:*682–684
Neuroimaging studies:
epilepsy diagnosis, *3:*407
3,4-methylenedioxymethamphetamine neurotoxicity, brain biochemical and functional changes, *2:*631–632
obsessive-compulsive disorders, *2:*219–220
psychostimulant abuse:
chronic exposure and sensitization effects, *2:*582–585
monoamine neuropharmacology, *2:*573–575
stroke management, *3:*360–361
Neuroinflammation:
antigen-presenting cells, *3:*626
arachidonic acid pathways, *3:*630
astrocytes, *3:*627
blood-derived inflammatory cells, *3:*628
chemokines, *3:*629–630
cytokines, *3:*628–629
endothelial cells, *3:*627
growth factors, *3:*639–641

humoral components, *3:*628–630
immunization approaches, *3:*644–645
microglia, *3:*626–627
neurons, *3:*628
pharmacological modification, *3:*645–646
radical formation and oxidative damage, *3:*630
stroke and, ischemic brain injury, *3:*351–353
Neurokinin 3 receptors, antipsychotic mechanisms with, *2:*430
Neurokinin antagonists, schizophrenia therapy, *2:*391
Neuroleptics, Tourette's syndrome and, *3:*273–276
Neurological disorders:
GABA transporters and, *1:*722
monoamine plasma membrane transporters, *1:*719–720
Neuromodulators, neuropeptides as, *1:*676–677
Neuromuscular transmission:
early research on, *1:*12–13
Eccles, Kuffler, and Katz research on, *1:*22–23, *1:*25–26
electric organ model of, *1:*22
Kuffler's research on, *1:*32–33
Loewi's experiments in, *1:*18–19
Nachmansohn's research on, *1:*23
Nobel Prize awarded for research on, *1:*21–22
voltage-gated sodium ion channel trafficking, *1:*638–639
Neuronal cell adhesion molecules (NCAM), anxiety neurobiology, *2:*30
Neuronal organization:
adult neurogenesis and, *1:*829
anxiety neurobiology and, *2:*15–18
knockout mice studies, *2:*24–26
mouse studies, *2:*19–20
calcitonin gene-related peptide sites and migraine therapy targeting, *2:*762
cognitive function and diversity in, *3:*461–463
developmental maturation, *3:*224
dopaminergic receptors, alcholol abuse studies, *2:*471–486
bed nucleus of stria terminalis, *2:*473–475
dopaminergic regulation, early research, *2:*472–473
extracellular dopamine, *2:*485–486

future research issues, 2:517–518
GABAergic interactions with, 2:486
lateral hypothalamus, 2:481–485
  D_2 dopaminergic regulation,
    hypothesized mechanisms,
    2:481–485
  ventral pallidum, 2:476–480
    dopaminargic regulation
    hypothesized mechanisms,
    2:478–480
histaminergic systems, 1:301–305
  afferents, 1:303–305
  histaminergic pathways, 1:303
  neuron activity and control, 1:317–322
    electrophysiology, 1:317
    pharmacological changes,
      1:321–322
    in vitro modulation, 1:317–319
    in vivo changes, 1:319–321
  perikarya, 1:301–303
KCNQ channel action on, 1:632–633
large-conductance calcium-activated
  potassium channels, structure and
  function, 1:630–631
modulation in adults, 3:224–225
narcolepsy therapy, dopaminergic effects,
  3:97–98
neurogenesis, survival mechanisms,
  3:204–206
neuroinflammation, 3:628
neurotrophins and, 3:239
nicotine dependence and withdrawal:
  nicotine reinforcement substrates,
    2:537–540
  withdrawal neurosubstrates, 2:541–543
pain management:
  anatomical drug interactions,
    2:718–720
  descending modulatory pathways,
    2:712–714
  neospinothalamic/paleospinothalamic
    pathways, 2:711–712
  overview, 2:709–710
stress and, 1:800
survival and differentation during
  development, 3:222–223
voltage-gated sodium ion channels,
  1:639–640
"Neuron doctrine," basic principles of,
  1:40–41
Neuropathy, human autoimmune
  neuropathies, 3:613–614

Neuropeptide FF, pain management and,
  2:716–717
Neuropeptides:
  administration, 1:693
  anxiety neurobiology, 2:16–17
  basic principles, 1:670–671
  behavioral techniques, 1:677–678
  biosynthesis and processing, 1:685–687
    preprohormones, 1:686
    prohormones, 1:686
    tissue specificity, 1:687
  blood-brain barrier, 1:692–693
  classification table, 1:672–673
  electrophysiological techniques,
    1:675–677
    neurohormones, 1:675–676
    neuromodulators, 1:676–677
    neurotransmitters, 1:676
  evolution, 1:679–685
    gene duplication, 1:680–685
    gene splicing, 1:685
    neurohypophyseal family, 1:682–684
    NPY family, 1:684
    opioid family, 1:680–682
    structural conservation, 1:679–680
  extracellular inactivation, 1:687–688
  future research issues, 1:695
  gene isolation and expression, 1:685
  genetic manipulations, 1:678–679
    knockout mice, 1:678
    transgenic animals, 1:678
  genomics, 1:678–679
  hypothalamic control of pituitary gland,
    1:691–692
  hypothalamic-pituitary pathways, 1:692
  hypothalamic release-stimulating/
    release-inhibiting actions, 1:691
  identification, 1:671–674
  inactivation, 1:687–688
  intercellular signaling, 1:44–45
  intracellular degradation, 1:687
  isolation and characterization, 1:674
  neurogenesis and, 3:210–211
  peptidomics, 1:675, 1:679
  perfusion and tissue culture studies, 1:677
  physiological/peptidomic/genomic
    techniques, 1:679
  prolactin release, 1:691–692
  psychostimulant abuse and, 2:578–579
  receptors:
    agonists/antagonists, 1:675
    arginine vasopressin, 1:689

cytokines, *1:*691
downregulation and desensitization,
    *1:*688–689
G-protein-coupled receptors, *1:*690
guanylate cyclase (cGMP) receptors,
    *1:*691
isoreceptors, *1:*689
melanocortin, *1:*690
neuropeptide Y system, *1:*689
phospholipase-phosphatidylinositol-
    linked messengers, *1:*690
second-messenger systems and,
    *1:*690–691
structure and function, *1:*688–690
tachykinin, *1:*689–690
tyrosine kinase-coupled receptors,
    *1:*691
upregulation and sensitization, *1:*689
redundancy, *1:*694
site-directed mutagenesis, *1:*679
stress/neuronal response, *1:*694–695
time- and tissue-sensitive responses to,
    *1:*693–694
Neuropeptide Y (NPY):
    alcholol abuse studies, in
        alcohol-preferring rats, *2:*471
    anxiety neurobiology and, *2:*17
        knockout mice studies, *2:*25–26
    gene duplication and divergence in, *1:*684
    ghrelin effects and, *3:*773
    hypocretin/orexin system and, *3:*132–134
    in knockout mice, *1:*678
    leptin signaling and and feeding
        regulation, *3:*742–743
    neuropeptide receptors, *1:*689
    physiology, *1:*679
    suprachiasmatic nucleus and, *3:*13–15
    white adipose tissue innervation,
        *3:*796–797
Neuropharmacology:
    Bovet's contributions to, *1:*25
    Forster's contributions in, *1:*9–11
    Gaskell and Langley's contributions to,
        *1:*11–13
    obsessive-compulsive disorders, *2:*225–235
        antipsychotic agents, *2:*229–234
        augmenting agents, *2:*225, *2:*229–234
        brain imaging studies, *2:*220–222
        current trials, *2:*234
        monotherapy trials, *2:*225
        serotonin uptake inhibitor efficacy,
            *2:*226–228

postwar trends in, *1:*24–25
schizophrenia dopamine hypothesis, *2:*287
Neuroplasticity, traumatic brain injury and,
    *3:*453–454
Neuroprotective agents:
    dementia disorders and, *3:*469
    3,4-methylenedioxymethamphetamine
        neurotoxicity and, *2:*625
    Parkinson's disease and, *3:*504–505
    stroke management:
        antioxidants, *3:*371–372
        apoptosis and caspase inhibitors,
            *3:*372–373
        development criteria, *3:*374
        downstream approaches, *3:*367–371
        glutamate release inhibitors, *3:*366–367
        metabotropic glutamate receptors,
            *3:*364–365
    Tat protein, *3:*702–703
    traumatic brain injury and, *3:*446–451
        anti-inflammatory agents, *3:*447–449
        free-radical scavengers, *3:*447
        neuroactive steroids/neurosteroids,
            *3:*450–451
        neurotransmitter agonists/antagonists,
            *3:*449–450
Neuropsychiatric disease. *See also* Mood
        disorders
    AMPA receptor allosteric potentiators,
        *1:*394–395
    $GABA_A$ subunit pharmacology, allosteric
        ligand modulation, *1:*505–506
    histaminergic neuron activity, *1:*321–322,
        *1:*327–329
        Alzheimer's disease, *1:*327–328
        Parkinson's disease, *1:*328
        schizophrenia and antipsychotics, *1:*326
    monoamine plasma membrane
        transporters, *1:*719–720
    plasma membrane glutamate transporter,
        *1:*718–719
    vesicular transporters and, *1:*723
Neuroreceptor imaging, schizophrenia,
    *2:*259–260
Neurosurgery, obsessive-compulsive
    disorders, *2:*235–237
Neurotensin agonist/antagonist:
    psychostimulant abuse and, *2:*579
    schizophrenia therapy, *2:*390
Neuroticism (N trait), anxiety neurobiology,
    *2:*5–6
    mouse behavior, *2:*6–9

Neurotoxic cascade, traumatic brain injury and, 3:444–446
Neurotoxicity:
  AMPA receptor orthosteric agonists, 1:376–377
  cannabinoid receptors and, 2:672–673
  human immunodeficiency virus:
    neuropathogenesis, chemokines and, 3:698–699
    proteins, 3:699–704
      glycoproteins gp120 and gp41, 3:699, 3:701
      Nef protein, 3:703
      neurobiology of, 3:700
      Rev protein, 3:704
      Tat protein, 3:701–703
      Vpr protein, 3:703
      Vpu protein, 3:704
  3,4-Methylenedioxymethamphetamine (MDMA), 2:619–628
    animal models, 2:620–621
    cytokines and microglia, 2:627–628
    hyperthermia, 2:624–625
    long-term neurochemical change, 2:619–620
    metabolite mechanisms, 2:621–622
    monoaminergic transporter, 2:625–627
    oxidative stress, 2:623–624
  Parkinson's disease, invertebrate models of cell death, 3:570–577
  sodium voltage-gated ion channels, 1:636
  voltage-gated calcium ion channels, Ca_v2 family, 1:649
  voltage-gated potassium channels, K_V subunits, structure and function, 1:630
  voltage-gated sodium channels and, 1:642–643
Neurotransmitters. See also specific Neurotransmitters
  addictive disorders, modulator therapy and, 2:458–459
  agonists/antagonists, traumatic brain injury and, 3:449–450
  anxiety neurobiology, knockout mice studies, 2:24–26
  anxiety neurobiology and, 2:15–18
  biosynthesis of, 1:42–43
  dementia disorders and, 3:462–463
  endocannabinoid system, 2:663
  $GABA_A$ receptor trafficking, 1:480
  human immunodeficiency virus dementia and, 3:711–712
  inactivation, 1:51–52
  3,4-methylenedioxymethamphetamine effects on, receptor/transporter effects, 2:617
  in myelin, 3:610
  neuropeptide electrophysiology, 1:675–676
  obsessive-compulsive disorders, metabolism studies, 2:223
  pain neuropharmacology, 2:714–717
    drug action localization, 2:718
  Parkinson's disease, neurochemistry, 3:482–483
  psychostimulant abuse, chronic exposure and sensitization effects, 2:580–581, 2:583–585
  stroke therapy and modulation of, 3:377
  transporters:
    clinical relevance, 1:718–723
      dopamine, 1:721
      GABA transporters, 1:721–722
      glycine transporters, 1:722–723
      monoamine transporters, 1:719–720
      norepinephrine, 1:721
      plasma membrane, 1:718–721
      serotonin, 1:720
      system interactions, 1:723
    early research, 1:706–707
    plasma membrane family, 1:707–715
      choline, 1:714–715
      clinical relevance, 1:718–723
      dopamine, 1:712–713, 1:721
      GABA transporters, 1:711–712, 1:721–722
      glutamate transporters, 1:708–711, 1:718–719
      glutamine, 1:715
      glycine transporters, 1:712, 1:722–723
      monoamine transporters, 1:719–720
      norepinephrine, 1:713–714, 1:721
      regulation, 1:724–728
      serotonin, 1:714, 1:720
      sodium/chloride-dependent transporters, 1:711–714
    vesicular transporters, 1:715–718
      acetylcholine and monoamine transporters, 1:716–718
      clinical relevance, 1:723

glutamate transporters, *1:*716
inhibitor amino acid transporters, *1:*718
voltage-gated calcium ion channels, Ca$_v$2 family, *1:*648–649
voltage-gated potassium channels, K$_V$ subunits, structure and function, *1:*628–630
Neurotrophic factor:
  adult neurogenesis, *3:*224
  drug discovery mechanisms, *3:*230–232
    biological antagonists, *3:*231
    direct receptor agonists/antagonists, *3:*231–232
    indirect modulators, *3:*232
  future research on, *3:*232–233
  history of, *3:*221–222
  HIV neuropathology, apoptosis and, *3:*705
  intercellular signaling, *1:*44–45
  mood disorders:
    antidepressants:
      BDNR expression and, *1:*804–806
      neurogenesis and, *1:*806–808
    behavioral effects, *1:*808–809
    brain-derived neurotrophic factor genetics, *1:*803
    depressed patients, *1:*800–802
      structural and cellular alterations, *1:*802–803
    intracellular signaling cascades, *1:*791–794
      fibroblast growth factor, *1:*793
      insulin/insulin-like growth factor, *1:*793
      nerve growth factor family, *1:*791–792
      transforming growth factor-beta, *1:*793–794
      vascular endothelial growth factor, *1:*792–793
    research background, *1:*790
    stress and, *1:*794–797
      adrenal glucocorticoids, *1:*796–797
      adult neurogenesis and morphology, *1:*797–800
        hippocampus, *1:*798
      alterations in, *1:*794–795
      brain-derived neurotrophic factor, *1:*794–796
      cytokines, *1:*797
      glial proliferation, *1:*800
      serotonin receptors, *1:*797
      vascular endothelial growth factor, *1:*797
  neuroinflammatory mechanisms, *3:*641
  neuronal function modulation, *3:*224–225
  neuronal maturation in development, *3:*224
  neuronal survival and differentiation, *3:*222–224
  physiological functions of, *3:*222–225
  therapeutic applications, *3:*225–230
    Alzheimer's disease and cognitive impairment, *3:*227–228
    amyotrophic lateral sclerosis, *3:*225–227
    depression, *3:*229–230
    obesity and weight control, *3:*229–230
    pain management, *3:*229
    Parkinson's disesase, *3:*228–229
    peripheral neuropathies, *3:*227
    traumatic brain injury and, *3:*452–453
Neurotrophic factor 3 (NT-3):
  discovery of, *3:*221–223
  neurogenesis regulation, *3:*224
  neuronal maturation regulation, *3:*224
  neuropathies and, *3:*227
  structure of, *3:*240
  in suprachiasmatic nucleus, melatonin receptor actions, *3:*50
Neurotrophic factor 4/5 (NT-4/5):
  discovery of, *3:*221–223, *3:*238
  obesity and weight control, *3:*229–230
  Parkinson's disease and, *3:*228–229
  structure of, *3:*240
Neurotrophic hypothesis, *3:*239
Neurotrophin-3 (NT-3), discovery of, *3:*238
Neurotrophins:
  history of, *3:*237–238
  intracellular signaling, *1:*791–792
  preference determinants, *3:*242
  receptors, *3:*238
    p75-TRK interactions, *3:*247–248
    signaling, *3:*242–247
    structure, *3:*240–242
  retrograde axonal signaling, *3:*248–249
  signaling functions, *3:*238–239
  structure, *3:*239–240
Neurovascular model, migraine therapy, calcitonin gene-related peptide, *2:*759–760
Neurturin (NRTN):
  discovery of, *3:*221–223
  Parkinson's disease and, *3:*228–229

Nev protein, HIV neurotoxicity, 3:703
NF-κB transcription factor:
   anxiety neurobiology and, 2:31
   HIV neuropathology and, 3:705
Nicotinamide adenine dinucleotide phosphate (NADPH) oxidase channel, structure and function, 1:649–650
Nicotine:
   basic properties, 2:535–536
   dementia disorders and, 3:463–465
   early research on, 1:11–12
   gum:
      nicotine dependence and withdrawal therapy, 2:547–548
      Tourette's syndrome, 3:277
   patches, obsessive-compulsive disorder therapy, 2:234
   pharmacology, 2:536–545
      absorption pharmacokinetics, 2:543–544
      dependence and withdrawal therapy:
         bupropion, 2:549–550
         cannabinoid antagonists, 2:550
         nicotinic antagonists, 2:548–549
         nicotinic partial agonists, 2:548
         nonnicotinic agents, 2:549–551
         opioid antagonists, 2:550–551
         overview, 2:545–546
         public health policy and, 2:551–552
         replacement medications, 2:546–548
         tricyclic antidepressants, 2:550
      distribution pharmacokinetics, 2:544
      metabolism and elimination pharmacokinetics, 2:544–545
      nicotine reinforcement neurosubstrates, 2:537–540
      nicotinic acetylcholine receptors, 2:537
         functional adaptations, 2:540–541
         withdrawal neurosubstrates, 2:541–543
Nicotine-N-oxide, nicotine dependence and withdrawal, metabolism and elimination pharmacokinetics, 2:544–545
Nicotinic acetylcholine receptor (nAChR):
   α_7nAChR subunit, 1:114–116
   action potential research and, 1:26–27
   agonist-induced upregulation, 1:127–130
   cloning of, 1:27–28
   dementia disorders and, 3:463–465
      agonist therapies, 3:467–468
   GABA$_A$ receptor structure and, 1:475
   heteromeric structures, 1:116–125
   history of, 1:107–110
   nicotine dependence and withdrawal:
      classification and function, 2:537
      functional adaptations mechanisms, 2:540–541
      nicotine reinforcement substrates, 2:538–540
      nicotinic partial agonist therapy, 2:548
      nicotinic partial antagonist therapy, 2:548–549
      overview, 2:536–537
      withdrawal substrates, 2:542–543
   NRG1 molecular interaction, 2:354–355
   overview, 1:110–111
   pharmacology of subtypes, 1:113–125
   regulation of, 1:125–130
      agonist-induced upregulation, 1:127–130
      desensitization and inactivation, 1:125–127
   schizophrenia pharmacotherapy, cholinergic agents, 2:393–394
   structure of, 1:111–113
   +TC actions and, 1:27
Nicotinic receptors:
   agonists:
      anxiety neurobiology and, receptor deficits and, 2:29–30
      dementia disorders and, 3:467–468
         neuroprotective aspects of, 3:469
         therapeutic targeting efficacy, 3:471–473
   antagonists, nicotine dependence and withdrawal therapy, 2:548
   histaminergic neuron activity, 1:321–322
   history of, 1:107–108
   overview, 1:110–111
   partial agonists, nicotine dependence and withdrawal therapy, 2:548
   pharmacology of subtypes, 1:113–125
Nigrostriatal system, human immunodeficiency virus and, 3:707–710
Nitric oxides:
   gaseous signaling:
      basic principles, 1:743–744
      neurodegeneration and, 1:754
      nitrosothiol detection, 1:747–748
      nitrosylation mechanism, 1:745–747
         cell survival, 1:752
         extracellular matrix, 1:751–752

gene transport, *1:*750–751
ion channels, *1:*748–749
Parkinson's disease and, *1:*755–756
protein-protein interactions,
   *1:*749–750
S nitrosylation physiology, *1:*752–754
vesicular transport, *1:*751
physiological role, *1:*745
neuroinflammation and, *3:*630
pharmacology of, *3:*636–637
parkin gene mutations and, *3:*532
traumatic brain injury and, *3:*447
Nitric oxide synthase (NOS) inhibitor:
3,4-methylenedioxymethamphetamine
   neurotoxicity, *2:*623–624
stroke management, *3:*370–371
Nitric oxide synthases (NOSs), nitric oxide
   synthesis, *1:*743–744
Nitrogen ohne radikal (NOR) metabolites,
   benzodiazepine receptor ligand
   metabolism, *2:*102
S-Nitrosocysteinyl glycine (CGSNO), nitric
   oxide nitrosilyation, *1:*747
S-Nitrosoglutathione (GSNO), nitric oxide
   nitrosilyation, *1:*747
S-Nitrosoglutathione reductase (GSNOR),
   nitric oxide nitrosilyation,
   *1:*747
Nitrosothiols:
nitric oxide gaseous signaling, *1:*747–748
S nitrosylation physiology and, *1:*753–754
Nitrosylation, nitric oxide gaseous signaling,
   *1:*745–747
cell survival, *1:*752
extracellular matrix, *1:*751–752
gene transport, *1:*750–751
ion channels, *1:*748–749
Parkinson's disease and, *1:*755–756
protein-protein interactions, *1:*749–750
S nitrosylation physiology, *1:*752–754
vesicular transport, *1:*751
NMDA (*N*-methyl-D-aspartic acid)
   receptors:
addictive disorder pharmacotherapy,
   methadone interactions, *2:*456–457
allosteric antagonists, *1:*386–390
allosteric potentiators, *1:*385–396
antiepileptic drugs and:
   felbamate, *3:*414–145
   topiramate, *3:*416–417
in bipolar disorder patients, *1:*863
lithium mechanisms, *1:*868–869

consolidated glutamate/dopamine
   hypotheses, *2:*295–296
dementia disorders and, *3:*470
GABA$_B$ receptor trafficking and
   heteromization, *1:*575–576
glutamate theory of schizophrenia:
history of, *2:*289–290
imaging studies, *2:*293
neurochemistry of, *2:*373–374
pathological evidence, *2:*291–292
pharmacological evidence, *2:*294–295
histamine receptor interaction, *1:*316–317
human immunodeficiency virus and:
   alcohol abuse and, *3:*716
   excitotoxicity cell death, *3:*705–706
ketamine effects on, *2:*636–637
mGlu5 allosteric antagonists, *1:*443–444
mGlu group I selective orthosteric
   agonists, *1:*424
neurogenesis and, *3:*208
neuroinflammation and, antioxidant
   modulation, *3:*637
nitric oxide physiology, *1:*745
nitrosylation, *1:*748–749
obsessive-compulsive disorders, glutamate
   genetic studies, *2:*223
orthosteric agonists, *1:*373
orthosteric antagonists, *1:*373–376
pain management and, *2:*717
schizophrenia pharmacotherapy:
   first- and second-generation
      antipsychotics, *2:*381
   targeted drug development for,
      *2:*391–392
schizophrenia psychosis, *2:*257–258
stress and neurogenesis and, *1:*799–800
stroke and:
   antagonist development, *3:*354–358
   side effects, *3:*359–360
   ischemic brain injury, *3:*351–353
   structure and function, *1:*367–370
   traumatic brain injury and, *3:*449–450
   voltage-gated potassium channels, K$_V$
      subunits, structure and function,
      *1:*629–630
NNC 09-0026 compounds, stroke
   management, *3:*367
Noceptin, histaminergic neuron activity,
   *1:*319
Nociception:
defined, *2:*710
drug action localization, *2:*718

GABA$_B$ receptor targeting, 1:595–596
histamine neuron physiology, 1:326
pain pathways and, 2:711–712
transient receptor potential V2 (TRPV2), 2:736–737
voltage-gated calcium ion channels, Ca$_v$2 family, 1:649
Nocturnal sleep studies, narcolepsy evaluation, 3:83
Nonopiate analgesics, migraine management, 2:765
Nonpeptide ligands, corticotropin-releasing factor receptor antagonists, 2:195–196
Nonpharmacological therapy, obsessive-compulsive disorders and, 2:235–237
Nonphotic stimuli, melatonin receptors, clock gene expression, 3:51
Nonsteroidal anti-inflammatory drugs, migraine management, 2:765, 2:768
Noradrenergic agents:
attention-deficit hyperactivity disorder therapy, 3:299–301
hypocretin/orexin system, arousal mechanisms, 3:141–142
psychostimulant abuse, chronic exposure and sensitization effects, 2:584
schizophrenia pharmacotherapy, 2:393
Norepinephrine (NE):
adipocyte proliferative capacity, 3:798–799
α-adrenergic receptors, α$_2$-adrenergic receptor, 1:204–209
β-adrenergic receptor activation, 1:209–210
alcohol abuse studies, dopaminergic receptor systems and substrates, 2:472–473
antidepressant influences on, hippocampal neurogenesis and, monoamines, 1:822–823
anxiety neurobiology, 2:15–17
basic properties, 1:193
dopamine synthesis, 1:56, 1:223–224
early research on, 1:29–30
historical perspective, 1:194–196
3,4-methylenedioxymethamphetamine effects on, 2:616
receptor/transporter effects, 2:617

mood disorders and, basic principles, 1:790
narcolepsy therapy, amphetamine targeting, 3:92–94
adverse effects, 3:98
anatomical substrates, 3:97–98
drug interactions, 3:98, 3:100
EEG arousal and, 3:94–97
neurochemistry, 1:198–199
neurogenesis regulation, 1:831–833
neurotransmitter transporters:
chronic substrate treatment, 1:726–727
clinical relevance, 1:721
structure and function, 1:713–714
physiology, 1:197–198
psychostimulant abuse:
chronic exposure and sensitization effects, 2:584
neuropharmacology, 2:570–575
schizophrenia pharmacotherapy, noradrenergic agent development, 2:393
Norepinephrine transporter (NET):
agent selectivity, 1:199–200
anxiety neurobiology and, knockout mice studies, 2:24–26
attention-deficit hyperactivity disorder therapy, 3:297–298
general characteristics, 1:199–200
genetic variations, 1:200–201
NS-649 compound, stroke management, 3:367
NS3763, kainate receptor allosteric antagonists, 1:397
Nuclear receptors, chemical release, 1:48–50
Nucleus accumbens (NAcc):
alcohol abuse studies:
in alcohol-preferring rats, 2:470–471
dopaminergic receptor systems and substrates, 2:471–472
GABA$_A$ benzodiazepine receptor complex manipulation, site-specific microinjection studies, 2:493–496
3,4-methylenedioxymethamphetamine (MDMA), reinforcing properties, 2:614–616
muscarinic acetylcholine receptor deficiency, dopamine efflux, 1:172–173
Nucleus basalis magnocellularis, H$_1$ receptors in, 1:311

NUDEL gene, DISC1 schizophrenia candidate gene, molecular interactions, 2:351–352
Null modulators, GABA$_A$ subunit pharmacology, 1:483
Nurr1 gene, familial Parkinson's disease and, 3:540
Nur transcription factors, schizophrenia therapy, dopamine neurotransmission and, 2:422

Obesity and weight control:
  adipose tissue:
    catecholamine signaling mechanisms, 3:801–803
    cell types and depots, 3:786–789
    future research issues, 3:804
    glyceroneogenesis, 3:799–801
    sympathetic nervous system innervation, 3:789–797
      adipocyte prolierative capacity, 3:797–799
      anterograde tract-testing, SNS to WAT, 3:792–797
      retrograde tracing neuroanatomical studies, 3:790–792
    white *vs.* brown adipocytes, 3:787–789
  epidemiology, 3:815–816
  leptin genetics and:
    early research, 3:733–734
    energy expenditure and, 3:743–744
    food intake regulation, 3:740–743
    OB gene expression and, 3:734–736
    peripheral nutrient utilization, 3:744–748
    receptor expression, 3:736–739
    signaling inhibition and resistance, 3:739–740
  neurotrophic factors and, 3:229–230
  pharmacotherapy, 3:816–821
    axokine, 3:822–824
    CCK$_A$ receptor agonists, 3:830–831
    future research issues, 3:831–833
    historic perspectives, 3:817–818
    MC4 receptor agonists, 3:828–829
    MCH receptor-1 antagonists, 3:829–830
    new drug development, 3:821–831
    orlistat, 3:820–821
    PYY3-36 peptide agonists, 3:831
    rimonabant, 3:824–828
    serotonin receptor 5-HT$_{2C}$ agonists, 3:828
    sibutramine, 3:818–820
OB gene, leptin secretion and expression of, 3:734–736
Obsessive-compulsive disorders (OCD):
  animal models, 2:224
  brain regions related to, 2:13–15
  clinical psychopharmacology, 2:225–235
    antipsychotic agents, 2:229–234
    augmenting agents, 2:225, 2:229–234
    current trials, 2:234
    monotherapy trials, 2:225
    serotonin uptake inhibitor efficacy, 2:226–228
  deep brain stimulation, 2:236–237
  defined, 2:216
  diagnostic criteria, 2:10–12, 2:216
  genetic studies, 2:222–224
    developmental genes, 2:223–224
    dopamine, 2:223
    glutamate, 2:223
    neurotransmitter metabolism, 2:223
    serotonin, 2:222–224
  immunomodulatory treatments, 2:235
  neurobiology, 2:216–224
    brain imaging studies, 2:217–222
    functional imaging studies, 2:219–220
    magnetic resonance spectroscopy, 2:220
  neuropharmacology, brain imaging studies, 2:220–222
  neurosurgery, 2:235–237
  nonpharmacological experimental treatments, 2:235–237
  pharmacotherapy, 2:77–78
  serotonin/noradrenaline reuptake inhibitors, 2:69
  serotonin transporters and, 1:720
  summary of therapeutic advances, 2:237
  symptom induction, 2:234
  Tourette's syndrome comorbidity, 3:266–268, 3:276–277
  transcranial magnetic stimulation, 2:236
  tricyclic antidepressants, 2:69–70
Ocapridone, schizophrenia therapy, 2:389
Ocinaplon, GABA$_A$ α_2 subunit pharmacology, 1:488
  allosteric ligand modulation, 1:505–506
8-OH-DPAT:
  nicotine dependence and withdrawal, withdrawal substrate specificity, 2:542–543

serotonin receptors 5-HT$_{2A}$-5-HT$_{2C}$
    interactions, *2:*422–424
Olanzapine:
    autism spectrum disorders, *3:*327–328
    D$_2$ receptor blockade, *2:*414–415
    neurogenesis and, *2:*430
    schizophrenia therapy:
        brain-derived neurotrophic factor and, *2:*421–422
        clinical profile, *2:*383–387
        D$_2$ receptor occupancy and effect, *2:*376–378
        safety and tolerability, *2:*388–389
        serotonin receptor 5-HT$_{2A}$, *2:*420–421
    Tourette's syndrome therapy, *3:*275–276
Olfactory bulb granule cell precursors, neurogenesis and, *3:*211–212
Oligodendrocyte myelin glycoprotein (OMgp), structure and function, *3:*607
Oligogenic anxiety-like conditions, anxiety neurobiology, mouse studies, *2:*32–33
Oocyte expression systems, heteromeric nicotinic acetylcholine, *1:*117–119
Open-field activity, mouse anxiety models, neurosteroid effects, *2:*148–149
Opiates/opioids:
    addiction and:
        buprenorphine studies, *2:*696–698
        drug discovery survey, *2:*699–700
        epidemiology, *2:*691–694
        future research issues, *2:*698–699
        treatment statistics, *2:*694–696
    HIV neuropharmacology and, *3:*715–716
    neuropeptide gene duplication in, *1:*680–682
    pain management, anatomical interactions, *2:*718–720
    Tourette's syndrome, *3:*272–273
Opioid agonists/antagonists:
    migraine management, *2:*765
    nicotine dependence and withdrawal therapy, *2:*550–551
Opioid receptors:
    addictive disorders, reward therapy and, *2:*458–459
    agonists, histaminergic neuron activity, *1:*321–322
    alcohol abuse studies, oral administration of βCCT/3PBC *vs.* agonists, *2:*507–511
    delta receptors, *2:*751
    dimerization, *2:*752
    endogenous opioids, *2:*746–748
    future research on, *2:*752
    kappa receptors, *2:*751–752
    mu receptors, *2:*748–751
    nicotine dependence and withdrawal, *2:*540
        withdrawal substrate specificity, *2:*543
    orphanin FQ/nociceptin and receptor, *2:*752
    overview, *2:*745–746
    pain management and, *2:*716–717
        targeting mechanisms, *2:*718
    psychostimulant abuse and, *2:*578–579
        chronic exposure and sensitization effects, *2:*584
    short-acting, addiction pharmacotherapy and, *2:*453–457
Orbitofrontal-dorsomedial thalamic loop, obsessive-compulsive disorders, neuropharmacology, *2:*221–222
Orexins, histaminergic neuron activity, *1:*318–319, *1:*320–322
Organic cation transporters (OCT), histamine inactivation, *1:*307
Orlistat, obesity therapy with, *3:*820–821
Orphanin FQ/nociceptin (OFQ/N) receptor:
    anxiety neurobiology and, knockout mice studies, *2:*25–26
    structure and function, *2:*748, *2:*752
Orthostatic hypotension, Parkinson's disease treatment and, *3:*500
    levodopa agents, *3:*486–487
Orthostatic intolerance, norepinephrine transporters and, *1:*721
Orthosteric agents:
    ionotropic glutamate receptors, *1:*373–385
        AMPA receptor agonists, *1:*376–377
        AMPA receptor antagonists, *1:*377–378
        kainate receptor agonists, *1:*378–381
        kainate receptor antagonists, *1:*381–385
        NMDA receptor agonists, *1:*373
        NMDA receptor antagonists, *1:*373–376
    metabotropic glutamate receptors:
        group III selective agonists, *1:*431–433
        group III selective antagonists, *1:*433–435
        group II selective agonists, *1:*426–429
        group II selective antagonists, *1:*429–431

group I selective agonists, *1:*423–424
group I selective antagonists, *1:*424–426
Osteogenic protein-1 (OP-1), stroke and, *3:*376–377
Output pathways, suprachiasmatic nucleus, *3:*12–13
Ovarian disease, prokineticins and, *3:*170
Oxidative stress:
  familial Parkinson's disease and, *DJ-1* gene mutation, *3:*536
  human immunodeficiency virus and, *3:*706
  methamphetamine/cocaine abuse and, *3:*714–715
  3,4-methylenedioxymethamphetamine neurotoxicity and, *2:*623–624
  Parkinson's disease pathogenesis and, *3:*545–547
Oxine derivatives, kainate receptor orthosteric antagonists, *1:*381–382
2-Oxoglutarate (2-OG), plasma membrane glutamate transporters, *1:*711
Oxycodone, abuse of, incidence and prevalence, *2:*692–694
Oxygen:
  nitric oxide gaseous signaling, nitrosylation, *1:*746–747
  S nitrosylation physiology and, *1:*752–754
Oxyhemoglobin, S nitrosylation physiology and, *1:*752–754
Oxytocin, neuropeptides and, *1:*682–684

p38 mitogen-activated protein kinase (MAPK) pathway, stroke management, *3:*369
p75 neurotrophin receptor:
  discovery of, *3:*238
  functional interactions, *3:*247–248
  signaling mechanisms, *3:*246–247
  structure and function, *3:*222–224, *3:*240–241
  synaptic function and, *3:*239
Painful dystonia, Parkinson's disease treatment and, *3:*499
Pain perception and management:
  calcitonin gene-related peptide for, *2:*768–769
  hypocretin/orexin system, *3:*136
  marijuana and, *2:*666–668
  mGlu1 allosteric antagonists, *1:*437
  neuronal pathways:
    descending modulatory pathways, *2:*712–714
    neospinothalamic/paleospinothalamic pathways, *2:*711–712
    overview, *2:*709–710
  neuropharmacology, *2:*714–717
    anatomically-based interactions, *2:*718–721
    drug targeting mechanisms, *2:*718
  neurotrophic factors and, *3:*229
  Parkinson's disease and, *3:*504
  prokineticins and, *3:*166–167
  transient receptor potential V1 (TRPV1) receptors:
    antagonists, *2:*733
    capsaicin, protons, and heat, *2:*730–732
    chemical activators, *2:*732–733
    cloning of, *2:*728–729
    desensitization, *2:*735–736
    expression, *2:*729
    knockout mouse models, *2:*736
    nociception channels, *2:*736–737
    sensitization, *2:*733–735
    voltage-gated calcium ion channels, Ca$_v$2 family, *1:*649
Paleospinothalamic pain pathways, classification of, *2:*711–712
Paliperodone, schizophrenia therapy, *2:*389
Pancreas function, ghrelin modulation, *3:*775–776
Pancreatic islets, muscarinic acetylcholine receptor deficiency, *1:*174–175
Panic disorders:
  anticonvulsant therapy, *2:*74–75
  anxiety disorder therapy, *2:*78
  brain regions related to, *2:*13–15
  diagnostic criteria, *2:*10–12
  neuroactive steroids, *2:*155
Paralytic disorders, voltage-gated sodium ion channels and, *1:*641–642
Paranodal proteins, structure and function, *3:*609
Parasympathetic nervous system, white adipose tissue in, *3:*792
Parkin gene:
  familial Parkinsonism and, PARK2 mutations and, *3:*529–532
  idiopathic Parkinson's disease and, *3:*542–543
  invertebrate models, *3:*576–577
Parkinsonism loci, familial Parkinson's disease and, *3:*540–541
Parkinson's disease (PD):
  classification, *3:*524–525

dopaminergic drugs, 1:236
dopamine transporters and, 1:721
etiology and classification, 3:480
familial (monogenetic) Parkinsonism,
    3:525–541
  causative mutations, 3:527–539
  non-PARK mutations, 3:540
  PARK1 loci, 3:527–529
  PARK2 (parkin) mutations, 3:529–532
  PARK3 mutations, 3:541
  PARK4 loci, 3:527–529
  PARK5 (UCH-L1) mutation,
    3:539–540
  PARK6 (PINK1) mutations, 3:532–535
  PARK7 (DJ-1) mutations, 3:535–536
  PARK8 (LRRK2) mutation, 3:536–539
  PARK9 mutations, 3:541
  PARK10 mutations, 3:541
  PARK11 mutations, 3:541
  Parkinsonism loci, 3:540–541
  PARK loci, 3:526–527
  potential causative mutations,
    3:539–541
future treatment options, 3:505–506
histaminergic neuron activity, 1:328
in HIV/AIDS, 3:718
idiopathic Parkinsonism:
  classification, 3:524
  environmental factors, 3:543–545
  genetics, 3:542–543
invertebrate models, dopamine neuron cell
    death, 3:569–577
mitochondria and oxidative stress,
    pathogenesis linked to, 3:545–547
motor fluctuations and dyskinesia,
    3:497–499
  delayed "on," 3:498–499
  diphasic dyskinesia, 3:499
  dose failure, 3:499
  painful dystonia, 3:499
  peak-dose dyskinesia, 3:499
  sudden "off," 3:498
  wearing off phenomenon, 3:497–498
  yo-yo-ing, 3:499
motor symptom treatments, 3:484–497
  amantadine, 3:496–497
  anticholinergics, 3:496
  antiglutamate agents, 3:496–497
  apomorphine, 3:493–494
  bromocriptine, 3:488, 3:490
  cabergoline, 3:491
  COMT inhibitors, 3:495

dihydroergocryptine, 3:491
  dopamine agonists, 3:488–494
  dopaminomimetic agents, 3:484–496
  entacapone, 3:496
  levodopa plus peripheral decarboxylase
    inhibitor, 3:484–487
  levodopa slow-release formulations,
    3:487–488
  lisuride, 3:491
  monoamine oxidase type B inhibitor,
    3:494
  nondopaminomimetic agents,
    3:496–497
  pergolide, 3:490–491
  piribedil, 3:493
  pramipexole, 3:491–492
  rasagiline, 3:495
  ropinirole, 3:492
  selegiline, 3:494–495
  stalevo, 3:496
  tolcapone, 3:495
neurochemistry, 3:481–483
neuroprotective therapy, 3:504–505
neurotrophic factor therapy and,
    3:228–229
nitric oxide and, 1:754–755
nitrosylation and, 1:755–756
nonmotor symptoms treatment,
    3:500–504
  dementia, 3:502
  depression and anxiety, 3:500–502
  nausea and vomiting, 3:500
  orthostatic hypotension, 3:500
  psychosis and hallucinations,
    3:502–503
pharmacotherapy:
  current treatments, 3:483–484
  history of, 3:480–481
plasma membrane glutamate transporter,
    1:719
Paroxetine:
  autism spectrum disorders, 3:324–325
  melatonin receptor targeting, 3:60–61
Parvicellular system, hypothalamic-pituitary
    pathways, 1:692
Pathogen-associated molecular patterns
    (PAMPs), neuroinflammation and,
    3:632
PD 6735 compound, melatonin receptor
    targeting, 3:58
PD90780, nerve growth factor inhibitor,
    3:232

Peak-dose dyskinesia, Parkinson's disease treatment and, 3:499
Pediatric autoimmune neuropsychiatric disorders associated with streptococcal infection (PANDAS), Tourette's syndrome, 3:268–269
Peptide ligands, corticotropin-releasing factor receptor antagonists:
  basic properties, 2:180–181
  CRF_1/CRF_2 binding mechanisms, 2:190–195
  CRF_1/CRF_2 pharmacology, 2:185–195
  CRF_1/CRF_2 receptor pharmacology, 2:185–195
  structure and function, 2:179–185
  subtypes and distribution, 2:181–185
Peptide toxins:
  large-conductance calcium-activated potassium channels, 1:631
  small-conductance calcium-activated potassium channels, 1:632
  voltage-gated potassium channels, K_V subunits, structure and function, 1:630
Peptide transmitters, intercellular signaling, 1:46
Peptide transport systems, blood-brain barrier neuropeptides and, 1:692–693
Peptide YY:
  antiobesity therapy, PYY3-36 peptide agonists, 3:831
  white adipose tissue innervation, 3:796–797
Peptidomics, neuropeptides, 1:675, 1:679
Per1 messenger RNA, benzodiazepines, 3:20–21
Perfusion and tissue culture studies, neuropeptides, 1:677
Pergolide:
  Parkinson's disease and, 3:490–491
  Tourette's syndrome therapy, 3:276
Periaqueductal gray (PAG) stimulation, cannabinoid analgesics and, 2:667–668
Period genes, melatonin receptors, 3:50–51
Periodic paralysis, voltage-gated sodium ion channels and, 1:641–642
Peripheral benzodiazepine receptors (PBRs), stress-induced behavior, neuroactive steroids, 2:155–156
Peripheral myelin protein-22, structure and function, 3:601–602
Peripheral nervous system (PNS):
  in bipolar disorder patients, 1:863–864
  kainate receptors, 1:372
  voltage-gated sodium ion channels, 1:640
Peripheral neuropathies, neurotrophic factor therapy, 3:227
Peripheral nutrient utilization, leptin and, 3:744–746
Peroxisomal proliferation activating receptors (PPARs), mGlu2 allosteric potentiators, 1:439
Peroxisome proliferator-activated receptor gamma (PPARγ), neuroinflammation, 3:635
Personality traits, continuous expression, anxiety neurobiology, 2:9–12
Persephin (PSPN), discovery of, 3:221–223
Pervasive developmental disorders (PDDs):
  aggression/self-injury, 3:334
  anxiety and depression, 3:334
  interfering repetitive behaviors, 3:334
  motor hyperactivity and inattention, 3:333–334
  overview, 3:320–321
  pharmacology, 3:321–333
    adrenergic agonists, 3:330
    amantidine, 3:332
    antiepileptic drugs, 3:332–333
    antipsychotics, 3:325–328
    atypical antipsychotics, 3:326
    clomipramine, 3:322
    clonidine, 3:330
    clozapine, 3:326
    d-cycloserine, 3:332
    dopaminergic medications, 3:325–330
    fluoxetine, 3:323–324
    fluvoxamine, 3:322–323
    glutamatergic medications, 3:331–332
    guanfacine, 3:330–331
    haloperidol, 3:325
    lamotrigine, 3:332
    methylphenidate, 3:329–330
    mirtazapine, 3:331
    olanzapine, quetiapine, ziprasidone, and aripipazole, 3:327–328
    pimozide, 3:325–326
    risperidone, 3:326–327
    serotonergic medications, 3:321–325
    sertraline, citalopram, escitalopram, and paroxetine, 3:324–325

stimulants, 3:328–330
venlafaxine, 3:331
syndromes within, 3:333–335
Pesticides, idiopathic Parkinson's disease and, 3:545
P-glycoprotein (P-gp), drug-resistant epilepsy, 3:425–426
Pharmacology, early research in, 1:11
Pharmacophore models, benzodiazepine activity, 2:116
Pharmacotherapy:
  addictive disorders:
    history of, 2:451–457
    reward modulation/countermodulation and, 2:458–459
    risk factors for addiction development, 2:457–458
  anxiety disorders:
    anxiolytic drugs, 2:62–75
      amino acid neurotransmission, 2:72–75
      anticonvulsants, 2:74–75
      antidepressants, 2:64–70
      antihistamines, 2:75
      antipsychotics, 2:71–72
      benzodiazepines, 2:73–74
      beta-blockers, 2:71
      lithium, 2:75
      monoamine neurotransmission, 2:63–72
      serotonin receptor agonists, 2:70–71
    depressive disorders, 2:80
    future research issues, 2:81
    generalized anxiety disorder, 2:77
    obsessive-compulsive disorder, 2:77–78
    overview, 2:60
    panic disorder/agoraphobia, 2:78
    phobias, 2:78, 2:80
    posttraumatic stress disorder, 2:79
    social anxiety disorder, 2:79–80
    treatments chart, 2:76
  obsessive-compulsive disorders, overview, 2:216
  schizophrenia:
    antipsychotic drug profiles:
      first-generation (conventional) agents, 2:383
      safety and tolerability, 2:387–388
      second-generation (atypical) agents, 2:383–387
    antipsychotic mechanisms of action, 2:376–382
      D_1 receptors, 2:380–381
      D_2/D_3 and D_4 antagonism and regional specificity, 2:380
      D_2 occupancy thresholds and rapid dissociation, 2:378–380
      D_2 receptor occupancy, 2:376–378
      dopamine release, 2:381
      NMDA receptor function, 2:381
      synthesis reactions, 2:381–382
    current developments and future directions, 2:388–394
      cannabinoid hypothesis, 2:394
      cholinergic agents, 2:393–394
      D_1 agonists and antagonists, 2:390
      D_3 antagonists, 2:390
      D_4 antagonists, 2:390
      dopamine system targeting, 2:389
      glutamate system targeting, 2:391–393
      neurokinin antagonists, 2:391
      neurosteroids, 2:394
      neurotensin agonist/antagonist, 2:390
      noradrenergic agents, 2:393
    future research issues, 2:394–395
    high $5\text{-}HT_{2A}$ vs. D_2 affinity, 2:378
    neurochemical hypotheses, 2:371–376
    overview, 2:370–371
PHCCC, mGlu4 allosteric antagonists, 1:440–441
Phencyclidine (PCP). See also Ketamine
  glutamate theory of schizophrenia:
    history of, 2:289–290
    neurochemistry of, 2:374
  ketamine derivative, 2:636–637
  mGlu II selective orthosteric agonists, 1:428–429
  mGlu II selective orthosteric antagonists, 1:430–431
  NMDA receptors, 1:368–370
  schizophrenia neurochemistry and, 2:260–262
Phen-Fen, history of, 3:818
Phenobarbital:
  as antiepileptic drug, 3:418–419
  focal/localization-related epilepsy therapy, 3:421, 3:423
Phenothiazines, schizophrenia therapy, clinical profiles, 2:383
Phenotype analysis:
  obsessive-compulsive disorders, 2:237
  schizophrenia, 2:262–263
    genetic epidemiology, 2:322–323

Phenotypic mice, muscarinic acetylcholine
  receptor deficiency, 1:167–177
 agonist-induced tremor and hypothermia,
   1:170–171
 amylase secretion, exocrine pancreas,
   1:175
 analgesia, 1:170
 autoreceptors, 1:171
 cardiovascular system, 1:175–176
 cytolytic T cells, 1:177
 drug abuse effects, 1:173
 epileptic seizures, 1:169
 food intake stimulation, 1:171
 gastric acid secretion, 1:175
 inhibitory hippocampal synapse
   suppression, 1:172
 learning and memory functions,
   1:168–169
 locomotor activity, 1:169–170
 nucleus accumbens, dopamine effects,
   1:172–173
 pancreatic islet insulin and glucagon
   secretion, 1:174–175
 peripheral autoreceptors and
   heteroreceptors, 1:176
 prepulse inhibition and
   haloperidol-induced catalepsy,
   1:172
 salivary secretion, 1:174
 skin functions, 1:177
 smooth muscle functions, 1:173–174
 striatal dopamine release modulation,
   1:171–172
Phentermine, as anti-obesity agent,
  3:817–818
Phenylalkylamines, 2:637–640
 addiction, 2:639–640
 mechanism of action, 2:638–639
 pharmacology, 2:638
α-Phenyl-N-tert-butylnitrone (PBN):
 3,4-methylenedioxymethamphetamine
   neurotoxicity, oxidative stress,
   2:623–624
 stroke management, 3:371–372
Phenyl-terazolyl acetophenone, mGlu2
  allosteric potentiators, 1:439
Phenytoin:
 development and testing, 3:419
 epilepsy efficacy, 3:417–418
Phobias:
 brain regions related to, 2:13–15
 pharmacotherapy, 2:79–80, 2:80

Phosphatase and tensin (PTEN)-induced
  putative kinase 1 (PINK1)
  mutation, familial Parkinson's
  disease and, 3:532–535
Phosphatase and tensin (PTEN) pathway:
 familial Parkinson's disease genetics and,
   3:532–535
 receptor-like PTPs, 1:94
Phosphodiesterases (PDEs),
  neuroinflammation and, 3:635–636
Phosphoenolpyruvate carboxykinase
  (PEPCK), leptin effect on,
  3:746–747
Phosphoenolpyruvate carboxykinase
  (PEPCK-C), glyceroneogenesis
  control, lipolysis and
  thermogenesis, 3:800–801
Phosphoinositide signaling molecules,
  intracellular signaling, 1:81–83
Phosphoinositol-4,5-bisphosphate (PIP_2),
  transient receptor potential V1
  (TRPV1) receptor sensitization,
  2:734–735
Phosphoinositol kinase (PI3), tyrosine
  kinase receptor signal
  transduction, 3:243
Phosphoinositol 3-kinase-AKT signaling
  pathway, dystrobrevin binding
  protein 1 (DTNBP1), molecular
  interactions, 2:353
Phospholipase C, transient receptor
  potential V1 (TRPV1) receptor
  sensitization, 2:734–735
Phospholipase Cγ-1, tyrosine kinase receptor
  signal transduction, 3:242–243
Phospholipase-phosphatidylinositol-linked
  messengers, neuropeptide
  receptors, 1:690
Phosphorus MRS, schizophrenia analysis,
  2:257
Phosphorylase, glycogen breakdown,
  1:31–32
Phosphorylation:
 cyclic nucleotide second messenger
   signaling, guanylyl cyclases,
   1:78–80
 $GABA_A$ receptor modulation, 1:481–482
 $GABA_B$ receptors, 1:584–585
 muscarinic acetylcholine receptors,
   1:164–166
 of proteins, intracellular signaling,
   synaptic transmission, 1:87–96

G-protein-coupled receptor kinases, 1:90–92
mitogen-activated protein kinase, 1:89–90
protein tyrosine kinase, 1:87–89
protein tyrosines phosphatases, 1:92–94
serine/threonine phosphatases, 1:94–96
Photic response:
  melatonin receptors, clock gene expression, 3:51
  suprachiasmatic nucleus and, 3:14–15
Phylogenetic tree, potassium channels, 1:623–625
Physostigmine, dementia disorders and, 3:464–465
Picrotoxin, alcohol abuse studies:
  $GABA_A$ benzodiazepine receptor complex, 2:487–488
  GABAergic modification of dopamine agonists, 2:496–497
Picrotoxin, $GABA_A$ receptor inhibition, 1:468–469
Pimozide, autism spectrum disorders, 3:325–326
Pineal gland, melatonin modulation of circadian rhythms, 3:55–57
Pinocytosis, blood-brain barrier neuropeptides and, 1:692–693
Piribendil, Parkinson's disease therapy, 3:493
Pituitary adenylate cyclase-activating peptide (PACAP):
  lithium mechanism in bipolar disorder and, 1:867–869
  neurogenesis and, 3:210–211
  neuropeptide hypothalamic control, 1:691–692
Pituitary gland, neuropeptide hypothalamic control of, 1:691–692
Pituitary hormones, histamine neuron physiology and secretion of, 1:324–325
PLA_2 enzymes, neuroinflammation, arachidonic acid/prostaglandin pathways, 3:634–635
Plant products:
  $GABA_A$ subunit pharmacology, allosteric ligand modulation, 1:505–506
  neuropharmacological research and role of, 1:6
  tubocurarine, small-conductance calcium-activated potassium channels, 1:632
Plasma membrane neurotransmitter transporter families, 1:707–715
  choline, 1:714–715
  clinical relevance, 1:718–723
    dopamine, 1:721
    GABA transporters, 1:721–722
    glycine, 1:722–723
    monoamine, 1:719–721
    norepinephrine, 1:721
    serotonin, 1:720
  dopamine, 1:712–713, 1:721
  GABA transporters, 1:467–468, 1:711–712, 1:721–722
  glutamate transporters, 1:708–711, 1:718–719
  glutamine, 1:715
  glycine transporters, 1:712, 1:722–723
  monoamine transporters, 1:719–720
  norepinephrine, 1:713–714, 1:721
  regulation, 1:724–728
    chronic substrate treatment, 1:726–727
    multiple transcription initiation sites, 1:725–726
    polymorphisms, 1:724–725
    second messengers, 1:727–728
  serotonin, 1:714, 1:720
  sodium/chloride-dependent transporters, 1:711–714
    dopamine transporters, 1:712–713
    GABA transporters, 1:711–712
    glycine transporters, 1:712
    norepinephrine transporters, 1:713–714
    serotonin transporters, 1:714
  structure and function, 1:707–708
Plasmolipin, structure and function, 3:608
Plic-1 protein, $GABA_A$ receptor trafficking, 1:480
p-MPPI receptor antagonist, nicotine dependence and withdrawal, withdrawal substrate specificity, 2:542–543
Polyamines:
  NMDA receptor allosteric antagonists, 1:389
  stroke and NMDA receptor, 3:357
Polymorphisms:
  dopamine, 1:234–236
  plasma membrane neurotransmitter transporter regulation, 1:724–725

Poly-Q repeats, Huntington's disease, invertebrate models, *3:*577–579
Polysomnography, narcolepsy evaluation, *3:*83
Population growth, impact on science of, *1:*7–9
Positional candidate genes, schizophrenia genetics, *2:*325
Positional cloning, schizophrenia genetics, *2:*324
Positive modulators:
 GABA$_A$ receptors:
  α$_1$ subunit pharmacology, *1:*488
  activation, allosteric ligands, *1:*503–506
  δ subunit pharmacology, *1:*492
  γ subunit pharmacology, *1:*491
  subunit pharmacology, *1:*483
Positron emission tomography (PET):
 obsessive-compulsive disorders, *2:*219–220
 schizophrenia, dopamine hypothesis, *2:*286
 schizophrenia analysis, *2:*257
Postmortem studies:
 bipolar disorder, *1:*860–861
 depressed patients, neurotrophic factors and, *1:*800–803
 schizophrenia, *2:*260–262
  dopamine hypothesis and, *2:*285
  future research issues, *2:*355–356
  overview, *2:*343–344
  susceptibility gene identification, *2:*344–351
  susceptibility gene interactions, *2:*351–355
Postpartum depression. *See also* Pregnancy
 neuroactive steroids, *2:*156–157
 neuroendocrine abnormalities and, *1:*848–849, *1:*851
Postsynaptic density protein (PSD), GABA$_B$ receptor modulation, *1:*586–587
Postsynaptic receptors:
 GABA$_A$ receptor distribution, *1:*474–475
 GABA$_B$ receptor subtypes, *1:*573–575
 intercellular signaling, *1:*48–50
Posttraumatic stress disorder (PTSD):
 anticonvulsant therapy, *2:*74–75
 brain regions related to, *2:*13–15
 diagnostic criteria, *2:*10–12
 mirtazapine therapy, *2:*70
 neuroactive steroids, *2:*154–155
 pharmacotherapy, *2:*79
 stress-monoamine convergence, *1:*826

Potassium channels:
 circadian rhythmicity and, *3:*9
 early research on, *1:*25
 GABA$_B$ receptors, effector systems, *1:*582
 histaminergic neuron activity, *1:*317–319
 leptin and nutrient utilization, *3:*745–746
 muscarinic acetylcholine receptor modulation, *1:*160–161
 neuroinflammation and, *3:*642
 voltage-gated ion channels, *1:*621–635
  calcium activation, *1:*630–632
  fast inactivation, *1:*627
  gating, *1:*626–627
  genetics, *1:*619–620
  interacting proteins, *1:*627–628
  inwardly-rectifying and two-P channels, *1:*634–635
  KCNH channels, *1:*633–634
  KCNQ family, *1:*632–633
  K$_V$ subunits, *1:*628–630
  K$_V$ subunits, structure and function, *1:*628–630
  physiology, disease and pharmacology, *1:*628–634
  selectivity, *1:*623–625
  voltage activation, *1:*625–626
PPP3CC gene, schizophrenia molecular genetics, *2:*328
PPT-LDT pathway, sedative/hypnotic action sites, *3:*183–184
Pramipexole, Parkinson's disease treatment, *3:*491–492, *3:*502
P rat line. *See* Alcohol-preferring rats
Prazosin, narcolepsy therapy, GABA inhibition, *3:*101–102
Predictive validity, animal anxiety-like behavior and, *2:*12
"Preemptive analgesia," pain management and, *2:*717
Prefrontal cortex (PFC), integrated glutamate/dopamine hypotheses of schizophrenia, *2:*374–376
Pregabalin:
 calcium channel modulation, *3:*413–414
 epilepsy efficacy, *3:*417–418
Pregnancy. *See also* Postpartum depression
 antiepileptic drugs in, *3:*424–425
 marijuana effects in, *2:*664–665
 3,4-methylenedioxymethamphetamine and, *2:*630–631
Pregnancy, depression in, neuroendocrine abnormalities and, *1:*846–847, *1:*851

Pregnanolone sulfate:
  GABA$_A$ δ subunit pharmacology, *1:*492
  GABA$_A$ receptor modulation, *1:*515
Pregnenolone sulfate (PREGS), in brain, *2:*137
Premenstrual cycle depressive disorder (PMDD). *See* Menstrual cycle depression
Prenatal development, marijuana effects on, *2:*664–665
Preprohormones, neuropeptide biosynthesis and, *1:*686
Prepulse inhibition:
  mGlu5 allosteric potentiators, *1:*443
  muscarinic acetylcholine receptor deficiency, *1:*172
Prescription drugs. *See also* Opiates
  abuse of, incidence and prevalence, *2:*692–694
Presenilin, Alzheimer's disease, invertebrate models, *3:*580–582
Presynaptic receptors:
  α$_2$ adrenergic receptor physiology, *1:*208–209
  GABA$_A$ receptor distribution, *1:*474–475
  GABA$_B$ receptor subtypes, *1:*573–575
  histaminergic neuron activity, *1:*321–322
  intercellular signaling, *1:*50–51
Preventive therapy, migraine management, *2:*766–768
Primary progressive multiple sclerosis (PPMS), classification, *3:*671–672
PRODH gene, schizophrenia molecular genetics, *2:*329–330
Prodromal period, schizophrenia therapy, second-generation antipsychotics, *2:*386–387
Progesterone:
  depression, neuroactive steroids, *2:*156–157
  traumatic brain injury and, *3:*450–451
Progressive multifocal leukoencephalitis (PML), neuroinflammation and, *3:*633
Prohormones, neuropeptide biosynthesis and, *1:*686
Proinflammatory pathways, neuroinflammation and, modulation of, *3:*638–639
Prokineticins:
  angiogenesis and reproduction, *3:*169–170
  basic properties, *3:*163, *3:*165
  circadian clock regulation, *3:*167–168
  feeding behavior, *3:*168–169
  future potential, *3:*172
  hematopoiesis, *3:*170–171
  neurogenesis and, *3:*171–172
  pain perception and management, *3:*166–167
  receptors, *3:*164
  smooth muscle contractility regulation, *3:*166
  structure and function, *3:*164, *3:*166
Prolactin release:
  depression and levels of:
    in menopause, *1:*850–851
    during menstrual cycle, *1:*846
    postpartum depression, *1:*848–849
    in pregnancy, *1:*847
  neuropeptides, *1:*691–692
Proliferation mechanisms, neurogenesis and, *3:*206–211
Promoter regions, plasma membrane transporter regulation, *1:*725
Proneurotrophins, structure, *3:*239–240
Pro-opiomelanocortin (POMC):
  antiobesity therapy, axokine, *3:*823–824
  gene organization and expression, *1:*685
  neuropeptide gene duplication, *1:*680–682
  nicotine dependence and withdrawal, *2:*540
3-Propoxy-β-carboline hydrochloride (3BPC), alcohol abuse studies:
  anxiety reduction with, *2:*510–511
  GABA$_{A1,2,3,5}$ receptor subunit modulation, *2:*499–501
  GABA$_{A1}$ receptor subunit selectivity, *2:*498–499
  microinjection techniques, *2:*505–507
  oral administration, *2:*507–511
  systemic administration, *2:*503–504
Propranolol, β-adrenergic receptor activation, *1:*210
Prostaglandin E-synthases (PGESs), neuroinflammation, *3:*635
Prostaglandins, neuroinflammation and, *3:*630
  pharmocological activation of, *3:*634–635
Protein 2, structure and function, *3:*603
Protein chemistry:
  GABA$_A$ receptor structure, sedative/hypnotic mechanisms, *3:*179–180
  myelin, *3:*594–609

Protein kinase A (PKA):
  adipose tissue signaling and, 3:802–803
  in bipolar disorder patients, 1:862
  cyclic nucleotide second messenger signaling, cAMP cellular targeting, 1:75, 1:78
  $GABA_A$ receptor phosphorylation, 1:481–482
  $GABA_B$ receptor desensitization and phosphorylation, 1:584–585
  transient receptor potential V1 (TRPV1) receptor sensitization, 2:733–735
Protein kinase C_γ, anxiety neurobiology and, 2:31
Protein kinase C (PKC):
  amino acid neurotransmitters, 1:43–44
  DAG activation, 1:85
  $GABA_A$ receptor phosphorylation, 1:481–482
  $GABA_B$ receptor desensitization and phosphorylation, 1:584–585
  GABA transporters, 1:467–468
  H_1 receptor signaling, 1:309–311
  heterotrimeric G proteins, 1:62–63
  muscarinic acetylcholine receptor phosphorylation, 1:164
  transient receptor potential V1 (TRPV1) receptor sensitization, 2:733–735
Protein-protein interactions. See also Interacting proteins
  G-protein coupled receptors, 1:70–71
  nitrosylation and, 1:749–750
Protein tyrosine kinases (PTKs), phosphorylation, 1:87–89
Protein tyrosine phosphatase 1B (PTP1B), leptin signaling inhibition and resistance, 3:739–740
Protein tyrosine phosphatases (PTPs), phosphorylation, 1:92–94
Protein zero, structure and function, 3:599–601
Proteolipid protein (PLP), structure and function, 3:596–598
Protons, transient receptor potential V1 (TRPV1) receptor expression, 2:730–732
Pseudogenes, D_1 receptor expression, 1:227
Pseudorabies virus (PSV), white adipose tissue innervation, 3:792–797
Psilocybin, schizophrenia therapy, serotonin receptor 5-HT_{2A}, 2:420–421

Psychoeducation, anxiety management with, 2:60–61
Psychological traits, anxiety neurobiology:
  continuous expression of normal personality, 2:9–10
  genetic basis of, 2:4–6
  mouse behavior extrapolation studies, 2:6–9
Psychosis:
  Parkinson's disease and, 3:502–503
  in schizophrenia, 2:253–254
    animal models, 2:264–265
    neural network studies, 2:257–258
    second-generation antipsychotics and, 2:386–387
Psychostimulants:
  abuse-related neuropharmacology, 2:569–579
    γ-aminobutyric acid, 2:576–577
    glutamate, 2:575–576
    hyopthalamic-pituitary-adrenal axis, 2:577–578
    monoamines, 2:570–575
    neuropeptides, 2:578–579
  addiction therapy development, 2:585–586
  chronic exposure-related neurobiology, 2:579–589
    neurotransmitter/neuroendocrine systems, 2:580–584
    signal transduction mechanisms and gene expression, 2:584–585
  future research issues, 2:588–589
  human immunodeficiency virus, nigrostriatal system and, 3:710
  therapeutic applications of, 2:567–569
Psychotropic drugs, neurogenesis and, 3:210
Public health policy, nicotine dependency and withdrawal therapy, 2:551–552
Puringergic receptors, neuroinflammation, adenosine pathway and, 3:643–644
Purines, packaging of, 1:46
Pyramidal neurons, 5-HT_{2A} receptors in, 1:270–271
Pyrazolopyrimidine, corticotropin-releasing factor receptor antagonists, anxiety/depression therapeutic potential, 2:197–198
Pyrazoloquinoline, alcohol abuse studies, $GABA_A$ benzodiazepine receptor complex, 2:490–493
Pyrethroid insecticides, voltage-gated sodium ion channels and, 1:643

Pyridoindole, GABA$_A$ subunit pharmacology, allosteric ligand modulation, *1:*504–506
Pyrrolidinones, AMPA receptor allosteric potentiators, *1:*390

QT prolongation, Tourette's syndrome therapy, *3:*274–276
Quaaludes, structure and function, *3:*187
Quantitative behavioral genetics, anxiety neurobiology, *2:*6
Quantitative trait locus (QTL) analysis, anxiety neurobiology, *2:*4
   emotionalty studies in mice, *2:*8–9
   mice studies, *2:*19
   oligogenic anxiety-like conditions, *2:*32–33
Quetiapine:
   autism spectrum disorders, *3:*327–328
   schizophrenia therapy:
      clinical profile, *2:*383–387
      safety and tolerability, *2:*389
   Tourette's syndrome therapy, *3:*275–276
Quinelorane, alcohol abuse studies, dopaminergic receptor systems and substrates, *2:*472–473
Quinidine, voltage-gated potassium channels, K$_V$ subunits, structure and function, *1:*630
Quinoazolines, AMPA receptor allosteric antagonists, *1:*395–396
Quinolinic acid, inflammation and, *3:*644
Quinoxalinediones:
   kainate receptor orthosteric antagonists, *1:*383
   stroke management, *3:*361–362
Quinoxalines, AMPA receptor orthosteric antagonists, *1:*377
Quinpirole, alcohol abuse studies, dopaminergic receptor systems and substrates, *2:*472–473
Quisqualate, mGlu group I selective orthosteric agonists, *1:*423

Raclopride:
   alcohol abuse studies, dopaminergic receptor systems and substrates, *2:*472–473
   chronic exposure and sensitization effects, *2:*582–585
^{11}C-Raclopride, striatal D$_2$ receptor blockade, *2:*414–415
Radioimmunoassay (RIA), neuropeptide identification, *1:*673
Radiolabeled peptides, corticotropin-releasing factor receptor antagonists, peptide ligand pharmacology, *2:*187–195
Ramelteon, melatonin receptor targeting, *3:*57–58
Rapid dissociation, schizophrenia pharmacotherapy, D$_2$ receptor occupancy thresholds, *2:*379–380
Rapid-eye-movement (REM) sleep:
   antidepressants and, *3:*17–18
   ghrelin effects, *3:*774
   melatonin modulation of circadian rhythms, *3:*56–57, *3:*58
   monoamine oxidase inhibitor reduction of, *3:*111
   narcolepsy pathophysiology, *3:*84–85
   hypocretin/orexin system, *3:*89
Reactive nitrogen species (RNS), neuroinflammation and, *3:*630
   pharmacology of, *3:*636–637
Reactive oxygen species (ROS):
   neuroinflammation and, pharmacology of, *3:*636–637
   Parkinson's disease pathogenesis and, *3:*546–547
Receptor activity modifying protein 1 (RAMP1), calcitonin gene-related peptide sites and migraine therapy targeting, *2:*762
Receptor activity modifying proteins (RAMPs), GABA$_B$ receptor modulation, *1:*585–586
Receptor agonists/antagonists:
   GABA$_A$ receptor activation, *1:*492–495
   allosteric ligand modulation, *1:*500–506
   GABA$_B$ receptors, *1:*590
   ghrelin receptors, *3:*777
   glutamate transporter regulation, *1:*728
   muscarinic acetylcholine receptor, ligand binding, *1:*152–153
   neuropeptide receptors, *1:*675
   neurotrophic factors as, *3:*231–232
   psychostimulant abuse therapy, *2:*586–587
   traumatic brain injury and, *3:*449–450
Receptor density assessment:
   schizophrenia, dopamine hypothesis and, *2:*285
   schizophrenia neuroreceptor imaging, *2:*259–260

Receptor for activated C kinase (RACK-1), GABA$_A$ phosphorylation, 1:482
Receptor ligand pharmacology, benzodiazepines, 2:97–102
  endogenous site, 2:98–99
  metabolism functions, 2:101–102
  single-cell GABA response modulation, 2:99–100
  therapeutic action, 2:97–98
  tolerance and dependence characteristics, 2:100–101
Receptor-like PTPs (RPTPs), phosphorylation, 1:92–94
Receptors, serotonin family, 1:262–264
Receptor tyrosine kinases (RTKs), signaling pathways, 1:88–89
Redundancy, of neuropeptides, 1:694
Reelin mRNA, in bipolar disorder patients, 1:862
Regional cerebral blood flow (rCBF), schizophrenia, 2:257–259
Regional specificity, schizophrenia therapy, D$_2$/D$_3$ and D$_4$ receptor antagonism and, 2:380
"Region-specific" neuroanatomical controls, alcohol abuse studies in alcohol-preferring rats, 2:469–470
Regulator of G-protein signaling 4 (RGS4), schizophrenia candidate gene, 2:328
  susceptibility identification, 2:351
Reinforcing mechanisms:
  alcohol abuse studies in alcohol-preferring rats, 2:469
  3,4-methylenedioxymethamphetamine (MDMA), 2:614–616
Relapsing remitting multiple sclerosis (RRMS):
  betaseron therapy, 3:674–675
  classification, 3:671–672
  multiple sclerosis therapy, 3:686
Release-inhibiting factor, neuropeptide hypothalamic control, 1:691–692
Release-stimulating hormones, neuropeptide hypothalamic control, 1:691–692
Remacemide, stroke management, 3:358–359
Repetitive behaviors, autism spectrum disorders, 3:334
Repolarization, voltage-gated potassium channels, K$_V$ subunits, structure and function, 1:628–630

Reproductive cycle depression, neuroendocrine studies:
  cross-reproductive cycle analysis, 1:851–853
  future research issues, 1:852–853
  menopause, 1:849–851
    cortisol, 1:850
    melatonin, 1:849–850
    prolactin, 1:850–851
    thyroid-stimulating hormone, 1:850
  menstrual cycle, 1:844–846
    cortisol, 1:845
    melatonin, 1:844–845
    prolactin, 1:846
    thyroid-stimulating hormone, 1:845
  postpartum depression, 1:848–849
    cortisol, 1:848
    estradiol, 1:849
    melatonin, 1:848
    prolactin, 1:848–849
    thyroid-stimulating hormone, 1:848
  pregnancy, 1:846–847
    cortisol, 1:847
    melatonin, 1:846–847
    prolactin, 1:847
    thyroid-stimulating hormone, 1:847
  research background, 1:844
Reproductive function, prokineticins and, 3:169–170
Resensitization, muscarinic acetylcholine receptor phosphorylation, 1:166
Reserpine, early research on, 1:30–31
Resinferatoxin (RTX):
  cloning of, 2:727–729
  transient receptor potential V1 (TRPV1) receptor expression, 2:733
Respiratory system, γ-hydroxybutyric acid (GHB) effects, 2:634
Resting membrane potentials, KCNH potassium channels, 1:633–634
Retinohypothalamic tract (RHT), suprachiasmatic nucleus and, 3:13–15
Retrograde axonal signaling, neurotrophins, 3:248–249
Reuptake inhibitors, psychostimulant abuse, monoamine neuropharmacology, 2:571–575
Reuptake mechanisms:
  dopamine synthesis, 1:55
  serotonin, 1:261–262

Reverse genetics, Parkinson's disease, invertebrate models, 3:573–577
Reversible inhibitor of monoamine oxidase A (RIMA), anxiety disorder therapy, 2:70
Rev protein, HIV neurotoxicity and, 3:704
Reward effects:
  addictive disorders, 2:458–459
  endocannabinoids and, 2:675–676
  3,4-methylenedioxymethamphetamine (MDMA), 2:614–616
  psychostimulant abuse, chronic exposure and sensitization effects, 2:581–585
RGS proteins:
  muscarinic acetylcholine receptors, 1:158
  structure and function, 1:65–66
RhoA, p75 neurotrophin receptor, 3:247
Rhodopsin, corticotropin-releasing factor receptor antagonists, ligand binding mechanisms, 2:191–195
Rhythmicity:
  cellular basis, 3:8
  Drosophila models, 3:7
Riluzole:
  obsessive-compulsive disorder therapy, 2:234
  stroke management, 3:367
Rimonabant:
  antiobesity therapy, 3:823–828
  appetite regulation, 2:670–672
  cannabinoid receptors and, 2:661–662
  cognition and, 2:669–670
  endocannabinoid physiology and, 2:665–675
  nicotine dependence and withdrawal therapy, 2:550
  opiate dependence therapy and, 2:699
  pain management and, 2:667–668
  reward, tolerance, and dependence, 2:675–676
Risk factors, idiopathic Parkinson's disease, 3:542–543
Risperidone:
  attention-deficit hyperactivity disorder therapy, 3:301
  autism spectrum disorders, 3:326–327
  neurogenesis and, 2:430
  schizophrenia therapy:
    clinical profile, 2:383–387
    safety and tolerability, 2:389
    serotonin receptor 5-HT$_{2A}$, 2:418–421
  Tourette's syndrome therapy, 3:274–276

Ritalin. *See* Methylphenidate
Ritanserin, 3,4-methylenedioxymethamphetamine effects on, 2:616
Rituximab, multiple sclerosis therapy, 3:687
RJR-2429 nicotinic agonist, dementia disorders and, 3:467–468
RNA editing, 5-HT$_{2C}$ receptors and, 1:272–273
Ro 15-4513, GABA$_A$ α_1 subunit pharmacology, 1:488
RO19-4603 inverse agonist, alcohol abuse studies, GABA$_A$ benzodiazepine receptor complex, 2:488–493
  site-specific microinjection techniques, 2:494–496
  systemic administration studies, 2:492–493
RO 67-7476/67-4853, mGlu1 allosteric potentiators, 1:435–436
RO 718218, mGlu2/3 allosteric antagonists, 1:439–440
Rohypnol. *See* Flunitrazepam
ROI15-4513 inverse agonist, alcohol abuse studies, GABA$_A$ benzodiazepine receptor complex, alcohol-modulator commonalities, 2:487–488
Romano-Ward syndrome, KCNQ channels and, 1:632–633
Ropinirole, Parkinson's disease treatment, 3:492
Rostral agranular insular cortex (RAIC), GABA$_B$ receptor targeting, 1:596
Rotenone exposure, Parkinson's disease and, invertebrate models, 3:577
Rotigotine, Parkinson's disease treatment, 3:505
RSSR signaling, GABA$_B$ receptor trafficking and heteromization, 1:575–578
RU34000 imidazopyrimidine inverse agonist, alcohol abuse studies, GABA$_A$ benzodiazepine receptor complex, 2:490–493
  site-specific microinjection techniques, 2:496
Running, neurogenesis and, 3:206
RY 023 inverse agonist, alcohol abuse studies, GABA$_{A5}$ receptor specificity, 2:512–516
Ryanodine, ion channel nitrosylation, 1:748–749

S20304 agonist, melatonin receptors,
    therapeutic targeting of, 3:59–61
Safety, schizophrenia therapy,
    second-generation antipsychotics,
    2:387–388
Salivary secretion, muscarinic acetylcholine
    receptor deficiency, 1:174
Samson test procedure, alcohol abuse studies
    in alcohol-preferring rats,
    2:468–470
Satiation, histaminergic neuron activity,
    1:325–326
Satiety signal, leptin and, 3:733–734
Saxitoxin (STX), voltage-gated sodium ion
    channels and, 1:642–643
SB271046, serotonin receptor 5-HT$_6$ and,
    2:426
SB-271046, serotonin receptor 5-HT$_6$ and,
    2:425–426
SB-399885, serotonin receptor 5-HT$_6$ and,
    2:426
Scaffolding proteins, voltage-gated
    potassium channels, 1:628
SCH 23390 compound, alcohol abuse
    studies:
  bed nucleus of stria terminalis system,
    2:475
  lateral hypothalamus, effects on,
    2:481–485
  ventral pallidum receptor blockade,
    2:477–480
Schizophrenia:
  animal models, 2:263–265
  biological mechanisms, 2:256–263
  brain imaging studies, 2:256–260
  characteristics of, 2:252
  clinical phenomenology and treatment,
    2:252–256
  cognitive dysfunction, 2:254–255
  dopamine hypothesis:
    cortical vs. striatal dopamine, 2:287–289
    genetic evidence, 2:286–287
    history, 2:284–285
    imaging evidence, 2:285–286
    pathological evidence, 2:285
    pharmacological evidence, 2:287
    pharmacotherapy, 2:371–373
  dopaminergic drugs, 1:237
  evolution of theories on, 2:283–284
  future research issues, 2:265–266
  genetic epidemiology, 2:321–323
    phenotype definition, 2:322–323

genetics and phenotypes, 2:262–263
glutamate theory of:
  genetic evidence for, 2:293–294
  history, 2:289–291
  imaging evidence for, 2:292–293
  pathological evidence for, 2:291–292
  pharmacological evidence for,
    2:294–295
  pharmacotherapy, 2:373–374
histaminergic neuron activity, 1:327
integrated glutamate/dopamine
  hypotheses, 2:295–297
  pharmacotherapy, 2:374–376
molecular genetics, 2:323–325
  candidate genes, 2:325–328
  chromosomal abnormalities, 2:328–331
  functional candidate genes, 2:331–332
  future research issues, 2:333
  susceptibility gene function, 2:332–333
negative affect, 2:255–256
neural network studies and, 2:255–259
neurochemistry, 2:260–262
neurogenesis in, 2:430
neuroreceptor imaging, 2:259–260
pharmacotherapy:
  antipsychotic drug profiles:
    first-generation (conventional)
      agents, 2:383
    safety and tolerability, 2:387–388
    second-generation (atypical) agents,
      2:383–387
  antipsychotic mechanisms of action,
    2:376–382
    D_1 receptors, 2:380–381
    D_2/D_3 and D_4 antagonism and
      regional specificity, 2:380
    D_2 occupancy thresholds and rapid
      dissociation, 2:378–380
    D_2 receptor occupancy, 2:376–378
    dopamine release, 2:381
    NMDA receptor function, 2:381
    synthesis reactions, 2:381–382
  current developments and future
    directions, 2:388–394
    cannabinoid hypothesis, 2:394
    chollinergic agents, 2:393–394
    D_1 agonists and antagonists, 2:390
    D_3 antagonists, 2:390
    D_4 antagonists, 2:390
    dopamine system targeting, 2:389
    glutamate system targeting,
      2:391–393

neurokinin antagonists, 2:391
neurosteroids, 2:394
neurotensin agonist/antagonist, 2:390
noradrenergic agents, 2:393
future research issues, 2:394–395
high 5-HT$_{2A}$ vs. D$_2$ affinity, 2:378
neurochemical hypotheses, 2:371–376
overview, 2:370–371
postmortem studies, 2:260–262
dopamine hypothesis and, 2:285
future research issues, 2:355–356
overview, 2:343–344
susceptibility gene identification, 2:344–351
susceptibility gene interactions, 2:351–355
prevalence, 2:252–253
psychosis and, 2:253–254
serotonin receptor 5-HT$_{2A}$ and, 1:270–271
symptom classification, 2:253
Scientific research:
Dale and Loewi's contributions in, 1:14–15
Forster's contributions in, 1:9–11
German universities and, 1:9
population growth and, 1:7–9
postwar trends in, 1:24–25
role of patronage in, 1:7–8
Wellcome's contributions to, 1:15
SCL17 transporter family, 1:716
SDZ EAA 494 antagonist, stroke management and, 3:356–357
Secondary lymphoid tissue, neuroinflammation and formation of, 3:629
Secondary progressive multiple sclerosis (SPMS):
betaseron therapy and, 3:675
classification, 3:671–672
Second-generation antipsychotics (SGAs), schizophrenia therapy:
clinical profile, 2:383–387
D$_2$/D$_3$ and D$_4$ receptor antagonism and regional specificity, 2:380
D$_2$ receptor occupancy thresholds and rapid dissociation, 2:378–380
history of, 2:370–371
NMDA receptor antagonists, 2:381
safety and tolerability, 2:387–388
Second-messenger systems:
early research on, 1:31–32

glutamate transporter regulation, 1:727–728
neuropeptide receptors, 1:690–691
Tourette's syndrome, 3:273
Secretin, hypocretin/orexin system and, 3:127
Sedative effects:
α$_2$ adrenergic receptor physiology, 1:207–208
GABA$_A$ β subunit pharmacology, 1:490–491
GABA$_A$ γ subunit pharmacology, 1:491
GABA$_A$ receptor activation, allosteric ligand modulation, 1:503–506
Sedatives:
barbiturate-like drugs, 3:187
barbiturates, 3:184–187
basic principles, 3:177–178
benzodiazepines, 3:187–188
brain sites of action, 3:181–184
GABA$_A$ receptors:
pharmacology, 3:180–181
structure, 3:178–180
mouse studies, 3:190–192
new agents, 3:188–190
non-GABA$_A$ receptor agents, 3:188
safe development of, 3:184–190
Seizure disorders. See also Epileptic seizures
acute seizures, 3:427–428
classification and definition, 3:404
GABA transporters and, 1:722
generalized seizures, classification, 3:404–405
histamine neuron physiology, 1:326
KCNQ channels and, 1:633
Selective serotonin reuptake inhibitors (SSRIs):
anxiety disorder therapy, 2:66–69
autism spectrum disorders, 3:322–325, 3:333–334
melatonin receptors, therapeutic targeting of, 3:58–61
obsessive-compulsive disorders, controlled trials, 2:225
panic disorder therapy, 2:78
Parkinson's disease and, 3:501
posttraumatic stress disorder therapy, 2:79
sleep effects, 3:17–18
social anxiety disorder therapy, 2:79–80
Selectivity:
potassium channels, 1:623–625
sodium voltage-gated ion channels, 1:637

Selegiline:
  cataplexy therapy, 3:111
  human immunodeficiency virus,
    nigrostriatal system and, 3:710
  narcolepsy therapy, 3:104
  schizophrenia therapy, 2:394
Self-injurious behaviors, autism spectrum
    disorders, 3:334
Selfotel, stroke management, 3:358–359
Sensitivity:
  psychostimulant abuse and reduction of,
    neurobiology of, 2:579–585
  transient receptor potential V1 (TRPV1)
    receptor expression, 2:733–735
Sensory neurons, pain pathways, 2:711–712
Separation-induced ultrasonic vocalizations,
    animal anxiety models,
    neurosteroid effects, 2:150
Sequence homology, corticotropin-releasing
    factor receptor antagonists, ligand
    binding mechanisms, 2:191–195
Serine/threonine phosphatases,
    phosphorylation, 1:94–96
Serotonergic neurons, model of, 1:264
Serotonin (5-HT) neurotransmitters:
  anatomy, 1:260
  antidepressant influences on, 1:806–808
    hippocampal neurogenesis and,
      monoamines, 1:822–823
    stress-monoamine convergence,
      1:825–826
  antipsychotic drugs and release of,
    2:426
  anxiety disorder anxiolytics, monoamine
    neurotransmission, 2:63–72
  anxiety neurobiology, 2:4
    genetic susceptibility studies, 2:18–19
    neurotransmission mechanisms,
      2:15–17
  autism spectrum disorders, 3:321–325
  basic properties, 1:257–259
  circadian rhythms and, antidepressant
    effects, 3:18–20
  degradation and reuptake, 1:261–262
  early history, 1:30–31, 1:259–260
  future research on, 1:276–277
  histaminergic neuron activity, 1:318–319
  hypocretin/orexin system, arousal
    mechanisms, 3:142
  melatonin production, 3:40–41
  3,4-methylenedioxymethamphetamine
    effects on, 2:616
    long-term neurochemical effects,
      2:619–620
    oxidative stress, 2:623–624
    receptor/transporter effects, 2:617
  mood disorders and, basic principles,
    1:790
  neurogenesis and, 3:209–210
  neurogenesis regulation, 1:831–833
  neurotransmitter transporters (SERTs):
    chronic substrate treatment, 1:726–727
    clinical relevance, 1:720
    glycosylation, 1:725–726
    multiple transcription initiation sites,
      1:725
    promoter region polymorphisms,
      1:725
    serotonin degradation and reuptake,
      1:261–262
    stress-monoamine convergence in
      depression, 1:825–826
    structure and function, 1:714
  neurotrophins and, stress influence on,
    1:797
  nicotine dependence and withdrawal,
    withdrawal substrates, 2:542–543
  obsessive-compulsive disorders, genetic
    studies, 2:222–224
  psychostimulant abuse,
    neuropharmacology, 2:570–575
  receptors, 1:262–276
  sedative/hypnotics and, 3:188
  suprachiasmatic nucleus and, 3:14–15
  synthesis, 1:260–261
  Tourette's syndrome, 3:272
Serotonin and noradrenaline reuptake
    inhibitors (SNRI), anxiety disorder
    therapy, 2:69
Serotonin hypothesis, obsessive-compulsive
    disorders, neuropharmacology,
    2:221–222
Serotonin receptor 5-HT/D_2 hypothesis,
    atypical antipsychotics, 2:417–418
  serotonin receptor 5-HT$_{2A}$, 2:419–421
Serotonin receptors:
  atypical antipsychotics:
    adrenergic mechanisms, 2:426–427
    serotonin receptor 5-HT$_{1A}$-5-HT$_{2A}$
      interactions, 2:421–425
    serotonin receptor 5-HT$_{2A}$, 2:418–421
      cortical dopamine efflux and
        cognitive function, 2:421–422
      extrapyramidal function, 2:422

serotonin receptor 5-HT$_{2A}$-5-HT$_{2C}$
  receptor interactions, 2:422–424
serotonin receptor 5-HT/D$_2$ hypothesis,
  2:417–418
melatonin receptors and, 3:38–39
schizophrenia neurochemistry and,
  2:261–262
schizophrenia pharmacotherapy,
  serotonin receptor 5-HT$_{2A}$, D$_2$
  antagonism and, 2:381
serotonin receptor 5-HT$_1$
  5-HT$_{1A}$ receptors, 1:263, 1:266–267
  5-HT$_{1B}$ and 5-HT$_{1D}$ receptors,
    1:267–268
  5-HT$_{1E}$ receptors, 1:268–269
  5-HT$_{1F}$ receptors, 1:269
  classification, 1:263–264
serotonin receptor 5-HT$_{1A}$:
  anxiety disorder therapy, 2:70–71
  anxiety neurobiology and, knockout
    mice deficit studies, 2:27–30
  nicotine dependence and withdrawal,
    2:542–543
serotonin receptor 5-HT$_{1B}$:
  anxiety neurobiology and, knockout
    mice deficit studies, 2:28–30
serotonin receptor 5-HT$_2$, 1:269–273
  5-HT$_{2A}$ receptors, 1:270–271
  5-HT$_{2B}$ receptors, 1:271
  5-HT$_{2C}$ receptors, 1:271–272
serotonin receptor 5-HT$_{2A}$:
  cortical dopamine efflux and cognitive
    function, 2:421–422
  extrapyramidal function, 2:422
  LSD downregulation of, 2:638–640
  schizophrenia pharmacotherapy, D$_2$
    antagonism and, 2:381
  sedative/hypnotics and, 3:190
serotonin receptor 5-HT$_{2C}$:
  agonist, antiobesity therapy,
    3:828
  psychostimulant abuse, 2:574–575
serotonin receptor 5-HT$_3$ family, structure
  and function, 1:273
serotonin receptor 5-HT$_4$ family, structure
  and function, 1:273–274
serotonin receptor 5-HT$_5$ receptor family,
  structure and function,
  1:274–275
serotonin receptor 5-HT$_6$:
  atypical antipsychotics, 2:425–426
  structure and function, 1:275

serotonin receptor 5-HT$_y$ family, structure
  and function, 1:275–276
triptan therapy for migraines, 2:764–765
Serotonin reuptake inhibitors (SRIs):
  depression therapy, hippocampal
    neurogenesis and, 1:827
  obsessive-compulsive disorders:
    brain neuropharmacology, 2:221–222
    neuropharmacology, 2:226–228
Serotonin transporter (SERT):
  antagonists, obsessive-compulsive
    disorders, 2:223
  anxiety neurobiology, environmental
    effects and, 2:34–35
  anxiety neurobiology and, knockout mice
    studies, 2:24–26
  3,4-methylenedioxymethamphetamine
    neurotoxicity and, 2:625–627
  obsessive-compulsive disorders:
    abnormalities, 2:219–220
    genetic studies, 2:222–224
Sertindole, schizophrenia therapy, clinical
  profile, 2:383–387
Sertraline, autism spectrum disorders,
  3:324–325
Serum analysis, brain-derived neurotrophic
  factor in depressed patients, 1:801
Serum response element (SRE) pathway,
  ghrelin receptor activity, 3:770
Severe myoclonic epilepsy of infancy
  (SMEI), voltage-gated sodium ion
  channels and, 1:642
Sex steroids, neurogenesis and, 3:207
Shc gene, tyrosine kinase receptor signal
  transduction, 3:243
Short-term potentiation (STP), muscarinic
  acetylcholine receptor deficiency,
  1:169
SIB-1533A nicotinic agonist, dementia
  disorders and, 3:467–468
SIB-1757, mGlu5 allosteric antagonists,
  1:443
SIB-1893, mGlu4 allosteric antagonists,
  1:440–441
Sibutramine, as obesity therapy, 3:818–820
Sickness behavior, circadian rhythms and,
  cytokines and, 3:21–23
Signaling mechanisms:
  leptin resistance and inhibition,
    3:739–740
  melatonin receptors, 3:44–46
  neurotrophic factors, 3:224–225

neurotrophins, *3:*238–239
tyrosine kinase receptors, *3:*242–244
Signaling molecules:
α₁ adrenergic receptor regulation, *1:*203
α₂-adrenergic receptor regulation, *1:*206
β-adrenergic receptor activation, *1:*210–211
calcium channels, *1:*83–85
dopamine, *1:*223–224
dopamine receptors, *1:*230–232
GABA$_A$ phosphorylation, *1:*482
gaseous signaling:
 carbon monoxide, *1:*756–757
 future research, *1:*757
 nitric oxide:
  basic principles, *1:*743–744
  neurodegeneration and, *1:*754
  nitrosothiol detection, *1:*747–748
  nitrosylation mechanism, *1:*745–747
   cell survival, *1:*752
   extracellular matrix, *1:*751–752
   gene transport, *1:*750–751
   ion channels, *1:*748–749
   Parkinson's disease and, *1:*755–756
   protein-protein interactions, *1:*749–750
   S nitrosylation physiology, *1:*752–754
   vesicular transport, *1:*751
  physiological role, *1:*745
  research background, *1:*743–744
H₁ receptors, *1:*309
H₂ receptor, *1:*312
H₃ receptor, *1:*314–315
IP₃ and phosphoinositides, *1:*81–83
muscarinic acetylcholine receptor modulation, *1:*158–159
voltage-gated calcium channels, *1:*647
Signal transducer and activator of transcription (STAT):
leptin receptor and expression, *3:*737–739
leptin signaling inhibition and resistance, *3:*739–740
Signal transduction mechanisms, psychostimulant abuse, chronic exposure and sensitization effects, *2:*584–585
Sinemet, Parkinson's disease treatment, *3:*484–487
slow-release formulations, *3:*487–488

Single-nucleotide polymorphisms (SNPs):
addictive disorders vulnerability, *2:*457–458
β-adrenergic receptor physiology, *1:*212–213
catechol-*O*-methyl transferase, as schizophrenia susceptibility gene, *2:*347–348
dopamine, *1:*234–236
familial Parkinson's disease and, PINK1 gene mutation and, *3:*534–535
plasma membrane neurotransmitter transporter regulation, *1:*724–725
schizophrenia genetics:
 DISC1 molecular interactions, *2:*352
 GRM3 gene, *2:*349
 positional candidate genes, *2:*325
Single-photon-emission computerized tomography (SPECT), schizophrenia analysis, *2:*257
Sipatrigine, stroke management, *3:*367
Site-directed mutagenesis:
melatonin receptor molecular structure, *3:*42
neuropeptides, *1:*679
neurotrophin structure and, *3:*240
Site-specific microinjection studies, alcohol abuse, GABA$_A$ benzodiazepine receptor complex manipulation, *2:*493–496
Sjogren's syndrome, AF102B agonist and, *3:*466
Skeletal muscle, voltage-gated sodium ion channels and, *1:*641–642
Skin function, muscarinic acetylcholine receptor deficiency, *1:*177
SLC1 family, plasma membrane glutamate transporters, *1:*708–711
SLC5 family, structure and function, *1:*714–715
SLC6 family of neurotransmitters, *1:*711–714
SLC32 transporter family, *1:*718
Sleep disorders:
antidepressants and, *3:*17–18
cataplexy:
 defined, *3:*82
 narcolepsy pathophysiology, *3:*85
  human leukocyte antigen and, *3:*85–86
 pharmacological treatment:
  future anticataplectics, *3:*113–114

historical overview, 3:106–107
monoamine oxidase inhibitors, 3:111
neurotransmission, animal studies,
　　3:109–110
receptor subtypes, 3:110–111
second- and third-generation
　　antidepressants, 3:108
sodium oxybate, 3:112
tricyclic antidepressants, 3:107–109
circadian rhythms:
　chronopharmacology, 3:15–23
　functional importance, 3:4
　future research issues, 3:23–24
　mammallian structural models, 3:10–13
　nonmammalian structural models,
　　3:6–10
　properties, 3:4–6
　superchiasmatic nucleus period and
　　phase, 3:13–15
disturbed nocturnal sleep, treatment of,
　3:112
melatonin receptors, therapeutic
　targeting, 3:57–58
narcolepsy:
　evaluation, 3:83–84
　　cerebrospinal fluid hypocretin-1
　　　assessment, 3:84
　　histocompatibility human leukocyte
　　　antigen testing, 3:84
　　polysomnography, 3:83
　future research issues, 3:114–115
　idiopathic hypersomnia, 3:84
　overview of, 3:80
　pathophysiology, 3:84–89
　　human leukocyte antigen analysis,
　　　3:85–86
　　hypocretin/orexin system and sleep
　　　regulation, 3:86–89
　　hypocretin transmission, animal
　　　models, 3:86
　　symptoms analysis, 3:84–85
　symptoms of, 3:80–83
　　cataplexy, 3:83
　　excessive daytime sleepiness, 3:82,
　　　3:84, 3:90–92
　　hypnagogic/hypnopompic
　　　hallucinations, 3:83
　　sleep paralysis, 3:83
　treatment of, 3:90–100
　　amphetamines, 3:90–100
　　　drug interactions with, 3:98, 3:100
　　　molecular targeting of, 3:93–94

　　　side effects, 3:98
　　bupropion, 3:103–105
　　caffeine, 3:104–105
　　dopamine neurotransmitters,
　　　substrates, 3:97–98
　　dopamine neurotransmitters and
　　　EEG arousal, 3:94–97
　　future stimulant development,
　　　3:105–106
　　mazindol, 3:103
　　modafinal, 3:100–103
　　nonamphetamine stimulants,
　　　3:99–105
　　selegiline, 3:104
Parkinson's disease and, 3:503
sleep paralysis:
　symptoms of, 3:83
　treatment of, 3:112
Sleep paralysis:
　symptoms of, 3:83
　treatment of, 3:112
Small-conductance calcium-activated
　potassium channels (SK channels),
　structure and function, 1:631–632
Small G proteins, structure and function,
　1:63–64
Small-molecular-weight peptide agonists,
　cataplexy therapy, 3:115
Smoking. See Nicotine
　idiopathic Parkinson's disease and, 3:544
Smooth muscle function:
　muscarinic acetylcholine receptor
　　deficiency, 1:173–174
　prokineticin regulation, 3:166
SNCA gene mutation:
　familial Parkinsonism and, 3:527–529
　idiopathic Parkinson's disease and,
　　3:542–543
S nitrosylation:
　nitric oxide, protein mechanisms, 1:747
　physiology of, 1:752–754
Social anxiety disorder, pharmacotherapy,
　2:79–80
Social interaction paradigm, 3,4-methylene-
　dioxymethamphetamine effects on,
　2:630–631
Social isolation:
　animal anxiety model, neurosteroid
　　effects, 2:151–152
　schizophrenia, animal models, 2:264
Sodium bromide, as antiepileptic drug,
　3:418–419

Sodium channels:
  early research on, 1:25
  epilepsy and modulation of, 3:411
  plasma membrane glutamate transporters, 1:709–711
  stroke management and modulation of, 3:367
  voltage-gated ion channels, 1:635–643
    α subunits, 1:636–637
    channelopathies, 1:641–642
    genetics, 1:619–620
    inactivation, 1:637–638
    pharmacology, 1:642–643
    physiological functions, 1:639–641
    selectivity, 1:637
    trafficking, 1:638–639
Sodium/chloride-dependent neurotransmitter transporters, 1:711–714
  dopamine transporters, 1:712–713
  GABA transporters, 1:711–712
  glycine transporters, 1:712
  norepinephrine transporters, 1:713–714
  serotonin transporters, 1:714
Sodium oxybate. See γ-hydroxybutyric acid (GHB)
  cataplexy therapy, 3:112
Soluble N-ethylmaleimide-sensitive factor attachment protein receptors (SNAREs):
  dystrobrevin binding protein 1 (DTNBP1), molecular interactions, 2:353
  plasma membrane transporter regulation, 1:728
  vesicle-dependent release, 1:46–47
  nitrosylation and, 1:751
Somatostatin (ST), neuropeptides and, 1:671
Somatotropin release-inhibiting factor (SRIF), neuropeptide hypothalamic control, 1:691–692
Sonic hedgehog (Shh) morphogen, stroke therapy, 3:378
SPD 502 antagonist, stroke management, 3:362
"Speedball" psychostimulant combination, neuropeptide pharmacology and, 2:578–579
Splice variants:
  corticotropin-releasing factor receptor antagonists, receptor subunits, 2:182–185

dopamine, 1:234–236
leptin receptor expression and, 3:738–739
tyrosine kinase receptors, 3:245–246
SR48692, psychostimulant abuse, neuropeptide pharmacology and, 2:579
SR144528 antagonist, cannabinoid receptors and, 2:661–662
Statins:
  multiple sclerosis therapy, 3:678–679
  novel drug development, 3:687–688
  neuroinflammation and, 3:643
Status epilepticus, 3:427–428
Stem cells:
  stroke therapy, 3:378–379
  traumatic brain injury and, 3:452–453
Steroids:
  GABA$_A$ α$_4$ subunit pharmacology, 1:488–489
  NMDA allosteric potentiators, 1:386
  stroke management, 3:371–372
  traumatic brain injury and, 3:450–451
Sterol regulatory element binding protein (SREBP1), leptin effect on, 3:747–748
Stimulant therapy:
  attention-deficit hyperactivity disorder, 3:293–298
    adverse effects, 3:298
    amphetamines, 3:296–298
    dexmethylphenidate, 3:296
    extended-release methylphenidate, 3:295
    immediate-release agents, 3:294
    methylphenidate hydrochloride, 3:294–296
  autism spectrum disorders, 3:328–330
  psychostimulants, 2:587–588
Stoichiometry, plasma membrane glutamate transporters, 1:709–711
Stress:
  addictive disorders and response to, 2:459
  cannabinoid analgesics and, 2:667–668
  histaminergic neuron activity, 1:320–322
    pituitary hormone secretion, 1:325
  hormones and, 1:679
  neurogenesis regulation, 1:829–830
  monoamine hypothesis of depression and, hippocampal neurogenesis and, 1:825–826

neuroactive steroid interactions:
   drug abuse relapse, 2:159–160
   HPA axis, 2:153–154
   overview, 2:152–153
neuroendocrine response, 1:694–695
neurogenesis and, 3:206–207
neurotrophic factors and, growth factors, 1:794–797
   adrenal glucocorticoids, 1:796–797
   adult neurogenesis and morphology, 1:797–800
      hippocampus, 1:798
   alterations in, 1:794–795
   brain-derived neurotrophic factor, 1:794–796
   cytokines, 1:797
   glial proliferation, 1:800
   serotonin receptors, 1:797
   vascular endothelial growth factor, 1:797
psychostimulant abuse:
   chronic exposure and sensitization effects, 2:580–585
   neuropharmacology and, 2:577–578
Striatal complex:
   dopamine release, muscarinic acetylcholine receptor deficiency, 1:171–172
   histaminergic neuron activity, Parkinson's disease, 1:328
Striatal dopamine receptors:
   atypical antipsychotic drugs, clozapine D_2 receptor blockade, 2:414–415
   schizophrenia dopamine hypothesis and, 2:287–288
Stroke:
   AMPA receptor antagonists, 3:361–363
   amphetamine and neurotransmitter modulators, 3:377
   antiadhesion molecules, 3:369–370
   anti-nogo (IN-1) inhibitors, 3:377–378
   antioxidants, 3:371–372
   apoptosis and caspase inhibitors, 3:372–373
   basic characteristics and symptoms, 3:348–349
   brain injury with:
      classification, 3:350
      mechanisms of, 3:351–353
      repair approaches, 3:377–379
   calcium channel blockers, 3:366–367
   chemokine inhibition, 3:369
   cytokine inhibition, 3:368–369
   decahydroisoguinolines, 3:362
   down-stream approaches, 3:367–368
   erythropoietin, 3:377
   GABA transporters and, 1:722
   global/focal ischemia, animal models, 3:353–354
   glutamate/glutamatergic receptors, 3:354–355, 3:361–366
   glutamate release inhibitors, 3:366–367
   glutamate transporters, 3:365–366
   growth factors, 3:375–377
   GYKI 52466/related benzodiazepines, 3:362
   inflammatory pathways, 3:368
   kainate receptor antagonists, 3:363
   metabotropic glutamate receptors, 3:363–365
   mGlu 2 selective orthosteric agonists, 1:428–429
   mGlu 2 selective orthosteric antagonists, 1:425
   NBQX/related quinoxalinediones, 3:361–362
   neuroprotective techniques, 3:366–373
   development criteria, 3:374
   neurotrophic factors and, 3:229–230
   nitric oxide synthase inhibition, 3:370–371
   NMDA receptor:
      antagonists, 3:354–359
         clinical trial data, 3:358–359
         competitive/noncompetitive agonists, 3:356–357
         glycine site antagonists, 3:357–358
         MK-801 compound, 3:355–356
         polyamine site antagonists, 3:357
         side effects, 3:359–360
      orthosteric antagonists, 1:375–377
   p38 inhibition, 3:369
   prevalence and incidence, 3:349–350
   sodium channel blockers, 3:367
   sonic hedgehog approach, 3:378
   stem cell approach, 3:378–379
   time window issues, 3:360–361
   upstream techniques, 3:366–373
Structural studies, obsessive-compulsive disorders, 2:217–218
Structure-activity relationships:
   benzodiazepines, 2:114–116
   dopamine, 1:232–234
   mGlu2 allosteric potentiators, 1:438–439

Structure-affinity relationships:
  dopamine, *1:*232–234
Substance P:
  anxiety neurobiology and, *2:*17
  neuropeptides and, *1:*670–671
  neurotransmitters, *1:*676
Substantia nigra, clozapine D_2 receptor blockade, *2:*414–415
Substantia nigra pars compacta (SNc), Parkinson's disease
  neurochemistry and, *3:*481–483
  invertebrate models of cell death, *3:*569–577
Substantia nigra pars reticularis (SNr), Parkinson's disease, neurochemistry, *3:*481–483
Subtype-selective ligands, $GABA_B$ receptors, *1:*592
Sucrose-fading technique, alcohol abuse studies in alcohol-preferring rats, *2:*467–470
Sulfate fraction, neuroactive steroids, in brain, *2:*137
6-Sulfatoxymelatonin (6-SMT), menopause therapy and, *1:*849–850
Sulpiride:
  alcohol abuse studies:
    dopaminergic receptor systems and substrates, *2:*472–473
    ventral pallidum receptor blockade, *2:*477–480
  Tourette's syndrome therapy, *3:*276
Sumatriptan:
  migraine management with, *2:*764–765
  obsessive-compulsive disorders, *2:*234
Superoxide dismutase (SOD):
  amyotrophic lateral sclerosis and, *3:*225–227
  stroke management, *3:*371–372
Supersensitization, melatonin receptors, *3:*54
Suprachiasmatic nucleus (SCN):
  animal models, *3:*10–11
  output pathways, *3:*12–13
  circadian rhythms and:
    antidepressant effects, *3:*18–20
    inputs and outputs, *3:*46–47
    period and phase, *3:*13–15
    prokineticin regulation, *3:*167–168
  in cockroach, *3:*10
  melatonin production, *3:*40–41
  melatonin receptors in:
    clock gene expression, *3:*50–51
    desensitization function, *3:*52–53
    localization, signaling, and function, *3:*47–50
    regulatory mechanisms, *3:*51–54
    supersensitization, *3:*54
    therapeutic targeting of, sleep mechanisms, *3:*57–58
Surface trafficking, $GABA_B$ receptors, *1:*575–578
Surgical treatment, epilepsy, *3:*426
Susceptibility genes, schizophrenia:
  future research issues, *2:*355–356
  gene linkage studies, *2:*324
  molecular genetics, functional implications, *2:*332–333
  molecular interactions, *2:*351–355
  postmortem studies:
    overview, *2:*343–344
    susceptibility gene identification, *2:*344–351
    susceptibility gene interactions, *2:*351–355
SVZ compound, neurogenesis and, *3:*209–210
Sweetened cocktail solution procedure, alcohol abuse studies in alcohol-preferring rats, *2:*468–470
Sympathetic nervous system (SNS):
  adipose tissue, *3:*789–797
    adipocyte prolifrative capacity, *3:*797–799
    anterograde tract-testing, SNS to WAT, *3:*792–797
    retrograde tracing neuroanatomical studies, *3:*790–792
  ghrelin effects, *3:*774
  leptin and energy expenditure, *3:*746
Synapses:
  curare's effect on, *1:*4–7
  early research on, *1:*13–14
  Eccles' research on, *1:*28–29
  electric organ model of, *1:*22
  Feldberg's research on, *1:*20–21
  $GABA_A$ receptor distribution on, *1:*473–475
  hypocretins at, *3:*130
  ion channels and, *1:*25
  Loewi's experiments on, *1:*18–19
  neurotrophins and, *3:*239

postwar research on, *1:*24–25
serotonergic neurons, *1:*264
Synapsin I progeins, dystrobrevin binding protein 1 (DTNBP1), molecular interactions, *2:*353
Synaptic release:
  vesicle-dependent release, *1:*46–47
  vesicle-independent release, *1:*47–48
  voltage-gated sodium ion channels, *1:*639–640
Synaptic transmission:
  AMPA receptor allosteric potentiators, *1:*394–395
  intercellular signaling:
    basic principles, *1:*40–41
    classical transmitters, *1:*45–46
    dopamine neurotransmitters, *1:*54–56
    endocannabinoids, purines, and gaseous transmitters, *1:*46
    glutamate neurotransmitters, *1:*52–54
    peptide transmitters and growth factors, *1:*46
    postsynaptic receptors, *1:*48–50
    presynaptic receptors, *1:*50–51
    synaptic release, *1:*46–48
    transmitter inactivation, *1:*51–52
    transmitter packaging, *1:*45–46
    transmitter synthesis, *1:*41–45
      amine transmitters, *1:*42–44
      endocannabinoids, *1:*45
      gaseous transmitters, *1:*45
      neuropeptides, neurotrophins, and growth factors, *1:*44–45
      vesicle-dependent release, *1:*46–47
      vesicle-independent release, *1:*47–48
  intracellular signaling:
    basic principles, *1:*59–60
    calcium channel calmodulin mediator, *1:*85–87
    calcium channel signaling molecules, *1:*83–85
    cyclic nucleotide second messengers, *1:*72–81
      adenylyl cyclase, *1:*72–77
      cAMP targets, *1:*75, *1:*78
      cGMP cellular targets, *1:*80–81
      guanylyl cyclase, *1:*78–80
    DAG activation of protein kinase C, *1:*85
    GPCR-G protein ion channel modulation, *1:*66–71
      downstream signaling molecules, *1:*69–70

$G\beta\gamma$ signaling, *1:*67–69
      protein-protein interactions, *1:*70–71
    G protein signal transducers, *1:*60–66
      cycle regulations, *1:*64–65
      disease and, *1:*67
      heterotrimeric protein structure, *1:*60–63
      RGS proteins, *1:*65–66
      small proteins, *1:*63–64
    IP_3 and phosphoinositide signaling molecules, *1:*81–83
    protein phosphorylation, *1:*87–96
      G-protein-coupled receptor kinases, *1:*90–92
      mitogen-activated protein kinase, *1:*89–90
      protein tyrosine kinase, *1:*87–89
      protein tyrosines phosphatases, *1:*92–94
      serine/threonine phosphatases, *1:*94–96
Synaptic vesicle protein SV2A:
  antiepileptic drug modulation, *3:*414
  epilepsy efficacy, *3:*417–418
Synaptic vesicles, early research on, *1:*27
Synaptosomal-associated protein 25 (SNAP25), dystrobrevin binding protein 1 (DTNBP1), molecular interactions, *2:*353
Synaptotagmin, vesicle-dependent release, *1:*46–47
Synphillin-1 point mutation, familial Parkinson's disease and, *3:*540
Synthesis:
  antipsychotics, schizophrenia pharmacotherapy, *2:*381–382
  endocannabinoid system, *2:*663–664
α-Synuclein mutations:
  familial Parkinsonism and, PARK 1 and PARK4 mutations, *3:*528–530
  parkin gene degradation, *3:*532
  Parkinson's disease genetics, invertebrate models, *3:*570–577
Systemic administration studies, alcohol abuse studies, $GABA_A$ benzodiazepine receptor complex, *2:*492–493
Systems biology theory, schizophrenia and, *2:*255–256
"Systems neuroscience," schizophrenia dopamine hypothesis and, *2:*288

T-182C polymorphism, norepinephrine
   transporter genetics, 1:201
Tachykinin, neuropeptide receptors,
   1:689–690
Tat protein, human immunodeficiency virus,
   3:701–703
   alcohol abuse and, 3:716
   apoptosis and, 3:705
   excitotoxicity cell death, 3:705–706
   methamphetamine/cocaine abuse and,
      3:714–715
   nigrostriatal system and, 3:709
   opioid abuse and, 3:715–716
+TC:
   actions of, 1:27
   postwar applications of, 1:25
Tele-methylhistamine (t-MeHA),
   histaminergic neuron activity,
   1:319–322
Temperature, circadian rhythms, 3:5
Temporal lobectomy, epilepsy, 3:426
Temsirolimus (CCI-779), multiple sclerosis
   therapy, 3:688
Teratogenecity, antiepileptic drugs,
   3:424–425
T-butyl agents, alcohol abuse studies,
   $GABA_A$ benzodiazepine receptor
   complex, site-specific
   microinjection techniques,
   2:494–496
Tetraethylammonium (TEA), voltage-gated
   potassium channels, K_V subunits,
   structure and function,
   1:630
Δ^9-Tetrahydrocannabinol:
   analgesic properties, 2:666–669
   antiobesity therapy, 3:825–828
   appetite regulation, 2:670–672
   cannabinoid receptor binding, 2:663
   cognition and, 2:669–670
   emesis modulation, 2:674–675
   endocannabinoid physiology and,
      2:665–675
   isolation off, 2:660–661
   neuroinflammation and, receptor
      modulation, 3:641–642
   neurotoxicity effects, 2:672–673
   prenatal development and, 2:664–665
   reward, tolerance, and dependence,
      2:675–676
Tetraspan proteins, structure and function,
   3:607–608

Tetrodotoxin (TTX), voltage-gated sodium
   ion channels and, 1:642–643
Thalamic relay neurons, histamine neuron
   physiology, arousal mechanisms,
   1:322–324
Thalamic reticular nucleus, $GABA_A$ α_3
   subunit pharmacology, 1:488
Therapeutic plasma exchange (TPE),
   multiple sclerosis acute relapse,
   treatment of, 3:673–674
Therapeutic targeting, $GABA_B$ receptors,
   1:592–593
Thermogenesis, glyceroneogenesis and,
   3:799–801
Thermoregulation, 3,4-methylenedioxy-
   methamphetamine effects on, 2:629
Thioxanthine, schizophrenia therapy,
   clinical profile, 2:383
THIP agonist:
   alcohol abuse studies, $GABA_A$
      benzodiazepine receptor complex,
      2:488–493
   as sedative/hypnotic, 3:190
Thyroid function, ghrelin modulation,
   3:775
Thyroid hormones, $GABA_A$ receptor
   modulation, 1:520
Thyroid-stimulating hormone (TSH):
   depression and levels of:
      in menopause, 1:850
      during menstrual cycle, 1:845
      postpartum depression, 1:848
      in pregnancy, 1:847
   neuropeptides and, 1:676–677
Thyrotropin-releasing hormone (TRH),
   narcolepsy therapy, 3:105–106
Tiagabine:
   epilepsy efficacy, 3:417–418
   $GABA_A$ receptor modulation,
      antiepileptic drugs, 3:412
   psychostimulant abuse therapy, 2:588
Tiapride, Tourette's syndrome therapy,
   3:276
Tics. See Tourette's syndrome
   Tourette's syndrome, 3:264–265,
      3:269–273
   suppressants, 3:277
Timeless gene, melatonin receptors, 3:51
Time-sensitive responses, to neuropeptides,
   1:693–694
Time window paradigm, stroke
   management, 3:360–361

Tissue culture studies:
  brain-derived neurotrophic factor in depressed patients, *1:*800–801
  neuropeptides, *1:*677
Tissue injury, transient receptor potential V1 (TRPV1) receptor expression, *2:*729–732
Tissue-specific processing, neuropeptides, *1:*687, *1:*693–694
TNF-related apoptosis-inducing ligand (TRAIL), inflammation mechanisms, *3:*625
  proinflammatory pathway modulation, *3:*639
Tolcapone, schizophrenia therapy, *2:*389
Tolerance mechanisms:
  benzodiazepines, *2:*100
  endocannabinoids, *2:*675–676
  psychostimulant abuse, neurobiology of, *2:*579–585
  schizophrenia therapy, second-generation antipsychotics, *2:*387–388
Toll-like receptors (TLR), inflammation and, *3:*631–632
Topiramate:
  as antiepileptic:
    ionotropic glutamate receptor modulation, *3:*413
    target interactions, *3:*415–416
  epilepsy efficacy, *3:*417–418
  migraine management, *2:*766
  psychostimulant abuse therapy, *2:*688
  for secondary generalized epilepsy, *3:*424
Topological analysis, corticotropin-releasing factor receptor antagonists, receptor subunits, *2:*183–185
Torpedo electric organ model:
  $GABA_A$ receptor structure, *1:*475
  sedative/hypnotic mechanisms, *3:*178–180
  nicotinic acetylcholine receptor, *1:*27–28
  history, *1:*108–110
  synapse research and, *1:*22–23
Torsade de pointes, KCNQ channels and, *1:*632–633
Tourette's syndrome:
  clinical course, *3:*266
  comorbid disorders, *3:*266
  diagnostic criteria, *3:*263–264
  dopaminergic drugs, *1:*237
  environmental factors, *3:*267–269
  epidemiology, *3:*266
  future research issues, *3:*278
  genetics, *3:*266–267
  obsessive-compulsive disorder comorbidity, *2:*216
  pathophysiology, *3:*269–273
    neuroanatomical abnormalities, *3:*269–270
    neurochemical abnormalities, *3:*270–273
    second-messenger systems, *3:*273
  phenomenology, *3:*264–265
  treatment, *3:*273–278
    adrenergic agonists, *3:*276–277
    antidopaminergic agents, *3:*276
    neuroleptics, *3:*273–276
    nonpharmacological treatments, *3:*277–278
    tic suppressants, *3:*277
Toxicity effects, antiepileptic drugs, *3:*420–421
Trafficking mechanisms:
  $GABA_A$ receptors, *1:*478–480
  $GABA_B$ receptors, *1:*575–578
  voltage-gated sodium ion channels, *1:*638–639
TRAM-34 analog, intermediate-conductance calcium-activated potassium channels, *1:*631
Tramadol, obsessive-compulsive disorder therapy, *2:*234
Tranquilizers, structure and function, *3:*187
Trans-aminocyclobutanedicarboxylate (ABCD), NMDA orthosteric agonists, *1:*373
Transcranial magnetic stimulation (TMS), obsessive-compulsive disorders, *2:*236
Transcriptional regulation:
  α_1 adrenergic receptors, *1:*202–203
  β-adrenergic receptor physiology, *1:*212–213
  anxiety neurobiology and, mouse studies, *2:*19, *2:*22
  lithium mechanism in bipolar disorder patients, *1:*867–869
  nitrosylation and, *1:*750–751
  plasma membrane transporters, *1:*725
Transdermal nicotine patch:
  mecamylamine in conjunction with, *2:*549

nicotine dependence and withdrawal therapy, 2:546–547
obsessive-compulsive disorder therapy, 2:234
Transforming growth factor-α (TGFα), suprachiasmatic nucleus, 3:13
Transforming growth factor-β (TGF-β):
intracellular signaling, 1:793–794
structure and function, 3:222–223
Transforming growth factor family, inflammation mechanisms, 3:640–641
Transgenic animals, neuropeptide genetic manipulations in, 1:678
Trans-Golgi network (TGN), GABA$_B$ receptor trafficking and heteromization, 1:577–578
Transient receptor potential (TRP) channels:
cyclic nucleotide second messenger signaling, adenylyl cyclase, 1:74–75
structure and function, 1:649–650
Transient receptor potential V1 (TRPV1) receptors:
analgesic properties, 2:668–669
antagonists, 2:733
capsaicin, protons, and heat, 2:730–732
chemical activators, 2:732–733
cloning of, 2:728–729
desensitization, 2:735–736
endocannabinoid ligands, 2:664
expression, 2:729
knockout mouse models, 2:736
nociception channels, 2:736–737
pain perception and management, 3:229
sensitization, 2:733–735
Transient receptor potential V2 (TRPV2), nociception and, 2:736–737
Transient receptor potential V3 (TRPV3), nociception and, 2:737
Transient receptor potential V4 (TRPV4), nociception and, 2:737
Transition metals, Parkinson's disease and, invertebrate models, 3:576–577
Translocation, plasma membrane glutamate transporters, 1:710–711
Transmembrane diffusion, blood-brain barrier neuropeptides and, 1:692–693
Transmembrane domains (TMDs):
AMPA receptors, 1:370–371
dopamine, 1:233–234

GABA$_A$ receptors:
allosteric sites in, 1:516–518
allosteric structural determinants, 1:508–509
channel gating binding, 1:495–497
desensitization and deactivation, 1:499
subunit gene splicing, 1:469–470
GABA transporters, 1:467–468
mGlu1 allosteric potentiators, 1:436
mGlu5 allosteric antagonists, 1:443–444
muscarinic acetylcholine receptor structure, 1:149–151
plasma membrane glutamate transporters, 1:709–711
sodium voltage-gated ion channels, 1:636
voltage-gated calcium channels, γ subunits, 1:646
Transmembrane segment (TMS) topology, voltage-gated ion channels, 1:619–620
Transmethylation, histamine inactivation, 1:306–307
Transmitter inactivation, intercellular signaling, 1:51–52
Transmitter packaging, classical transmitters, 1:45–46
Transmitter synthesis, intercellular signaling and, 1:41–45
amine transmitters, 1:42–44
endocannabinoids, 1:45
gaseous transmitters, 1:45
neuropeptides, neurotrophins, and growth factors, 1:44–45
TRAR4 gene, schizophrenia molecular genetics, 2:328
Traumatic brain injury (TBI):
characteristics and classification, 3:443–446
future research issues, 3:454
neural regeneration, 3:452–453
neuroplasticity, 3:453–454
neuroprotective agents, 3:446–451
anti-inflammatory agents, 3:447–449
free-radical scavengers, 3:447
neuroactive steroids/neurosteroids, 3:450–451
neurotransmitter agonists/antagonists, 3:449–450
Treatment Episode Data Set (TEDS), opiate treatment statistics, 2:694–696
Tremor induction, muscarinic acetylcholine receptor deficiency, 1:170–171

Tricarboxylic acid (TCA) cycle, plasma membrane glutamate transporters, *1:*711
Trichloroethanol, GABA$_A$ receptor modulation, *1:*516
Tricyclic antidepressants (TCAs):
  anxiety disorder therapy, *2:*69–70
  attention-deficit hyperactivity disorder therapy, *3:*299
  early research on, *1:*30–31
  nicotine dependence and withdrawal therapy, *2:*550
  panic disorder therapy, *2:*78
  Parkinson's disease and, *3:*501
  psychostimulant abuse therapy, *2:*586–587
Trigeminal ganglion, migraine therapy targeting of, *2:*760
Trigeminovasculature system, calcitonin gene-related peptide sites and migraine therapy targeting, *2:*761–762
Trihexyphenidyl, Parkinson's disease treatment, *3:*496
Triptans, migraine management with, *2:*764–765
TrkA receptors:
  cognitive function and, *3:*228
  neurotrophins and, *3:*238
  pain perception and management, *3:*229
  TrkAIII splice variants, *3:*245–246
TrkB receptors:
  amyotrophic lateral sclerosis and, *3:*226–227
  anxiety neurobiology, receptor deficits and, *2:*29–30
  neurotrophic factor expression, *3:*222–224
  obesity and weight control, *3:*229–230
  Parkinson's disease and, *3:*228–229
  splice variants, *3:*245–246
  synaptic function and, *3:*239
TrkC receptors:
  neuropathies and, *3:*227
  splice variants, *3:*245–246
Tryptophan, inflammation and metabolism of, *3:*644
Tryptophan hydroxylase (TPH):
  3,4-methylenedioxymethamphetamine effects on, *2:*616–617
  serotonin synthesis, *1:*260–261
Tuberomammillary nucleus:
  histamine neuron physiology:
    arousal mechanisms, *1:*323–324
    cognitive function, *1:*324
    histaminergic neuron activity, *1:*319–322
    histaminergic neurons, *1:*301–303
Tubocurarine, small-conductance calcium-activated potassium channels, *1:*632
Tumor cell growth and migration:
  GABA$_B$ receptor targeting, *1:*596
  KCNH potassium channels, *1:*634
Tumor necrosis factor-α (TNFα), human immunodeficiency virus, nigrostriatal system and, *3:*710
Tumor necrosis factor (TNF):
  neuroinflammation, proinflammatory pathway modulation, *3:*638–639
  p75 neurotrophin receptor structure and, *3:*240–241
Two-bottle water choice procedure, alcohol abuse studies in alcohol-preferring rats, *2:*468–470
Two-P (KCNK) channels, structure and function, *1:*634–635
Tyrosine-hydroxylase, schizophrenia dopamine hypothesis and, *2:*288–289
Tyrosine kinase receptors. *See also* specific receptors, e.g. TrkA receptor
  chemical release, *1:*48–50
  functional interactions, *3:*247–248
  GABA$_A$ phosphorylation, *1:*482
  glutamate transporter regulation, *1:*727–728
  neuropeptide receptors, *1:*691
  neurotrophic factors and, *3:*231–232
  neurotrophins and, *3:*238
  signaling mechanisms, *3:*242–246
    preference determinants, *3:*242
    protein binding, *3:*243–245
    signal transduction pathways, *3:*242–243
  splice variants and, *3:*245–246
  structure of, *3:*241–242

Ubiquitin carboxyl terminal hydrolase L1 (UCH-L1) mutation, familial Parkinson's disease and, *3:*539–540
Uncoupling protein, adipose tissue cell types and depots, *3:*786–789
Uncoupling reactions, muscarinic acetylcholine receptors, *1:*162
Upregulation, neuropeptide receptors, *1:*689

Upstream techniques, stroke management, 3:366–373
Uridine-diphosphoglucose-N-acetyl-glucosamine (UDP-GlcNAc), leptin secretion and, 3:736
Urocortins, corticotropin-releasing factor receptor antagonists, ligand structure, 2:180–181

Vagal nerve stimulation (VNS), epilepsy management, 3:427
Val66Met substitution polymorphism:
  anxiety neurobiology, genetic susceptibility studies, 2:18–19
  schizophrenia, serotonin receptor 5-HT$_{2A}$ receptor and, 2:421–422
val alleles, BDNF in mood disorders, 1:803
Valproate:
  anxiety disorder therapy, 2:75
  development and testing, 3:419
  epilepsy efficacy, 3:417–418
  migraine management, 2:765–766
  for secondary generalized epilepsy, 3:424
Vanilloid receptors:
  cloning, 2:727–729
  transient receptor potential V1 expression, 2:729
    antagonists, 2:733
    capsaicin, protons, and heat, 2:730–732
    chemical activators, 2:732–733
    desensitization, 2:735–736
    knockout mouse models, 2:736
    nociception channels, 2:736–737
    sensitization, 2:731–735
    tyrosine kinase receptor signaling, 3:245
Varenicline, nicotine dependence and withdrawal therapy, 2:548
Variable number of tandem repeats (VNTRs):
  plasma membrane transporter regulation, 1:725
  serotonin transporters and, 1:720
Variable numbers of tandem repeats (VNTR), obsessive-compulsive disorders, dopamine genetics, 2:223
Vascular cell adhesion molecule-1 (VCAM-1), inflammation mechanisms, 3:624–625
Vascular endothelial growth factor (VEGF):
  antidepressant influences on, 1:805–806
  adult neurogenesis and, 1:807–808
  depression models and, 1:809
  intracellular signaling, 1:792–793
  prokineticins and, 3:169–170
  stress influence on, 1:797
  neurogenesis and, 1:799–800
Vascular monoamine transporter (VMAT), narcolepsy therapy, amphetamine targeting, 3:94
Vascular tone, α_1 adrenergic receptor physiology, 1:203–204
Vasoactive intestinal polypeptide (VIP), neuropeptides and, 1:670–671
  modulation actions, 1:677
Vasopressin, neuropeptides and:
  gene duplication and, 1:682–684
  modulation, 1:677
Vasopressinergic neurons, H$_1$ receptor signaling, 1:309
Velocardiofacial syndrome gene, schizophrenia:
  chomosome mapping, 2:346
  COMT catabolism and, 2:329
Venlafaxine:
  anxiety disorder therapy, 2:69
  attention-deficit hyperactivity disorder therapy, 3:301
  autism spectrum disorders, 3:331
  obsessive-compulsive disorder therapy, 2:234
Ventral hippocampal lesions, in schizophrenia, animal models, 2:265
Ventral pallidum, alcohol abuse studies, 2:476–480
  dopaminergic regulation hypotheses, 2:478–480
  GABA$_{A1}$ subunit probe selectivity, 2:501–503
  GABAergic modification of dopamine agonists, 2:497–498
Ventral tegmental area (VTA):
  alcohol abuse studies, dopaminergic receptor systems and substrates, 2:472–473
  alcohol abuse studies in alcohol-preferring rats, control substrates in, 2:470
  atypical antipsychotic drug mechanisms in, clozapine D$_2$ receptors, 2:414–415
  cannabinoid receptors in, 2:675–676
  integrated glutamate/dopamine hypotheses of schizophrenia, 2:375–376

nicotine dependence and withdrawal:
　nicotine reinforcement substrates,
　　2:538–540
　withdrawal substrates, 2:542–543
Parkinson's disease neurochemistry and,
　3:481–483
psychostimulant abuse:
　monoamine neuropharmacology,
　　2:571–575
　neuropeptide pharmacology, 2:578–579
Ventrolateral preoptic nucleus (VLPO):
　histaminergic neuron activity,
　　1:319–322
　histaminergic neurons, 1:305
　narcolepsy therapy, modafinil, 3:102–103
Vesicle-dependent synaptic release, 1:46–47
Vesicle-independent synaptic release,
　1:47–48
Vesicular GABA transporters (VGATs):
　function of, 1:466
　GABA affinity, 1:467–468
Vesicular glutamate transporter (VGLUT):
　glutamate synthesis and storage, 1:366
　glutamate theory of schizophrenia,
　　pathological evidence, 2:292
　neurotransmitter functions, 1:716, 1:723
Vesicular inhibitory amino acid transporters,
　structure and function, 1:718
Vesicular monoamine transporter 2
　(VMAT2):
　attention-deficit hyperactivity disorder
　　therapy, 3:297–298
　chronic substrate treatment, 1:726–727
　histamine metabolism, 1:306
　neurotransmitter functions, 1:716–717,
　　1:723
Vesicular monoamine transporter (VMAT)
　protein, dopamine hypothesis of
　schizophrenia, 2:284–285
Vesicular neurotransmitter transporters,
　1:715–718
　acetylcholine and monoamine
　　transporters, 1:716–718
　clinical relevance, 1:723
　glutamate transporters, 1:716
　inhibitor amino acid transporters, 1:718
　nitrosylation and, 1:751
Vigabatrin:
　epilepsy efficacy, 3:417–418
　$GABA_A$ receptor modulation, 3:412
Visual system, γ-hydroxybutyric acid (GHB)
　effects, 2:634

Vitamin D, neuroinflammation and,
　3:642–643
Vitamin D receptor agonists,
　neuroinflammation and, 3:643
Vitamin D receptor (VDR), anxiety
　neurobiology and, 2:32
Vitamin E, neuroinflammation and,
　antioxidant modulation, 3:637
Vitamins, idiopathic Parkinson's disease
　and, 3:544–545
VLPO nucleus, sedative/hypnotic action
　sites, 3:182–184
Vogel conflict test:
　mGlu5 allosteric antagonists, 1:444
　mouse models of anxiety, neurosteroid
　　effects, 2:145–146
Vogel punished drinking test, emotionality
　studies in mice, 2:8–9
Voltage-gated ion channels:
　calcium channels, 1:643–650
　　α subunits, 1:644–645
　　$\alpha\delta$ subunits, 1:646
　　auxiliary subunit modulators, 1:650
　　β subunits, 1:645–646
　　Ca_v1 family, 1:647–648
　　Ca_v2 family, 1:648–649
　　Ca_v3 family, 1:649–650
　　downstream signaling, 1:69–70
　　γ subunits, 1:646
　　general blockers, 1:647
　　miscellaneous channels, 1:650–651
　　signal modulation, 1:68–69
　cloning and evolutionary relationships,
　　1:619–620
　nomenclature, 1:621
　potassium channels, 1:621–635, 1:625–626
　　calcium activation, 1:630–632
　　fast inactivation, 1:627
　　gating, 1:626–627
　　interacting proteins, 1:627–628
　　inwardly-rectifying and two-P channels,
　　　1:634–635
　　KCNH channels, 1:633–634
　　KCNQ family, 1:632–633
　　K_v subunits, 1:628–630
　　physiology, disease and pharmacology,
　　　1:628–634
　　selectivity, 1:623–625
　　voltage activation, 1:625–626
　research background, 1:618–619
　sodium channels, 1:635–643
　　α subunits, 1:636–637

channelopathies, 1:641–642
epilepsy and modulation of, 3:411
inactivation, 1:637–638
pharmacology, 1:642–643
physiological functions, 1:639–641
selectivity, 1:637
trafficking, 1:638–639
Vpr protein, HIV neurotoxicity and, 3:703
Vpu protein, HIV neurotoxicity, 3:704

WAY-100635 compound:
  5-HT$_{2A}$-5-HT$_{2C}$ receptor interactions, 2:422–424
  nicotine dependence and withdrawal, withdrawal substrate specificity, 2:542–543
Weibel Palade bodies, nitrosylation and, 1:751
White adipose tissue (WAT):
  classification, 3:786–789
  glyceroneogenesis control, lipolysis and thermogenesis, 3:799–801
  molecular features, 3:787–789
  sympathetic nervous system innervation, 3:789–797
    anterograde tract-tracing, 3:792–797
    retrograde neuroanatomical studies, 3:790–792
Willardiines:
  AMPA receptor orthosteric agonists, 1:376–377
  kainate receptor orthosteric agonists, 1:380–381
  kainate receptor orthosteric antagonists, 1:384–385
WIN 55,212-2:
  analgesic properties, 2:666–668
  convulsant effects of, 2:673
  pain management and, 2:667–668
Wisconsin card sort task (WCST), schizophrenia dopamine hypothesis, genetic evidence, 2:286–287

Withdrawal, antiepileptic drugs, 3:419–420
Withdrawal syndrome:
  benzodiazepines, 2:74
  nicotine dependence and withdrawal, withdrawal neurosubstrates, 2:541–543
  opiate addiction and, 2:699

Yellow fluorescent protein (YFP), Huntingdon's disease trinucleotide repeats, invertebrate model, 3:577–579
YM-872 antagonist, stroke management, 3:361–362
Yo-yo-ing dyskinesia, Parkinson's disease treatment and, 3:499

Zaleplon, GABA$_A$ subunit pharmacology, allosteric ligand modulation, 1:504–506
ZDHHC8 candidate gene, schizophrenia molecular genetics, 2:330
Zeitgeber time:
  circadian rhythms and, 3:20–21
  narcolepsy pathophysiology, hypocretin/orexin system, 3:88–89
Ziconotide, voltage-gated calcium ion channels, Ca$_v$2 family, 1:649
Ziprasidone:
  autism spectrum disorders, 3:327–328
  schizophrenia therapy, safety and tolerability, 2:389
  Tourette's syndrome therapy, 3:275–276
Zolpidem:
  alcohol abuse studies, GABA$_{A1}$ receptor subunit selectivity, 2:499
  GABA$_A$ subunit pharmacology:
    allosteric ligand modulation, 1:504–506
    benzodiazepine binding sites, 1:510–511
  GABA$_A$ subunit selectivity, 1:484
Zonisamide, T-type calcium channel modulation, 3:413